Handbook of Experimental Pharmacology

Continuation of Handbuch der experimentellen Pharmakologie

Vol. 58/II

Cyclic Nucleotides

Part II: Physiology and Pharmacology

Contributors

D. A. Ausiello · N. Barden · P. Barrett · M. Beaulieu · M. J. Berridge
P. Borgeat · B. L. Brown · J. Cote · J. Drouin · R. van Driel
E. A. Duell · T. V. Dunwiddie · J. H. Exton · J. N. Fain · D. B. Farber
L. Ferland · J. B. Field · D. L. Friedman · V. Giguere · M. Godbout
B. J. Hoffer · S. D. Holmes · E. D. Jacobson · A. M. Katz · F. Labrie
L. Lagace · J. Lepine · C. J. Lingle · D. McMahon · E. Marder
J. Massicotte · H. Meunier · D. C. B. Mills · D. H. Namm
J. A. Nathanson · J. Orloff · H. Rasmussen · V. Raymond
G. C. Rosenfeld · G. R. Siggins · W. J. Thompson · R. Veilleux
J. J. Voorhees · H. J. Wedner · M. Zatz

Editors

John W. Kebabian and James A. Nathanson

Springer-Verlag Berlin Heidelberg New York 1982

Dr. John W. Kebabian

Biochemical Neuropharmacology Unit, National Institutes of Health, Room 5c 108/Bldg. 10, Bethesda, MD 20205/USA

Professor Dr. James A. Nathanson

Neuropharmacology Research Laboratory, Departments of Neurology and Pharmacology, Harvard Medical School, Massachusetts General Hospital, Fruit Street, Boston, MA 02114/USA

With 101 Figures

ISBN-13: 978-3-642-68395-4 e-ISBN-13: 978-3-642-68393-0
DOI: 10.1007/978-3-642-68393-0

Softcover reprint of the hardcover 1st edition 1982

2122/3130-543210

Preface

Cyclic nucleotides are intimately involved in the consequences of either stimulation or blockade of receptors; therefore, an understanding of the biochemistry of cyclic nucleotides ought to be important for pharmacologists. Pharmacology is a science that among other things investigates chemical compounds that affect the physiology of cells, tissues and organs. Frequently pharmacologists account for the effect of low concentrations of a drug upon a tissue by invoking the presence of a receptor upon the surface of the cell. Traditional pharmacologists excelled at identifying and classifying the properties of receptors. A. J. CLARK's monograph in the earlier series of the Handbook of Experimental Pharmacology (CLARK 1937) summarized the mathematics underlying the traditional pharmacological approach towards receptors. By its nature, however, classic pharmacology provided little useful information about the intracellular events occurring as a consequence of occupying a receptor; for example, ALQUIST (1948) identified the beta-adrenoceptor, but he did not provide any insight into how stimulation of the receptor produces tissue-specific physiological responses. The discovery of cyclic AMP by RALL and SUTHERLAND (see RALL, Vol. I) led to biochemical investigations of many different receptors (including ALQUIST's beta-adrenoceptor) that share a cyclic nucleotide as a common factor in the biochemical mechanisms that translate the occupancy of receptors into physiological effects.

Ten years ago, in the introduction to their monograph on cyclic nucleotides, ROBISON et al. (1971) commented on the rapid growth of interest in cyclic nucleotides over the preceding years. In the last decade, cyclic nucleotides has remained a "growth industry." The proliferation of the cyclic nucleotide literature, a problem for ROBISON, BUTCHER, and SUTHERLAND 10 years ago, has continued at an ever increasing rate. Today the topic of cyclic nucleotides is so large that three individuals would not even consider writing a comprehensive summary of the topic. In preparing the initial outline of this volume, it seemed more efficient to go to the experts in the many different areas of cyclic nucleotide research and ask them to summarize how the general principles of cyclic nucleotide biochemistry presented in the accompanying volume have been applied to a physiological process common to many different tissues (e.g., secretion) or to a specific tissue (e.g., the adrenal cortex). Each author was requested to separate the seeds of useful information from the mass of chaff comprising the bulk of the cyclic nucleotide literature and report the status of his topic as of 1981.

References

Alquist, RP (1948) A study of the adrenotopic receptor. Am J Physiol 153:586–600
Clark AJ (1937) General Pharmacology. In: Handbuch der Experimentellen Pharmakologie, Vol. 4. Springer-Verlag, Berlin, Heidelberg, New York.
Robison GA, Butcher RW, and Sutherland EW (1971) Cyclic AMP. Academic Press, New York, London.

Bethesda and Boston J.W. KEBABIAN and J.A. NATHANSON

List of Contributors

D. A. AUSIELLO, Medical Services (Renal Unit), Massachusetts General Hospital and Harvard Medical School, Boston, MA 02114/USA

N. BARDEN, Centre de Recherches en Endocrinologie Moléculaire, Le Centre Hospitalier de l'Université Laval, Québec, G1V 4G2/CDN

P. BARRETT, Department of Internal Medicine, Division of Endocrinology, Yale University, New Haven, CT 06510/USA

M. BEAULIEU, Centre de Recherches en Endocrinologie Moléculaire, Le Centre Hospitalier de l'Université Laval, Québec, G1V 4G2/CDN

M. J. BERRIDGE, A.R.C. Unit of Invertebrate Chemistry and Physiology, Department of Zoology, University of Cambridge, Cambridge/GB

P. BORGEAT, Centre de Recherches en Endocrinologie Moléculaire, Le Centre Hospitalier de l'Université Laval, Québec, G1V 4G2/CDN

B. L. BROWN, Department of Human Metabolism and Clinical Biochemistry, University of Sheffield, Medical School. Beech Hill Road, Sheffield, S10 2RX/GB

J. COTE, Centre de Recherches en Endocrinologie Moléculaire, Le Centre Hospitalier de l'Université Laval, Québec, G1V 4G2/CDN

J. DROUIN, Centre de Recherches en Endocrinologie Moléculaire, Le Centre Hospitalier de l'Université Laval, Québec, G1V 4G2/CDN

R. VAN DRIEL, Universiteit van Amsterdam, Vakgroep Biochemie, B.C.P. Jansen Instituut, Plantage Muidergracht 12, NL-1018 TV Amsterdam-C

E. A. DUELL, University of Michigan Medical School, Departments of Dermatology and Biological Chemistry, R 6558 Kresge Medical Research Building, Ann Arbor, MI 48109/USA

T. V. DUNWIDDIE, University of Colorado, Health Sciences Center, Department of Pharmacology, 4200 E. 9th Ave. Denver, CO 80262/USA

J. H. EXTON, Howard Hughes Medical Institute and Department of Physiology, Vanderbilt University, Nashville, TN 37232/USA

J. N. FAIN, Section of Physiological Chemistry, Division of Biology and Medicine, Brown University, Providence, RI 02912/USA

D. B. Farber, Jules Stein Eye Institute, University of California, School of Medicine, Los Angeles, CA 90024/USA and Developmental Neurology Laboratory, Veterans Administration Medical Center, Sepulveda, CA 91343/USA

L. Ferland, Centre de Recherches en Endocrinologie Moléculaire, Le Centre Hospitalier de l'Université Laval, Québec, G1V 4G2/CDN

J. B. Field, Diabetes Research Laboratory, St. Luke's Hospital, P.O. Box 20269, Houston, TX 77025/USA

D. L. Friedman, Department of Molecular Biology, Vanderbilt University, Nashville, TN 37235/USA

V. Giguere, Centre de Recherches en Endocrinologie Moléculaire, Le Centre Hospitalier de l'Université Laval, Québec, G1V 4G2/CDN

M. Godbout, Centre de Recherches en Endocrinologie Moléculaire, Le Centre Hospitalier de l'Université Laval, Québec, G1V 4G2/CDN

B. J. Hoffer, University of Colorado, Health Sciences Center, Department of Pharmacology, 4200 E. 9th Ave., Denver, CO 80262/USA

S. D. Holmes, Diabetes Research Laboratory, St. Luke's Hospital, P.O. Box 20269, Houston, TX 77025/USA

E. D. Jacobson, College of Medicine, University of Cincinnati, Cincinnati, OH/USA

A. M. Katz, Division of Cardiology, Department of Medicine, University of Connecticut, Health Center, Farmington, CT 06032/USA

F. Labrie, Centre de Recherches en Endocrinologie Moléculaire, Le Centre Hospitalier de l'Université Laval, Québec, G1V 4G2/CDN

L. Lagace, Centre de Recherches en Endocrinologie Moléculaire, Le Centre Hospitalier de l'Université Laval, Québec, G1V 4G2/CDN

J. Lepine, Centre de Recherches en Endocrinologie Moléculaire, Le Centre Hospitalier de l'Université Laval, Québec, G1V 4G2/CDN

C. J. Lingle, Department of Biology, Brandeis University, Waltham, MA 02254/USA

D. McMahon, Molecular Genetics, Washington State University, Pullman, WA 99164/USA

E. Marder, Department of Biology, Brandeis University, Waltham, MA 02254/USA

J. Massicotte, Centre de Recherches en Endocrinologie Moléculaire, Le Centre Hospitalier de l'Université Laval, Québec, G1V 4G2/CDN

H. Meunier, Centre de Recherches en Endocrinologie Moléculaire, Le Centre Hospitalier de l'Université Laval, Québec, G1V 4G2/CDN

D. C. B. MILLS, Thrombosis Research Center, Temple University Health Sciences Center, 3400 North Broad Street, Philadelphia, PA 19140/USA

D. H. NAMM, Department of Pharmacology, Wellcome Research Laboratories, Burroughs Wellcome Co., Research Triangle Park, NC 27709/USA

J. A. NATHANSON, Departments of Neurology and Pharmacology, Harvard Medical School, Massachusetts General Hospital, Boston, MA 02114/USA

J. ORLOFF, Heart, Lung, and Blood Institute, National Institutes of Health, Bethesda, MA 20205/USA

H. RASMUSSEN, Department of Internal Medicine and Cell Biology, Yale University, New Haven, CT 06510/USA

V. RAYMOND, Centre de Recherches en Endocrinologie Moléculaire, Le Centre Hospitalier de l'Université Laval, Québec, G1V 4G2/CDN

G. C. ROSENFELD, Department of Pharmacology, University of Texas Medical School, Houston, TX 77025/USA

G. R. SIGGINS, The Salk Institute, P.O. Box 85800, San Diego, CA 92138/USA

W. J. THOMPSON, Department of Pharmacology, University of Texas Medical School, Houston, TX 77025/USA

R. VEILLEUX, Centre de Recherches en Endocrinologie Moléculaire, Le Centre Hospitalier de l'Université Laval, Québec, G1V 4G2/CDN

J. J. VOORHEES, University of Michigan Medical School, Departments of Dermatology and Biological Chemistry, R 6558 Kresge Medical Research Building, Ann Arbor, MI 48109/USA

H. J. WEDNER, Department of Internal Medicine, Washington University School of Medicine, St. Louis, MO 63110/USA

M. ZATZ, Laboratory of Clinical Science, National Institutes of Mental Health, Bethesda, MD 20205/USA

Contents

Section III. Physiology and Pharmacology of Cellular Regulatory Processes

CHAPTER 16

Regulation of Carbohydrate Metabolism by Cyclic Nucleotides.
J. H. EXTON. With 26 Figures

CHAPTER 18

Regulation of the Cell Cycle and Cellular Proliferation by Cyclic Nucleotides
D. L. Friedman

CHAPTER 19

Regulation of Development by Cyclic Nucleotides and Inorganic Ions.
D. McMahon

CHAPTER 22

Regulation of Cellular Excitability by Cyclic Nucleotides.
G. R. SIGGINS. With 2 Figures

CHAPTER 23

Regulation of Cardiac Contractile Activity by Cyclic Nucleotides.
A.M. KATZ. With 3 Figures

CHAPTER 24

Cyclic Nucleotides as First Messengers. R. VAN DRIEL. With 6 Figures

CHAPTER 23

Regulation of Cardiac Contractile Activity by Cyclic Nucleotides.
A.M. KATZ. With 3 Figures

CHAPTER 24

Cyclic Nucleotides as First Messengers. R. VAN DRIEL. With 6 Figures

M. Godbout, J. Massicotte, L. Ferland, N. Barden, M. Beaulieu, J. Cote, J. Lepine, H. Meunier, and R. Veilleux. With 20 Figures

CHAPTER 28

The Role of Cyclic Nucleotides in the Thyroid Gland.
S. D. Holmes and J. B. Field

CHAPTER 29

Parathyroid Hormone, Bone and Cyclic AMP. P. BARRETT and H. RASMUSSEN

CHAPTER 32

The Role of Cyclic Nucleotides in the Vasculature. D. H. NAMM

CHAPTER 33

The Role of Cyclic Nucleotides in the Pineal Gland. M. ZATZ. With 6 Figures

CHAPTER 34

The Role of Cyclic Nucleotides in Epithelium. E. A. Duell and J. J. Voorhees

CHAPTER 35

The Role of Cyclic Nucleotides in Platelets. D. C. B. Mills. With 7 Figures

CHAPTER 36

Cyclic Nucleotides in the Immune Response. H. J. WEDNER

CHAPTER 37

The Role of Cyclic Nucleotides in Invertebrates.
C.J. LINGLE, E. MARDER, and J.A. NATHANSON

Contents of Companion Volume 58, Part I
Cyclic Nucleotides: Biochemistry

Section II: Biochemistry of Protein Phosphorylation

Section III:
Physiology and Pharmacology of Cellular Regulatory Processes

CHAPTER 16

Regulation of Carbohydrate Metabolism by Cyclic Nucleotides

J. H. EXTON

Overview

The regulation of mammalian carbohydrate metabolism occurs by hormonal and non-hormonal mechanisms; the hormonal mechanisms may be cyclic AMP-dependent or cyclic AMP-independent. The regulation may be rapid involving covalent modification (usually phosphorylation) of enzymes or alterations in the concentrations of allosteric effectors. Alternatively, regulation may involve slower changes in enzyme concentrations due to alterations in enzyme synthesis or degradation.

Glucagon and β-adrenergic agonists regulate liver carbohydrate metabolism by promoting intracellular cyclic AMP accumulation and hence activation of cyclic AMP-dependent protein kinase. This enzyme phosphorylates and activates phosphorylase *b* kinase which, in turn, phosphorylates and activates phosphorylase leading to glycogenolysis. Cyclic AMP-dependent protein kinase also phosphorylates and inactivates glycogen synthase and pyruvate kinase resulting in inhibition of glycogen synthesis and stimulation of gluconeogenesis, respectively. Other mechanisms, including increased mitochondrial pyruvate carboxylation, inhibition of P-fructokinase, stimulation of fructose bisphosphatase and of amino acid transport and induction of P-enolpyruvate carboxykinase appear to be involved in the action of glucagon on gluconeogenesis.

Insulin inhibits the effects of glucagon on hepatic glycogen metabolism and gluconeogenesis by decreasing the intracellular level of cyclic AMP. Glucocorticoids exert a permissive effect on the actions of glucagon on these processes, apparently by acting on steps beyond the activation of cyclic AMP-dependent protein kinase. α-Adrenergic agonists, vasopressin and angiotensin II produce changes in liver carbohydrate metabolism which resemble those of glucagon. However, these agents do not increase cyclic AMP, but apparently act by raising cytosolic Ca^{2+}. Insulin and glucocorticoids modulate α-adrenergic responses in the liver perhaps by altering catecholamine receptors.

Catecholamines acting through β-adrenergic receptors activate phosphorylase and inactivate glycogen synthase in heart and skeletal muscle through mechanisms similar to those for glucagon in liver, except that additional control through alterations in the activity of P-protein phosphatase(s) may be involved. The changes in the phosphorylation and kinetics of glycogen synthase and phosphorylase *b* kinase induced by cyclic AMP-dependent or other protein kinases are known in much greater detail in muscle than in liver.

Insulin does not alter cyclic AMP or cyclic AMP-dependent protein kinase in muscle, but activates glycogen synthase through an unknown mechanism(s). β-Adrenergic stimulation reverses the stimulatory effects of insulin on glucose uptake and glycogen synthase in skeletal muscle.

Catecholamines produce β-receptor-mediated changes in glycogen metabolism in adipose tissue similar to those occurring in muscle. Insulin counteracts these changes by lowering cyclic AMP. However, added alone, insulin activates glycogen synthase and pyruvate dehydrogenase by unknown, cyclic AMP-independent mechanisms.

A. Regulation of Hepatic Glycogenolysis

I. Glucagon Stimulation of Hepatic Glycogenolysis

1. Evidence That Glucagon Exerts Physiological Control on Hepatic Glycogenolysis

The studies of CHERRINGTON et al. (1976, 1978), LILJENQUIST et al. (1977), FELIG et al. (1976), and GERICH et al. (1976) have established that glucagon plays a major role in the regulation of hepatic glucose output in vivo. As shown in Fig. 1 (left panel) from CHERRINGTON et al. (1976), induction of glucagon deficiency in dogs by infusion of insulin plus somatostatin causes a rapid decline in splanchnic glucose production with a resultant fall in blood glucose. Restoration of physiological concentrations of glucagon by infusion of the hormone into the portal vein results in normal glucose production and normoglycemia (not shown). On the other hand, when glucagon is infused without insulin (Fig. 1, right panel), glucose production increases and blood glucose rises.

These effects of glucagon are due to stimulation of both glycogenolysis and gluconeogenesis in the liver. Stimulation of hepatic glycogenolysis and gluconeogenesis by concentrations of glucagon within the range found in portal venous blood in vivo (JASPAN et al. 1977) can be demonstrated in vitro using the perfused rat liver (EXTON et al. 1971) or isolated liver parenchymal cells (CHERRINGTON and EXTON 1976; CHERRINGTON et al. 1977; Fig. 2).

2. Role of Cyclic AMP in Glucagon Action

There is abundant evidence supporting the original proposal of SUTHERLAND and co-workers (RALL et al. 1957; RALL and SUTHERLAND 1958; SUTHERLAND and RALL 1958, 1960) that cyclic AMP is the intracellular mediator of glucagon action on hepatic glycogenolysis. Although some investigators have presented data in support of another mechanism(s) for glucagon action (OKAJIMA and UI 1976; BIRNBAUM and FAIN 1977; COTE and EPAND 1979), their studies can be criticized on methodological or theoretical grounds (CHERRINGTON et al. 1977).

Figure 3 depicts a current version of the cyclic AMP or "second messenger" hypothesis of glucagon action on hepatic glycogen breakdown. As discussed in detail in Vol. 1 [see BIRNBAUMER and IYENGAR (1982)], glucagon binds to specific receptors on the external surface of the plasma membrane of the hepatic parenchymal cell leading to activation of the enzyme adenylate cyclase. The catalytic site of this

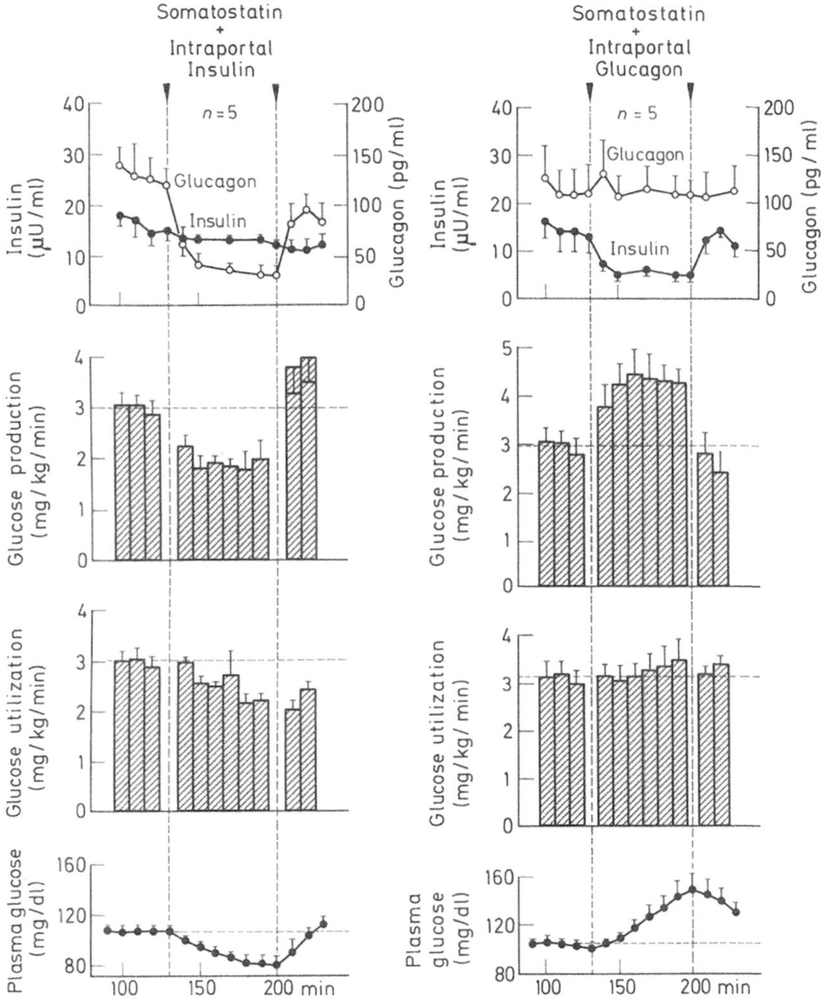

Fig. 1. *Left panel.* Effects of somatostatin infusion combined with intraportal insulin replacement on arterial plasma immunoreactive insulin and immunoreactive glucagon levels and on the production, utilization and concentration of plasma glucose in normal dogs. *Right panel.* Effects of somatostatin infusion combined with intraportal glucagon replacement on these parameters. (CHERRINGTON et al. 1976)

enzyme is located on the inner surface of the plasma membrane and its activation leads to increased conversion of ATP to cyclic AMP.

3. Role of Cyclic AMP-Dependent Protein Kinase

The increased concentration of cyclic AMP in the liver cell induced by glucagon leads to activation of the enzyme cyclic AMP-dependent protein kinase. The mechanism of activation is described in detail in Vol. 1 (see BEAVO), but the following is a brief description. In the basal state of the cell, i.e., in the absence of hormonal

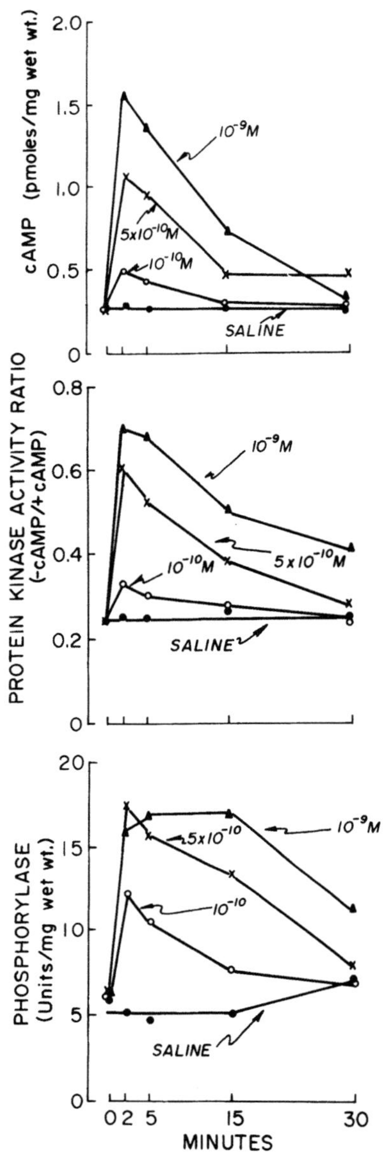

Fig. 2. Effects of physiological concentrations of glucagon on the level of cyclic AMP and the activation states of cyclic AMP-dependent protein kinase and phosphorylase in isolated rat hepatocytes. (CHERRINGTON and EXTON 1976)

stimulation, cyclic AMP-dependent protein kinase exists predominantly in a "holo" form (R_2C_2) in which a regulatory subunit dimer (R_2) is bound to two catalytic (C) subunits (Fig. 3). In this form, the enzyme is inactive since the regulatory dimer exerts an inhibitory effect on the activity of the catalytic subunits. When the cyclic AMP concentration of the cytosol increases, the nucleotide interacts with cyclic AMP binding sites on the regulatory dimer and this causes a conformational change in the protein such that its binding to, and inhibitory action on, the catalytic subunits is decreased (Fig. 3). Consequently, there is an increase in the activity of

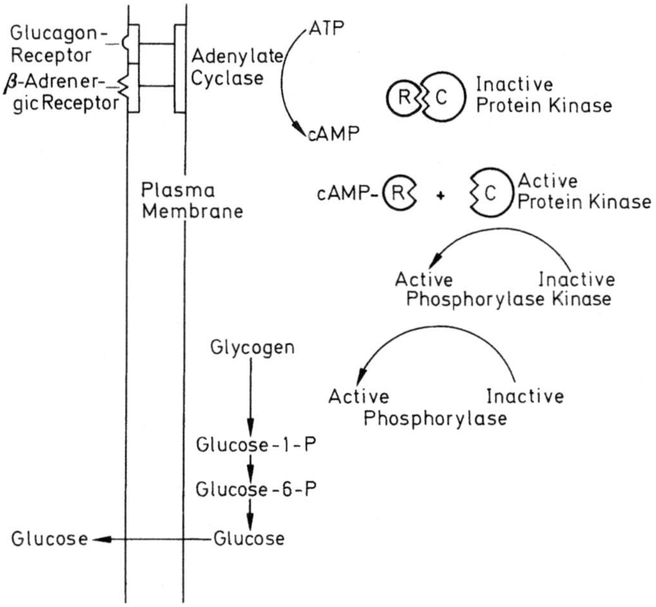

Fig. 3. Diagram of the mechanisms involved in the stimulation of glycogenolysis in the liver cell by glucagon and β-adrenergic agents

the catalytic subunits, which is reflected in vitro as an increase in the −cAMP/+cAMP activity ratio of the enzyme. This is illustrated in Fig. 2 which presents data from experiments with isolated liver cells.

The catalytic subunits of cyclic AMP-dependent protein kinase catalyze the phosphorylation of a variety of intracellular enzymes and other proteins using ATP as the phosphoryl donor. This phosphorylation alters the functional activity of many of the enzymes, i.e., causes either activation or inactivation, and the activity changes, in turn, are responsible for many of the physiological actions of glucagon. The cascade of phosphorylation reactions initiated by activation of adenylate cyclase results in amplification of the primary signal, i.e., a small increase in cyclic AMP results in large effects on enzymes (e.g., Fig. 2). Part of the cyclic AMP-dependent protein kinase in liver is bound to the plasma membrane and other intracellular membranes and thus may act more directly on enzymes and other proteins attached to or present in the membranes (Corbin et al. 1977; Sommarin and Jergil 1978; Henriksson and Jergil 1979).

4. Role of Phosphorylase *b* Kinase

Following the initial demonstration by Sutherland and Cori (1948) that phosphorylase activity was rate-limiting for glycogen breakdown in liver and that glucagon stimulated glycogenolysis by activating phosphorylase (Sutherland and Cori 1951), Rall et al. (1956) showed that activation of phosphorylase by the hormone involved incorporation of phosphate into the enzyme. The enzyme catalyzing the reaction, phosphorylase *b* kinase, was partially purified and the reaction was shown to involve ATP and Mg^{2+}. It is generally assumed, by analogy with the phosphorylase activation cascade in muscle, that cyclic AMP acts on liver phosphorylase *b* kinase via cyclic AMP-dependent protein kinase (Fig. 3).

Glucagon causes a rapid, stable increase in phosphorylase *b* kinase activity in intact liver preparations (VANDENHEEDE et al. 1976; VAN DE WERVE et al. 1977; CHAN et al. 1979c). Cyclic AMP-dependent protein kinase also activates the enzyme in crude liver extracts (VANDENHEEDE et al. 1977) and in liver glycogen pellets (CHRISMAN and EXTON 1980). However, attempts to demonstrate that the purified enzyme is activated or phosphorylated by cyclic AMP-dependent protein kinase have been variably successful. SAKAI et al. (1979) were unable to see any effects of cyclic AMP-dependent protein kinase, protein kinase inhibitor or alkaline phosphatase on the activity of liver phosphorylase *b* kinase purified about 100-fold. On the other hand, VANDENHEEDE et al. (1979) reported that addition of cyclic AMP and Mg[γ-^{32}P] ATP to partially purified preparations of the enzyme caused a 20- to 30-fold activation accompanied by incorporation of [^{32}P] into polypeptides which comigrated with the α- and β-subunits of skeletal muscle phosphorylase *b* kinase in sodium dodecylsulfate gel electrophoresis. These changes were attributed to activation of cyclic AMP-dependent protein kinase present in the preparations, since they were blocked by the heat-stable inhibitor of the protein kinase.

Purified liver phosphorylase *b* kinase resembles the muscle enzyme in that it has a molecular weight of 1.3 million and is very sensitive to stimulation by Ca^{2+} (K_a, 3×10^{-7} *M*) (SAKAI et al. 1979; VANDENHEEDE et al. 1979). However, unlike the muscle enzyme, the pH optimum of the unactivated form is about 6 and that of the activated form is above 7 (VANDENHEEDE et al. 1979). Also unlike the muscle enzyme, it is only partly (70%) inhibited by the divalent cation chelator EGTA.

5. Activation of Phosphorylase

Liver phosphorylase *b* kinase activates phosphorylase by phosphorylating phosphorylase *b* thereby converting it to the more active form phosphorylase *a* (Fig. 3). Activation involves the incorporation of 1 mole of phosphate per mole of enzyme subunit, but does not alter the dimeric structure of the enzyme (WOLF et al. 1970). Phosphorylation occurs on a specific serine in a sequence similar to that at the phosphorylation site in the muscle enzyme. Consequently muscle phosphorylase *b* kinase acts readily on liver phosphorylase *b* and liver phosphorylase *b* kinase acts on muscle phosphorylase *b*. Liver phosphorylase *b* exhibits little or no basal activity depending on the mammalian species (STALMANS and HERS 1975). Like the muscle enzyme, it can be stimulated by AMP, but never to the activity of phosphorylase *a*. AMP also affects phosphorylase *a*: it does not alter the V_{max} of the enzyme, but reduces its K_m for all three of its substrates (MADDIAH and MADSEN 1966a; STALMANS et al. 1974b). MADDIAH and MADSEN (1966a, b) have examined the kinetics of liver phosphorylase *a* in detail and have found that it is inhibited by UDP glucose, which is competitive with Pi. Caffeine and glucose also inhibit the enzyme in a synergistic, competitive and nonexclusive manner (KASVINSKY et al. 1978c). The mechanisms involved in the actions of these effectors are described in detail in Sect. D.I.3.

Phosphorylase *a* catalyzes the formation of glucose-1-P from glycogen and Pi (Fig. 3). The glucose-1-P is converted to glucose-6-P by the enzyme phosphoglucomutase and the glucose-6-P is converted to glucose in the liver by the enzyme glucose-6-phosphatase (Fig. 3). This enzyme is absent in muscle, and thus increased glycogenolysis is this tissue results in enhanced glycolysis and not glucose formation. Liver possesses an insulin-insensitive glucose transport system with a K_m of at least 17 m*M* and a very high V_{max} (180 μmoles/min · *g* liver) (T. WILLIAMS et al. 1968). Thus intracellular and extracellular glucose concentrations are rapidly equilibrated and glucose formed from glycogen breakdown is immediately released (Fig. 3).

6. Possible Role of Phosphoprotein Phosphatase

Several phosphoprotein phosphatases exist in the liver which dephosphorylate the enzymes and other proteins acted on by cyclic AMP-dependent protein kinase (LEE et al. 1978). Dephosphorylation leads to reversal of the changes in enzyme activities induced by the kinase. Isolation and characterization of these phosphatases is far from complete. A multifunctional phosphoprotein phosphatase which acts on phosphorylase *a*, glycogen synthase *b*, activated phosphorylase *b* kinase, phosphorylated histone and certain other phosphorylated proteins has been isolated from liver (BRANDT et al. 1967a; KHANDELWAL et al. 1976; KILLILEA et al. 1976, 1979). This enzyme has a molecular weight of 35,000, but may represent the catalytic subunit of a larger complex (LEE et al. 1978; KILLILEA et al. 1979). It appears to be regulated in three ways: a) competition between substrates, b) interaction of the enzyme with protein modifiers, and c) interaction of ligands with the substrates of the enzyme (KREBS and BEAVO 1979). The protein modifiers of this multifunctional phosphatase include heat-stable inhibitors isolated from muscle or liver (BRANDT et al. 1975b; F. HUANG and GLINSMANN 1975, 1976, G. NIMMO and COHEN 1978; LEE et al. 1978, KHANDELWAL and ZINMAN 1978; GORIS et al. 1978). One of the inhibitors from muscle requires phosphorylation by cyclic AMP-dependent protein kinase for activity (F. HUANG and GLINSMANN 1975, 1976; G. NIMMO and COHEN 1878). F. HUANG et al. (1977) were unable to find a phosphorylatable inhibitor in rat liver, but GORIS et al. (1978) reported such an inhibitor in dog liver.

Specific hepatic phosphoprotein phosphatases probably exist for glycogen synthase *b*, phosphorylase *a* and perhaps other phosphorylated proteins (KIKUCHI et al. 1977; LALOUX et al. 1978). They probably have molecular weights higher than 200,000 and may consist of a catalytic subunit combined with regulatory subunits which confer selectivity (LEE et al. 1978; KILLILEA et al. 1979). LALOUX et al. (1978) have reported the presence of a "native" form of phosphorylase phosphatase in mouse liver which behaves differently from synthase phosphatase during several treatments. It is not influenced by the heat-stable protein inhibitors described above and is bound to particulate glycogen. Glucagon treatment of rats does not alter the activity of phosphorylase phosphatase in gel filtrates of liver (LALOUX et al. 1978) or liver glycogen pellets (GILBOE and NUTTALL 1978). Thus the possibility that glucagon activation of liver phosphorylase is partly due to inhibition of phosphorylase phosphatase has yet to be proved.

7. Evidence Against a Role for Ca^{2+} in Glucagon Stimulation of Glycogenolysis

Several investigators (Friedmann and Park 1968; Keppens et al. 1977; Assimacopoulos-Jeannet et al. 1977; Blackmore et al. 1978; 1979b, Chen et al. 1978; Foden and Randle 1978) have shown that high concentrations of glucagon alter Ca^{2+} fluxes in the perfused rat liver and isolated rat hepatocytes, and some workers have proposed that these changes are related to certain actions of the hormone on hepatic metabolism (Friedmann and Rasmussen 1970; Chen et al. 1978). It is clear that the glycogenolytic action of glucagon is largely independent of any effect of the hormone on cellular Ca^{2+}. This is because: a) depletion of hepatocyte Ca^{2+} by the chelator EGTA does not impair phosphorylase activation induced by glucagon or exogenous cyclic AMP (Assimacopoulos-Jeannet et al. 1977; Chan and Exton 1977; Blackmore et al. 1979b), b) mobilization of cell calcium is barely detectable with concentrations of glucagon (10^{-9} *M*) which maximally activate phosphorylase (Blackmore et al. 1978), and c) mobilization of cell calcium by glucagon appears to involve components of the endoplasmic reticulum, but not mitochondria (Blackmore et al. 1979b).

II. Catecholamine Stimulation of Hepatic Glycogen Breakdown

1. Role of Catecholamines and the Sympathetic Nervous System in the Control of Hepatic Glycogenolysis

Bernard (1849) first demonstrated through piqûre stimulation of the medulla oblongata that the nervous system regulates glucose mobilization from the liver. Studies of the effects of electrical stimulation and microinjection of certain areas of the hypothalamus on hepatic glycogen levels (Rosenberg and Distefano 1962; Shimazu et al. 1966) have confirmed this classic observation. The neural pathway mediating the response is the splanchnic sympathetic outflow as shown by stimulation of splanchnic or hepatic nerves in several mammalian species (Shimazu and Amakawa 1968; Edwards and Silver 1970; Edwards 1971, 1972; Seydoux et al. 1979; Lautt 1979).

Several observations indicate that the sympathetic stimulation is exerted directly on the liver, in part at least: The hyperglycemic or glycogenolytic response to splanchnic or hepatic nerve stimulation is extremely rapid (occurs within 10 s) and persists after pancreatectomy and adrenalectomy (Shimazu and Amakawa 1968; Edwards and Silver 1970; Edwards 1971, 1972). It is demonstrable in calves in which the portal effluent blood flow is collected, and is reduced when the liver is partly denervated (Edwards and Silver 1970). Finally, Seydoux et al. (1979) and Lautt (1979) have shown that electrical stimulation of the hepatic nerves elicits glycogenolysis in the isolated perfused liver (Fig. 4).

There is much evidence that the sympathetic nervous system is importantly involved in the increased hepatic glucose output seen during exercise (Wahren et al. 1971; Galbo et al. 1975), insulin-induced hypoglycemia (Garber et al. 1976a; Sacca et al. 1977) and other stress situations requiring rapid fuel mobilization. In the case of insulin hypoglycemia, some reports indicate that sympathetic stimulation of the liver plays a major role in the response (Garber et al. 1976a; Sacca et al. 1977), although a fall in blood glucose can increase hepatic glucose output directly

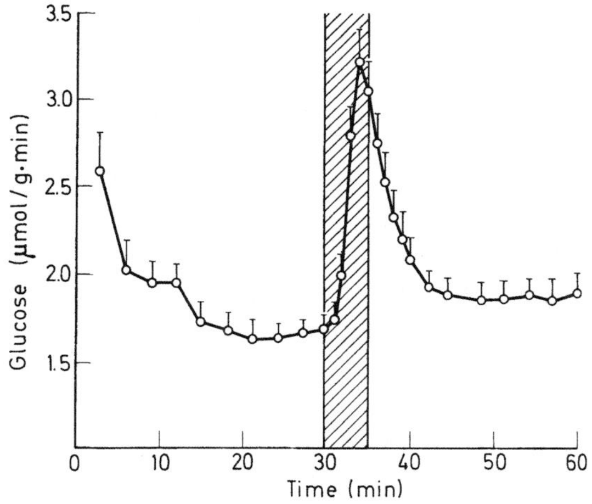

Fig. 4. Effect of electrical stimulation of perivascular nerves on glucose output by the mouse liver perfused in situ. The hatched area indicates electrical stimulation (29 Hz, 5 min). (SEYDOUX et al. 1979)

(GLINSMANN et al. 1969; CHERRINGTON et al. 1979) or indirectly through stimulation of glucagon secretion. As indicated above, glucagon release does not seem to be important in the hepatic glycogenolytic response to sympathetic stimulation in calves, but this may not be true for all species. In man, the effect of epinephrine on hepatic glucose output appears to be both direct and indirect (via glucagon) (GARBER et al. 1976a; SACCA et al. 1977, 1978; GERICH et al. 1976b; CHIDECKEL et al. 1977; RIZZA et al. 1979, 1980).

The effects of catecholamines on hepatic glucose output in vitro and in vivo are very rapid, but transient (EXTON et al. 1971; EXTON and HARPER 1975; BLACKMORE et al. 1979b; ALTSZULER et al. 1967; SACCA et al. 1978; RIZZA et al. 1979). This is because of the nature of the time courses of their effects on intracellular Ca^{2+} (mediated by α_1-adrenergic receptors) and cyclic AMP (mediated by β-adrenergic receptors) (see Sect. B.II.3). Down regulation of hepatic adrenergic receptors may also account for the non-persistence of the response. Another factor, especially in vivo, is the suppressive effect of hyperglycemia on hepatic glucose output.

The contribution of epinephrine released from the adrenal medulla to the hepatic glycogenolysis and hyperglycemia resulting from activation of the sympathetic nervous system appears to vary depending on the species. Rabbits are very sensitive to infusion of catecholamines (HIMMS-HAGEN 1967). However in man, rat, dog, and mouse, the concentrations of epinephrine required to elicit hyperglycemic responses in vivo or in the isolated perfused liver are high relative to those seen in plasma normally, and may only be achieved during insulin hypoglycemia, hemorrhagic shock or vigorous exercise (SILVERBERG et al. 1978; SOKAL and SARCIONE 1964; EXTON et al. 1971; SEYDOUX et al. 1979; HJEMDAHL et al. 1979; GALBO et al. 1975; GARBER et al. 1976a). In these species, the local release of norepinephrine from adrenergic nerve endings within the liver (FORSSMANN and ITO 1977) may mediate most of the effects of the sympathetic nervous system on this organ.

2. The Nature of the Adrenergic Receptors Mediating Catecholamine Effects on the Liver

It is now clear that both α_1- and β-receptors can mediate the effects of catecholamines on the liver (SHERLINE et al. 1972; TOLBERT et al. 1973; HUTSON et al. 1976). This clarifies previous uncertainty regarding the nature of the hepatic adrenergic receptor (HORNBROOK 1970; JENKINSON 1973). SUTHERLAND and co-workers (for review see SUTHERLAND and RALL 1960) first discovered that epinephrine acting through β-adrenergic receptors activates adenylate cyclase in many tissues. Except for a very few situations, these receptors mediate the stimulatory effects of catecholamines on cyclic AMP accumulation, and cyclic AMP mediates the effects of β-adrenergic stimulation. One exception is certain areas of the brain where there is some evidence that α-receptors are involved in the cyclic AMP response to adrenergic agonists (see SCHWABE and DALY 1977). However, recent experiments suggest that prostaglandins of the E series mediate this response (PARTINGTON et al. 1980). Another exception is the inhibitory effect of β-agonists on Mg^{2+} uptake by S 49 lymphoma cells which appears not to involve cyclic AMP (MAGUIRE and ERDOS 1980). The mechanisms by which β-adrenergic agonists activate adenylate cyclase are described in detail in another chapter and will not be presented here.

Cyclic AMP accumulation induced by β-adrenergic stimulation appears to be important in the hepatic effects of catecholamines in the dog (HIMMS-HAGEN 1967), but in many other species (rat, mouse, rabbit, cat, and guinea pig) α-adrenergic mechanisms not involving cyclic AMP appear to play a more predominant role (EXTON 1979). For example, the cyclic AMP response to catecholamines in perfused rat livers and isolated rat hepatocytes (Fig. 5) is transient and very small compared to that elicited by glucagon (EXTON et al. 1971; EXTON and HARPER 1975; HUTSON et al. 1976). Consequently the hepatic responses mediated by the β-receptor-cyclic AMP system in this species are very small (CHERRINGTON et al. 1977) and the system may contribute little to the overall hepatic effects of catecholamines. Furthermore, higher concentrations of epinephrine are required to elicit β-adrenergic responses (cAMP accumulation and protein kinase activation) than α_1-adrenergic responses (Ca^{2+} mobilization and phosphorylase activation) in rat hepatocytes (CHAN and EXTON 1977, CHERRINGTON et al. 1977; BLACKMORE et al. 1978). In man, it appears that β-adrenergic receptors are mainly involved in the hepatic responses to catecholamines (RIZZA et al. 1980; DEIBERT and DEFRONZO 1980).

3. Mechanisms Involved in Adrenergic Stimulation of Hepatic Glycogenolysis

The mechanisms by which cyclic AMP accumulation generated by β-adrenergic stimulation results in hepatic glycogen breakdown are almost certainly identical to those by which glucagon acts (SUTHERLAND and RALL 1960; CHERRINGTON et al. 1977) and will therefore not be described.

As indicated above, it is becoming increasingly clear that α_1-adrenergic receptors are the major mediators of hepatic catecholamine effects in rat and mouse (HUTSON et al. 1976; SEYDOUX et al. 1979) and play a significant role in these effects in guinea pig, cat, and rabbit (HAYLETT and JENKINSON 1972; OSBORN 1978; KUO et al. 1977; PROOST et al. 1979). These receptors are also important in neural stimulation of hepatic glycogenolysis in mouse and cat (SEYDOUX et al. 1979; LAUTT

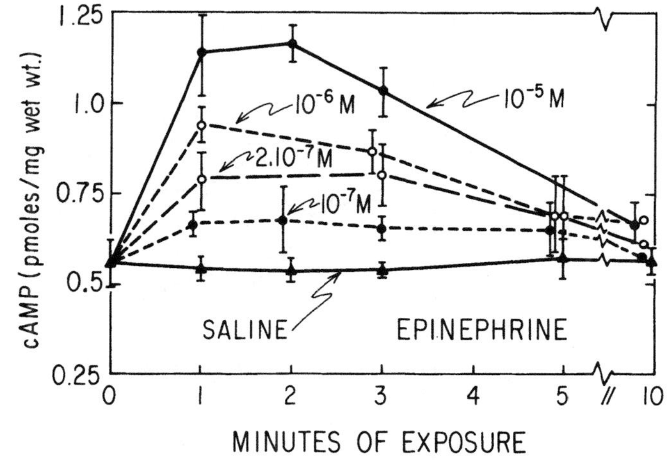

Fig. 5. Effects of different concentrations of epinephrine on cyclic AMP levels in isolated rat hepatocytes. (S. C. HARPER and J. H. EXTON, unpublished work)

1979) and appear to be involved in the early phase of liver glycogen mobilization seen during exercise in the rat (WINDER et al. 1979).

The mechanism(s) by which α_1-adrenergic stimulation activates hepatic phosphorylase and glycogenolysis has been shown by many workers not to involve cyclic AMP accumulation or activation of cyclic AMP-dependent protein kinase (CHERRINGTON et al. 1976; BIRNBAUM and FAIN 1977; KEPPENS et al. 1977; VAN DE WERVE et al. 1977; HUE et al. 1978; GARRISON et al. 1979). It also does not involve a *stable* activation of phosphorylase kinase, in contrast to the situation with glucagon (VAN DE WERVE et al. 1977; KEPPENS et al. 1977). On the other hand, there is much evidence that it results from a rise in cytosolic Ca^{2+} due to mobilization of Ca^{2+} from intracellular stores and perhaps an influx of extracellular Ca^{2+} (ASSIMACOPOULOS-JEANNET et al. 1977; KEPPENS et al. 1977; VAN DE WERVE et al. 1977; BLACKMORE et al. 1978, 1979b; CHEN et al. 1978; GARRISON 1978; GARRISON et al. 1979). Mitochondria have been shown to be a major source of the intracellular Ca^{2+} mobilized during α-adrenergic stimulation (Fig. 6; BLACKMORE et al. 1979b; BABCOCK et al. 1979; W. TAYLOR et al. 1980) and the site of Ca^{2+} action on phosphorylase activation is almost certainly phosphorylase *b* kinase since the enzyme is inhibited by EGTA and stimulated by concentrations of Ca^{2+} within the probable cytosolic range (SHIMAZU and AMAKAWA 1975; KHOO and STEINBERG 1975; SAKAI et al. 1979; CHRISMAN and EXTON 1980).

SHIMAZU and AMAKAWA (1975) have claimed that splanchnic nerve stimulation, but not epinephrine administration, decreases phosphorylase phosphatase activity in rabbit liver. However, this observation has not been confirmed (PROOST et al. 1979). Several workers have also been unable to see effects of cytosolic concentrations of Ca^{2+} on phosphorylase phosphatase (KHOO and STEINBERG 1975; BRANDT et al. 1975a), but it is possible that any inhibition is mediated by Ca^{2+}-dependent changes in a protein modifier of the enzyme.

The α-adrenergic receptors mediating the activation of hepatic phosphorylase have been shown to be of the α_1 subtype and have been localized to the liver plasma

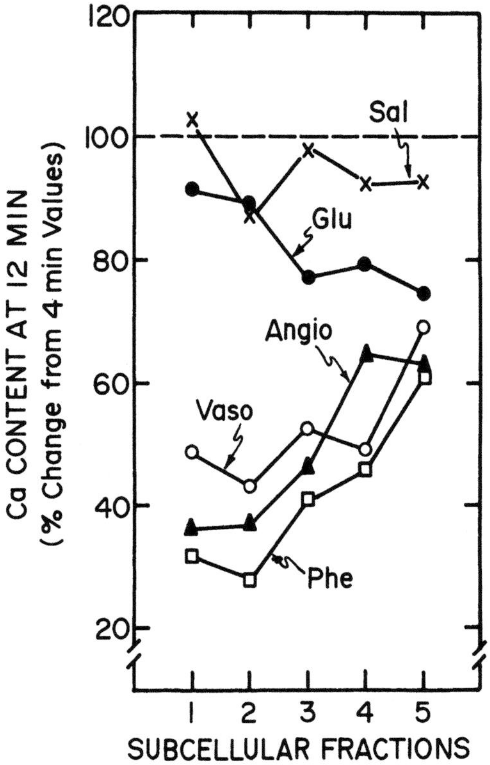

Fig. 6. Effects of infusion of saline (Sal), glucagon (Glu, 10^{-7} *M*), angiotensin II (Angio, 10^{-8} *M*), vasopressin (Vaso, 10^{-8} *M*), and phenylephrine (Phe, 10^{-5} *M*) on the Ca content of subcellular fractions isolated from perfused rat livers. Fractions 1–3 are enriched in mitochondria, and fractions 4 and 5 are enriched with microsomes. Values shown are percentage changes in fractions prepared from liver samples taken 8 min after commencement of infusions. (BLACKMORE et al. 1979b)

membrane (GUELLAEN et al. 1978; W. CLARKE et al. 1978; EL-REFAI et al. 1979; EL-REFAI and EXTON 1980; HOFFMAN et al. 1980; AGGERBECK et al. 1980). DEHAYE et al. (1980) have also demonstrated that epinephrine immobilized by covalent linkage to a large polymer rapidly and potently elicits α-adrenergic responses in hepatocytes without penetrating the cell membrane or releasing epinephrine. These findings imply the existence of an intracellular second messenger for the α-adrenergic system which is generated at the plasma membrane by activation of α-adrenergic receptors and causes mitochondrial Ca^{2+} release and perhaps other intracellular changes.

Interestingly, treatment of livers with epinephrine, which activates both β- and α-adrenergic receptors, results in decreased mitochondrial Ca^{2+}, but increased microsomal Ca^{2+} (DEHAYE et al. 1980). The increase in microsomal Ca^{2+} is mediated by β-receptors since it is completely blocked by propranolol. It is also partly decreased by phentolamine, but this is probably because some release of Ca^{2+} from the mitochondria into the cytosol is necessary for full β-adrenergic stimulation of Ca^{2+} uptake by components of the endoplasmic reticulum.

III. Actions of Vasopressin, Angiotensin II and Oxytocin on Hepatic Glycogenolysis

Liver glycogen breakdown is rapidly stimulated by vasopressin, oxytocin and angiotensin II due to phosphorylase activation (HEMS and WHITTON 1973; HEMS et al. 1976, 1978; KEPPENS et al. 1977; VAN DE WERVE et al. 1977; BLACKMORE et al. 1978, 1979b; GARRISON et al. 1979). The action of these peptides resembles that of α_1-adrenergic agonists in that it is independent of cyclic AMP and cyclic AMP-dependent protein kinase (KIRK and HEMS 1974; KEPPENS et al. 1977; GARRISON et al. 1979), but is dependent on Ca^{2+} (STUBBS et al. 1976; KEPPENS et al. 1977; GARRISON et al. 1979). Like α-agonists, the peptides rapidly mobilize intracellular (mitochondrial) Ca^{2+} (Fig. 6; BLACKMORE et al. 1978, 1979b; CHEN et al. 1978) which presumably leads to stimulation of phosphorylase *b* kinase. Studies with antagonists indicate that the hepatic receptors for angiotensin II and vasopressin are different from the hepatic α-adrenergic receptors (BLACKMORE et al. 1979b; GARRISON et al. 1979).

The physiological significance of the hepatic effects of the vasoactive peptides is debatable. HEMS et al. (1976) present data supporting the claim that the plasma concentrations of vasopressin and angiotensin II can reach levels sufficient to activate glycogenolysis during hemorrhagic shock and certain other stress states. More recently, HAUSTRAETE and DEWULF (1979) have reported the occurrence of very high levels of vasopressin in alloxan-diabetic rats and have suggested that these contribute to the hyperglycemia. Uncontrolled human diabetics also show large elevations of plasma vasopressin which are decreased by insulin therapy (ZERBE et al. 1979).

IV. Insulin Inhibition of Hepatic Glycogenolysis

1. Action Against Glucagon

It has been demonstrated in vivo and in vitro that insulin inhibits the action of low concentrations of glucagon and catecholamines on hepatic glucose output. Figure 1 from the studies of CHERRINGTON et al. (1976) illustrates the inhibitory action of insulin in vivo on splanchnic glucose output in dogs. When insulin deficiency is induced by infusion of somatostatin plus glucagon (right panel), there is a prompt, marked rise in hepatic glucose production which results in hyperglycemia. When normal concentrations of insulin are restored by portal infusion (not shown), glucose production and blood sugar are normalized. Thus, these data and similar findings in other in vivo studies (CHERRINGTON et al. 1978; EL-REFAI and BERGMAN 1979) indicate that basal concentrations of insulin normally restrain the glycogenolytic action of glucagon in vivo. When insulin is restored in the absence of glucagon in somatostatin-infused dogs, there is no significant effect (CHERRINGTON et al. 1976). Thus basal insulin appears to have no detectable action on liver glucose metabolism in the absence of glucagon in vivo. SACCA et al. (1979) have shown that infusion of glucagon into a peripheral vein in dogs in vivo at a rate sufficient to produce a peak *peripheral* venous plasma concentration of 5×10^{-11} *M* reverses the effects of insulin on hepatic glucose output. However, it is not known what concentrations of portal venous glucagon were achieved in this study.

Most in vitro studies have also shown negligible or very small effects of insulin on hepatic glycogen metabolism in the absence of other hormones (EXTON and PARK 1972; VAN DE WERVE et al. 1977; BLACKMORE et al. 1979a). WITTERS and AVRUCH (1978) have reported that insulin causes a slow inactivation of phosphorylase in hepatocytes incubated with high concentrations of glucose.

Insulin restraint of glucagon-stimulated hepatic glycogenolysis has been repeatedly demonstrated in the perfused rat liver and isolated rat hepatocytes (GLINSMANN and MORTIMORE 1968; JEFFERSON et al. 1968; MACKRELL and SOKAL 1969; EXTON and PARK 1972; EXTON et al. 1972b; VAN DE WERVE et al. 1977; MASSAGUE and GUINOVART 1977; BLACKMORE et al. 1979a). The effect is attributable to a reduction in phosphorylase *a* levels (MACKRELL and SOKAL 1969; VAN DE WERVE et al. 1977; BLACKMORE et al. 1979a) and is mainly, if not entirely, the result of a decrease in cyclic AMP (Fig. 7; JEFFERSON et al. 1968; EXTON and PARK 1972; EXTON et al. 1972b; BLACKMORE et al. 1979a) with associated reductions in the activities of cyclic AMP-dependent protein kinase and phosphorylase *b* kinase (VAN DE WERVE et al. 1977). Insulin is ineffective against glucagon concentrations higher than 10^{-9} *M* in isolated rat hepatocytes (VAN DE WERVE et al. 1977; BLACKMORE et al. 1979a) and is of similar limited effectiveness in the perfused liver (GLINSMANN and MORTIMORE 1968; MACKRELL and SOKAL 1969; EXTON et al. 1972b). These findings suggest that the major role of insulin is to suppress the glycogenolytic action of the low levels of glucagon seen normally in portal blood.

The decrease in hepatic cyclic AMP induced by insulin may be due to stimulation of the low K_m form of cyclic AMP phosphodiesterase (LOTEN et al. 1978). When administered to intact liver cells, physiological levels of the hormone produce a rapid, but stable, increase in the activity of a membrane-bound form of the enzyme. The magnitude of the effect is small, but evidence has been produced that it is sufficient to account for the reduction in cyclic AMP observed in intact cells (LOTEN et al. 1978). The mechanism(s) involved remains obscure. Surprisingly, glucagon and cyclic AMP produce similar effects to insulin on the enzyme (LOTEN et al. 1978). Insulin has also been reported to inhibit hepatic adenylate cyclase, but this effect has been difficult to reproduce (for references, see LOTEN et al. 1978).

2. Action Against Catecholamines

Insulin exerts a small, but significant inhibitory action against epinephrine-induced glycogenolysis in the rat liver in vitro (EXTON et al 1972b; BLACKMORE et al. 1979a). This is attributable largely to its inhibition of α-adrenergic activation of phosphorylase (VAN DE WERVE 1977; BLACKMORE et al. 1979a; MASSAGUE and GUINOVART 1978). Insulin inhibits the mobilization of intracellular Ca^{2+} from mitochondria induced by α-adrenergic stimulation in hepatocytes (BLACKMORE et al. 1979a; DEHAYE et al. 1981). It is probable that this leads to a reduction in cytosolic Ca^{2+} thus decreasing phosphorylase *b* kinase activity and hence phosphorylase *a* levels. Insulin does not inhibit glycogenolysis induced by vasopressin or angiotensin II (MA et al. 1978; BLACKMORE et al. 1979a; DEHAYE et al. 1981), nor does it alter the intracellular mobilization of Ca^{2+} induced by these agents (BLACKMORE et al. 1979a; DEHAYE et al. 1981). This selectivity of insulin action implies that the hormone acts by inhibiting the binding of agonists to the α_1-receptor

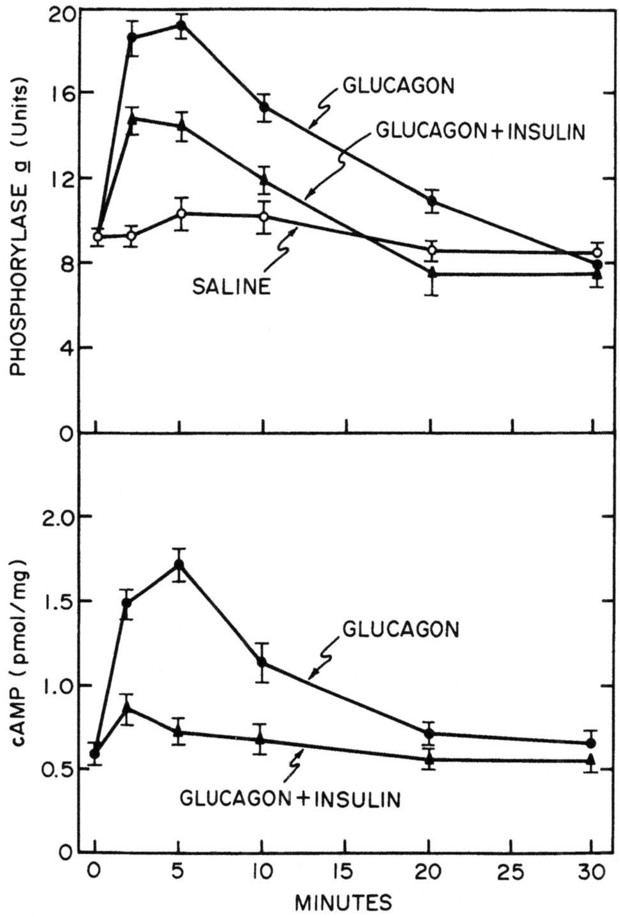

Fig. 7. Time courses of effects of glucagon (2×10^{-10} *M*) and glucagon plus insulin (6×10^{-9} *M*) on the levels of phosphorylase *a* and cyclic AMP in isolated rat hepatocytes. (BLACKMORE et al. 1979a)

or the early events leading to the generation of the putative intracellular messenger of the α_1-adrenergic system. Preliminary observations by P. F. BLACKMORE and J. H. EXTON have indicated that insulin inhibits α-agonist binding to hepatocytes.

Since insulin antagonizes the actions of glucagon in the liver by inhibiting the accumulation of cyclic AMP, it would also be expected to inhibit the β-adrenergic effects of catecholamines by a similar mechanism. However, this has not been demonstrated (VAN DE WERVE et al. 1977).

V. Glucose Modulation of Hormone Effects on Hepatic Glycogenolysis

Hepatic glucose production in vivo is importantly regulated by variations in the blood glucose level (SHULMAN et al. 1978; CHERRINGTON et al. 1979). Hyperglycemia induced by infusion of glucose into dogs depresses hepatic glucose output markedly under conditions in which glucagon and insulin do not change, and causes uptake of glucose by the liver when glucagon is withdrawn (SHULMAN et al. 1978). Likewise, when the hypoglycemia following induction of selective glucagon deficiency in dogs is prevented by glucose infusion, hepatic glucose output is reduced further (CHERRINGTON et al. 1979). Thus changes in blood glucose can modify the action of glucagon on glucose production in vivo. The inhibitory effect of hyperglycemia on phosphorylase activation by glucagon and other agents can also be demonstrated in the perfused rat liver (BUSCHIAZZO et al. 1970) and in hepatocytes (STRICKLAND et al. 1980).

Hers and associates (STALMANS et al. 1970, 1971, 1974a, b) have provided evidence that glucose acts by binding to phosphorylase *a* favoring its conversion to phosphorylase *b* by phosphorylase phosphatase. MADSEN et al. (1978) have observed structural changes in muscle phosphorylase *a* caused by glucose binding (see Sect. D.I.2). There is transition of the enzyme from a relaxed to a taut conformation in which the phosphorylated serine residue 14 becomes exposed to the action of phosphorylase phosphatase. When phosphorylase *a* is converted to phosphorylase *b*, it binds the phosphatase poorly. It is proposed that the phosphatase thus becomes free to activate glycogen synthase.

VI. Permissive Effects of Glucocorticoids on Hormone Activation of Liver Phosphorylase

The actions of glucagon and epinephrine on hepatic phosphorylase and glycogenolysis are impaired in adrenalectomized rats and can be restored by glucocorticoid treatment (SCHAEFFER et al. 1969a; EXTON et al. 1972a; SAITOH and UI 1975; CHAN et al. 1979b, 1979c). These changes are a manifestation of the permissive effect of glucocorticoids and are illustrated in Fig. 8. Since cyclic AMP accumulation in response to glucagon is normal in livers from adrenalectomized rats (Fig. 8; EXTON et al. 1972a; CHAN et al. 1979c), it is clear that the steroids are not acting at the level of the glucagon receptor, adenylate cyclase or cyclic AMP phosphodiesterase. There is also much evidence that the effect of the nucleotide on cyclic AMP-dependent protein kinase is not impaired. This is shown by the normal activation of the enzyme by glucagon in intact hepatocytes (Fig. 8; CHAN et al. 1979c) and by cyclic AMP in broken cell preparations (ZAPF et al. 1973; ROUSSEAU et al. 1976). There is also no alteration in the subcellular distribution of the kinase (ROUSSEAU et al. 1976) or in the activity of its thermostable protein inhibitor (ROUSSEAU 1977).

CHAN et al. (1979c) have obtained evidence that phosphorylase *b* kinase activation by glucagon is impaired in adrenalectomized rats (Fig. 8) and this would explain the defect in hormone activation of glycogenolysis. Whether the decreased activation of phosphorylase *b* kinase is due to alterations in the action of cyclic AMP-dependent protein kinase on the enzyme, or is due to increased activity of the phosphatase which inactivates phosphorylase *b* kinase is unknown.

The effects of glucocorticoids on catecholamine actions in the liver are complicated since the steroids suppress β-adrenergic actions (WOLFE et al. 1976; CHAN et al. 1979b) and enhance α-adrenergic actions (CHAN et al. 1979b). Thus the effects of adrenalectomy and steroid replacement depend on the relative roles of the two receptors in mediating hepatic responses to catecholamines. In adrenalectomized

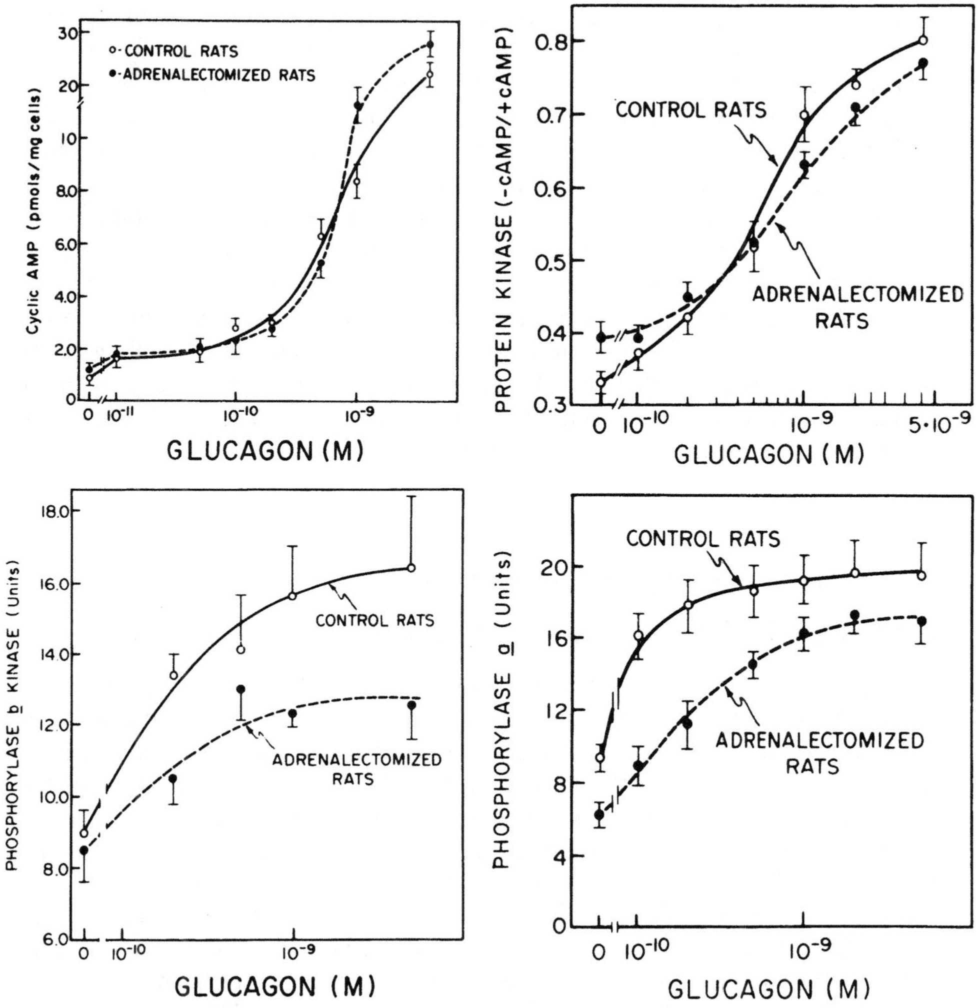

Fig. 8. Effects of adrenalectomy on glucagon stimulation of cyclic AMP accumulation *(top left panel)*, cyclic AMP-dependent protein kinase *(top right panel)*, phosphorylase *b* kinase *(bottom left panel)*, and phosphorylase *(bottom right panel)*. (CHAN et al. 1979c)

rats, the net result is an impaired response to epinephrine (SCHAEFFER et al. 1969a; EXTON et al. 1972a; SAITOH and UI 1975; CHAN et al. 1979b). Although glucocorticoid deficiency enhances the hepatic cyclic AMP response to β-agonists (EXTON et al. 1972; LERAY et al. 1973; WOLFE et al. 1976; CHAN et al. 1979b) due to an increase in β-receptors (WOLFE et al. 1976; GUELLAEN et al. 1978), the response of the liver to cyclic AMP is reduced (SCHAEFFER et al. 1969a; EXTON et al. 1972a; CHAN et al. 1979c). Furthermore, α-adrenergic responses are impaired (CHAN et al. 1979b). Preliminary data have indicated that adrenalectomy does not alter the number or affinity of α-receptors in liver (GUELLAEN et al. 1978; CHAN et al. 1979b) and it has been suggested that there is a defect in the generation or action of the putative intracellular messenger of the α-adrenergic system (CHAN et al. 1979b). However, more recent studies (M.F. EL-REFAI and J.H. EXTON, unpublished work) have indicated a loss of high affinity epinephrine binding sites in plasma membranes from adrenalectomized rats. Further work is required to resolve the situation. Interestingly, hypothyroidism, like adrenalectomy, also increases hepatic β-adrenergic responses (MALBON et al. 1978).

BLAIR et al. (1979a, b) have shown that in juvenile rats (27–35 days old), β-adrenergic receptors play a significant role in the hepatic responses to catecholamines, whereas in mature rats the β-receptor-mediated component is lost and catecholamines act primarily through α-receptors. Human diabetics also have an increased hyperglycemic response to epinephrine due to enhanced hepatic glucose output (SHAMOON et al. 1980), but it is not known which adrenergic component(s) is changed. The hormonal or other basis for the changes in adrenergic responses in aging and diabetic animals has not been explored.

B. Regulation of Hepatic Glycogen Synthesis

I. Glucagon Inhibition of Hepatic Glycogen Synthesis

Glucagon reduces the incorporation of isotopically labeled glucose and gluconeogenic substrates into liver glycogen in vivo and in vitro. The effect is due not only to activation of phosphorylase, but also to phosphorylation and inactivation of glycogen synthase (Fig. 9; BISHOP and LARNER 1967; DEWULF and HERS 1968a, b). Cyclic AMP-dependent protein kinase has been shown to phosphorylate the active or *a* form of liver glycogen synthase, converting it to the inactive form *b* (DEWULF and HERS 1968a; KILLILEA and WHELAN 1976; JETT and SODERLING 1979). The *a* form of the enzyme is almost fully active in the absence of glucose-6-P, whereas the *b* form is largely dependent on glucose-6-P for activity. Liver glycogen synthase *a* has a molecular weight of about 170,000 and is a dimer of apparently identical subunits (KILLILEA and WHELAN 1976; JETT and SODERLING 1979). It can be phosphorylated by cyclic AMP-dependent protein kinase to the extent of 2 or 3 moles of phosphate per mole of subunit with a reduction of the −glucose-6-P/+glucose-6-P activity ratio from approximately 0.9 to approximately 0.2 (JETT and SODERLING 1979). As is the case for muscle glycogen synthase *a*, it can also be phosphorylated by a cyclic AMP-independent kinase with a greater reduction in the activity ratio (JETT and SODERLING 1979).

Liver phosphorylase *b* kinase has been reported to phosphorylate and inactivate muscle glycogen synthase (SODERLING et al. 1979a) and recently PAYNE and SODERLING (1980) have identified in liver a separate, calmodulin-dependent synthase kinase using muscle glycogen synthase as substrate. Presumably both these kinases act on liver glycogen synthase, but this has not been demonstrated. It also seems likely that phosphorylation of liver glycogen synthase *a* by either cyclic AMP-dependent or -independent protein kinases produces alterations in the responsiveness of the enzyme to adenine nucleotide and other allosteric effectors similar to those reported for the muscle enzyme (ROACH and LARNER 1976; BROWN et al. 1977).

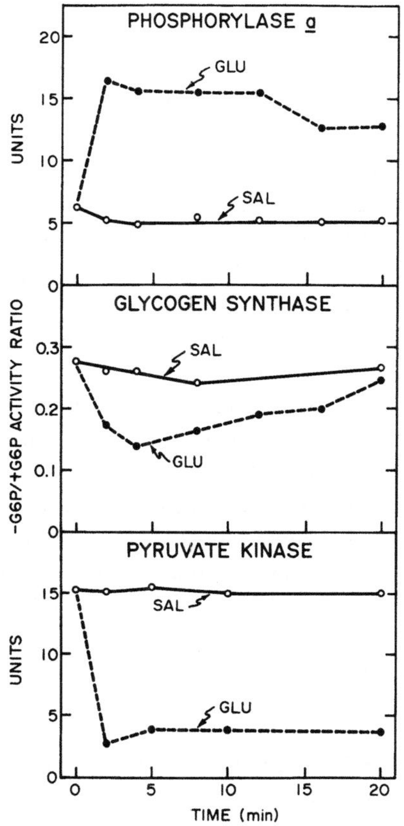

Fig. 9. Effects of glucagon (10^{-9} *M*) on the activities of phosphorylase *a*, glycogen synthase and pyruvate kinase in isolated rat hepatocytes. (N. J. HUTSON, T. M. CHAN, and J. H. EXTON, unpublished work)

The kinetic properties of liver glycogen synthase *a* and *b* are similar to those of the muscle enzyme, which is considered in more detail in Sect. E.I. The dephosphorylated form of the liver enzyme (*a*) has a K_m for UDP-glucose of about 1 m*M* in the absence of glucose-6-P and of about 0.1 m*M* in the presence of glucose-6-P (LARNER and VILLAR-PALASI 1971). It also has a K_a for glucose-6-P of about 0.06 m*M*. On the other hand, the phosphorylated form of the enzyme (*b*) has a K_m for UDP-glucose of 0.6 m*M* in the presence of glucose-6-P, and a K_a for glucose-6-P of about 1 m*M*.

HERS and his co-workers (STALMANS et al. 1971) have proposed an additional mechanism by which glucagon can control glycogen synthase activity in liver. As described in Sect. A.VI above, glycogen synthase *b* can be dephosphorylated and activated by a phosphoprotein phosphatase which also acts on phosphorylase *a* (KILLILEA et al. 1976). When phosphorylase *a* levels rise in response to hormonal stimulation, dephosphorylation of synthase *b* by the phosphatase is competitively inhibited. It is uncertain to what extent this effect contributes to the overall conversion of synthase *a* to *b* catalyzed by cyclic AMP-dependent protein kinase.

II. Catecholamine Inhibition of Hepatic Glycogen Synthesis

Epinephrine inactivates glycogen synthase in the liver in vivo (DEWULF and HERS 1968 b) and in vitro (HUTSON et al. 1976; HOSTMARK 1973; STRICKLAND et al. 1980). The effect is mediated by both α- and β-receptors. The β-receptor-cyclic AMP mechanism is presumably similar to that utilized by glucagon. The α-receptor mechanism in cAMP-independent, but involves phosphorylation of the enzyme (GARRISON et al. 1979). Several lines of evidence suggest a role for Ca^{2+} (GARRISON et al. 1979; STRICKLAND et al. 1980). For example, agents such as ionophore A23187, vasopressin and angiotensin II, which act like α-agonists in mobilizing intracellular Ca^{2+}, also cause phosphorylation and inactivation of glycogen synthase in a Ca^{2+}-dependent manner (GARRISON et al. 1979; STRICKLAND et al. 1980).

The mechanism by which α-adrenergic stimulation causes phosphorylation of glycogen synthase is unknown. A likely possibility is stimulation of a Ca^{2+}-dependent protein kinase by a rise in cytosolic Ca^{2+}. As noted above, it is not known whether liver phosphorylase *b* kinase can phosphorylate and inactive liver glycogen synthase. However, it has been reported that liver phosphorylase kinase can phosphorylate and inactive muscle glycogen synthase (SODERLING et al. 1979 b). The data of STRICKLAND et al. (1980) suggest that α-adrenergic inactivation of hepatic glycogen synthase is attributable to other changes besides phosphorylase *a*-mediated inhibition of synthase phosphatase (see Sect. B.I above).

III. Insulin, Glucose, and Glucocorticoid Stimulation of Hepatic Glycogen Synthesis

Insulin stimulates hepatic glycogen synthesis and activates glycogen synthase in vivo (BISHOP and LARNER 1967; KREUTNER and GOLDBERG 1967; BISHOP et al. 1971; BLATT and KIM 1971; T. MILLER and LARNER 1973) and in vitro (T. MILLER and LARNER 1973; WITTERS and AVRUCH 1978). It also inhibits or reverses the inactivation of liver glycogen synthase induced glucagon or epinephrine (HOSTMARK 1973; T. MILLER and LARNER 1973; STRICKLAND et al. 1980). Part of its action against these hormones is attributable to a reduction in cytosolic cyclic AMP and Ca^{2+} levels (see Sect. A.IV above). However, the effect of insulin added alone on glycogen synthase and glycogen synthesis in isolated liver preparations seems to be unrelated to changes in cyclic AMP (T. MILLER and LARNER 1973; WITTERS and AVRUCH 1978) and its mechanism(s) remains obscure.

Hepatic glycogen synthesis is reduced in fed diabetic animals and there have been many reports showing that the activation of glycogen synthase which occurs spontaneously during incubation of liver homogenates is reduced or absent in fed diabetic rats (GOLD 1970; BISHOP 1970; TAN and NUTTALL 1976; T. MILLER 1978 a, 1979; GOLDEN et al. 1979). This change is associated with a reduction in the activity of the *a* form of the enzyme which can be reversed by insulin treatment in vivo. Starvation also decreases the activity of the *a* form, but the spontaneous activation in homogenates is not altered (GOLDEN et al. 1979). These findings have been interpreted as indicating a reduction in hepatic glycogen synthase phosphatase activity in diabetic, but not fasted, animals (BISHOP 1970; T. MILLER 1978 a; GOLDEN et al. 1979).

Cyclic AMP is increased in livers of diabetic and fasted rats (JEFFERSON et al. 1968; EXTON et al. 1973; T. MILLER 1978a). The increase in diabetic livers is reversed by insulin treatment in vivo. There is also a small increase in the −cyclic AMP/+cyclic AMP activity ratio of protein kinase in diabetic liver. However, since the total activity of cAMP-dependent protein kinase is decreased, the −cyclic AMP activity does not change (T. MILLER 1978a). Phosphorylase *a* is increased in diabetic liver (T. MILLER 1978a), but this may be due to decreased P-protein phosphatase activity. Further work is needed to define the changes in cAMP-dependent and cAMP-independent protein kinase, P-protein phosphatases and phosphorylase in diabetic and insulin-treated rats.

Glucose activates liver glycogen synthase and promotes glycogen synthesis in vivo and in vitro (DEWULF and HERS 1968b; HUE et al. 1975; KATZ et al. 1979). HERS and his co-workers attribute the effect to a reduction in phosphorylase *a* (see Sect. VI). This is because they have demonstrated that phosphorylase *a* inhibits the action of synthase phosphatase to dephosphorylate and activate glycogen synthase (STALMANS et al. 1971), and that a decrease in phosphorylase *a* is a prerequisite for glucose activation of glycogen synthase in intact animals or isolated hepatocytes (STALMANS et al. 1974a; HUE et al. 1975). However, additional explanations for the action of glucose seem necessary (KATZ et al. 1979; STRICKLAND et al. 1980).

T. MILLER et al. (1973) and T. MILLER (1978a) have shown that the stimulatory effect of glucose on liver glycogen synthase is lost in diabetic rats, but can be restored by insulin treatment after 2 h. T. MILLER has suggested that the defect may be due to a decrease in glycogen synthase phosphatase activity or a change in the synthase molecule itself (T. MILLER 1978a, 1979). The effect of insulin on glycogen synthase phosphatase and on the activating effect of glucose both develop slowly and are blocked by cycloheximide (T. MILLER 1979).

Glucocorticoid administration in vivo increases liver glycogen levels and activates liver glycogen synthase (DEWULF and HERS 1968b; NICHOLS and GOLDBERG 1972), but there have been no reports of similar changes in vitro, and one group has obtained evidence that insulin release may mediate the changes (KREUTNER and GOLDBERG 1967; NICHOLS and GOLDBERG 1972). The increase in glycogen synthase *a* is slow and can be explained by enhanced glycogen synthase phosphatase activity (NICHOLS and GOLDBERG 1972). It has been suggested that glucocorticoids increase phosphorylase phosphatase activity thus diminishing the inhibitory action of phosphorylase *a* on synthase phosphatase (STALMANS et al. 1970). As described on Sect. A.VI, there is much evidence that glucocorticoids do not alter cAMP levels or the activity of cyclic AMP-dependent protein kinase in liver.

C. Regulation of Hepatic Gluconeogenesis

I. Glucagon Stimulation of Hepatic Gluconeogenesis

1. Evidence That Glucagon Exerts Physiological Control on Gluconeogenesis

Experiments in vivo in which physiological levels of glucagon have been replaced in animals infused with somatostatin have demonstrated that glucagon exerts physiological control on hepatic gluconeogenesis (JENNINGS et al. 1977; CHERRING-

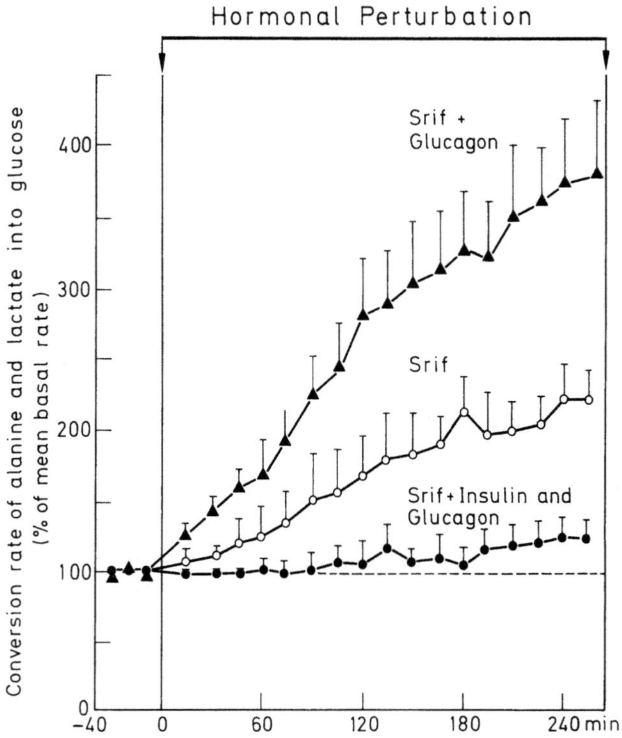

Fig. 10. Effects of somatostatin, somatostatin plus intraportal glucagon replacement, and somatostatin plus intraportal insulin and glucagon replacement on the conversion of circulating alanine and lactate into glucose in normal conscious dogs. (CHERRINGTON et al. 1978)

TON et al. 1978). Figure 10 from CHERRINGTON et al. (1978) shows the conversion of circulating alanine and lactate into glucose in conscious dogs infused with either somatostatin alone (to suppress endogenous secretion of glucagon and insulin) or somatostatin in combination with glucagon or glucagon plus insulin. The latter hormones were infused intraportally to restore normal arterial levels. The figure illustrates that basal glucagon stimulates gluconeogenesis markedly and that basal insulin completely suppresses the stimulation.

The in vivo findings cited above are supported by numerous studies showing that concentrations of glucagon within the range normally found in portal blood (10^{-10} to 10^{-9} *M*) stimulate gluconeogenesis from lactate, pyruvate, alanine, and certain other gluconeogenic amino acids in the isolated perfused liver and isolated hepatocytes (EXTON and PARK 1968; MALLETTE et al. 1969a; CLAUS et al. 1975; PILKIS et al. 1975; FELIU et al. 1976).

Since the liver consumes alanine and lactate, and converts them to glucose under most conditions in vivo (JENNINGS et al. 1977; CHIASSON et al. 1979; RABIN et al. 1979; FELIG et al. 1969; WAHREN et al. 1971, 1972, 1973; AHLBORG et al. 1974; FELIG and WAHREN 1971; Cherrington et al. 1978, 1979) and in vitro (for references, see EXTON 1972), it is customary to think of hormone effects on gluconeogenesis rather than on glycolysis. However, under certain conditions e.g. high blood glucose and insulin levels and low glucagon levels, the liver may release lactate formed by glycolysis. In this situation, glucagon's action would be thought of as inhibiting glycolysis, as originally proposed by SCHIMASSEK and MITZKAT (1963). As will be discussed in Sect. C.I.2 and C.I.5, this effect is probably attributable to inhibition of pyruvate kinase and P-fructokinase.

2. Glucagon Inhibition of Hepatic Pyruvate Kinase

Many mechanisms have been suggested for the stimulatory effect of glucagon on hepatic gluconeogenesis (for references, see PILKIS et al. 1978), but only four are reasonably well-established. These are: inhibition of pyruvate kinase and P-fructokinase and stimulation of mitochondrial pyruvate carboxylation, which occur rapidly, and induction of P-enolpyruvate carboxykinase, which is slower. ENGSTROM and his co-workers first reported that L-type pyruvate kinase from liver is phosphorylated by cyclic AMP-dependent protein kinase (LJUNGSTROM et al. 1974). Phosphorylation causes a decrease in enzyme activity at low concentrations of the substrate P-enolpyruvate and of the allosteric effector fructose-1,6-P_2.

Kinetic analysis shows that phosphorylation increases the concentration of P-enolpyruvate required for half-maximal activity of the enzyme ($K_{0.5}$) and increases the Hill coefficient for this substrate. It results in the incorporation of up to 1 mole of phosphate per mole of subunit and does not alter the tetrameric structure of the enzyme which has a molecular weight of 228,000. Neither the K- or M-types (isozymes) of the enzyme (which are found mainly in kidney and muscle, respectively) are phosphorylated or inhibited cyclic AMP-dependent protein kinase. Analogous to the situation with glycogen synthase, phosphorylation of L-type pyruvate kinase alters its sensitivity to allosteric regulators such as fructose-1,6-P_2, which is an activator, and alanine and ATP which are inhibitors (PILKIS et al. 1978). These changes may represent the major mechanism(s) by which the enzyme is controlled by cyclic AMP-dependent protein kinase in vivo (CLAUS et al. 1979).

Addition of glucagon to intact rats, perfused rat livers or isolated rat hepatocytes results in increased phosphorylation (LJUNGSTROM and EKMAN 1977; RIOU et al. 1978; ISHIBASHI and COTTAM 1978) and inactivation of pyruvate kinase (Fig. 9; BLAIR et al. 1976; FELIU et al. 1976). The decrease in the assayed activity of the enzyme is associated with decreased flux through pyruvate kinase in situ as determined by isotopic means (ROGNSTADT and KATZ 1977), and is well-correlated with the stimulatory effect of the hormone on gluconeogenesis (FELIU et al. 1976). The reason for this is that the gluconeogenic pathway is primarily regulated at the two substrate cycles located between pyruvate and P-enolpyruvate and between fructose 1,6-P_2 and fructose-6-P (Fig. 11). Thus inhibition of the reconversion of P-enolpyruvate to pyruvate due to the action of glucagon on pyruvate kinase will stimulate gluconeogenesis since it will result in greater flow of P-enolpyruvate to glucose.

3. Glucagon Stimulation of Hepatic Pyruvate Carboxylation

HAYNES and others (ADAMS and HAYNES 1969; GARRISON and HAYNES 1975; CHAN et al. 1979a) have presented evidence that glucagon stimulates pyruvate entry and

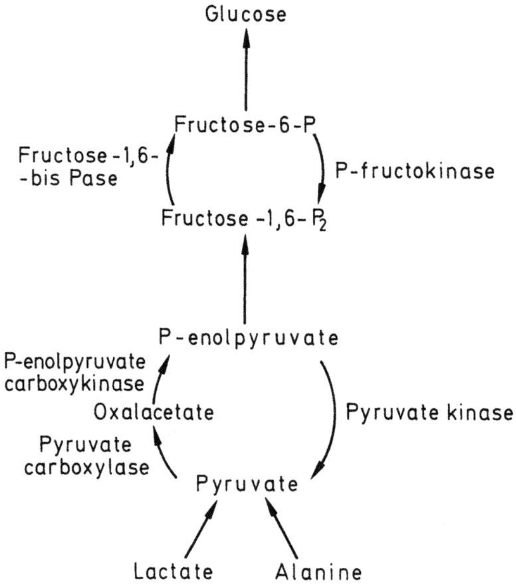

Fig. 11. Diagram of the gluconeogenic pathway showing substrate cycles between pyruvate and P-enolpyruvate and between fructose-1,6-P_2 and fructose-6-P

carboxylation in rat liver mitochondria. The effect is seen when the hormone is administered to whole animals or intact hepatocytes, and is mimicked by cyclic AMP. Glucagon treatment also increases respiration from several substrates, ATP generation, and ion movements in liver mitochondria. The primary change responsible for these alterations appears to be a stimulation of mitochondrial respiratory activity (YAMAZAKI 1975; TITHERADGE et al. 1978, 1979) due to increased electron flow between cytochromes c_1 and c (HALESTRAP 1978a). ZAHLTEN et al. (1972) have obtained evidence that glucagon increases the phosphorylation of liver inner mitochondrial membranes. Since cytochrome c_1 is located on the outer surface of the inner mitochondrial membrane, it may be available for phosphorylation by cyclic AMP-dependent protein kinase.

HALESTRAP (1978a, b) and others (PRPIC et al. 1978) have observed several changes reflecting an increase in the pH of the matrix of mitochondria from glucagon-treated rats and Halestrap has proposed that this is responsible for the stimulation of pyruvate transport. The increase in proton motive force is presumably due to the increased respiratory chain activity. Although the evidence that glucagon stimulates mitochondrial pyruvate uptake is extensive, CHAN et al. (1979a) have recently obtained results indicating a separate stimulatory effect of the hormone on intramitochondrial pyruvate carboxylation.

As noted in Sect. A.I.7 above, several groups have shown that high concentrations of glucagon alter Ca^{2+} fluxes in the perfused rat liver and isolated hepatocytes, and some have suggested that the changes may be related to the action of glucagon on gluconeogenesis (FRIEDMANN and RASMUSSEN 1970; CHEN et al. 1978). However this seems unlikely since gluconeogenesis can be activated by glucagon concentrations much lower than those required to stimulate Ca^{2+} fluxes.

4. Apparent Non-Involvement of Pyruvate Dehydrogenase in Glucagon Stimulation of Hepatic Gluconeogenesis

Pyruvate entering liver mitochondria can be converted to oxalacetate by pyruvate carboxylase or to acetyl-CoA by pyruvate dehydrogenase. Thus changes in the activity of pyruvate dehydrogenase can potentially alter the rate of gluconeogenesis from 3-carbon substrates. This enzyme is located within the inner mitochondrial membrane and is a high molecular weight complex (7–10,000,000 daltons) comprised of three types of catalytic components. These are: pyruvate decarboxylase (Enz. 1), dihydrolipoyl transacetylase (Enz. 2) and dihydrolipoyl dehydrogenase (Enz. 3). The reactions catalyzed by these enzymes are:

(1) $Pyruvate + TPP \cdot Enz_1 \rightarrow CO_2 + 2\alpha\text{-hydroxyethyl-}TPP \cdot Enz_1$

(2) $2\text{-}\alpha\text{-hydroxyethyl-}TPP \cdot Enz_1 + Lip\ S \cdot S \cdot Enz_2 \rightarrow TPP \cdot Enz_1 + Lip\ SH \cdot S\ acetyl \cdot Enz_2$

(3) $Lip\ SH \cdot S\ acetyl \cdot Enz_2 + CoA \rightarrow acetyl\ CoA + Lip\ SH \cdot SH \cdot Enz_2$

(4) $Lip\ SH \cdot SH \cdot Enz_2 + FAD \cdot Enz_3 \rightarrow Lip\ S \cdot S \cdot Enz_2 + FADH_2 \cdot Enz_3$

(5) $FADH_2 \cdot Enz_3 + NAD^+ \rightarrow FAD \cdot Enz_3 + NADH + H^+$.

The overall regulation of the complex is exerted at the first reaction i.e. pyruvate decarboxylation. This reaction is thermodynamically very favorable and cannot be reversed, unlike the other steps.

In the native complex, there are 60 subunits of dihydrolipoyl transacetylase (52,000 daltons) to which 20–30 pyruvate carboxylases ($\alpha_2\beta_2$ composition: α, 41,000 daltons, β, 36,000 daltons) and 5–6 dihydrolipoyl dehydrogenases (55,000 daltons) are attached (REED 1969; REED et al. 1974). The complex also contains a cAMP-independent kinase attached to the transacetylase core which phosphorylates the α-subunits of pyruvate decarboxylase thereby inhibiting the two reactions involving 2 α-hydroxyethyl TPP. A less tightly bound phosphatase which reverses the reaction is also present. This enzyme requires Mg^{2+} and Ca^{2+} for full activity.

In general, the kinase is inhibited by the substrates of pyruvate dehydrogenase (pyruvate, NAD^+, CoA, TPP) and is activated by the products (NADH, acetyl CoA) (DENTON et al. 1975). In addition, the kinase is inhibited by ADP which competes with ATP. Because of these effects, pyruvate dehydrogenase is controlled under physiological conditions by the $NADH/NAD^+$ and acetyl CoA/CoA ratios. For example, under conditions of enhanced fatty acid oxidation when these ratios increase, the enzyme is inhibited and pyruvate oxidation is suppressed. It is probable that some of the effects of hormones on the enzyme are secondary to changes in fatty acid metabolism.

The α-subunit of the pyruvate carboxylase component of the enzyme can be phosphorylated by the kinase at 3 different serine residues. There is rapid incorporation of 0.5 mole of phosphate per mole of subunit at one site and this is associated with complete inactivation. The two other sites are phosphorylated much more slowly (DAVIS et al. 1977; YEAMAN et al. 1978; SUGDEN and RANDLE 1978). A possible function of these two sites is to control dephosphorylation. As expected, dephosphorylation of the first site is associated with reactivation. When the other two sites are phosphorylated, the rate of dephosphorylation of the first site is reduced (SUDGEN et al. 1978).

The foregoing description of the structure and regulation of pyruvate dehydrogenase has been based on data from several tissues. The liver enzyme appears similar to that described above. It has a similar structure (REED 1969; REED et al. 1974) and is regulated in the same manner by substrates and products of the reaction (REED 1969; REED et al. 1974; WIELAND et al. 1972; PORTENHAUSER and WIELAND 1972; WALAJTYPS et al. 1974; S. TAYLOR et al. 1975; SIESS and WIELAND 1976). Hormone actions which increase hepatic fatty acid oxidation could therefore alter pyruvate dehydrogenase activity (WIELAND et al. 1972; PATZELT et al. 1973).

Dichloroacetate, an activator of pyruvate dehydrogenase, has variable effects on gluconeogenesis in hepatocytes depending on the substrate, incubation conditions and nutritional state of the liver donors (CRABB et al. 1976; CLAUS and PILKIS 1977). However, it does not modify the effects of glucagon on gluconeogenesis even though it markedly stimulates pyruvate oxidation (CLAUS and PILKIS 1977). This indicates that changes in pyruvate dehydrogenase are not involved in the action of glucagon on gluconeogenesis. YAMAZAKI and HAYNES (1975) and MAPES and HARRIS (1976) have reached a similar conclusion using different approaches.

Several groups have shown that pyruvate oxidation is increased in liver mitochondria from rats injected with glucagon or epinephrine in vivo (ADAM and HAYNES 1969; YAMAZAKI and HAYNES 1975; TITHERADGE and COORE 1976a, b; CHAN et al. 1979a). This effect is probably related to a stimulation of pyruvate uptake by the mitochondria (see Sect. C.I.3). Efforts to demonstrate a change in pyruvate dehydrogenase actively in homogenates of rat hepatocytes or liver treated with glucagon have been unsuccessful (CLAUS and PILKIS 1977; DENTON et al. 1981). In addition, it has not been shown that glucagon alters pyruvate oxidation in *intact* hepatocytes or perfused livers. Although ZAHLTEN et al. (1973) reported that glucagon decreased [^{14}C]-CO_2 formation from [1-^{14}C] pyruvate in hepatocytes by 20%, this effect has been attributed to the decrease in gluconeogenesis which occurred in their experiments (PILKIS et al. 1978). In overall summary, there is no evidence that the effect of glucagon on mitochondrial pyruvate oxidation in vitro plays any role in the effects of the hormone on gluconeogenesis in the intact liver cell. There is also no clear evidence that insulin regulates pyruvate oxidation in liver in vivo or in vitro (PATZELT et al. 1973; STANSBIE et al. 1976).

5. Glucagon Inhibition of Hepatic P-Fructokinase

Several studies have indicated that glucagon stimulates flux through the gluconeogenesis pathway at the fructose-6-P-fructose-1,6-P_2 substrate cycle (CLARK et al. 1974; ROGNSTAD and KATZ 1977; VAN SCHAFTINGEN et al. 1980a). Stimulation at this site as well at the pyruvate-P-enolpyruvate substrate cycle would explain the stimulatory effect of glucagon on substrates entering gluconeogenesis at the level of triose-P (PILKIS et al. 1976) and also the changes in metabolic intermediates induced by glucagon in livers perfused with gluconeogenic substrates (EXTON and PARK 1969). Several groups have recently shown glucagon inhibition of hepatic P-fructokinase when the enzyme is assayed with limiting fructose-6-P concentrations (CASTANO et al. 1979, PILKIS et al. 1979; NIETO and CASTANO 1980; VAN SCHAFTINGEN et al. 1980b). One group has shown that the enzyme can be phosphorylated by cyclic AMP-dependent protein kinase (KAJIMOTO and UYEDA 1979). However, it appears that this phosphorylation is not responsible for the inhibitory action of glucagon on the enzyme, and VAN SCHAFTINGEN et al. 1980a, b) have obtained evidence that glucagon acts by reducing the intracellular concentration of fructose-2,6-P_2, an activator of the enzyme. Their findings have been confirmed by PILKIS et al. (1981a) and UYEDA et al. (1981).

6. Glucagon Induction of P-Enolpyruvate Carboxykinase

In addition to causing rapid changes in enzyme activity which are attributable to enzyme phosphorylation, glucagon produces slower alterations in liver enzyme levels. Amongst the enzymes whose synthesis or degradation is altered by the hormone is P-enolpyruvate carboxykinase which catalyzes the conversion of oxalacetate to P-enolpyruvate in the gluconeogenic pathway. This enzyme is located in the cytosol and/or mitochondria depending on the species, but only the cytosolic form is subject to hormonal and dietary changes (NORDLIE et al. 1965). Both forms of the enzyme have a molecular weight of about 80,000, but are immunologically distinct (BALLARD and HANSON 1969). The cytosolic enzyme is activated by divalent transition metal ions (Fe^{2+}, Mn^{2+}, Co^{2+}, and Cd^{2+}) and it has been shown by LARDY and co-workers (BENTLE et al. 1976; BENTLE and LARDY 1977; MACDONALD et al. 1978) that the effect of Fe^{2+} on the enzyme requires a cytosolic protein called the ferroactivator. This is a tetramer of approximately 100,000 daltons which has a tissue distribution similar to that of P-enolpyruvate carboxykinase (highest in liver and kidney). Starvation and diabetes increase the amount of ferroactivator in liver (MACDONALD et al. 1978), but it is not known whether the effect is mediated by glucagon or if the hormone alters the activity of the ferroactivator.

Glucagon and cyclic AMP increase the synthesis of P-enolpyruvate carboxykinase in liver (SHRAGO et al. 1963; YEUNG and OLIVER 1968; WICKS 1969, 1971; WICKS et al. 1972; GUNN et al. 1975) and this is probably responsible for the "long-term" effect of the hormone on gluconeogenesis. The hormone acts through cyclic AMP to increase the amount of functional messenger RNA coding for the enzyme on the ribosomes (IYNEDJIAN and HANSON 1977). It is not known whether the increase is due to increased production or decreased degradation of the message. Cyclic AMP-dependent protein kinase has been shown to phosphorylate and activate DNA-dependent RNA polymerase II from calf thymus (KRANIAS et al. 1977). but whether a similar action is involved in glucagon induction of enzymes in liver is unknown.

7. Other Mechanisms Possibly Involved in Glucagon Stimulation of Gluconeogenesis

Glucagon and epinephrine stimulate the transport of the model amino acid α-aminoisobutyrate into perfused livers or incubated hepatocytes (MALLETTE et al. 1969b; LECAM and FREYCHET 1976; FEHLMANN et al. 1979; EDMONDSON et al. 1979). There is also evidence that glucagon stimulates the uptake of alanine and other gluconeogenic amino acids (MALLETTE et al. 1969b; EDMONDSON et al. 1979). Although it is not certain that membrane transport is rate-limiting for amino acid gluconeogenesis under physiological circumstances, these findings point to this process as a possible site for hormonal control of gluconeogenesis. Surprisingly, the transport of α-aminobutyrate into hepatocytes is also stimulated by insulin, which inhibits gluconeogenesis (LeCam and Freychet 1978; Fehlmann et al. 1979).

Another gluconeogenic enzyme which has been implicated in the short-term glucagon stimulation of gluconeogenesis is fructose 1,6-bisphosphatase. Riou et al. (1977) have found that cyclic AMP-dependent protein kinase can phosphorylate this enzyme and cause a slight increase in its activity. The enzyme has also been shown to be phosphorylated in vivo (Riou et al. 1977). The major action of glucagon on the enzyme is probably mediated by the decrease in fructose-2,6-P_2 since this is an inhibitor of the enzyme (Van Schaftingen and Hers 1981; Pilkis et al. 1981b).

Glucagon produces slow changes in the activity of a number of enzymes involved in carbohydrate and amino acid metabolism in liver in addition to P-enolpyruvate carboxykinase (Rosenfeld and Barrieux 1979). Some of these changes have been shown to result from alterations in enzyme synthesis. It is not clear what role, if any, they play in the gluconeogenic action of glucagon in vivo.

II. Catecholamine Stimulation of Hepatic Gluconeogenesis

Epinephrine and norepinephrine stimulate hepatic gluconeogenesis, but are less potent than glucagon (Exton and Park 1968; Tolbert et al. 1973; Feliu et al. 1976; Hutson et al. 1976). Although it was earlier thought that the action of the catecholamines was due to the rise in cyclic AMP induced by activation of β-receptors (Exton and Park 1968; Exton et al. 1971), Tolbert et al. (1973) showed that it was also due to cyclic AMP-independent mechanisms mediated by α-receptors. Their findings have been confirmed repeatedly, although the mechanisms involved are not well understood. α-Adrenergic stimulation of liver cells results in rapid inactivation of pyruvate kinase (Chan and Exton 1978; Kemp and Clark 1978; Blair et al. 1979b; Garrison et al. 1979; Claus et al. 1979) which is associated with phosphorylation of the enzyme (Garrison et al. 1979; Steiner et al. 1980). Garrison et al. (1979) have speculated that the phosphorylation is Ca^{2+}-dependent. They have found that vasopressin and angiotensin II also produce phosphorylation and inhibition of pyruvate kinase in hepatocytes. Like α-adrenergic agonists, these peptides do not stimulate cyclic AMP accumulation and their actions on pyruvate kinase are Ca^{2+}-dependent (Garrison et al. 1979).

Epinephrine has been shown to stimulate hepatic mitochondrial pyruvate carboxylation via an α-adrenergic, cyclic AMP-independent mechanism (Garrison and Borland 1979). The hormone also has a small inhibitory effect on P-fructokinase activity in hepatocytes (Pilkis et al. 1979), which is probably mediated by β-receptors.

Kneer et al. (1979) have recently demonstrated that Ca^{2+} ions are required for α-adrenergic stimulation of gluconeogenesis from substrates which enter the gluconeogenic pathway prior to P-enolpyruvate and from reduced substrates that enter at triose-P or fructose-6-P (glycerol or polyols). However, the ions are not necessary for the stimulation by α-agonists of gluconeogenesis from substrates entering at triose-P which increase the oxidation state of cytosolic NAD. Kneer et al.

(1979) have proposed that Ca^{2+} acts by increasing the rate of reoxidation of cytosolic NADH by mitochondria, and have suggested that the effect may involve stimulation of α-glycerophosphate dehydrogenase.

Vasopressin, angiotensin II and oxytoxin have been reported to stimulate gluconeogenesis from several substrates in the perfused rat liver and rat hepatocytes (HEMS and WHITTON 1973; WHITTON et al. 1978). However the changes are relatively small (10–40% increases). Vasopressin and angiotensin II have also been shown to inhibit pyruvate kinase activity in liver (CHAN and EXTON 1978; GARRISON et al. 1979) apparently by a Ca^{2+}-dependent phosphorylation mechanism(s) (GARRISON et al. 1979). This inhibition could explain the effects of these agents on gluconeogenesis. Collaborative experiments between the groups of D. A. HEMS and R. M. DENTON (cited in DENTON et al. 1981) have shown that pyruvate dehydrogenase activity is increased about 2-fold in rat livers perfused with vasopressin or in rat hepatocytes incubated with the agent. Angiotensin, epinephrine and phenylephrine, an α-adrenergic agonist, have been reported to have similar effects (cited in DENTON et al. 1981; ADAM and HAYNES 1969). The biochemical basis for these changes and their possible relation to the gluconeogenic action of these agents remain to be defined.

Exercise results in the mobilization of lactate and alanine from muscle, and glycerol and fatty acids from adipose tissue, in part because of increased sympathetic stimulation. Despite the large increase in glucose uptake occurring in muscle during exercise, the arterial concentration of this substrate remains remarkably constant. This is because hepatic glucose output is concurrently increased (ISSEKUTZ et al. 1970; VRANIC and WRENSHALL 1969), due mainly to glycogenolysis, but also to gluconeogenesis, especially during prolonged exercise (AHLBORG et al. 1974; WAHREN et al. 1971). Enhancement of the splanchnic uptake of lactate, pyruvate, and glycerol occurs rapidly (WAHREN et al. 1971) and there is also increased splanchnic fractional extraction of alanine and other glucogenic amino acids (AHLBORG et al. 1974; FELIG and WAHREN 1971; WAHREN et al. 1973). Splanchnic uptake of gluconeogenic precursors increases further during prolonged exercise and, under such conditions, gluconeogenesis would account for almost half of hepatic glucose output if there was total conversion of extracted gluconeogenic precursors to glucose (AHLBERG et al. 1974).

III. Insulin Inhibition of Hepatic Gluconeogenesis

As described earlier in this section, insulin can suppress the stimulatory effect of glucagon on gluconeogenesis in vivo (Fig. 10). Insulin inhibition of glucagon or epinephrine stimulation of gluconeogenesis can also be demonstrated in in vitro preparations such as isolated hepatocytes (PILKIS et al. 1975; FELIU et al. 1976; CLAUS and PILKIS 1976). FELIU et al. (1976) have shown effects of insulin on pyruvate kinase activity which correspond to those on gluconeogenesis. In the case of insulin antagonism of glucagon action, the changes can be ascribed to alterations in the level of cyclic AMP (EXTON et al. 1972b; PILKIS et al. 1975; BLACKMORE et al. 1979a) and in the activity of cyclic AMP-dependent protein kinase (VAN DE WERVE 1977; CLAUS et al. 1979). In the case of insulin inhibition of epinephrine action in rat liver, the changes are largely independent of cyclic AMP and cyclic

AMP-dependent protein kinase (CHAN and EXTON 1978; CLAUS et al. 1979) since they mainly involve modulation of α-adrenergic responses (BLACKMORE et al. 1979a). It is not known whether insulin inhibition of α-adrenergic stimulation of gluconeogenesis is attributable to a decrease in cytosolic Ca^{2+} (BLACKMORE et al. 1979a; DEHAYE et al. 1981), but this is possible. There have been no published reports of the effects of insulin on β-adrenergic stimulation of hepatic gluconeogenesis in any species.

In addition to exerting direct inhibitory effects on hepatic gluconeogenesis, insulin can also reduce glucose synthesis in vivo by reducing the supply of gluconeogenic substrates to the liver from the periphery. It has been well demonstrated that insulin inhibits the release of glycerol from adipose tissue and of gluconeogenic amino acids from skeletal muscle.

Diabetes and starvation are characterized by enhanced gluconeogenesis with muscle protein wasting and mobilization of adipose tissue triglyceride (EXTON et al. 1973; WAHREN et al. 1972; GARBER et al. 1974; POZEFSKY et al. 1976). Amino acids and glycerol are released from these tissues into the bloodstream at an accelerated rate. There is increased hepatic utilization of gluconeogenic amino acids (FELIG et al. 1969; WAHREN et al. 1972; GARBER et al. 1974) leading to a decrease in their plasma concentrations. However, branched-chain amino acids accumulate in the bloodstream since their hepatic uptake is minimal (WAHREN et al. 1972).

It is probable that the enhancement of gluconeogenesis in the liver during diabetes and starvation is due to insulin lack and glucagon excess. This would be consistent with the effects of these hormones on the liver in vivo and in vitro as described in preceding sections, and with the rises in hepatic cyclic AMP observed in starvation and diabetes (JEFFERSON et al. 1968; GOLDBERG et al. 1969; EXTON et al. 1973). The high rate of gluconeogenesis from amino acids seen in the early stages of starvation in man declines during prolonged starvation i.e. after 5–6 weeks (FELIG et al. 1969). This has been attributed to the large decline in plasma alanine, but other factors may be involved.

There is no doubt that alterations in enzyme levels underlie the changes in hepatic gluconeogenesis during diabetes and starvation. Many gluconeogenic enzymes are increased in activity and, in addition, glucokinase and pyruvate kinase are decreased. Measurements of tissue metabolic intermediates have identified the sequences between pyruvate and P-pyruvate and between glucose-6-P and glucose as the major sites at which changes occur (EXTON et al. 1973). Thus, the known increases in P-enolpyruvate carboxykinase and glucose-6-phosphatase and decreases in glucokinase and pyruvate kinase in diabetes and starvation probably play significant roles. However, since metabolite analyses may not identify all the enzyme changes contributing to alterations in metabolic flux, there may be important effects at other sites.

The gluconeogenic enzyme which probably plays a major role in the changes in gluconeogenesis in diabetes and starvation is P-enolpyruvate carboxykinase. LARDY and his associates (SHRAGO et al. 1963; YOUNG et al. 1964) first demonstrated the large increases in cytosolic P-enolpyruvate carboxykinase that occur during starvation and diabetes. Since inhibitors of protein synthesis block the rise in the enzyme in these conditions, it is generally assumed that increased enzyme formation is involved. A role for cyclic AMP in the induction of P-enolpyruvate carboxykinase and the enhancement of gluconeogenesis during diabetes and starvation has been proposed by EXTON et al. (1973). These workers found a correlation between the ability of insulin to lower cyclic AMP levels and reduce lactate gluconeogenesis and P-enolpyruvate carboxykinase activity in diabetic livers. KRONE et al. (1976) have also found a good correlation between liver cyclic AMP levels and P-enolpyruvate carboxykinase activity during starvation. As noted earlier (Sect. C.I.5), it has been amply demonstrated that cyclic AMP or its derivatives, and agents which promote cyclic AMP accumulation induce several gluconeogenic enzymes including P-enolpyruvate carboxykinase in the liver in vivo, in liver explants or in hepatoma cells (BARNETT and WICKS 1971; SHRAGO et al. 1963; WICKS 1969, 1971; WICKS et al. 1972; YEUNG and OLIVER 1968).

The increase in glycerol release from adipose tissue during diabetes and starvation is attributable to insulin lack and/or insensitivity. A role for glucagon in this phenomenon in insulin-deficient diabetics is also possible (SCHADE et al. 1979). The enhanced release of amino acids from muscle in these situations is explicable in terms of decreased insulin levels and sensitivity since this hormone stimulates protein synthesis and inhibits protein breakdown in muscle (CAHILL et al. 1972) leading to a decrease in amino acid release (POZEFSKY et al. 1969).

IV. Permissive Effects of Glucocorticoids on Hormone Activation of Hepatic Gluconeogenesis

FRIEDMANN et al. (1967) first demonstrated that glucocorticoids were required for the stimulation of hepatic gluconeogenesis by glucagon. Subsequent work showed that the steroid hormones did not act by modifying the cyclic AMP- cyclic AMP-dependent protein kinase system (EXTON et al. 1972a; ROUSSEAU et al. 1976; CHAN et al. 1979c).

The biochemical basis of the permissive effects of glucocorticoids on gluconeogenesis remains obscure and there is no evidence at present which indicates that these hormones act by altering the action of cyclic AMP-dependent protein kinase on specific hepatic gluconeogenic enzymes. Glucocorticoids are also permissive for catecholamine activation of hepatic gluconeogenesis (EXTON et al. 1972a). This may be attributed in part to their potentiation of α-adrenergic responses in the liver (CHAN et al. 1979b), but other factors are probably involved.

Glucocorticoids also stimulate gluconeogenesis in vivo, by virtue of their permissive effects on the stimulation of glycerol release by lipolytic hormones (for references, see EXTON et al. 1972a) and their stimulatory action on net amino acid release from muscle protein (CALDWELL et al. 1978).

D. Regulation of Muscle Glycogenolysis

I. Catecholamine Stimulation of Muscle Glycogenolysis

1. Physiological Aspects

The classic metabolic response of muscle to epinephrine is glycogen breakdown. This is more prominent in fast-contracting white skeletal muscle than in cardiac or slower-contracting red muscle, which probably relates to the that fast-contracting muscle relies more on glycolysis for ATP production, whereas the latter muscles rely more on oxidative metabolism for their energy needs (ELLIS 1956; MAYER 1970; HORNBROOK and BRODY 1963; WILLIAMSON 1975). White skeletal muscle has a higher content of glycogen and glycogen-metabolizing enzymes and a lower mitochondrial content than slow-contracting red muscle (PETTE and BUCHER 1963). Consequently, it responds rapidly to epinephrine by increasing glycogenolysis and glycolysis thus generating ATP for fast anaerobic contractions (HELMREICH and Cori 1965). In man, most skeletal muscles are of an intermediate type, but glycogenolysis provides ATP production during short bursts of intense activity. It also contributes to energy production during the brief period before blood flow to contracting skeletal muscles is increased during exercise.

The stimulation of muscle glycogenolysis by catecholamines is due to activation of phosphorylase by phosphorylase *b* kinase (Fig. 12), and both these enzymes are present in higher concentrations in fast-contracting muscles than in slower-contracting muscles. The response in skeletal muscle is mediated entirely by β-adrenergic receptors (Fig. 13; DIETZ et al. 1980). These receptors also play the major role in the action of epinephrine on the heart (B. WILLIAMS and MAYER 1966; NAMM and MAYER 1968), but there is some evidence for a minor contribution via α-receptors in this tissue (KEELY et al. 1977). As noted below, catecholamines stimulate glycogen breakdown in smooth muscle, but the mechanism depends on the type(s) of adrenergic receptor stimulated.

Epinephrine activation of glycogenolysis without concurrent stimulation of P-fructokinase leads to accumulation of hexose phosphates in skeletal or cardiac muscle, but minimal increases in lactate and energy production or in O_2 consumption (KARTAPKIN et al. 1964; HELMREICH and CORI 1965; WILLIAMSON 1964, 1966; DIETZ et al. 1980; O. WALAAS and WALAAS 1950). In contrast, during contraction of these muscle types, when glycogenolysis is accompanied by increased glycolysis, due to the effects of adenine nucleotide changes on P-fructokinase activity, there is rapid energy production, O_2 consumption and lactate release (FISHER and WILLIAMSON 1961; KARTAPKIN et al. 1964; HELMREICH and CORI 1965; WILLIAMSON 1966).

The role of the sympathetic nervous system in regulating glycogen metabolism in contracting skeletal muscle is not well defined. Contraction per se appears to provide sufficient activation of glycogenolysis, and addition of epinephrine to contracting frog sartorius muscle does not lead to further increases in lactate production (HELMREICH and CORI 1965). However, epinephrine has been reported to delay muscle fatigue in frogs and increase the responsiveness of glycogenolysis to repetitive stimulation (HELMREICH and CORI 1966). In view of the generally held view that epinephrine contributes to the performance of athletes, this area needs further investigation.

In heart, where epinephrine increases the force of contraction (inotropism), the concentrations of adenine nucleotides change due to the increased work and this causes facilitation of P-fructokinase (WILLIAMSON 1966). At low epinephrine concentrations the substrate utilized in cardiac glycolysis is blood glucose, whereas at higher concentrations both glucose and endogenous glycogen are used (MAYER 1963; WILLIAMSON 1964). Epinephrine causes an initial burst of lactate production

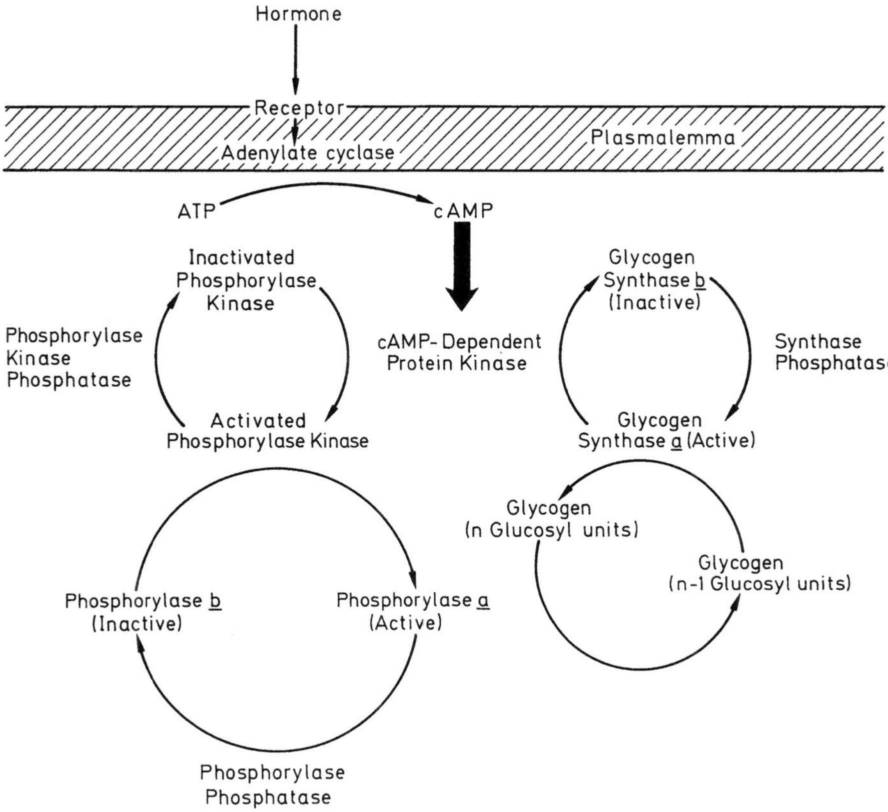

Fig. 12. Diagram of the mechanisms involved in epinephrine activation of phosphorylase and inactivation of glycogen synthase in skeletal muscle

due to glycogenolysis, followed by a more prolonged increase in oxidative metabolism which is probably the result of increased work (WILLIAMSON 1964, 1966). The inotropic and glycogenolytic effects of epinephrine can be dissociated (WILLIAMSON 1964; WILLIAMSON and JAMIESON 1965, 1966) although they probably both arise from the increase in cAMP (ROBISON et al. 1965). Phosphorylation of cardiac troponin I can be shown in vitro with cyclic AMP-dependent protein kinase (COLE and PERRY 1975) and in rat or rabbit hearts perfused with epinephrine (ENGLAND 1975; SOLARO et al. 1976). There is evidence that this phosphorylation alters the Ca^{2+}-sensitivity of the ATPase activity of cardiac contractile proteins and may thus be partly responsible for the inotropic action of epinephrine (ENGLAND 1975; RAY and ENGLAND 1976; SOLARO et al. 1976; RUBIO et al. 1975; MCCLELLAN and WINEGRAD 1978). However, it seems that other changes are involved (ENGLAND 1976; FREARSON et al. 1976; EZRAILSON et al. 1977).

Initiation of the action potential in muscle causes a depolarization of the sarcolemma which spreads to the transverse tubular system (T system) of the muscle fiber. By some unknown mechanism, this causes release of Ca^{2+} from the cisternae of the sarcoplasmic reticulum (EBASHI and ENDO 1968; ENDO 1977). The rise in

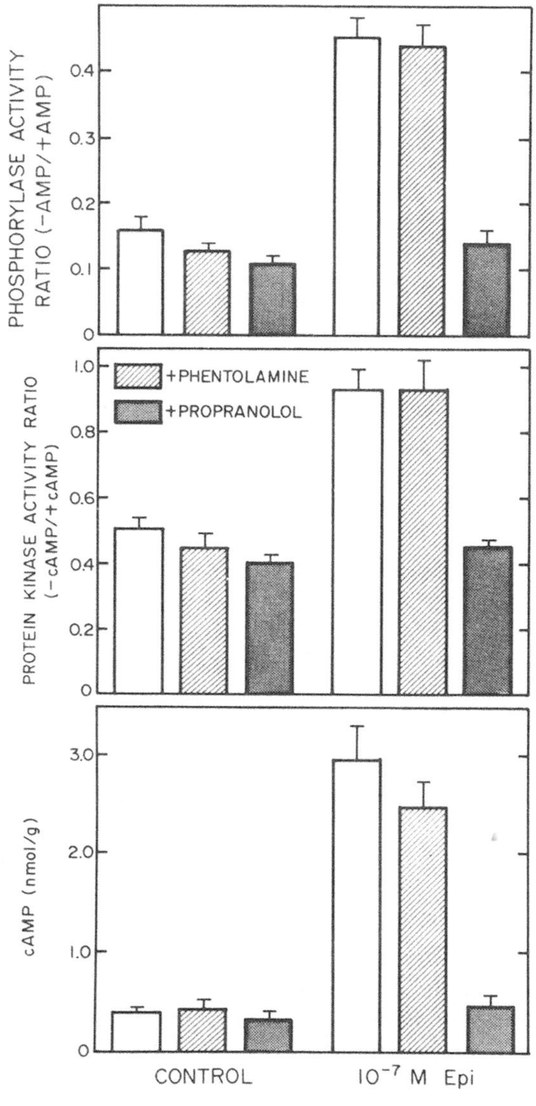

Fig. 13. Effects of adrenergic blockade on epinephrine actions on cyclic AMP, cyclic AMP-dependent protein kinase and phosphorylase in perfused rat skeletal muscle. (DIETZ et al. 1980)

myoplasmic Ca^{2+} arising from these changes results in increased binding of Ca^{2+} to troponin C and this decreases the inhibitory effect of the troponin-tropomyosin complex on the interaction of actin and myosin. Thus actin and myosin interact resulting in contraction. Since the Ca^{2+} concentration changes which influence the contractile process are similar to those which stimulate muscle phosphorylase *b* kinase (BROSTROM et al. 1971), contraction is accompanied by phosphorylase activation. With relaxation, Ca^{2+} is pumped back into the sarcoplasmic reticulum and phosphorylase *b* kinase activity declines. Interestingly, the activation of phosphorylase in continuously or intermittently stimulated muscle is transient (CONLEE et al. 1979). This may be due to the rise in glucose-6-P (see Sect. D.I.3).

In smooth muscle, the effects of epinephrine are determined by the type of adrenergic receptor principally affected. Activation of β-receptors causes relaxation and phosphorylase activation, whereas activation of α-receptors causes contraction (except for intestinal smooth muscle where relaxation occurs) and also phosphorylase activation. The β-adrenergic activation of phosphorylase probably occurs by the same phosphorylation cascade as in skeletal muscle (Fig. 12), and relaxation is probably the result of the action of cAMP-dependent protein kinase on myosin light chain kinase (ADELSTEIN et al. 1978). Smooth muscle contraction results from the phosphorylation of the light chains of myosin by the Ca^{2+}-calmodulin-sensitive enzyme, myosin light chain kinase (CHACKO et al. 1977; DABROWSKA et al. 1978; BARRON et al. 1980). When this enzyme is phosphorylated by cAMP-dependent protein kinase its sensitivity to Ca^{2+}, and hence activity, is decreased (ADELSTEIN et al. 1978) and relaxation ensues. β-Adrenergic relaxation of smooth muscle may also result from enhanced uptake of cytosolic Ca^{2+} by endoplasmic reticulum due to cyclic AMP-dependent phosphorylation of a specific protein (BOLTON 1979; NISHIKORI et al. 1977; NISHIKORI and MAENO 1979; MUELLER and VAN BREEMEN 1979; CASTEELS and RAEYMAEKERS 1979), or from increased Ca^{2+} efflux as a result of stimulation of the Na^+/K^+ pump in the plasma membrane (for detailed mechanism, see SCHEID et al. 1979). The α-adrenergic responses are probably due to a rise in cytosolic Ca^{2+} resulting from the influx of extracellular Ca^{2+} and mobilization of Ca^{2+} from intracellular pools (ENDO 1977; BOLTON 1979). It is probable that smooth muscle phosphorylase *b* kinase is regulated by mechanisms similar to those in skeletal muscle.

Epinephrine exerts direct, but opposite, effects on the contractility of fast-contracting and slow-contracting skeletal muscle. Both effects are mediated by β-adrenergic receptors. Fast-contracting muscles respond to the catecholamine by augmented twitch tension, increased total duration of contraction, and slightly decreased rate of rise of tension (TOMITA 1975; MORAN 1975). Slow-contracting muscles respond by decreased twitch tension and shortening of the contraction duration. In heart, activation of β-receptors results in increased rate and force of contraction (chronotropic and inotropic effects). The effects of epinephrine on muscle contractility probably relate to changes in Ca^{2+} release or uptake by the sarcoplasmic reticulum. In heart, there is also an increase in the inward Ca^{2+} current during the plateau phase of the action potential (WILLIAMSON 1975; STULL and MAYER 1979; WINEGRAD 1979). The biochemical basis of these effects is not well-defined, except for the enhancement of cardiac relaxation. It has been found that cyclic AMP increases Ca^{2+} uptake and Ca^{2+}-activated ATP-ase activity in cardiac sarcoplasmic reticulum (ENTMAN et al. 1969; WRAY et al. 1973; TADA et al. 1974; KIRCHBERGER et al. 1974) and this has been attributed to phosphorylation by cyclic AMP-dependent protein kinase of phospholamban, a 22,000 dalton protein in sarcoplasmic reticulum (TADA et al. 1974, 1975; KIRCHBERGER and TADA 1976; LE PEUCH et al. 1979). Recently, it has been found that phospholamban can also be phosphorylated by a Ca^{2+}-calmodulin-dependent protein kinase (LE PEUCH et al. 1979). In this way the activity of the sarcoplasmic Ca^{2+}-ATP-ase pump can be controlled by the cytosolic Ca^{2+} concentration. KIRCHBERGER and TADA (1976) have also reported that cyclic AMP-dependent protein kinase phosphorylates microsomes from slow-contracting skeletal muscle and causes increased Ca^2 uptake. They noted that microsomes from fast-contracting muscle were not affected. However, SCHWARTZ et al. (1976) and BORNET et al. (1977) have reported that the kinase does increase Ca^{2+} accumulation in such microsomes.

There have been reports that cyclic AMP stimulates the phosphorylation of proteins in cardiac sarcolemmal preparations and increases the accumulation of Ca^{2+} in these preparations (for references, see ST. LOUIS and SULAKHE 1979; D. WALSH et al. 1979). Such changes could be related to the epinephrine-induced increase in Ca^{2+} inflow during the cardiac action potential. However, these findings have been questioned on the basis of the impurity of the sarcolemmal preparations used (STULL and MAYER 1979).

Because of the evidence that catecholamines alter Ca^{2+} movements in the heart and the possibility that they do so in skeletal muscle (KIRCHBERGER and TADA 1976; SCHWARTZ et al. 1976), the mechanisms by which they control glycogenolysis in these tissues may be complex, i.e. through phosphorylation of phosphorylase *b* kinase and alterations in Ca^{2+} fluxes due to phosphorylation of intracellular membrane constituents. The effects of epinephrine on cytosolic Ca^{2+} probably account for some of the reported discrepancies between catecholamine action on the assayed activities of phosphorylase *b* kinase and phosphorylase *a* in cardiac and skeletal muscle (NAMM et al. 1968; STULL and MAYER 1971).

Infusion of epinephrine in dogs, rats, and man in vivo decreases glucose clearance (ALTSZULER et al. 1967; SHIKAMA and UI 1975a, b; SACCA et al. 1978, 1979; RIZZA et al. 1979, 1980; DEIBERT and DEFRONZO 1980). This is probably due to several factors including decreased insulin release mediated by α-adrenergic receptors in the endocrine pancreas (PORTE 1967) and inhibition of insulin-stimulated glucose uptake in muscle (see below). However, the reduced clearance is also seen when insulin secretion is suppressed by somatostatin infusion (RIZZA et al. 1979) and appears to be mediated by β-receptors (SHIKAMA and UI 1975b).

Studies of the effects of epinephrine on glucose uptake by isolated muscle have given variable results (HIMMS-HAGEN 1967). In early experiments utilizing isolated diaphragm, the hormone was reported to inhibit glucose uptake (O. WALAAS and E. WALAAS 1950; ELLIS 1956), and it was suggested that this occurred because glycogenolysis caused the accumulation of hexose phosphates which inhibit hexokinase (CRANE and SOLS 1954; NEWSHOLME and RANDLE 1961; MAYER 1963; REGEN et al. 1964; E. WALAAS 1955). However, the significance of these effects is uncertain since they were observed in phosphate-buffered media, but not consistently in bicarbonate-buffered media.

More recently, epinephrine (10^{-8} to 10^{-5} *M*) has been reported to inhibit 3-O-methylglucose transport in rat diaphragm and soleus through β-adrenergic mechanisms (BIHLER et al. 1978; SLOAN et al. 1978). At higher concentration (10^{-5} to 10^{-3} *M*) the catecholamine has also been shown to stimulate 3-O-methylglucose transport in diaphragm (BIHLER et al. 1978; SAITOH et al. 1974), but this effect seems unlikely to be of physiological significance. As described earlier, epinephrine can stimulate glucose uptake by the heart because of increased contractility (inotropism) which stimulates glucose transport (NELLY et al. 1967, 1969) and alters

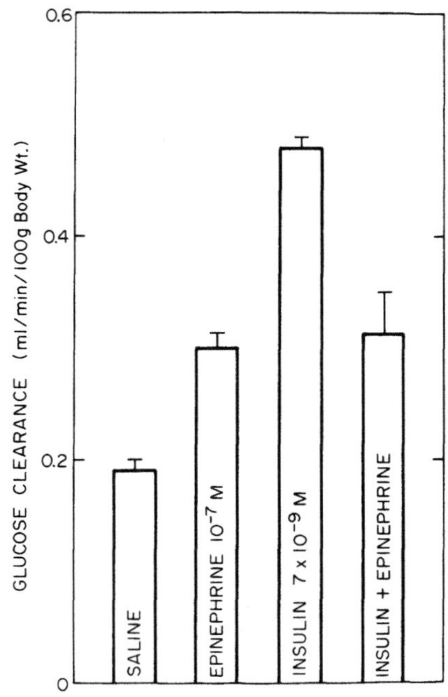

Fig. 14. Effects of epinephrine and insulin (alone or in combination) on glucose clearance in perfused rat hindlimbs. (J. L. CHIASSON, H. SHIKAMA, and J. H. EXTON,, unpublished work)

the tissue levels of adenine nucleotides leading to activation of P-fructokinase (WILLIAMSON 1966).

In some experiments, the effects of epinephrine on muscle glucose uptake have been studied in the presence of controlled levels of insulin. Under these conditions, epinephrine inhibits the stimulation of glucose uptake in vivo (SACCA et al. 1979; RIZZA et al. 1980; DEIBERT and DEFRONZO 1980) and in vitro (E. WALAAS 1955; CHIASSON et al. 1981; Fig. 14). This effect is mediated by β-adrenergic receptors (CHIASSON et al. 1981; RIZZA et al. 1980; DEIBERT and DEFRONZO 1980) and enhances the ability of catecholamines to reverse insulin-induced hypoglycemia (SACCA et al. 1979). Since glucagon has no effects on peripheral glucose utilization (CHERRINGTON and VRANIC 1974; POZEFSKY et al. 1976; SHERWIN et al. 1976), its reversal of insulin hypoglycemia is attributable mainly, if not entirely, to its hepatic actions (SACCA et al. 1979). The mechanism by which epinephrine inhibits insulin-stimulated glucose uptake in muscle has been explored by CHIASSON et al. (1981) who have shown that it is not due to inhibition of glucose transport, but to restraint of glucose phosphorylation because of the accumulation of hexose phosphates which inhibit hexokinase (see above).

2. Roles of Cyclic AMP, Cyclic AMP-Dependent Protein Kinase, and Phosphorylase b Kinase

Epinephrine promotes glycogen breakdown in striated, smooth and cardiac muscle through a cascade of phosphorylation reaction triggered by activation of the β-ad-

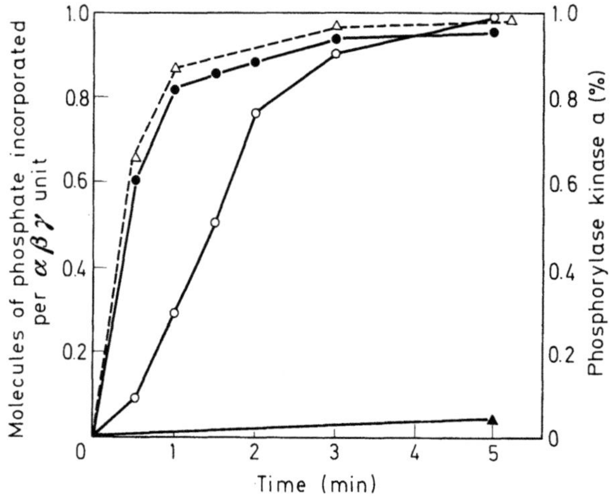

Fig. 15. Phosphorylation of muscle phosphorylase *b* kinase in vitro by cAMP-dependent protein kinase. Phosphorylation of α-subunit *(open circles)*, β-subunit *(solid circles)*, and γ-subunit *(solid triangle)* as well as changes in the pH 6.8/8.2 activity ratio *(open triangles* and *broken line)* are shown. (P. COHEN 1978)

renergic receptor-adenylate cyclase system of the sarcolemma and resulting finally in the conversion of phosphorylase *b* to *a*. Various aspects of the sequence are considered in detail in other chapters and only the general scheme will be presented here (Fig. 12). The accumulation of cyclic AMP induced by epinephrine in muscle tissues is very rapid (detectable within a few seconds in heart and skeletal muscle) and is accompanied by prompt activation of cyclic AMP-dependent protein kinase, phosphorylase *b* kinase and phosphorylase (DANFORTH et al. 1962; DRUMMOND et al. 1966, 1969; B. WILLIAMS and MAYER 1966; ROBISON et al. 1965; POSNER et al. 1965; NAMM and MAYER 1968; LYON and MAYER 1969; DIETZ et al. 1980). The mechanism by which cyclic AMP activates cyclic AMP-dependent protein kinase is described briefly in Sect. A.I.3, and in more detail in Vol. 1 (see BEAVO and MUMBY 1982).

Phosphorylase *b* kinase is a major substrate of cyclic AMP-dependent protein kinase in fast-twitch glycolytic skeletal muscle and cardiac muscle. It is a high molecular weight complex (1.3 million daltons) composed of four distinct subunits (α, β, γ, and δ) associated as $\alpha_4\beta_4\gamma_4\delta_4$. The α subunit from white muscle differs from that from red muscle (JENNISSEN and HEILMEYER 1974). It is unknown whether this is associated with functional differences in the enzymes. Cyclic AMP-dependent protein kinase phosphorylates the enzyme to the extent of 2 moles of phosphate per mole of αβγδ monomer. Phosphate is incorporated into specific serine residues in both the α and β subunits, (Fig. 15; P. COHEN 1973; YEAMAN et al. 1977). The other subunits are not phosphorylated. Phosphorylation of the β-subunit occurs more rapidly and is associated with activation of the enzyme, whereas phosphorylation of the α-subunit is slower and does not directly alter enzyme activity (Fig. 15).

The δ-subunit has recently been shown to be identical to calmodulin, the calcium-dependent regulator protein of cAMP phosphodiesterase (P. COHEN et al.

1978; WOLFF and BROSTROM 1979). It is probably the site at which Ca^{2+} ions bind to and stimulate the enzyme (Fig. 16). Phosphorylase *b* kinase can also bind, with less affinity, a second molecule of calmodulin per monomer accounting for the stimulatory effect of added calmodulin on the enzyme (SHENOLIKAR et al. 1979; K. WALSH et al. 1980).

There is dispute as to whether the catalytic activity of the enzyme resides in the β- or γ-subunit. GRAVES and co-workers have obtained strong evidence that the γ-subunit is the catalytic moiety of phosphorylase *b* kinase from rabbit muscle (SKUSTER et al. 1980). However, results from FISCHER'S group working with the enzyme from dogfish indicate that the β-subunit is catalytically active (FISCHER et al. 1976). The two enzymes differ in that the dogfish enzyme does not undergo phosphorylation-dephosphorylation.

Phosphorylase *b* kinase undergoes intermolecular autophosphorylation in the presence of Mg-ATP and Ca^{2+}, and this results in a large increase in activity. Phosphate is incorporated into both the α- and β-subunits up to a total of 9 moles per mole of monomer (WANG et al. 1976). It appears that most of the phosphate is incorporated into the α-subunit. There is evidence that some of the sites which are autophosphorylated are different from those phosphorylated by cAMP-dependent kinase, but there also seem to be some common sites (SINGH and WANG 1977). Activation by either process involves a large (50-fold) increase in activity at pH 6.8 (due to a decrease in the K_m for phosphorylase *b*) and a smaller (2-fold) increase at pH 8.2. The ratio of activities at pH 6.8 and 8.2 is routinely used as a measure of the activation state of the enzyme.

There is abundant evidence that epinephrine activates muscle phosphorylase through the cAMP-dependent phosphorylation mechanism (e.g. Fig. 13). Furthermore, phosphorylation of muscle phosphorylase *b* kinase by cyclic AMP-dependent protein kinase has been well demonstrated in vitro. However, only recently has it been clearly shown that epinephrine stimulates the phosphorylation of the enzyme in vivo (YEAMAN and COHEN 1975; MCCULLOUGH and WALSH 1979a). YEAMAN and COHEN (1978) isolated the enzyme from rabbits injected with epinephrine using a homogenizing medium containing EDTA and NaF. The activation state of the enzyme was largely preserved through purification. The phosphate content of the enzyme from untreated rabbits was 2.5–3 moles per mole of αβγδ subunit, while that of the enzyme from epinephrine-treated animals was 3.5–4 moles per mole of subunit. Analysis of tryptic peptides isolated from the enzyme from epinephrine-treated animals showed phosphate in the same sites in the α- and β-subunits as those found when the enzyme is phosphorylated by cAMP-dependent protein kinase in vitro. No significant phosphorylation of these sites was found in the enzyme from control rabbits.

MCCULLOUGH and WALSH (1979a) examined the incorporation of $[^{32}P]$ into the enzyme in rat hearts perfused with $[^{32}P]$i and different concentrations of epinephrine. They found a linear correlation between $[^{32}P]$ content of the enzyme and its activation state. $[^{32}P]$ was incorporated into both the α- and β-subunits.

Mice of the I strain have been shown to have only 0.2% of normal phosphorylase *b* kinase activity in their skeletal muscles (GROSS and MAYER 1974; P. T. W. COHEN and COHEN 1973). This is due to an alteration in the amino acid sequence in the β-subunit (P. T. W. COHEN and COHEN 1973). During muscle contraction in I

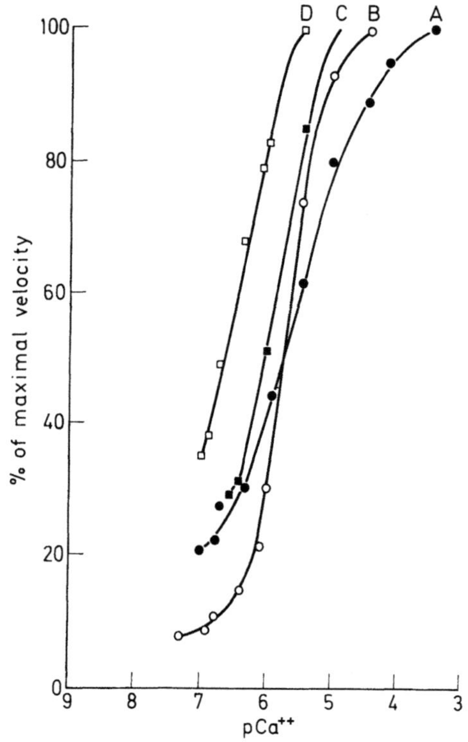

Fig. 16. Effects of Ca^{2+} on the activity of muscle phosphorylase *b* kinase. Non-activated phosphorylase *b* kinase is represented at pH 6.8 by curve *A* and at pH 8.2 by curve *B*. Activated phosphorylase *b* kinase is represented at pH 6.8 by curve *C* and at pH 8.2 by curve *D*. (Brostrom et al. 1971)

strain mice, there is no conversion of phosphorylase *b* to *a* as seen in normal mice (Danforth and Lyon 1964). However, glycogenolysis occurs after a lag (Danforth and Lyon 1964) due probably to the increase in AMP during contraction.

Figure 16 illustrates that, like the liver enzyme, muscle phosphorylase *b* kinase is stimulated by concentrations of Ca^{2+} within the range (10^{-7} *M* to 10^{-6} *M*) prevailing in muscle cytosol (Brostrom et al. 1971; Ebashi and Endo 1968). Both non-activated and activated phosphorylase *b* kinase are stimulated by Ca^{2+}, but the activated form is more sensitive to the cation (Fig. 16; Brostrom et al. 1971). Ca^{2+} probably acts by interacting with the δ subunit and any additional calmodulin bound to the enzyme. As stated earlier, there is much evidence that the release of Ca^{2+} from the sarcoplasmic reticulum plays a major role in the activation of phosphorylase seen during the contraction of skeletal muscle (Drummond et al. 1969; Stull and Mayer 1971).

Phosphorylase *b* kinase can be activated in vitro by cGMP-dependent protein kinase (Lincoln and Corbin 1977) and by a Ca^{2+} dependent protease present in muscle (Huston and Krebs 1968). It is doubtful whether the proteolytic mechanism of activation operates under physiological conditions since it is irreversible. The possible physiological role of cGMP-dependent kinase is unknown.

Phosphorylase *b* kinase can be dephosphorylated by at least two separate phosphatases in muscle (Antoniw and Cohen 1976). One enzyme has greater activity towards the β-subunit, is also active towards phosphorylated histone, phosphorylase and glycogen synthase, and is inhibited by at least two heat-stable proteins isolated from muscle (P. COHEN 1978). The other enzyme dephosphorylates the α-subunit, is more specific, and is not affected by the inhibitory proteins (P. COHEN 1978). The control of the dephosphorylation of phosphorylase *b* kinase may be very complex, particularly since the activity of one of the inhibitor proteins is increased when it is phosphorylated by cyclic AMP-dependent protein kinase (see Sect. D.I.4). P. COHEN (1978) and his colleagues (H. NIMMO and COHEN 1977; FOULKES and COHEN 1979) have proposed some complex schemes by which phosphorylase *b* kinase activity can be controlled by cyclic AMP-dependent protein kinase, but it is uncertain how many of these operate in vivo.

For many years it was thought that phosphorylase *b* was the sole substrate of muscle phosphorylase *b* kinase, but recently it has been found that the enzyme phosphorylates troponin T, troponin I and sarcoplasmic reticulum (STULL et al. 1972; PERRY and COLE 1974; SCHWARTZ et al. 1976; HORL et al. 1978), and phosphorylates and inactivates glycogen synthase (ROACH et al. 1978; DEPAOLI-ROACH et al. 1979a, b; SODERLING et al. 1979a, b; K. WALSH et al. 1979; EMBI et al. 1979). It is unclear whether phosphorylase *b* kinase acts on these other substrates in vivo or that its action on them is of physiological significance. In the case of phosphorylation of troponin I, there is evidence that this is not important in vitro (PERRY and COLE 1974). Furthermore, since epinephrine has normal chronotropic and inotropic effects in I strain mice (ENGLAND 1977), its possible phosphorylation by phosphorylase *b* kinase seems not to be physiologically significant.

3. Activation of Phosphorylase

Phosphorylase is a large component of the soluble protein of muscle, especially in fast-twitch glycolytic fibers (H. NIMMO and COHEN 1977). The *b* form of the muscle enzyme is a dimer of approximately 200,000 daltons containing 2 sites for pyridoxal 5-P, a ligand which is essential for activity (FISCHER et al. 1971). This form of the enzyme is dependent upon AMP for activity. The nucleotide greatly increases the affinity of the enzyme for its substrates (HELMREICH and CORI 1964; HEDRICK et al. 1969) and its stimulatory effect is competitively inhibited by ATP, ADP, and glucose-6-P (MORGAN and PARMEGGIANI 1964). On the other hand, glucose-1-P and Pi increase the affinity of phosphorylase *b* for AMP (FISCHER et al. 1971). The stimulation of muscle glycogenolysis seen during anoxia is attributable to the effects of altered concentrations of adenine nucleotides and glucose-6-P on phosphorylase *b* (MORGAN and PARMEGGIANI 1964). These changes may also contribute to the stimulation of glycogenolysis which occurs during muscle contraction. For example, muscles of I strain mice produce lactate during contraction despite the absence of phosphorylase *a* formation (DANFORTH and LYON 1964).

The activation of phosphorylase *b* to *a* catalyzed by phosphorylase *b* kinase results in the incorporation of 1 mole of phosphate per mole of monomer. Phosphorylation occurs on a single specific amino acid (serine 14) and results in a large increase in activity in the absence of any allosteric effectors. Phosphorylase *a* can exist in both tetrameric and dimeric forms. Originally it was thought that activation depended on the formation of the tetrameric form, but this view is no longer ten-

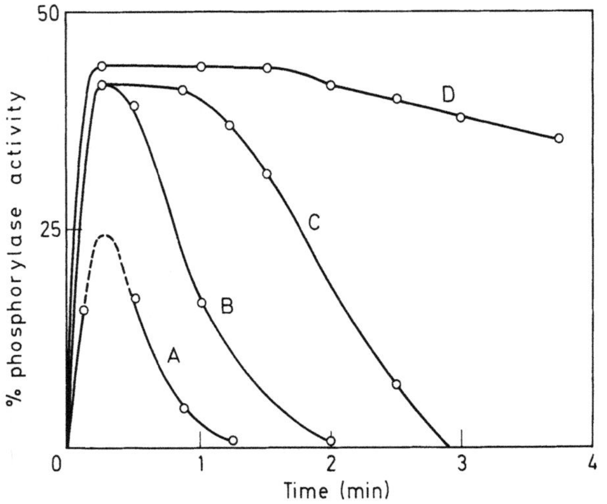

Fig. 17. Effects of various ATP concentrations on the "flash activation" of phosphorylase in muscle glycogen particles. Activation was determined at the following ATP concentrations: *A*, 0.5 m*M*; *B*, 1 m*M*; *C*, 2 m*M*; and *D*, 4 m*M*. In each case, the Mg^{2+} concentration was 3 times that of ATP. (HEILMEYER et al. 1970)

able (FISCHER et al. 1971). For example, rabbit muscle phosphorylase *a* dissociates from a tetramer to a dimer in the presence of glucose or glycogen with a concomitant increase in activity (METZGER et al. 1968). FISCHER et al. (1971) have obtained evidence that phosphorylation or dephosphorylation of phosphorylase does not occur in an all-or-none fashion in which only fully phosphorylated or fully dephosphorylated forms are produced. It seems, rather, that dimeric or tetrameric phospho-dephospho hybrids are formed during these interconversions. Such hybrids are more sensitive to positive or negative allosteric effectors (FISCHER et al. 1971).

Muscle phosphorylase has been sequenced (TITANI et al. 1977). Furthermore, JOHNSON et al. (1974, 1977) and WEBER et al. (1978) have examined the crystal structure of phosphorylase *b*, and FLETTERICK et al. (1976a, b), SYGUSCH et al. (1977), and KASVINSKY et al. (1978a, b, c) have described the structure of phosphorylase *a*. X-ray studies have shown that the 97,000 dalton subunit of the enzyme has its polypeptide chain organized largely into alternating α- and β-structures, like all other glycolytic enzymes analyzed so far (BLAKE 1979). The subunit is folded into three domains: a 320 residue domain at the N-terminus, a 160 residue central domain, and a 360 residue domain at the C-terminus. The three domains are located approximately at the apices of an equilateral triangle.

Phosphorylase *a* in vivo is complexed with AMP and substrates so that the phosphorylation site is tucked into a fold in the protein and is unavailable to phosphorylase phosphatase (MADSEN et al. 1978). Binding of glucose or glucose-6-P to the active site of the enzyme alters its configuration from a relaxed (R) to a taut (T) conformation (MADSEN et al. 1978) and exposes the phosphorylated site to the action of phosphorylase phosphatase (KASVINSKY et al. 1978c). A similar effect is produced by binding of caffeine to the "nucleoside site," whereas binding of AMP to the "nucleotide site" or interaction of glucose-1-P with the active site causes the phosphorylated site to become inaccessible to the phosphatase. These substrate-directed changes explain the effects of glucose and caffeine on the phosphorylase phosphatase reaction (HURD et al. 1966; HOLMES and MANSOUR 1968; STALMANS et al. 1970; BAILEY and WHELAN 1972; MARTENSEN et al. 1973a, b; DETWILER et al. 1977). These effects are important in the regulation of liver phosphorylase, but their role in the physiological control of the muscle enzyme is unclear at present.

In muscle, a large fraction of glycogen phosphorylase and synthase and the enzymes which control their activities are found in a protein-glycogen particulate complex in which glycogen forms the matrix (MEYER et al. 1970). The glycogen are also accompanied by elements of the sarcoplasmic reticulum. When the particles are isolated in the presence of chelating agents, phosphorylase is in the *b* form. However, when Mg-ATP and Ca^{2+} are added, phosphorylase is very rapidly activated (Fig. 17; HEILMEYER et al. 1970). Upon exhaustion of the ATP due to ATPase activity, phosphorylase *a* is rapidly reconverted to phosphorylase *b*. Readdition of ATP again causes another "flash activation." The protein-glycogen particles found in skeletal muscle correspond to the cardiac sarcoplasmic reticulum fractions described earlier, except that they do not show changes when cAMP or epinephrine is added.

4. Possible Role of Phosphorylase Phosphatase

Although it is well established that epinephrine regulates phosphorylase *a* levels in muscle through activation of phosphorylase *b* kinase, evidence is accumulating in support of additional control through inhibition of phosphorylase phosphatase (F. HUANG and GLINSMANN 1976; P. COHEN 1978; TAO et al. 1978). Several groups (KATO and BISHOP 1972; NAKAI and THOMAS 1974; BRANDT et al. 1975a; ANTONIW and COHEN 1976; ANTONIW et al. 1977; ZIEVE and GLINSMANN 1973; GRATECOS et al. 1977; H. LI et al. 1978) have purified from skeletal muscle a P-protein phosphatase of low molecular weight (35,000) which exhibits activity towards the phosphorylated forms of phosphorylase, phosphorylase kinase and glycogen synthase. This multifunctional phosphatase can be inhibited by several heat-stable proteins from muscle (F. HUANG and GLINSMANN 1975, 1976; P. COHEN et al. 1977; G. NIMMO and COHEN 1978). One of these inhibitory proteins (P-protein phosphatase inhibitor-I) is active only when it is phosphorylated by cyclic AMP-dependent protein kinase (F. HUANG and GLINSMANN 1976; G. NIMMO and COHEN 1978). Thus epinephrine has the potential of activating phosphorylase (and inactivating glycogen synthase) through an additional mechanism i.e. by increasing the activity of P-protein phosphatase inhibitor-I through phosphorylation (P. COHEN 1978). Evidence in support of this mechanism has recently been obtained in vitro (TAO et al. 1978; KHATRA et al. 1980) and in vivo (FOULKES and COHEN 1979).

A possible role for phosphorylase phosphatase in the activation of phosphorylase during muscle contraction was also suggested by HASCHKE et al. (1970). This suggestion arose because the phosphorylase phosphatase activity of the muscle protein-glycogen complex appeared to be inhibited by Ca^{2+}. However, it now seems more likely that a Ca^{2+}-dependent kinase similar to phosphorylase *b* kinase is the major mediator of Ca^{2+} effects in the complex (HORL et al. 1978; HORL and HEILMEYER 1978; VARSANYI et al. 1978).

As described in the previous section, several effectors (AMP, glucose-6-P, glucose) can modulate phosphorylase phosphatase activity by interacting with phosphorylase *a* and causing conformational changes which alter the accessibility of the phosphorylated site to the phosphatase.

5. Permissive Effects of Glucocorticoids on Catecholamine Stimulation of Muscle Glycogenolysis

Glucocorticoids play a permissive role in catecholamine activation of glycogenolysis in skeletal and cardiac muscle (SCHAEFFER et al. 1969b; T. MILLER et al. 1971). This is illustrated by Fig. 18 taken from the report of T. MILLER et al. (1971). As in the case of the liver, the action of these steroid hormones is exerted at a step beyond the formation of cyclic AMP and activation of cyclic AMP-dependent protein kinase (T. MILLER et al. 1971). The step appears to be between phosphorylase *b* kinase and phosphorylase (T. MILLER et al. 1971), but further work is needed to establish this clearly.

There has been very little study of the effects of glucocorticoids per se on muscle glycogen metabolism. However, it is known that these hormones exert minimal effects on glycogen levels in muscle compared with liver (LONG et al. 1960). Glucocorticoids do not appear to exert direct effects on glucose uptake by muscle (MUNCK 1971, CALDWELL et al. 1978). It is well documented that they reduce the sensitivity of muscle to insulin action (STEELE 1975), but the mechanism(s) involved is unclear.

E. Regulation of Muscle Glycogen Synthesis

I. Regulation of Glycogen Synthase by Phosphorylation

In addition to stimulating glycogen breakdown in muscle, catecholamines inhibit glycogen synthesis by inactivating glycogen synthase which catalyzes the rate-limiting reaction in the process.

Studies in vitro with purified glycogen synthase have led to the concept that the enzyme can exist in two basic forms. One form has a low phosphate content and is relatively independent of cofactors for activity. This is termed the I or *a* form. It can be converted through phosphorylation by several protein kinases to the D or *b* form which is dependent on glucose-6-P (or other cofactors) for activity (SODERLING and PARK 1974). The *b* form also has a higher K_m for UDP-glucose than the *a* form in the absence of glucose-6-P (BROWN et al. 1977).

Glycogen synthase *a* appears to exist under physiological conditions as a dimer or tetramer with a monomer weight of 90,000 daltons (SODERLING 1976). Cyclic AMP-dependent protein kinase catalyzes rapid incorporation of 1 mole of phosphate per mole of subunit and slower incorporation of more phosphate (SODERLING 1975). Complete conversion of the enzyme to the *b* form by this kinase requires phosphorylation to greater than 1 mole of phosphate per mole of subunit (SODERLING 1975; Fig. 19).

Analysis of the synthase domains phosphorylated by cyclic AMP-dependent protein kinase indicates that the enzyme acts preferentially at two sites in a domain

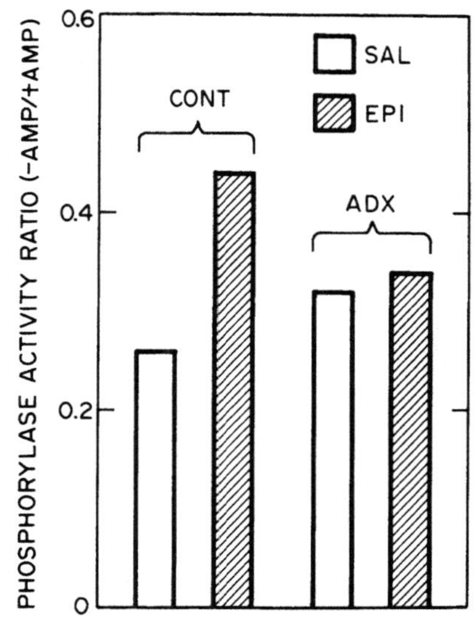

Fig. 18. Effects of epinephrine on phosphorylase activity in perfused hearts from control *(CONT)* and adrenalectomized *(ADX)* rats. Hearts were perfused for 8 min without hormone and then for 3 min with saline *(SAL)* or epinephrine *EPI*, 10^{-8} *M)* before freeze clamping for phosphorylase assay. (T. MILLER et al. 1971)

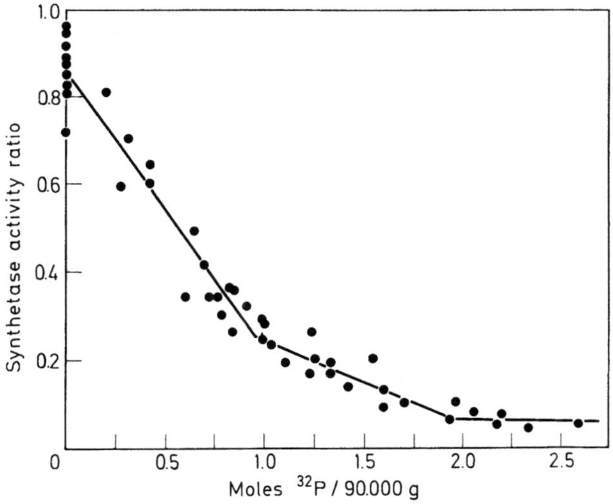

Fig. 19. Correlation of glycogen synthase activity ratio (−glc-6-P/+glc-6-P) with phosphate content in enzyme preparations incubated with cyclic AMP-dependent protein kinase. Low concentrations of ATP (0.1–0.3 m*M*) and reaction times of 1 h or less were used in the phosphorylation incubations. (SODERLING 1975)

of 17,000 daltons which is located at the C terminus and is trypsin-sensitive (SODERLING et al. 1977; PROUD et al. 1978; T. HUANG and KREBS 1977). As expected, the two sites have two basic residues on the N-terminus side of the phosphorylated serine, i.e. have the recognition determinants for cyclic AMP-dependent protein kinase. The kinase additionally incorporates up to 1 mole of phos-

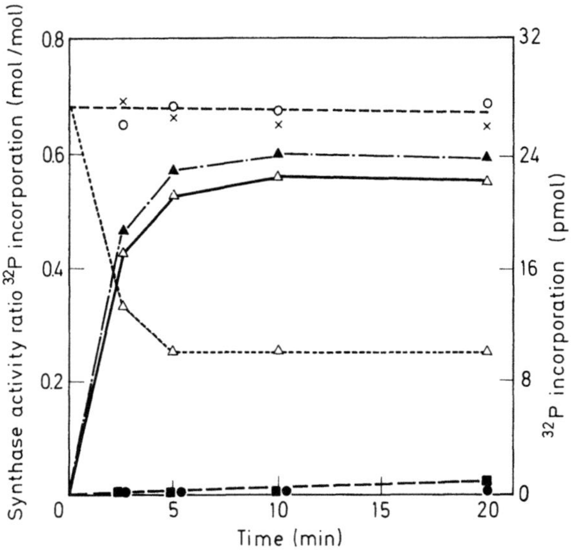

Fig. 20. Phosphorylation *(solid symbols)* and alteration of the activity ratio (−glc-6-P/+glc-6-P) of glycogen synthase incubated with phosphorylase *b* kinase. Phosphorylation was determined in the presence of phosphorylase *b* kinase and glycogen synthase (▲), absence of phosphorylase *b* kinase (●), and absence of glycogen synthase (■). Phosphorylation is expressed as pmol of ^{32}P incorporated per 10 μl of reaction mixture (---) or as mol of ^{32}P incorporated per mol of 90,000 dalton synthase subunit (———). Alterations in the activity ratio are shown in the presence of phosphorylase *b* kinase and glycogen synthase with ATP (▲) and without ATP (×) or in the absence of phosphorylase *b* kinase (○). (SODERLING et al. 1979a)

phate in a relatively trypsin-insensitive domain of 10,000 daltons situated at the amino terminus (SODERLING et al. 1977). The sites have recently been sequenced (EMBI et al. 1981; PARKER et al. 1981).

Recently it has been found that muscle glycogen synthase can be phosphorylated and inactivated by phosphorylase *b* kinase (ROACH et al. 1978; DEPAOLI-ROACH et al. 1979a, b; SODERLING et al. 1979a; K. WALSH et al. 1979; EMBI et al. 1979). The phosphorylation site (serine 7) is located near the N terminus in the trypsin-insensitive domain and thus differs from the sites acted on by low concentrations of cyclic AMP-dependent protein kinase (SODERLING et al. 1979b; EMBI et al. 1979; RYLATT et al. 1980). The surrounding sequence is homologous to that around the phosphorylation site of phosphorylase (RYLATT et al. 1980). As expected, the effect of phosphorylase *b* kinase on glycogen synthase is stimulated by Ca^{2+} and calmodulin. Phosphorylation occurs more slowly than with phosphorylase *b*, reaches a plateau of 0.5–0.7 mole of phosphate per subunit and results in partial inactivation of the enzyme (Fig. 20, SODERLING et al. 1979a, b; EMBI et al. 1979; DEPAOLI-ROACH et al. 1979a).

Muscle glycogen synthase can also be phosphorylated by cyclic AMP-independent protein kinases which are separate from phosphorylase *b* kinase. These enzymes have been partially purified from muscle and other tissues (SCHLENDER et al. REIMANN 1975, 1977; H. NIMMO et al. 1976; SODERLING et al. 1977; ITARTE et al. 1977; BROWN et al. 1977; JETT and SODERLING 1979; K. HUANG et al. 1979; EMBI et al. 1980). It is uncertain to what extent they may be identical. The enzymes purified by H. NIMMO et al. (1976), SODERLING et al. (1977), BROWN et al. (1977), SCHLENDER and REIMANN (1975, 1977), and EMBI et al. (1980) have many similar properties, but it is uncertain that they are identical. They incorporate 1–1.5 mole of phosphate per mole of subunit and produce a relatively greater inactivation of the synthase than that caused by cyclic AMP-dependent protein kinase (Table 1). Three serine residues located in a 9 amino acid segment are phosphorylated by the enzyme isolated by EMBI et al. (1980). These sites differ from those acted on by phosphorylase *b* kinase and low concentrations of cyclic AMP-dependent protein kinase (RYLATT et al. 1980). The cAMP-independent enzyme isolated by ITARTE et al. (1977) and K. HUANG et al. 1979) is probably different from the preceding enzyme(s) because it incorporates 4 moles of phosphate per mole of glycogen synthase subunit. K. HUANG et al. (1979) have proposed that their enzyme phosphorylates synthase sequentially at 4 sites. Phosphorylation of the first site is associated with a rapid decrease in the activity ratio and a rapid increase in the K_m for UDP-glucose (in the absence of glucose-6-P). Phosphorylation of the remaining 3 sites is associated with an increase in the K_a for glucose-6-P. They postulate that the first site controls the binding of UDP-glucose and the conversion of synthase *a* to *b*, whereas the other sites control sensitivity to glucose-6-P. There are no known regulators of the cyclic AMP-independent synthase kinases.

Purified glycogen synthase *a* has a −glucose-6-P/+glucose-6-P activity ratio of about 0.8 and a K_a for glucose-6-P of about 10 μM (H. NIMMO et al. 1976; BROWN et al. 1977; Table 1). When cyclic AMP-dependent protein kinase phosphorylates it to the extent of approximately 1 mole of phosphate per mole of subunit, the resulting glycogen synthase *b* has an activity ratio of about 0.2 and a K_a of about 200 μM (H. NIMMO et al. 1976; BROWN et al. 1977; SODERLING et al. 1977). A similar extent of phosphorylation by cyclic AMP-independent protein kinase purified by BROWN et al. (1977) yields a glycogen synthase *b* with an activity ratio of about 0.05 and a K_a of about 500 μM. Similar changes are produced by the cyclic AMP-independent kinase prepared by SODERLING et al. (1977) and EMBI et al. (1980). When the enzyme is further phosphorylated by either cAMP-dependent or cAMP-independent kinase or by both together, the activity ratio declines further and the K_a increases more (H. NIMMO et al. 1976; BROWN et al. 1977; EMBI et al. 1980). Phosphorylation of synthase by phosphorylase *b* kinase results in the incorporation of less than 1 mole of phosphate per subunit and causes smaller kinetic changes i.e. a decrease in the activity ratio to about 0.4 and an increase in the K_a to about 25 μM (DEPAOLI-ROACH et al. 1979a; SODERLING et al. 1979a, b; EMBI et al. 1979). The kinetic changes induced by the four kinases are summarized in Table 1 and lead to the general conclusion that phosphorylation of the relatively trypsin-insensitive domain is mainly responsible for the decrease in activity measured in the absence of glucose-6-P (SODERLING 1979).

The primary effect of glucose-6-P on glycogen synthase *b* is to increase the V_{max} of the reaction (LARNER and VILLAR-PALASI 1971). The metabolite also decreases the K_m for UDP-glucose of the *a* form from about 300 μM to about 25 μM (BROWN et al. 1977). This efect is probably important in vivo where the concentration of UDP-glucose in muscle is 30–50 μM (CHIASSON et al. 1980; PIRAS and STANELONI 1969). Adenine and uridine nucleotides and inorganic phosphate are in-

Table 1. Properties of muscle glycogen synthase phosphorylated by different protein kinases

Phosphorylating kinase	Phosphate content (mol/subunit)	Trypsin action on phosphate content: sensitive (mol/subunit)	Trypsin action on phosphate content: insensitive (mol/subunit)	K_m for UDPG: −G1c6P μ*M*	K_m for UDPG: +G1c6P μ*M*	Activity ratio −G1c6P/+G1c6P	K_a for G1c6P μ*M*	References
None	<0.1			≃ 300	≃ 25	≃0.8	≃ 10	DIETZ et al. (1980) K. HUANG et al. (1979) BROWN et al. (1977) SODERLING et al. (1977)
cAMP-dependent kinase	≃1	0.7	0.3		50	≃0.2	≃ 200	DIETZ et al. (1980) SODERLING et al. (1977) H. NIMMO et al. (1976) EMBI et al. (1980)
	≃2	1	1		≃ 50	≃0.05	≃ 300	BROWN et al. (1977) SODERLING et al. (1977) H. NIMMO et al. (1976)
	≃3	2	1			0.05	400	SODERLING 1979
Phosphorylase *b* kinase	≃0.5	0	0.5			≃0.4	≃ 25	ROACH et al. (1978) SODERLING et al. (1979a, b) D. WALSH et al. (1979) EMBI et al. (1979)
cAMP-independent kinase(s) I	≅1	0.2	0.8		≃ 40	≃0.05	≃ 500	BROWN et al. (1977) SODERLING et al. (1977) H. NIMMO et al. (1976) EMBI et al. (1980)
cAMP-independent kinase II	≃1			1,500		0.08	≃ 200	
	≃2			2,000		≃0.05	≃ 500	ITARTE et al. (1977)
	≃3			> 3,000		≃0.02	≃2,000	K. HUANG et al. (1979)
	≃4			≃20,000	800	<0.02	4,500	
cAMP-dependent kinase + cAMP-independent kinase I	≃3				61	0.01	1,500–2,000	BROWN et al. (1977)

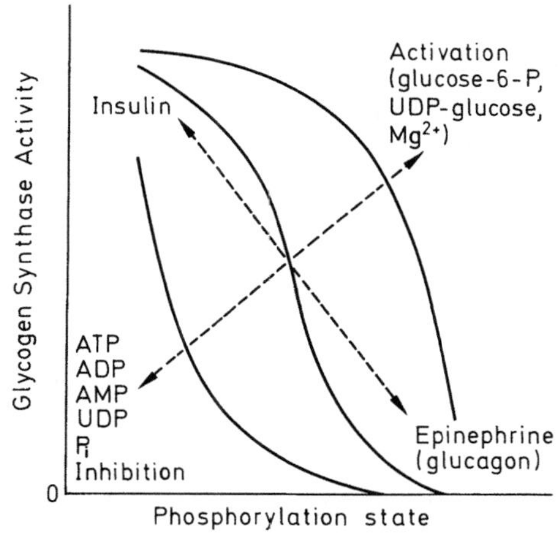

Fig. 21. Diagram showing schematically the effects of allosteric effectors on glycogen synthase in relation to the phosphorylation state of the enzyme. The activity of the enzyme is viewed as the resultant of two regulating inputs, one through changes in allosteric effectors, and the other through changes in the phosphorylation state induced by hormones. The hormonal influences and allosteric influences act along the respective *solid lines*. (ROACH and LARNER 1976)

hibitory to both forms of glycogen synthase and their action is relieved by glucose-6-P (PIRAS et al. 1968). However, the allosteric inhibitors have a more marked effect on the *b* form of the enzyme than the *a* form. Furthermore, higher concentrations of glucose-6-P are required to relieve the inhibition of the *b* form than the *a* form (ROACH and LARNER 1976; PIRAS et al. 1968; ROACH et al. 1976). As a result, phosphorylation of the enzyme renders it less active in the presence of physiological levels of its allosteric modifiers. This is illustrated in Fig. 21 from ROACH and LARNER (1976).

As noted earlier (Sect. D.I.4), ANTONIW et al. (1977) and others have purified a low molecular weight, general (multifunctional) phosphatase from muscle which dephosphorylates several phosphorylated proteins including glycogen synthase, and which can be regulated by inhibitory proteins from muscle (F. HUANG and GLINSMANN 1976; G. NIMMO and COHEN 1978). KHATRA and SODERLING (1978) have also isolated a muscle phosphatase with broad specificity. However, this is of higher molecular weight than that isolated by Cohen's group, and is not affected by the inhibitory proteins. Interestingly, it dephosphorylates the trypsin-insensitive domain of glycogen synthase more rapidly than the trypsin-sensitive domain (HUTSON et al. 1978 a; KHATRA and SODERLING 1978). Dephosphorylation of the trypsin-insensitive domain correlates very well with activation of the enzyme, supporting the view that this domain is an important determinant of synthase activity. Interestingly, the V_{max} of the phosphatase differs with the extent of phosphorylation of the synthase. Dephosphorylation of synthase which has 2 moles of phosphate per mole of subunit mainly in the trypsin-insensitive domain is more rapid than that of synthase which has 1 mole of phosphate mainly in the trypsin-sensitive domain. The reason for the difference resides in the fact that the phosphatase dephosphorylates the trypsin-insensitive domain more rapidly than the trypsin-sensitive domain. With further phosphorylation of synthase in the trypsin-sensitive domain, the V_{max} declines because the "trypsin-sensitive phosphate" behaves as a competitive inhibitor. The regulation of phosphatase activity by the degree of phosphorylation of synthase may represent an important mechanism by which synthase activity is regulated (see Sect. D.III).

II. Catecholamine Inhibition of Muscle Glycogen Synthesis

In resting skeletal muscle, glycogen synthase appears to exist in a partially phosphorylated form which has a −glucose-6-P/+glucose-6-P activity ratio of 0.1–0.3 and a K_a for glucose-6-P of 150–250 μM (B. WILLIAMS and MAYER 1966; P. COHEN 1978; DIETZ et al. 1980; SODERLING 1979). DIETZ et al. (1980) and SODERLING (1979) have speculated that the phosphorylation of the enzyme in resting muscle is due to the activity of phosphorylase kinase and another cAMP-independent protein kinase. Following epinephrine treatment, glycogen synthase becomes more dependent upon glucose-6-P for activity, having a −glucose-6-P/+glucose-6-P activity ratio of 0.1 and a K_a for glucose-6-P of greater than 1 mM (CRAIG and LARNER 1964; B. WILLIAMS and MAYER 1966; P. COHEN 1978; DIETZ et al. 1980). This is illustrated in Fig. 22. The view that these changes are due to increased activity of cyclic AMP-dependent protein kinase is supported by the following evidence. (1) The changes in the kinetics of the enzyme caused by epinephrine treatment in vitro are well correlated with the alterations in the activation state of the kinase and are completely abolished when the increase in cyclic AMP is abolished by the β-blocker propranolol (Figs. 13, 22); DIETZ et al. 1980). (2) P. COHEN (1978) has reported the enzyme isolated from rabbits treated with epinephrine in vivo has a higher phosphate content than that from untreated rabbits. (3) The alterations in kinetics caused by epinephrine in vivo or in vitro are very similar to those seen when the purified enzyme is phosphorylated by cyclic AMP-dependent protein kinase (DIETZ et al. 1980).

The effects of epinephrine on glycogen synthase activity in cardiac muscle differ from those in skeletal muscle. In the heart, epinephrine at low concentrations increases phosphorylase *a*, but does not change glycogen synthase a activity or causes a transient increase, in contrast to its action in skeletal muscle (B. WILLIAMS and MAYER 1966; ROBISON et al. 1965; MCCULLOUGH and WALSH 1979b). With higher epinephrine concentrations, the hormone causes an increase and then a decrease in cardiac glycogen synthase *a* (B. WILLIAMS and MAYER 1966). There is also relatively less glycogen mobilization in cardiac muscle than in skeletal muscle in response to epinephrine (B. WILLIAMS and MAYER 1966). The lesser changes in glycogen synthase *a* in heart have been attributed to the inhibitory action of glycogen on the activity of glycogen synthase *a* (DANFORTH 1965). Alternatively it could relate to the increased work done by the heart in response to epinephrine (B. WILLIAMS and MAYER 1966). Efforts to demonstrate an epinephrine effect on glycogen synthase phosphorylation in perfused rat hearts have not been successful so far (MCCULLOUGH and WALSH 1979b).

Since activation of phosphorylase *b* kinase accompanies activation of cyclic AMP-dependent protein kinase in muscle, it is possible that the changes in glycogen synthase induced by epinephrine are attributable to some extent to the action

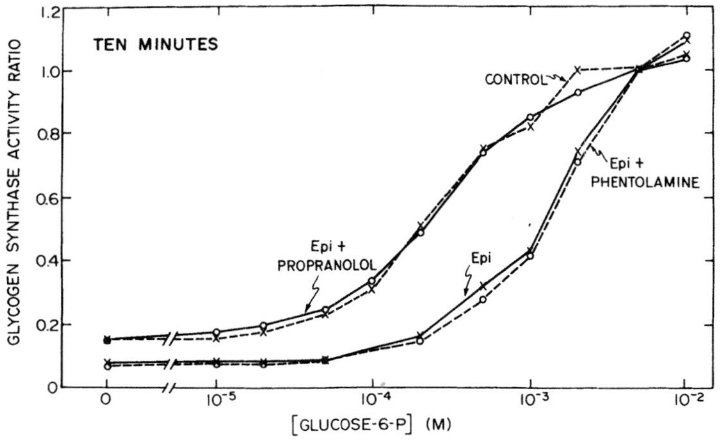

Fig. 22. Effect of glucose-6-P concentration on the activity of glycogen synthase from rat hindlimb muscle perfused with epinephrine and adrenergic blockers. Epinephrine (10^{-7} *M*) was infused for 10 min. Blockers (10^{-6} *M*) were added to the perfusion medium 10 min prior to infusion of epinephrine. (DIETZ et al. 1980)

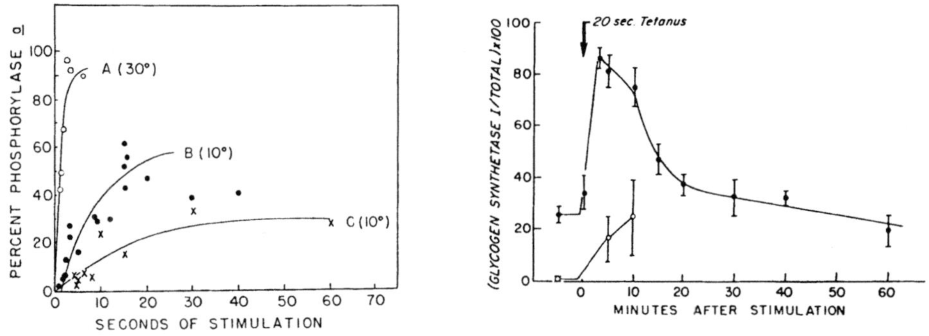

Fig. 23. *Left panel.* Increase in phosphorylase *a* in frog sartorius muscle during isometric contraction. Stimulation was by 12-volt shocks, 1.5 ms in duration. Curve *A*, muscles tetanized with 35 Hz at 30°; curve *B*, muscles tetanized with 15 Hz at 10°; curve *C*, single twitches at 1 Hz at 10°. (DANFORTH et al. 1962). *Right panel.* Effect of electrical stimulation on the activity ratio of glycogen synthase (expressed as % of enzyme in the I or *a* form) in mouse muscle. The *arrow* indicates a 20 s tetanic stimulation (110 V, 5 ms duration at 40 Hz). No pretreatment (●); pretreatment with 5 μg of epinephrine/10 g of body weight, given subcutaneously 5 min prior to stimulation (○). (DANFORTH 1965)

of phosphorylase *b* kinase. However, it is unlikely that phosphorylase *b* kinase controls glycogen synthase under physiological conditions in vivo. This is because of the fact that glycogen synthase *a* is very low in the muscle of I-strain mice (LYON and PORTER 1963) and because of the findings of two groups (DANFORTH 1965; DANFORTH and LYON 1964; DANFORTH et al. 1962; PIRAS and STANELONI 1969) who examined the changes in glycogen synthase in electrically stimulated muscle. Whereas phosphorylase was mainly in the *b* form in resting muscle, glycogen synthase appeared to be largely in a phosphorylated form since its activity ratio was 0.2 (DANFORTH 1965; DIETZ et al. 1980). As illustrated in Fig. 23, tetanic stimulation caused rapid activation of phosphorylase, and phosphorylase *b* was rapidly reformed on cessation of the stimulus (DANFORTH 1965; DANFORTH et al. 1962; PIRAS and STANELONI 1969). In contrast, the activity ratio of glycogen synthase increased very slowly (relative to phosphorylase *a*) during stimulation, continued to rise for several minutes and then declined slowly (DANFORTH 1965). The rise was blocked by epinephrine treatment (DANFORTH 1965).

The time course of the glycogen synthase changes during electrical stimulation and their and dissociation from the changes in phosphorylase render it unlikely that they arise from an increase in cytosolic Ca^{2+}. DANFORTH (1965) has noted an inverse correlation between muscle glycogen content and glycogen synthase activity ratio and has suggested that the glycogen synthase changes during electrical stimulation may be secondary to alterations in glycogen level due to phosphorylase activity. Muscle contraction does not alter cyclic AMP levels in muscle or convert phosphorylase *b* kinase to the activated from (DRUMMOND et al. 1969; STULL and MAYER 1971).

III. Insulin Stimulation of Muscle Glycogen Synthesis

It is well-established that insulin stimulates glucose uptake in muscle and adipose tissue by increasing the transport of glucose across the plasma membrane. This transport occurs by facilitated diffusion and is non-active i.e. non ATP-dependent (PARK et al. 1968). Insulin acts to increase the V_{max} of transport, but does not appear to alter the K_m i.e. the affinity of the putative carrier for glucose. The precise mechanism(s) by which insulin acts is unknown, but recent studies suggest that it involves translocation of intracellular transport systems to the plasma membrane (SUZUKI and KONO 1980; CUSHMAN and WARDZALA 1980).

It is also well-established that insulin promotes glycogen synthesis in muscle through activation of glycogen synthase. The hormone increases the activity ratio of the enzyme and reduces its K_a for flucose-6-P (VILLAR-PALASI and LARNER 1960; CHIASSON et al. 1980). These changes are consistent with dephosphorylation of the enzyme. As shown in Fig. 24, the effect is not mediated by a change in the level of cyclic AMP or in the assayed activity of cyclic AMP-dependent protein kinase (KEELY et al. 1975; CRAIG and LARNER 1964; CRAIG et al. 1969; CHIASSON et al. 1980, 1981; GOLDBERG et al. 1967; T. MILLER 1978 b), nor is it accompanied by any alteration in phosphorylase activity or total synthase activity (CHIASSON et al. 1980; B. WILLIAMS and MAYER 1966; ADOLFSSON et al. 1972; T. MILLER 1978 b). It is also independent of the stimulatory effect of insulin on glucose transport in this tissue since it is observed in the absence of extracellular glucose (VILLAR-PALASI and LARNER 1960; CHIASSON et al. 1980; LE MARCHAND-BRUSTEL and FREYCHET 1979). Furthermore, in skeletal muscle, it develops more slowly than the stimulation of glucose transport (CHIASSON et al. 1980). In heart, it occurs more rapidly, but is not sustained (ADOLFSSON et al. 1972; T. MILLER 1978 b).

T. MILLER (1978 b) has obtained evidence that synthase phosphatase is involved in the action of insulin on glycogen synthase in heart. In addition, Larner's group has proposed that insulin induces the formation of a factor(s) which is an inhibitor of cAMP-dependent protein kinase and an activator of glycogen synthase phosphatase, and have presented evidence in favor of this hypothesis (WALKENBACH et

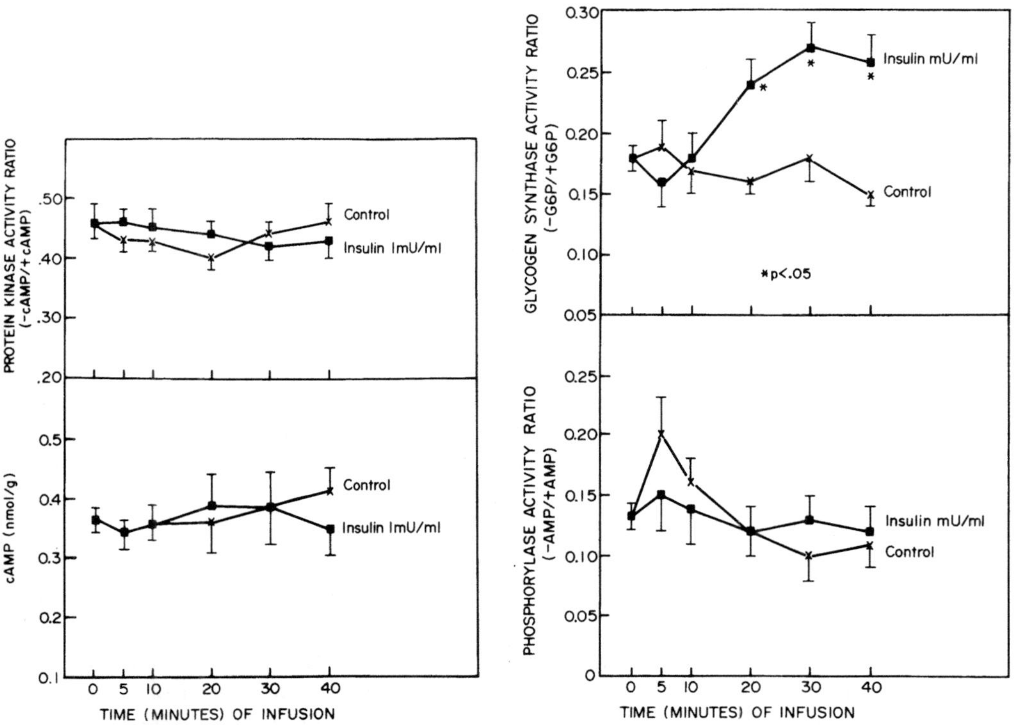

Fig. 24. Effects of insulin on cyclic AMP levels and the activities of cyclic AMP-dependent protein kinase, phosphorylase and glycogen synthase in perfused rat hindlimb muscle. (M. R. DIETZ and J. H. EXTON, unpublished work)

al. 1978, 1980; LARNER et al. 1979). More recently, FOULKES et al. (1980) have reported that insulin decreases the phosphorylation, and hence activity, of P-protein phosphatase inhibitor-I in muscle. However, this observation has not been confirmed (KHATRA et al. 1980). It should be noted that if insulin were to act by generating an inhibitor of cAMP-dependent protein kinase, changes in phosphorylase *b* kinase and phosphorylase would be expected. Likewise, if it acted by stimulating a P-protein phosphatase, this enzyme would have to be specific for glycogen synthase. As noted above, P-protein phosphatase inhibitor-I acts on the multifunctional P-protein phosphatase and would therefore be expected to regulate other enzymes of glycogen metabolism.

Epinephrine has been shown to reverse the effects of insulin on glycogen synthase in muscle (CRAIG et al. 1969; SHIKAMA et al. 1981), but there has been relatively little study of the interaction between these two hormones in the control of muscle glycogen metabolism. Although some workers have reported that insulin partly blocks the rise in cAMP and the activation of phosphorylase *b* kinase and phosphorylase induced by epinephrine in rat diaphragm (CRAIG et al. 1969), these observations have not been confirmed in skeletal muscle (SHIKAMA et al. 1981). In this type of muscle, insulin does not inhibit the effects of epinephrine on cyclic AMP, cyclic AMP-dependent protein kinase, phosphorylase or glycogen synthase (SHIKAMA et al. 1981). These observations cast strong doubt on the hypothesis that

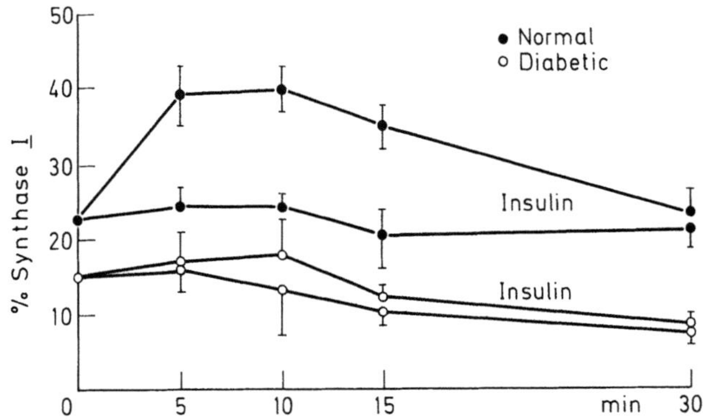

Fig. 25. Effect of insulin (10^{-8} *M*) on glycogen synthase in perfused hearts from normal and alloxan-diabetic rats. Glycogen synthase activity is expressed as % of enzyme in the I or *a* form. In hearts from normal rats, the increases with insulin at 5, 10, and 15 min were significant. (T. MILLER 1978b)

insulin acts by inhibiting cyclic AMP-dependent protein kinase or by stimulating a multifunctional P-protein phosphatase.

Recently, LE MARCHAND-BRUSTEL et al. (1979) have demonstrated that insulin causes normal activation of glycogen synthase in the muscle of phosphorylase *b* kinase-deficient (I-strain) mice. This indicates that phosphorylase *b* kinase is not involved in this action of insulin. A role for cyclic GMP-dependent protein kinase is also improbable since insulin does not alter the level of cyclic GMP in muscle (TARUI et al. 1976). Clearly much more work is needed to elucidate the mechanism of this important action of insulin.

Fasting and diabetes are classically considered to inhibit glycogen synthesis in muscle. This is due primarily to reduced glucose transport which is attributable to lack of insulin stimulation (MORGAN et al. 1961 a; KIPNIS 1959; RANDLE et al. 1964; CHIASSON et al. 1980; cf LE MARCHAND-BRUSTEL et al. 1979; GOODMAN and RUDERMAN 1979). In hearts and diaphragms of diabetic animals, there is also evidence of decreased phosphorylation of glucose and this has been attributed to indirect effects of pituitary and adrenal cortical hormones which can be slowly reversed by insulin (MORGAN et al. 1961 a, b; PARK et al. 1961; KIPNIS 1959; GARLAND and RANDLE 1964; NEWSHOLME and RANDLE 1964). The inhibition of phosphorylation is secondary to an increase in tissue glucose-6-P due to a restraint of P-fructokinase (REGEN et al. 1964; NEWSHOLME and RANDLE 1964) which has been ascribed to increased levels of citrate which inhibit the enzyme (GARLAND et al. 1963). It has been postulated that the increase in citrate is due to increased tissue fatty acid oxidation (RANDLE et al. 1964, NEWSHOLME and RANDLE 1964). This explanation may be correct for cardiac muscle, but there is no clear evidence to support it in skeletal muscle (RUDERMAN et al. 1969; GOODMAN et al. 1974; BERGER et al. 1976).

There have been few studies of the effects of fasting or diabetes on muscle glycogen synthase and these have not given consistent results. T. MILLER (1978 a) has found a lower glycogen synthase activity ratio and a markedly impaired effect of insulin on the enzyme in hearts from diabetic animals (Fig. 25). Cyclic AMP levels and the activation of cyclic AMP-dependent protein kinase and phosphorylase were not altered. LE MARCHAND-BRUSTEL and FREYCHET (1979 b) found in soleus muscle, on the other hand, that glycogen synthase was more sensitive to insulin activation in diabetic and 48-h-fasting rats, although the basal activity ratio and maximum response to the hormone were unchanged. In contrast, CHIASSON et al. (1980) reported that the perfused hindlimb muscle of 24-h-fasting rats has a higher basal glycogen synthase activity ratio and an increased maximum response to insulin.

SODERLING (1980) has made the interesting suggestion that the effect of the phosphorylation state of glycogen synthase on synthase phosphatase activity may explain the apparently reduced activity of the phosphatase in tissues from diabetic animals (GOLD 1970; BISHOP 1970; TAN and NUTTALL 1976; T. MILLER 1978 a, b; 1979; GOLDEN et al. 1979). As described in Sect. E.I, highly phosphorylated glycogen synthase may be a relatively poor substrate for synthase phosphatase. EICHNER (1976) has obtained kinetic evidence of a high degree of phosphorylation of glycogen synthase in adipose tissue from diabetic and fasting rats.

F. Regulation of Pyruvate Metabolism in Muscle

Pyruvate metabolism in skeletal muscle is influenced by many metabolic events. As indicated in the preceding sections, pyruvate production from blood glucose and tissue glycogen is under complex control, being influenced by hormones such as epinephrine and insulin, changes in muscular contraction, changes in the blood and O_2 supply, and changes in substrates in the blood. In addition, regulation of pyruvate disposal via oxidation to acetyl-CoA, reduction to lactate and transamination to alanine is similarly complex. A key enzyme controlling pyruvate metabolism in muscle is pyruvate dehydrogenase. The structure and regulation of this enzyme have been described in Sect. C.I.4.

RANDLE and co-workers (GARLAND et al. 1962, 1963, 1964; NEWSHOLME and RANDLE 1964; RANDLE et al. 1964; GARLAND and RANDLE 1964; RANDLE and TUBBS 1979) and others (GOODMAN et al. 1974; BERGER et al. 1976) have demonstrated in great detail the effects of diabetes, starvation, fatty acids and ketone bodies on pyruvate metabolism in rat heart, diaphragm and skeletal muscle. They showed that these factors impair pyruvate utilization in these tissues. This impairment is attributable to the effects of increased tissue ratios of acetyl-CoA/CoA and $NADH/NAD^+$ which inhibit the pyruvate dehydrogenase reaction directly or via stimulation of pyruvate dehydrogenase kinase (COOPER et al. 1974; KERBEY et al. 1976; and see Sect. C.I.4). This mechanism is supported by measurements of the proportions of active (dephosphorylated) and inactive (phosphorylated) pyruvate dehydrogenase in muscle from diabetic and fasting animals in vivo (KERBEY et al. 1976, 1977; HAGG et al. 1976; HENNIG et al. 1975) or in hearts perfused with fatty acids in vitro (WIELAND et al. 1971). There have also been reports of alterations in the activity of pyruvate dehydrogenase kinase in these conditions (KERBEY et al. 1976; HUTSON and RANDLE 1978). In addition, HUTSON et al. (1978 b) have reported that pyruvate dehydrogenase phosphatase activity is inhibited in cardiac mitochondria from diabetic or fasting rats. These workers suggested that phosphorylation of sites in pyruvate dehydrogenase additional to the inactivating site may be responsible for the decreased activity of the phosphatase in these mitochondria (see Sect. C.I.4). This would be analogous to the situation for glycogen synthase in muscle from diabetic and fasting animals (see Sect. E.III).

Epinephrine increases lactate formation and the oxidation of [U-^{14}C] glucose to [^{14}C]-CO_2 in perfused rat hearts (WILLIAMSON 1964). There is an initial decrease in cytosolic NADH, followed by a more pronounced, but transient, increase in this parameter (WILLIAMSON and JAMIESON 1966). The initial decrease is probably due to the response of mitochondrial respiration to ADP formed by the increased work of the heart, while the later increase is probably due to greater production of NADH by glyceraldehyde-3-P dehydrogenase because of increased glycogenolysis and glycolysis (WILLIAMSON and JAMIESON 1966). Some of this NADH may be utilized in the conversion of pyruvate to lactate. Although there may be a transient decrease in pyruvate dehydrogenase activity due to the increase in the NADH/NAD^+ ratio, pyruvate oxidation in the citric acid cycle is increased at later times as shown by increased respiration and increased oxidation of [2-^{14}C] acetate to [^{14}C]-CO_2 (WILLIAMSON 1964). The effects of epinephrine on the pyruvate dehydrogenase reaction in the heart appear to be explicable in terms of changes in the levels of effectors of the pyruvate dehydrogenase kinase reaction. As noted in Sect. C.I.4, the kinase is unaffected by cyclic AMP. Insulin does not seem to influence muscle pyruvate dehydrogenase activity directly. It may cause alterations secondary to its control of fatty acid release from adipose tissue.

Catecholamines inhibit alanine release from skeletal muscle in vitro (GARBER et al. 1976b; J. LI and JEFFERSON 1977). The effect is mediated by β-receptors and is attributable in part to decreased protein degradation (J. LI and JEFFERSON 1977). Increased alanine utilization via oxidative metabolism may also be involved (BUSE et al. 1973; J. LI and JEFFERSON 1977). Alanine release from skeletal muscle in vitro is also inhibited by insulin (JEFFERSON et al. 1977). This is due to inhibition of protein breakdown and stimulation of protein synthesis (FULKS et al. 1975; JEFFERSON et al. 1977).

G. Regulation of Carbohydrate Metabolism in Adipose Tissue

I. Catecholamine Effects on Glycogen and Pyruvate Metabolism in Adipose Tissue

Epinephrine profoundly alters carbohydrate metabolism in adipose tissue. Some of the changes are exerted directly on carbohydrate metabolism, whereas others are attributable to alterations in lipid metabolism i.e. increased lipolysis. The hormone activates phosphorylase and inactivates glycogen synthase in adipose tissue (KHOO et al. 1973; HONEYMAN et al. 1979), but the very low levels of glycogen make it doubtful that these effects are important. The properties of adipose tissue phosphorylase, glycogen synthase and phosphorylase phosphatase appear to be similar to those of the muscle enzymes (F. MILLER et al. 1975; R. MILLER et al. 1975) except that EICHNER (1976) has also found forms of glycogen synthase which have different kinetic properties to those of muscle glycogen synthase. As in the case of liver, adipose tissue phosphorylase *b* kinase has been shown to be stimulated by Ca^{2+}, but the effects of cyclic AMP-dependent protein kinase are unclear (KHOO et al. 1973; KHOO 1976). HONEYMAN et al. (1979) have reported the puzzling finding that, although serotonin elevates cyclic AMP and activates protein kinase and phosphorylase in adipose tissue, it does not stimulate lipolysis in adipose tissue.

LAWRENCE and LARNER (1977) have shown that the changes in phosphorylase and glycogen synthase induced by epinephrine in adipose tissue are mediated by a_1, α_2- and β-receptors and are independent of glucose. Activation of β-receptors produces the expected rise in cAMP, whereas activation of the α_2-receptors leads to a decrease in the accumulation of cyclic AMP induced by β-receptor stimulation. However α_1-receptor stimulation induces cyclic AMP-independent changes in phosphorylase and glycogen synthase (LAWRENCE and LARNER 1977, 1978a) which are additive to those caused by β-receptor stimulation. It has been suggested that the α_1-adrenergic effects are due to an increase in cytosolic Ca^{2+} analogous to that observed in liver (LAWRENCE and LARNER 1977, 1978a). Some evidence in support of this hypothesis has been presented (LAWRENCE and LARNER 1978a).

As in the case of muscle in vivo, adipose tissue glycogen synthase appears to be mainly in a glucose-6-P-dependent form in unstimulated tissues (KASLOW et al. 1979). Epinephrine causes the conversion of glycogen synthase to a form which is more dependent on glucose-6-P i.e. has a higher K_a for this metabolite.

Epinephrine can stimulate or inhibit glucose uptake in adipose tissue depending on the experimental conditions. If the accumulation of free fatty acids is not marked, there is stimulation of glucose uptake and oxidation, and of glyceride glycerol and lactate formation (CAHILL et al. 1960; BALL and JUNGAS 1964; FLATT and BALL 1965). These effects are also seen in the presence of insulin (HAGEN and BALL 1961; BALL and JUNGAS 1964; FLATT and BALL 1965). If excessive accumulation of tissue free fatty acids occurs, glucose utilization is inhibited (HAGEN and BALL 1961). This may be because of inhibition of glucose transport by the high concentrations of fatty acids (RANDLE et al. 1964; NEELY et al. 1969) and restraint of glycolysis due to the accumulation of citrate which inhibits P-fructokinase (PARMEGGIANI and BOWMAN 1963; GARLAND et al. 1963; DENTON and RANDLE 1966).

Stimulation of glucose uptake appears to be the more physiological response to epinephrine. This has been attributed to enhanced reesterification of liberated free fatty acids (CAHILL et al. 1960) and to stimulation of P-fructokinase by cyclic AMP (DENTON et al. 1966), but may also involve α-adrenergic receptors (LUZIO et al. 1974). Recently, LUDVIGSEN et al. (1980) have presented evidence for β-adrenergic stimulation of glucose transport in adipose tissue. Clearly the mechanisms involved in catecholamine stimulation of glucose uptake in adipose tissue need further exploration.

The action of epinephrine on adipose tissue lipolysis is clearly attributable to activation of cyclic AMP-dependent protein kinase due to cyclic AMP accumulation (for references see SODERLING et al. 1973). The kinase is postulated to phosphorylate and activate a hormone-sensitive lipase (CORBIN et al. 1970, 1972; HUTTUNEN et al. 1970; HUTTUNEN and STEINBERG 1971). The effects of epinephrine on triglyceride synthesis in adipose tissue depend upon the presence or absence of endogenous or exogenous carbohydrate. When glucose is available, triglyceride synthesis is stimulated and this has been attributed to the increased availability of free fatty acids generated by lipolysis (BALL and JUNGAS 1964; FLATT and BALL 1965).

In the absence of carbohydrate, epinephrine can inhibit triglyceride synthesis (DENTON and HALPERIN 1968; SOORANNA and SAGGERSON 1975). This appears to be due to decreased activity of glycerolphosphate acyltransferase (SOORANNA and SAGGERSON (1976). There is some evidence that cyclic AMP-dependent protein kinase can phosphorylate and inactive this enzyme (H. NIMMO and HOUSTON 1978). This would provide another instance where cyclic AMP affects both breakdown and synthesis of storage forms of metabolic fuels in tissues.

Epinephrine can inhibit pyruvate dehydrogenase activity in adipose tissue especially when the enzyme is activated by insulin (for references, see SMITH and SAGGERSON 1978). In the absence of insulin, the effects of epinephrine and other lipolytic hormones are variable (JUNGAS 1971; COORE et al. 1971; SICA and CUATRECASAS 1973; S. TAYLOR et al. 1973; WEISS et al. 1974; SOORANNA and SAGGERSON 1976; SMITH and SAGGERSON 1978). In a detailed study of the action of epinephrine in the presence of insulin, SMITH and SAGGERSON (1978) found a good correlation between the inhibitory action of hormone on pyruvate dehydrogenase and its stimulatory effect on lipolysis. However its effect on the enzyme could not be mimicked by addition of albumin-bound palmitate. The mechanism(s) by which epinephrine alters pyruvate dehydrogenase thus remains obscure. However, SEVERSON et al. (1976) have observed that epinephrine decreases the uptake of [^{45}Ca] into the mitochondria of fat pads incubated with insulin. They suggest epinephrine may act by decreasing mitochondrial Ca^{2+} thereby reducing the activity of pyruvate dehydrogenase phosphatase and hence inactivating pyruvate dehydrogenase. The postulated change in mitochondrial Ca^{2+} observed with epinephrine resembles that mediated by α-adrenergic receptors in liver (BLACKMORE et al. 1979b; BABCOCK et al. 1979).

II. Insulin Effects on Glycogen Metabolism in Adipose Tissue

The actions of insulin on glycogen metabolism in adipose tissue are related to changes in both glucose uptake and cyclic AMP levels (LAWRENCE et al. 1977; LAWRENCE and LARNER 1978a, b, 1979). Administered alone, insulin causes rapid activation of glycogen synthase, but produces no detectable change in cyclic AMP, cyclic AMP-dependent protein kinase or phosphorylase (LAWRENCE et al. 1977; BUTCHER et al. 1966; SODERLING et al. 1973). Its action to decrease the K_a of the enzyme for glucose-6-P is more prominent than its effect on the activity ratio (KASLOW et al. 1979). It activates glycogen synthase half-maximally at 1 min and completely at 4 min, and is effective at a concentration of 8 μ units per ml (5×10^{-11} *M*) (LAWRENCE et al. 1977). Glucose addition causes a transient activation of the enzyme and greatly potentiates the stimulatory effect of insulin (Fig. 26). Studies utilizing other hexoses have shown that part of insulin's action is related to increased glucose transport, whereas part is independent of glucose (LAWRENCE et al. 1977; LAWRENCE and LARNER 1978b). The part related to glucose transport may be due to increased formation of glucose-6-P which inhibits glycogen synthase phosphatase (LAWRENCE and LARNER 1977).

Starvation and diabetes inhibit glycogen synthesis in adipose tissue and alter glycogen synthase (EICHNER 1976; KASLOW and MAYER 1979). They cause the appearance of a form of the enzyme with a very low affinity for glucose-6-P

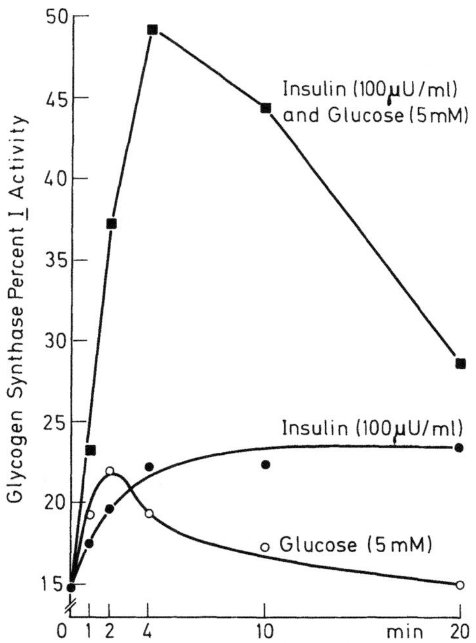

Fig. 26. Stimulatory effect of insulin on fat cell glycogen synthase in the presence and absence of glucose. (LAWRENCE et al. 1977)

(K_a, 3 mM) and a K_m for UDP-glucose of 0.3 mM in the presence of glucose-6-P. EICHNER (1976) considers that this form differs from the *b* form of the enzyme. Comparison with the data of Table I suggests that it is phosphorylated to a high degree.

Insulin has been shown by many investigators to decrease cyclic AMP levels in adipose tissue when these are increased by lipolytic agents (for references see KONO and BARHAM 1973). This decrease is associated with inactivation of cyclic AMP-dependent protein kinase (SODERLING et al. 1973) and has been attributed to activation of cyclic AMP phosphodiesterase (for references see KONO et al. 1975). There have also been some reports of insulin inhibition of adenylate cyclase (HEPP 1971; ILLIANO and CUATRECASAS 1972), but this effect has proved difficult to reproduce. Changes in cyclic AMP levels presumably account for the ability of insulin to inhibit the activation of phosphorylase and inactivation of glycogen synthase induced by epinephrine, although this has not been demonstrated directly (KHOO et al. 1973).

Studies of the effects of insulin on Ca^{2+} fluxes and other parameters in fat cells and adipose tissue segments have led to opposing views about the role of Ca^{2+} in insulin action. The group of JARETT (MCDONALD et al. 1976a, b, 1978) has obtained evidence that insulin increases the uptake of Ca^{2+} by endoplasmic reticulum and also increases the binding of Ca^{2+} to plasma membranes. Several groups, on the other hand, have interpreted the effects of insulin on [$^{45}Ca^{2+}$] fluxes and glycogen synthase activity as indicating a mobilization of intracellular Ca^{2+} (KISSEBAH et al. 1975; P. CLARKE et al. 1975; HOPE-GILL et al. 1976; SCHUDT et al. 1976; CLAUSEN and MARTIN 1977; CLAUSEN et al. 1979). However, the interpretation of

[$^{45}Ca^{2+}$] flux data is seldom unequivocal and the claim that Ca^{2+} activates glycogen synthase (Hope-Gill et al. 1976) is not well substantiated. By analogy with findings in liver (Blackmore et al. 1979a; Dehaye et al. 1981), one would expect insulin to decrease cytosolic Ca^{2+}.

III. Insulin Effects on Pyruvate Metabolism in Adipose Tissue

It is well established that insulin activates pyruvate dehydrogenase in adipose tissue (Denton et al. 1971; Jungas 1971; Coore et al. 1971; Sica and Cuatrecasas 1973; S. Taylor et al. 1973; Weiss et al. 1974; Sooranna and Saggerson 1976; Smith and Saggerson 1978). The effect can be dissociated from the action of the hormone on lipolysis or glucose transport (Martin et al. 1972; Weiss et al. 1974; Coore et al. 1971), and is due to conversion of the inactive (phosphorylated) form of the enzyme to the active (dephosphorylated) form (Coore et al. 1971; Weiss et al. 1971; Denton et al. 1971; S. Taylor et al. 1973; S. Taylor and Jungas 1974). There is substantial evidence that insulin acts by stimulating the dephosphorylation and activation of the enzyme rather than by inhibiting its phosphorylation (Sica and Cuatrecasas 1973; Mukherjee and Jungas 1975; Severson et al. 1976). It has also been proposed that pyruvate dehydrogenase phosphatase is activated by insulin (Mukherjee and Jungas 1975; Denton et al. 1972; Severson et al. 1974, 1976; Seals et al. 1979a, b; Jarett and Seals 1979; Seals and Jarett (1980) and that this is due to a rise in mitochondrial Ca^{2+} which stimulates the phosphatase (Linn et al. 1969a, b; Hucho et al. 1972; Siess and Wieland 1972; Denton et al. 1972).

Reduced incorporation of [^{32}P] into the α-subunit of the pyruvate decarboxylase moiety of pyruvate dehydrogenase has been shown to occur in response to insulin in adipocytes incubated with ^{32}Pi (W. Hughes and Denton 1976). This subunit has also been identified as the 42,000 dalton mitochondrial protein whose labeling is decreased when crude adipocyte plasma membranes are incubated in a medium containing Mg[$\gamma^{32}P$] ATP and insulin, or when isolated plasma membranes are incubated together with mitochondria in this medium (Seals et al. 1979a, b; Jarett and Seals 1979). Since mitochondria incubated alone with medium containing insulin did not show changes in phosphorylation of the protein, Jarett and his colleagues have proposed that insulin interacts with plasma membranes to generate a "second messenger" which decreases the phosphorylation of the α-subunit of pyruvate dehydrogenase in mitochondria, thereby activating the enzyme. They have presented evidence that the effect is due to activation of the Ca^{2+}-sensitive pyruvate dehydrogenase phosphatase (Seals et al. 1979b; Jarett and Seals 1979; Seals and Jarett 1980; Popp et al. 1980; Kiechle et al. 1980).

Very interestingly, it has been shown that fractions of muscle extracts containing the factor(s) generated in response to insulin which apparently inhibits cyclic AMP-dependent protein kinase and activates glycogen synthase phosphatase (Larner et al. 1979) also causes activation of pyruvate dehydrogenase when added to isolated adipocyte mitochondria (Jarett and Seals 1979). There has also been a report of the partial purification of an insulin-dependent activator of pyruvate dehydrogenase phosphatase from adipose tissue (Kiechle et al. 1980). As noted in Sect. A.IV.2, evidence has been obtained which shows that insulin can reduce the release of Ca^{2+} from liver mitochondria under conditions where the ion is mobilized (DEHAYE et al. 1981). It is therefore possible that the primary action of the putative "second messenger" of insulin is to cause an increase in the concentration of free Ca^{2+} in mitochondria. This would be consistent with observations of mitochondrial Ca^{2+} changes in insulin-treated adipocytes (McDONALD et al. 1976a) and could account for the reported effects of insulin on pyruvate dehydrogenase phosphatase.

References

Adam PAJ, Haynes RC Jr (1969) Control of hepatic mitochondrial CO_2 fixation by glucagon, epinephrine, and cortisol. J Biol Chem 244:6440–6450

Adelstein RS, Conti MA, Hathaway DR, Klee CB (1978) Phosphorylation of smooth muscle myosin light chain kinase by the catalytic subunit of adenosine 3′:5′-monophosphate-dependent protein kinase. J Biol Chem 253:8347–8350

Adolfsson S, Isaksson O, Hjalmarson A (1972) Effect of insulin on glycogen synthesis and synthetase activity in the perfused rat heart. Biochim Biophys Acta 279:146–156

Aggerbeck M, Guellaen G, Hanoune J (1980) Adrenergic receptor of the $alpha_1$ subtype mediates the activation of the glycogen phosphorylase in normal rat liver. Biochem Pharmacol 29:643–645

Ahlborg G, Felig P, Hagenfeldt L, Hendler R, Wahren J (1974) Substrate turnover during prolonged exercise in man. J Clin Invest 53:1080–1090

Altszuler N, Steele R, Rathgeb I, Debodo RC (1967) Glucose metabolism and plasma insulin level during epinephrine infusion in the dog. Am J Physiol 212:677–682

Antoniw JF, Cohen P (1976) Separation of two phosphorylase kinase phosphatases from rabbit skeletal muscle. Eur J Biochem 68:45–54

Antoniw JF, Nimmo HG, Yeaman SJ, Cohen P (1977) Comparison of the substrate specificities of protein phosphatases involved in the regulation of glycogen metabolism in rabbit skeletal muscle. Biochem J 162:423–433

Assimacopoulos-Jeannet FD, Blackmore PF, Exton JH (1977) Studies in α-adrenergic activation of hepatic glucose output. Studies on role of calcium in α-adrenergic activation of phosphorylase. J Biol Chem 252:2662–2669

Babcock DF, Chen J-LJ, Yip BP, Lardy HA (1979) Evidence for mitochondrial localization of the hormone- responsive pool of Ca^{2+} in isolated hepatocytes. J Biol Chem 254:8117–8120

Bailey JM, Whelan WJ (1972) The roles of glucose and AMP in regulating the conversion of phosphorylase *a* into phosphorylase *b*. Biochem Biophys Res Commun 46:191–197

Ball EG, Jungas RL (1964) Some effects of hormones on the metabolism of adipose tissue. Recent Prog Horm Res 20:183–213

Ballard FJ, Hanson RW (1969) Purification of phospho-enolpyruvate carboxykinase from the cytosol fraction of rat liver and the immunochemical demonstration of differences between this and the mitochondrial phosphoenolpyruvate carboxykinase. J Biol Chem 244:5625–5630

Barnett CA, Wicks WD (1971) Regulation of phosphoenol- pyruvate carboxykinase and tyrosine transaminase in hepatoma cell cultures. I. Effects of glucocorticoids, N^6, $O^{2'}$-dibutyryl cyclic adenosine 3′,5′-monophosphate and insulin in Reuber H35 cells. J Biol Chem 246:7201–7206

Barron JT, Barany M, Barany K, Storti RV (1980) Reversible phosphorylation and dephosphorylation of the 20,000-dalton light chain of myosin during the contraction-relaxation-contraction cycle of arterial smooth muscle. J Biol Chem 255:6238–6244

Beavo JA, Mumby MC (1982) Cyclic AMP-dependent protein phosphorylation. In: Nathanson JA; Kebabian JW (eds) Cyclic nucleotides. Springer, Berlin Heidelberg New York (Handbook of experimental pharmacology, vol 58/I)

Bentle LA, Lardy HA (1977) P-Enolpyruvate carboxykinase ferroactivator. Purification and some properties. J Biol Chem 252:1431–1440

Bentle LA, Snoke RE, Lardy HA (1976) A protein factor required for activation of phosphoenolpyruvate carboxykinase by ferrous ions. J Biol Chem 251:2922–2928

Berger M, Hagg SA, Goodman MN, Ruderman NB (1976) Glucose metabolism in perfused skeletal muscle. Biochem J 158:191–202

Bernard C (1849) Chiens rendus diabetiques. C R Soc Biol (Paris) 1:60

Bihler I, Sarvh PC, Sloan IG (1978) Dual effect of adrenaline on sugar transport in rat diaphragm muscle. Biochim Biophys Acta 510:349–360

Birnbaumer L, Iyengar R (1982) Coupling of receptors adenylate cyclases. In: Nathanson JA, Kebabian JW (eds) Cyclic nucleotides. Springer, Berlin Heidelberg New York (Handbook of experimental pharmacology, vol 58/I)

Birnbaum MJ, Fain JN (1977) Activation of protein kinase and glycogen phosphorylase in isolated rat liver cells by glucagon and catecholamines. J Biol Chem 252:528–535

Bishop JS (1970) Inability of insulin to activate liver glycogen transferase D phosphatase in the diabetic pancreatectomized dog. Biochim Biophys Acta 208:202–218

Bishop JS, Larner J (1967) Rapid activation-inactivation of liver UDPG-glycogen transferase and phosphorylase by insulin and glucagon in vivo. J Biol Chem 242:1354–1356

Bishop JS, Goldberg ND, Larner J (1971) Insulin regulation of hepatic glycogen metabolism in the dog. Am J Physiol 220:499–506

Blackmore PF, Brumley FT, Marks JL, Exton JH (1978) Studies on α-adrenergic activation of hepatic glucose output. Relationship between α-adrenergic stimulation of calcium efflux and activation of phosphorylase in isolated rat liver parenchymal cells. J Biol Chem 253:4851–4858

Blackmore PF, Assimacopoulos-Jeannet FD, Chan TM, Exton JH (1979a) Studies on α-adrenergic activation of hepatic glucose output. Insulin inhibition of α-adrenergic and glucagon actions in normal and calcium-depleted hepatocytes. J Biol Chem 254:2828–2834

Blackmore PF, Dehaye J-P, Exton JH (1979b) Studies on α-adrenergic activation of hepatic glucose output. The role of mitochondrial calcium release in α-adrenergic activation of phosphorylase in perfused rat liver. J Biol Chem 254:6945–6950

Blair JB, Cimbala MA, Foster JL, Morgan RA (1976) Hepatic pyruvate kinase. Regulation by glucagon, cyclic adenosine 3′:5′-monophosphate and insulin in the perfused rat liver. J Biol Chem 251:3756–3762

Blair JB, James ME, Foster JL (1979a) Adrenergic control of glucose output and adenosine 3′:5′-monophosphate levels in hepatocytes from juvenile and adult rats. J Biol Chem 254:7579–7584

Blair JB, James ME, Foster JL (1979b) Adrenergic control of glycolysis and pyruvate kinase activity in hepatocytes from young and old rats. J Biol Chem 254:7585–7590

Blake CCF (1979) Structure and control of phosphorylase. Nature 280:448

Blatt LM, Kim K-H (1971) Regulation of rat liver glycogen synthetase. Relationship of the hormonal activation and the time-dependent in vitro activation. J Biol Chem 246:7256–7264

Bolton TB (1979) Mechanisms of action of transmitters and other substances on smooth muscle. Physiol Rev 59:606–718

Bornet EP, Entman ML, Van Winkle WB, Schwartz A, Lehotay DC, Levey GS (1977) Cyclic AMP modulation of calcium accumulation by sarcoplasmic reticulum from fast skeletal muscle. Biochim Biophys Acta 468:188–193

Brandt H, Capulong ZL, Lee EYC (1975a) Purification and properties of rabbit liver phosphorylase phosphatase. J Biol Chem 250:8038–8044

Brandt H, Lee EYC, Killilea SD (1975b) A protein inhibitor of rabbit liver phosphorylase phosphatase. Biochem Biophys Res Commun 63:950–956

Brostrom CO, Hunkeler FL, Krebs EG (1971) The regulation of skeletal muscle phosphorylase kinase by Ca^{2+}. J Biol Chem 246:1961–1967

Brown JH, Thompson B, Mayer SE (1977) Conversion of skeletal muscle glycogen synthase to multiple glucose-6-phosphate dependent forms by cyclic adenosine monophosphate dependent and independent protein kinases. Biochemistry 16:5501–5508

Buschiazzo H, Exton JH, Park CR (1970) Effect of glucose on glycogen synthetase, phosphorylase and glycogen deposition in the perfused rat liver. Proc Natl Acad Sci USA 65:383–387

Buse MG, Biggers JF, Drier C, Buse JF (1973) The effect of epinephrine, glucagon, and the nutritional state on the oxidation of branched chain amino acids and pyruvate by isolated hearts and diaphragms of the rat. J Biol Chem 248:697–706

Butcher RW, Sneyd JGT, Park CR, Sutherland EW Jr (1966) Effect of insulin on adenosine 3′,5′-monophosphate in the rat epididymal fat pad. J Biol Chem 241:1652–1653

Cahill GF Jr, LeBoeuf B, Flinn RB (1960) Studies on rat adipose tissue in vitro. VI. Effect of epinephrine on glucose utilization. J Biol Chem 235:1246–1250

Cahill GF Jr, Aoki TT, Marliss EB (1972) Insulin and muscle protein. In: Steiner DF, Freinkel N (eds) Endocrine pancreas. American Physiological Society, Washington; DC (Handbook of physiology, sect 7, Endocrinology, vol 1)

Caldwell MD, Lacy WW, Exton JH (1978) Effects of adrenalectomy on the amino acid and glucose metabolism of perfused rat hindlimbs. J Biol Chem 253:6837–6844

Castano JG, Nieto A, Feliu JE (1979) Inactivation of phosphofructokinase by glucagon in rat hepatocytes. J Biol Chem 254:5576–5579

Casteels R, Raeymaekers L (1979) The action of acetylcholine and catecholamines on an intracellular calcium store in the smooth muscle cells of the guinea pig taenia coli. J Physiol (Lond) 294:51–68

Chacko S, Conti MA, Adelstein RS (1977) Effect of phosphorylation of smooth muscle myosin on actin activation and Ca^{2+} regulation. Proc Nat Acad Sci USA 74:129–133

Chan TM, Exton JH (1977) α-Adrenergic-mediated accumulation of adenosine 3′,5′-monophosphate in calcium-depleted hepatocytes. J Biol Chem 252:8645–8651

Chan TM, Exton JH (1978) Studies on α-adrenergic activation of hepatic glucose output. Studies on α-adrenergic inhibition of hepatic pyruvate kinase and activation of gluconeogenesis. J Biol Chem 253:6393–6400

Chan TM, Bacon CB, Hill SA (1979a) Glucagon stimulation of liver mitochondrial CO_2 fixation utilizing pyruvate generated inside the mitochondria. J Biol Chem 254:8730–8732

Chan TM, Blackmore PF, Steiner KE, Exton JH (1979b) Effects of adrenalectomy on hormone action on hepatic glucose metabolism. Reciprocal change in α- and β-adrenergic activation of hepatic glycogen phosphorylase and calcium mobilization in adrenalectomized rats. J Biol Chem 254:2428–2433

Chan TM, Steiner KE, Exton JH (1979c) Effects of adrenalectomy on hormone action on hepatic glucose metabolism. Impaired glucagon activation of glycogen phosphorylase in hepatocytes from adrenalectomized rats. J Biol Chem 254:11374–11378

Chen J-LJ, Babcock DF, Lardy HA (1978) Norepinephrine, vasopressin, glucagon, and A23187 induce efflux of calcium from an exchangeable pool in isolated rat hepatocytes. Proc Natl Acad Sci USA 75:2234–2238

Cherrington AD, Exton JH (1976) Studies on the role of cAMP-dependent protein kinase in the actions of glucagon and catecholamines on liver glycogen metabolism. Metabolism 25:1351–1354

Cherrington AD, Vranic M (1974) Effect of interaction between insulin and glucagon on glucose turnover and FFA concentration in normal and depancreatized dogs. Metabolism 23:729–744

Cherrington AD, Chiasson J-L, Liljenquist JE, Jennings AS, Keller U, Lacy WW (1976) The role of insulin and glucagon in the regulation of basal glucose production in the postabsorptive dog. J Clin Invest 58:1407–1418

Cherrington AD, Hundley RF, Dolgin S, Exton JH (1977) Studies on the role of beta-adrenergic receptors in the activation of phosphorylase in rat hepatocytes by catecholamines. J Cyclic Nucleotide Res 3:263–273

Cherrington AD, Lacy WW, Chiasson J-L (1978) Effect of glucagon on glucose production during insulin deficiency in the dog. J Clin Invest 62:664–677

Cherrington AD, Liljenquist JE, Shulman GI, Williams PE, Lacy WW (1979) The importance of hypoglycemia-induced glucose production during isolated glucagon deficiency. Am J Physiol 236:E263–E271

Chiasson J-L, Atkinson RL, Cherrington AD, Keller U, Sinclair-Smith BC, Lacy WW, Liljenquist JE (1979) Effects of fasting on gluconeogenesis from alanine in non-diabetic man. Diabetes 28:56–60
Chiasson JL, Dietz MR, Shikama H, Wootten M, Exton JH (1980) Insulin regulation of skeletal muscle glycogen metabolism. Am J Physiol 239:E69–E74
Chiasson J-L, Shikama H, Exton JH (1981) Inhibitory effect of epinephrine on insulin-stimulated glucose uptake in skeletal muscle. J Clin Invest 68:706–713
Chideckel EW, Goodner CJ, Koerker DJ, Johnson DG, Ensinck JW (1977) Role of glucagon in mediating metabolic effects of epinephrine. Am J Physiol 232:E464–E470
Chrisman TD, Exton JH (1980) Activation of endogenous phosphorylase kinase in liver glycogen pellet by cAMP-dependent protein kinase. J Biol Chem 255:3270–3273
Clark MG, Kneer NM, Bosch AL, Lardy HA (1974) The fructose 1,6-diphosphate-phosphofructokinase substrate cycle. A site of regulation of hepatic gluconeogenesis by glucagon. J Biol Chem 249:5695–5703
Clarke PV, Kissebah AH, Hope-Gill H, Vydelingum N, Tulloch B, Fraser TR (1975) The role of calcium in insulin action. Eur J Clin Invest 5:351–358
Clarke WR, Jones LR, Lefkowitz RJ (1978) Hepatic α-adrenergic receptors. Identification and subcellular localization using [^{3}H]dihydroergocryptine. J Biol Chem 253:5975–5979
Claus TH, Pilkis SJ (1976) Regulation by insulin of gluconeogenesis in isolated rat hepatocytes. Biochim Biophys Acta 421:246–262
Claus TH, Pilkis SJ (1977) Effect of dichloroacetate and glucagon on the incorporation of labeled substrates into glucose and on pyruvate dehydrogenase in hepatocytes from fed and starved rats. Arch Biochem Biophys 182:52–63
Claus TH, Pilkis SJ, Park CR (1975) Stimulation by glucagon of the incorporation of U-^{14}C-labeled substrates into glucose by isolated hepatocytes from fed rats. Biochim Biophys Acta 404:110–123
Claus TH, El-Maghrabi MR, Pilkis SJ (1979) Modulation of the phosphorylation state of rate liver pyruvate kinase by allosteric effectors and insulin. J Biol Chem 254:7855–7864
Clausen T, Martin BR (1977) The effect of insulin on the washout of [^{45}Ca] calcium from adipocytes and soleus muscle of the rat. Biochem J 164:251–255
Clausen T, Dahl-Hansen AB, Elbrink J (1979) The effect of hyperosmolarity and insulin on resting tension and calcium fluxes in rat liver soleus muscle. J Physiol (Lond) 292:505–526
Cohen P (1973) The subunit structure of rabbit-skeletal muscle phosphorylase kinase and molecular basis of its activation reaction. Eur J Biochem 34:1–14
Cohen P (1978) The role of cyclic-AMP-dependent protein kinase in the regulation of glycogen metabolism in mammalian skeletal muscle. Curr Top Cell Regul 14:117–196
Cohen P, Nimmo GA, Antoniw JF (1977) Specificity of a protein phosphatase inhibitor from rabbit skeletal muscle. Biochem J 162:435–444
Cohen P, Burchell A, Foulkes JG, Cohen PTW, Vanaman TC, Nairn AC (1978) Identification of the Ca^{2+}-dependent modulator protein as the fourth subunit of rabbit skeletal muscle phosphorylase kinase. FEBS Lett 92:287–293
Cohen PTW, Cohen P (1973) Skeletal muscle phosphorylase kinase deficiency: detection of a protein lacking any activity in ICR/IAW mice. FEBS Lett 29:113–116
Cole HA, Perry SV (1975) The phosphorylation of troponin I from cardiac muscle. Biochem J 149:525–533
Conlee RK, McLane JA, Rennie MJ, Winder WW, Holloszy JO (1979) Reversal of phosphorylase activation in muscle despite continued contractile activity. Am J Physiol 237:R291–R296
Cooper RH, Randle PJ, Denton RM (1974) Regulation of heart muscle pyruvate dehydrogenase kinase. Biochem J 143:625–641
Coore HG, Denton RM, Martin BR, Randle PJ (1971) Regulation of adipose tissue pyruvate dehydrogenase by insulin and other hormones. Biochem J 125:115–127
Corbin JD, Reimann EM, Walsh DA, Krebs EG (1970) Activation of adipose tissue lipase by skeletal muscle cyclic adenosine 3′,5′-monophosphate-stimulated protein kinase. J Biol Chem 245:4849–4851
Corbin JD, Brostrom CO, Alexander RL, Krebs EG (1972) Adenosine 3′,5′-monophosphate-dependent protein kinase from adipose tissue. J Biol Chem 247:3736–3743

Corbin JD, Sugden PH, Lincoln TM, Keely SL (1977) Compartmentalization of adenosine 3′:5′-monophosphate and adenosine 3′:5′-monophosphate-dependent protein kinase in heart tissue. J Biol Chem 252:3854–3861

Cote TE, Epand RM (1979) N^{a}-trinitrophenyl glucagon. An inhibitor of glucagon-stimulated cyclic AMP production and its effects on glycogenolysis. Biochim Biophys Acta 582:295–306

Crabb DW, Mapes JP, Boersma RW, Harris RH (1976) Effect of dichloroacetate on carbohydrate and lipid metabolism of isolated hepatocytes. Arch Biochem Biophys 173:658–665

Craig JW, Larner J (1964) Influence of epinephrine and insulin on uridine diphosphate glucose-α-glucose transferase and phosphorylase in muscle. Nature 202:971–973

Craig JW, Rall TW, Larner J (1969) The influence of insulin and epinephrine on adenosine 3′,5′-phosphate and glycogen transferase in muscle. Biochim Biophys Acta 177:213–219

Crane RK, Sols A (1954) The noncompetitive inhibition of brain hexokinase by glucose-6-phosphate and related compounds. J Biol Chem 210:597–606

Cushman SW, Wardzala LJ (1980) Potential mechanism of insulin action on glucose transport in the isolated rat adipose cell. Apparent translocation of intracellular transport systems to the plasma membrane. J Biol Chem 255:4758–4762

Dabrowska R, Sherry JMF, Aromatorio DK, Hartshorne DJ (1978) Modulator protein as a component of the myosin light chain kinase from chicken gizzard. Biochemistry 17:253–258

Danforth WH (1965) Glycogen synthetase activity in skeletal muscle. Interconversion of two forms and control of glycogen synthesis. J Biol chem 240:588–593

Danforth WH, Lyon JB (1964) Glycolysis during tetanic contraction of isolated mouse muscles in the presence and absence of phosphorylase *a*. J Biol Chem 239:4047–4050

Danforth WH, Helmreich E, Cori CF (1962) The effect of contraction and of epinephrine on the phosphorylase activity of frog sartorius muscle. Proc Natl Acad Sci USA 48:1191–1199

Davis PF, Pettit FH, Reed LJ (1977) Peptides derived from pyruvate dehydrogenase as substrates for pyruvate dehydrogenase kinase and phosphatase. Biochem Biophys Res Commun 75:541–549

Dehaye J-P, Blackmore PF, Venter JC, Exton JH (1980) Studies on the α-adrenergic activation of hepatic glucose output. α-Adrenergic activation of phosphorylase by immobilized epinephrine. J Biol Chem 253:3905–3910

Dehaye J-P, Blackmore PF, Exton JH (1981) Studies on α-adrenergic activation of hepatic glucose output. Insulin inhibition of α-adrenergic mobilization of mitochondrial calcium in the perfused liver. Biochem J 194:949–956

Deibert DC, DeFronzo RA (1980) Epinephrine-induced insulin resistance in man. J Clin Invest 65:717–721

Denton RM, Halperin ML (1968) The control of fatty acid and triglyceride synthesis in rat epididymal adipose tissue: roles of coenzyme A derivatives, citrate and L-glycerol 3-phosphate. Biochem J 110:27–38

Denton RM, Randle PJ (1966) Citrate and the regulation of adipose tissue phosphofructokinase. Biochem J 100:420–423

Denton RM, Yorke RE, Randle PJ (1966) Measurements of concentrations of metabolites in adipose tissue and effects of insulin, alloxan-diabetes and adrenaline. Biochem J 100:407–419

Denton RM, Coore HG, Martin BR, Randle PJ (1971) Insulin activates pyruvate dehydrogenase in rat epididymal adipose tissue. Nature 231:115–116

Denton RM, Randle PJ, Martin BR (1972) Stimulation by calcium ions of pyruvate dehydrogenase phosphate phosphatase. Biochem J 128:161–163

Denton RM, Randle PJ, Bridges BJ et al. (1975) Regulation of mammalian pyruvate dehydrogenase. Mol Cell Biochem 9:27–53

Denton RM, McCormack JG, Oviasu OA (1981) Short-term regulation of pyruvate dehydrogenase activity in the liver. In: Hue L, Van der Werve G (eds) Short term regulation of liver metabolism. Elsevier/North-Holland, Amsterdam Oxford New York

DePaoli-Roach AA, Roach PJ, Larner J (1979a) Rabbit skeletal muscle phosphorylase kinase. Comparison of glycogen synthase and phosphorylase as substrates. J Biol Chem 254:4212–4219
DePaoli-Roach AA, Roach PJ, Larner J (1979b) Multiple phosphorylation of rabbit skeletal muscle glycogen synthase. J Biol Chem 254:12062–12068
Detwiler TC, Gratecos D, Fischer EH (1977) Rabbit muscle phosphorylase phosphatase. 2. Kinetic properties and behavior in glycogen particles. Biochemistry 16:4818–4823
DeWulf H, Hers H-G (1968a) The interconversion of liver glycogen synthetase *a* and *b* in vitro. Eur J Biochem 6:552–557
DeWulf H, Hers H-G (1968b) The role of glucose, glucagon and glucocorticoids in the regulation of liver glycogen synthesis. Eur J Biochem 6:558–564
Dietz MR, Chiasson J-L, Soderling TR, Exton JH (1980) Epinephrine regulation of skeletal muscle glycogen metabolism. Studies utilizing the perfused rat hindlimb preparation. J Biol Chem 255:2301–2307
Drummond GI, Duncan L, Hertzman E (1966) Effect of epinephrine on phosphorylase *b* kinase in perfused rat hearts. J Biol Chem 241:5899–5903
Drummond GI, Harwood JP, Powell CA (1969) Studies on the activation of phosphorylase in skeletal muscle by contraction and by epinephrine. J Biol Chem 244:4235–4240
Ebashi S, Endo M (1968) Calcium ion and muscle contraction. Prog Biophys Mol Biol 18:123–183
Edmondson JW, Lumenz L, Li T-K (1979) Comparative studies of alanine and α-aminoisobutyric acid uptake by freshly isolated rat liver cells. J Biol Chem 254:1653–1658
Edwards AV (1971) The glycogenolytic response to stimulation of the splanchnic nerves in adrenalectomized calves, sheep, dogs, cats and pigs. J Physiol (Lond) 213:741–759
Edwards AV (1972) The sensitivity of the hepatic glycogenolytic mechanism to stimulation of the splanchnic nerves. J Physiol (Lond) 220:315–334
Edwards AV, Silver M (1970) The glycogenolytic response to stimulation of the splanchnic nerves in adrenalectomized calves. J Physiol (Lond) 211:109–124
Eichner RD (1976) Rat adipose tissue glycogen synthase. Evidence for multiple discrete kinetic species and their interconversion. J Biol Chem 251:2316–2322
Ellis S (1956) The metabolic effects of epinephrine and related amines. Pharmacol Rev 8:485–562
El-Refai M, Bergman RN (1979) Glucagon-stimulated glycogenolysis: time-dependent sensitivity to insulin. Am J Physiol 236:E246–E254
El-Refai MF, Exton JH (1980) Subclassification of two types of α-adrenergic binding sites in rat liver. Eur J Pharmacol 62:201–204
El-Refai MF, Blackmore PF, Exton JH (1979) Evidence for two α-adrenergic binding sites in liver plasma membranes. Studies with [^{3}H]epinephrine and [^{3}H]dihydroergocryptine. J Biol Chem 254:4375–4386
Embi N, Rylatt DB, Cohen P (1979) Glycogen synthase kinase-2 and phosphorylase kinase are the same enzyme. Eur J Biochem 100:339–347
Embi N, Rylatt DB, Cohen P (1980) Glycogen synthase kinase-3 from rabbit skeletal muscle. Separation from cyclic AMP-dependent protein kinase and phosphorylase kinase. Eur J Biochem 107:519–527
Embi N, Parker PJ, Cohen P (1981) A reinvestigation of the phosphorylation of rabbit skeletal-muscle glycogen synthase by cyclic-AMP-dependent protein kinase. Identification of the third site of phosphorylation as serine-7. Eur J Biochem 115:405–413
Endo M (1977) Calcium release from sarcoplasmic reticulum. Physiol Rev 57:71–108
England PJ (1975) Correlation between contraction and phosphorylation of the inhibitory subunit of troponin in perfused rat heart. FEBS Lett 50:57–60
England PJ (1976) Studies on the phosphorylation of the inhibitory subunit of troponin in perfused rat heart. Biochem J 160:295–304
England PJ (1977) Phosphorylation of the inhibitory subunit of troponin in perfused hearts of mice deficient in phosphorylase kinase: evidence for the phosphorylation of troponin by adenosine 3′:5′-phosphate-dependent protein kinase in vivo. Biochem J 168:307–310
Entman ML, Levey GS, Epstein SE (1969) Mechanism of action of epinephrine and glucagon on the canine heart. Evidence for increase in sarcotubular calcium stores mediated by cyclic 3′,5′-AMP. Circ Res 25:429–438

Exton JH (1972) Gluconeogenesis. Metabolism 21:945–990
Exton JH (1979) Mechanisms involved in alpha-adrenergic effects of catecholamines on liver metabolism. J Cyclic Nucleotide Res 5:277–287
Exton JH, Harper SC (1975) Role of cyclic AMP in the actions of catecholamines on hepatic carbohydrate metabolism. Adv Cyclic Nucleotide Res 5:519–532
Exton JH, Park CR (1968) Control of gluconeogenesis in liver. II. Effects of glucagon, catecholamines, and adenosine 3′,5′-monophosphate on gluconeogenesis in the perfused rat liver. J Biol Chem 243:4189–4196
Exton JH, Park CR (1969) Control of gluconeogenesis in liver. III. Effects of L-lactate, pyruvate, fructose, glucagon, epinephrine and adenosine 3′,5′-monophosphate on gluconeogenic intermediates in the perfused rat liver. J Biol Chem 244:1424–1433
Exton JH, Park CR (1972) Interaction of insulin and glucagon in the control of liver metabolism. In: Steiner DF, Freinkel N (eds) Endocrine pancreas. American Physiological Society, Washington; DC (Handbook of physiology, sect 7, Endocrinology, vol 1)
Exton JH, Robison GA, Sutherland EW, Park CR (1971) Studies on the role of adenosine 3′,5′-monophosphate in the hepatic actions of glucagon and catecholamines. J Biol Chem 246:6166–6177
Exton JH, Friedmann N, Wong EYA, Brineaux JP, Corbin JD, Park CR (1972a) Interaction of glucocorticoids with glucagon and epinephrine in the control of gluconeogenesis and glycogenolysis in liver and of lipolysis in adipose tissue. J Biol Chem 247:3579–3588
Exton JH, Lewis SB, Ho RJ, Park CR (1972b) The role of cyclic AMP in the control of hepatic glucose production by glucagon and insulin. Adv Cyclic Nucleotide Res 1:91–101
Exton JH, Harper SC, Tucker AL, Ho R-Y (1973) Effects of insulin on gluconeogenesis and cyclic AMP levels in perfused livers from diabetic rats. Biochim Biophys Acta 329:23–40
Ezrailson EG, Potter JD, Michael L, Schwartz A (1977) Positive inotropy induced by ouabain, increased frequency, X537A, calcium and isoproterenol: the lack of correlation with phosphorylation of TN-I. J Mol Cell Cardiol 9:693–698
Fehlmann M, LeCam A, Freychet P (1979) Insulin and glucagon stimulation of amino acid transport in isolated rat hepatocytes. Synthesis of a high affinity component of transport. J Biol Chem 254:10431–10437
Felig P, Wahren J (1971) Amino acid metabolism in exercising man. J Clin Invest 50:2703–2714
Felig P, Owen OE, Wahren J, Cahill GF Jr, (1969) Amino acid metabolism during prolonged starvation. J Clin Invest 48:584–594
Felig P, Wahren J, Hendler R (1976) Influence of physiologic hyperglucagonemia on basal and insulin-inhibited glucose output in normal man. J Clin Invest 58:761–765
Feliu JE, Hue L, Hers H-G (1976) Hormonal control of pyruvate kinase activity and of gluconeogenesis in isolated hepatocytes. Proc Natl Acad Sci USA 73:2762–2766
Fischer EH, Heilmeyer LMG Jr, Haschke RH (1971) Phosphorylase and the control of glycogen degradation. Curr Top Cell Regul 4:211–251
Fischer EH, Blum HE, Byers B et al. (1976) Concerted regulation of glycogen metabolism and muscle contraction. In: Wieland O, Helmreich E, Holzer H (eds) metabolic interconversion of enzymes. Springer, Berlin Heidelberg New York
Fisher RB, Williamson JR (1961) The effects of insulin, adrenaline and nutrients on the oxygen consumption of the perfused rat heart. J Physiol (Lond) 158:102–112
Flatt JP, Ball EG (1965) Pathways of glucose metabolism. In: Renold AE, Cahill GF Jr (eds) Adipose tissue. American Physiological Society, Washington, DC (Handbook of physiology, sect 5)
Fletterick RJ, Sygusch J, Murray N, Madsen NB, Johnson LN (1976a) Low resolution structures of the glycogen phosphorylase *a* monomer and comparison with phosphorylase *b*. J Mol Biol 103:1–13
Fletterick RJ, Sygusch J, Semple M, Madsen NB (1976b) The structure of glycogen phosphorylase *a* at 3.0 A resolution and its ligand binding sites at 6 A. J Biol Chem 251:6142–6146
Foden S, Randle PJ (1978) Calcium metabolism in rat hepatocytes. Biochem J 170:615–625
Forssmann WG, Ito S (1977) Hepatocyte innervation in primates. J Cell Biol 74:299–313

Foulkes JG, Cohen P (1979) The hormonal control of glycogen metabolism. Phosphorylation of protein phosphatase inhibitor-1 in vivo in response to epinephrine. Eur J Biochem 97:251–256
Foulkes JG, Jefferson LS, Cohen P (1980) The hormonal control of glycogen metabolism: dephosphorylation of protein phosphatase inhibitor-1 in vivo in response to insulin. FEBS Lett 112:21–24
Frearson N, Solaro RJ, Perry SV (1976) Changes in phosphorylation of P light chain of myosin in perfused rabbit heart. Nature 264:801–802
Friedmann N, Park CR (1968) Early effects of 3′,5′-adenosine monophosphate on the fluxes of calcium and potassium in the perfused liver of normal and adrenalectomized rats. Proc Natl Acad Sci USA 61:504–508
Friedmann N, Rasmussen H (1970) Calcium, manganese and hepatic gluconeogenesis. Biochim Biophys Acta 222:41–52
Friedmann N, Exton JH, Park CR (1967) Interaction of adrenal steroids and glucagon on gluconeogenesis in perfused rat liver. Biochem Biophys Res Commun 29:113–119
Fulks RM, Li JB, Goldberg AL (1975) Effects of insulin, glucose, and amino acids on protein turnover in rat diaphragm. J Biol Chem 250:290–298
Galbo H, Holst JJ, Christensen NJ (1975) Glucagon and plasma catecholamine responses to graded and prolonged exercise in man. J Appl Physiol 38:70–76
Garber A, Menzel PH, Boden G, Owen OE (1974) Hepatic ketogenesis and gluconeogenesis in humans. J Clin Invest 54:981–989
Garber AJ, Cryer PE, Santiago JV, Haymond MW, Pagliara AS, Kipnis DM (1976a) The role of adrenergic mechanisms in the substrate and hormonal response to insulin-induced hypoglycemia in man. J Clin Invest 58:7–15
Garber AJ, Karl IE, Kipnis DM (1976b) Alanine and glutamine synthesis and release from skeletal muscle. J Biol Chem 251:851–857
Garland PB, Randle PJ (1964) Regulation of glucose uptake by muscle. Biochem J 93:678–687
Garland PB, Newsholme EA, Randle PJ (1962) Effect of fatty acids, ketone bodies, diabetes and starvation on pyruvate metabolism in rat heart and diaphragm muscle. Nature 195:381–383
Garland PB, Randle PJ, Newsholme EA (1963) Citrate as an intermediary in the inhibition of phosphofructokinase in rat heart muscle by fatty acids, ketone bodies, pyruvate, diabetes and starvation. Nature 200:169–170
Garland PB, Newsholme EA, Randle PJ (1964) Regulation of glucose uptake by muscle. Biochem J 93:665–678
Garrison JC (1978) The effects of glucagon, catecholamines, and the calcium ionophore A23187 on the phosphorylation of rat hepatocyte cytosolic proteins. J Biol Chem 253:7091–7100
Garrison JC, Borland MK (1979) Regulation of mitochondrial pyruvate carboxylation and gluconeogenesis in rat hepatocytes via an α-adrenergic, adenosine 3′:5′-monophosphate-independent mechanism. J Biol Chem 254:1129–1133
Garrison JC, Haynes RC Jr (1975) The hormonal control of gluconeogenesis by regulation of mitochondrial pyruvate carboxylation in isolated rat liver cells. J Biol Chem 250:2769–2777
Garrison JC, Borland MK, Florio VA, Twible DA (1979) The role of calcium ion as a mediator of the effects of angiotensin II, catecholamines and vasopressin on the phosphorylation and activity of enzymes in isolated hepatocytes. J Biol Chem 254:7147–7156
Gerich JE, Lorenzi M, Bier DM, Tsalikian E, Schneider V, Karam JH, Forsham PH (1976a) Effects of physiologic levels of glucagon and growth hormone on human carbohydrate and lipid metabolism. J Clin Invest 57:875–884
Gerich JE, Lorenzi M, Tsalikian E, Karam JH (1976b) Studies on the mechanism of epinephrine-induced hyperglycemia in man. Evidence for participation of pancreatic glucagon secretion. Diabetes 25:65–71
Gilboe DP, Nuttall FO (1978) In vivo glucose-, glucagon-, and cAMP-induced changes in liver glycogen synthase phosphatase activity. J Biol Chem 253:4078–4081
Glinsmann WH, Mortimore GE (1968) Influence of glucagon and 3′,5′-AMP in insulin responsiveness of the perfused rat liver. Am J Physiol 215:553–559

Glinsmann WH, Hern EP, Lynch A (1969) Intrinsic regulation of glucose output by rat liver. Am J Physiol 216:698–703
Gold AH (1970) The effect of diabetes and insulin on liver glycogen synthetase activation. J Biol Chem 245:903–906
Goldberg ND, Villar-Palasi C, Sasko H, Larner J (1967) Effects of insulin treatment on muscle 3′,5′-cyclic adenylate levels in vivo and in vitro. Biochim Biophys Acta 148:665–672
Goldberg ND, Dietz SB, O'Toole AG (1969) Cyclic guanosine 3′,5′-monophosphate in mammalian tissues and urine. J Biol Chem 244:4458–4460
Golden S, Wals PA, Okajima F, Katz J (1979) Glycogen synthesis by hepatocytes from diabetic rats. Biochem J 182:727–734
Goodman MN, Ruderman NB (1979) Insulin sensitivity of rat skeletal muscle: Effects of starvation and aging. Am J Physiol 236:E519–E523
Goodman MN, Berger M, Ruderman NB (1974) Glucose metabolism in rat skeletal muscle at rest. Diabetes 23:881–888
Goris J, Defreyn G, Vandenheede JR, Merlevede W (1978) Protein inhibitors of dog liver phosphorylase phosphatase dependent on and independent of protein kinase. Eur J Biochem 91:457–464
Gratecos D, Detwiler TC, Hurd S, Fischer EM (1977) Rabbit muscle phosphorylase phosphatase. I. Purification and chemical properties. Biochemistry 16:4812–4817
Gross SR, Mayer SE (1974) Characterization of the phosphorylase *b* to *a* converting activity in skeletal muscle extracts of mice with the phosphorylase *b* kinase deficiency mutation. J Biol Chem 249:6710–6718
Guellaen G, Yates-Aggerbeck M, Gauguelin G, Strosberg D, Hanoune J (1978) Characterization with [^{3}H]dihydroergocryptine of the α-adrenergic receptor of the hepatic plasma membrane. J Biol Chem 253:1114–1120
Gunn JM, Tilgham SM, Hanson RW, Reshef L, Ballard FJ (1975) Effects of cyclic adenosine monophosphate, dexamethasone and insulin on phosphoenolpyruvate carboxykinase. Biochemistry 14:2350–2357
Hagen JH, Ball EG (1961) Studies on the metabolism of adipose tissue. VI. The effect of adrenaline on oxygen consumption and glucose utilization. Endocrinology 69:752–760
Hagg SA, Taylor SI, Ruderman NB (1976) Glucose metabolism in perfused skeletal muscle. Biochem J 158:203–210
Halestrap AP (1978a) Stimulation of the respiratory chain of rat liver mitochondria between cytochrome C_1 and cytochrome C by glucagon treatment of rats. Biochem J 172:399–405
Halestrap AP (1978b) Stimulation of pyruvate transport in metabolizing mitochondria through changes in the transmembrane pH gradient induced by glucagon treatment of rats. Biochem J 172:389–398
Haschke RH, Heilmeyer LMG Jr, Meyer F, Fischer EH (1970) Control of phosphorylase activity in a muscle glycogen particle. J Biol Chem 245:6657–6663
Haustraete F, DeWulf H (1979) Vasopressin levels in alloxan diabetic rats. Ann Endocrinol (Paris) 40:255–256
Haylett DG, Jenkinson DH (1972) The receptors concerned in the actions of catecholamines on glucose release, membrane potential and ion movements in guinea-pig liver. J Physiol (Lond) 255:751–772
Hedrick JL, Shaltiel S, Fischer EH (1969) Conformational changes and the mechanism of resolution of glycogen phosphorylase *b*. Biochemistry 8:2422–2429
Heilmeyer LMG Jr, Meyer F, Haschke RH, Fischer EH (1970) Control of phosphorylase activity in a muscle glycogen particle. J Biol Chem 245:6649–6656
Helmreich E, Cori CF (1964) The role of adenylic acid in the activation of phosphorylase. Proc Natl Acad Sci USA 51:131–138
Helmreich E, Cori CF (1965) Regulation of glycolysis in muscle. Adv Enzyme Regul 3:91–107
Helmreich E, Cori CF (1966) The activation of glycolysis in frog sartorius muscle by epinephrine. Pharmacol Rev 18:189–196
Hems DA, Whitton PD (1973) Stimulation by vasopressin of glycogen breakdown and gluconeogenesis in the perfused rat liver. Biochem J 136:705–709

Hems DA, Rodrigues LM, Whitton PD (1976) Glycogen phosphorylase, glucose output and vasoconstriction in the perfused rat liver. Concentration-dependence of actions of adrenaline, vasopressin and angiotensin II. Biochem J 160:367–374
Hems DA, Rodrigues LM, Whitton PD (1978) Rapid stimulation by vasopressin, oxytocin and angiotensin II of glycogen degradation in hepatocyte suspensions. Biochem J 172:311–317
Hennig G, Loffler G, Wieland OH (1975) Active and inactive forms of pyruvate dehydrogenase in skeletal muscle as related to the metabolic and functional state of the muscle cell. FEBS Lett 59:142–145
Henriksson T, Jergil B (1979) Protein kinase activity and endogenous phosphorylation in subfractions of rat liver mitochondria. Biochim Biophys Acta 588:380–391
Hepp KD (1971) Inhibition of glucagon-stimulated adenyl cyclase by insulin. FEBS Lett 12:263–266
Himms-Hagen J (1967) Sympathetic regulation of metabolism. Pharmacol Rev 19:367–471
Hjemdahl P, Belfrage E, Daleskog M (1979) Vascular and metabolic effects of circulating epinephrine and norepinephrine. J Clin Invest 64:1221–1228
Hoffman BB, Michel T, Kilpatrick DM, Lefkowitz RJ, Tolbert MEM, Gilman H, Fain JN (1980) Agonist versus antagonist binding to α-adrenergic receptors. Proc Natl Acad Sci USA 77:4569–4573
Holmes PA, Mansour TE (1968) Glucose as a regulator of glycogen phosphorylase in rat diaphragm. Biochim Biophys Acta 156:266–274
Honeyman TW, Levy LK, Goodman HM (1979) Independent regulation of phosphorylase and lipolysis in adipose tissue. Am J Physiol 237:E11–E17
Hope-Gill H, Kissebah A, Tulloch B, Clarke P, Vydelingum N, Fraser TR (1976) The effects of insulin on adipocyte calcium flux and the interaction with the effects of dibutyryl cyclic AMP and adrenaline. Horm Metab Res 7:195–196
Horl WH, Heilmeyer LMG (1978) Evidence for the participation of a Ca^{2+}-dependent protein kinase and protein phosphatase in the regulation of the Ca^{2+} transport ATPase of the sarcoplasmic reticulum. 2. Effect of phosphorylase kinase and phosphorylase phosphatase. Biochemistry 17:766–772
Horl WH, Jennisen HP, Heilmeyer LMG (1978) Evidence for the participation of a Ca^{2+}-dependent protein kinase and a protein phosphatase in the regulation of the Ca^{2+} transport ATPase of the sarcoplasmic reticulum. 1. Effect of inhibitors of the Ca^{2+}-dependent protein kinase and protein phosphatase. Biochemistry 17:759–766
Hornbrook KR (1970) Adrenergic receptors for metabolic responses in the liver. Fed Proc 29:1381–1385
Hornbrook KR, Brody TM (1963) The effect of catecholamines on muscle glycogen and phosphorylase activity. J Pharmacol Exp Ther 140:295–307
Hostmark AT (1973) The effect of insulin on epinephrine and glucagon inactivated glycogen synthase I in the isolated perfused rat liver. Acta Physiol Scand 88:248–255
Huang FL, Glinsmann WH (1975) Inactivation of rabbit muscle phosphorylase phosphatase by cyclic AMP-dependent kinase. Proc Natl Acad Sci USA 72:3004–3008
Huang FL, Glinsmann WH (1976) Separation and characterization of two phosphorylase phosphatase inhibitors from rabbit skeletal muscle. Eur J Biochem 70:419–426
Huang FL, Tao S, Glinsmann WH (1977) Multiple forms of protein phosphatase inhibitors in mammalian tissues. Biochem Biophys Res Commun 78:615–623
Huang K-P, Lee S-L, Huang FL (1979) Phosphorylation of rabbit skeletal muscle glycogen synthase I by a cyclic AMP-independent synthase kinase. J Biol Chem 254:9867–9870
Huang TS, Krebs EG (1977) Amino acid sequence of a phosphorylation site in skeletal muscle glycogen synthetase. Biochem Biophys Res Commun 75:643–650
Hucho F, Randall DD, Roche TE, Burgett MW, Pelley JW, Reed LJ (1972) α-Keto acid dehydrogenase complexes. Arch Biochem Biophys 151:328–340
Hue L, Bontemps F, Hers H-G (1975) The effect of glucose and of potassium ions on the interconversion of the two forms of phosphorylase and of glycogen synthetase in isolated rat liver preparations. Biochem J 152:105–114
Hue L, Feliu JE, Hers H-G (1978) Control of gluconeogenesis and of enzymes of glycogen metabolism in isolated rat hepatocytes. Biochem J 176:791–797

Hughes BP, Barritt GJ (1978) Effects of glucagon and $N^6,O^{2'}$-dibutyryladenosine 3':5'-cyclic monophosphate on calcium transport in isolated rat liver mitochondria. Biochem J 176:295–304
Hughes WA, Denton RM (1976) Incorporation of ^{32}Pi into pyruvate dehydrogenase phosphate in mitochondria from control and insulin-treated adipose tissue. Nature 264:471–473
Hurd SS, Teller D, Fischer EH (1966) Probable formation of partially phosphorylated intermediates in the interconversions of phosphorylase *a* and *b*. Biochem Biophys Res Commun 24:79–84
Huston RB, Krebs EG (1968) Activation of skeletal muscle phosphorylase kinase by Ca^{2+}. II. Identification of the kinase activating factor as a proteolytic enzyme. Biochemistry 7:2116–2122
Hutson NJ, Randle PJ (1978) Enhanced activity of pyruvate dehydrogenase kinase in rat heart mitochondria in alloxan-diabetes or starvation. FEBS Lett 92:73–76
Hutson NJ, Brumley FT, Assimacopoulos FD, Harper SC, Exton JH (1976) Studies on the α-adrenergic activation of hepatic glucose output. Studies on the α-adrenergic activation of phosphorylase and gluconeogenesis and inactivation of glycogen synthase in isolated rat liver parenchymal cells. J Biol Chem 251:5200–5208
Hutson NJ, Khatra BS, Soderling TR (1978a) Regulation of glycogen synthase. Dephosphorylation of the skeletal muscle enzyme. J Biol Chem 253:2540–2545
Hutson NJ, Kerbey AL, Randle PJ, Sugden PH (1978b) Conversion of inactive (phosphorylated) pyruvate dehydrogenase complex into active complex by the phosphatase reaction in heart mitochondria is inhibited by alloxan diabetes or starvation in the rat. Biochem J 173:669–680
Huttunen JK, Steinberg D (1971) Activation and phosphorylation of purified adipose tissue hormone-sensitive lipase by cyclic AMP-dependent protein kinase. Biochim Biophys Acta 239:411–427
Huttunen JK, Steinberg D, Mayer SE (1970) ATP-dependent and cyclic AMP-dependent activation of rat adipose tissue lipase by protein kinase from rabbit skeletal muscle. Proc Natl Acad Sci USA 67:290–295
Illiano G, Cuatrecasas P (1972) Modulation of adenylate cyclase activity in liver and fat cell membranes by insulin. Science 175:906–908
Ishibashi H, Cottam GL (1978) Glucagon-stimulated phosphorylation of pyruvate kinase in hepatocytes. J Biol Chem 253:8767–8771
Issekutz B Jr, Issekutz AC, Nash D (1970) Mobilization of energy sources in exercising dogs. J Appl Physiol 29:691–697
Itarte E, Robinson JC, Huang KP (1977) Total conversion of glycogen synthase from the I- to the D-form by a cyclic AMP-dependent protein kinase from rabbit skeletal muscle. J Biol Chem 252:1231–1234
Iynedjian PB, Hanson RW (1977) Increase in liver of functional messenger RNA coding for phosphoenolpyruvate carboxykinase (GTP) during induction by cyclic adenosine 3':5'-monophosphate. J Biol Chem 252:655–662
Jarett L, Seals JR (1979) Pyruvate dehydrogenase activation in adipocyte mitochondria by an insulin-generated mediator from muscle. Science 206:1407–1408
Jaspan JB, Huen AHJ, Morley CG, Moossa AR, Rubenstein AH (1977) The role of the liver in glucagon metabolism. J clin Invest 60:421–428
Jefferson LS, Li JB, Rannels SR (1977) Regulation by insulin of amino acid release and protein turnover in the perfused rat hemicorpus. J Biol Chem 252:1476–1483
Jefferson LS, Exton JH, Butcher RW, Sutherland EW, Park CR (1968) Role of adenosine 3',5'-monophosphate in the effects of insulin and antiinsulin serum on liver metabolism. J Biol Chem 243:1031–1038
Jenkinson DH (1973) Classification and properties of peripheral adrenergic receptors. Br Med Bull 29:142–147
Jennings AS, Cherrington AD, Liljenquist JE, Keller U, Lacy WW, Chiasson JL (1977) The roles of insulin and glucagon in the regulation of gluconeogenesis in the postabsorptive dog. Diabetes 26:847–856

Jennissen HP, Heilmeyer LMG (1974) Multiple forms of phosphorylase kinase in red and white skeletal muscle. FEBS Lett 42:77–80

Jett MF, Soderling TR (1979) Purification and phosphorylation of rat liver glycogen synthase. J Biol Chem 254:6739–6745

Johnson LN, Madsen NB, Mosley J, Wilson KS (1974) The crystal structure of glycogen phosphorylase *b* at 6 A resolution. J Mol Biol 90:703–717

Johnson LN, Weber IT, Wild DL, Wilson KS, Yeates DGR (1977) The crystal structure of glycogen phosphorylase *b*. In: Esmann V (ed) Regulatory mechanisms of carbohydrate metabolism. Pergamon, Oxford New York

Jungas RL (1971) Hormonal regulation of pyruvate dehydrogenase. Metabolism 20:43–53

Kajimoto T, Uyeda K (1979) Hormone-stimulated phosphorylation of liver phosphofructokinase in vivo. J Biol Chem 254:5584–5587

Kartapkin S, Helmreich E, Cori CF (1964) Regulation of glycolysis in muscle. II. Effect of stimulation and epinephrine in isolated frog sartorius muscle. J Biol Chem 239:3139–3145

Kaslow HR, Mayer SE (1979) Adaptations of glycogen metabolism in rat epididymal adipose tissue during fasting and refeeding. J Biol Chem 254:4678–4683

Kaslow HR, Eicher RD, Mayer SE (1979) Interconversion between multiple glucose-6-phosphate-dependent forms of glycogen synthase in intact adipose tissue. J Biol Chem 254:4674–4677

Kasvinsky PJ, Madsen NB, Fletterick RJ, Sygusch J (1978a) X-ray crystallographic and kinetic studies of oligosaccharide binding to phosphorylase. J Biol Chem 253:1290–1296

Kasvinsky PJ, Madsen NB, Sygusch J, Fletterick RJ (1978b) The regulation of glycogen phosphorylase *a* by nucleotide derivatives. Kinetics and x-ray crystallographic studies. J Biol Chem 253:3343–3351

Kasvinsky PJ, Schechovsky S, Fletterick RJ (1978c) Synergistic regulation of phosphorylase *a* by glucose and caffeine. J Biol Chem 253:9102–9106

Kato K, Bishop JS (1972) Glycogen synthetase-D phosphatase. J Biol Chem 247:7420–7429

Katz J, Golden S, Wals PA (1979) Glycogen synthesis by rat hepatocytes. Biochem J 180:389–402

Keely SL, Corbin JD, Park CR (1975) Regulation of adenosine 3′:5′-monophosphate-dependent protein kinase. J Biol Chem 250:4832–4840

Keely SL, Corbin JD, Lincoln T (1977) Alpha adrenergic involvement in heart metabolism: effects on adenosine cyclic 3′,5′-monophosphate, adenosine cyclic 3′,5′-monophosphate-dependent protein kinase, guanosine cyclic 3′,5′-monophosphate, and glucose transport. Mol Pharmacol 13:965–975

Kemp BE, Clark MG (1978) Adrenergic control of the cyclic AMP-dependent protein kinase and pyruvate kinase in isolated hepatocytes. Application of a synthetic peptide substrate for measuring protein kinase activity. J Biol Chem 253:5147–5154

Keppens S, Vandenheede JR, DeWulf H (1977) On the role of calcium as second messenger in liver for the hormonally induced activation of glycogen phosphorylase. Biochim Biophys Acta 496:448–457

Kerbey AL, Randle PJ, Cooper RH, Whitehouse S, Pask HT, Denton RM (1976) Regulation of pyruvate dehydrogenase in rat heart. Biochem J 154:327–348

Kerbey AL, Radcliffe PM, Randle PJ (1977) Diabetes and the control of pyruvate dehydrogenase in rat heart mitochondria by concentration ratios of adenosine triphosphate/adenosine diphosphate, of reduced/oxidized nicotinamide-adenine dinucleotide and of acetyl-coenzyme A/coenzyme A. Biochem J 164:509–519

Khandelwal RL, Zinman SM (1978) Purification and properties of a heat-stable protein inhibitor of phosphoprotein phosphatase from rabbit liver. J Biol Chem 253:560–565

Khandelwal RL, Vandenheede JR, Krebs EG (1976) Purification, properties, and substrate specificities of phosphoprotein phosphatase(s) from rabbit liver. J Biol Chem 251:4850–4858

Khatra BS, Soderling TR (1978) Relationship between dephosphorylation and D to I conversion of rabbit skeletal muscle glycogen synthase. J Biol Chem 253:5247–5250

Khatra BS, Chiasson J-L, Shikama H, Exton JH, Soderling TR (1980) Effect of epinephrine and insulin on the phosphorylation of phosphorylase inhibitor 1 in perfused rat skeletal muscle. FEBS Lett 114:253–256

Khoo JC (1976) Ca^{2+}-dependent activation of phosphorylase by phosphorylase kinase in adipose tissue. Biochim Biophys Acta 422:87–97
Khoo JC, Steinberg D (1975) Stimulation of rat liver phosphorylase kinase by micromolar concentrations of Ca^{2+}. FEBS Lett 57:68–72
Khoo JC, Steinberg D, Thompson B, Mayer SE (1973) Hormonal regulation of adipocyte enzymes. J Biol Chem 248:3823–3830
Kiechle FL, Jarett L, Popp DA, Kotagal N (1980) Isolation from rat adipocytes of a chemical mediator for insulin activation of pyruvate dehydrogenase. Diabetes 29:852–855
Kikuchi K, Tamura S, Hiraga A, Tsuiki S (1977) Glycogen synthase phosphatase of rat liver. Its separation from phosphorylase phosphatase on DE-52 colums. Biochem Biophys Res Commun 75:29–37
Killilea SD, Whelan WJ (1976) Purification and properties of rabbit liver glycogen synthase. Biochemistry 15:1349–1356
Killilea SD, Brandt H, Lee EYC, Whelan WJ (1976) Evidence for the coordinate control of activity of liver glycogen synthase and phosphorylase by a single protein phosphatase. J Biol Chem 251: 2363–2368
Killilea SD, Mellgren RL, Aylward JH, Metieh ME, Lee EYC (1979) Liver protein phosphatases: Studies of the presumptive native forms of phosphorylase phosphatase activity in liver extracts and their dissociation to a catalytic subunit of MW 35,000. Arch Biochem Biophys 193:130–139
Kipnis DM (1959) Regulation of glucose uptake by muscle: functional significance of permeability and phosphorylating activity. Ann NY Acad Sci 82:354–365
Kirchberger MA, Tada M (1976) Effects of adenosine 3′:5′-monophosphate-dependent protein kinase on sarcoplasmic reticulum isolated from cardiac and slow and fast contracting skeletal muscles. J Biol Chem 251:725–729
Kirchberger MA, Tada M, Katz AM (1974) Adenosine 3′:5′-monophosphate dependent protein kinase-catalyzed phosphorylation reaction and its relationship to calcium transport in cardiac sarcoplasmic reticulum. J Biol Chem 249:6166–6173
Kirk CJ, Hems DA (1974) Hepatic action of vasopressin: lack of a role for adenosine 3′:5′-cyclic monophosphate. FEBS Lett 47:128–131
Kissebah AH, Clarke P, Vydelingum N, Hope-Gill H, Tulloch B, Fraser TR (1975) The role of calcium in insulin action. Eur J Clin Invest 5:339–349
Kneer NM, Wagner MJ, Lardy HA (1979) Regulation by calcium of hormonal effects on gluconeogenesis. J Biol Chem 254:12160–12168
Kono T, Barham FW (1973) Effects of insulin on the levels of adenosine 3′:5′-monophosphate and lipolysis in isolated rat epididymal fat cells. J Biol Chem 248:7417–7426
Kono T, Robinson FW, Sarver JA (1975) Insulin-sensitive phosphodiesterase. J Biol Chem 250:7826–7835
Kranias EG, Schweppe JS, Jungmann RA (1977) Phosphorylative and functional modifications of nucleoplasmic RNA polymerase II by homologous adenosine 3′:5′-monophosphate-dependent protein kinase from calf thymus and by heterologous phosphatase. J Biol Chem 252:6750–6758
Krebs EG, Beavo JA (1979) Phosphorylation-dephosphorylation of enzymes. Annu Rev Biochem 48:923–929
Kreutner W, Golgberg ND (1967) Dependence on insulin of the apparent hydrocortisone activation of hepatic glycogen synthetase. Proc Natl Acad Sci USA 58:1515–1519
Krone W, Hubner WB, Seitz HJ, Tarnowski W (1976) Induction of rat liver phosphoenolpyruvate carboxykinase (GTP) by cyclic AMP during starvation. The permissive action of glucocorticoids. Biochim Biophys Acta 437:62–70
Kuo S-H, Kamaka JK, Lum BKB (1977) Adrenergic receptor mechanisms involved in the hyperglycemia and hyperlacticacidemia produced by sympathomimetic amines in the cat. J Pharmacol Exp Ther 202:301–309
Laloux M, Stalmans W, Hers H-G (1978) Native and latent forms of liver phosphorylase phosphatase. Eur J Biochem 92:15–24
Larner J, Villar-Palsi C (1971) Glycogen synthase and its control. Curr Top Cell Regul 3:195–236
Larner J, Galasko G, Cheng K, DePaoli-Roach J (1979) Generation by insulin of a chemical mediator that controls protein phosphorylation and dephosphorylation. Sience 206:1408–1410

Lautt WW (1979) Neural activation of α-adrenoreceptors in glucose mobilization from liver. Can J Physiol Pharmacol 58:1037–1039
Lawrence JC Jr, Larner J (1977) Evidence for alpha adrenergic activation of phosphorylase and inactivation of glycogen synthase in rat adipocytes. Mol Pharmacol 13:1060–1075
Lawrence JC Jr, Larner J (1978a) Effects of insulin, methoxamine, and calcium on glycogen synthase in rat adipocytes. Mol Pharmacol 14:1079–1091
Lawrence JC Jr, Larner J (1978b) Activation of glycogen synthase in rat adipocytes by insulin and glucose involves increased glucose transport and phosphorylation. J Biol Chem 253:2104–2113
Lawrence JC Jr, Larner J (1979) Control of glycogen synthase and phosphorylase by insulin in rat adipocytes which is unreleated to the concentration of cyclic AMP. Biochim Biophys Acta 582:402–411
Lawrence JC Jr, Guiovart JJ, Larner J (1977) Activation of rat adipocyte glycogen synthase by insulin. J Biol Chem 252:444–450
LeCam A, Freychet P (1976) Glucagon stimulates the A system for neutral amino acid transport in isolated hepatocytes of adult rat. Biochem Biophys Res Commun 72:893–901
LeCam A, Freychet P (1978) Effect of insulin on amino acid transport in isolated rat hepatocytes. Diabetologia 15:117–123
Lee EYC, Mellgren RL, Killilea SD, Aylward JH (1978) Properties and regulation of liver protein phosphatases. In: Regulatory mechanisms of carbohydrate metabolism. Pergamon, Oxford New York
Le Marchand-Brustel Y, Freychet P (1979) Effect of fasting and streptozotocin diabetes on insulin binding and action in the isolated mouse soleus muscle. J Clin Invest 64:1505–1515
Le Marchand-Brustel Y, Cohen PTW, Cohen P (1979) Insulin activates glycogen synthase in phosphorylase kinase deficient mice. FEBS Lett 105:235–238
Le Peuch CJ, Haiech J, De Maille JG (1979) Concerted regulation of cardiac sarcoplasmic reticulum transport by cyclic adenosine monophosphate dependent and calcium-calmodulin-dependent phosphorylations. Biochemistry 18:5150–5157
Leray F, Chambaut A-M, Perrenoud M-L, Hanoune J (1973) Adenylate cyclase activity of rat liver plasma membranes. Hormonal stimulations and effect of adrenalectomy. Eur J Biochem 38:185–192
Li H-C, Hsiao K-J, Chan WWS (1978) Purification and properties of phosphoprotein phosphatases with different substrate and divalent cation specificities from canine heart. Eur J Biochem 84:215–225
Li JB, Jefferson LS (1977) Effect of isoproterenol on amino acid levels and protein turnover in skeletal muscle. Am J Physiol 232:E243–E249
Liljenquist JE, Mueller GL, Cherrington AD et al. (1977) Evidence for an important role of glucagon in the regulation of hepatic glucose production in normal man. J Clin Invest 59:369–374
Lincoln TM, Corbin JD (1977) Adenosine 3′:5′-cyclic monophosphate- and guanosine 3′:5′-cyclic monophosphate-dependent protein kinases: possible homologous proteins. Proc Natl Acad Sci USA 74:3239–3243
Linn TC, Pettit FH, Reed LJ (1969a) α-Keto acid dehydrogenase complexes. X. Regulation of the activity of the pyruvate dehydrogenase complex from beef kidney mitochondria by phosphorylation and dephosphorylation. Proc Natl Acad Sci USA 64:234–241
Linn TC, Pettit FH, Hucho F, Reed LJ (1969b) α-Keto acid dehydrogenase complexes. XI. Comparative studies of regulatory properties of the pyruvate dehydrogenase complexes from kidney, heart, and liver mitochondria. Proc. Natl Acad Sci USA 64:227–234
Ljungstrom O, Hjelmquist G, Engstrom L (1974) Phosphorylation of purified rat liver pyruvate kinase by cyclic 3′,5′-AMP-stimulated protein kinase. Biochim Biophys Acta 358:289–298
Ljungstrom O, Ekman P (1977) Glucagon-induced phosphorylation of pyruvate kinase (type L) in rat liver slices. Biochem Biophys Res Commun 78:1147–1155
Long CNH, Fry EG, Bonnycastle M (1960) The effect of cortisol on carbohydrate deposition and urea nitrogen excretion in the adrenalectomized rat. Acta Endocrinol [Suppl] 51:819

Loten EG, Assimacopoulos-Jeannet FD, Exton JH, Park CR (1978) Stimulation of a low K_m Phosphodiesterase from liver by insulin and glucagon. J Biol Chem 253:746–757
Ludvigsen C, Jarett L, McDonald JM (1980) The characterization of catecholamine stimulation of glucose transport by rat adipocytes and isolated plasma membranes. Endocrinology 106:786–790
Luzio PJ, Jones RC, Siddle K, Hales CN (1974) Dissociation of the effect of adrenalin on glucose uptake from that on adenosine cyclic 3′,5′-monophosphate levels and on lipolysis in isolated rat-fat cells. Biochim Biophys Acta 362:29–36
Lyon JB Jr, Mayer SE (1969) Epinephrine induced formation of adenosine 3′,5′-monophosphate in mouse skeletal muscle. Biochem Biophys Res Commun 34:459–464
Lyon JB Jr, Porter J (1963) The relation of phosphorylase to glycogenolysis in skeletal muscle and heart of mice. J Biol Chem 238:1–11
Ma GY, Gove CD, Hems DA (1978) Effects of glucagon and insulin on fatty acid synthesis and glycogen degradation in the perfused liver of normal and genetically obese (ob/ob) mice. Biochem J 174:761–768
MacDonald MJ, Bentle LA, Lardy HA (1978) P-enolpyruvate carboxykinase ferroactivator. Distribution and the influence of diabetes and starvation. J Biol Chem 253:116–124
Mackrell DJ, Sokal JE (1969) Antagonism between the effects of insulin and glucagon on the isolated liver. Diabetes 18:724–732
Maddiah VT, Madsen NB (1966a) Kinetics of purified liver phosphorylase. J Biol Chem 241:3873–3881
Maddiah VT, Madsen NB (1966b) Studies on the biological control of glycogen metabolism in liver. I. State and activity pattern of glycogen phosphorylase. Biochim Biophys Acta 121:261–268
Madsen NB, Kasvinsky PJ, Fletterick RJ (1978) Allosteric transitions of phosphorylase *a* and the regulation of glycogen metabolism. J Biol Chem 253:9097–9101
Maguire ME, Erdos JJ (1980) Inhibition of magnesium uptake by β-adrenergic agonists and prostaglandin E_1 is not mediated by cyclic AMP. J Biol Chem 255:1030–1035
Malbon CC, Li S-Y, Fain JN (1978) Hormonal activation of glycogen phosphorylase in hepatocytes from hypothyroid rats. J Biol Chem 253:8820–8825
Mallette LE, Exton JH, Park CR (1969a) Control of gluconeogenesis from amino acids in the perfused rat liver. J Biol Chem 244:5713–5723
Mallette LE, Exton JH, Park CR (1969b) Effects of glucagon on amino acid transport and utilization in the perfused rat liver. J Biol Chem 244:5724–5728
Mapes JP, Harris RA (1976) Inhibition of gluconeogenesis and lactate formation from pyruvate by $N^6,O^{2\prime}$-dibutyryl adenosine 3′:5′-monophosphate. J Biol Chem 251:6189–6196
Martensen TM, Brotherton JE, Graves DJ (1973a) Kinetic studies of the activation of muscle phosphorylase phosphatase. J Biol Chem 248:8329–8336
Martensen TM, Brotherton JE, Graves DJ (1973b) Kinetic studies of the inhibition of muscle phosphorylase phosphatase. J Biol Chem 248:8323–8328
Martin BR, Denton RM, Pask HT, Randle PJ (1972) Mechanisms regulating adipose tissue pyruvate dehydrogenase. Biochem J 129:763–773
Massague J, Guinovart JJ (1977) Insulin control of rat hepatocyte glycogen synthase and phosphorylase in the absence of glucose. FEBS Lett 82:317–320
Massague J, Guinovart JJ (1978) Insulin counteraction of α-adrenergic effects on liver glycogen metabolism. Biochim Biophys Acta 543:269–272
Mayer SE (1963) Action of epinephrine on glucose uptake and glucose-6-phosphate in the dog heart in situ. Biochem Pharmacol 12:193–201
Mayer SE (1970) Regulation of cardiac and skeletal muscle glycogen metabolism by biogenic amines. In: Biogenic amines as Physiological regulators. Prentice-Hall, Englewood Cliffs, New Jersey
McClellan G, Winegrad S (1978) The regulation of the calcium sensitivity of the contractile system in mammalian cardiac muscle. J Gen Physiol 72:737–764
McCullough TE, Walsh DA (1979a) Phosphorylation and dephosphorylation of phosphorylase kinase in the perfused rat heart. J Biol Chem 254:7345–7352
McCullough TE, Walsh DA (1979b) Phosphorylation and glycogen synthase in the perfused rat heart. J Biol Chem 254:7336–7344

McDonald JM, Bruns DE, Jarett L (1976a) The ability of insulin to alter the stable calcium pools of isolated adipocyte subcellular fractions. Biochem Biophys Res Commun 71:114–121
McDonald JM, Bruns DE, Jarett L (1976b) Ability of insulin to increase calcium binding by adipocyte plasma membranes. Proc Natl Acad Sci USA 73:1542–1546
McDonald JM, Bruns DE, Larett L (1978) Ability of insulin to increase calcium uptake by adipocyte endoplasmic reticulum. J Biol Chem 253:3504–3508
Metzger BE, Helmreich E, Glaser L (1968) The mechanism of activation of skeletal muscle phosphorylase *a* by glycogen. Proc Natl Acad Sci USA 57:994–1001
Meyer F, Heilmeyer LMG Jr, Haschke RH, Fischer EH (1970) Control of phosphorylase activity in a muscle glycogen particle. J Biol Chem 245:6642–6648
Miller E, Fredholm B, Miller RE, Steinberg D, Mayer SE (1975) Enzymes regulating glycogen metabolism in swine subcutaneous adipose tissue. I. Phosphorylase and phosphorylase phosphatase. Biochemistry 14:2470–2480
Miller RE, Miller EA, Fredholm B, Yellin JB, Eichner RD, Mayer SE, Steinberg D (1975) Enzymes regulating glycogen metabolism in swine subcutaneous adipose tissue. II. Glycogen synthase. Biochemistry 14:2481–2488
Miller TB Jr (1978a) Effects of diabetes on glucose regulation of enzymes involved in hepatic glycogen metabolism. Am J Physiol 234:E13–E19
Miller TB Jr (1978b) A dual role for insulin in the regulation of cardiac glycogen synthase. J Biol Chem 253:5389–5394
Miller TB Jr (1979) Glucose activation of liver glycogen synthetase. Insulin-mediated restoration of glucose effect in diabetic rats is blocked by protein synthesis inhibitor. Biochim Biophys Acta 583:36–46
Miller TB Jr, Larner J (1973) Mechanism of control of hepatic glycogenesis by insulin. J Biol Chem 248:3483–3488
Miller TB Jr, Exton JH, Park CR (1971) A block in epinephrine-induced glycogenolysis in hearts from adrenalectomized rats. J Biol Chem 246:3672–3678
Miller TB Jr, Hazen R, Larner J (1973) An absolute requirement for insulin in the control of hepatic glycogenesis by glucose. Biochem Biophys Res Commun 53:466–474
Moran NC (1975) Adrenergic receptors. In: Blaschko H, Sayers G, Smith AD (eds) Adrenal gland. American Physiological Society, Washington, DC (Handbook of physiology, sect 7, Endocrinology, vol 6)
Morgan HE, Parmeggiani A (1964) Regulation of glycolysis in muscle. III. Control of muscle glycogen phosphorylase activity. J Biol Chem 239:2440–2445
Morgan HE, Cardenas E, Regen DM, Park CR (1961a) Regulation of glucose uptake in muscle. J Biol Chem 236:262–268
Morgan HE, Regen DM, Henderson MJ, Sawyer TK, Park CR (1961b) Regulation of glucose uptake in muscle. J Biol Chem 236:2162–2168
Mueller E, Van Breemen C (1979) Role of intracellular Ca^{2+} sequestration in β-adrenergic relaxation of a smooth muscle. Nature 281:682–683
Mukherjee C, Jungas RL (1975) Activation of pyruvate dehydrogenase in adipose tissue by insulin. Biochem J 148:229–235
Munck A (1971) Glucocorticoid inhibition of glucose uptake by peripheral tissues: old and new evidence, molecular mechanisms, and physiological significance. Perspect Biol Med 14:265–289
Nakai C, Thomas JA (1974) Properties of a phosphoprotein phosphatase from bovine heart with activity on glycogen synthase, phosphorylase and histone. J Biol Chem 249:6459–6467
Namm DH, Mayer SE (1968) Effects of epinephrine on cardiac cyclic 3′,5′-AMP, phosphorylase kinase, and phosphorylase. Mol Pharmacol 4:61–69
Namm DH, Mayer SE, Maltbie M (1968) The role of potassium and calcium ions in the effect of epinephrine on cardiac cyclic adenosine 3′,5′-monophosphate, phosphorylase kinase and phosphorylase. Mol Pharmacol 4:522–530
Neely JR, Liebermeister H, Morgan HE (1967) Effect of pressure development on membrane transport of glucose in isolated rat heart. Am J Physiol 212:815–822

Neely JR, Bowman RH, Morgan HG (1969) Effects of ventricular pressure development and palmitate on glucose transport. Am J Physiol 216:804–811

Newsholme EA, Randle PJ (1961) Regulation of glucose uptake by muscle. Biochem J 80:655–662

Newsholme EA, Randle PJ (1964) Regulation of glucose uptake by muscle. Biochem J 93:641–651

Nichols WK, Goldberg ND (1972) The relationship between insulin and apparent glucocorticoid-promoted activation of hepatic glycogen synthetase. Biochim Biophys Acta 279:245–259

Nieto A, Castano JG (1980) Control in vivo of rat liver phosphofructokinase by glucagon and nutritional changes. Biochem J 186:953–957

Nimmo GA, Cohen P (1978) The regulation of glycogen metabolism. Phosphorylation of inhibitor-1 from rabbit skeletal muscle and its interaction with protein phosphatases-III and II. Eur J Biochem 87:353–365

Nimmo HG, Cohen P (1977) Hormonal control of protein phosphorylation. Adv Cyclic Nucleotide Res 8:145–266

Nimmo HG, Houston B (1978) Rat adipose-tissue glycerol phosphate acyltransferase can be inactivated by cyclic AMP-dependent protein kinase. Biochem J 176:607–610

Nimmo HG, Proud CG, Cohen P (1976) The phosphorylation of rabbit skeletal muscle glycogen synthase by glycogen synthase kinase-2 and adenosine-3′:5′-monophosphate-dependent protein kinase. Eur J Biochem 68:31–44

Nishikori K, Maeno H (1979) Close relationship between adenosine 3′:5′-monophosphate-dependent endogenous phosphorylation of a specific protein and stimulation of calcium uptake in rat uterine microsomes. J Biol Chem 254:6099–6106

Nishikori K, Tekenaka T, Maeno H (1977) Stimulation of microsomal calcium uptake and protein phosphorylation by adenosine cyclic 3′,5′-monophosphate in rat uterus. Mol Pharmacol 13:671–678

Nordlie RC, Varricchio FE, Holten DD (1965) Effects of altered hormonal states and fasting on rat liver mitochondrial phosphoenolpyruvate carboxykinase levels. Biochim Biophys Acta 97:214–221

Okajima F, Ui M (1976) Lack of correlation between hormonal effects on cyclic AMP and glycogenolysis in rat liver. Arch Biochem Biophys 175:549–557

Osborn D (1978) The alpha adrenergic receptor mediated increase in guinea-pig liver glycogenolysis. Biochem Pharmacol 27:1315–1320

Park CR, Morgan HE, Henderson MJ, Regen DM, Cadenas E, Post RL (1961) The regulation of glucose uptake in muscle as studied in the perfused rat heart. Recent Prog Horm Res 17:493–538

Park CR, Crofford OB, Kono T (1968) Mediated (nonactive) transport of glucose in mammalian cells and its regulation. J Gen Physiol 52:296–318

Parker PJ, Aitken A, Bilham T, Embi N, Cohen P (1981) Amino acid sequence of a region in rabbit skeletal muscle glycogen synthase phosphorylated by cyclic AMP-dependent protein kinase. FEBS Lett 123:332–336

Parmeggiani A, Bowman RH (1963) Regulation of phosphofructokinase activity by citrate in normal and diabetic muscle. Biochem Biophys Res Commun 12:268–273

Partington CR, Edwards MW, Daly JW (1980) Regulation of cyclic AMP formation in brain tissue by α-adrenergic receptors: requisite intermediary of prostaglandins of the E series. Proc Natl Acad Sci USA 77:3024–3028

Patzelt C, Loffler G, Wieland OH (1973) Interconversion of pyruvate dehydrogenase in the isolated perfused rat liver. Eur J Biochem 33:117–122

Payne E, Soderling TR (1980) Calmodulin-dependent glycogen synthase kinase. J Biol Chem 255:8054–8056

Perry SV, Cole HA (1974) Phosphorylation of troponin and the effects of interactions between the components of the complex. Biochem J 141:733–743

Pette D, Bucher T (1963) Proportions-konstante Gruppen in Beziehung zur Differenzierung der Enzymaktivitätsmuster von skeletal Muskeln des Kaninchens. Hoppe Seylers Z Physiol Chem 331:180–195

Pilkis SJ, Claus TH, Johnson RA, Park CR (1975) Hormonal control of cyclic 3′:5′-AMP levels and gluconeogenesis in isolated hepatocytes from fed rats. J Biol Chem 250:6328–6336
Pilkis SJ, Riou JP, Claus TH (1976) Hormonal control of [^{14}C]glucose synthesis from [U-^{14}C]dihydroxyacetone and glycerol in isolated rat hepatocytes. J Biol Chem 251:7841–7852
Pilkis SJ, Park CR, Claus TH (1978) Hormonal control of hepatic gluconeogenesis. Vitam Horm 36:383–460
Pilkis S, Schlumpf J, Pilkis J, Claus TH (1979) Regulation of phosphofructokinase activity by glucagon in isolated rat hepatocytes. Biochem Biophys Res Commun 88:960–967
Pilkis SJ, El-Maghrabi MR, Pilkis J, Claus TH, Cumming DA (1981a) Fructose 2,6-biphosphate. A new activator of phosphofructokinase. J Biol Chem 256:3171–3174
Pilkis SJ, El-Maghrabi MR, Pilkis J, Claus TH (1981b) Inhibition of fructose-1,6,biphosphatase by fructose 2,6-bisphosphate. J Biol Chem 256:3619–3622
Piras R, Staneloni R (1969) *In vivo* regulation of rat muscle glycogen synthetase activity. Biochemistry 8:2153–2160
Piras R, Rothman LB, Cabib E (1968) Regulation of muscle glycogen synthetase by metabolites. Differential effects on the I and D forms. Biochemistry 7:56–66
Popp DA, Kiechle FL, Kotagal N, Jarett L (1980) Insulin stimulation of pyruvate dehydrogenase in an isolated plasma membrane mitochondrial mixture occurs by activation of pyruvate dehydrogenase phosphatase. J Biol Chem 255:7540–7543
Porte D Jr (1967) A receptor mechanism for the inhibition of insulin release by epinephrine in man. J Clin Invest 46:86–94
Portenhauser R, Wieland O (1972) Regulation of pyruvate dehydrogenase in mitochondria of rat liver. Eur J Biochem 31:308–314
Posner JB, Stern R, Krebs EG (1965) Effects of electrical stimulation and epinephrine on muscle phosphorylase, phosphorylase *b* kinase, and adenosine 3′,5′-phosphate. J Biol Chem 240:982–985
Pozefsky T, Felig P, Tobin JD, Soeldner JS, Cagill GF Jr (1969) Amino acid balance across tissues of the forearm in postabsorptive man. Effects of insulin at two dose levels. J Clin Invest 48:2273–2282
Pozefsky T, Tancredi RG, Moxley RT, Dupre J, Tobin JD (1976) Effects of brief starvation on muscle amino acid metabolism in nonobese man. J Clin Invest 57:444–449
Proost C, Carton H, Dewulf H (1979) The α-adrenergic control of rabbit liver glycogenolysis. Biochem Pharmacol 28:2187–2191
Proud CCG, Rylatt DB, Yeaman SJ, Cohen P (1978) Amino acid sequences at the two sites on glycogen synthase phosphorylated by cyclic AMP-dependent protein kinase and their dephosphorylation by protein phosphatase-III. FEBS Lett 80:435–442
Prpić V, Spencer TL, Bygrave FL (1978) Stable enhancement of calcium retention in mitochondria isolated from rat liver after administration of glucagon to the intact animal. Biochem J 176:705–714
Rabin D, Mueller GL, Lacy WW, Liljenquist JE (1979) Splanchnic metabolism of alanine in intact man. Diabetes 28:486–490
Rall TW, Sutherland EW (1958) Formation of a cyclic adenine ribonucleotide by tissue particles. J Biol Chem 232:1065–1076
Rall TW, Sutherland EW, Wosilait WD (1956) The relationship of epinephrine and glucagon to liver phosphorylase in slices and in extracts. J Biol Chem 218:483–495
Rall TW, Sutherland EW, Berthet J (1957) The relationship of epinephrine and glucagon to liver phosphorylase. IV. Effect of epinephrine and glucagon on the reactivation of phosphorylase in liver homogenates. J Biol Chem 224:463–475
Randle PJ, Tubbs PK (1979) Carbohydrate and fatty acid metabolism. In: Hamilton WF (ed) Circulation. American Physiological Society, Bethesda, Maryland (Handbook of physiology, sect 2, vol 1)
Randle PJ, Newsholme EA, Garland PB (1964) Regulation of glucose uptake by muscle. Biochem J 93:652–665
Ray KP, England PJ (1976) The identification and properties of phosphatases in skeletal muscle with activity towards the inhibitory subunit of troponin, and their relationship to other phosphoprotein phosphatases. Biochem J 157:369–380

Reed LJ (1969) Pyruvate dehydrogenase complex. Curr Top Cell Regul 1:233–251
Reed LJ, Pettit FH, Roche TE, Butterworth PJ, Barrera CR, Tsai CS (1974) Structure, function and regulation of the mammalian pyruvate dehydrogenase-complex. In: Wieland O, Helmreich E, Holzer H (eds) Metabolic interconversion of enzymes. Springer, Berlin Heidelberg New York
Regen DM, Davis WW, Morgan HE, Park CR (1964) The regulation of hexokinase and phosphofructokinase activity in heart muscle. J Biol Chem 239:43–49
Riou J-P, Claus TH, Flockhart DA, Corbin JD, Pilkis SJ (1977) In vivo and in vitro phosphorylation of rat liver fructose-1,6-bisphosphatase. Proc Natl Acad Sci USA 74:4615–4619
Riou JP, Claus TH, Pilkis SJ (1978) Stimulation by glucagon of in vivo phosphorylation of rat hepatic pyruvate kinase. J Biol Chem 253:656–659
Rizza R, Haymond M, Cryer P, Gerich J (1979) Differential effects of epinephrine on glucose production and disposal in man. Am J Physiol 237:E356–E362
Rizza RA, Cryer PE, Haymond MW, Gerich JE (1980) Adrenergic mechanisms for the effects of epinephrine on glucose production and clearance in man. J Clin Invest 65:682–689
Roach PJ, Larner J (1976) Rabbit skeletal muscle glycogen synthase. 2. Enzyme phosphorylation state and effector concentrations as interacting control parameters. J Biol Chem 251:1920–1925
Roach PJ, Takeda Y, Larner J (1976) Rabbit skeletal muscle glycogen synthase. 1. Relationship between phosphorylation state and kinetic properties. J Biol Chem 251:1913–1919
Roach PJ, DePaoli-Roach AA, Larner J (1978) Ca^{2+}-stimulated phosphorylation of muscle glycogen synthase by phosphorylase *b* kinase. J Cyclic Nucleotide Res 4:245–257
Robison GA, Butcher RW, Oye I, Morgan HE, Sutherland EW (1965) The effect of epinephrine on adenosine-3′,5′-phosphate levels in the isolated perfused rat heart. Mol Pharmacol 1:168–177
Rognstad R, Katz J (1977) Role of pyruvate kinase in the regulation of gluconeogenesis from L-lactate. J Biol Chem 252:1831–1833
Rosenberg FJ, Distefano V (1962) A central nervous system component of epinephrine hyperglycemia. Am J Physiol 203:782–788
Rosenfeld MG, Barrieux A (1979) Regulation of protein synthesis by polypeptide hormones and cyclic AMP. Adv Cyclic Nucleotide Res 11:205–264
Rousseau GG (1977) Activity of protein kinase dependent on adenosine 3′:5′-monophosphate and of its thermostable protein inhibitor in rat hepatoma (HTC) cells. Unlikely role in the permissive action of glucocorticoids. Eur J Biochem 76:309–316
Rousseau GG, Martial J, Devisscher M (1976) Activity and subcellular distribution of protein kinase dependent on adenosine 3′:5′-monophosphate in liver from normal and adrenalectomized rats. Eur J Biochem 66:499–506
Rubio R, Bailey C, Villar-Palasi C (1975) Effects of cyclic AMP dependent protein kinase on cardiac actomyosin: increase in Ca^{2+} sensitivity and possible phosphorylation of troponin I. J Cyclic Nucleotide Res 1:143–150
Ruderman NB, Toews CJ, Shafrir E (1969) Role of free fatty acids in glucose homeostasis. Arch Intern Med 123:299–313
Rylatt DB, Aitken A, Bilham T, Condon GD, Embi N, Cohen P (1980) Glycogen synthase from rabbit skeletal muscle. Amino acid sequence at the sites phosphorylated by glycogen synthase kinase-3, and extension of the N-terminal sequence containing the site phosphorylated by phosphorylase kinase. Eur J Biochem 107:529–537
Sacca L, Perez G, Carteni G, Rengo F (1977) Evaluation of the role of the sympathetic nervous system in the gluco-regulatory response to insulin-induced hypoglycemia in the rat. Endocrinology 101:1016–1022
Sacca L, Sherwin R, Felig P (1978) Effect of sequential infusions of glucagon and epinephrine on glucose turnover in the dog. Am J Physiol 235:E287–E290
Sacca L, Eigler N, Cryer PE, Sherwin RS (1979) Insulin antagonistic effects of epinephrine and glucagon in the dog. Am J Physiol 237:E487–E492
Saitoh Y, Ui M (1975) Activation and inactivation of phosphorylase and glycogen synthetase during perfusion of rat liver as influenced by epinephrine, glucagon and hydrocortisone. Biochim Biophys Acta 404:7–17

Saitoh Y, Itaya K, Ui M (1974) Adrenergic α-receptor-mediated stimulation of the glucose utilization by isolated rat diaphragm. Biochim Biophys Acta 343:492–499
Sakai K, Matsumara S, Okimura Y, Yamamura H, Nishizuka Y (1979) Liver glycogen phosphorylase kinase. Partial purification and characterization. J Biol Chem 254:6631–6637
Schade DS, Woodside W, Eaton PR (1979) The role of glucagon in the regulation of plasma lipids. Metabolism 28:874–886
Schaeffer LD, Chenoweth M, Dunn A (1969a) Adrenal corticosteroid involvement in the control of liver glycogen phosphorylase activity. Biochim Biophys Acta 192:292–303
Schaeffer LD, Chenoweth M, Dunn A (1969b) Adrenal corticosteroid involvement in the control of phosphorylase in muscle. Biochim Biophys Acta 192:304–309
Scheid CR, Honeyman TW, Fay FS (1979) Mechanism of β-adrenergic relaxation of smooth muscle. Nature 277:32–36
Schimassek H, Mitzkat HJ (1963) Über eine spezifische Wirkung des Glucagon auf die Embden-Meyerhof-Kette in der Leber. Biochem Z 337:510–518
Schlender KK, Reimann EM (1975) Isolation of a glycogen synthase I kinase that is independent of adenosine 3':5'-monophosphate. Proc Natl Acad Sci USA 72:2197–2201
Schlender KK, Reimann EM (1977) Glycogen synthase kinases. Distribution in mammalian tissues of forms that are independent of cyclic AMP. J Biol Chem 252:2384–2389
Schudt C, Gaertner U, Pette D (1976) Insulin action on glucose transport and calcium fluxes in developing muscle cells in vitro. Eur J Biochem 68:103–111
Schwabe U, Daly JW (1977) The role of calcium ions in accumulations of cyclic adenosine monophosphate elicited by alpha and beta adrenergic agonists in rat brain slices. J Pharmacol Exp Ther 202:134–143
Schwartz A, Entman ML, Kanike K, Lane LA, Van Winkle WB, Bornet EP (1976) The role of calcium uptake into sarcoplasmic reticulum of cardiac muscle and skeletal muscle. Effects of cyclic AMP-dependent protein kinase and phosphorylase *b* kinase. Biochim Biophys Acta 426:57–72
Seals JR, Jarett L (1980) Activation of pyruvate dehydrogenase by direct addition of insulin to an isolated plasma membrane/mitochondria mixture: evidence for generation of insulin's second messenger in a subcellular system. Proc Natl Acad Sci USA 77:77–81
Seals JR, McDonald JM, Jarett L (1979a) Insulin effect on protein phosphorylation of plasma membranes and mitochondria in a subcellular system from rat adipocytes. J Biol Chem 254:6991–6996
Seals JR, McDonald JM, Jarett L (1979b) Insulin effect on protein phosphorylation of plasma membranes and mitochondria in a subcellular system from rat adipocytes. J Biol Chem 254:6997–7001
Severson DL, Denton RM, Pask HT, Randle PJ (1974) Calcium and magnesium ions as effectors of adipose tissue pyruvate dehydrogenase phosphate phosphatase. Biochem J 140:225–237
Severson DL, Denton RM, Bridges BJ, Randle PJ (1976) Exchangeable and total calcium pools in mitochondria of rat epididymal fat-pads and isolated fat cells. Biochem J 154:209–233
Seydoux J, Brunsmann MJA, Jeanrenaud B, Girardier L (1979) α-Sympathetic nerve control of glucose output of mouse liver perfused in situ. Am J Physiol 236:E323–E327
Shamoon H, Hendler R, Sherwin RS (1980) Altered responsiveness to cortisol, epinephrine and glucagon in insulin-infused juvenile-onset diabetics. A mechanism for diabetic instability. Diabetes 29:284–291
Shenolikar S, Cohen PTW, Cohen P, Nairn AC, Perry SV (1979) The role of calmodulin in the structure and regulation of phosphorylase kinase from rabbit skeletal muscle. Eur J Biochem 100:329–337
Sherline P, Lynch A, Glinsmann WH (1972) Cyclic AMP and adrenergic control of rat liver glycogen metabolism. Endocrinology 91:680–690
Sherwin RS, Fisher M, Hendler R, Felig P (1976) Hyperglucagonemia and blood glucose regulation in normal, obese, and diabetic subjects. N Engl J Med 294:455–461
Shikama H, Ui M (1975a) Metabolic background for glucose tolerance: mechanism for epinephrine-induced impairment. Am J Physiol 229:955–961

Shikama H, Ui M (1975b) Adrenergic receptor and epinephrine-induced hyperglycemia and glucose tolerance. Am J Physiol 229:962–966

Shikama H, Chiasson J-L, Chu D, Exton JH (1981) Studies of the interactions between insulin and epinephrine in the control of skeletal muscle glycogen metabolism. J Biol Chem 256:4450–4454

Shimazu T, Amakawa A (1968) Regulation of glycogen metabolism in liver by the autonomic nervous system. II. Neural control of glycogenolytic enzymes. Biochim Biophys Acta 165:335–348

Shimazu T, Amakawa A (1975) Regulation of glycogen metabolism in liver by the autonomic system. Biochim Biophys Acta 385:242–256

Shimazu T, Fukuda A, Ban T (1966) Reciprocal influences of the ventromedial and lateral hypothalamic nuclei on blood glucose level and liver glycogen content. Nature 120:1178–1179

Shrago E, Lardy HA, Nordlie RC, Foster DO (1963) Metabolic and hormonal control of phosphoenolpyruvate carboxykinase and malic enzyme in rat liver. J Biol Chem 238:3188–3192

Shulman GI, Liljenquist JE, Williams PE, Lacy WW, Cherrington AD (1978) Glucose disposal during insulinopenia in somatostatin-treated dogs. The roles of glucose and glucagon. J Clin Invest 62:487–491

Sica V, Cuatrecasas P (1973) Effects of insulin, epinephrine, and cyclic adenosine monophosphate on pyruvate dehydrogenase in adipose tissue. Biochemistry 12:2282–2291

Siess EA, Wieland OH (1972) Purification and characterization of pyruvate-dehydrogenase phosphatase from pig-heart muscle. Eur J Biochem 26:96–105

Siess EA, Wieland OH (1976) Phosphorylation state of cytosolic and mitochondrial adenosine nucleotides and of pyruvate dehydrogenase in isolated rat liver cells. Biochem J 156:91–102

Silverberg AB, Shah SD, Haymond MW, Cryer PE (1978) Norepinephrine: hormone and neurotransmitter in man. Am J Physiol 234:E252–E256

Singh TS, Wang JH (1977) Effect of Mg^{2+} concentration on the cAMP-dependent protein kinase-catalyzed activation of rabbit skeletal muscle phosphorylase kinase. J Biol Chem 252:625–632

Skuster JR, Chan KFJ, Graves DJ (1980) Isolation and properties of the catalytically active γ subunit of phosphorylase kinase. J Biol Chem 255:2203–2210

Sloan IG, Sawn PC, Bihler I (1978) Influence of adrenalin on sugar transport in soleus, a red skeletal muscle. Mol Cell Endocrinol 10:3–12

Smith SJ, Saggerson ED (1978) Regulation of pyruvate dehydrogenase activity in rat epididymal fat-pads and isolated adipocytes by adrenaline. Biochem J 174:119–130

Soderling TR (1975) Regulation of glycogen synthetase. J Biol Chem 250:5407–5412

Soderling TR (1976) Regulation of glycogen synthetase. J Biol Chem 251:4359–4364

Soderling TR (1979) Regulatory functions of protein multisite phosphorylation. Mol Cell Endocrinol 16:157–179

Soderling TR, Park CR (1974) Recent advances in glycogen metabolism. Adv Cyclic Nucleotide Res 4:283–333

Soderling TR, Corbin JD, Park CR (1973) Regulation of adenosine 3′,5′-monophosphate-dependent protein kinase. J Biol Chem 248:1822–1829

Soderling TR, Jett MF, Hutson NJ, Khatra BS (1977) Regulation of glycogen synthase. Phosphorylation specificities of cAMP-dependent and cAMP-independent kinase for skeletal muscle synthase. J Biol Chem 252:7517–7524

Soderling TR, Svrivastava AK, Bass MA, Khatra BS (1979a) Phosphorylation and inactivation of glycogen synthase by phosphorylase kinase. Proc Natl Acad Sci USA 76:2536–2540

Soderling TR, Sheorain VS, Ericsson LH (1979b) Phosphorylation of glycogen synthase by phosphorylase kinase. Stoichometry, specificity and site of phosphorylation. FEBS Lett 106:181–184

Sokal JE, Sarcione EJ (1964) Failure of physiological concentrations of epinephrine to affect glycogen levels in the isolated rat liver. Nature 204:881–882

Solaro RJ, Moir AJG, Perry SV (1976) Phosphorylation of troponin I and the inotropic effect of adrenaline in the perfused rabbit heart. Nature 262:615–617

Sommarin M, Jergil B (1978) Protein kinase of rat liver endoplasmic reticulum. Eur J Biochem 88:49–60
Sooranna SR, Saggerson ED (1975) Studies on the role of insulin in the regulation of glyceride synthesis in rat epididymal adipose tissue. Biochem J 150:441–451
Sooranna SR, Saggerson ED (1976) Interactions of insulin and adrenaline with glycerol phosphate acylation processes in fat-cells from rat. FEBS Lett 64:36–39
Stalmans W, Hers H-G (1975) The stimulation of liver phosphorylase *b* by AMP, fluoride and sulfate. Eur J Biochem 54:341–350
Stalmans W, DeWulf H, Lederer B, Hers H-G (1970) The effect of glucose and of a treatment by glucocorticoids on the inactivation in vitro of liver glycogen phosphorylase. Eur J Biochem 15:9–12
Stalmans W, DeWulf H, Hers H-G (1971) The control of liver glycogen synthase phosphatase by phosphorylase. Eur J Biochem 18:582–587
Stalmans W, DeWulf H, Hue L, Hers HG (1974a) The sequential inactivation of glycogen phosphorylase and activation of glycogen synthetase in liver after the administration of glucose to mice and rats. Eur J Biochem 41:127–134
Stalmans W, Laloux M, Hers H-G (1974b) The interaction of liver phosphorylase *a* with glucose and AMP. Eur J Biochem 49:415–427
Stansbie D, Brownsey RW, Crettaz M, Denton RM (1976) Acute effects in vivo of anti-insulin serum on rates of fatty acid synthesis and activities of acetyl-coenzyme A carboxylase and pyruvate dehydrogenase in liver and epididymal adipose tissue of fed rats. Biochem J 160:413–416
Steele R (1975) Influences of corticosteroids on protein and carbohydrate metabolism. In: Blaschko H, Sayers G, Smith AD (eds) Adrenal gland. Physiological Society, Washington; DC (Handbook of physiology, sect 7, Endocrinology, vol 6)
Steiner KE, Chan TM, Claus TH, Exton JH, Pilkis SJ (1980) The role of phosphorylation in the α-adrenergic-mediated inhibition of rat hepatic pyruvate kinase. Biochim Biophys Acta 632:366–374
St Louis PJ, Sulakhe PV (1979) Phosphorylation of cardiac sarcolemma by endogenous and exogenous protein kinases. Arch Biochem Biophys 198:227–240
Strickland WG, Blackmore PF, Exton JH (1980) The role of calcium in α-adrenergic inactivation of glycogen synthase in rat hepatocytes and its inhibition by insulin. Diabetes 29:617–622
Stubbs M, Kirk CJ, Hems DA (1976) Role of extracellular calcium in the action of vasopressin on hepatic glycogenolysis. FEBS Lett 69:199–202
Stull JT, Mayer SE (1971) Regulation of phosphorylase activation in skeletal muscle in vivo. J Biol Chem 246:5716–5723
Stull JT, Mayer SE (1979) Biochemical mechanisms of adrenergic and cholinergic regulation of myocardial contractility. In: Hamilton WF (ed) Circulation. American Physiological Society, Bethesda, Maryland (Handbook of physiology, sect 2, vol 1)
Stull JT, Brostrom CO, Krebs EG (1972) Phosphorylation of the inhibitor component of troponin by phosphorylase kinase. J Biol Chem 247:5272–5274
Sugden PH, Randle PJ (1978) Regulation of pig heart pyruvate dehydrogenase. Biochem J 173:659
Sugden PH, Hutson NJ, Kerbey AL, Randle PJ (1978) Phosphorylation of additional sites on pyruvate dehydrogenase inhibits its re-activation by pyruvate dehydrogenase phosphate phosphatase. Biochem J 169:433–435
Sutherland EW, Cori CF (1948) Effects of insulin preparations on glycogenolysis in liver slices. J Biol Chem 172:737–750
Sutherland EW, Cori CF (1951) Effect of hyperglycemic-glycogenolytic factor and epinephrine on liver phosphorylase. J Biol Chem 188:531–543
Sutherland EW, Rall TW (1958) Fractionation and characterization of a cyclic adenine ribonucleotide formed by tissue particles. J Biol Chem 232:1077–1091
Sutherland EW, Rall TW (1960) The relation of adenosine 3′,5′-phosphate and phosphorylase to the actions of catecholamines and other hormones. Pharmacol Rev 12:265–299
Suzuki K, Kono T (1980) Evidence that insulin causes translocation of glucose transport activity to the plasma membrane from an intracellular storage site. Proc Nat. Acad Sci 77:2542–2545

Sygusch PJ, Madsen NB, Kasvinsky PJ, Fletterick RJ (1977) Location of pyridoxal phosphate in glycogen phosphorylase *a*. Proc Natl Acad Sci USA 74:4757–4761
Tada M, Kirchberger MA, Repke DI, Katz AM (1974) The Stimulation of calcium transport in cardiac sarcoplasmic reticulum by adenosine 3':5'-monophosphate dependent protein kinase. J Biol Chem 249:6174–6180
Tada M, Kirchberger MA, Katz AM (1975) Phosphorylation of a 22,000-dalton component in the cardiac sarcoplasmic reticulum by adenosine 3':5'-monophosphate-dependent protein kinase. J Biol Chem 250:2640–2647
Tan AWH, Nuttall FQ (1976) Regulation of synthase phosphatase and phosphorylase phosphatase in rat liver. Biochim Biophys Acta 445:118–130
Tao SH, Huang FL, Lynch A, Glinsmann WH (1978) Control of rat skeletal-muscle phosphorylase phosphatase by adrenaline. Biochem J 176:347–350
Tarui S, Saito Y, Fujimoto M, Okabayashi T (1976) Effects of insulin on diaphragm muscle independent of the variation of tissue levels of cyclic AMP and cyclic GMP. Arch Biochem Biophys 174:192–198
Taylor SI, Jungas RL (1974) Regulation of lipogenesis in adipose tissue: the significance of the activation of pyruvate dehydrogenase by insulin. Arch Biochem Biophys 164:12–19
Taylor SI, Mukherjee C, Jungas RL (1973) Studies on the mechanism of activation of adipose tissue pyruvate dehydrogenase by insulin. J Biol Chem 248:73–81
Taylor SI, Mukherjee C, Jungas RL (1975) Regulation of pyruvate dehydrogenase in isolated rat liver mitochondria. J Biol Chem 250:2028–2035
Taylor WM, Prpić V, Exton JH, Bygrave FL (1980) Stable changes to calcium fluxes in mitochondria isolated from rat livers perfused with α-adrenergic agonists and with glucagon. Biochem J 188:443–450
Titani K, Koide A, Hermann J et al. (1977) Complete amino acid sequence of rabbit muscle glycogen phosphorylase. Proc Natl Acad Sci USA 74:4762–4766
Titheradge MA, Coore HG (1976a) The mitochondrial pyruvate carrier, its exchange properties and its regulation by glucagon. FEBS Lett 63:45–50
Titheradge MA, Coore HG (1976b) Hormonal regulation of liver mitochondrial pyruvate carrier in relation to gluconeogenesis and lipogenesis. FEBS Lett 71:73–78
Titheradge MA, Binder SB, Yamazaki RK, Haynes RC Jr (1978) Glucagon treatment stimulates the metabolism of hepatic submitochondrial particles. J Biol Chem 253:3357–3360
Titheradge MA, Stringer JL, Haynes RC Jr (1979) The stimulation of the mitochondrial uncoupler-dependent ATPase in isolated hepatocytes by catecholamines and glucagon and its relationship to gluconeogenesis. Eur J Biochem 102:117–124
Tolbert MEM, Butcher FR, Fain JN (1973) Lack of correlation between catecholamine effects on cyclic adenosine 3':5'-monophosphate and gluconeogenesis in isolated rat liver cells. J Biol Chem 48:5686–5692
Tomita T (1975) Action of catecholamines on skeletal muscle. In: Blaschko H, Sayers G, Smith AD (eds) Adrenal gland. American Physiological Society, Washington; DC (Handbook of physiology, sect 7, Endocrinology, vol 6)
Uyeda K, Furuya E, Luby LJ (1981) The effect of natural and synthetic D-fructose 2,6-bisphosphate on the regulatory kinetic properties of liver and muscle phosphofructokinases. J Biol Chem 256:8394–8399
Vandenheede JR, Keppens S, DeWulf H (1976) The activation of liver phosphorylase *b* kinase by glucagon. FEBS Lett 61:213–217
Vandenheede JR, Khandelwal RL, Krebs EG (1977) Studies on the role of adenosine 3':5'-monophosphate in the activation of liver phosphorylase. J Biol Chem 252:7488–7494
Vandenheede JR, DeWulf H, Merlevede W (1979) Liver phosphorylase *b* kinase. Cyclic AMP-mediated activation and properties of the partially purified rat-liver enzyme. Eur J Biochem 101:51–58
Van de Werve G, Hue L, Hers H-G (1977) Hormonal and ionic control of the glycogenolytic cascade in rat liver. Biochem J 162:135–142
Van Schaftingen E, Hers H-G (1981) Inhibition of fructose-1,6-bisphosphatase by fructose 2,6-bisphosphate. Proc Natl Acad Sci USA 78:2861–2863
Van Schaftingen E, Hue L, Hers H-G (1980a) Control of the fructose 6-phosphate/fructose 1,6-bisphosphate cycle in isolated hepatocytes by glucose and glucagon. Biochem J192:887–895

Van Schaftingen E, Hue L, Hers H-G (1980b) Fructose 2,6-bisphosphate, the probable structure of the glucose and glucagon sensitive stimulator of phosphofructokinase. Biochem J 192:897–901
Varsanyi M, Groschel-Stewart U, Heilmeyer LMG Jr (1978) Characterization of a Ca^{2+}-dependent protein kinase in skeletal muscle membrane in I-strain and wild-type mice. Eur J Biochem 87:331–340
Villar-Palasi C, Larner J (1960) Levels of activity of the enzymes of the glycogen cycle in rat tissues. Arch Biochem 86:270–273
Vranic M, Wrenshall GA (1969) Exercise, insulin, and glucose turnover in dogs. Endocrinology 85:165–171
Wahren J, Felig P, Ahlborg G, Jorfeldt L (1971) Glucose metabolism during leg exercise in man. J Clin Invest 50:2715–2725
Wahren J, Felig P, Cerasi E, Luft R (1972) Splanchnic and peripheral glucose and amino acid metabolism in diabetes mellitus. J Clin Invest 51:1870–1878
Wahren J, Felig P, Hendler R, Ahlborg G (1973) Glucose and amino acid metabolism during recovery after exercise. J Appl Physiol 34:838–845
Walaas E (1955) The effect of adrenaline on the uptake of glucose, mannose and fructose in the rat diaphragm. Acta Physiol Scand 35:109–125
Walaas O, Walaas E (1950) Effect of epinephrine on rat diaphragm. J Biol Chem 187:769–776
Walajtys EJ, Gottesman DP, Wiliamson JR (1974) Regulation of pyruvate dehydrogenase in rat liver mitochondria by phosphorylation-dephosphorylation. J Biol Chem 249:1857–1865
Walkenbach RJ, Hazen R, Larner J (1978) Reversible inhibition of cyclic AMP-dependent protein kinase by insulin. Mol Cell Biochem 19:31–41
Walkenbach RJ, Hazen R, Larner J (1980) Hormonal regulation of glycogen synthase. Insulin decreases protein kinase sensitivity to cyclic AMP. Biochim Biophys Acta 629:421–430
Walsh DA, Clippinger MS, Sivaramakrishman S, McCullough TE (1979) Cyclic adenosine monophosphate dependent and independent phosphorylation of sarcolemma membrane proteins in perfused rat heart. Biochemistry 18:871–877
Walsh KX, Millikin DM, Schlender KK, Reimann EM (1979) Calcium-dependent phosphorylation of glycogen synthase by phosphorylase kinase. J Biol Chem 254:6611–6616
Walsh KX, Millikin DM, Schlender KK, Reimann EM (1980) Stimulation of phosphorylase *b* kinase by the calcium-dependent regulator. J Biol Chem 255:5036–5042
Wang, JH, Stull JT, Huang TS, Krebs EG (1976) A study on the autoactivation of rabbit muscle phosphorylase kinase. J Biol Chem 251:4521–4527
Weber IT, Johnson LN, Wilson KS, Yeates DGR, Wild DL, Jenkins JA (1978) Crystallographic studies on the activity of glycogen phosphorylase *b*. Nature 274:433–437
Weiss L, Loffler G, Schirmann A, Wieland O (1971) Control of pyruvate dehydrogenase interconversion in adipose tissue by insulin. FEBS Lett 15:229–231
Weiss L, Loffler G, Wieland OH (1974) Regulation by insulin of adipose tissue pyruvate dehydrogenase. Hoppe Seylers Z Physiol Chem 355:363–377
Whitton PD, Rodrigues LM, Hems DA (1978) Stimulation by vasopressin, angiotensin and oxytocin of gluconeogenesis in hepatocyte suspensions. Biochem J 176:893–898
Wicks WD (1969) Induction of hepatic enzymes by adenosine 3′,5′-monophosphate in organ culture. J Biol Chem 252:7202–7213
Wicks WD (1971) Differential effects of glucocorticoids and adenosine 3′:5′-monophosphate on hepatic enzyme synthesis. J Biol Chem 246:217–233
Wicks WD, Lewis W, McKibbin JB (1972) Induction of phosphoenolpyruvate carboxykinase by N^6,$O^{2'}$-dibutyryl cyclic AMP in rat liver. Biochim Biophys Acta 264:177–185
Wieland O, Funcke HV, Loffler G (1971) Interconversion of pyruvate dehydrogenase in rat heart muscle upon perfusion with fatty acids or ketone bodies. FEBS Lett 15:295–298
Wieland OH, Patzelt C, Loffler G (1972) Active and inactive forms of pyruvate dehydrogenase in rat liver. Eur J Biochem 26:426–433
Williams BJ, Mayer SE (1966) Hormonal effects on glycogen metabolism in the rat heart in situ. Mol Pharmacol 2:454–464
Williams TF, Exton JH, Park CR, Regen DM (1968) Stereospecific transport of glucose in the perfused rat liver. Am J Physiol 215:1200–1209

Williamson JR (1964) Metabolic effects of epinephrine in the isolated perfused rat heart. I. Dissociation of the glycogenolytic from the metabolic stimulatory effect. J Biol Chem 239:2721–2729
Williamson JR (1966) Metabolic effects of epinephrine in the perfused rat heart. II. Control steps of glucose and glycogen metabolism. Mol Pharmacol 2:206–220
Williamson JR (1975) Effects of epinephrine on glycogenolysis and myocardial contractility. In: Blaschko H, Sayers G, Smith AD (eds) Adrenal gland. American Physiological Society, Washington, DC (Handbook of physiology, sect 7, Endocrinology, vol 6)
Williamson JR, Jamieson D (1965) Dissociation of the inotropic from the glycogenolytic effect of epinephrine in the isolated rat heart. Nature 206:364–367
Williamson JR, Jamieson D (1966) Metabolic effects of epinephrine in the perfused rat heart. I. Comparison of intracellular redox states, tissue PO_2 and force of contraction. Mol Pharmacol 2:191–205
Winder WW, Boullier J, Fell RD (1979) Liver glycogenolysis during exercise without a significant increase in cAMP. Am J Physiol 237:R147–R152
Winegrad S (1979) Electromechanical coupling in heart muscle. In: Hamilton WF (ed) Circulation. American Physiological Society, Bethesda, Maryland (Handbook of physiology, sect 2, vol 1)
Witters LA, Avruch J (1978) Insulin regulation of hepatic glycogen synthase and phosphorylase. Biochemistry 17:406–410
Wolf DP, Fischer EH, Krebs EG (1970) Amino acid sequence of the phosphorylated site in rabbit liver glycogen phosphorylase. Biochemistry 9:1923–1929
Wolfe BB, Harden TK, Molinoff PB (1976) β-Adrenergic receptors in rat liver: effects of adrennalectomy. Proc Natl Acad Sci USA 73:1343–1347
Wolff DJ, Brostrom CO (1979) Properties and functions of the calcium-dependent regulator protein. Adv Cyclic Nucleotide Res 11:27–88
Wray HL, Gray RR, Olsson RA (1973) Cyclic adenosine 3′,5′-monophosphate-stimulated protein kinase and a substrate associated with cardiac sarcoplasmic reticulum. J Biol Chem 248:1496–1498
Yamazaki RK (1975) Glucagon stimulation of mitochondrial respiration. J Biol Chem 250:7924–7930
Yamazaki RK, Haynes RC Jr (1975) Dissociation of pyruvate dehydrogenase from the glucagon stimulation of pyruvate carboxylation in rat liver mitochondria. Arch Biochem Biophys 166:575–583
Yeaman SJ, Cohen P (1975) The hormonal control of activity of skeletal muscle phosphorylase kinase. Eur J Biochem 51:93–104
Yeaman SJ, Cohen P, Watson DC, Dixon GH (1977) The substrate specificity of adenosine 3′:5′-cyclic monophosphate-dependent protein kinase of rabbit skeletal muscle. Biochem J 162:411–421
Yeaman SJ, Hutcheson EF, Roche TE et al. (1978) Studies of phosphorylation on pyruvate dehydrogenase from bovine kidney and heart. Biochemistry 17:2364–2370
Yeung D, Oliver IT (1968) Induction of phosphopyruvate carboxylase in neonatal rat liver by adenosine 3′,5′-cyclic phosphate. Biochemistry 7:3231–3239
Young JW, Shrago E, Lardy HA (1964) Metabolic control of enzymes involved in lipogenesis and gluconeogenesis. Biochemistry 3:1687–1692
Zahlten RN, Hochberg AA, Stratman FW, Lardy HA (1972) Glucagon-stimulated phosphorylation of mitochondrial and lysosomal membranes of rat liver in vivo. Proc Natl Acad Sci USA 69:800–804
Zahlten RN, Stratman FW, Lardy HA (1973) Regulation of glucose synthesis in hormone-sensitive isolated rat hepatocytes. Proc Natl Acad Sci USA 70:3213–3218
Zapf J, Waldvogel M, Froesch ER (1973) Protein kinase and cyclic AMP-binding activities in liver and adipose tissue of normal, streptozotocin-diabetic and adrenalectomized rats. FEBS Lett 36:253–256
Zerbe RL, Vinicor F, Robertson GL (1979) Plasma vasopressin in controlled diabetes mellitus. Diabetes 28:503–508
Zieve FJ, Glinsmann WH (1973) Activation of glycogen synthase and inactivation of phosphorylase kinase by the same phosphoprotein phosphatase. Biochem Biophys Res Commun 50:872–878

CHAPTER 17

Regulation of Lipid Metabolism by Cyclic Nucleotides

J. N. FAIN

Overview

The intracellular concentration of cyclic AMP regulates triglyceride breakdown in adipocytes. However, it remains to be established whether hormones which activate lipolysis exert their effects solely through cyclic AMP. Under appropriate conditions, all agents which increase lipolysis in adipocytes increase cyclic AMP formation. Catecholamines and other activators of adipocyte lipolysis also increase the activity of adenylate cyclase, protein kinase and triacylglycerol lipase. Cholera toxin, after a lag period of 30–90 min, increases cyclic AMP accumulation in adipocytes and accelerates triglyceride breakdown. Cholera toxin inhibits the guanosine triphosphatase involved in conversion of active to inactive adenylate cyclase through NAD ribosylation of a plasma membrane protein. The addition of adenosine deaminase to rat adipocytes rapidly activates adenylate cyclase by removing membrane-bound adenosine which exerts an inhibitory constraint on basal adenylate cyclase activity. Thyroid hormones regulate adenylate cyclase activity of adipocytes by affecting the coupling of the hormone-receptor complexes to adenylate cyclase. Growth hormone also activates adenylate cyclase through a process involving synthesis of a protein(s).

Methyl xanthines and other inhibitors of cyclic AMP phosphodiesterase increase lipolysis. However, there are no hormones whose effects on lipolysis can be attributed to regulation of cyclic AMP phosphodiesterase. The effects of methyl xanthines on cyclic AMP accumulation in rat adipocytes may be due primarily to antagonism of adenosine inhibition of adenylate cyclase. Insulin activates cyclic AMP phosphodiesterase activity of rat adipocytes; it is unlikely that this accounts for the anti-lipolytic action of insulin. Similarly, the lipolytic action of glucocorticoids does not appear to involve regulation of cyclic AMP metabolism. There is even evidence that agents such as ACTH and catecholamines may activate some process in addition to adenylate cyclase which contributes to their activation of lipolysis. One possibility is hormonal regulation of the availability of triglyceride stores in the central triglyceride droplet of adipocytes to the triacylglycerol lipase in the cytosol.

α_2-Adrenergic agonists inhibit hormone-activated adenylate cyclase activity of adipocytes from hamsters and man. This appears to be a direct effect not mediated through calcium. There is an α_1-adrenergic effect in rat adipocytes which results in an increase in cytosol calcium. The increase in phosphatidylinositol turnover seen with α-adrenergic agonists is exclusively an α_1-

effect and may be involved in some unknown fashion with the release of bound intracellular calcium and entry of extracellular calcium. Alterations in the level of cytosol calcium have little effect on lipolysis; but an elevation of cytosol calcium inactivates glycogen synthase and activates glycogen phosphorylase. Insulin activates glycogen synthase in adipocytes but its action does not appear to involve either cytosol calcium, cyclic AMP, cyclic GMP, or H_2O_2. Insulin probably regulates mitochondrial pyruvate dehydrogenase and glycogen synthase through generation of an unknown second messenger. An attractive hypothesis is that the interaction of insulin with plasma membrane receptors results in activation of a protease which forms a polypeptide messenger.

The regulation of fatty acid synthesis by agents altering cyclic AMP is well recognized. Recent evidence supports the hypothesis that the key regulatory enzymes are subject to cyclic AMP dependent phosphorylation through protein kinase. Hormones activating triglyceride breakdown inhibit fatty acid synthesis; this is another example of reciprocal metabolic regulation.

A. Cyclic Nucleotides in Regulation of Triglyceride Breakdown in Adipocytes

I. Role of Lipid Mobilization from Adipocytes

GORDON and CHERKES (1956) and DOLE (1956) discovered that stored lipid is mobilized as free fatty acids during periods of stress and caloric deprivation and thereby focused attention on triglyceride breakdown in adipose tissue. The level of plasma free fatty acids is regulated primarily by the rate of their release to the bloodstream rather than by the rate of their uptake. The rate of release of free fatty acids by adipocytes is the difference between the rate of triglyceride breakdown to free fatty acids and the rate of esterification of fatty acids and α-glycerophosphate, derived from glucose metabolism. Both breakdown and esterification are under hormonal control. Insulin, whose release from the pancreas is regulated by the plasma glucose concentration, stimulates fatty acid esterification. The ingestion of a meal after a period of starvation results in increased uptake of glucose by adipose tissue which is utilized for de novo fatty acid synthesis and esterification. In addition, insulin inhibits lipolysis, the primary process regulating fatty acid release. Insulin is the only *hormone* which inhibits triglyceride breakdown; other putative *regulators of metabolism*, such as prostaglandins of the E series and adenosine, also inhibit lipolysis. In contrast a bewildering array of hormones can activate lipolysis; these include (in probable order of physiological importance) catecholamines, thyroid hormones, growth hormone, glucocorticoids, glucagon, ACTH, and other peptides.

BUTCHER et al. (1965) demonstrated that lipolytic hormones elevate the concentration of cyclic AMP in adipose tissue. The literature on adipose tissue metabolism covering the period between the discovery of triglyceride breakdown in adipose tissue and the discovery of the involvement of cyclic AMP in this process was reviewed in a volume of the Handbook of Physiology (containing over 4,000 references) exclusively devoted to adipose tissue (RENOLD and CAHILL 1965). Another volume devoted to adipose tissue was published 5 years later (JEANRENAUD and HEPP 1970) along with an excellent review on the mobilization, transport and utilization of free fatty acids (*Scow* and CHERNICK 1970). A number of reviews with primary emphasis on adipose tissue lipolysis and its regulation have been published since 1970 (FAIN 1973B, 1977, 1970; FAIN et al. 1978; KUPIECKI 1971; BJORNTORP and OSTMAN 1971, JUNGAS 1975; STEINBERG 1976; MEISNER and CARTER 1977, HALES et al. 1978; FREDHOLM 1978).

II. Adenylate Cyclase Regulation

Cyclic AMP is the only known factor which regulates triglyceride lipolysis by the adipocytes. The role of cyclic AMP in the regulation of lipolysis by catecholamines is shown in Fig. 1. The evidence for an involvement of cyclic AMP in the lipolytic action of catecholamines is as follows:

(1) Catecholamines activate adenylate cyclase in broken cell preparations.
(2) Cyclic AMP activates the protein kinase and triglyceride lipase activities of broken cell preparations.
(3) β-Adrenergic antagonists block the elevation of cyclic AMP and of lipolysis due to catecholamines.
(4) All agents which elevate intracellular cyclic AMP also activate lipolysis.
(5) Prostaglandin E_1, adenosine and cyclic carboxylic acids inhibit both cyclic AMP accumulation and lipolysis.

RODBELL (1964) prepared pure adipocytes by digestion of adipose tissue with bacterial collagenase. RODBELL (1967) subsequently prepared hormonally-responsive adipocyte ghosts by lysis of isolated adipocytes with hypotonic buffer in the presence of ATP. The presence of ATP during the lysis of the fat cells and the preparation of plasma membranes enhances the response to hormones (COMBRET and LAUDAT 1972; SAHYOUN and CUATRECASAS 1975; RODBELL 1975).

BIRNBAUMER and RODBELL (1969) found that at least five different hormones activate the same adenylate cyclase enzyme. Different hormone-specific sites (receptors) bind catecholamines, corticotropin (ACTH), glucagon, thyrotropin (TSH) and luteinizing hormone (LH). BUTCHER et al. (1968) had originally shown that these hormones stimulated cyclic AMP accumulation by rat adipocytes in the presence of methyl xanthines. The combination of any two hormones did not produce a greater accumulation of cyclic AMP than could be observed with a maximal concentration of a single hormone in intact adipocytes in the presence of methylxanthines or of adenylate cyclase activation in adipocyte ghosts.

BIRNBAUMER and RODBELL (1969) suggested that each hormone interacted with a separate receptor, and that the different hormone-receptor complexes activated the same population of adenylate cyclase enzymes. The current formulation of this hypothesis is that the activation of adenylate cyclase by hormone receptor complexes involves lateral diffusion of these complexes until they collide with adenylate cyclase; RIMON et al. (1978) have described this as a collision theory for activation of adenylate cyclase and CUATRECASAS et al. 1975), as a mobile receptor hypothesis.

Many different hormones activate adipocyte adenylate cyclase. Among these hormones are: corticotropin or ACTH (WHITE and ENGEL 1958); glucagon (HAGEN 1961; VAUGHAN 1961); secretin (BUTCHER and CARLSON 1970, RODBELL et al.

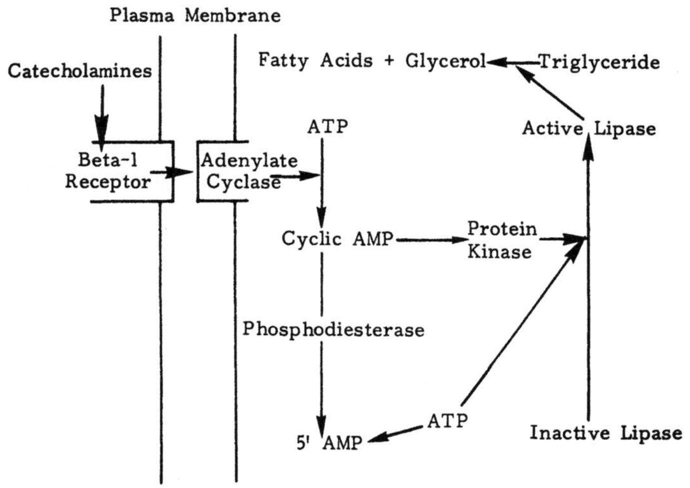

Fig. 1. Role of cyclic AMP in the activation of lipolysis by catecholamines. Catecholamines interact with the β_1-adrenergic receptor which results in activation of adenylate cyclase. Adenylate cyclase increases ATP conversion to cyclic AMP which activates protein kinase. The inactive triglyceride lipase is converted to its active form by protein kinase in the presence of ATP and triglycerides are hydrolyzed to give free fatty acids and glycerol

1970); parathormone (WERNER and LÖW 1973; GOZARIU et al. 1974; THAJCHAYAPONG et al. 1976); serotonin (BIECK et al. 1966); thyrotropin or TSH (FREINKEL 1961); luteinizing hormone or LH (BUTCHER et al. 1968); α- and β-melanotropin and vasopressin (RUDMAN 1963); neurophysins (ASTWOOD 1965; FOSS et al. 1973), and lipotropin (LOHMAR and LI 1968; BIELMANN et al. 1972). The references just cited are the initial reports which in some cases were based on measurements of lipolysis; subsequent studies have shown that the agents also activate adenylate cyclase. A sufficiently high concentration of any of these hormones will activate adipocyte adenylate cyclase and lipolysis. Except for catecholamines, no other hormone appears to be a physiological regulator of adenylate cyclase or lipolysis under normal conditions.

Lipotropin, a polypeptide not involved in lipid mobilization, is a prohormone giving rise to β-endorphin, β-melanotropin and met-enkephalin (LI 1978). TSH, ACTH and LH activate adenylate cyclase in their target cells at lower concentrations than are required for activation of adipocyte adenylate cyclase; this probably reflects a relative difference in receptor concentrations. For example, the adipocyte and the adrenal cortex differ in that the adrenal cortex has far more receptors for ACTH per cell than the adipocyte; this difference is reflected as a far greater sensitivity of the adrenal cortex to ACTH.

GTP can both activate and inhibit adipocyte adenylate cyclase. A stimulatory effect of GTP on the activation of hepatic adenylate cyclase by hormone-receptor complexes was described by RODBELL et al. (1971). However, CRYER et al. (1969) had previously reported that as little as 0.5 μ*M* GTP actually inhibited adipocyte adenylate cyclase activation by hormones. YAMAMURA et al. (1977) found that 0.1 μ*M* GTP activated adipocyte adenylate cyclase assayed with low ATP [0.1 m*M*, which is important because many commercially available ATP preparations are contaminated with GTP as shown by KIMURA and NAGATA (1977)], high

Mg^{2+} (10 mM) and 1 mM dithiothreitol. If the concentration of GTP was increased to 1 μM, there was a complete loss of GTP activation of adipocyte adenylate cyclase. The inhibitory effect of high GTP concentrations appeared to involve a protein which was much more trypsin-sensitive than the proteins involved in activation of adenylate cyclase. COOPER et al (1979) subsequently demonstrated that the inhibitory effects of GTP could be abolished by treatment of adipocyte membranes with cholera toxin in the presence of NAD^+. The inhibitory effect of GTP on adipocyte adenylate cyclase probably reflects an activation of GTPase by high levels of GTP. This GTPase is quite trypsin sensitive and can also be inhibited as a result of ADP ribosylation by cholera toxin. CASSEL and SELINGER (1977) proposed that continuous hydrolysis of GTP, bound to the regulatory guanine nucleotide binding site is a mechanism for inactivation of adenylate cyclase. Cholera toxin irreversibly inhibits the GTPase enzyme involved in this process.

The suggestion that adipocytes have high levels of a phosphotransferase (GTPase) activated by GTP was supported by studies with guanyl 5′-yl imidodiphosphate, a guanine nucleotide analog which cannot participate in these reactions. LONDOS et al. (1974) found that the guanyl 5′-yl imidodiphosphate [Gpp(NH)p] was a potent activator of adenylate cyclase in many eukaryotic cells, including adipocytes. The long-lasting activation of adenylate cyclase by Gpp(NH)p is similar to that of cholera toxin in that both agents inhibit the conversion of active to inactive adenylate cyclase (Fig. 2). The studies of RODBELL (1975) with rat adipocyte membranes and those of KATHER and GEIGER (1977) and COOPER et al. (1975) with human adipocyte membranes demonstrate that Gpp(NH)p is just as potent an activator of adipocyte adenylate cyclase as it is in other eukaryotic cells.

Adipocyte adenylate cyclase is more sensitive to inhibition by GTP than the enzyme from other tissues. COOPER et al. (1979) demonstrated that treatment of adipocyte membranes with p-hydroxymercuriphenyl sulfonic acid eliminated the stimulatory effect of low concentrations of GTP upon adenylate cyclase without affecting the inhibitory response to high concentrations of GTP. A stimulatory effect of GTP, at concentrations above 1 μM, on the GTPase reaction involved in deactivation of adenylate cyclase may distinguish adipocytes from other cells; whether this is linked in some way to the inhibition of adipocyte adenylate cyclase by adenosine and prostaglandins remains to be demonstrated. COOPER et al. (1979) and LONDOS et al. (1978) found that adenosine inhibited adipocyte adenylate cyclase only in the presence of inhibitory amounts of GTP (1 μM or greater). FAIN and MALBON (1979) suggested that the inhibition of adenylate cyclase by adenosine requires the presence of appreciable amounts of adenylate cyclase in a state between a very active form containing GTP and an inactive form which can be activated by hormones. This intermediate state of adenylate cyclase might contain bound GDP and be partially active. Adenosine and prostaglandins of the E series may increase the breakdown of this intermediate to an inactive form of the cyclase which can be activated by hormones. This hypothesis is supported by the findings of COOPER et al. (1979) that adenosine inhibition did not occur in the presence of cholera toxin which blocked conversion from the highly active to a less active form of the cyclase. Whether or not the putative GDP form of adenylate cyclase exists, the available data suggest that adenosine inhibition of adenylate cyclase involves increased deactivation of adenylate cyclase (Fig. 2).

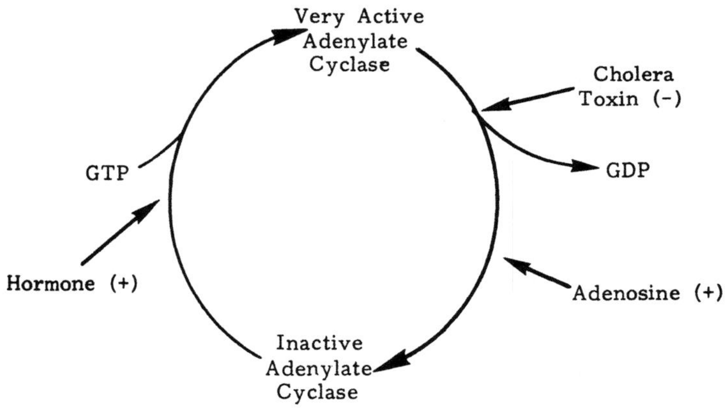

Fig. 2. Adenylate cyclase regulation by hormones and cholera toxin. The figure emphasizes that active adenylate cyclase is in equilibrium with inactive adenylate cyclase and that regulation can occur on either side of the cycle. Hormones are postulated to act by converting inactive to active adenylate cyclase through a process dependent on the continuous presence of hormone. Cholera toxin on the other hand inhibits the de-activation of the active adenylate cyclase through a reaction involving ADP ribosylation which results in irreversible inhibition of the GTPase. Adenosine is postulated to have effects which are the opposite of cholera toxin on the de-activation of adenylate cyclase

1. Short-Acting Hormones Which Activate Adenylate Cyclase Through Receptor Binding: Catecholamines

The structure-activity relationships for catecholamine binding to β-adrenergic receptor, adenylate cyclase activation and lipolysis are similar. No dissociation has yet been found between the effects of catecholamines on any of these parameters. Figure 1 depicts a model for lipolysis; catecholamines interact with a β_1-adrenergic receptor to activate adenylate cyclase and to accelerate lipolysis. The classical differentiation of catecholamine effects into α- and β-effects by AHLQUIST (1948) was subsequently supported by the demonstration that the β-effects are associated with an activation of adenylate cyclase while α-effects, are generally associated with either an inhibition of adenylate cyclase or with cyclic AMP-independent effects (ROBISON et al. 1971). In later sections of this chapter, the hypothesis is presented that α-effects of catecholamines on adipocytes can be divided into α_2-effects which are due to inhibition of adenylate cyclase and α_1-effects which are due to an increase in intracellular calcium.

LANDS et al. (1967) suggested, on the basis of structure activity relationships for agonists, that the β-adrenergic receptors of heart and adipocytes were β_1 while those of lung were β_2. Subsequent studies have confirmed this hypothesis (FAIN 1973b) but there are some differences in sensitivity to antagonists between the β_1-receptors of heart and adipocytes (HARMS et al. 1974). These may be due to slight differences between the β_1-sites of adipocytes and heart resulting in a greater inhibitory effect of practolol on cardiac than on adipocyte β-receptors (KATHER and SIMON 1977). In contrast, propranolol inhibits both β_1- and β_2-effects; while butoxamine, a β_2-antagonist, has little effect on adipocyte lipolysis (FAIN et al. 1966). However, MILLER and ALLEN (1971) demonstrated that practolol can inhibit catecholamine activation of adipocyte lipolysis.

ARIENS et al. (1979) suggested that the β_1-receptors are actually those for the neurotransmitter β-effects of catecholamines mediated through release of norepinephrine at nerve endings. In contrast, the β_2-receptors are those for the β-effect of the hormone epinephrine released by the adrenal medulla. This classification is the best available explanation for the data and fits with the concept that β-effects of catecholamines on adipocytes involve sympathetic release of norepinephrine at nerve endings present in adipose tissue (SCOW and CHERNICK 1970; FAIN 1973b; HALES et al. 1978).

The ability of different amines to stimulate lipolysis is compatible with a β_1-response based on the following points: 1. Norepinephrine and epinephrine are equipotent as activators of either adipocyte lipolysis (FAIN et al. 1966) or adenylate cyclase (WILLIAMS et al. 1976) and are equipotent as inhibitors of dihydroalprenolol binding to adipocyte membranes (WILLIAMS et al. 1976). In contrast, epinephrine is often 10 to 60 times more potent than norepinephrine as a stimulator of β_2-receptors (BURGES and BLACKBURN 1972). 2. Isoproterenol is only 5- to 10-fold more potent than norepinephrine in inhibiting dihydroalprenolol binding to adipocyte membranes and as an activator of adenylate cyclase and lipolysis. In contrast, isoproterenol is 100-fold more effective than norepinephrine as a stimulator of β_2-receptors. 3. The addition of bulkier groups to the amine group of norepinephrine results in compounds as potent as isoproterenol on β_2-receptors but have only 1% of the activity of isoproterenol on adipocyte lipolysis (WENKE et al. 1966; FAIN et al. 1973b; WENKEOVA et al. 1976) or adenylate cyclase (KATHER and SIMON 1977). There is little difference between the β_1-receptors of human as compared to rat adipocytes except for a greater sensitivity of human adipocytes to inhibition of catecholamine action by β-antagonists (HARMS 1976).

The effects of catecholamines on adenylate cyclase and dihydroalprenolol binding in adipocyte membranes are stereospecific with the (+) isomers of adrenergic agonists being 30- to 300-fold less potent than the (−) stereoisomers (WILLIAMS et al. 1976). A similar specificity was also noted for activation of lipolysis (SHONK et al. 1971). The structural requirements of the β_1-receptor for binding of catecholamines include a catechol binding site and an anionic binding site (FAIN 1973b; FELLER et al. 1978); a hydroxyl binding site is not an absolute requirement if there is a large hydrophobic group on the ligand. An example is trimetoquinol, a cyclized N-substituted catecholamine, in which the lack of an alcoholic hydroxyl group is compensated for by a bulky ara-alkyl group on the amine nitrogen. The structural requirements for activation of lipolysis have been reviewed by FAIN (1973b). Although trimetoquinol is structurally similar to papaverine, trimetoquinol did not inhibit cyclic AMP phosphodiesterase; the elevation in cyclic AMP due to trimetoquinol was inhibited by propranolol and correlated with lipolysis (PIASCIK et al. 1978).

β-Adrenergic antagonists bind to the β-receptors with considerably greater affinity than the catecholamine agonists and have proven more satisfactory for binding studies. Iodinated hydroxybenzylpindolol bound to turkey erythrocytes with considerably greater affinity than catecholamines (AURBACH et al. 1974). However, YAMAMURA et al. (1976) found that while hydroxybenzylpindolol bound with a 25- to 40-fold greater affinity to rat adipocyte membranes than did isoproterenol, it was also a partial agonist. At a concentration of 0.01 μM, hydroxybenzylpindolol was more potent than isoproterenol as an activator of either lipolysis or cyclic AMP accumulation. However, the maximal effect of hydroxybenzylpindolol was considerably less than that of isoproterenol; hydroxybenzylpindolol also inhibited the effects of isoproterenol. These are the properties of an antagonist which binds tightly to the receptor site and is a partial agonist.

The most useful compound for examining β-adrenergic binding sites in adipocytes is(−)-(^{3}H)dihydroalprenolol. WILLIAMS et al. (1976) using adipocyte membranes and CABELLI and MALBON (1979) using intact adipocytes demonstrated specific binding sites with properties similar to those of the physiological β-adrenergic receptors. The binding of dihydroalprenolol to both membranes and intact adipocytes was rapid, reversible and displayed stereospecificity; the relative potency of agonists to compete with dihydroalprenolol was similar to their relative potency for activation of adenylate cyclase or lipolysis (WILLIAMS et al. 1976; MALBON et al. 1978; CABELLI and MALBON 1979). Kinetic analysis of the binding of dihydroalprenolol to adipocyte β-receptors gave Scatchard plots with upward concavity. Negative cooperativity explains this type of non-classical binding in some systems; however the β-receptors of adipocytes displayed no cooperative site-to-site interactions (MALBON and CABELLI 1979).

Dihydroalprenolol bound primarily to the adipocyte plasma membranes possessing catecholamine-responsive adenylate cyclase (WILLIAMS et al. 1976). The specific binding of dihydroalprenolol to mitochondria and to microsomes was 20% and less than 12%, respectively, of binding to plasma membrane. In the mitochondrial fraction, there was no catecholamine activation of adenylate cyclase and binding appeared to be to low affinity sites which could not be saturated. These data support the hypothesis that the β-adrenergic receptors are specialized entities found primarily in the plasma membrane.

GIUDICELLI et al. (1979a, b) found that prior exposure of rat adipocyte membranes to agonists (catecholamines) and antagonists (propranolol) reduced the subsequent specific binding of dihydroalprenolol. An unusual feature of this study was the claim that prior binding of propranolol to membranes did not affect the subsequent activation of adenylate cyclase by 100 μ*M* isoproterenol (GIUDICELLI et al. 1979b). In fact, prior exposure of adipocyte membranes to either propranolol or isoproterenol produced identical, and rather strange, kinetics when binding of dihydroalprenolol was measured over a 60 min incubation. At 5 to 10 min, binding was half of the control values in pre-exposed membranes; at 20 min it was 5% or less of control; but at 45 to 60 min, it was 150–200% of control binding (GIUDICELLI et al. 1979b). It is not clear what these findings mean or even whether the process should be referred to as desensitization. Whether prior exposure of adipocytes to catecholamines results in appreciable desensitization at the receptor level remains to be demonstrated. Studies in my laboratory (unpublished) have as yet failed to demonstrate such effects in adipocytes incubated for periods of up to four hours. However, in human adipocytes incubated for 4 days, such effects are observed (SMITH et al. 1976). There are other mechanisms which contribute to catecholamine resistance, including long-term increases in cyclic AMP phosphodiesterase (SMITH et al. 1977) and nonspecific inhibitory factors released to the medium (SJÖSTRÖM et al. 1977).

The presence of catecholamine binding sites and the ability of the catecholamine-β_1 receptor complex to activate adenylate cyclase is not necessarily associated with an activation of lipolysis by catecholamines (GIUDICELLI and PECQUERY 1978). Adipocytes from 30 month old rats contain 7,000 high-affinity dihydroalprenolol binding sites per cell; adipocytes from 1 month old rats contain 11,000 binding sites per cell. In response to 1 μM catecholamine, adenylate cyclase activation in membranes of adipocytes from 30 month old rats was only slightly less than in membranes from 1 month old rats. However, lipolysis was not activated by 0.1 μM norepinephrine in adipocytes from 30 month old rats while there was a 300% increase in adipocytes from 1 month old rats.

In adipocytes from obese, hyperglycemic mice there is a relatively unimpaired lipolytic response to catecholamines. However, the activation of cyclic AMP accumulation in intact cells and adenylate cyclase in fat cell ghosts from obese mice was virtually abolished as compared to their lean littermates. The catalytic activity of adenylate cyclase was unimpaired since fluoride and guanylimidodiphosphate had similar effects in adipocytes from lean and obese mice (SHEPHERD er al. 1977).

2. Regulation of the Coupling of Hormone-Receptor Complexes to Adenylate Cyclase: Thyroid Hormones

In adipocytes from obese or hypothyroid animals, the ability of hormones to accelerate cyclic AMP accumulation is markedly impaired. This effect is due to defective coupling of the hormone-receptor complexes to the common adenylate cyclase; regulation of cyclic AMP phosphodiesterase is involved to a lesser extent, the changes observed appear to be relatively minor. SHEPHERD et al. (1977) found an elevation in total cyclic AMP phosphodiesterase activity of adipocyte preparations from obese-hyperglycemic mice as compared to their lean littermates; however, membrane-bound enzyme activity was actually less in preparations from obese mice. The sensitivity of the particulate cyclic AMP phosphodiesterase activity to methyl xanthines was unaltered by obesity (SHEPHERD et al. 1977); in contrast, soluble enzyme activity was much less sensitive to inhibition by methyl xanthines if derived from adipocytes of obese mice. KAPLAN et al. (1973) found increases in the high K_m cyclic nucleotide phosphodiesterase of obese mice. It is doubtful that this enzyme is involved in breakdown of physiological concentrations of cyclic AMP. BEGIN-HEICK and HEICK (1977) found that the administration of thyroid hormone to obese hyperglycemic mice had no effect on cyclic AMP phosphodiesterase activity but did increase hormone-responsive adenylate cyclase activation.

ARMSTRONG et al. (1974) and VAN INWEGEN et al. (1975) found increases in the particulate, but not the soluble, low K_m cyclic AMP phosphodiesterase activity of homogenates prepared from hypothyroid rats. In contrast, CORREZE et al. (1976) found increases in both soluble and particulate cyclic AMP phosphodiesterase activity of hypothyroid rats. MALBON et al. (1978) found no alteration in the cyclic AMP phosphodiesterase activity of fat cell ghosts which should contain the plasma membrane bound activity. The changes in cyclic AMP phosphodiesterase activity are probably adaptive responses of hypothyroid status which contribute to, but are not the primary cause of, the defective accumulation of cyclic AMP.

GORMAN et al. (1973) found that the ability of hormones to activate adenylate cyclase in membrane preparations derived from rats fed a high fat diet was markedly impaired. The defect in adenylate cyclase activation could be corrected by transferring the rats from the high-fat to a high-carbohydrate diet three days prior to the experiment. This dietary shift might work through an increase in active thyroid hormone. In adipocytes from obese hyperglycemic mice the adminstration of thyroid hormone partially restored the defective hormone-responsive adenylate cyclase. There is some evidence that obese hyperglycemic mice have an impaired peripheral response to thyroid hormone which might result from defective nuclear binding of triiodothyronine (GUERNSEY and MORISHIGE 1979).

A defective responsiveness of adipocytes to triiodothyronine is probably not causally related to the alterations of metabolism in adipocytes from obese-hyperglycemic mice. The alterations in metabolism noted in adipocytes from obese animals are primarily, adaptive responses to an increased deposition of triglyceride. Furthermore, the lipolytic response of adipocytes from obese, hyperglycemic mice is only slightly impaired while that of adipocytes from hypothyroid rats is markedly impaired.

The stimulation of lipid mobilization by thyroid hormones was first demonstrated by RICH et al. (1959) who found that triiodothyronine administration to humans elevated plasma free fatty acids. DEBONS and SCHWARTZ (1961) subsequently demonstrated that epinephrine-induced lipolysis was impaired in adipose tissue obtained from hypothyroid rats; hormone-responsiveness could be restored to normal by prior administration of thyroid hormone. The sensitivity of fat cell lipolysis to all hormones was reduced by hypothyroidism (GOODMAN and BRAY 1966; CORREZE et al. 1974). All reports agree that the accumulation of cyclic AMP and lipolysis are markedly impaired in adipocytes from hypothyroid rats. However, beyond this there is substantial disagreement which probably results from the use of different types of preparations, the inability to control conditions precisely, and our lack of understanding of the primary site of thyroid hormone action. The available evidence is compatible with the hypothesis that triiodothyronine regulates the ability of the hormone-receptor complex to regulate adenylate cyclase activity of adipocytes. The maximal catalytic activity of adenylate cyclase as measured in the presence of fluoride is unaltered by thyroid status (MALBON et al. 1978).

Even the demonstration of an impaired ability of hormones to activate adenylate cyclase activity in broken-cell preparations of adipocytes from hypothyroid rats has been a variable finding. ARMSTRONG et al. (1974) observed no effect of hypothyroidism on adenylate cyclase; CORREZE et al. (1974) observed a 20% decrease and MALBON et al. (1978) observed a 50% decrease in the maximal response to catecholamines. CALDWELL and FAIN (1971) observed that administration of 25 μg of triiodothyronine to euthyroid rats, 8–18 h prior to sacrifice, markedly potentiated catecholamine stimulated elevations in cyclic AMP without affecting adenylate cyclase activity of fat cell ghosts. One explanation for these divergent findings is mediation of triiodothyronine action through unrecognized factors involved in regulation of adenylate cyclase activity which are sometimes lost during disruption of adipocytes and isolation of hormonally-responsive plasma membrane fractions.

Oxygen consumption is reduced and carbohydrate and lipid metabolism are depressed by hypothyroidism to the same extent in liver as in adipose tissue (BAQUER et al. 1976). The redox equilibrium is more oxidized in mitochondria as contrasted to cytosol in hypothyroid animals. In the hyperthyroid state there are increases in fatty acid synthesis as well as in breakdown and oxidation (DIAMANT et al. 1972). The link between energy status of adipocytes, redox equilibrium, and cyclic AMP accumulation remains to be established.

Naphthoquinones, such as menadione, act as shuttles transferring reducing equivalents between cytosol and mitochondria and thus affect energy status of adipocytes (FAIN 1971). Menadione enhances the ability of catecholamines to stimulate cyclic AMP accumulation in intact rat adipocytes but has little effect on adenylate cyclase activity of fat cell ghosts (FAIN 1971). Menadione also increases respiration, glucose oxidation and fatty acid synthesis from glucose. Menadione alters adipocyte metabolism in a manner similar to hyperthyroidism except that lipolysis is inhibited by menadione.

Both the hypothyroid and the insulin-deficient states are characterized by a reduced rate of fatty acid synthesis. In hypothyroidism, lipolysis is impaired but hexose transport is accelerated; in insulin deficiency, lipolysis is accelerated but hexose transport is impaired (CZECH et al. 1980). The complexity of insulin-thyroid interrelationships is underscored since hypothyroidism enhances the entry of glucose into adipocytes via the hexose carrier process while, at the same time, reducing the activity of the NADPH-dependent cytoplasmic enzymes involved in biosynthetic processes. Thus, depending on experimental conditions and the relative rate of turnover of the proteins involved in hexose transport, as contrasted to hexose metabolism either an increase or decrease in glucose metabolism might be observed. CORREZE et al. (1977) actually found an enhanced rate of glucose metabolism and lipogenesis in adipocytes obtained from rats which had been thyroidectomized 14 days previously. Ordinarily the oxidation of glucose and synthesis of fatty acids is markedly reduced by hypothyroidism (BAQUER et al. 1976; CZECH et al. 1980). Future experiments should determine whether any of these effects are mediated through changes in the redox equilibrium between the intracellular compartments of adipocytes.

Increased respiration occurs in adipocytes from hyperthyroid rats (FAIN and ROSENTHAL 1971). The calorigenic action of thyroid hormones is insensitive to 1 m*M* ouabain which markedly reduces respiration in liver slices from hyperthyroid rats (ISMAIL-BEIGI and EDELMAN 1970). Ouabain reduces the lipolytic action of catecholamines to the same extent in euthyroid and hyperthyroid rats. These effects of ouabain are probably secondary to decreases in intracellular K^+ arising from inhibition of the Na^+/K^+ ATPase by ouabain (FAIN and ROSENTHAL 1971). The calorigenic action of thyroid hormones on adipocytes may be secondary to an uncoupling of mitochondrial oxidative phosphorylation (i.e. proton conductance from electron transport). The ATP content of adipocytes from euthyroid rats is unaffected by thyroid treatment or the addition of catecholamines. However, in adipocytes from hyperthyroid rats the addition of catecholamines reduces total ATP content (FAIN and ROSENTHAL 1971).

Among the explanations put forth to explain the reduced lipolytic responsiveness of adipocytes from hypothyroid rats is an increase in adenosine (OHISALO and STOUFFER 1979). However, FAIN and MALBON (1979) found a decrease rather than an increase in adenosine accumulation in hypothyroid rats. The metabolism of labelled ATP in adipocytes from hypothyroid rats was the opposite of what was seen in hyperthyroid rats. In adipocytes from euthyroid rats lipolytic agents cause a drop in ATP and rise in AMP; this effect was not observed in adipocytes from hypothyroid rats (FAIN and MALBON 1979). However, a marked drop in the oxidative degradation of adenosine and inosine occurred in cells from hypothyroid rats.

The hypothesis that adipocytes from hypothyroid rats might have an increased release of, or response to, adenosine was based on the observation that adenosine deaminase increased lipolysis (OHISALO and STOUFFER 1979). However, this study did not compare the effect of adenosine deaminase on the lipolytic sensitivity of cells from both euthyroid and hypothyroid rats. My experience is that adenosine deaminase increases the response of adipocytes from normal, hypothyroid, adrenalectomized or hyperthyroid rats to about the same extent. What would be desirable is an agent which will increase the lipolytic sensitivity of adipocytes from hypothyroid rats without affecting that of adipocytes from euthyroid controls.

Another, somewhat implausible, explanation for the reduced lipolytic sensitivity seen in hypothyroidism is an increase in cytosolic Ca^{2+} (GOSWAMI and ROSENBERG 1978). Thus, A 23187, a divalent cation ionophore, is slightly less inhibitory on maximal lipolysis by adipocytes from hypothyroid rats than on maximal lipolysis by adipocytes from euthyroid or hyperthyroid rats. However, intracellular Ca^{2+} does not have a major role in the regulation of lipolysis (FAIN 1980). Glycogen synthase activity in adipocytes is reduced by α-adrenergic agonists secondary to elevation of cytosol Ca^{2+} (LAWRENCE and LARNER 1977, 1978b). The increase in cytosol Ca^{2+} due to epinephrine is mediated through α_1-adrenergic receptors and is associated with phosphatidylinositol turnover in rat adipocytes (GARCIA-SAINZ and FAIN 1980a). The inactivation of glycogen synthase and elevation of phosphatidylinositol turnover in α_1-agonists was unaffected by hypothyroidism (GARCIA-SAINZ and FAIN 1980b). These data indicate that hypothyroidism does not affect the α_1-responses of adipocytes under circumstances in which β responsiveness is markedly reduced.

ROSENQVIST et al. (1971) suggested that the impaired lipolytic sensitivity of adipocytes from hypothyroid humans was due to an increased α-adrenergic responsiveness. However, unaltered α-adrenergic responsiveness accompanied by a markedly decreased β-adrenergic responsiveness seems more plausible. Human adipocytes possess α_2-receptors which directly inhibit adenylate cyclase; affects of thyroid status on the sensitivity of this receptor remain to be demonstrated. However, the effects of thyroid status on human adipocytes are similar to those on rat adipocytes (ARNER et al. 1979; RECKLESS et al. 1976).

The reduced β-adrenergic responsiveness in adipocytes from hypothyroid animals does not involve changes in the number or affinity of β-adrenergic receptors; indeed the responsiveness to polypeptide hormones is also reduced (MALBON et al. 1979; GOSWAMI and ROSENBERG 1978). The administration of triiodothyronine to normal rats had no effect on the number of β-adrenergic antagonist binding sites (MALBON et al. 1978; GOSWAMI and ROSENBERG 1978; GIUDICELLI 1978). GIUDICELLI (1978) claimed that thyroidectomy at 3 weeks of age reduced binding of dihydroalprenolol to adipocyte membranes prepared from 150 g rats. Controls in this study were large male rats weighing 320–350 g. The binding was increased by giving triiodothyronine for 10 days; however, this may be related to general growth

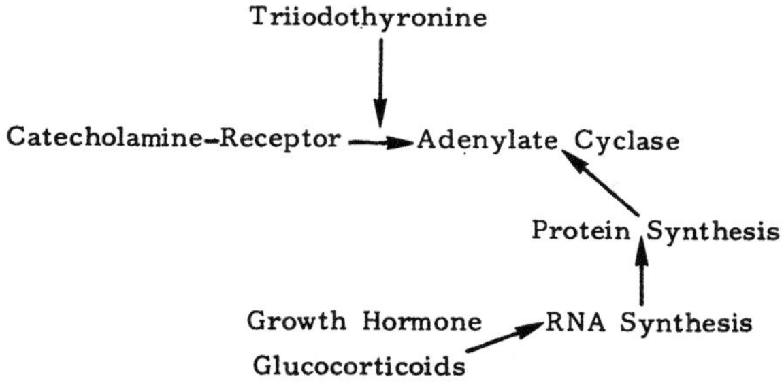

Fig. 3. Regulation of adenylate cyclase by triiodothyronine, glucocorticoids and growth hormone. Triiodothyronine is postulated to regulate the coupling of hormone-receptor complexes to adenylate cyclase through an unknown mechanism. Triiodothyronine does not affect the number of β-catecholamine receptors or the fluoride-activatable adenylate cyclase but regulates the ability of hormones and cholera toxin to activate adenylate cyclase. Growth hormone and glucocorticoids work through to process involving RNA and protein synthesis which results in an increase in the amount of adenylate cyclase. The lag period before lipolysis is activated by these hormones is one to two hours. There may be a somewhat longer lag period for thyroid hormone action which involves protein synthesis

of the cretinous rats. MALBON et al. (1978) made adult female rats hypothyroid in order to separate the effects of hypothyroidism on growth from those on general body metabolism. Possibly growth retardation associated with hypothyroidism may decrease the number of adipocyte β-adrenergic receptors. This possibility is supported by GIUDICELLI's (1978) inability to demonstrate any change in the number of β-adrenergic receptors after administration of large doses of triiodothyronine to euthyroid rats for 10 days. Probably thyroid status does not affect the number or affinity of β-adrenergic receptors but rather the ability of all hormone-receptor complexes to elevate cyclic AMP accumulation (Fig. 3).

3. Adenylate Cyclase Regulation by Inhibition of Deactivation: Cholera Toxin

Cholera toxin, like catecholamines and other activators of adenylate cyclase, enhances adipocyte lipolysis. VAUGHAN et al. (1970) first reported that, after a 1–2 h lag period, lipolysis was activated by cholera toxin. The lag period for cholera toxin action is similar to that noted in other tissues and does not involve processes which are blocked by inhibitors of RNA and protein synthesis (CUATRECASAS 1973). Ganglioside GM_1 acts as the receptor for cholera toxin. Initially, KANFER et al. (1976) were unable to detect ganglioside GM_1 in rat adipocytes but more recently PACUSKA et al. (1978) were able to find trace amounts of this compound. EVANS et al. (1972), HEWLETT et al. (1974), and BENNET et al. (1975) found that adenylate cyclase activity was elevated in membranes from adipocytes previously incubated with cholera toxin.

The mechanism by which cholera toxin activates adenylate cyclase is depicted in Fig. 2. GILL and MEREN (1978) found that the active subunit of the toxin ribosylated a pigeon erythrocyte membrane protein with a molecular weight of 42,000 daltons in the presence of NAD, thereby blocking the phosphotransferase reaction in which GTP is cleaved to GDP (GTPase). MALBON and GILL (1979) found that cholera toxin ADP-ribosylated a protein of molecular weight 42,000 in adipocyte membrane. The effect of cholera toxin on adipocyte adenylate cyclase is primarily to convert a GTP inhibition of adenylate cyclase to an activation as originally noted by BENNET et al. (1975).

The basal adenylate cyclase activity was also elevated by cholera toxin but neither the activation of the enzyme by epinephrine or by Gpp(NH)p were affected (MALBON and GILL 1979). Similar results had previously been reported by MANGANIELLO et al. (1976) for catecholamine activation of adenylate cyclase. These data suggest that the GTPase activity of adipocyte membrane preparations does not contribute appreciably to hormonal regulation of adenylate cyclase except in the presence of added GTP.

Regulation of adenylate cyclase activity by thyroid hormone might involve GTP binding proteins. Thus Gpp(NH)p, did not activate adenylate cyclase in adipocyte membranes from hypothyroid rats to the same extent as in membranes from euthyroid controls (MALBON and GILL 1979). Cholera toxin and Gpp(NH)p were equally effective on membranes from euthyroid and hypothyroid rats (MALBON and GILL 1979); but the maximal cyclase activity was less in membranes from hypothyroid rats. While, the total amount of adenylate cyclase activity activated by hormones, Gpp(HN)p or cholera toxin was reduced, the incorporation of labelled ADP-ribose due to cholera toxin addition was some 20–30% higher in membranes from hypothyroid as compared to euthyroid rat adipocyte ghosts (MALBON and GILL 1979).

4. Regulation Through Synthesis of Components of Adenylate Cyclase: Growth Hormone and Glucocorticoids

GOODMAN and SCHWARTZ (1974) and RAO and RAMACHANDRAN (1977) have published reviews on the regulation of lipid mobilization and lipolysis by growth hormone and FAIN (1979b) has reviewed the effects of glucocorticoids. Growth hormone and glucocorticoids inhibit glucose metabolism and accelerate lipolytic sensitivity; therefore their effects are opposite to those of insulin. RABEN and HOLLENBERG (1959) demonstrated that the plasma free fatty acids were elevated after administration of growth hormone to dogs. WHITE and ENGEL (1958) were unable to obtain an immediate lipolytic effect of growth hormone but were able to accelerate lipolysis by addition of ACTH which had little effect on plasma free fatty acids in vivo.

FAIN et al. (1965) demonstrated in vitro a lipolytic effect of growth hormone upon adipose tissue. Lipolysis was accelerated by growth hormone only after a one to two hour lag period and was dependent on the presence of glucocorticoids in the incubation medium, Previously, FAIN (1962) had found that the fatty acid release by parametrial adipose tissue from acutely adrenalectomized rats was markedly elevated if the animals received the combination of growth hormone and glucocorticoid. The prior administration of either hormone alone had a small effect, as had been previously shown in vivo by LEVIN and FARBER (1952). The lipolytic actions of both growth hormone and glucocorticoids appear to be permissive in nature since they regulate the sensitivity of adipocytes to activators of lipolysis.

Both growth hormone and glucocorticoids have a 1–2 h lag period prior to enhancing lipolysis; their lipolytic effects are blocked by inhibitors of RNA or protein synthesis (FAIN et al. 1965; FAIN 1967a; FAIN and SAPERSTEIN 1970; GOODMAN 1970; FAIN et al. 1971). However, growth hormone affects cyclic AMP formation while glucocorticoids have little effect on cyclic AMP.

MOSKOWITZ and FAIN (1970) found that cyclic AMP accumulation in adipocytes was elevated by incubation with growth hormone plus glucocorticoid. The increases in cyclic AMP were blocked by puromycin or cycloheximide which are inhibitors of protein synthesis. The elevations of cyclic AMP were due to growth hormone since growth hormone alone was effective and glucocorticoids alone had little effect on cyclic AMP accumulation (FAIN and SAPERSTEIN 1970; FAIN et al. 1971). Exposure to either growth hormone or glucocorticoid caused a 40% increase in catecholamine-responsive adenylate cyclase activity of adipocyte ghosts (FAIN and CZECH 1975). Thus, glucocorticoids elevated adipocyte ghost adenylate cyclase but had little effect on cyclic AMP accumulation by intact cells. More recently FAIN (1980) confirmed that adenylate cyclase activity of adipocyte ghosts was enhanced by exposure to either growth hormone or glucocorticoid. However in the experiment of FAIN (1980), the elevation in maximal adenylate cyclase activity was expressed in the presence of fluoride or Gpp(NH)p. The results suggest that both hormones can increase the synthesis of proteins which regulate adenylate cyclase activity (Fig. 3).

The elevation in adenylate cyclase due to growth hormone is associated with an enhancement of glycogen phosphorylase. EISEN and GOODMAN (1969) and MOSKOWITZ and FAIN (1970) found that prior exposure of adipocytes to growth hormone plus glucocorticoid potentiated the ability of methyl xanthines to elevate glycogen phosphorylase. This effect of growth hormone plus glucocorticoids was blocked by cycloheximide (MOSKOWITZ and FAIN 1970). The nature of the proteins whose synthesis is regulated by these hormones is unknown.

Another similarity in the actions of growth hormone and glucocorticoids is their ability to inhibit glucose transport in adipocytes. The glucocorticoid inhibition is readily demonstrated after 2–3 h incubation of adipocytes with steroid (FAIN 1979b) but the effect of growth hormone requires a longer incubation period (NYBERG and SMITH 1977). SCHOENLE et al. (1979) have shown that adipocytes from hypophysectomized rats have a high rate of basal glucose transport which could be restored to normal values by pre-treatment with growth hormone. FAIN (1962) found that the basal rate of glucose uptake by incubated adipose tissue was elevated by adrenalectomy and restored to normal values by administration of either growth hormone or glucocorticoid. Treatment with either hormone alone did not affect fatty acid release by the adipose tissue but the combination produced a marked increase (FAIN 1962). These data suggest that growth hormone and glucocorticoids have inhibitory effects on glucose transport which are independent of their actions on lipolysis. The combination of the two hormones has effects on lipolysis which are usually far greater than those of either hormone alone while either hormone alone has a maximal inhibitory effect on glucose transport.

Whether the inhibitory effects of growth hormone on glucose transport by adipocytes are linked to the increases in adenylate cyclase activity remain to be demonstrated. It is also possible that growth hormone and glucocorticoids stimulate the synthesis of proteins which restrain the glucose transport system in adipocytes. Insulin could accelerate transport by binding to these inhibitory proteins. SCHOEN-

LE et al. (1979) observed that glucose transport in adipocytes from hypophysectomized rats was similar to that in adipocytes from normal rats incubated with a maximal concentration of insulin.

There are cytosol receptors which bind glucocorticoids entering adipocytes and transport them to the nucleus where the hormones regulate the synthesis of certain proteins (FAIN 1979b). However, growth hormone needs an as yet unidentified second messenger to transmit a signal into the nucleus if it binds with receptors on the surface of adipocytes. Alternatively, growth hormone could be taken up by adipocytes and, in some fashion, transported to the nucleus. However, this second possibility seems unlikely, because HECHT et al. (1972) demonstrated that the delayed lipolytic response to growth hormone bound to Sepharose beads was 40% of the response to native hormone.

A third possibility is that the binding of growth hormone to its receptor activates a protease and thereby liberates an active protein which transmits a signal to the nucleus. This hypothesis is based on analogy to the complement system (KISHIMOTO et al. 1979). The binding of growth hormone to the receptor might activate either latent protease activity of the receptor itself or change the conformation of the receptor which is then cleaved by endogenous proteases.

No evidence is available that an active core of the growth hormone molecule can interact directly with the adipocyte receptors (WIESER et al. 1974). The two major fragments obtained after limited tryptic digestion were less active than growth hormone as lipolytic agents. These data do not eliminate the possibility that an active fragment is cleaved from growth hormone after the interaction of the native growth hormone with adipocytes since such a fragment might lack the site for binding by adipocytes. At present, no data support the idea that either a fragment of growth hormone or some other molecule formed after interaction of growth hormone with receptors is involved in transmission of information to the nucleus.

5. Inhibition of Adenylate Cyclase

a) Free Fatty Acids

Fatty acids can serve as product inhibitors of lipolysis and feedback regulators of adenylate cyclase (Fig. 4). The important factor is not the total concentration of free fatty acids but rather the free fatty acid to albumin ratio in the medium. RODBELL (1965) found that lipolysis by adipocytes virtually ceases when the fatty acid to albumin ratio exceeds 3. BURNS et al. (1975) using human adipocytes and FAIN and SHEPHERD (1975) using rat adipocytes found that cyclic AMP accumulation in the presence of lipolytic agents was markedly inhibited at fatty acid to albumin ratios above 2. The addition of sodium oleate to the medium inhibited cyclic AMP accumulation if the fatty acid to albumin ratio was above 2 and maximal inhibition was seen at a ratio of 6 (FAIN and SHEPHERD 1975).

Either dialyzed medium previously incubated with adipocytes in the presence of lipolytic agents or fatty acids inhibited the adenylate cyclase activity of adipocyte ghosts if the fatty acid to albumin ratio was above 2 (FAIN and SHEPHERD 1975). Long chain fatty acids ranging from palmitate to arachidonate inhibited adenylate cyclase. Oleate, during the first 6 min after its addition to the assay system, inhibited basal and hormone-stimulated adenylate cyclase but had no effect of

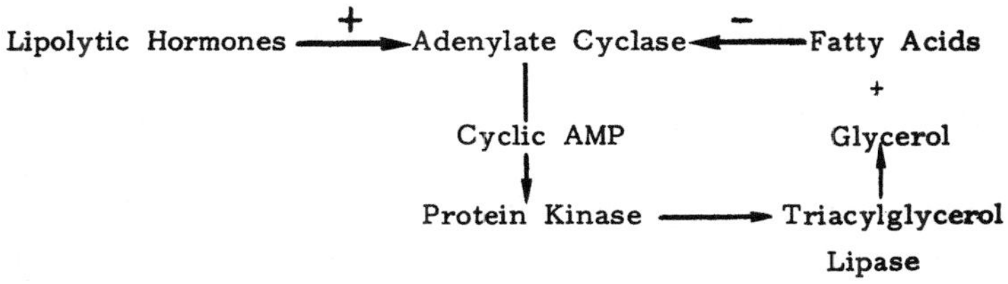

Fig. 4. Feedback regulation of adenylate cyclase by free fatty acids. Lipolytic hormones regulate adenylate cyclase through closed loop control in which the end products of lipolysis act as inhibitors of adenylate cyclase. A further illustration of the circularity of biological control is product inhibition of the triacylglycerol lipase by free fatty acids. The important feature is the intracellular free fatty acid content which is in equilibrium with fatty acids bound to albumin and other proteins. Inhibition is seen when the medium fatty acid to albumin ratio exceeds 2

fluoride-activated cyclase and potentiated guanyl-5′-imido-diphosphate activated adenylate cyclase activity (FAIN and SHEPHERD 1979).

Chicken adipocytes are relatively insensitive to feedback regulation of adenylate cyclase by free fatty acids. The addition of oleate to chicken adipocytes did not inhibit glucagon-induced elevations in cyclic AMP. The glucagon-activated adenylate cyclase activity of chicken adipocytes was not inhibited by addition of oleate even at molar ratios of fatty acid to albumin of 12 (MALGIERI et al. 1975).

The feedback regulation of adenylate cyclase by free fatty acids is a good example of the closed-loop control characteristic of most biological systems (RASMUSSEN and GOODMAN 1977). Figure 4 suggests that the final products of lipolysis inhibit the first steps in lipolytic activation when the primary binding sites on medium albumin are saturated. The intracellular free fatty acids are in equilibrium with the fatty acids bound to medium albumin and high levels of intracellular fatty acids have deleterious effects on fat cell energy metabolism (ANGEL et al. 1971).

b) Prostaglandins

ILLIANO and CUATRECASAS (1971) postulated that prostaglandins were physiologically important feedback regulators of lipolysis based on studies with indomethacin, an inhibitor of prostaglandin formation. However, others have been unable to find any potentiation of lipolysis or cyclic AMP accumulation in adipocytes by indomethacin (FAIN et al. 1973 a; DALTON and HOPE 1973; FREDHOLM and HEDQVIST 1975; CHANG et al. 1977). Further evidence against the prostaglandin theory of feedback regulation was the report by FREDHOLM and ROSELL (1970) that the amounts of E-type prostaglandins released during and after stimulation of nerves supplying canine subcutaneous adipose tissue were lower than the amounts required for inhibition of lipolysis. BOWERY and LEWIS (1973) found that indomethacin inhibited prostaglandin formation and functional vasodilation in rabbit adipose tissue but did not affect lipolysis during ACTH infusion. These data do not support the hypothesis that prostaglandins are important feedback regulators of adenylate cyclase in fat cells.

The major factor regulating prostaglandin formation in many cells is the availability of arachidonic acid derived from the breakdown of cellular phospholipids which contain high amounts of arachidonic acid. However, in adipocytes the prostaglandins formed during activation of lipolysis can be derived from arachidonic acid released during triglyceride breakdown. Christ and Nugteren (1970) reported that arachidonic acid accounted for about $\alpha/1\%$ of the fatty acids released during hormone-stimulated lipolysis in incubated adipose tissue. Dalton and Hope (1974) found that about 0.1 nmole of prostaglandin E_2 per gram of adipocytes was released during incubation of fat cells with lipolytic agents; basal release was about one-tenth of this value. Dalton and Hope (1974) suggested that the prostaglandin E_2 came from cyclic AMP activation of a phospholipase since arachidonic acid accounts for 18% of phospholipid fatty acids. However, arachidonic acid could have arisen during triglyceride hydrolysis since 2,400 nanomoles of arachidonic acid would have accumulated if the amount of fatty acid released in the presence of hormones was 240 micromoles per gram over 1 h and 1% of triglyceride fatty acids were accounted for by arachidonic acid (Dalton and Hope 1974). The prostaglandins formed from arachidonic acid released during lipolysis may act as vasodilators to increase blood flow through adipose tissue. This might enhance lipolysis by preventing saturation of plasma albumin with fatty acids.

Prostaglandin endoperoxides might be feedback regulators of adenylate cyclase. Gorman et al. (1975) found that 0.3 μM to 30 μM PGH_2 (15-hydroxy-9-peroxidoprosta-5,13-dienoic acid) inhibited adenylate cyclase. However, Fredholm (1978) has pointed out that PGH_2 is about 10 times less potent than PGE_2 as an inhibitor of catecholamine-induced elevations of cyclic AMP in intact adipocytes. In fact, conversion of PGH_2 to PGE_2 by adipocytes may account for all or part of its effects. Fredholm (1978) has also pointed out that neither thromboxane A_2 nor PGI_2 are formed by adipocytes. The available studies do not suggest that local release of prostaglandins is important in the short term regulation of lipolysis and cyclic AMP accumulation.

c) Alpha$_2$-Adrenergic Agonists

Robison et al. (1971) suggested that stimulation of α-adrenoceptors may inhibit adenylate cyclase. α_1-effects of catecholamines are not related directly to adenylate cyclase; rather these effects involve increased turnover of phosphatidylinositol and elevation of cytosol Ca^{2+} (section C). However, in rabbit and human, but not pig platelets there is a direct inhibitory effect of α_2-catecholamines on adenylate cyclase (Jakobs 1978).

In hamster and human adipocytes catecholamines inhibit adenylate cyclase through α_2-receptors (Fig. 5). Burns and Langley (1975), using human adipocyte ghosts, and Aktories et al. (1979), using hamster adipocyte ghosts found an inhibition of adenylate cyclase by epinephrine. Burns et al. (1981) concluded that the α-adrenergic inhibition by epinephrine of adenylate cyclase and lipolysis was mediated through α_2-receptor activation based on the finding of α_2-binding sites (receptors) in human adipocytes, an inhibition of lipolysis and cyclic AMP accumulation by clonidine but not by methoxamine and a specific inhibition of epinephrine action on adenylate cyclase activity by yohimbine but not by prazosin. In hamster adipocytes, α-catecholamines such as clonidine which preferentially interact with α_2-receptors inhibited the accumulation of cyclic AMP stimulated either by ACTH

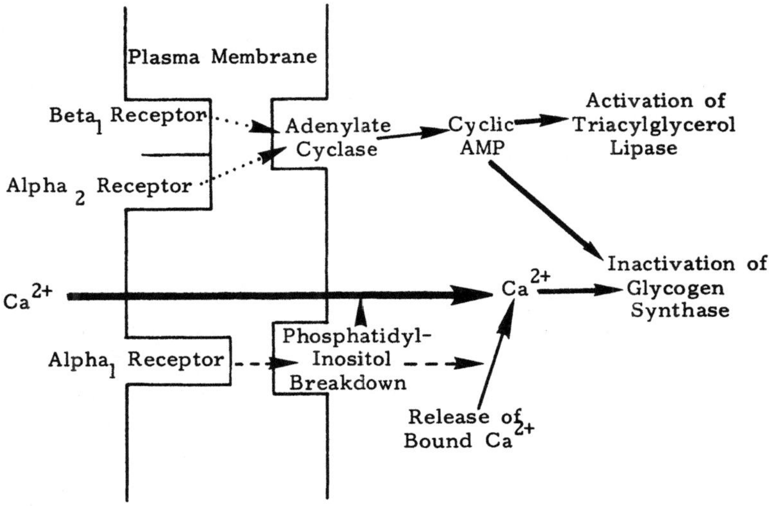

Fig. 5. Regulation of adipocyte metabolism via α- and βadrenoreceptors. The activation of adenylate cyclase is postulated to occur in adipocytes of all species via activation of adrenoreceptors of the β_1 type which result in activation of adenylate cyclase and of triacylglycerol lipase. In certain species (hamster and man) there are inhibitory α_2-receptors whose activation results in non-specific inhibition of adenylate cyclase activation by all hormones. The mechanism is not known but is unlikely to be through changes in Ca^{2+}. There are α-effects which result in the release of bound intracellular Ca^{2+} and the entry of extracellular Ca^{2+} but they are mediated through receptors of the α_1-type. The α_1 but not α_2-effects of catecholamines are associated with increased turnover of phosphatidylinositol and the elevation of cytosol Ca^{2+} has little effect on cyclic AMP metabolism or lipolysis but does regulate glycogen synthase activity

or by catecholamines (Schimmel 1979; Garcia-Sainz et al. 1980). These data suggest that α_2-adrenergic agonists interact with receptors which inhibit adenylate cyclase at a site beyond β-catecholamine-receptor interactions. The effect of α_2-agonists on adenylate cyclase activity of platelets (Jakobs 1978) and of hamster adipocytes (Aktories et al. 1979) are best seen in the presence of GTP. Possibly α_2-agonists inhibit adenylate cyclase by stimulating the deactivation of adenylate cyclase. One possibility is that GTPase activity is accelerated by α_2-agonists. This hypothesis suggest that cholera toxin and α_2-agonists regulate the same enzyme but in opposite directions. An interesting difference between platelets and adipocytes is that adenosine stimulates adenylate cyclase in platelets and antagonizes it in adipocytes.

d) Adenosine

Dole (1961) first reported that lipolysis was inhibited by adenosine. Similar results were found by Kappeler (1966), Raben and Matsuzaki (1966), Pereira and Holland (1966), and Davies (1968). Adenosine also inhibited cyclic AMP accumulation by adipocytes through a mechanism involving inhibition of adenylate cyclase (Fain et al. 1972; Schwabe et al. 1973). Conversely, adenosine deaminase activates lipolysis and increases cyclic AMP accumulation (Fain 1973a, Schwabe and Ebert 1974; Fain and Wieser 1975).

The physiological role of adenosine in adipocyte metabolism remains to be established. Neither SCHWABE et al. (1973), FREDHOLM and HJEMDAHL (1979), nor FAIN (1979 a) could detect any effect of hormones on adenosine release. Adenosine seems to be an endogenous, inhibitory regulator of adenylate cyclase. In rat adipocytes, lipolytic agents cause a large increase in cyclic AMP accumulation only in the presence of adenosine deaminase or methyl xanthines.

The remarkable sensitivity of adipocytes to adenosine is illustrated by the ability of 0.01 to 0.1 μM N^6(phenylisopropyl)adenosine to inhibit the lipolytic action of catecholamines (WESTERMANN et al. 1969). FAIN (1973 a) found that as little as 0.05 μM N^6(phenylisopropyl)adenosine or 0.2 μM adenosine inhibited cyclic AMP accumulation by rat adipocytes. TURPIN et al. (1977) found an inhibition by 0.01 μM adenosine of hormone stimulated lipolysis in perifused adipocytes. The sensitivity of adipocytes to adenosine supports the suggestion that it could have a physiological role in the regulation of cyclic AMP metabolism in adipocytes.

The concept that methyl xanthines are primarily adenosine antagonists is slowly becoming appreciated. FAIN and MALBON (1979) have reviewed the evidence that, in contrast to other inhibitors of cyclic AMP phosphodiesterase such as papaverine or RO 20-1724, the methyl xanthines antagonize the inhibitory action of adenosine upon adenylate cyclase. SCHWABE and EBERT (1972) found that if dilute suspensions of adipocytes were incubated with lipolytic hormones, high levels of cyclic AMP accumulated. However, if more concentrated suspensions of cells were used, lipolytic agents were relatively ineffective except in the presence of methyl xanthines. These results suggested that an inhibitor, whose action is antagonized by methyl xanthines, accumulates during incubation of adipocytes. SCHWABE et al. (1973) subsequently identified the inhibitor as adenosine.

Chicken adipocytes respond to glucagon with a marked rise in cyclic AMP which is not potentiated by methyl xanthines (MALGIERI et al. 1975; KITABGI et al. 1976). Chicken adipocytes have a high level of endogenous adenosine deaminase (FAIN and SHEPHERD 1979) and there is little effect of added adenosine deaminase (BOYD et al. 1975). An adenosine analog which cannot be deaminated [such as N^6-(phenylisopropyl)adenosine] inhibited the rise in cyclic AMP due to glucagon; this inhibition could be blocked by methyl xanthines. The available data support the hypothesis that inhibition of adenosine action by methyl xanthines may be more significant than inhibition of cyclic AMP phosphodiesterase.

Phenylisopropyl adenosine is a potent inhibitor of lipolysis either in vivo or in vitro (WESTERMANN et al. 1969). FAIN et al. (1972) observed that phenylisopropyl adenosine was a potent inhibitor of cyclic AMP accumulation in intact adipocytes but had little effect on adenylate cyclase activity. In contrast, 2′,5′-dideoxy adenosine inhibited adenylate cyclase activity to the same extent as it did cyclic AMP accumulation by intact cells (FAIN et al. 1972, 1979). However, the inhibition of cyclic AMP accumulation due to dideoxy adenosine was not accompanied by any inhibition of lipolysis (FAIN et al. 1972, 1979).

The divergent effects of adenosine analogs are best accounted for by the hypothesis of LONDOS and WOLFF (1977) that two separate sites exist for adenosine regulation of adenylate cyclase. The "R" site, located on the extracellular surface of the plasma membrane, is stimulated by low concentrations of adenosine and is antagonized by methyl xanthines. Agonists for this site require an intact ribose group (hence the designation as the "R" site). Phenylisopropyladenosine, an

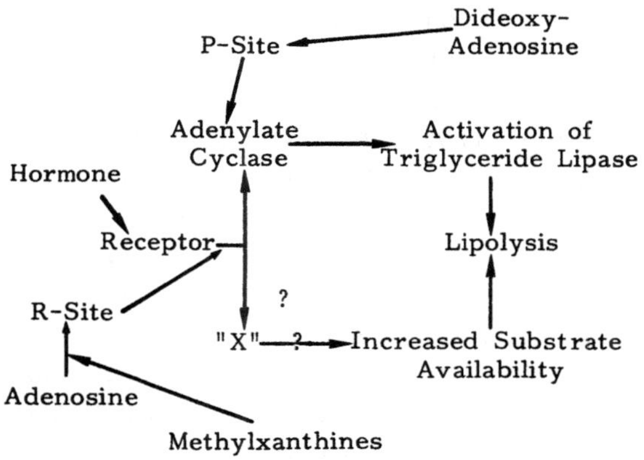

Fig. 6. Regulation of adenylate cyclase by adenosine at this sites. Adenosine is an endogenous regulator of adenylate cyclase which reacts with receptors on the external surface of adipocytes. Methylxanthines are postulated to block adenosine interaction at this extracellular or R-site. Compounds which react at this site have an intact ribose moiety (hence R-site) and compounds such as N^6(phenylisopropyl)adenosine interact as this site. The intracellular or P-site in contrast requires an intact purine moiety (hence P-site) but can react with analogs such as 2′,5′-dideoxyadenosine. The inhibitory effects at this site are limited to adenylate cyclase inhibition and are not antagonized by adenosine. Adenosine interaction at the R-site is postulated the block all effects of hormones including an unknown or "X" pathway which increases substrate availability for the triacylglycerol lipase

adenosine analog which is neither deaminated nor phosphorylated to nucleotides, reacts with the "R" site.

The intracellular "P" site is stimulated by high concentrations of adenosine, but this site is not antagonized by methyl xanthines. Agonists for this site require an intact purine (hence the designation as the "P" site); the most potent agonist upon the "P" site is 2′,5′-dideoxy-adenosine. The physiological regulator of this site may be 5′-AMP. Inhibition of adenylate cyclase at the "P" site is readily demonstrated in broken cell preparations. A two site model for adenosine regulation of fat cell metabolism and lipolysis is shown in Fig. 6. The true adenosine or R-site is difficult to demonstrate in cell-free preparations, while the AMP or P-site is easily seen in these systems. However, inhibition of adenylate cyclase at the adenosine or R-site can be seen under special conditions (LONDOS et al. 1978; FAIN and MALBON 1979).

The interaction between an agonist and the R-site is antagonized by methylxanthines; in contrast, the interaction between an agonist and the P-site is not antagonized by methyl xanthines (FAIN et al. 1978). The marked drop in cyclic AMP accumulation due to 2′,5′-dideoxyadenosine, an agonist upon the P-site, is not accompanied by any inhibition of hormone-activated lipolysis. Inhibition of cyclic AMP accumulation by N^6(phenylisopropyl)adenosine, an agonist upon the R-site, is accompanied by an inhibition of lipolysis (FAIN et al. 1979). These data suggest that stimulation of the R-site inhibits the signal transfer between the hormone-receptor complex and all processes regulating lipolysis in the fat cell. In contrast, stimulation of the P-site inhibits only activation of the adenylate cyclase system without affecting the other hormone-receptor mediated events regulating lipolysis (Fig. 6). Alternatively, the pool of cyclic AMP measured in these studies is unrelated to lipolysis.

The R-site appears to be on the exterior of the adipocyte. The inhibition by adenosine of cyclic AMP accumulation in intact cells is not antagonized by inhibitors of adenosine uptake, such as dipyridamole (EBERT and SCHWABE 1973; FAIN 1973a). Adenosine, covalently linked to stachyose, is equipotent with adenosine as an inhibitor of cyclic AMP accumulation by intact rat and chicken adipocytes (FAIN and SHEPHERD 1979). The adenosine-stachyose compounds are thought not to enter fat cells; OLSSON et al. (1976) demonstrated that the adenosine-stachyose complex was a coronary vasodilator in dogs.

In conclusion, adenosine is a potent endogenous regulator of cyclic AMP accumulation by rat adipocytes. Removal of adenosine with exogenous adenosine deaminase elevates cyclic AMP and activates lipolysis. Adenosine or N^6(phenylisopropyl)adenosine inhibit lipolysis and cyclic AMP accumulation at an extracellular site which inhibits the ability of hormone-receptor complexes to activate both adenylate cyclase and lipolysis.

III. Cyclic AMP Phosphodiesterase Regulation

BUTCHER and SUTHERLAND (1962) reported the irreversible hydrolysis of cyclic AMP by an enzyme from heart designated cyclic AMP phosphodiesterase. The K_m for cyclic AMP was about 0.1 m*M*; the enzyme was inhibited by methyl xanthines. Most cells contain at least two forms of phosphodiesterase activity with rather different affinities for cyclic AMP. One form can hydrolyze both cyclic AMP and cyclic GMP, but with relatively low affinities for either nucleotide; this form is sometimes called cyclic GMP phosphodiesterase. Another form, designated as the low K_m form, has a higher affinity for cyclic AMP and does not hydrolyze cyclic GMP (THOMPSON and APPLEMAN 1971). The second enzyme appears to be of physiological significance in the degradation of cyclic AMP (APPLEMAN et al. 1973; WELLS and HARDMANN 1977).

LOTEN and SNEYD (1970) reported that cyclic AMP phosphodiesterase activity was elevated in homogenates prepared from either fat pads or cells of rats previously exposed to insulin. This effect of insulin has been confirmed; only the low K_m, particulate enzyme is affected (MANGANIELLO and VAUGHAN 1973; ZINMAN and HOLLENBERG 1974; KONO et al. 1975; SOLOMON et al. 1977). The activation of cyclic AMP phosphodiesterase by insulin does not occur in broken cell preparations; attempts to purify the enzyme have resulted in loss of the insulin effect. KONO et al. (1975) suggested that the insulin-activated enzyme was located on particles derived from the endoplasmic reticulum, rather than the plasma membrane. The cyclic AMP phosphodiesterase activity of rat fat cells is also elevated by prior exposure to lipolytic agents (PAWLSON et al. 1974; ZINMAN and HOLLENBERG 1974; SOLOMON 1975). Since lipolytic agents elevate cyclic AMP while insulin is an antilipolytic agent, the mechanisms for activation must be different. The physiological significance of the activation of cyclic AMP phosphodiesterase by insulin is unknown; PAWLSON et al. (1974) reported that during the first 20 min after the addition of insulin, no change in basal cyclic AMP accumulation occurred despite a marked increase in cyclic AMP phosphodiesterase.

The increases in cyclic GMP due to lipolytic hormones, insulin, the divalent cation ionophore A 23187 and cholinergic agents were dependent on extracellular calcium (FAIN and BUTCHER 1976). Possibly, the rise in cyclic AMP phosphodiesterase in fat was secondary to a rise in calcium; but no effects of the ionophore A 23187 or cholinergic agents on cyclic AMP phosphodiesterase activity occur and the activation by insulin was unaltered by the absence of calcium from the extracellular medium (FAIN, unpublished work). DESAI and HOLLENBERG (1975) reported that extracellular calcium was required for the activation of cyclic AMP phosphodiesterase by insulin. However, the same laboratory found that the anti-lipolytic action of insulin was unaffected by the absence of calcium (DESAI et al. 1976); this is in agreement with other studies on lipolysis (HALES et al. 1977; FAIN and BUTCHER 1976). Further progress in understanding how hormones regulate cyclic AMP phosphodiesterase awaits purification of the enzyme in a form which maintains the increases due to hormones.

IV. Protein Kinase Regulation by Cyclic AMP

CORBIN and KREBS (1969) and CORBIN et al. (1970) found that protein kinase activity in rat adipocytes was stimulated several-fold by cyclic AMP. The mechanism by which cyclic AMP activates adipocyte protein kinase is similar to the mechanism in other tissues. SODERLING et al. (1973) found a good correlation between the effects of hormones on total cyclic AMP and protein kinase activity measured in extracts obtained by homogenization in the presence of high salt concentrations (CORBIN et al. 1973). The protein kinase present in adipose tissue appears to be type II isozyme differing in some respects form the type II enzyme of heart (CORBIN et al. 1976). The so-called type II protein kinases are eluted from DEAE-cellulose columns by high salt, dissociate slowly upon addition of histone, reassociate rapidly and undergo self-phosphorylation (ROSEN et al. 1977).

V. Activation of Triacylglycerol Lipase by Protein Kinase

CORBIN et al. (1970) and HUTTUNEN et al. (1970a) found that rabbit muscle protein kinase, in the presence of cyclic AMP and ATP enhanced triglyceride lipase activity. Subsequently HUTTUNEN et al. (1970b) and HUTTUNEN and STEINBERG (1971) found that during such activation, the γ-phosphate of ATP was transferred to the lipase; the time course for this phosphorylation paralled the time course for activation of the lipase.

STEINBERG (1976), in a comprehensive review on the activation of triglyceride lipase by protein kinase, suggested that activation is direct in contrast to the activation of glycogen phosphorylase, which involves an intermediate enzyme. This conclusion was based on the finding by HUTTUNEN and STEINBERG (1971) that activation by protein kinase was just as great using the most highly purified preparations of triglyceride lipase as with impure preparations. Furthermore, KHOO et al. (1974) found that in human adipose tissue homogenates the activation of lipase was immediately stopped by the addition of a protein kinase inhibitor and restored upon the addition of exogenous protein kinase without an appreciable lag phase.

The soluble, triglyceride lipase activity of chicken adipose tissue was enhanced by protein kinase to a much greater extent than is the lipase of rat adipose tissue (KHOO and STEINBERG 1974). The activation of triglyceride lipase was rapidly reversed after removal of cyclic AMP; a second addition of protein kinase in the presence of cyclic AMP and ATP resulted in elevation of activity. Several cycles of this activation-deactivation process could be carried (STEINBERG et al. 1975). The reversible, deactivation appeared to be catalyzed by a Mg^{2+}-dependent lipase phosphatase. SEVERSON et al. (1977) subsequently reported that a variety of phosphoprotein phosphatase preparations from different tissues would reversibly deactivate hormone-sensitive lipase.

An inactivation of hormone-sensitive triglyceride lipase activity has also been observed in the presence of ATP, Mg^{2+} and ascorbic acid (TSAI et al. 1973). Inactivation required only 0.3–3 μM ascorbic acid and was relatively specific since other reducing agents did not work. The importance of this pathway remains to be established. It is possibly related to cyclic AMP-independent pathways for activation of hormone-sensitive lipase which depend upon the oxidation-reduction of the enzyme.

The addition of cyclic AMP and protein kinase to soluble extracts of adipose tissue resulted in the activation of cholesterol ester hydrolase, diglyceride hydrolase, and monoglyceride hydrolase in addition to triglyceride lipase (KHOO et al. 1976). Whether or not these activities are the product of a single hormone-sensitive hydrolase is unclear but the activities do co-purify. However, both the absolute activities and relative degree of activation by protein kinase vary for the different hydrolase activities.

A reciprocal relationship exists between the activity of lipoprotein lipase and hormone-sensitive triglyceride lipase. Lipoprotein lipase is active in the fed state under the influence of insulin; its physiological role is the uptake of circulating triglycerides. In contrast, the hormone-sensitive lipase is involved in the hydrolysis of endogenous triglyceride in the starved state; this enzyme is inhibited by insulin.

The hypothesis that the protein kinase involved in activation of triglyceride lipase has a reciprocal effect on lipoprotein lipase was once popular. This hypothesis was based on analogy to glycogen phosphorylase and glycogen synthase since both enzymes are phosphorylated by protein kinase; phosphorylation results in the activation of glycogen phosphorylase and inactivation of glycogen synthase. However, KHOO et al. (1976) were unable to find any effect of added protein kinase and cyclic AMP on the activity of lipoprotein lipase obtained from chicken adipose tissue.

Lipoprotein lipase activity can be separated from cyclic AMP activated triglyceride lipases by chromatography on heparin-Sepharose columns (KHOO et al. 1976). Antibodies against the lipoprotein lipase had no effect on hormone-sensitive lipase activities. These data indicate that the enzymes responsible are distinct entities. The reciprocal relationship between the two enzymes may involve cyclic AMP-independent pathways which activate hormone-sensitive lipase and inactivate lipoprotein lipase.

VI. Lipoprotein Lipase Regulation

NIKKILÄ and PYKÄLISTÖ (1968) noted that in adipose tissue lipoprotein lipase activity is inversely correlated to free fatty acid accumulation. Possibly, lipoprotein lipase is more sensitive to product inhibition by free fatty acids than is the triacylglycerol lipase activated by lipolytic agents. In the presence of insulin, lipoprotein lipase is active and there is a marked increase in fatty acid esterification, secondary to increased α-glycerophosphate derived from glucose metabolism; these enzymes prevent intracellular accumulation of free fatty acids.

PATTEN (1970) suggested that the accumulation of free fatty acids due to lipolytic hormones inhibited the synthesis of lipoprotein lipase by causing a drop in ATP. More recently, ASHBY et al. (1978) found that, in the presence of cycloheximide, respiratory poisons and lipolytic agents lower ATP and decrease lipoprotein lipase activity; thus, lipolytic agents may actually inactivate lipoprotein lipase. All the available data suggest that high concentrations of lipolytic agents decrease lipoprotein lipase but the mechanisms involved have proven difficult to elucidate.

The activity of lipoprotein lipase may be regulated by the rate of synthesis of a pro-enzyme as well as by post-translational activation through processes involving glycosylation (ASHBY et al. 1978). Insulin may affect synthesis of the enzyme, while glucose may affect glycosylation. This possibility is based on the finding by ASHBY et al. (1978) that insulin does not affect the enzyme activity if protein synthesis is blocked; however, glucose can still activate enzyme activity under these conditions. Since lipoprotein lipase is a glycosylated enzyme (BENSADOUN et al. 1974; IVERIUS and OSTLUND-LINDQVIST 1976) its formation in adipocytes may be linked to the rate of glucose metabolism which is regulated by insulin. This glycosylation may be regulated by insulin secondary to a stimulation of glucose uptake.

The studies on cultured 3T3 mouse fibroblasts during their conversion to adipocytes (ECKEL et al. 1977; WISE and GREEN 1978; SPOONER et al. 1979) suggest that an increase in lipoprotein lipase occurs prior to triglyceride accumulation and may be one of the first markers to 3T3 adipocytes. WISE and GREEN (1978) found that the increase in lipoprotein lipase activity occurred even in the absence of lipoprotein triglycerides in the culture medium. In 3T3 adipocytes, insulin greatly enhances both the lipoprotein lipase activity and the activity of the enzymes for fatty acid synthesis prior to the accumulation of triglyceride.

Possibly in the presence of insulin, synthesis of the enzyme is increased and the acceleration of glucose metabolism results in glycosylation of the enzyme to the active form. This theory suggests that the hexose units used to glycosylate the enzyme are derived from glucose and that formation of glycosylated enzyme is limited by the availability of glucose. The inhibition of lipoprotein lipase activity by fatty acids and lipolytic agents may be due to interference with the formation of the precursors required for glycosylation of the enzyme. This could be due to diversion of glucose metabolites into glyceride-glycerol formation. Lipolytic agents increase the intracellular accumulation of free fatty acids; this increases fatty acid esterification and decreases hexosemonophosphate shunt activity (FAIN and ROSENBERG 1972). Figure 7 summarizes the main features of the proposed hypothesis for the reciprocal regulation of lipoprotein lipase. Future experimentation will decide whether the antagonistic effects of lipolytic agents and insulin on glucose metabolism explain their regulation of lipoprotein lipase. The effects of lipolytic agents may involve cyclic AMP in addition to free fatty acids. FAIN and ROSENBERG (1972) found that lipolytic agents and dibutyryl cyclic AMP inhibited lactate formation from glucose while free fatty acids actually stimulated lactate formation. Free fatty

Regulation of lipoprotein lipase.

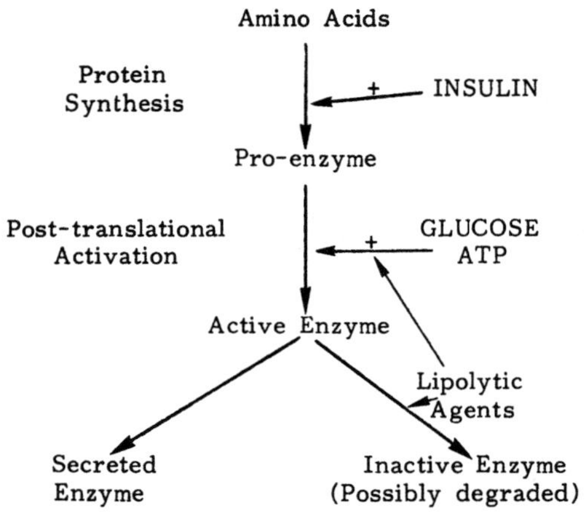

Fig. 7. Regulation of lipoprotein lipase. Active lipoprotein lipase turns over rapidly with a T½ of about 30 min. Lipoprotein lipase like other secretory proteins is synthesized as a largely inactive pro-enzyme which is glycosylated to an active form prior to secretion by adipocytes. Insulin is postulated to increase synthesis of the pro-enzyme while the rate of glucose metabolism regulates glycosylation. Lipolytic agents may inactivate the enzyme or inhibit glycosylation

acids and dibutyryl cyclic AMP inhibited glucose-1-[^{14}C]oxidation and fatty acid synthesis. These results suggest that cyclic AMP inhibits glycolysis independent of any activation of lipolysis.

VII. Role of Cyclic AMP Independent Processes in Triglyceride Breakdown

1. Calcium and Catecholamine Activation of Lipolysis

Lipolytic agents, other than ACTH, do not require extracellular calcium in order to activate lipolysis. LOPEZ et al. (1959), FASSINA and CONTESSA (1967), and SCHIMMEL (1973, 1976) found that the lipolytic action of high concentrations of epinephrine was unaffected by the absence of calcium. However, there is evidence that the response to low concentrations of epinephrine or norepinephrine is depressed in the absence of calcium. FASSINA and CONTESSA (1967) and SCHIMMEL (1973, 1976) found that the lipolytic effect of epinephrine, norepinephrine, isoproterenol or TSH (thyrotropin) was significantly reduced in the absence of calcium but the response to theophylline or dibutyryl cyclic AMP was unaffected. In calcium-free buffer, the increase in cyclic AMP due to low concentrations of epinephrine was totally abolished while the increases in lipolysis were reduced but still significant (SCHIMMEL 1976).

Experiments with A 23187, the divalent calcium ionophore, minimize the importance of calcium in lipolysis. FAIN and BUTCHER (1976) and HALES et al. (1977) did not detect any effects of A 23187 on lipolysis or cyclic AMP metabolism in the presence of catecholamines. The ionophore A 23187 had little effect on fat cell phosphorylase a activity but did decrease glycogen synthase activity by a mechanism similar to that for α-adrenergic agonists (LAWRENCE and LARNER 1978b). There is no evidence that A 23187 has any appreciable effect on cyclic AMP accumulation by rat adipocytes (LAWRENCE and LARNER 1978b; HALES et al. 1977).

2. Calcium, Phospholipase A_2 Activation, and the Lipolytic Action of ACTH

The presence of calcium is required for ACTH activation of lipolysis (LOPEZ et al. 1959), the elevation of cyclic AMP by low concentrations of ACTH in rat adipocytes (KUO 1970), and activation of adenylate cyclase in rat adipocyte ghosts (BÄR and HECHTER 1969; BIRNBAUMER and RODBELL 1969). Futhermore, if fat cells are perifused for 30 min with catecholamines or ACTH the rate of lipolysis rapidly returns to basal values after removal of epinephrine but remains elevated after the removal of ACTH (KATOCS et al. 1974). The elevated lipolysis due to prior exposure to ACTH is rapidly reduced to control values by changing to calcium-free buffer.

WONG et al. (1978) suggested that all effects of ACTH are mediated through cyclic AMP; however they found that low concentrations of ACTH accelerated lipolysis without affecting total cyclic AMP accumulation. The data presented by WONG et al. (1978) demonstrate that measurements of total cyclic AMP in fat cells do not always correlate with lipolysis. This can be interpreted as indicating that a very small part of the total pool of cyclic AMP is involved in the regulation of lipolysis in fat cells. The data of WONG et al. (1978) do not prove or disprove the presence of a cyclic AMP-independent pathway for activation of lipolysis by ACTH. However, the data with ACTH analogs support the concept of a cyclic AMP-independent pathway (LANG et al. 1976). LANG et al. (1976) reported that the N(α-benzyloxycarbonyl)derivative of ACTH lacking the first six amino acids ($ACTH_{7-24}$) was able to stimulate adenylate cyclase activity of rat fat cell ghosts to the same extent as ACTH lacking the first four amino acids ($ACTH_{5-24}$). However, only $ACTH_{5-24}$ was able to increase lipolysis in intact fat cells (LANG et al. 1976). Possibly $ACTH_{5-24}$ is readily inactivated by fat cell ghosts but not by intact fat cells. However, it seems more likely that ACTH activation of lipolysis involves, in addition to cyclic AMP, a Ca^{2+}-dependent process. The concept of ACTH as a dual effector was first suggested by CARCHMAN et al. (1971) to explain the effects of ACTH on the adrenal gland. Definition of a dual effector system for ACTH has been difficult because an elevation in cyclic AMP is sufficient to activate lipolysis or steroidogenesis. The alternative pathway "X" may be more important in the presence of low concentrations of ACTH where there is no detectable elevation in cyclic AMP. SCHWYZER (1978) has suggested that cyclic AMP is necessary but insufficient to account for the action of ACTH.

The calcium-dependency for ACTH action does not involve binding of hormone to receptor. The binding of tritiated ACTH to rat fat cell ghosts was unaffected by the absence of calcium (LANG and SCHWYZER 1976). Similar observations were reported for the binding of ACTH to adrenal cells (LEFKOWITZ et al. 1970). These data suggest that calcium is more likely to be involved in the ability of the hormone-receptor complexes to regulate metabolism than in hormone binding to receptors.

LAYCHOCK et al. (1977) suggested that the cyclic AMP-dependent process in which ACTH acts on the adrenal may involve activation of phospholipases. For a while it was thought that the increase in prostaglandin E formation by adrenal cells in the presence of ACTH might account for steroidogenesis. However, inhibition of the formation of prostaglandins with indomethacin does not affect ACTH-induced steroidogenesis (RUBIN and LAYCHOCK 1978). Rather it appears that the prostaglandins are formed because of an increase in free arachidonic acid release due to increased breakdown of phospholipids. Possibly the primary event is an increase in phospholipase activity which results in the release of arachidonic acid. SCHREY and RUBIN (1979) found that ACTH selectively increased turnover of arachidonic acid linked to phosphatidylinositol. This suggests that ACTH activates a phospholipase C specific for phosphatidylinositol which results in release of arachidonic acid and elevation of cytosol Ca^{2+}.

LEWIS et al. (1979) recently reported that the addition of ACTH to rabbit adipocyte ghosts increased the release of arachidonic acid from phospholipids. Whether ACTH activated phospholipase A_2 or phospholipase C remains to be demonstrated. However, we have been unable to see any effect of ACTH on formation of lysophospholipids in rat or hamster adipocytes (unpublished studies, 1980).

3. Regulation of Lipolysis via Substrate Availability

WISE and JUNGAS (1978) suggested that a cyclic AMP-independent pathway exists for the activation of lipolysis by catecholamines. They found that homogenates prepared from adipose tissue previously exposed to epinephrine had a markedly enhanced breakdown of endogenous substrate. The soluble supernatant derived from these homogenates did not demonstrate any elevation in the rate at which added exogenous triolein emulsion was hydrolyzed. However, the addition of beef heart protein kinase along with ATP and cyclic AMP increased the ability of the adipose tissue soluble supernatant to hydrolyze exogenous triolein. WISE and JUNGAS (1978) found that a factor is formed in response to catecholamines which associates with endogenous substrate and facilitates its breakdown by triacylglycerol lipase (Fig. 6). This factor could be a phospholipid or a protein like colipase (BLÄCKBERG et al. 1979).

Melittin is an amphipathic polypeptide containing 26 amino acid residues which is the main lytic factor present in bee venom (HABERMANN 1972). The hydrolysis of unsonicated liposomes of egg phosphatidylcholine by phospholipase A_2 is markedly enhanced by the addition of melittin (YUNES et al. 1977). Melittin apparently binds to phospholipids provided the lipid is the fluid state (MOLLAY and KREIL 1973, 1974). SESSA et al. (1969) initially suggested that melittin effects upon biomembranes are due to alterations in the arrangement of membrane phospholipids. Possibly the alterations in structure increase the access of phospholipids to cytosol phospholipase A_2 which results in the formation of lysophospholipids. The cytotoxic effects of melittin on cells may be due to increased permeability of the membrane as the result of the loss of key phospholipids and accumulation of lysophospholipids. SHIER (1979) has shown that melittin addition to cultured cells resulted in the activation of endogenous phospholipase A_2 activity. However, in adipocytes pure melittin, even at concentrations toxic to the cells, does not result in the accumulation of appreciable amounts of lysophospholipids (FAIN et al. 1981). In fact, melittin was toxic to adipocytes even in the absence of Ca^{2+} where no detectable accumulation of lysophospholipids in cells or medium can be demonstrated.

The presence of phospholipase A_2 activity (pH optimum of around 8) in fat cell homogenates was originally demonstrated by DE CINGOLANI et al. (1972) who also found that the addition of 1 mg/ml of cyclic AMP increased the activity in homogenates. In contrast, BEREZIAT et al. (1978) suggested that insulin activates phospholipase A_2 in adipocytes. FAIN et al. (1981) found no evidence that melittin was an insulin-like agent with respect to either inhibition of lipolysis or stimulation of glucose oxidation. Furthermore, adipocytes seem to have very low amounts of phospholipase A_2 since little accumulation of lysophospholipids can be detected in fat cells. In fact, with concentrations of melittin which cause appreciable breakdown of phosphatidylcholine or phosphatidylethanolamine there is very little accumulation of lysophospholipids (FAIN et al. 1981). Apparently the phospholipase A_1 activity is appreciable in relationship to A_2 and there is complete breakdown of the phospholipids. The initial impetus for the hypothesis of BEREZIAT et al. (1978) probably arose from the findings of BLECHER (1967, 1969) and RODBELL et al. (1968), who demonstrated that addition of lysophospholipids or phospholipase A_2 to fat cells incubated in the absence of albumin was able to mimic the stimulation of glucose metabolism and inhibition of lipolysis by insulin. However, BLECHER (1967) pointed out that the increase in glucose oxidation was not seen in the presence of albumin which presumably bound the lysophospholipids and blocked their detergent-like activation of glucose oxidation.

B. Catecholamine Activation of Thermogenesis in Brown Adipose Tissue via Cyclic Nucleotides

Brown fat is readily distinguished from white fat by the presence of many mitochondria containing tightly packed cristae and multiple lipid droplets. The large number of mitochondria is related to the thermogenic function of brown fat. In white fat, the fatty acids released during lipolysis are utilized by other tissues; in brown fat, the fatty acids formed during lipolysis are directly oxidized. Fatty acids are mobilized from white fat by caloric deprivation; in contrast, lipolysis in brown fat is activated by a drop in ambient temperature. Catecholamines are the primary signal for the acceleration of lipolysis and respiration by brown fat in cold-stressed animals. A model for activation of thermogenesis in brown adipocytes is depicted in Fig. 8.

I. Role of the Na^+/K^+ Plasma Membrane Pump in Thermogenic Action of Catecholamines

In brown fat the thermogenic action of catecholamines involves an uncoupling of oxidative phosphorylation by mitochondria which occurs secondary to activation of triglyceride breakdown by cyclic AMP. However, GIRARDIER et al. (1968) and

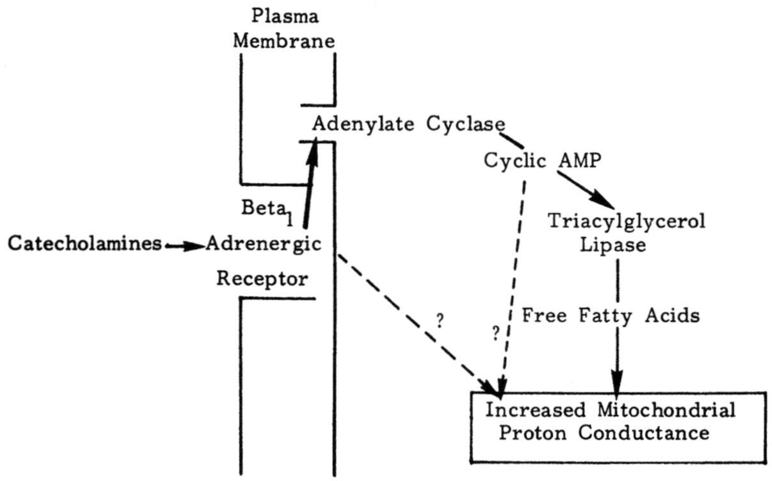

Fig. 8. A 1980 model for the thermogenic action of catecholamines on brown adipose tissue. Catecholamines are postulated to interact with β_1-adrenergic receptors in the plasma membrane of brown adipocytes which results in activation of adenylate cyclase. The resulting increase in cyclic AMP activates protein kinase which convert inactive to active triacylglycerol lipase. The free fatty acids provide substrate for mitochondrial oxidation and also uncouple mitochondrial oxidative phosphorylation by increasing the proton conductance of the inner mitochondrial membrane. The figure also depicts the possibility that cyclic AMP might directly bind to or increase the phosphorylation of mitochondrial membrane proteins which regulate proton conductance. There is also the possibility that the catecholamine-receptor complex activates other processes which are involved in lipolysis and thermogenesis

HORWITZ (1973) postulated that an increase in energy utilization for active ion transport across the plasma membrane of brown adipocytes might account for the thermogenic action of catecholamines. More recently, HORWITZ (1979) suggested that the catecholamine-receptor complex regulates mitochondrial proton conductance through generation of a signal which is related to the activity of the Na^+/K^+ membrane pump. I believe that the plasma membrane Na^+/K^+ membrane pump regulates the intracellular K^+ concentration which plays a permissive but not regulatory function in catecholamine-induced thermogenesis. The inhibition of thermogenesis by ouabain is due to a decreased activation of adenylate cyclase by catecholamines and the unique K^+ permeability of brown adipocyte mitochondria.

FAIN et al. (1973b) and HERD et al. (1973) using brown adipocytes from rats and HORWITZ (1973) using brown adipocytes from hamsters observed that 1 m*M* ouabain was able to inhibit catecholamine-activated respiration. FAIN et al. (1973b) also noted that ouabain markedly inhibited the rise in cyclic AMP accumulation of rat brown adipocytes; the decreased accumulation of cyclic AMP could account for the inhibition of lypolysis and oxygen consumption. In contrast, ouabain did not inhibit the increase in respiration stimulated by fatty acids or theophylline. Previously, REED and FAIN (1968b) found that omission of K^+ prevented the increase in respiration stimulated by fatty acids or lipolytic agents; in the absence of K^+, high concentrations of lipolytic agents caused appreciable lipolysis without an increase in respiration. NICHOLLS and LINDBERG (1973) found that mitochondria from hamster brown adipose tissue are much more permeable to K^+

than are liver mitochondria. FLATMARK and PEDERSEN (1975) suggested that, in view of the unique permeability of brown adipocyte mitochondria to K^+, a high level of K^+ is required for fatty acids or lipolytic agents to increase respiration. This would explain the finding that under certain conditions the stimulation of respiration by added fatty acids or cyclic AMP analogs is inhibited by ouabain (HORWITZ 1973). I believe that the drop in cytosol K^+ due to inhibition of Na^+/K^+ plasma membrane pump by ouabain accounts for the inhibitory effects of ouabain on respiration; I do not believe that an appreciable part of the catecholamine-induced thermogenesis is secondary to an increase in cytosol K^+ due to activation of the Na^+/K^+ membrane pump. GIRARDIER and SEYDOUX (1971) found an influx of Na^+ and efflux of K^+ after the addition of catecholamines to brown adipocytes; the efflux of K^+ may oppose the thermogenic action of catecholamines and act as a feedback signal. However, GIRARDIER and SEYDOUX (1971) found that in phosphate buffer catecholamines could stimulate respiration without affecting the membrane potential or the intracellular K^+ content.

II. Mitochondrial Uncoupling by Fatty Acids in the Regulation of Thermogenesis

The hypothesis that free fatty acids mediate the thermogenic action of catecholamines is depicted in Fig. 8. The figure also indicates alternative mechanisms by which catecholamines could uncouple mitochondrial oxidative phosphorylation through a direct action of cyclic AMP on mitochondria or a cyclic AMP-independent mechanism involving unknown second messengers. REED and FAIN (1970) suggested that free fatty acids provide the substrate for the increase in mitochondrial oxygen consumption and act as uncoupling agents via a K^+-dependent process. REED and FAIN (1968b), using rat brown adipocytes, and PRUSINER et al. (1968), using hamster adipocytes, found that fatty acids mimicked the increase in respiration caused by lipolytic agents.

The most probable mechanism for uncoupling of oxidative phosphorylation in brown fat mitochondria by fatty acids is a short circuiting of the proton conductance involved in oxidative phosphorylation (NICHOLLS 1976, 1977; HEATON et al. 1978). The hypothesis of MITCHELL (1979) links proton entry, driven by the respiratory chain to ATP formation via adenosine triphosphatase. In brown adipocytes, such a mechanism operates under basal conditions, but hormones activate a unique, controllable pathway of proton conductance across the inner mitochondrial membrane and permit respiration to occur without ATP synthesis. In effect, fatty acids collapse the proton-electrochemical gradient across the inner mitochondria membrane in a similar fashion to classical uncouplers, such as FCCP and dinitrophenol.

HEATON et al. (1978) have shown that the 32,000-M_r protein, with a high-affinity binding site for nucleotides, accounts for 10% of the protein of inner membrane of mitochondria from hamster brown fat; this protein is absent from liver mitochondria. This protein may be involved in the uncoupling action of free fatty acids or other messengers during catecholamine-activated thermogenesis. The nucleotide-binding protein may enable the uniport to change from a potential-dependent uniport, with low conductance, to a high-conductance, ion uniport allowing H^+ to cross the inner mitochondrial membrane without obligatory ATP synthesis.

Brown fat mitochondria also have a low ATPase activity and limited capacity to increase respiration in response to added ADP (LINDBERG et al. 1976; DRAHOTA and HOUSTEK 1976). Brown fat mitochondria apparently have a high respiratory rate but only a limited capacity to synthesize ATP. Additionally, the coupling of proton motive force to ATP formation is readily disrupted by uncoupling agents including fatty acids.

Brown fat mitochondria are isolated in an uncoupled state even if isolation procedures resulting in tightly coupled liver mitochondria are used. GUILLORY and RACKER (1968) found that the addition of albumin resulted in tightly coupled brown adipocyte mitochondria; albumin was thought to bind free fatty acids which were uncoupling the mitochondria. Under certain conditions, the addition of nucleotide di- or triphosphates is required in addition to albumin. Subsequently, tightly coupled mitochondria were obtained if endogenous fatty acids were removed by the addition of carnitine plus ATP (DRAHOTA et al. 1968). The unique features of brown adipocyte mitochondria have been reviewed by FLATMARK and PEDERSEN (1975) and by NICHOLLS (1976).

Fatty acids may be the physiological uncouplers as proposed by REED and FAIN (1968 b), PRUSINER et al. (1968) and more recently affirmed by LINDBERG et al. (1976). However, NICHOLS (1977) has raised two objections to this hypothesis. First, BIEBER et al. (1975) failed to see an increase, over the high basal values, for cell-associated free fatty acids after the additions of catecholamines. However, the important concern is the fraction of total intracellular fatty acids which is free, rather than bound to intracellular proteins; the latter is so large that it is difficult to demonstrate an increase in the free pool. In fact, BIEBER et al. (1975) found the total intracellular free fatty acid concentration to be around 20 mM; palmitate, at a concentration of 3 µM, was required to stimulate respiration half-maximally in isolated brown adipocyte mitochondria. The second objection of NICHOLLS (1977) was based on his conclusion from the report by PRUSINER et al. (1968) that high concentrations of fatty acids were required to stimulate cells respiration. In fact, BIEBER et al. (1975) found that the addition of palmitate to fatty acid-free albumin, yielding a molar ratio of fatty acid to albumin of only 0.25, was able to markedly potentiate respiration in the presence of epinephrine. REED and FAIN (1968 b) originally reported that the addition of palmitate to medium containing fatty acid-free albumin, at a molar ratio of fatty acid to albumin of 4, was able to stimulate respiration over a four hour incubation. REED and FAIN (1968 a) had failed to see any effect of palmitate on respiration when the molar ratio of fatty acid to albumin was 5.8; however, such conditions abolished the lipolytic action of added catecholamines. The triglyceride lipase of white adipocytes is inhibited at molar ratios of fatty acid to albumin above 3; furthermore, feedback regulation of adenylate cyclase is observed under these conditions (FAIN and SHEPHERD 1975). I conclude that acceleration of respiration is caused by very low concentrations of free fatty acids; but other factors may be involved as well.

Free fatty acids mimic the enhanced thermogenesis caused by lipolytic agents. Cyclic AMP could also directly uncouple mitochondrial respiration and provide substrate for oxidation secondary to activation of triacylglycerol lipase; both effects of cyclic AMP could be mediated through protein kinase if phosphorylated proteins were to regulate proton conductance in mitochondria. Alternatively, cyclic AMP might bind directly to nucleotide-binding proteins which regulate proton conductance.

III. Cyclic AMP as the Mediator of Catecholamine-Activated Lipolysis

In brown fat, catecholamines interact with a β_1-adrenergic receptor and activate triacylglycerol lipase through cyclic AMP. The dibutyryl derivative of cyclic AMP activates lipolysis and respiration in rat brown adipocytes (REED and FAIN 1968a). Catecholamines elevate cyclic AMP in brown adipocytes from rat (FAIN et al. 1973b) or hamster (HITTELMAN et al. 1974), and brown adipose tissue from rabbit (KNIGHT 1974). In rat adipocytes (in the presence of ouabain) and in rabbit brown fat (in the presence of propranolol or insulin), catecholamines activate lipolysis without any detectable increases in cyclic AMP. This suggests that either the active pool of cyclic AMP is a small part of the total intracellular cyclic AMP or that something else, besides cyclic AMP, is involved in the activation of lipolysis. Protein kinase is present in brown adipose tissue; the extent of its activation correlates well with lipolysis and cyclic AMP concentrations (SKALA and KNIGHT 1977).

C. Calcium, Cyclic Nucleotides, and Glycogen Synthase Regulation

I. Calcium-Dependent Regulation of Glycogen Metabolism by Alpha$_1$-Catecholamins

Stimulation of the α_1-adrenergic receptor of the rat adipocyte activates glycogen phosphorylase through cyclic AMP-independent mechanisms (LAWRENCE and LARNER 1977, 1978b); such stimulation also inactivates glycogen synthase I activity (GARCIA-SAINZ and FAIN 1980b). The α-adrenergic inactivation of glycogen synthase was abolished in the absence of extracellular calcium and was mimicked by the ionophore A 23187 (LAWRENCE and LARNER 1978b). However, glycogen phosphorylase, cyclic AMP accumulation and lipolysis in rat adipocytes are not affected by the ionophore A 23187 and are independent of extracellular calcium (LAWRENCE and LARNER 1977, 1978b). This suggests that calcium is probably not the putative "X" intermediate postulated as the mediator of cyclic AMP independent activation of lipolysis and glycogenolysis (Fig. 6). Effects of calcium on glycogen phosphorylase in adipose tissue may be mediated through regulation of phosphorylase kinase, a calcium dependent enzyme (KHOO 1976).

II. Relationship Between Alpha$_1$-Adrenergic Stimulation of Phosphatidylinositol Turnover and Ca^{2+}

STEIN and HALES (1972) first demonstrated that α-adrenergic stimulation enhances [^{32}P]incorporation into phosphatidylinositol and phosphatidic acid in adipose tissue. GARCIA-SAINZ and FAIN (1980a) confirmed this finding and established that the receptors involved are of the α_1-subtype. This conclusion was based on the potency of adrenergic antagonists (prazosin»phentolamine > yohimbine) and the ability of methoxamine, but not clonidine, to increase phosphatidylinositol turnover. Similar results have been seen in rat pineal glands where prazosin was a potent inhibitor of the catecholamine-induced increases in phosphatidylinositol synthesis (SMITH et al. 1979).

The α-adrenergic increase in phosphatidylinositol labeling by adipocytes occurs in Ca^{2+}-free medium containing EGTA (GARCIA-SAINZ and FAIN 1980 a); in other tissues, it does not appear to be secondary to entry of extracellular Ca^{2+} (MICHELL 1975, 1979; BERRIDGE and FAIN 1979; FAIN and BERRIDGE 1979). Alternatively, catecholamine effects on Ca^{2+} gating and phosphatidylinositol metabolism may be independent. However, there is a close association between α-adrenergic regulation of phosphatidylinositol turnover and Ca^{2+} entry in many systems (MICHELL 1975, 1979; MICHELL et al. 1977; JONES and MICHELL 1978).

STEIN and HALES (1974) found that insulin increased the incorporation of phosphate into rat adipocyte phospholipids, which was attributed to an increase in the specific radioactivity of ATP. Similar results were obtained by GARCIA-SAINZ and FAIN (1980 a) using adipocytes incubated in Ca^{2+}-containing or in Ca^{2+}-free buffers. However, GARCIA-SAINZ and FAIN (1980 a) found that in medium containing 1 m*M* EGTA plus 2.6 m*M* Ca^{2+} insulin did not, but α-catecholamines did, increase the labeling of phosphatidylinositol. Their results indicate that α-adrenergic agonists increase phosphatidylinositol labeling by mechanisms separate from those involved in any effect of insulin on phospholipid labeling.

GARCIA-SAINZ and FAIN (1980 b) found that thyroid status had little influence on $[^{32}P]P_i$ incorporation into phosphatidylinositol stimulated by α-catecholamines. Similar results were also seen with respect to glycogen synthase inactivation which they found to be an α_1-catecholamine effect. The suggestion by KUNOS (1977) that β-adrenoceptors are converted to α-adrenoreceptors does not appear to be applicable to the situation in rat adipocytes. It is striking that hypothyroidism selectively inhibited the ability of β-catecholamines and insulin to affect cyclic AMP metabolism and glycogen synthase.

The effects of α- and β-adrenergic regulation in fat cells are summarized in Fig. 5. β-Effects of catecholamines are associated with activation of adenylate cyclase and cyclic AMP activates triglyceride lipase. α_2-Adrenergic effects are secondary to a non-specific inhibition of adenylate cyclase. α_1-Adrenergic effects may involve increased entry of extracellular calcium and possibly the release of bound or "trigger" calcium within cells through a mechanism involving breakdown of phosphatidylinositol. The elevation in cytosol calcium or cyclic AMP results in inactivation of glycogen synthase. However, calcium and cyclic AMP may not account for all the effects of catecholamines on fat cells.

D. Mode of Insulin Action Through Cyclic Nucleotides, Ca^{2+} and Special Mediators

The mechanisms involved in insulin action remain unknown despite all the research over the 60 years since the discovery of insulin. No unique second messenger for insulin has yet been isolated. Insulin affects a bewildering array of enzymatic reactions; it has been difficult to separate causes from effects. Whatever is currently in style in biochemical investigations has been invoked to explain insulin action. In the 1940's insulin was thought to directly alter hexokinase and other enzymes in a fashion similar to that of coenzymes. In the 1950's great emphasis was placed on the ability of insulin to directly alter membrane transport of glucose; all effects of insulin were thought to be secondary to this process. In the 1960's emphasis was placed on regulation of protein and RNA synthesis; insulin was found to affect these processes. The 1970's were the decade for cyclic nucleotides and Ca^{2+}; under appropriate conditions, insulin alters the intracellular concentration of cyclic AMP, cyclic GMP or Ca^{2+}. The 1980's emphasis remains to be seen but will probably represent renewed activity in elucidating the mechanisms by which insulin affects hexose transport and intracellular enzymatic processes through unique second messengers.

The literature on insulin action is so extensive as to be overwhelming. The literature prior to 1970 is reviewed by KRAHL (1961) and STEINER and FREINKEL (1972). Several specialized review articles with emphasis on insulin action in adipocytes have been published (FAIN 1974; JUNGAS 1975; CZECH 1977, 1980, 1981).

No hormone appears to be more important in the regulation of adipocyte metabolism than insulin. The increase in fatty acid release by adipocytes during fasting may result from a drop in plasma insulin rather than to an elevation in lipolytic hormones. In the transition from the starved to the fed state, insulin shifts the adipocyte from the release of lipid to the uptake of lipid. Insulin inhibits fatty acid release both by inhibiting lipolysis and by stimulating re-esterification of fatty acids with α-glycerophosphate derived from glucose metabolism. Insulin also activates the steps involved in uptake of plasma lipoproteins by adipocytes.

I. Insulin Action on Adipocytes. Regulation of Glycogen Synthase and Pyruvate Dehydrogenase

The effects of anabolic hormones such as insulin are antagonistic to those of catabolic hormones such as catecholamines. Much of our thinking about mode of insulin action has been colored by the discovery that cyclic AMP serves as a second messenger for the β-adrenergic effects of catecholamines. However, a second messenger for insulin has not been discovered. The effects of insulin have been attributed to a reduction in cyclic AMP accumulation; a simple view is that insulin lowers, and catecholamines elevate cyclic AMP. However, insulin can regulate five enzymes in adipocytes (Table 1). Effects 1 and 2 directly lower cyclic AMP through inhibition of its formation and stimulation of its degradation. The inhibition of cyclic AMP-dependent protein kinase is independent of the first two effects and blocks cyclic AMP action. The fourth and fifth effects could involve cyclic AMP-independent phosphorylation of proteins or activation of phosphoprotein phosphatases. Whether all five of these effects are involved in the physiological regulation of adipocyte metabolism remains to be established. All the effects depicted in Table 1 are independent of insulin action on hexose entry. However, insulin-stimulated uptake of glucose results in increases in fatty acid synthesis, fatty acid re-esterification and activation of glycogen synthase phosphatase.

Table 1. Adipocyte enzymes affected by Insulin

1. Inhibition of Adenylate Cyclase (Illiano and Cuatrecasas 1972; Hepp and Renner 1972)
2. Activation of Cyclic AMP Phosphodiesterase (Loten and Sneyd 1970; Manganiello and Vaughan 1973; Zinman and Hollenberg 1974; Sakai et al. 1974; Solomon 1975; Kono et al. 1975)
3. Inhibition of the Activation of Cyclic AMP-Dependent Protein Kinase (Guinovart et al. 1978; Walkenbach et al. 1978)[a]
4. Activation of Mitochondrial Pyruvate Dehydrogenase (Coore et al. 1971; Taylor et al. 1973; Weiss et al. 1971; Seals and Jarett 1980), Glycogen Synthase (Lawrence and Larner 1978a, b; Larner et al. 1978), and Acetyl CoA Carboxylase (Halestrop and Denton 1973)[a]
5. Phosphorylation of ATP Citrate Lyase (Alexander et al. 1979; Ramakrishna and Benjamin 1979)[a]

[a] These effects are independent of cyclic nucleotides and Ca^{2+} and may be mediated through a peptide messenger generated in the presence of insulin

Table 2. Regulation of Adipocyte Glycogen Synthase

1. Activated by insulin through a mechanism independent of Ca^{2+} or cyclic nucleotides
2. Inhibited by an elevation of cyclic AMP in the presence of beta-adrenergic agonists
3. Inhibited by an elevation in cytosol Ca^{2+} due to α_1-adrenergic agonists or the calcium ionophore A-23187

It has been difficult to demonstrate an association between insulin effects on cyclic AMP accumulation and adipocyte metabolism. Fain and Rosenberg (1972); Khoo et al. (1973); Knight and Iliffe (1973; Fain (1977) and Fain et al. (1979) observed antilipolytic effects of insulin under circumstances in which cyclic AMP was unaffected. Under appropriate conditions, an inhibition of cyclic AMP accumulation by insulin can be demonstrated (Jungas 1966; Butcher et al. 1966; Desai et al. 1973; Kono and Barham 1973; Siddle and Hales 1974). However, the inhibition by insulin of cyclic AMP elevation by lipolytic agents is far smaller than that of agents such as adenosine, prostaglandins of the E series or nicotinic acid (Fain 1974, 1977, 1980; Wieser and Fain 1975). I view adenosine and prostaglandins of the E series as being primarily inhibitors of cyclic AMP accumulation; I feel insulin works through regulation of cyclic AMP action and mechanisms independent of cyclic AMP.

The stimulation of glycogen synthase by insulin is an excellent example of both the cyclic AMP-dependent and the cyclic AMP-independent actions of insulin. Three major mechanisms by which adipocyte glycogen synthase is regulated are presented in Table 2 which is based on the work of Lawrence et al. (1977) and Lawrence and Larner (1977, 1978a, b). The inhibition of glycogen synthase by β-adrenergic agonists is mediated through cyclic AMP activation of protein kinase which phosphorylates active glycogen synthase, converting it to a relatively inactive form. The inhibition by α-adrenergic agonists results from elevated cytosol Ca^{2+} which increases calcium-dependent protein phosphorylation of synthase. Insulin activates glycogen synthase through at least three different mechanisms. Insulin increases glucose entry and conversion to glucose-6-phosphate which is able

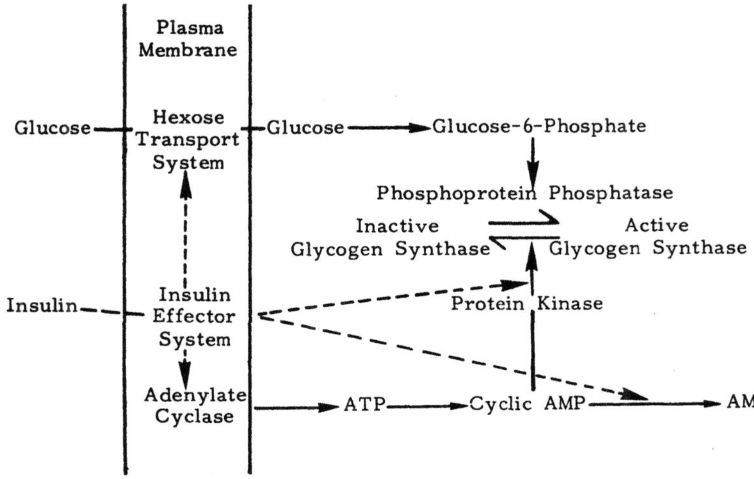

Fig. 9. Insulin regulation of adipocyte glycogen synthase. Insulin is postulated to react with an effector system which results in activation of hexose transport and inhibition of adenylate cyclase in plasma membrane. A putative second messenger is formed which activates cyclic AMP phosphodiesterase and inhibits cyclic AMP-dependent protein kinase conversion of active to inactive glycogen synthase. The effects of insulin on phosphoprotein phosphatase are primarily mediated through changes in the levels of glucose-6-phosphate but there may be other effects as well

to activate the enzymes (LAWRENCE and LARNER 1978 a). Insulin also increases glycogen synthase in the absence of glucose; this effect may involve both cyclic AMP-dependent and cyclic AMP-independent effects unrelated to Ca^{2+} (LAWRENCE and LARNER 1978 b). Possible sites at which insulin regulates glycogen synthase are depicted in Fig. 9.

In adipocytes, activation of glycogen synthase is not secondary to inactivation of glycogen phosphorylase (LAWRENCE and LARNER 1978 a). The effects of insulin involving increased formation of glucose-6-phosphate can be mimicked by other factors which increase glucose uptake by adipocytes such as H_2O_2 or concanavalin A. However, the activation of glycogen synthase due to insulin in the absence of glucose was not duplicated by concanavalin A (LAWRENCE and LARNER 1978 a). In contrast, SEALS and JARETT (1980) found that concanavalin A could mimic the insulin activation of pyruvate dehydrogenase in intact adipocytes. The discrepancies could be due to separate glucose-independent mechanisms for regulation of glycogen synthase and pyruvate dehydrogenase.

The regulation by insulin of mitochondrial pyruvate dehydrogenase is as complex as the regulation of glycogen synthase. Insulin activates, and lipolytic agents inhibit, pyruvate dehydrogenase, the antagonism does not appear to involve cyclic AMP. The activation by insulin of pyruvate dehydrogenase involves effects independent of, but also secondary to, hexose uptake. Figure 10 outlines various possibilities for pyruvate dehydrogenase regulation by insulin. The most interesting aspect of this enzyme is its location in the mitochondria; effects of insulin must involve second messengers formed as a result of an interaction with the plasma membrane.

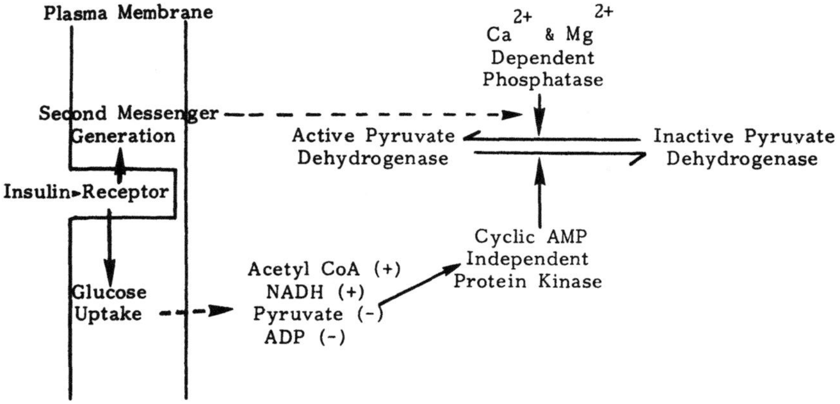

Fig. 10. Regulation of adipocyte pyruvate dehydrogenase by insulin. The regulation of pyruvate dehydrogenase by insulin may involve activation of a phosphatase through an unknown messenger and inhibition of a cyclic AMP-independent protein kinase. This protein kinase may be activated by increases in acetyl CoA or NADH and inhibited by increases in pyruvate or ADP

Regulation of pyruvate dehydrogenase is thought to be controlled by phosphorylation of the α-subunit with a cyclic AMP-independent protein kinase (Denton and Hughes 1978). The inactive, phosphorylated form of the enzyme is activated by a Mg^{2+} and Ca^{2+}-dependent phosphatase. There is end product inhibition of the pyruvate dehydrogenase and of the kinase by NADH and acetyl CoA. Thus, changes in the ratio of the products to the substrates (expressed as the $NADH/NAD^{+}$ or acetyl CoA/CoA) appears to be the major site of regulation.

Regulation of pyruvate dehydrogenase is of physiological significance because the conversion of pyruvate to acetyl CoA is essentially irreversible in mammals. Thus, the activity of this enzyme must be reduced to low levels during starvation in order to prevent loss of carbohydrate reserves. In the fed state, the pyruvate dehydrogenase complex converts pyruvate to acetyl CoA which is oxidized via the citric acid cycle as in muscle, brain, and kidney. However, in tissues such as liver and adipose tissue much of the acetyl CoA is used for formation of triglycerides. In conditions associated with reduced lipogenesis (such as starvation, diabetes or high fat diet) there is a marked reduction in pyruvate dehydrogenase activity (Denton et al. 1978). Dichloroacetate is an analog of pyruvate which like insulin activates pyruvate dehydrogenase (White-House and Randle 1973). However, there are marked differences between the two agents; the activation by dichloroacetate was blocked by fatty acid addition to adipocytes, while that due to insulin was not affected (Sooranna and Saggerson 1979).

The activation by insulin of pyruvate dehydrogenase due to increased glucose metabolism may result from a decrease in intracellular fatty acids secondary to increased re-esterification and inhibition of lipolysis. Palmitate, at concentrations sufficient to give a final FFA/albumin ratio between 1 and 3, markedly inhibited pyruvate dehydrogenase; this effect could be reversed by insulin in the presence of glucose (Sooranna and Saggerson 1979). The insulin protection was primarily due to an acceleration of fatty acid esterification with α-glycerophosphate derived from glucose. No effect of insulin on fatty acid inhibition was noted in the absence of glucose (SOORANNA and SAGGERSON 1975).

Agents such as nicotinic acid or prostaglandin E_1 inhibit lipolysis and cyclic AMP accumulation and do not appreciably stimulate glucose uptake by adipocytes; however they are able to activate pyruvate dehydrogenase (TAYLOR et al. 1973). This suggests that, under appropriate conditions, the anti-lipolytic action of insulin could contribute to activation of pyruvate dehydrogenase.

One mechanism by which pyruvate dehydrogenase can be activated is by uncoupling agents which lower mitochondrial ATP. However, insulin activation of mitochondrial pyruvate dehydrogenase is not accompanied by any change in ATP/ADP ratio (PAETZKE-BRUNNER et al. 1978). However, insulin activation was associated with a marked drop in the mitochondrial acetyl-CoA/CoASH ratio from 0.69 to 0.20. There were also significant increases in CoA-SH in the cytosol and mitochondria, but acetyl CoA only increased in the cytosol (PAETZKE-BRUNNER et al. 1978).

DENTON and HUGHES (1978) reported that adipocytes incorporate labelled inorganic phosphate into the α-subunit of pyruvate dehydrogenase and net incorporation is markedly decreased in the presence of insulin. SEALS et al. (1979 a, b) obtained similar results in a system containing mitochondria and plasma membranes of rat adipocytes. The decrease in phosphorylation of pyruvate dehydrogenase was not seen after the addition of insulin to purified mitochondria. Interestingly, the effect of insulin was unaltered by the absence or presence of Ca^{2+} in the buffer. SEALS and JARETT (1980) subsequently demonstrated that insulin addition to plasma membranes incubated with mitochondria activated pyruvate dehydrogenase. The effect of insulin could be mimicked by concanavalin A and antiinsulin receptor antibody; and the effect of insulin did not occur if only mitochondria were present.

These results suggest that interaction of insulin or other agents with the plasma membrane of adipocytes results in formation of a chemical mediator which alters mitochondrial pyruvate dehydrogenase; it is unlikely that this mediator is a cyclic nucleotide or Ca^{2+}. JARETT and SEALS (1979) have shown that the putative second messenger for insulin obtained from muscle by LARNER et al. (1979) activated adipocyte mitochondrial pyruvate dehydrogenase. The isolation of the insulin second messenger, as a pure substance, and the elucidation of its structure will advance our understanding of mode of insulin action.

SEALS and JARETT (1980) suggested that insulin activates a phosphatase since the insulin effect on pyruvate dehydrogenase activity was observed in the absence of added ATP. The available data are compatible with the suggestions of SICA and CUATRECASAS (1973) and of MUKHERJEE and JUNGAS (1975) that insulin caused a persistent activation of pyruvate dehydrogenase phosphatase activity in mitochondria of adipose tissue.

II. Insulin, Cyclic GMP, and Calcium

ILLIANO et al. (1973), FAIN and BUTCHER (1976) and VYDELINGUM et al. (1978) found that insulin elevated the level of adipocyte cyclic GMP. However, no known effect of insulin on adipocyte metabolism is mediated by cyclic GMP. Norepinephrine, carbachol, the divalent cation ionophore, A 23187, and added free fatty acids all elevated cyclic GMP in adipocytes (FAIN and BUTCHER 1976). The elevation of cyclic GMP required Ca^{2+} in the incubation medium. Some agents might elevate cyclic GMP secondary to an elevation of cytosol Ca^{2+}; others may act through increases in intracellular free fatty acids or lysophospholipids or by altering redox regulation.

ASAKAWA et al. (1978) found that the epinephrine-stimulated elevation in cyclic GMP was blocked by a β-adrenergic antagonist, propranolol; but not by an α-adrenergic antagonist, phentolamine. Free fatty acids also elevate cyclic GMP accumulation; SHIER et al. (1976) found that lysolecithin activated guanylate cyclase and inhibited adenylate cyclase activity of fibroblasts. Similarly free fatty acids elevate cyclic GMP accumulation but inhibit cyclic AMP accumulation and adenylate cyclase activity of adipocytes (FAIN and SHEPHERD 1975).

Cyclic GMP was also elevated by acetylcholine or carbamylcholine in adipocytes (ILLIANO et al. 1973; FAIN and BUTCHER 1976; TAKEDA and NAKAYA 1976). This is especially intriguing since cholinergic agonists do not affect adipocyte lipolysis. These results like those with the ionophore A-23187 indicate that agents which have no effect of adipocyte lipolysis or glucose metabolism can elevate cyclic GMP. The significance of cyclic GMP in adipocytes remains to be established.

The basal values for cyclic GMP and the increases due to added agents are small in comparison to cyclic AMP. Furthermore, cyclic GMP stimulates, rather than inhibits, adipocyte triglyceride lipase. In the presence of purified lung cyclic GMP-dependent protein kinase, cyclic GMP activated triacylglycerol lipase and phosphorylase kinase (KHOO et al. 1977). Thus, separate protein kinases for cyclic AMP and cyclic GMP apparently phosphorylate the same substrates (KHOO and GILL 1979). I believe in view of the low levels of cyclic GMP and the lack of correlation between cyclic GMP and metabolism, that cyclic GMP is unimportant to adipocytes.

The role of calcium in insulin action is unclear. KISSEBAH et al. (1975) suggested that insulin might elevate cytosol Ca^{2+}; but MCDONALD et al. (1976a, b, 1978) suggested that the effect of insulin is a reduction in cytosol Ca^{2+} since insulin accelerated uptake of Ca^{2+} by the endoplasmic reticulum of adipocytes. LAWRENCE and LARNER (1978b) found that insulin activates, while α-adrenergic agonists and the ionophore A-23187 inhibit, glycogen synthase activity. The inhibition due to α-adrenergic agonists and A-23187 was dependent on the presence of extracellular calcium; the activation by insulin was independent of extracellular Ca^{2+}. Furthermore, insulin activated glycogen synthase even in the presence of A23187.

The paucity of data supporting the view that cyclic GMP, cyclic AMP or Ca^{2+} are the second messengers for insulin has stimulated the search for a unique messenger. LARNER (1972) suggested that such a mediator regulates glycogen synthase by altering the sensitivity of protein kinase to cyclic AMP. Progress has been slow but recently LARNER et al. (1979) have partially purified a material from muscle of insulin-treated animals with a greater effect on protein kinase than similar extracts from control animals. The partially purified extracts from insulin-treated animals also mimicked the activation of adipocyte mitochondrial pyruvate dehydrogenase seen in the presence of insulin and plasma membranes (JARETT and SEALS 1979). This suggests that the interaction of insulin with plasma membranes results in generation of a second messenger whose effects can be duplicated by extracts from muscle of insulin-treated animals.

The insulin-generated mediator is a small, heat stable substance weighing 1,000–1,500 daltons; that is stable at acid pH but labile at alkaline pH. The mediator is prepared by first heating muscle at 100 °C in dilute acetic acid which removes the bulk of the proteins. Further purification has involved paper and Sephadex G-25 chromatography. The substance may be a small peptide since it is trypsin-labile (LARNER et al. 1979).

III. Insulin and Hexose Transport

The uptake by adipocytes of glucose occurs through a facilitated diffusion process; uptake, the rate-limiting step for glucose metabolism, is activated by insulin (CZECH 1976a, b, 1980). Plasma membrane vesicles derived from adipocytes previously incubated with insulin take up glucose at an elevated rate (CARTER et al. 1972). The finding that the effect of insulin survived the procedures used for cell disruption and vesicle isolation suggested that some kind of covalent modification was involved. Four possibilities seem likely but none have been proven. One possibility is that insulin resulted in oxidation of key sulphydryl groups in the membrane as suggested by CZECH et al. (1974a) and more recently by HOLMGREN (1979). A second possibility is that insulin activated phosphorylation (CHANG and CUATRECASAS 1974) or dephosphorylation of plasma membrane proteins (SEALS et al. 1979a, b). A third possibility is that insulin changes membrane fluidity; the addition to adipocyte vesicles of membrane fluidizers, such as cis-vaccenic acid, mimicked the effects of prior exposure to insulin (PILCH et al. 1980). A fourth possibility is that insulin activates a protease which generates a second messenger. Possibly the insulin receptor is a protease which is activated by the binding of insulin; this protease, in turn, inactivates a short-lived protein which inhibits hexose transport.

While we know little about how insulin activates the hexose transport system, rapid progress has been made in the elucidation of the adipocyte hexose carrier system. The increase in glucose uptake by vesicles derived from adipocytes previously exposed to insulin is retained even after extraction of 80% of the membrane proteins with dimethylmaleic anhydride (SHANAHAN and CZECH 1977a, b). A protein fraction extracted with sodium cholate from adipocyte membranes, previously extracted with dimethylmaleic anhydride, when combined with exogenous phospholipids, resulted in artificial vesicles with a stereospecific uptake of D-glucose. More recently, CARTER-SU et al. (1980) have obtained evidence, that the hexose transport protein is present in adipocyte membrane in very small quantities; it exhibits an apparent Stokes radius of 60–80 Å in sodium cholate.

A wide variety of agents mimic the stimulatory effect of insulin upon hexose transport. Antibodies raised against the intrinsic proteins of rat adipocyte plasma membranes have an insulin-like effect on hexose uptake (PILLON and CZECH 1978; PILLION et al. 1979); monovalent antibody fragments are inactive (PILLION et al. 1979). Antibodies have been found in the sera of patients with certain types of insulin resistance which stimulate hexose uptake and metabolism of adipocytes (FLIER et al. 1976; KAHN et al. 1977). Antibodies against the adipocyte membrane glycoproteins do not affect insulin binding to adipocytes, while those present in the sera of insulin-resistant patients block insulin binding. Likewise, concanavalin A also binds to adipocyte glycoproteins and stimulates glucose metabolism by adipocytes (CZECH and LYNN 1973; CZECH 1976b).

There is no evidence that cyclic AMP, cyclic GMP or Ca^{2+} mediate the action of insulin on hexose uptake. Lipolytic agents inhibit the stimulation by insulin of glucose metabolism; FAIN and ROSENBERG (1972) suggested that the intracellular accumulation of free fatty acids in the presence of high concentration of lipolytic agents, rather than cyclic AMP, is responsible for this inhibition. TAYLOR et al. (1976) and TAYLOR and HALPERIN (1979) concluded that cyclic AMP inhibits glucose transport; this conclusion was based on the assumption that (1-^{14}C)glucose oxidation by adipocytes incubated with 10 m*M* fluoride and 20 μ*M* phenazine methosulfate reflects glucose transport. Before this conclusion can be accepted studies will have to be performed in which hexose transport is measured directly in the absence of fluoride and phenazine methosulfate; TAYLOR and HALPERIN (1979) noted that glucose oxidation was 60% higher and basal cyclic AMP was 30% lower in the absence of fluoride.

Agents which lower cyclic AMP potentiate insulin-stimulated glucose oxidation when basal values for cyclic AMP are fairly high as in the presence of fluoride (TAYLOR and HALPERIN 1979) or when incubations use dilute concentrations of adipocytes (WIESER and FAIN 1975). However, in both conditions, insulin inhibits lipolysis without significantly affecting cyclic AMP. In contrast, agents which inhibit cyclic AMP accumulation and lipolysis (e.g. adenosine or nicotinic acid) had little stimulatory effect on glucose oxidation. These data suggest that the effects of insulin on glucose oxidation and lipolysis are mediated through cyclic AMP-independent pathways; however, high levels of cyclic AMP inhibit the effects of insulin on either parameter.

IV. Menadione, Insulin, and H_2O_2

In many cells, menadione (2-methyl-1,4-naphthoquinone) is readily reduced by NADH or NADPH. In adipocytes menadione increases the pentose shunt activity by short circuiting the normal control mechanisms regulating NADPH formation. Menadione competes favorably with flavoproteins for electrons from NADH or NADPH and donates these electrons to cytochromes in the respiratory chain; alternatively menadione is oxidized by molecular oxygen back to the quinone with the liberation of H_2O_2.

In isolated rat pancreatic islets, menadione (10 μ*M*) severely inhibited the ability of glucose to stimulate insulin release, increased glucose metabolism via the pentose shunt and lowered both NADH and NADPH (MALAISSE et al. 1978). MALAISSE et al. (1978) suggested that the cytoplasmic redox ratio of pyridine nucleotides regulate insulin secretion by modulating Ca^{2+} entry. Whether any of the effects of menadione in islets are mediated through changes in cyclic AMP remains to be elucidated. However, in islets as in adipocytes the menadione effects are opposite to those of cyclic AMP.

In adipocytes, menadione stimulated cyclic AMP accumulation and inhibited lipolysis (FAIN 1971). However, menadione actually inhibited adenylate cyclase activity of adipocyte ghosts. These data suggest that a reduction in cytosol redox ratio of pyridine nucleotides increases cyclic AMP accumulation while inhibiting lipolysis. Unfortunately little information is available about mechanisms by which redox status could regulate either process. The data suggest that factors other than cyclic AMP could be involved in the regulation of lipolysis.

Menadione also mimics the ability of insulin to increase glucose oxidation via the pentose pathway (FAIN 1971). This suggests that increased oxidation of glucose can directly activate hexose entry either directly through effects on membrane sulfhydryl oxidation or indirectly through increased H_2O_2 formation (CZECH 1976b, 1980). Other insulin-like agents such as thiols in the presence of Cu^{2+} (CZECH et al. 1974b) and polyamines (LIVINGSTON et al. 1977) increase the formation of H_2O_2 which increases glucose transport and metabolism of adipocytes. MAY and DE HAEN (1979a, b) suggested that insulin-induced formation of H_2O_2 mediates membrane sulfhydryl oxidation and is responsible for the increase in glucose transport due to insulin. MUKHERJEE and LYNN (1977) claim that insulin or sulfhydryl agents activate a reduced pyridine nucleotide oxidase in the plasma membrane which produces H_2O_2. I doubt that H_2O_2 is the long sought for second messenger for insulin. However, the ability of oxidants and H_2O_2 to activate adipocyte hexose transport (CZECH 1976b) indicate that alterations of the cytosol redox status do regulate hexose entry.

Insulin and oxidants like menadione have different effects on adipocytes. Insulin does not affect oxygen consumption and stimulates fatty acid synthesis to a much greater extent than do oxidants (FAIN 1971). Conversely, menadione has profound effects on cyclic AMP accumulation; under similar conditions, insulin has little effect on cyclic AMP (FAIN 1971). However, both menadione and insulin are equipotent as inhibitors of lipolysis.

The effects on hexose transport of menadione and other oxidants are probably secondary to changes in cytosol redox status. Possibly the effects of H_2O_2 are also secondary to a drop in the cytosol NADPH/NADP ratio. Adipocyte metabolism of H_2O_2 probably involves peroxidation of reduced glutathione to oxidized glutathione, followed by reduction of the oxidized glutatione by NADPH in the presence of glutathione reductase (MUKHERJEE et al. 1978). It remains to be established if the effects of insulin or lipolytic hormones upon adipocytes involve changes in cytosol redox status.

V. Insulin, Catecholamines, and Protein Phosphorylation

Insulin and catecholamines affect the incorporation of [^{32}P] into adipocyte proteins (AVRUCH et al. 1976; FORN and GREENGARD 1976, BENJAMIN and SINGER 1975). Insulin enhances the phosphorylation of two protein groups (subunit $M_r =$ 128,000 to 140,000 and 50,000 to 75,000) and inhibits the phosphorylation of one group of proteins (62,000 to 70,000). Epinephrine increased [^{32}P] incorporation into many proteins. The effects of both agents together were antagonistic with respect to phosphorylation of some proteins and additive with respect to other proteins. Recently, the identification of some of these phosphorylated proteins has clarified the possible physiological significance of protein phosphorylation. However, the identity of only a few phosphorylated proteins is known.

Benjamin and Clayton (1978) found that a protein of $M_r = 60{,}000$ was phosphorylated in the presence of insulin and dephosphorylated by lipolytic hormones. This protein was the only labelled phosphoprotein found associated with the bulk triglycerides of adipocyte homogenates. The 62,000 M_r protein might represent the subunits of lipoprotein lipase which have a similar M_r. This enzyme is subject to reciprocal regulation by insulin and lipolytic hormones. Furthermore, cyclic AMP-dependent protein kinase does not affect phosphorylation of this enzyme (Khoo et al. 1976). Possibly, insulin stimulates phosphorylation of this enzyme through a cyclic AMP-independent kinase and lipolytic agents increase dephosphorylation by activating a phosphatase.

ATP-citrate lyase is probably the other protein whose phosphorylation is stimulated by insulin (Alexander et al. 1979; Ramakrishna and Benjamin 1979). Paradoxically, agents which elevate cyclic AMP also increase phosphorylation of ATP-citrate lyase in both adipocytes and hepatocytes. However, Janski et al. (1979) found no effect of glucagon on the biological activity of this enzyme in hepatocytes. In hepatocytes of fed animals, ATP-citrate lyase activity is elevated; fasting and refeeding increases the [^{32}P] present in ATP citrate lyase and acetyl CoA carboxylase (Alexander et al. 1979).

Lipolytic agents enhance phosphorylation of acetyl CoA carboxylase (M_r = 220,000 to 230,000) in adipocytes (Lee and Kim 1979; Brownsey et al. 1979; Witters et al. 1979). The increased phosphorylation of this enzyme is associated with a decrease in its activity. Prior exposure of adipocytes to insulin enhances their acetyl CoA carboxylase activity (Halestrap and Denton 1973) and insulin does stimulates protein phosphorylation (Brownsey et al. 1977). The enzyme is regulated by the levels of ATP, citrate and especially long chain fatty acyl CoA esters. Insulin reduces the level of acyl CoA esters by inhibiting lipolysis and stimulating fatty acid re-esterification; these two effects may contribute to the activation by insulin of acetyl CoA carboxylase.

Glycerol phosphate acyltransferase in adipose tissue is inactivated by protein kinase and cyclic AMP and activated by treatment with alkaline phosphatase (Nimmo and Houston 1978). Exposure to epinephrine inactivates this enzyme (Sooranna and Saggerson 1976); the physiological significance of this decrease in glycerol phosphate acyltransferase activity is not known. In intact fat pads, epinephrine enhances the net rate of fatty acid re-esterification (Vaughan and Steinberg 1963).

Catecholamines inhibit and insulin activates adipocyte Mg^{2+}-dependent phosphatidate phosphohydrolase (Cheng and Saggerson 1978a, b). No studies on [^{32}P] incorporation into this enzyme have been reported. This enzyme is possibly involved in the regulation of lipid formation since it stands at the branch-point between triglyceride and phospholipid synthesis. The activation by insulin of this enzyme along with ATP-citrate lyase and acetyl CoA carboxylase is consistent with the ability of insulin to accelerate triglyceride formation.

Belfrage et al. (1980) have shown that the hormone-sensitive lipase is phosphorylated in intact adipocytes from rats; the enzyme has a molecular weight of 84,000 daltons. The purified lipase is also phosphorylated by the catalytic subunit of cyclic AMP dependent protein kinase isolated from adipose tissue. The demonstration that the minor phosphorylated band associated with 84,000 dalton proteins is triacylglycerol lipase required the development of new procedures for purification of the enzyme. This involved homogenization of adipose tissue in isotonic sucrose followed by high speed centrifugation. The supernatant was brought to pH 5.2 with acetic acid; the resulting precipitate was solubilized with a nonionic detergent and subjected to gradient sievorptive chromatography on QAE Sephadex. The pooled enzyme fractions were further purified by adsorption chromatography on Ultrogel AcA 34. The enzyme purity was 50%; this is the best purification reported to date (FREDRIKSON et al. 1981).

NILSSON et al. (1980) demonstrated that norepinephrine increased the incorporation of [^{32}P] into the 84,000 dalton band containing triacylglycerol lipase. Previously, FORN and GREENGARD (1976) noted small increases in incorporation of [^{32}P] into a phosphoprotein of molecular weight 86,000 daltons which was a minor, unidentified component in their gels. The same concentration of norepinephrine (20 n*M*) half maximally stimulated [^{32}P] incorporation into hormone-sensitive lipase and half-maximally activated free fatty acid release (NILSSON et al. 1980). The addition of 10–100 microunits/ml of insulin to cells previously incubated with norepinephrine for 7–10 min resulted in a rapid loss of [^{32}P] from the hormone-sensitive lipase and inhibited lipolysis (NILSSON et al. 1980). The half-maximal concentration of insulin required for both effects was between 0.1 and 1 microunit/ml, a remarkable sensitivity to insulin. These results suggest that insulin may be activating a phosphoprotein phosphatase resulting in rapid dephosphorylation of the lipase. However, further studies are required to determine whether insulin effects in this system are mediated through inhibition of protein phosphorylation (by lowering cyclic AMP) or through activation of protein dephosphorylation (possibly through a polypeptide messenger).

E. Conclusion

The activation of triglyceride hydrolysis by lipolytic hormones involves a cyclic AMP dependent phosphorylation of a triacylglycerol lipase. However, CHASIN et al. (1977) and FAIN et al. (1979) have pointed out conditions in which total cyclic AMP levels can be dissociated from lipolysis. Derivatives of glucagon have been described which activate hepatic glycogenolysis without affecting cyclic AMP (COTE and EPAND 1979). Similarly, derivatives of ACTH have been obtained which activate steroidogenesis in adrenal cells (MOYLE et al. 1973) and lipolysis in adipocytes (LANG et al. 1976) without affecting cyclic AMP. These studies do not contradict the extensive evidence that cyclic AMP can activate glycogenolysis, steroidogenesis and lipolysis. Rather they suggest that the hormone-receptor complex is able to activate other processes in addition to adenylate cyclase or that the active pool of cyclic AMP involved in phosphorylation of the hormone-sensitive lipase is compartmentalized from total cyclic AMP in adipocytes.

Insulin action canot be explained as being secondary to its effects on adipocyte H_2O_2, cyclic GMP or cytosol Ca^{2+}. It appears that insulin increases the formation of a unique second messenger whose effects are usually antagonistic to those of cyclic AMP. However, some effects of insulin may be secondary to inhibition of cyclic AMP accumulation in adipocytes.

References

Ahlquist RP (1948) A study of the adrenotropic receptors. Am J Physiol 153:586–600
Aktories K, Jakobs KH, Schultz G (1979) Influence of sodium chloride on the inhibition of hamster fat cells adenylate cyclase by GTP and on the inhibitory effects of alpha-adrenergic agonists and prostaglandin E_1 (Abstr). Arch Pharmacol 308:R 15
Alexander MC, Kowaloff EM, Witters LA, Dennihy DT, Avruch J (1979) Purification of a hepatic 123,000-dalton hormone-stimulated ^{32}P-peptide and its identification as ATP-citrate lyase. J Biol Chem 254:8052–8056
Angel A, Desai KS, Halperin ML (1971) Reduction in adipocyte ATP by lipolytic agents: relation to intracellular free fatty acid accumulation. J Lipid Res 12:203–211
Appleman MM, Thompson WJ, Russell TR (1973) Cyclic nucleotide phosphodiesterase. Adv Cyclic Nucleotide Res 3:65–98
Ariens EJ, Beld AJ, Miranda JFR, Simonis AM (1979) The pharmacon-receptor-effector concept. In: O'Brien RD (ed) Receptors: vol 1, General principles and procedures. Plenum, New York London, pp 33–91
Armstrong KJ, Stouffer JE, Van Inwegen RG, Thompson WJ, Robison GA (1974) Effect of thyroid hormone deficiency on cyclic adenosine 3′,5′-monophosphate and control of lipolysis in fat cells. J Biol Chem 249:4226–4231
Arner P, Wennlund A, Ostman J (1979) Regulation of lipolysis by human adipose tissue in hyperthyroidism. J Clin Endocrinol Metab 48:415–419
Asakawa T, Ruiz J, Ho R-J (1978) Epinephrine-induced elevation of guanosine 3′,5′-cyclic monophosphate in isolated fat cells of rat. Proc Natl Acad Sci USA 75:2684–2688
Ashby P, Bennett DP, Spencer IM, Robinson D (1978) Post-translational regulation of lipoprotein lipase activity in adipose tissue. Biochem J 176:865–872
Astwood EB (1965) The pituitary gland and the mobilization of fat. In: Renold AE, Cahill GF Jr (eds) Adipose tissue. American Physiological Society, Washington, DC (Handbook of physiology, sect 5, pp 529–532)
Aurbach GD, Fedak SA, Woodard CJ, Palmer JS, Hauser D, Troxler F (1974) Beta-adrenergic receptor: stereospecific interaction of iodinated beta-blocking agent with high afinity site. Science 186:1223–1224
Avruch J, Leone GR, Martin DB (1976) Effects of epinephrine and insulin on phosphopeptide metabolism in adipocytes. J Biol Chem 251:1511–1515
Bär HP, Hechter O (1969) Adenyl cyclase and hormone action. III. Calcium requirement for ACTH stimulation of adenyl cyclase. Biochem Biophys Res Commun 35:681–686
Baquer NZ, Cascales M, McLean P, Greenbaum AL (1976) Effects of thyroid hormone deficiency on the distribution of hepatic metabolites and control of pathways of carbohydrate metabolism in liver and adipose tissue of the rat. Eur J Biochem 68:403–413
Begin-Heick N, Heick HM (1977) Increased response of adipose tissue of the ob/ob mouse to the action of adrenaline after treatment with thyroxin. Can J Physiol Pharmacol 55:1320–1329
Belfrage P, Fredrikson G, Nilsson NO, Stralfors P (1980) Regulation of adipose tissue lipolysis: phosphorylation of hormone-sensitive lipase in intact rat adipocytes. FEBS Lett 111:120–124
Benjamin WB, Clayton N-L (1978) Action of insulin and catecholamines on the phosphorylation of proteins associated with the cytosol, membranes, and "fat cake" of rat fat cells. J Biol Chem 253:1700–1709
Benjamin WB, Singer I (1975) Actions of insulin, epinephrine and dibutyryl cyclic adenosine 5′ monophosphate on fat cell protein phosphorylations. Cyclic adenosine 5′-monophosphate dependent and independent mechanisms. Biochemistry 14:3301–3309
Bennet V, Mong L, Cuatrecasas P (1975) Mechanism of activation of adenylate cyclase by Vibrio cholera enterotoxin. J Membr Biol 24:107–129
Bensadoun A, Ehnholm C, Steinberg D, Brown WV (1974) Purification and characterization of lipoprotein lipase from pig adipose tissue. J Biol Chem 249:2220–2227
Bereziat G, Wolf C, Colard O, Polonovski J (1978) Phospholipases of plasmic membranes of adipose tissue. Possible intermediaries for insulin action. Adv Exp Biol 101:191–199

Berridge MJ, Fain JN (1979) Inhibition of phosphatidylinositol synthesis and the inactivation of calcium entry after prolonged exposure of the blowfly salivary gland to 5-hydroxytryptamine. Biochem J 178:59–69
Bieber LL, Petterson B, Lindberg O (1975) Studies on norepinephrine-induced efflux of free fatty acid from hamster brown adipose tissue cells. Eur J Biochem 58:375–381
Bieck P, Stock K, Westermann E (1966) Lipolytic action of serotonin in vitro. Life Sci 5:2157–2163
Bielmann P, Chretien M, Gattereau A (1972) Lipogenic activity of a potent lipolytic hormone: Sheep beta-lipotropin (β-LPH). II. Further effects of sheep β-LPH on specifically labeled glucose and the localization of the lipogenic active center of the molecule. Horm Metab Res 4:22–25
Birnbaumer L, Rodbell M (1969) Adenyl cyclase in fat cells. II. Hormone receptors. J Biol Chem 244:3477–3482
Bjorntorp P, Ostman J (1971) Human adipose tissue dynamics and regulation. Adv Metab Disord 5:277–327
Bläckberg, Hernell O, Bengtsson G, Olivecrona T (1979) Colipase enhances hydrolysis of dietary triglycerides in the absence of bile salts. J Clin Invest 64:1303–1308
Blecher M (1967) The effects of insulin and phospholipase A on glucose transport across the plasma membrane of free adipose cells. Biochim Biophys Acta 137:557–571
Blecher M (1969) Insulin-like, antilipolytic actions of phospholipase A in isolated rat adipose cells. Biochim Biophys Acta 187:380–384
Bowery B, Lewis GP (1973) Inhibition of functional vasodilation and prostaglandin formation in rabbit adipose tissue by indomethacin and aspirin. Br J Pharmacol 47:305–314
Boyd TA, Wieser PB, Fain JN (1975) Lipolysis and cyclic AMP accumulation in isolated fat cells from chicks. Gen Comp Endocrinol 26:243–247
Brownsey RW, Hughes WA, Denton RM, Mayer RJ (1977) Demonstration of the phosphorylation of acetyl-coenzyme A carboxylase within intact rat epididymal fat cells. Biochem J 168:441–445
Brownsey RW, Hughes WA, Denton RM (1979) Adrenaline and the regulation of acetyl-coenzyme A carboxylase in rat epididymal adipose tissue. Biochem J 184:23–32
Burges RA, Blackburn KJ (1972) Adenyl cyclase and the differentiation of β-adrenoreceptors. Nature 235:249–250
Burns TW, Langley PE (1975) The effect of alpha- and beta-adrenergic receptor stimulation on the adenylate cyclase activity of human adipocytes. J Cyclic Nucleotide Res 1:321–328
Burns TW, Langley PE, Robison GA (1975) Site of free-fatty acid inhibition of lipolysis by human adipocytes. Metabolism 24:265–276
Burns TW, Langley PE, Terry BE, Bylund DB, Hoffman BB, Tharp MD, Lefkowitz RJ, Garcia-Sainz JA, Fain JN (1981) Pharmacological characterization of adrenergic receptors in human adipocytes. J Clin Invest 67:467–475
Butcher RW, Carlson LA (1970) Effects of secretin on fat mobilizing lipolysis and cyclic AMP levels in rat adipose tissue. Acta Physiol Scand 79:559–563
Butcher RW, Sutherland EW (1962) Adenosine 3′,5′-phosphate in biological materials. I. Purification and properties of cyclic 3′,5′-nucleotide phosphodiesterase and use of this enzyme to characterize adenosine 3′,5′-phosphate in human urine. J Biol Chem 237:1244–1250
Butcher RW, Ho RJ, Meng HC, Sutherland EW (1965) Adenosine 3′,5′-monophosphate in biological materials. II. The measurement of adenosine 3′5′-monophosphate in tissues and the role of the cyclic nucleotide in the lipolytic response of fat to epinephrine. J Biol Chem 240:4515–4523
Butcher RW, Sneyd JGT, Park CR, Sutherland EW Jr (1966) Effect of insulin on adenosine 3′:5′-monophosphate in the rat epididymal fat pad. J Biol Chem 241:1651–1653
Butcher RW, Baird CE, Sutherland EW (1968) Effects of lipolytic and antilipolytic substances on adenosine 3′,5′-monophosphate levels in isolated fat cells. J Biol Chem 243:1705–1712
Cabelli RJ, Malbon CC (1979) Characterization of (−)-[^{3}H]dihydroalprenolol binding sites on isolated rat fat cells. J Biol Chem 254:8903–8908

Caldwell A, Fain JN (1971) Triiodothyronine stimulation of cyclic adenosine 3′,5′-monophosphate accumulation in white fat cells. Endocrinology 89:1195–1204
Carchman RA, Janus SC, Rubin RP (1971) The role of adrenocorticotropin and calcium in adenosine cyclic 3′,5′-phosphate production and steroid release from the isolated perfused cat adrenal gland. Mol Pharmacol 7:491–499
Carter JR Jr, Avruch J, Martin DB (1972) Glucose transport in plasma membrane vesicles from rat adipose tissue. J Biol Chem 247:2682–2688
Carter-Su C, Pillion DJ, Czech MP (1980) Reconstituted D-glucose transport from the adipocyte plasma membrane. Chromatographic resolution of transport activity from membrane glycoproteins using immobilized concanavalin A. Biochemistry 19:2374–2385
Cassel D, Selinger Z (1977) Mechanism of adenylate cyclase activation by cholera toxin: inhibition of GTP hydrolysis at the regulatory site. Proc Natl Acad Sci USA 74:3307–3311
Chang J, Lewis GP, Piper PJ (1977) Inhibition by glucocorticoids of prostaglandin release from adipose tissue in vitro. Br J Pharmacol 59:425–432
Chang KJ, Cuatrecasas P (1974) Adenosine triphosphate-dependent inhibition of insulin-stimulated glucose transport in fat cells. Possible role of membrane phosphorylation. J Biol Chem 249:3170–3180
Chasin M, Mamrak F, Koshelnyk K, Rispoli M (1977) Dissociation of lipolysis from the levels of cyclic AMP in rat epididymal fat cells. Arch Int Pharmacodyn Ther 227:180–194
Cheng CHK, Saggerson ED (1978a) Rapid effects of noradrenaline on Mg^{2+}-dependent phosphatidate phosphohydrolase activity in rat adipocytes. FEBS Lett 87:65–68
Cheng CHK, Saggerson ED (1978b) Rapid antagonistic actions of noradrenaline and insulin on rat adipocyte phosphatidate phosphohydrolase activity. FEBS Lett 93:120–124
Christ EJ, Nugteren DH (1970) The biosynthesis and possible function of prostaglandins in adipose tissue. Biochim Biophys Acta 218:296–307
Combret Y, Laudat P (1972) Adenyl cyclase activity in a plasma membrane fraction purified from "ghosts" of rat fat cells. FEBS Lett 21:45–48
Cooper B, Partilla JS, Gregerman RT (1975) Expression of epinephrine-sensitive activation revealed by 5′-guanylyl-imidodiphosphate. Clin Invest 56:1350–1353
Cooper MF, Schlegel W, Lin MC, Rodbell M (1979) The fat cell adenylate cyclase system. J Biol Chem 254:8927–8931
Coore HG, Denton RM, Martin BR, Randle PJ (1971) Regulation of adipose tissue pyruvate dehydrogenase by insulin and other hormones. Biochem J 125:115–127
Corbin JD, Krebs EG (1969) A cyclic AMP – stimulated protein kinase in adipose tissue. Biochem Biophys Res Commun 36:328–338
Corbin JD, Reimann EM, Walsh DA, Krebs EG (1970) Activation of adipose tissue lipase by skeletal muscle cyclic adenosine-3′,5′-monophosphate-stimulated protein kinase. J Biol Chem 245:4849–4851
Corbin JD, Soderling TR, Park CR (1973) Regulation of adenosine 3′,5′-monophosphate-dependent protein kinase. 1. Preliminary characterization of the adipose tissue enzyme in crude extracts. J Biol Chem 248:1813–1821
Corbin JD, Soderling TR, Sugden PH, Keely SL, Park CR (1976) Control of metabolic processes by cAMP-dependent protein phosphorylation. In: Dumont JE, Brown BL, Marshall NJ (eds) Eukaryotic cell function and growth. Plenum, New York London, pp 231–247
Correze C, Laudat MH, Laudat P, Nunez J (1974) Hormone-dependent lipolysis in fat cells from thyroidectomized rats. Mol Cell Endocrinol 1:309–327
Correze C, Auclair R, Nunez J (1976) Cyclic nucleotide phosphodiesterases, insulin and thyroid hormones. Mol Cell Endocrinol 5:67–79
Correze C, Nunez J, Gordon A (1977) Thyroid hormones and lipogenesis from glucose in rat fat cells. Mol Cell Endocrinol 9:133–144
Cote TE, Epand RM (1979) N^{α}-trinitrophenyl glucagon. An inhibitor of glucagon-stimulated cyclic AMP production and its effects on glycogenolysis. Biochim Biophys Acta 582:295–306
Cryer PE, Jarett L, Kipnis DM (1969) Nucleotide inhibition of adenyl cyclase activity in fat cell membranes. Biochim Biophys Acta 177:586–590

Cuatrecasas P (1973) Cholera toxin-fat cell interaction and the mechanism of activation of the lipolytic response. Biochemistry 12:3567–3577
Cuatrecasas P, Hollenberg MD, Chang K, Bennett V (1975) Hormone receptor complexes and their modulation of membrane function. Recent Prog Horm Res 31:37–94
Czech MP (1976a) Differential effects of sulfhydryl reagents on activation and deactivation of the fat cell hexose transport system. J Biol Chem 251:1164–1170
Czech MP (1976b) Regulation of the D-glucose transport system in isolated fat cells. Mol Cell Biochem 11:51–63
Czech MP (1977) Molecular basis of insulin action. Annu Rev Biochem 46:359–384
Czech MP (1980) Insulin action and the regulation of hexose transport. Diabetes 29:399–409
Czech MP (1981) Insulin action: second messengers. In: Brownlee M (ed) Handbook of diabetes mellitus: Vol. 2. Jarland STPM Press, New York, pp. 117–149
Czech MP, Lynn WS (1973) Stimulation of glucose metabolism by lectins in isolated white fat cells. Biochim Biophys Acta 297:368–377
Czech MP, Lawrence JC Jr, Lynn WS (1974a) Evidence for the involvement of sulfhydryl oxidation in the regulation of fat cell hexose transport by insulin. Proc Natl Acad Sci USA 71:4173–4177
Czech MP, Lawrence JC, Lynn WS (1974b) Evidence for electron transfer reactions involved in the Cu^{2+}-dependent thiol activation of fat cell glucose utilization. J Biol Chem 249:1001–1006
Czech MP, Malbon C, Kerman K, Gitomer W, Pilch PF (1980) Effect of thyroid status on insulin action in rat adipocytes and skeletal muscle. J Clin Invest 66, 574–582
Dalton C, Hope HR (1973) Inability of prostaglandin synthesis inhibitors to affect adipose tissue lipolysis. Prostaglandins 4:641–651
Dalton C, Hope WC (1974) Cyclic AMP regulation of prostaglandin biosynthesis in fat cells. Prostaglandins 6:227–242
Davies JI (1968) In vitro regulation of the lipolysis of adipose tissue. Nature 218:349–352
Debons AF, Schwartz IL (1961) Dependence of the lipolytic action of epinephrine in vitro upon thyroid hormone. J Lipid Res 2:86–89
De Cingolani GEC, Van Den Bosch H, Van Deenen LLM (1972) Phospholipase A and lysophospholipase activities in isolated fat cells: effect of cyclic 3′,5′-AMP. Biochim Biophys Acta 260:387–393
Denton RM, Hughes WA (1978) Pyruvate dehydrogenase and the hormonal regulation of fat synthesis in mammalian tissues. Int J Biochem 9:545–552
Denton RM, Hughes WA, Bridges BJ, Brownsey RW, McCormack JG, Stansbie D (1978) Regulation of mammalian pyruvate dehydrogenase by hormones. In: Dumont J, Nunez J (eds) Hormones and cell regulation. Elsevier/North-Holland Biomedical, Amsterdam Oxford New York, pp 121–208
Desai K, Hollenberg CH (1975) Regulation, by insulin, of lipoprotein lipase and phosphodiesterase activities in rat adipose tissue. Isr J Med Sci 11:540–550
Desai KS, Li KC, Angel A (1973) Bimodal effect of insulin on hormone-stimulated lipolysis. Relation to intracellular 3′,5′-cyclic adenylic acid and free fatty acid levels. J Lipid Res 14:647–655
Desai K, Zinman B, Hollenberg CH (1976) Role of calcium in insulin induced inhibition of lipolysis and activation of phosphodiesterase. Clin Res 24:680A
Diamant S, Gorin E, Shafrir E (1972) Enzyme activities related to fatty acid synthesis in liver and adipose tissue of rats treated with triiodothyroinine. Eur J Biochem 26:553–559
Dole VP (1956) A relation between non-esterified fatty acids in plasma and the metabolism of glucose. J Clin Invest 35:150–154
Dole VP (1961) Effect of nucleic acid metabolites on lipolysis in adipose tissue. J Biol Chem 236:3125–3130
Drahota Z, Houstek J (1976) Biochemical aspects of non-shivering thermogenesis in brown adipose tissue. In: Jansky L, Musacchia XJ (eds) Regulation of depressed metabolism and thermogenesis. Thomas, Springfied, pp 213–224
Drahota Z, Honova E, Han P (1968) The effect of ATP and carnitine on the endogenous respiration of mitochondria from brown adipose tissue. Experientia 24:431–432

Ebert R, Schwabe U (1973) Antilipolytic effect of adenosine and purine bases in isolated fat cells. Arch Pharm (Weinheim) 278:247–259
Eckel RH, Fujimoto WY, Brunzell JD (1977) Development of lipoprotein lipase in cultured 3T3-L1 cells. Biochem Biophys Res Commun 78:288–293
Eisen HJ, Goodman HM (1969) Growth hormone and phosphorylase activity in adipose tissue. Endocrinology 84:414–416
Evans DJ Jr, Chen LC, Curlin GT, Evans DG (1972) Stimulation of adenyl cyclase by escherichia coli enterotoxin. Nature New Biol 236:137–138
Fain JN (1962) Effects of dexamethasone and growth hormone on fatty acid mobilization and glucose utilization in adrenalectomized rats. Endocrinology 71:633–635
Fain JN (1967a) Adrenergic blockade of hormone-induced lipolysis in isolated fat cells. Ann NY Acad Sci 139:879–890
Fain JN (1967b) Studies on the role of RNA and protein synthesis in the lipolytic action of growth hormone in isolated fat cells. Adv Enzyme Regul 5:39–51
Fain JN (1971) Effects of menadione and vitamin K_5 on glucose metabolism, respiration, lipolysis, cyclic 3′,5′-adenylic acid accumulation, and adenyl cyclase in white fat cells. Mol Pharmacol 7:465–479
Fain JN (1973a) Inhibition of cyclic adenosine 3′,5′-monophosphate accumulation in fat cells by adenosine N^6-(phenylisopropyl)adenosine and related compounds. Mol Pharmacol 9:595–604
Fain JN (1973b) Biochemical aspects of drug and hormone action on adipose tissue. Pharmacol Rev 25:67–118
Fain JN (1974) Mode of action of insulin. MTP Int Rev Sci Ser. One Biochem. 8:1–24
Fain JN (1977) Cyclic nucleotides in adipose tissue. In: Cramer H, Schultz J (eds) Cyclic nucleotides: mechanisms of action, John Wiley and Sons, New York Chichester, pp 207–228
Fain JN (1979a) Effect of lipolytic agents on adenosine and AMP formation by fat cells. Biochim Biophys Acta 573:510–520
Fain JN (1979b) Inhibition of glucose transport in fat cells and activation of lipolysis by glucocorticoids. Monogr Endocrinol 12:547–560
Fain JN (1980) Hormonal regulation of lipid mobilization from adipose tissue. In: Litwack G (ed) Biochemical actions of hormones, vol 7. Academic Press, New York London, pp 119–204
Fain JN, Berridge MJ (1979) Relationship between hormonal activation of phosphatidylinositol hydrolysis, fluid secretion and calcium flux in the blowfly salivary gland. Biochem J 178:45–58
Fain JN, Butcher FR (1976) Cyclic guanosine 3′,5′-monophosphate and the regulation of lipolysis in rat fat cells. J Cyclic Nucleotide Res 2:71–78
Fain JN, Czech MP (1975) Glucocorticoid effects on lipid mobilization and adipose tissue metabolism. In: Blasehko H, Sayers G, Smith D (eds) adrenal gland American Physiological Society, Washington, DC (Handbook of physiology, sect 7, vol 6, pp 169–178)
Fain JN, Malbon CC (1979) Regulation of adenylate cyclase by adenosine. Mol Cell Biochem 25:143–169
Fain JN, Rosenberg L (1972) Antilipolytic action of insulin on fat cells. Diabetes 21:414–425
Fain JN, Rosenthal JW (1971) Calorigenic action of triiodothyronine on white fat cells: effects of ouabain oligomycin, and catecholamines. Endocrinology 89:1205–1211
Fain JN, Saperstein R (1970) The involvement of RNA synthesis and cyclic AMP in the activation of fat cell lipolysis by growth hormone and glucocorticoids. In: Jeanrenaud B, Hepp D (eds) Adipose tissue: regulation and metabolic functions. Academic Press, New York London, pp 20–27
Fain JN, Shepherd RE (1975) Free fatty acids as feedback regulators of adenylate cyclase and cyclic AMP accumulation in rat fat cells. J Biol Chem 250:6586–6592
Fain JN, Shepherd RE (1979) Hormonal regulation of lipolysis: role of cyclic nucleotides, adenosine and free fatty acids. Adv Exp Biol Med 111:43–78
Fain JN, Wieser PB (1975) Effects of adenosine deaminase on cyclic adenosine monophosphate accumulation, lipolysis and glucose metabolism of fat cells. J Biol Chem 250:1027–1034

Fain JN, Kovacev VP, Scow RO (1965) Effect of growth hormone and dexamethasone on lipolysis and metabolism in isolated fat cells of the rat. J Biol Chem 240:3522–3529
Fain JN, Galton DJ, Kovacev VP (1966) Effect of drugs on the lipolytic action of hormones in isolated fat cells. Mol Pharmacol 2:237–247
Fain JN, Dodd A, Novak L (1971) Relationship of protein synthesis and cyclic AMP to lipolytic action of growth hormone and glucocorticoids. Metabolism 20:109–118
Fain JN, Pointer RH, Ward WF (1972) Effects of adenosine nucleotides on adenylate cyclase, phosphodiesterase, cyclic adenosine monophosphate accumulation, and lipolysis in fat cells. J Biol Chem 247:6866–6872
Fain JN, Psychoyos S, Czernik AJ, Frost S, Cash WD (1973a) Indomethacin, lipolysis and cyclic AMP accumulation in white fat cells. Endocrinology 93:632–639
Fain JN, Jacobs MD, Clement-Cormier YC (1973b) Interrelationship of cyclic AMP, lipolysis and respiration in brown fat cells. Am J Physiol 224:346–351
Fain JN, Shepherd RE, Malbon CC, Moreno FJ (1978) Hormonal Regulation of the breakdown of triglyceride. In: Dietschy JN (ed) Disturbances in lipids and lipoprotein metabolism. American Physiological Society, Washington DC, pp 213–228
Fain JN, Li S-Y, Moreno FJ (1979) Regulation of cyclic AMP metabolism and lipolysis in isolated rat fat cells by insulin, N^6-(phenylisopropyl)adenosine and 2′,5′-dideoxyadenosine. J Cyclic Nucleotide Res 5:189–196
Fain JN, Kabnick KS, Li S-Y (1981) Effects of melittin on adipocyte metabolism unrelated to lysophospholipid accumulation. Biochim Biophys Acta 677:274–279
Fassina G, Contessa AR (1967) Digitoxin and prostaglandin E_1 as inhibitors of catecholamine-stimulated lipolysis and their interaction with Ca^{2+} in the process. Biochem Pharmacol 16:1447–1453
Feller DR, Piascik MT, Miller DD (1978) Activation of adrenoceptors and adenylate cyclase in adipocytes by catecholamines and tetrahydroisoquinolines. In: Szabadi E, Bradshaw CM, Bevan P (eds) Recent advances in the pharmacology of adrenoceptors. Elsevier/North-Holland Biomedical, Amsterdam Oxford New York, pp 111–120
Flatmark T, Pedersen JI (1975) Brown adipose tissue mitochondria. Biochim Biophys Acta 416:53–103
Flier JS, Kahn CR, Jarrett DB, Roth J (1976) Characterization of antibodies to the insulin receptor: a cause of insulin-resistant diabetes in man. J Clin Invest 58:1442–1449
Forn J, Greengard P (1976) Regulation by lipolytic and antilipolytic compounds of the phosphorylation of specific proteins in isolated intact fat cells. Arch Biochem Biophys 176:721–733
Foss I, Sletten K, Trygstad O (1973) Studies on the primary structure and biological activity of a human neurophysin. FEBS Lett 30:151–156
Fredholm BB (1978) Local regulation of lipolysis in adipose tissue by fatty acids, prostaglandins and adenosine. Med Biol 59:249–261
Fredholm BB, Hedqvist P (1975) Indomethacin and the role of prostaglandins in adipose tissue. Biochem Pharmacol 24:61–66
Fredholm BB, Hjemdahl P (1979) Uptake and release of adenosine in isolated rat fat cells. Acta Physiol Scand 105:257–267
Fredholm BB, Rosell S (1970) Release of prostaglandin-like material from canine subcutaneous adipose tissue by nerve stimulation. Acta Physiol Scand 79:18 A
Fredrikson G, Stralfors P, Nilsson NO, Belfrage P (1981) Hormone-sensitive lipase of rat adipose tissue: purification and some properties. J Biol Chem 256:6311–6320
Freinkel N (1961) Extrathyroidal actions of pituitary thyrotropin: effects on the carbohydrate, lipid and respiratory metabolism of rat adipose tissue. J Clin Invest 40:476–489
Garcia-Sainz JA, Fain JN (1980a) Effect of insulin, catecholamines and calcium on phospholipid metabolism in isolated white fat cells. Biochem J 186:781–789
Garcia-Sainz JA, Fain JN (1980b) Effect of adrenergic amines on phosphatidylinositol labelling and glycogen synthase activity in fat cells from euthyroid and hypothyroid rats. Mol Pharmacol 18:116–121
Garcia-Sainz JA, Hoffmann BB, Li S-H, Lefkowitz RJ, Fain JN (1980) Role of $alpha_1$ adrenoceptors in the turnover of phosphatidylinositol and $alpha_2$ adrenoceptors in the regulation of cyclic AMP accumulation in hamster adipocytes. Life Sci 27:953–961

Gill DM, Meren R (1978) ADP-ribosylation of membrane proteins catalyzed by cholera toxin: basis of the activation of adenylate cyclase. Proc Natl Acad Sci USA 75:3050–3054

Girardier L, Seydoux J (1971) Cytomembrane phenomena during stimulation of brown fat thermogenesis by norepinephrine in non-shivering thermogenesis. In: Jansky L (ed) Nonshivering thermogenesis. Academia, Prague, pp 255–270

Girardier L, Seydoux J, Clausen T (1968) Membrane potential of brown adipose tissue. J Gen Physiol 52:925–940

Giudicelli Y (1978) Thyroid hormone modulation of the number of β-adrenergic receptors in rat fat cell membranes. Biochem J 176:1007–1010

Giudicelli Y, Pecquery R (1978) Beta-adrenergic receptors and catecholamine-sensitive adenylate cyclase in rat fat cell membranes: influence of growth, cell size and aging. Eur J Biochem 90:413–419

Giudicelli Y, Agli B, Lacasa D (1979a) Beta-adrenergic receptor desensitization in rat adipocyte membranes. Biochim Biophys Acta 585:85–93

Giudicelli Y, Lacasa D, Agli B (1979b) Evidence for a second desensitized state of beta-adrenergic receptor with low affinity for beta-antagonists and normal reactivity towards beta-agonists in adipocyte membranes previously exposed to beta-antagonists. Eur J Biochem 99:457–462

Goodman HM (1970) Permissive effects of hormones of lipolysis. Endocrinology 86:1064–1074

Goodman HM, Bray GA (1966) Role of thyroid hormones in lipolysis. Am J Physiol 210:1053–1058

Goodman HM, Schwartz J (1974) Growth hormone and lipid metabolism. In: Knobil E, Sawyer (eds). The pituitary gland and its neuroendocrine Catral. American Physiological Society, Washington, DC (Handbook of Physiology, sect 7, vol 4, part 2, pp 211–231)

Gordon RS Jr, Cherkes A (1956) Unesterified fatty acids in human blood plasma. J Clin Invest 35:206–212

Gorman RR (1975) Prostaglandin endoperoxides: possible new regulators of cyclic nucleotide metabolism. J Cyclic Nucleotide Res 1:1–9

Gorman RR, Tepperman HM, Tepperman J (1973) Epinephrine binding and the selective restoration of adenylate cyclase activity in fat-fed rats. J Lipid Res 14:279–285

Gorman RR, Hamberg M, Samuelsson B (1975) Inhibition of basal and hormone-stimulated adenylate cyclase in adipocyte ghosts by the prostaglandin endoperoxide prostaglandin H_2. J Biol Chem 250:6460–6463

Goswami A, Rosenberg IN (1978) Thyroid hormone modulation of epinephrine-induced lipolysis in rat adipocytes: a possible role of calcium. Endocrinology 103:2223–2233

Gozariu L, Forster K, Faulhaber JD, Minne H, Ziegler R (1974) Parathyroid hormone and calcitonin: influences upon lipolysis of human adipose tissue. Horm Metab Res 6:243–245

Guernsey DL, Morishige WK (1979) Na^+ pump activity and nuclear T_3 receptors in tissues of genetically obese (ob/ob) mice. Metabolism 28:629–632

Guillory RJ, Racker E (1968) Oxidative phosphorylation in brown adipose mitochondria. Biochim Biphys Acta 153:490–493

Guinovart JJ, Lawrence JC Jr, Larner J (1979) Hormonal effects on fat cell adenosine 3′,5′-monophosphate dependent protein kinase. Biochim Biophys Acta 539:181–194

Habermann E (1972) Bee and wasp venoms. Science 177:314–322

Hagen JH (1961) Effect of glucagon on the metabolism of adipose tissue. J Biol Chem 236:1023–1027

Hales CN, Campbell AK, Luzio JP, Siddle K (1977) Calcium as mediator of hormone action. Biochem Soc Trans 5:866–872

Hales CN, Luzio JP, Siddle K (1978) Hormonal control of adipose tissue lipolysis. Biochem Soc Symp 43:97–135

Halestrap AP, Denton RM (1973) Insulin and the regulation of adipose tissue acetyl-coenzyme A carboxylase. Biochem J 132:509–517

Harms HH (1976) Stereochemical Aspects of β-adrenoceptor antagonist-receptor interaction in adipocytes. Differentiation of β-adrenoceptors in human and rat adipocytes. Life Sci 19:1447–1452
Harms HH, Zaagsma J, Van der Wal B (1974) Beta-adrenoceptor studies. III. On the beta-adrenoceptors in rat adipose tissue. Eur J Pharmacol 25:87–91
Heaton GM, Wagenvoord RJ, Kemp A Jr, Nicholls DG (1978) Brown adipose tissue mitochondria: photoaffinity labelling of the regulatory site of energy dissipation. Eur J Biochem 82:515–521
Hecht JP, Dellacha JM, Santome JA, Paladini AC, Hurwitz E, Sela M (1972) Lipolytic activity of bovine growth hormone bound to Sepharose beads. FEBS Lett 20:83–86
Hepp KD, Renner R (1972) Insulin action on the adenyl cyclase system: antagonism to activation of lipolytic hormones. FEBS Lett 20:191–194
Herd PA, Hammond RP, Hamolsky MW (1973) Sodium pump activity during norepinephrine-stimulated respiration in brown adipocytes. Am J Physiol 224:1300–1304
Hewlett EL, Guerrant RL, Evand DJ Jr, Greenough WB III (1974) Toxins of vibrio cholerae and escherichia coli stimulate adenyl cyclase in rat fat cells. Nature 249:371–373
Hittelman KJ, Bertin R, Butcher RW (1974) Cyclic AMP metabolism in brown adipocytes of hamsters exposed to different temperatures. Biochim Biophys Acta 338:398–407
Holmgren A (1979) Reduction of disulfides by thioredoxin. Exceptional reactivity of insulin and suggested functions of thioredoxin in mechanism of hormone action. J Biol Chem 254:9113–9119
Horwitz B (1973) Ouabain-sensitive component of brown fat thermogenesis. Am J Physiol 224:352–355
Horwitz BA (1979) Cellular events underlying catecholamine-induced thermogenesis: cation transport in brown adipocytes. Fed Proc 38:2170–2176
Huttunen JK, Steinberg D (1971) Activation and phosphorylation of purified adipose tissue hormone-sensitive lipase by cyclic AMP-dependent protein kinase. Biochim Biophys Acta 239:411–427
Huttunen JK, Steinberg D, Mayer SE (1970a) ATP-dependent and cyclic AMP-dependent activation of rat adipose tissue lipase by protein kinase from rabbit skeletal muscle. Proc Natl Acad Sci USA 67:290–295
Huttunen JK, Steinberg D, Mayer SE (1970b) Protein kinase activation and phosphorylation of purified hormone-sensitive lipase. Biochem Biophys Res Commun 41:1350–1356
Illiano G, Cuatrecasas P (1971) Endogenous prostaglandins modulate lipolytic processes in adipose tissue. Nature New Biol 234:72–74
Illiano G, Cuatrecasas P (1972) Modulation of adenylate cyclase activity in liver and fat cell membranes by insulin. Science 175:906–908
Illiano G, Tell GPE, Siegel MI, Cuatrecasas P (1973) Guanosine 3′,5′-cyclic monophosphate and the action of insulin. Proc Natl Acad Sci USA 70:2443–2447
Ismail-Beigi F, Edelman IS (1970) Mechanism of thyroid calorigenesis: role of active sodium transport. Proc Natl Acad Sci USA 67:1071–1078
Iverius PH, Ostlund-Lindqvist AM (1976) Lipoprotein lipase from bovine milk. J Biol Chem 251:7791–7795
Jakobs KH (1978) Inhibition of platelet adenylate cyclase by alpha-adrenergic agonists. In: Folco G, Paoletti (eds) Molecular biology and pharmacology of cyclic nucleotides. Elsevier, Amsterdam Oxford New York, pp 265–277
Janski AM, Srere PA, Cornell NW, Veech RL (1979) Phosphorylation of ATP citrate lyase in response to glucagon. J Biol Chem 254:9365–9368
Jarett L, Seals JR 1979) Pyruvate dehydrogenase activation in adipocyte mitochondria by an insulin generated mediator from muscle. Science 206:1407–1408
Jeanrenaud B, Hepp D (eds) (1970) Adipose-tissue, regulation and metabolic functions. Thieme, Stuttgart
Jones LM, Michell RH (1978) Stimulus-response coupling at alpha-adrenergic receptors. Biochem Soc Trans 6:673–688
Jungas RL (1966) Role of cyclic 3′,5′-AMP in the response of adipose tissue to insulin. Proc Natl Acad Sci USA 56:757–763

Jungas RL (1975) Metabolic effects on adipose tissue in vitro. In: Hasselblatt A, Bruchhausen FV (eds) Insulin action. Springer, Berlin Heidelberg New York (Handbook of experimental pharmacology, vol XXXII/2, pp 371–412)

Kahn CR, Baird K, Flier JS, Jarrett DB (1977) Effects of autoantibodies to the insulin receptor on isolated adipocytes. J Clin Invest 60:1094–1106

Kanfer JN, Carter TP, Katzen HM (1976) Lipolytic action of cholera toxin on fat cells. Reexamination of the concept implicating GM_1 ganglioside as the native membrane receptor. J Biol Chem 251:7610–7619

Kaplan JC, Pichard AL, Laudat MH, Laudat P (1973) Kinetic and electrophoretic abnormality of cyclic AMP phosphodiesterase in genetically obese mouse adipocytes. Biochem Biophys Res Commun 51:1008–1014

Kappeler H (1966) Zur Pharmakologie der Lipolysehemmung. I. Wirkungsweise adenosinhaltiger Nucleoside und Nucleotide auf die Lipolyse des Fettgewebes in vitro. Diabetologia 2:52–61

Kather H, Geiger M (1977) Adrenaline-sensitive adenylate cyclase of human fat cell ghosts: properties and hormone-sensitivity. Eur J Clin Invest 7:363–371

Kather H, Simon B (1977) Catecholamine-sensitive adenylate cyclase of human fat cell ghosts: a comparative study using different beta-adrenergic agents. Metabolism 26:1179–1184

Katocs AS Jr, Largis EE, Allen DO (1974) Role of Ca^{2+} in adrenocorticotropic hormone-stimulated lipolysis in the perifused fat cell system. J Biol Chem 249:2000–2004

Khoo JC (1976) Ca^{2+}-dependent activation of phosphorylase by phosphorylase kinase in adipose tissue. Biochim Biophys Acta 422:87–97

Khoo JC, Gill GN (1979) Comparison of cyclic nucleotide specificity of guanosine 3′:5′-monophosphate-dependent protein kinase and adenosine 3′:5′-monophosphate-dependent protein kinase. Biochim Biophys Acta 584:21–32

Khoo JC, Steinberg D (1974) Reversible protein kinase activation of a hormone-sensitive lipase from chicken adipose tissue. J Lipid Res 15:602–610

Khoo JC, Steinberg D, Thompson B, Mayer SE (1973) Hormonal regulation of adipocyte enzymes: the effects of epinephrine and insulin on the control of lipase, phosphorylase kinase, phosphorylase, and glycogen synthase. J Biol Chem 248:3823–3830

Khoo JC, Aguino AA, Steinberg D (1974) The mechanism of activation of hormone-sensitive lipase in human adipose tissue. J Clin Invest 53:1124–1131

Khoo JC, Steinberg D, Huang JJ, Vagelos PR (1976) Triglyceride, diglyceride, monoglyceride, and cholesterol ester hydrolases in chicken adipose tissue activated by adenosine 3′,5′-monophosphate-dependent protein kinase. J Biol Chem 251:2882–2890

Khoo JC, Sperry PJ, Gill GN, Steinberg D (1977) Activation of hormone-sensitive lipase and phosphorylase kinase by purified cyclic GMP-dependent protein kinase. Proc Natl Acad Sci USA 74:4843–4847

Kimura N, Nagata N (1977) The requirement of guanine nucleotides for glucagon stimulation of adenylate cyclase in rat liver plasma membranes. J Biol Chem 252:3829–3835

Kishimoto T, Kikutani H, Nishizawa Y, Sakaguchi N, Yamamura Y (1979) Involvement of anti-Ig-activated serine protease in the generation of cytoplasmic factor(s) that are responsible for the transmission of Ig-receptor-mediated signals. J Immunol 123:1504–1510

Kissebah AH, Hope-Gill H, Vydelingum N, Tulloch BR, Clarke PV, Fraser TR (1975) Mode of insulin action. Lancet 144–147

Kitabgi P, Rosselin G, Bataille D (1976) Interactions of glucagon and related peptides with chicken adipose tissue. Horm Metab Res 8:266–270

Knight BL (1974) Adenosine 3′,5′-cyclic phosphate, lipolysis and oxygen consumption in brown adipose tissue from newborn rabbits. Biochem Biophys Acta 343:287–296

Knight BL (1975) Adenosine 3′:5′-cyclic monophosphate-dependent protein kinase in brown fat from newborn rabbits. Biochim J 152:577–583

Knight BL, Iliffe J (1973) The effect of glucose, insulin and noradrenaline on lipolysis, and on the concentrations of adenosine 3′:5′-monophosphate and adenosine 5′-triphosphate in adipose tissue. Biochem J 132:77–82

Kono T, Barham FW (1973) Effects of insulin on the levels of adenosine 3′:5′-monophosphate and lipolysis in isolated rat epididymal fat cells. J Biol Chem 248:7417–7426
Kono T, Robinson FW, Sarver JA (1975) Insulin-sensitive phosphodiesterase: its localization, hormonal stimulation, and oxidative stabilization. J Biol Chem 250:7826–7835
Krahl ME (1961) The action of insulin on cells. Academic Press, New York London
Kunos G (1977) Thyroid hormone-dependent interconversion of myocardial alpha- and beta-adrenoreceptors in the rat. Br J Pharmacol 59:177–189
Kuo JF (1970) Differential effects of Ca^{2+}, EDTA, and adrenergic blocking agents on the actions of some hormones on adenosine 3′,5′-monophosphate levels in isolated adipose cells as determined by prior labeling with (8-^{14}C)adenine. Biochim Biophys Acta 208:509–516
Kupiecki FP (1971) Pharmacological control of free fatty acids. Prog Biochem Pharmacol 6:274–316
Lands AM, Arnold A, McAuliff JP, Luduena FP, Brown TG (1967) Differentiation of receptor systems activated by sympathomimetic amines. Nature 214:597–598
Lang U, Schwyzer R (1976) The ACTH fat cell system as a model for hormone-receptor interaction. In: Parsons JA (ed) Peptide hormones. Macmillan, London, pp 337–348
Lang U, Fauchere J-L, Pelican G-M, Karlaganis G, Schwyzer R (1976) Hormone-receptor interactions. Adrenocorticotrophin-(7-24)-octadecapeptide stimulates adipocyte membrane adenylate cyclase without causing lipolysis in fat cells. FEBS Lett 66:246–249
Larner J (1972) Insulin and glycogen synthase. Diabetes 21:428–438
Larner J, Lawrence JC, Walkenbach RJ, Roach PJ, Hazen RJ, Huang LC (1978) Insulin control of glycogen synthesis. Adv Cyclic Nucleotide Res 9:425–439
Larner J, Galasko J, Cheng G, DePaoli-Roach AA, Huang L, Daggy LP, Kellogg J (1979) Generation by insulin of a chemical mediator that controls protein phosphorylation and dephosphorylation. Science 206:1408–1410
Lawrence JC Jr, Larner J (1977) Evidence for alpha-adrenergic activation of phosphorylase and inactivation of glycogen synthase in rat adipocytes. Mol Pharmacol 13:1060–1075
Lawrence JC Jr, Larner J (1978 a) Activation of glycogen synthase in rat adipocytes by insulin and glucose involves increased glucose transport and phosphorylation. J Biol Chem 253:2104–2113
Lawrence JC Jr, Larner J (1978 b) Effects of insulin, methoxamine, and calcium on glycogen synthase in rat adipocytes. Mol Pharmacol 14:1079–1091
Lawrence JC Jr, Guinovart JJ, Larner J (1977) Activation of rat adipocyte glycogen synthase by insulin. J Biol Chem 252:444–450
Laychock SG, Franson RC, Weglicki WB, Rubin RP (1977) Identification and partial characterization of phospholipases in isolated adrenocortical cells. Biochem J 164:753–756
Lee K-H, Kim K-H (1979) Stimulation by epinephrine of in vivo phosphorylation and inactivation of acetyl coenzyme A carboxylase of rat epididymal adipose tissue. J Biol Chem 254:1450–1453
Lefkowitz RJ, Roth J, Pastan I (1970) Effects of calcium on ACTH stimulation of the adrenal: separation of hormone binding from adenyl cyclase activation. Nature 228:864–866
Levin L, Farber RK (1952) Hormones and metabolism. Hormonal factors which regulate the mobilization of depot fat to the liver. Recent Prog Horm Res 7:399–435
Lewis GP, Piper PJ, Vigo C (1979) The effects of glucocorticoids on the distribution and mobilization of arachidonic acid in fat cell ghosts. Br J Pharmacol 67:393–400
Li CH (1978) Hormonal proteins and peptides, vol 5: Lipotropin and related peptides. Academic Press, New York London
Lindberg O, Bieber LL, Houstek J (1976) Brown adipose tissue metabolism; an attempt to apply results from in vitro experiments on tissue in vivo. In: Jansky L, Musacchia XJ (eds) Regulation of depressed metabolism and thermogenesis. Thomas, Springfield, pp 117–136
Livingston JN, Gurny PA, Lockwood DH (1977) Insulin-like effects of polyamines in fat cells. J Biol Chem 252:560–562
Lohmar P, Li CH (1968) Biological properties of ovine beta lipotropin hormone. Endocrinology 82:898–904

Londos C, Wolff J (1977) Two distinct adenosine-sensitive sites on adenylate cyclase. Proc Natl Acad Sci USA 74:5482–5486
Londos C, Salomon Y, Lin MC, Harwood JP, Schramm M, Wolff J, Rodbell M (1974) 5′-Guanylylimidodiphosphate, a potent activator of adenylate cyclase systems in eukaryotic cells. Proc Natl Acad Sci USA 71:3087–3090
Londos C, Cooper DMF, Schlegel W, Rodbell M (1978) Adenosine analogs inhibit adipocyte adenylate cyclase by a GTP-dependent process: basis for actions of adenosine and methylxanthines on cyclic AMP production and lipolysis. Proc Natl Acad Sci USA 75:5362–5366
Lopez E, White JE, Engel FL (1959) Contrasting requirements for the lipolytic action of corticotropin and epinephrine on adipose tissue in vitro. J Biol Chem 234:2254–2258
Loten EG, Sneyd JGT (1970) An effect of insulin on adipose tissue adenosine 3′:5′-cyclic monophosphate phosphodiesterase. Biochem J 120:187–193
Malaisse WJ, Hutton JC, Kawazu S, Sener A (1978) The stimulus-secretion coupling of glucose-induced insulin release. Metabolic effects of menadione in isolated islets. Eur J Biochem 87:121–130
Malbon CC, Cabelli RJ (1978) Evaluation of the negative cooperativity model for fat cell beta-adrenergic receptors. Biochim Biophys Acta 544:93–101
Malbon CC, Gill DM (1979) ADP-ribosylation of membrane proteins and activation of adenylate cyclase by cholera toxin in fat cell ghosts from euthyroid and hypothyroid rats. Biochim Biophys Acta 586:518–527
Malbon CC, Moreno FJ, Cabelli RJ, Fain JN (1978) Fat cell adenylate cyclase and beta-adrenergic receptors in altered thyroid states. J Biol Chem 253:671–678
Malgieri JA, Shepherd RE, Fain JN (1975) Lack of feedback regulation of cyclic 3′:5′-AMP accumulation by free fatty acids in chicken fat cells. J Biol Chem 250:6593–6598
Manganiello V, Vaughan M (1973) An effect of insulin on cyclic adenosine 3′.5′-monophosphate phosphodiesterase activity in fat cells. J Biol Chem 248:7164–7170
Manganiello VC, Lovell-Smith CJ, Vaughan M (1976) Effects of choleragen on hormonal responsiveness of adenylate cyclase in human fibroblasts and rat fat cells. Biochim Biophys Acta 451:62–71
May JM, de Haen C (1979 a) Insulin-stimulated intracellular hydrogen peroxide production in rat epididymal fat cells. J Biol Chem 254:2214–2220
May JM, de Haen C (1979 b) The insulin-like effect of hydrogen peroxide on pathways of lipid synthesis in rat adipocytes. J Biol Chem 254:9017–9021
McDonald JM, Bruns DE, Jarett L (1976 a) Characterization of calcium binding to adipocyte plasma membranes. J Biol Chem 251:5345–5351
McDonald JM, Bruns DE, Jarett L (1976 b) Ability of insulin to increase calcium binding to adipocyte plasma membranes. Proc Natl Acad Sci USA 73:1542–1546
McDonald JM, Bruns DE, Jarett L (1978) Ability of insulin to increase calcium uptake by adipocyte endoplasmic reticulum. J Biol Chem 253:3504–3508
Meisner H, Carter JR Jr (1977) Regulation of lipolysis in adipose tissue. Horiz Biochem Biophys 4:91–129
Michell RH (1975) Inositol phospholipids and cell surface receptor function. Biochim Biophys Acta 415:81–147
Michell RH (1979) Inositol phospholipids in membrane function. Trends Biochem Sci 4:128–131
Michell RH, Jafferji SS, Jones LM (1977) The possible involvement of phosphatidylinositol breakdown in the mechanism of stimulus-response coupling at receptors which control cell-surface calcium gates. Adv Exp Med Biol 83:447–465
Miller DW, Allen DW (1971) Antilipolytic activity of 4-(2-hydroxy-3-isopropylaminopropoxy) acetanilide (practolol). Proc Soc Exp Biol Med 136:715–718
Mitchell P (1979) Keilin's respiratory chain concept and its chemiosomatic consequences. Science 206:1148–1159
Mollay C, Kreil G (1973) Fluorimetric measurements on the interaction of mellitin with lecithin. Biochim Biophys Acta 316:196–203
Mollay C, Kreil G (1974) Enhancement of bee venom phospholipase A_2, activity by melittin, direct lytic factor from cobra venom and polymyxin B. FEBS Lett 46:141–144

Moskowitz J, Fain JN (1970) Stimulation by growth hormone and dexamethasone of labeled cyclic adenosine 3′,5′-monophosphate accumulation by white fat cells. J Biol Chem 245:1101–1107
Moyle WR, Kong YC, Ramachandran J (1973) Steroidogenesis and cyclic AMP accumulation in rat adrenal cells. J Biol Chem 248:2409–2417
Mukherjee C, Jungas RL (1975) Activation of pyruvate dehydrogenase in adipose tissue by insulin. Evidence for an effect of insulin on pyruvate dehydrogenase phosphate phosphatase. Biochem J 148:229–235
Mukherjee SP, Lynn WS (1977) Reduced nicotinamide adenine dinucleotide phosphate oxidase in adipocyte plasma membrane and its activation by insulin. Arch Biochem Biophys 184:69–76
Mukherjee SP, Lane RH, Lynn WS (1978) Endogenous hydrogen peroxide and peroxidative metabolism in adipocytes in response to insulin and sulfhydryl reagents. Biochem Pharmacol 27:2589–2594
Nicholls DG (1976) The bioenergetics of knows adipose tissue mitochondria. FEBS Lett 61:103–110
Nicholls DG (1977) Hormonal control of brown adipose tissue metabolism. Biochem Soc Trans 5:908–912
Nicholls DG, Lindberg O (1973) Brown adipose tissue mitochondria. The Influence of albumin and nucleotides on passive ion permeabilities. Eur J Biochem 37:523–530
Nikkilä EY, Pykälistö O (1968) Regulation of adipose tissue lipoprotein lipase synthesis by intracellular free fatty acid. Life Sci 7:1303–1309
Nilsson NO, Stralfors P, Fredrikson G, Belfrage P (1980) Regulation of adipose tissue lipolysis: effects of noradrenaline and insulin on phosphorylation of hormonesensitive lipase and on lipolysis in intact rat adipocytes. FEBS Lett 111:125–130
Nimmo HG, Houston B (1978) Rat adipose tissue glycerol phosphate acyltransferase can be inactivated by cyclic AMP-dependent protein kinase. Biochem J 176:607–610
Nyberg G, Smith U (1977) Human adipose tissue in culture. VII. The long-term of effect of growth hormone. Horm Metab Res 9:22–27
Ohisalo JJ, Stouffer JE (1979) Adenosine, thyroid status and regulation of lipolysis. Biochem J 178:249–251
Olsson RA, Davis CJ, Khouri EM, Patterson RE (1976) Evidence for an adenosine receptor on the surface of dog coronary myocytes. Circ Res 39:93–98
Pacuszka T, Moss J, Fishman PH (1978) A sensitive method for the detection of GM_1-ganglioside in rat adipocyte preparations based on its interaction with choleragen. J Biol Chem 253:5103–5108
Paetzke-Brunner K, Schön H, Wieland OH (1978) Insulin activates pyruvate dehydrogenase by lowering the mitochondrial acetyl-CoA/CoA ratio as evidenced by digitonin fractionation of isolated fat cells. FEBS Lett 93:307–311
Patten RL (1970) The reciprocal regulation of lipoprotein lipase activity and hormone-sensitive lipase activity in rat adipocytes. J Biol Chem 245:5577–5584
Pawlson LG, Lovell-Smith CJ, Manganiello VC, Vaughan M (1974) Effects of epinephrine, adrenocorticotrophic hormone, and theophylline on adenosine 3′,5′-monophosphate phosphodiesterase activity in fat cells. Proc Natl Acad Sci USA 71:1639–1642
Pereira JN, Holland GF (1966) The effect of nicotinamide adenine dinucleotide on lipolysis in adipose tissue in vitro. Experientia 22:658–659
Piascik MT, Osei-Gyimah P, Miller DD, Feller DR (1978) Stereoselective interaction of tetrahydroisoquinolines in β-adrenoceptor systems. Eur J Pharmacol 48:393–401
Pilch PF, Thompson PA, Czech MP (1980) Coordinate modulation of D-glucose transport activity and bilayer fluidity in plasma membranes derived from control and insulin-treated adipocytes. Proc Natl Acad Sci USA 77:915–918
Pillion DJ, Czech MP (1978) Antibodies against intrinsic adipocyte plasma membrane proteins activate D-glucose transport independent of interaction with insulin binding sites. J Biol Chem 253:3761–3764
Pillion DJ, Grantham JR, Czech MP (1979) Biological properties of antibodies against rat adipocyte intrinsic membrane proteins. J Biol Chem 254:3211–3220

Prusiner SB, Cannon B, Lindberg O (1968) Oxidative metabolism in cells isolated from brown adipose tissue. 1. Catecholamine and fatty acid stimulation of respiration. Eur J Biochem 6:15–22
Raben MS, Hollenberg CH (1959) Effect of growth hormone on plasma fatty acids. J Clin Invest 38:484–488
Raben MS, Matsuzaki F (1966) Effect of purines on epinephrine-induced lipolysis in adipose tissue. J Biol Chem 241:4781–4786
Ramakrishna S, Benjamin WB (1979) Fat cell protein phosphorylation: identification of phosphoprotein-2 as ATP-citrate lyase. J Biol Chem 254:9232–9236
Rao AJ, Ramachandran J (1977) Growth hormone and the regulation of lipolysis. In: Li H (ed) Hormonal proteins and peptides, vol IV. Academic Press, New York London, pp 43–60
Rasmussen H, Goodman DBP (1977) Relationships between calcium and cyclic nucleotides in cell activation. Physiol Rev 57:421–509
Reckless JPD, Gilbert CH, Galton DJ (1976) Alpha-adrenergic receptor activity, cyclic AMP and lipolysis in adipose tissue of hypothyroid man and rat. J Endocrinol 68:419–430
Reed N, Fain JN (1968 a) Stimulation of respiration in brown fat cells by epinephrine, dibutyryl-3′,5′-adenosine monophosphate, and m-chloro(carbonyl cyanide)phenylhydrazone. J Biol Chem 243:2843–2848
Reed N, Fain JN (1968 b) Potassium-dependent stimulation of respiration in brown fat cells by fatty acids and lipolytic agents. J Biol Chem 243:6077–6083
Reed N, Fain JN (1970) Hormonal regulation of the metabolism of free brown fat cells. In: Lindberg O (ed) Brown adipose tissue, Elsevier, Amsterdam Oxford New York, pp 207–224
Renold AE, Cahill GF Jr (sect eds) (1965) Handbook of physiology, sect 5: Adipose tissue. American Physiological Society, Washington, DC
Rich C, Bierman EL, Schwartz IL (1959) Plasma nonesterified fatty acids in hyperthyroid states. J Clin Invest 38:275–278
Rimon G, Hanski E, Braun S, Levitzki A (1978) Mode of coupling between hormone receptors and adenylate cyclase elucidated by modulation of membrane fluidity. Nature 276:394–396
Robison GA, Butcher RW, Sutherland EW (1971) Cyclic AMP. Academic Press, New York London
Rodbell M (1964) Metabolism of isolated fat cells. 1. Effects of hormone on glucose metabolism and lipolysis. J Biol Chem 239:375–380
Rodbell M (1965) Modulation of lipolysis in adipose tissue by fatty acid concentration in fat cell. Ann NY Acad Sci 131:302–333
Rodbell M (1967) Metabolism of isolated fat cells. V. Preparation of "ghosts" and their properties; adenyl cyclase and other enzymes. J Biol Chem 242:5744–5750
Rodbell M (1975) On the mechanism of activation of fat cell adenylate cyclase by guanine nucleotides. An explanation for the biphasic inhibitory and stimulatory effects of the nucleotides and the role of hormones. J Biol Chem 250:5826–5834
Rodbell M, Jones AB, Cingolani GEC, Birnbaumer L (1968) The actions of insulin and catabolic hormones on the plasma membrane of the fat cells. Recent Prog Horm Res 24:215–254
Rodbell M, Birnbaumer L, Pohl SL (1970) Adenyl cyclase in fat cells, III. Stimulation by secretin and the effects of trypsin on the receptors for lipolytic hormones. J Biol Chem 245:718–722
Rodbell M, Birnbaumer L, Pohl SL, Krans H (1971) The glucagon-sensitive adenyl cyclase system in plasma membranes of rat liver. V. An obligatory role of guanyl nucleotides in glucagon action. J Biol Chem 246:1877–1882
Rosen OM, Rangel-Aldao R, Ehrlichman NJ (1977) Soluble cyclic AMP-dependent protein kinase: review of the enzyme isolated from bovine cardiac muscle. Curr Top Cell Regul 12:39–74
Rosenqvist U, Efendic S, Jereb B, Ostman J (1971) Influence of the hypothyroid state on lipolysis in human adipose tissue in vitro. Acta Med Scand 189:381–384

Rubin RP, Laychock SG (1978) Prostaglandins and calcium-membrane interactions in secretory glands. Ann NY Acad Sci 307:377–390
Rudman D (1963) The adipokinetic action of polypeptide and amine hormones upon the adipose tissue of various animal species. J Lipid Res 4:119–129
Sahyoun N, Cuatrecasas P (1975) Mechanism of activation of adenylate cyclase by cholera toxin. Proc Natl Acad Sci USA 72:3438–3442
Sakai T, Thompson WJ, Lavis VR, Williams RH (1974) Cyclic nucleotide phosphodiesterase activities from isolated fat cells: correlation of subcellular distribution with effects of nucleotides and insulin. Arch Biochem Biophys 162:331–339
Schimmel RJ (1973) The influence of extracellular calcium ion on hormone-activated lipolysis. Biochim Biophys Acta 326:262–278
Schimmel RJ (1976) The role of calcium ion in epinephrine activation of lipolysis. Horm Metab Res 8:195–201
Schimmel RJ (1979) Inhibition of lipolysis in hamster epididymal adipocytes by selective alpha-adrenergic agents. Evidence for cyclic AMP-dependent and independent mechanisms. Biochim Biphys Acta 587:217–226
Schoenle C, Zapf J, Froesch ER (1979) Effect of insulin on glucose metabolism and glucose transport in fat cells of hormone-treated hypophysectomized rats: evidence that growth hormone restricts glucose transport. Endocrinology 105:1237–1242
Schrey MP, Rubin RP (1979) Characterization of a calcium-mediated activation of arachidonic acid turnover in adrenal phospholipids by corticotropin. J Biol Chem 254:11234–11241
Schwabe U, Ebert R (1972) Different effects of lipolytic hormones and phosphodiesterase inhibitors on cyclic 3′,5′-AMP levels in isolated fat cells. Arch Pharm (Weinheim) 274:287–298
Schwabe U, Ebert R (1974) Stimulation of cyclic adenosine 3′,5′-monophosphate accumulation and lipolysis in fat cells by adenosine deaminase. Arch Pharm (Weinheim) 282:33–44
Schwabe U, Ebert R, Erbler HC (1973) Adenosine release from isolated fat cells and its significance for the effects of hormones on cyclic 3′,5′-AMP levels and lipolysis. Arch Pharm (Weinheim) 276:133–148
Schwyzer R (1978) Studies on polypeptide receptors. A critical view on the mechanism of ACTH action. Bull Schweiz Akad Med Wiss 34:263–274
Scow RO, Chernick SS (1970) Transport and utilization of free fatty acids. In: Florkin M, Stotz EH (eds) Comprehensive biochemistry, vol 18. Elsevier, Amsterdam Oxford New York, pp 19–50
Seals JR, Jarett L (1980) Activation of pyruvate dehydrogenase by direct addition of insulin to an isolated plasma membrane-mitochondria mixture: evidence for generation of insulin's second messenger in a subcellular system. Proc Natl Acad Sci USA 77:77–81
Seals JR, McDonald JM, Jarett L (1979 a) Insulin effect on protein phosphorylation of plasma membranes and mitochondria in a subcellular system from rat adipocytes. I. Identification of insulin-sensitive phosphoproteins. J Biol Chem 254:6991–6996
Seals JR, McDonald JM, Jarett L (1979 b) Insulin effect on protein phosphorylation of plasma membranes and mitochondria in a subcellular system from rat adipocytes. II. Characterization of insulin-sensitive phosphoproteins and conditions for observation of the insulin effect. J Biol Chem 254:6997–7001
Sessa G, Freer JH, Colacicco G, Weissmann G (1969) Interaction of a lytic polypeptide, mellitin, with lipid membrane systems. J Biol Chem 244:3375–3582
Severson DL, Khoo JC, Steinberg D (1977) Role of phosphoprotein phosphatases in reversible deactivation of chicken adipose tissue hormone-sensitive lipase. J Biol Chem 252:1484–1489
Shanahan MF, Czech MP (1977 a) Partial purification of the D-glucose transport system in rat adipocyte plasma membranes. J Biol Chem 252:6554–6561
Shanahan MF, Czech MP (1977 b) Purification and reconstitution of the adipocyte plasma membrane D-glucose transport system. J Biol Chem 252:8341–8343
Shepherd RE, Malbon CC, Smith CJ, Fain JN (1977) Lipolysis and adenosine 3′,5′-cyclic AMP metabolism in isolated white fat cells from genetically obese hyperglycemic mice (ob/ob). J Biol Chem 252:7242–7248

Shier WT (1979) Activation of high levels of endogenous phospholipase A_2 in cultured cells. Proc Natl Acad Sci USA 76:195–199

Shier WT, Baldwin JH, Nilsen-Hamilton M, Hamilton RT, Thanassi N (1976) Regulation of guanylate and adenylate cyclase activities by lysolecithin. Proc Natl Acad Sci USA 73:1586–1590

Shonk RF, Miller DD, Feller DR (1971) Influence of substituted tetrahydroisoquinolines and catecholamines on lipolysis in vitro. Biochem Pharmacol 20:3403–3412

Sica V, Cuatrecasas P (1973) Effects of insulin, epinephrine, and cyclic adenosine monophosphate on pyruvate dehydrogenase of adipose tissue. Biochemistry 12:2282–2291

Siddle K, Hales CN (1974) The relationship between the concentration of adenosine 3':5'-cyclic monophosphate and the anti-lipolytic ation of insulin in isolated rat fat cells. Biochem J 142:97–103

Sjöström L, Smith U, Björntorp P, Jacobsson B, Hallgren P (1977) Human adipose tissue maintained in a continuous flow system. J Biol Chem 252:8833–8839

Skala JP, Knight RL (1977) Protein kinases in brown adipose tissue of developing rats; state of activation of protein kinase during development and cold exposure and its relationship to adenosine 3':5'-monophosphate, lipolysis and heat production. J Biol Chem 252:1064–1070

Smith U, Isaksson O, Nyberg G, Sjöstrom L (1976) Human adipose tissue in culture. IV. Evidence for the formation of a hormone antagonist by catecholamines. Eur J Clin Invest 6:35–42

Smith U, Sternström G, Sjöström L, Isaksson O, Jacobsson B (1977) Studies on the catecholamine resistance in fat cells from patients with phaeochromocytoma. Eur J Clin Invest 7:355–361

Smith TL, Eichberg J, Hauser G (1979) Postsynaptic localization of the alpha receptor-mediated stimulation of phosphatidylinositol turnover in pineal gland. Life Sci 24:2179–2184

Soderling TR, Corbin JD, Park CR (1973) Regulation of adenosine 3',5'-monophosphate-dependent protein kinase. II. Hormonal regulation of the adipose tissue enzyme. J Biol Chem 248:1822–1829

Solomon SS (1975) Effect of insulin and lipolytic hormones on cyclic AMP phosphodiesterase activity in normal and diabetic rat adipose tissue. Endocrinology 96:1366–1373

Solomon SS, Palazzolo M, King LE Jr (1977) Cyclic nucleotide phosphodiesterase. Insulin activation detected in adipose tissue by gel electrophoresis. Diabetes 26:967–972

Sooranna SR, Saggerson ED (1975) Studies on the role of insulin in the regulation of glyceride synthesis in rat epididymal adipose tissue. Biochem J 150:441–451

Sooranna SR, Saggerson ED (1976) Interactions of insulin and adrenaline with glycerol phosphate acylation processes in fat cells from rat- FEBS Lett 64:36–39

Sooranna SR, Saggerson ED (1979) Inactivation of rat adipocyte pyruvate dehydrogenase by palmitate. Biochem J 184:59–62

Spooner PM, Chernick SS, Garrison MM, Scow RO (1979) Development of lipoprotein lipase activity and accumulation of triacylglycerol in differentiating 3T3-L1 adipocytes. J Biol Chem 254:1305–1311

Stein JM, Hales CN (1972) The effect of adrenaline and of adrenergic blocking agents on ^{32}P incorporation into fat cell phospholopids. Biochem J 28:531–541

Stein JM, Hales CN (1974) The effect of insulin on ^{32}Pi incorporation into rat fat cell phospholipids. Biochim Biophys Acta 337:41–49

Steinberg D (1976) Interconvertible enzymes in adipose tissue regulated by cyclic AMP-dependent protein kinase. Adv Cyclic Nucleotide Res 7:157–198

Steinberg D, Mayer SE, Khoo JC, Miller EA, Miller RE, Fredholm B, Eichner R (1975) Hormonal regulation of lipase, phosphorylase, and glycogen synthase in adipose tissue. Adv Cyclic Nucleotide Res 5:549–568

Steiner DF, Freinkel N (eds) (1972) Handbook of Physiology, sect 7, Endocrinology, vol 1, Endocrine pancreas. American Physiological Society, Washington, DC

Takeda M, Nakaya Y (1976) Effect of guanosine 3':5'-monophosphate on glucose oxidation and epinephrine-stimulated lipolysis in isolated rat epididymal fat cells. J Biochem (Tokyo) 80:717–722

Taylor SI, Mukherjee C, Jungas RL (1973) Studies on the mechanism of activation of adipose tissue pyruvate dehydrogenase by insulin. J Biol Chem 248:73–81
Taylor WM, Halperin ML (1979) Stimulation of glucose transport in rat adipocytes by insulin, adenosine, nicotinic acid and hydrogen peroxide. Biochem J 178:381–389
Taylor WM, Mak ML, Halperin ML (1976) Effect of 3′:5′-cyclic AMP on glucose transport in rat adipocytes. Proc Natl Acad Sci USA 73:4359–4363
Thajchayapong P, Queener SF, McClintock R, Allen DO, Bell NH (1976) Demonstration that cyclic adenosine 3′,5′-monophosphate mediates the lipolytic action of parathyroid hormone. Horm Metab Res 8:190–195
Thompson WJ, Appleman MM (1971) Characterization of cyclic nucleotide phosphodiesterases of rat tissues. J Biol Chem 246:3145–3150
Tsai S-C, Fales HM, Vaughan M (1973) Inactivation of hormone-sensitive lipase from adipose tissue with adenosine triphosphate, magnesium, and ascorbic acid. J Biol Chem 248:5278–5281
Turpin BP, Duckworth WC, Solomon SS (1977) Perifusion of isolated adipose cells. Modulation of lipolysis by adenosine. J Clin Invest 60:442–448
Van Inwegen RG, Robison GA, Thompson WJ, Armstrong KJ, Stouffer JE (1975) Cyclic nucleotide phosphodiesterase and thyroid hormones. J Biol Chem 250:2452–2456
Vaughan M, (1961) Effect of hormones on glucose metabolism in adipose tissue. J Biol Chem 236:2196–2199
Vaughan M, Steinberg D (1963) Effect of hormones on lipolysis and exterification of free fatty acids during incubation of adipose tissue in vitro. J Lipid Res 4:193–199
Vaughan M, Pierce NF, Greenough WB III (1970) Stimulation of glycerol production in fat cells by cholera toxin. Nature 226:658–659
Vydelingum N, Kissebah AH, Wynn V (1978) The role of calcium in insulin action. V. Importance of cyclic guanosine 3′5′-monophosphate and calcium ions in insulin stimulation of lipoprotein lipase activity and protein synthesis in adipose tissue. Horm Metab Res 10:38–46
Walkenbach RJ, Hazen R, Larner J (1978) Reversible inhibition of cyclic AMP-dependent protein kinase by insulin. Mol Cell Biochem 19:31–41
Weiss L, Loffler G, Schirmann A, Wieland O (1971) Control of pyruvate dehydrogenase interconversion in adipose tissue by insulin. FEBS Lett 15:229–231
Wells JN, Hardmann JG (1977) Cyclic nucleotide phosphodiesterases. Adv Cyclic Nucleotide Res 8:119–144
Wenke M, Lincová D, Černohorsky M, Čepelik J (1966) The relation between tracheorelaxant and fat mobilizing action of some derivatives of noradrenaline and 2-amino-1-p-hydroxyphenylethanol. J Pharm Pharmacol 18:190–191
Wenkeova J, Kuhn E, Wenke M (1976) Some adrenomimetic drugs affecting lipolysis in human adipose tissue in vitro. Eur J Pharmacol 35:1–6
Werner S, Löw H (1973) Stimulation of lipolysis and calcium accumulation by parathyroid hormone in rat adipose tissue in vitro after adrenalectomy and administration of high doses of cortisone acetate. Horm Metab Res 5:292–296
Westermann E, Stock K, Bieck P (1969) Phenylisopropyl-adenosine (PIA): ein potenter Hemmstoff der Lipolyse in vivo und in vitro. Med Ernaehr 10:143–147
White JE, Engel FL (1958) Lipolytic action of corticotropin on rat adipose tissue in vitro. J Clin Invest 37:1556–1563
Whitehouse S, Randle PJ (1973) Activation of pyruvate dehydrogenase in perfused rat heart by dichloroacetate. Biochem J 134:651–653
Wieser PB, Fain JN (1975) Insulin, prostaglandin E_1, phenylisopropyl adenosine and nicotinic acid as regulators of fat cell metabolism. Endocrinology 96:1221–1225
Wieser PB, Malgieri JA, Ward WF, Pointer RH, Fain JN (1974) Effects of bovine growth hormone preparations, fragments of growth hormone and pituitary anti-insulin peptide on lipolysis and glucose metabolism of isolated fat cells and adipose tissue. Endocrinology 95:206–212
Williams LT, Jarett L, Lefkowitz RJ (1976) Adipocyte β-adrenergic receptors. Identification and subcellular localization by (−)-[^{3}H]dihydroalprenolol. J Biol Chem 251:3096–3104
Wise LS, Green H (1978) Studies of lipoprotein lipase during the adipose conversion of 3T3 cells. Cell 13:233–242

Wise LS, Jungas RL (1978) Evidence for a dual mechanism of lipolysis activation by epinephrine in rat adipose tissue. J Biol Chem 253:2624–2627

Witters LA, Kowaloff EM, Avruch J (1979) Glucagon regulation of protein phosphorylation. Identification of acetyl coenzyme A carboxylase as a substrate. J Biol Chem 254:245–248

Wong EHA, Loten EG, Park CR (1978) The correlation of cyclic AMP and protein kinase activity in adipocytes with lipolysis stimulated by ACTH: the effect of adenosine deaminase and actinomycin. J Cyclic Nucleotide Res 4:359–374

Yamamura H, Rodbell M, Fain JN (1976) Hydroxybenzylpindolol and hydroxybenzylpropranolol: partial beta-adrenergic agonists of adenylate cyclase in the rat adipocyte. Mol Pharmacol 12:693–700

Yamamura H, Lad PM, Rodbell M (1977) GTP stimulates and inhibits adenylate cyclase in fat cell membranes through distinct regulatory processes. J Biol Chem 252:7964–7966

Yunes R, Goldhammer AR, Garner WK, Cordes EH (1977) Phospholipases: melittin facilitation of bee venom phospholipase A_2-catalyzed hydrolysis of unsonicated lecithin liposomes. Arch Biochem Biophys 183:105–112

Zinman B, Hollenberg CH (1974) Effect of insulin and lipolytic agents on rat adipocyte low K_m cyclic adenosine 3′:5′-monophosphate phosphodiesterase. J Biol Chem 249:2182–2187

CHAPTER 18

Regulation of the Cell Cycle and Cellular Proliferation by Cyclic Nucleotides

D. L. FRIEDMAN

Overview

The involvement of cyclic nucleotides in the regulation of cell proliferation has been a focus of considerable interest for almost a decade. Unfortunately, studies in this area have engendered a great deal of confusion, resulting in part from a number of experimental pitfalls (FRIEDMAN et al. 1976a), and in part from the observation of varied and multiple effects of cyclic nucleotides. The growth of certain cell types is stimulated by cAMP while that of others is inhibited. In some instances a single cell type may be either stimulated or inhibited depending on conditions, or it may be inhibited at two different points in its cell division cycle.

Since cyclic nucleotides participate in different ways depending upon the tissue, this review will consider particular cell types separately. An attempt will then be made to generalize on the types of regulation cyclic nucleotides may exert on cell proliferation. Most attention will focus upon the studies that have appeared during the past four years since there have been a number of critical reviews covering prior studies (ABELL and MONAHAN 1973; RYAN and HEIDRICK 1974; PASTAN and JOHNSON 1974; PASTAN et al. 1975; CHLAPOWSKI et al. 1975; FRIEDMAN et al. 1976a; FRIEDMAN 1976; REBHUN 1977). This review will be further confined to studies in higher organisms.

A. Role of Cyclic Nucleotides in Cell Proliferation

I. Cultured Fibroblasts

1. The G_+–G_0 Interconversion

Non-growing normal cells usually contain a 2N complement of chromosomes, indicating that their growth is arrested in the G_1 phase. Evidence has been presented by PARDEE (1974) to suggest that a variety of conditions which induce growth arrest all block cells at the same locus in G_1. He has termed this the restriction point and

Abbreviations: dbcAMP, N^6,2′-O-dibutyryl cAMP; MIX, 1-methyl, 3-isobutylxanthine; PGE_1, prostaglandin E_1; EGF, epidermal growth factor; ACTH, Adrenocorticotropic hormone (corticotropin); TSH, thyroid-stimulating hormone (thyrotropin); MSH, melanocyte-stimulating hormone; G_+, the dividing or cycling state; G_0, the quiescent, or non-cycling state; M, mitosis; S phase, stage of the cell cycle in which DNA is replicated; G_1, cell cycle stage following M and preceeding S phase; G_2, cell cycle stage following S phase and preceeding M suggests that this is a physiological resting point in the cell cycle. There are two controversial hypotheses on the nature of growth arrest. One states that when cell growth is arrested cells enter a new state, termed G_0, in which they display a variety of biochemical properties different from G_1 cells (BECKER and STANNERS 1972; SALAS and GREEN 1971; Levine et al. 1965). The second hypothesis (SMITH and MARTIN 1973) states that all dividing cells become arrested transiently in G_1 during every cell cycle and must accomplish some special process before proceeding to S phase. The ability to carry out this process has a constant probability, which accounts for the variability of transit rates from M to S consistently seen in proliferating cells. The probability constant for this process depends on conditions such as serum or other growth factors. According to this hypothesis, arrested cells are characterized by an extremely low probability constant. For simplicity, in the following discussion we will assume that there is a distinct G_0 state rather than an altered probability constant for G_1 transit.

Cultured "normal" fibroblasts have been studied extensively as models of the interconversion between quiescent (G_0) and growing (G_+) states. Unfortunately, little attempt has been made to relate this in vitro model to the regulation of fibroblast growth in vivo and the physiological significance of this model remains unknown. A variety of conditions cause cultured fibroblasts to cease dividing, e.g., high cell density (density-dependent inhibition) (TODARO and GREEN 1963, 1964), serum deprivation (DULBECCO 1970; HOLLEY and KIERNAN 1968), growth in suspension (MACPHERSON and MONTAGNIER 1964), or various deficiency states PARDEE 1974; HOLLEY and KIERNAN 1974; DULBECCO and ELKINGTON 1975; TOBEY and LEY 1971). Under all conditions, the entrance into a quiescent state is clearly from the G_1 phase (NILHAUSIN and GREEN 1965), since activation of cells results in the synthesis of DNA prior to cell division. While cells are in the quiescent state they remain viable, but exhibit diminished rates of glucose and amino acid transport (PARDEE and ROZENGURT 1975), protein synthesis, and RNA synthesis (GREEN 1974; L. JOHNSON et al. 1974; TODARO et al. 1965). Upon stimulation these functions rapidly revert. Stimulation is achieved by serum addition, proteolytic treatment, replacement of missing nutrients, or addition of various hormones.

a) Regulation by cAMP

When normal rodent fibroblasts enter the quiescent state as a result of serum deprivation there is usually an accompanying rise in cAMP levels (OEY et al. 1974; KRAM et al. 1973; MOENS et al. 1975; Rudland et al. 1974b; SEIFERT and PAUL 1972). Fibroblasts from other species, such as humans, may (AHN et al. 1978; RECHLER et al. 1977; D'Armiento et al. 1973) or may not (HASLAM and GOLDSTEIN 1974; KELLY and BUTCHER 1974; KURTZ et al. 1974; DELL'ORCO et al. 1977) show such a rise. In those instances where elevations in cAMP occur during serum deprivation, they generally do so with about the expected time frame, consistent with a role for cAMP in the mediation of quiescence. Quiescent stimuli other than serum restriction, such as density dependent inhibition, often are not accompanied by elevations in cAMP (BURSTIN et al. 1974; MOENS et al. 1975; OEY et al. 1974; SHEPPARD 1972), though in several studies elevations have been observed (ANDERSON et al. 1973a; BANNAI and SHEPPARD 1974; HEIDRICK and RYAN 1971; OTTEN et al. 1971, 1972a). In at least one instance where a rise was observed, the temporal relationships were highly questionable (BANNAI and SHEPPARD 1974). It has been suggested (OEY et al. 1974) that the differences in the results in studies on density dependent inhibition arise because inadvertent serum deprivation may accompany cell crowding in some experiments.

Regardless of the quiescent stimulus, upon release from quiescence, cellular levels of cAMP usually fall within minutes (BURGER et al. 1972; FROEHLICH and RACHMELER 1972; KRAM et al. 1973; MOENS et al. 1975; OEY et al. 1974; OTTEN et al. 1972a; RUDLAND et al. 1974a, b; SEIFERT and PAUL 1972; SEIFERT and RUDLAND 1974a; SHEPPARD 1972; PLEDGER et al. 1979). The levels stay low for a time period which varies widely, between minutes and many hours, in the different studies.

Addition of cAMP analogs, or of agents which induce elevations in cAMP, to cells at the time of release from quiescence usually blocks cells from entering DNA synthesis (BOMBIK and BURGER 1973; BURGER et al. 1972; FRANK 1972; FROEHLICH and RACHMELER 1972, 1974; KURTZ et al. 1974; WILLINGHAM et al. 1972; ZIMMERMAN and RASKA 1972). Moreover, if exponentially growing cultures are treated for long time periods with such agents, cells become reversibly blocked in $G_1(G_0)$ phase (FROEHLICH and RACHMELER 1972; FRANK 1972; ROZENGURT and PARDEE 1972). Evidence has been presented in BHK and NIL 8 cells that the point within G_1 phase at which cells are blocked by cAMP is the same point at which they are blocked during serum restriction, nutritional deficiencies, or density inhibition, i.e., the restriction point (PARDEE 1974).

The above findings lead to the tentative conclusion that (1) high levels of cAMP can induce and keep cells in a physiological quiescent state, and (2) a rise in cAMP may mediate the induction of G_0 by certain environmental conditions.

Even these limited conclusions regarding a role for cAMP have been seriously challenged recently. RECHLER et al. (1977) have reported results with human fibroblasts which are difficult to rationalize in terms of a model wherein cAMP is a physiological inducer of G_0. The cells used in these experiments showed typical findings: a 3- to 4-fold rise in cAMP during density dependent inhibition of growth, a rapid fall in cAMP levels upon stimulation of quiescent cells with serum, and inhibition by dbcAMP of serum-stimulated DNA synthesis in quiescent cells. However, if the fall in cAMP levels following serum stimulation was totally prevented for the first 4 h, there was no detectable change in the timing or intensity of DNA synthesis. Similar results were obtained if the fall in cAMP was prevented by addition of dbcAMP or by pretreatment of cells with MIX. In contrast, experimental elevations in cAMP during the period from 4–8 h after serum addition resulted in a 4–8 h delay in DNA synthesis. These results suggest that an early fall in cAMP is not essential for growth activation, and are in conflict with earlier studies (FROEHLICH and RACHMELER 1972, 1974) which were also with human cells.

BOYNTON et al. (1978) compared serum-restriction of Balb/3T3 cells in the presence of normal levels of calcium with that in low calcium medium, with interesting results. In both cases the cells became quiescent, and addition of complete medium containing 20% serum induced a release from quiescence. The kinetics of DNA synthesis were identical in the two cultures. However, the fluctuations in cAMP differed with the two experimental protocols. In the cells that had been made quiescent in normal calcium, cAMP levels rapidly fell upon addition of serum whereas in the cultures that had been made quiescent in low calcium, the levels of cAMP remained constant. The reason for this difference is unclear. In both cultures cAMP levels rose at a later time, prior to DNA synthesis. The authors conclude that a fall in cAMP is not essential for initiation of DNA synthesis. As will be discussed later, they believe that the later rise in cAMP *is* essential.

CHLAPOWSKI et al. (1978) studied the effects of PGE_1 on cAMP levels and cell growth in WI-38 fibroblasts. Continuous treatment with 1 μM PGE_1 led to elevations in cAMP which remained above normal for several days. The elevated cAMP activated cAMP-dependent protein kinase. Accumulation of protein was used as a measure of growth. There was little difference in protein content between untreated controls and cells treated with PGE_1 for 48 h, leading to the conclusion that elevations in cAMP do not inhibit cell growth. At higher concentrations of PGE_1 or at high levels of MIX, there was significant inhibition of growth, but there were also morphological signs of toxicity to the cells. To circumvent this problem, combinations of low levels of PGE_1 and MIX were used, resulting in potentiated effects on cAMP levels with little apparent toxicity. Under these conditions the elevated cAMP had no affect on cell protein accumulation. The authors conclude that in WI-38 cells cAMP does not inhibit growth at levels which markedly activate protein kinase. However, the significance of the activation of protein kinase is difficult to assess because total protein kinase activity decreased by as much as 50% during the prolonged increases in cAMP.

PRUSS and HERSCHMAN (1979) reported a surprising result upon addition of cholera toxin to 3T3 cells. The toxin, at low concentrations, actually stimulated cell division in quiescent cells. In addition, it potentiated the stimulatory action of EGF. Following a short lag period, the toxin induced a 40-fold increase in cAMP which lasted at least 4 h, the longest period assayed. Other agents which elevate cAMP did not activate growth, and in fact were inhibitory. The mechanism of cholera toxin action in these cells is unclear and may be unrelated to cAMP metabolism. However, these observations indicate that DNA synthesis can be effectively activated in the presence of high levels of cAMP.

DELL'ORCO et al. (1977) studied serum restriction in human diploid foreskin fibroblasts (HPF strain of CF-2). When these cells became quiescent in response to either serum restriction or density inhibition, no elevation of cAMP was observed. However, the cells could be induced into a quiescent state by 0.5 mM dbcAMP. A comparison, however, of cells induced to quiescence by dbcAMP with those induced by serum-restriction suggested marked differences in the state of the cells. On electron microscopy the dbcAMP treated cells displayed morphology indistinguishable from that of untreated cells growing in medium with 10% serum. In contrast, serum restricted cultures showed a marked decrease in the numbers of free ribosomes and mitochondria, changes in morphology of the mitochondria and the rough endoplasmic reticulum, and an absence of Golgi apparatus. The serum-restricted cells also underwent a 20% decrease in protein content in 14 days of quiescence whereas there was no change in the dbcAMP arrested cells. This latter finding is consistent with studies by HENDEL (1977), who found that both high density inhibited cells and serum restricted cells, in contrast to cAMP arrested cells, exhibit an increased rate of protein degradation. These findings suggest that the nature of the quiescent state in cAMP arrested cells is different from that of serum-restricted or density-inhibited cultures. Unfortunately in these studies it was not determined if the cells were inhibited in G_1 or G_2 phase by cAMP. This is pertinent because, as will be seen in Sect. A.I.2, cAMP can also block fibroblasts in G_2 phase.

In summary, the role of cAMP in the induction of G_0 has been questioned on a number of grounds: (1) it is clear that certain conditions can induce the G_0 state without the mediation of cAMP; (2) even conditions, such as serum deprivation, which are usually accompanied by a rise in cAMP, may not be mediated by cAMP, since the fall in cAMP levels seen upon readdition of serum may not be essential for DNA synthesis; (3) high levels of cAMP induce a state which exhibits different characteristics than the G_0 state induced by other conditions.

In spite of these considerations, it is premature to discount an important role for cAMP in the induction of G_0 for several reasons. First, all of the criticisms noted above must be confirmed with other cell lines and by other laboratories. Second, the quiescent state induced by cAMP appears to be localized to precisely the same cell cycle locus as that of other inducers of G_0. Third, the consistent fall in cAMP upon release from G_0 and the consistent finding that experimental elevations in cAMP inhibit DNA synthesis require alternative explanations.

b) Regulation by cGMP or cAMP/cGMP Ratio

Early studies on levels of cGMP during quiescence and growth stimulation gave rise to the theory that growth stimulation is induced by a brief elevation in cGMP that occurs concomitant with a fall in cAMP (RUDLAND et al. 1974a, b; SEIFERT and RUDLAND 1974a; MOENS et al. 1975). This idea was challenged by Z. MILLER et al. (1975) who found that in their system the levels of both cGMP and cAMP decline following stimulation of serum restricted Balb/3T3 cells. Recent reports have continued to yield conflicting data. The finding that cGMP levels do not rise and, in fact, fall following stimulation with serum has been reproduced by BOYNTON et al. (1978) and WRAY and GLINOS (1978), whereas an elevation has been observed by AHN et al. (1978) and by YASUDA et al. (1978). Contrasting results also have been obtained regarding the changes in cellular cGMP levels during serum deprivation (MOENS et al. 1975; AHN et al. 1978). Finally, there are conflicting reports regarding the effects of experimentally elevated cGMP. SEIFERT and RUDLAND (1974a) reported partial success in stimulating fibroblasts to enter DNA synthesis with cGMP and its analogs. However, these findings have not been confirmed, and PASTAN and co-workers (CARCHMAN et al. 1974; PASTAN et al. 1975) have noted their negative attempts with 3T3 cells. Clearly, no conclusions can presently be drawn concerning a role for cGMP in growth regulation of fibroblasts.

2. Other Cell Cycle Effects of cAMP in Fibroblasts

Although prolonged elevations in cAMP induce growth arrest in G_0, other effects of cAMP on cell division, apparently unrelated to the G_0–G_+ transition, have also been observed.

Fluctuations in cAMP levels during the cell cycle were first reported by BURGER et al. (1972) in 3T3 Swiss mouse fibroblasts. Upon release from quiescence there was an initial fall in cAMP levels, but they subsequently rose in G_1. Time points were taken too infrequently to determine when the maximum levels were obtained, but a clear fall in cAMP levels was observed coincident with the peak of mitosis.

Using Balb/C 3T3 cells, similar results were obtained by SEIFERT and RUDLAND (1974a, b) except that the levels were monitored into a second cell cycle. In the second G_1 phase after the release from quiescence, two peaks of cAMP were observed, an early G_1 peak which was very sharp and a broad peak late in G_1 phase. The significance of the sharp peak and its relationship to the cell cycle must be seriously questioned because of the poor synchrony in these studies. HIBASAMI et al. (1977) reported cell cycle fluctuations in BHK fibroblasts synchronized with excess thymidine. They also found minimum levels in G_2 and M phases and a single G_1 peak with maximum near the G_1/S border. BOYNTON et al. (1978) confirmed a late G_1 maximum in cAMP levels in Balb/3T3 cells.

Consistent with a decline in cAMP content at G_2 and mitosis, prolonged treatment with dbcAMP and theophylline blocks the growth of virally transformed 3T3 cells in G_2 phase rather than in G_1, as indicated by their 4N content of DNA (PAUL 1973; SMETS 1972).

The results of WILLINGHAM et al. (1972) suggest that normal fibroblasts are also blocked in G_2 by high levels of cAMP, in addition to the $G_1(G_0)$ block. 3T3 cells were synchronized by release from quiescence and dbcAMP was added for varying time intervals thereafter. If this analog was present continuously cells were inhibited in G_1. However, if it was added during S phase, a potent inhibition in G_2 was observed.

Stimulatory effects of cAMP in fibroblasts have also been noted. WILLINGHAM et al. (1972) observed that if dbcAMP was added at 3 h or 6 h after the release from quiescence, there was an advanced wave of DNA synthesis, i.e., a shortening of G_1. This result is consistent with the hypothesis that the peak in cAMP observed during G_1 phase is an essential step for the progress of cells through the cell cycle. Unfortunately, butyrate and 5′AMP were not tested in these studies, and other workers have reported such stimulatory effects with a variety of purine nucleosides and nucleotides (CLARK and SMITH 1973; HOVI and VAHERI 1973; LANDAU and SACHS 1971; MONTAGNIER 1971; SCHOR and ROZENGURT 1973).

II. Liver Cells

1. Liver Regeneration

Adult hepatocytes normally divide at an extremely slow rate and can be thought of as a quiescent, G_0, cell population. Following partial hepatectomy, the surviving cells rapidly enter the growing state and, after about 14–20 h, begin DNA synthesis and subsequently cell division. Two waves of cAMP accumulation have been consistently observed following partial hepatectomy, one with a peak at about 2 h and a second with a peak at about 12 h (MACMANUS et al. 1972; SHORT et al. 1975; THROWER and ORD 1974). In one report (THROWER and ORD 1974), a third peak in cAMP was seen during DNA synthesis. Both 2 h and 12 h peaks in cAMP can be inhibited with DL-propranolol. Inhibition of the earlier peak does not significantly alter the progress of cells towards DNA synthesis (MACMANUS et al. 1973). However, if propranolol is injected 8 h after partial hepatectomy there is a 6–8 h delay in the second cAMP peak, correlated with a delay of a remarkably similar duration in the onset of DNA synthesis. Curiously, the second wave of cAMP and

DNA synthesis is also blocked by α-adrenergic blocking agents. These results suggest that a late G_1 peak in cAMP is required for the initiation of DNA synthesis.

A stimulatory role for cAMP in liver regeneration is suggested also by the investigations of LIEBERMAN and co-workers, who found that infusion of mixtures of triiodothyronine, amino acids, glucagon, and heparin induces DNA synthesis in intact rat liver (SHORT et al. 1972). Of the four components of this mixture, glucagon and triiodothyronine are most essential. Glucagon can be replaced by dbcAMP plus theophylline, but not dbcGMP (± theophylline) or by insulin plus high glucose (SHORT et al. 1975). In the absence of the other components of the mixture dbcAMP plus theophylline stimulates two growth related phenomena: RNA polymerase activity and ribosome synthesis (BAILEY et al. 1975).

BUCHER and SWAFFIELD (1975) examined liver regeneration in rats from which the gastrointestinal tract, pancreas, and spleen had been removed. They found that the proliferative response is both considerably reduced and delayed in these rats, but can be effectively restored by infusion of a combination of insulin and glucagon. Either hormone separately is ineffective. The results of hormone treatment are the same if infusion is begun at the time of partial hepatectomy or 6–7 h later. This suggests that the hormones are not "initiators" of regeneration, but rather act some later time as "promoters".

In the studies described above, the action of insulin and glucagon could have been directly upon the liver or could have been indirect, via effects on other tissues. The studies of RICHMAN et al. (1976) on primary monolayer cultures of adult rat hepatocytes strongly support a direct action. It was shown that insulin, glucagon, and a third hormone, EGF, act synergistically to stimulate DNA synthesis in hepatocytes from partially hepatectomized rats. Similar findings have been obtained recently with cultured cells from intact livers. cAMP plus MIX, epinephrine or isoproterenol can effectively replace glucagon in the mixture (FRIEDMAN et al. 1981). The ability of EGF to act in concert with glucagon and insulin has been confirmed in vivo by BUCHER et al. (1978), supporting the possibility of a physiological role of this hormone mixture. The in vitro studies have also been confirmed (MCGOWAN et al. 1979; T. CHRISTOFFERSEN, personal communication). Furthermore, in studies with cultured neonatal rat hepatocytes, as well as hepatocytes from young rats, cAMP (0.15 mM) or dbcAMP (1 μM) has been reported to stimulate DNA synthesis and mitosis. cGMP, though less effective than cAMP, also produced a positive effect in this system (ARMATO et al. 1976, 1977).

In summary, a number of lines of evidence support the idea that cAMP plays a stimulatory role in hepatocyte proliferation, though it is only one component in a complex multifactor system. The precise function of cAMP is not known, but evidence suggests that it may be involved in regulating RNA synthesis (BAILEY et al. 1975). Consistent with such a role are the immunocytochemical findings of STEINER et al. (1978; see also this volume) which suggest the nuclear accumulation of catalytic and regulatory (especially R II) subunits of cAMP-dependent protein kinase during liver regeneration. KALLOS (1977) has also presented evidence for the nuclear translocation of cAMP in liver cells.

Cyclic GMP also may participate in liver regeneration. Although measurements of cGMP levels during regeneration reveal no significant fluctuations (STEINER et al. 1978; WHITFIELD et al. 1976), changes in cGMP compartmentalization have been suggested by the use of fluorescent antibodies to cGMP (STEINER et al. 1978). Between 8 and 12 h after hepatectomy a number of changes occur. The fluorescence staining of plasma membrane, nuclear membrane and nucleoplasm become greatly enhanced. These cytochemical changes coincide with an increase in biochemically determined particulate guanylate cyclase activity (STEINER et al. 1978; KIMURA and MURAD 1975). The significance of these alterations with regard to cell proliferation remains unknown.

2. Continuous Cultures of Liver Cells

Possible roles of cyclic nucleotides in the cell cycle of liver cells have been investigated in several liver cell lines. VAN WIJK et al. (1972, 1973) have shown that dbcAMP (0.5 m*M*) and other analogs of cAMP inhibit DNA synthesis per se (i.e., within S phase) in Reuber H35 hepatoma cells. The inhibition appears to result from decreased levels of pyrimidine nucleotides, since it is reversed by addition of thymidine or deoxycytidine. The finding of S phase inhibition by cAMP may represent an unusual situation, possibly relating to the requirement of this cell line for a specific pyrimidine precursor, the uptake of which is inhibited by dbcAMP. In another transformed liver cell line, NOSE and KATSUTA (1975) reported a reversible G_2 inhibition by dbcAMP (0.25 m*M*) and theophylline (1 m*M*). Cultures were treated for four days with agents and analyzed by cytophotometric techniques.

BOYNTON and WHITFIELD (1979) have carried out studies with T51B rat liver epithelioid cells which support a stimulatory action of cAMP in liver growth. In the presence of medium containing low Ca^{++} (0.015 m*M*), these cells apparently become arrested near the beginning of S phase. Addition of Ca^{++} induces a transient elevation in cAMP levels which is followed by the initiation of DNA synthesis. If the elevation in cAMP is prevented by use of imidazole, which is thought to activate phosphodiesterase, the cells do not enter DNA synthesis. Furthermore cAMP itself, but not 5′AMP, induces Ca^{++} deprived cells to enter DNA synthesis in the absence of extra Ca^{++}.

ZEILIG and GOLDBERG (1977) have analyzed cAMP and cGMP levels in synchronized Novikoff hepatoma cells. They found that cAMP levels reach a minimum level as cells accumulate in colcemid-blocked mitosis. Following reversal of the colcemid block, cAMP levels rise coincident with the exit of cells from metaphase. They continue to rise to a peak in G_1 phase 2-fold greater than mitotic levels. cGMP levels are high in colcemid-blocked cells and drop 80% almost immediately upon reversal of the colcemid block. With the possible exception of a small rise at S phase, the levels of cGMP remain low until the next mitosis. By using bleomycin to block cells in G_2 it was shown that colcemid did not affect cyclic nucleotide levels unless cells first reached mitosis, indicating that the alterations were due to cell cycle changes rather than to the action of colcemid. These results suggest the possibility of effects of both cAMP and cGMP in or near mitosis. The results are also consistent with a stimulatory role for cAMP in G_1 phase.

III. Neuroblastoma Cells

An extensive literature suggests a role for cAMP in the morphological and biochemical differentiation of cultured neuroblastoma cells. In response to dbcAMP or other cAMP-elevating agents, cells develop extensions ("neurites") up to 3 mm in length, and their cell bodies and nuclei enlarge (FURMANSKI et al. 1971; PRASAD and HSIE 1971; PRASAD 1972b; PRASAD and KUMAR 1974). These morphological changes are reversible during the first few days of treatment, but, after 4 days, become irreversible, (PRASAD and KUMAR 1974) and cells become less tumorigenic (PRASAD 1972a). In addition to morphological differentiation, a number of enzymes involved in neurotransmitter metabolism are altered. For example, elevations in tyrosine hydroxylase (WAYMIRE et al. 1972), choline acetyltransferase (PRASAD and KUMAR 1974), and acetylcholinesterase (PRASAD and VERNADAKIS 1972) are observed. The role of cAMP in neuroblastoma cell differentiation has been reviewed by PRASAD (1977).

In addition to an increased expression of differentiated functions the growth rate and final cell density of cultures are markedly diminished by dbcAMP. However, recent studies by WAYMIRE et al. (1978) suggest that closer scrutiny of this effect is needed. Their studies suggest that growth inhibition by dbcAMP may result from the release of butyrate rather than to activation of protein kinase. Sodium butyrate mimicked the action of dbcAMP upon growth though it had no effect on either neurite extension or enzyme levels. Moreover, 8-Br-cAMP was a potent stimulator of differentiation but did not inhibit cell proliferation. In fact, at concentrations of 0.1 m*M*, 8-Br-cAMP caused a 60% stimulation of growth. These results indicate that the effect of agents on growth can be dissociated from those on differentiation, and the question is raised as to whether cAMP inhibits growth in these cells at all. There is independent evidence that cAMP can inhibit growth. cAMP-elevating agents other than dbcAMP, for example, PGE_1 plus papaverine (LAZO and RUDDON 1977), have been reported to inhibit growth. NOMURA et al. (1978) showed potentiation between theophylline and dbcAMP in the inhibition of growth in a cell line from rat brain tumor, further supporting the view that high levels of cAMP do inhibit growth. Additional studies are required to clarify the role of cAMP. Correlation between growth inhibition and the activation state of cAMP dependent protein kinase would be useful in this regard.

Early studies suggested that the inhibition of cell growth by dbcAMP was localized to G_1 phase. This conclusion was based on the low average DNA content per cell in blocked cultures (PRASAD and KUMAR 1974), A G_1 inhibition was confirmed in a recent analysis of the cell cycle in rat brain tumor cells using autoradiography and microfluorometry (NOMURA et al. 1978). In addition it was shown that the progress of cells was considerably slowed in G_2 prior to becoming blocked in G_1 phase.

IV. Adrenal Cortical Cells

Although it is well known that the action of ACTH results in adrenal cortical proliferation in vivo (FARESE and REDDY 1963; GARREN et al. 1971; IMRIE et al. 1965; MASUI and GARREN 1970), both ACTH and cAMP have been found consistently to inhibit growth of adrenal cells in culture. Growth inhibition is accompanied by alterations in morphology and increased steroidogenesis. This result has been seen in both adrenal tumor cells (MASUI and GARREN 1971) and in normal primary cultures (RAMACHANDRAN and SUYAMA 1975).

The cell cycle locus of inhibition has been studied by WEIDMAN and GILL (WEIDMAN and GILL 1976; GILL and WEIDMAN 1977) in Y-1 functional mouse adrenal tumor cells using flow microfluorometry. Both ACTH and 8-Br-cAMP inhibit cells in G_1 phase. 8-Br-cAMP, but not ACTH, also blocks in G_2 phase. A comparison of the G_1 blocks induced by 8-Br-cAMP, ACTH, and serum restriction revealed a major distinction similar to that noted above in a study on fibroblasts (Sect. A.I.1.a). Cells blocked with ACTH or 8-Br-cAMP exhibit markedly increased cell volume, protein, and RNA content relative to serum-restricted cells. Moreover, when ACTH or 8-Br-cAMP are added with serum to serum-deprived cells they inhibit the onset of DNA synthesis, but not the increases in protein and RNA content, rates of leucine and uridine incorporation, or RNA polymerase I activity. It is concluded that ACTH and 8-Br-cAMP are not negative pleiotypic mediators (KRAM et al. 1973) in these cells, but rather that they specifically inhibit the initiation of DNA synthesis. In spite of these differences, cells that are arrested with ACTH or 8-Br-cAMP undergo an 8–10 h lag following reversal of the block, and then enter DNA synthesis exponentially. These kinetics are very similar to those seen with serum readdition to serum-deprived cells. This result is consistent with the idea that ACTH and 8-Br-cAMP block the cell cycle at the restriction point. However, certain growth related metabolic processes are unaffected by these agents and unbalanced growth results.

cAMP resistant mutants of Y-1 cells have been selected by virtue of their resistance to growth inhibition by 8-Br-cAMP (RAE et al. 1979). These mutants exhibit both reduced growth inhibition and reduced steroidogenesis in response to 8-Br-cAMP or ACTH. One class of mutants has altered cytosolic cAMP-dependent protein kinase activity and a second class shows decreased sensitivity of adenylate cyclase to ACTH stimulation. The production of the latter class of mutants is surprising, in view of the selective pressure (8-Br-cAMP). The different protein kinase mutants display variable activation constants for kinase stimulation by cAMP which parallels the dose response curves for stimulation of steroidogenesis with both cAMP and ACTH. Taken together, these findings strongly support the idea that cAMP and protein kinase mediate ACTH action in steroidogenesis in these cells, and that the kinase also mediates growth inhibition. Cytosol from Y-1 cells exhibits the two classical cAMP-dependent protein kinase peaks on DEAE cellulose (CORBIN et al. 1975). The alterations in these activities were investigated in one of the mutants (GUTMANN et al. 1978). A 5-fold increase in the apparent K_a for cAMP was observed in the peak I enzyme of the mutant, whereas, there was no change in the peak II enzyme. These results suggest the involvement of peak I protein kinase in growth inhibition.

V. Thyroid Cells

When normal thyroid cells are dispersed with trypsin and placed into culture, the addition of TSH induces the cells to rearrange into structural patterns which strikingly resemble the follicular thyroid gland (FAYET and LISSITZKY 1970; LISSITZKY et al. 1971). The lumen of the follicular structures concentrates iodide and contains colloidlike substances that react with thyroglobulin antisera. This remarkable effect of TSH is mimicked by dbcAMP (0.017–0.2 m*M*), cAMP (about 1 m*M*), and theophylline (0.05 m*M*), but not by 5′AMP or cGMP.

The regulation of cell growth in this system is controversial. Both stimulatory and inhibitory effects of TSH have been reported. WINAND and KOHN (1975) showed a clear stimulation by TSH of cell number in sparse monolayers of thyroid cells, conditions which do not lead to follicle formation. On the other hand, WESTERMARK et al. (1979) have seriously questioned the ability of TSH to promote growth. They studied cultures from both normal thyroid and benign nodular goiter and observed only inhibition of growth and DNA synthesis by TSH. They argue that the trophic action of TSH in vivo is a very late effect of the hormone (6 days or longer), and that data are lacking in the literature to support a direct trophic action of TSH. PAWLIKOWSKI et al. (1979) have presented evidence for both stimulatory and inhibitory effects of TSH. They measured the effect of TSH on mitotic index in thyroid explants and found inhibition at 14 h of culture and stimulation after 24 h.

DUMONT et al. (1978) have reviewed arguments that only certain of the actions of TSH are mediated by cAMP (β effects) and that others (α) involve alterations in Ca^{++}. With regard to the growth effects, there is as yet little evidence that either the inhibitory or the stimulatory actions of TSH are mediated by cAMP. Further studies are needed to determine if TSH is a positive or negative regulator of growth and whether its action is mediated by cAMP.

VI. Melanoma Cells

PAWELEK and co-workers (WONG and PAWELEK 1973; PAWELEK et al. 1973) first showed that melanotropin (MSH), or other conditions that raise cAMP levels, increase melanin deposition and tyrosinase activity, while slowing cell growth. The cells also increase in size and develop exaggerated dendrites in response to these agents. The ability of MSH to increase cAMP and of cAMP-elevating agents to induce differentation and growth inhibition has been demonstrated repeatedly using a number of different melanoma cell lines (G. JOHNSON and PASTAN 1972a; KREIDER et al. 1973; WHITE et al. 1979; WADE and BURKART 1978; NILES and MAKARSKI 1978; SANTORO et al. 1977; KNECHT and LIPKIN 1977). Other treatments, such as high cell density (WADE and BURKART 1978) and retinoids (LOTAN et al. 1978) induce similar changes, without apparent alterations in cAMP.

Growth inhibition which may be mediated by cAMP has also been reported in melanomas growing in vivo. SANTORO et al. (1977) showed that injection of a stable derivative of PGE_2 resulted in a markedly decreased tumor size and increased survival of rats that carried B-16 melanoma. The tumors isolated from drug-treated animals contained elevated levels of both cAMP and cGMP.

While it is clear that both MSH and cAMP inhibit melanoma cell growth and MSH elevates cAMP levels, it nonetheless appears that MSH and cAMP may act by separate mechanisms. LERNER and co-workers (HALABAN and LERNER 1977; PAWELEK 1976) have presented considerable evidence that the inhibitory action of MSH results from the production of autotoxic substances which are intermediates in the formation of melanin. Thus MSH inhibition does not occur if tyrosinase is inhibited, if cells are grown in the absence of tyrosine, or in cell lines with low tyrosinase activity. The inhibition of growth by MSH occurs after 5 or 6 days of treatment compared with less than 1 day for cAMP (DIPASQUALE and MCGUIRE 1977). A possible explanation for these results is that the elevation in cAMP induced by MSH is not of a magnitude that will rapidly inhibit growth. With prolonged elevations in cAMP, inhibition occurs due to accumulation of toxic materials. Further evidence that MSH and cAMP act by different mechanisms has been presented by DIPASQUALE and MCCUIRE (1977), who showed that the rapid inhibitory effects of dbcAMP are independent of tyrosine metabolism. They further showed that dbcAMP blocks cells in late S or G_2 phase rather than in G_1. Previous evidence, based upon DNA content of blocked cells, had indicated that MSH blocks melanoma cells in G_1 phase (PAWELEK et al. 1975b).

While there is strong evidence for an inhibitory action of cAMP and MSH in melanoma cells, there is equally strong evidence for a stimulatory action of these agents, conceivably at another stage of the cell cycle. In this instance cAMP apparently mediates the action of MSH. In 1975 PAWELEK et al. (1975a) reported the isolation of temperature sensitive mutants of melanoma cells in which cAMP and MSH dramatically stimulate the growth rate. The doubling time of these cells in normal medium at 37 °C is 96 h compared with 41 h for the wild type. Addition to the mutant cells of either MSH plus theophylline, PGE_1 (4×10^{-5} *M*), dbcAMP (2×10^{-4} *M*) or cholera toxin (0.5 µg/ml) reduces the doubling time to about 48 h. These same agents inhibit rather than stimulate the growth of wild type cells at 37 °C or mutant cells at 40 °C.

A reexamination of wild type cells led to the discovery that low concentrations of dbcAMP (10^{-5} *M*) also stimulate growth in these cells, in contrast to the inhibitory effects of high doses (2×10^{-4} *M*). Under the proper conditions MSH also can be shown to stimulate growth of melanomas both in vitro (HALABAN and LERNER 1977) and in vivo (PAWELEK et al. 1973).

PAWELEK (1979) has recently reported that the cAMP-requiring mutant cell line has an alteration in the type I cAMP-dependent protein kinase. The partially purified enzyme displays a markedly increased thermolability and a 1.8-fold increase in its K_a for cAMP. Type II kinase is present in low, sometimes negligible amounts in wild type and mutant cells. These results suggest that the type I protein kinase is a positive regulator of proliferation in these cells. However, the kinase defect does not appear to explain all of the differences between mutant and wild type cells. For example, the mutants are stimulated to a much greater extent by low levels of dbcAMP than are wild type cells. Yet at high levels of cAMP both mutant and wild type cell growth are equally inhibited by cAMP. The concentration dependence for inhibition is the same in both cell types. It is difficult to explain these results in terms of a single cAMP receptor. Further studies on R_2 or other possible cAMP binding proteins would be of great interest.

It is enigmatic as to why MSH and cAMP both inhibit and stimulate growth of the same cell type. It is possible that opposing effects are signaled at different concentrations of hormone and that this has physiological relevance. Alternatively these observations could reflect diverse roles of cAMP in the regulation of the cell cycle at different stages (see Sect. A.XII).

VII. Schwann Cells

RAFF et al. (1978a) reported that cAMP analogs or inducers markedly stimulate growth of cultures of purified Schwann cells prepared from newborn rat sciatic nerve. These cells divide very slowly (one doubling every 7–8 days) in medium containing 10% fetal calf serum. Cholera toxin dramatically decreases the generation time to 48 h. dbcAMP also increases the rate of cell division though to a lesser extent than cholera toxin. Using incorporation of radioactive precursors into DNA as an assay, it was found that cholera toxin (0.01 pg/ml), dbcAMP (10^{-5} to 10^{-4}), or MIX all stimulate this parameter and that MIX potentiates the action of dbcAMP. Choleragenoid, a biologically inactive derivative of cholera toxin, is without effect, as are dbcGMP, cAMP, 5′AMP, sodium butyrate, PGE_1, and isoprenaline. These latter hormones do not raise cAMP in these cells whereas cholera toxin does.

RAFF et al. (1978b) have also described a pituitary factor, distinct from previously known growth factors, which stimulates Schwann cell growth. This factor does not elevate cAMP levels. When maximal stimulatory levels of the pituitary factor and cholera toxin are added together the stimulation is essentially additive, suggesting that the two act through different mechanisms.

A plausible physiological role for the regulation of Schwann cell replication is suggested by these authors, namely nerve regeneration. Schwann cell division is observed following nerve injury and stimulation of division in cell culture has been reported to be induced by contact of cells with sensory or sympathetic neurons. cAMP could conceivably play a role in the regenerative process.

It is interesting that these authors note that, in contrast to normal Schwann cells, growth of a malignant Schwannoma cell line was inhibited rather than stimulated by cholera toxin (RAFF et al. 1978a). SHEPPARD, while not noting effects on growth rate, had previously reported morphological differentiation of Schwannoma cells in response to agents which elevate cAMP (SHEPPARD et al. 1975).

VIII. S49 Lymphoma Cells

COFFINO and co-workers have carried out elegant studies on growth regulation of a lymphoma cell line, S49. These cells undergo cytolysis shortly after their growth is inhibited by dbcAMP or isoproterenol. Using this serendipity, mutants which did not respond to these agents were isolated. Mutants both lacking in adenylyl cyclase and with altered cAMP-dependent protein kinase were characterized. These studies have been reviewed recently (COFFINO et al. 1978) and only pertinent aspects will be summarized here.

Exponentially growing wild type S49 cells are blocked exclusively in G_1 phase by dbcAMP (0.1 mM) plus theophylline (0.2 mM), by dbcAMP (0.5 mM) plus RO 20–1724 (30 µM) or by cholera toxin (100 ng/ml) plus RO 20–1724 (30 µM) (COFFINO et al. 1975; COFFINO and GRAY 1978). By following cells during the drug treatment using a flow cytometer, it was shown that cells in the blocked state do not increase in size; nor does cell size decrease before cells become blocked in G_1 phase, i.e., unbalanced growth does not occur as has been reported in fibroblasts and adrenal cells (see Sect. A.I.1.a and A.IV). Cells resume growth when cAMP levels are allowed to fall. No evidence is cited for any effect on the cell cycle other than a G_1 block.

Three kinase mutants were characterized with different kinetics of activation by cAMP (HOCHMAN et al. 1975; INSEL et al. 1975). These mutants exhibit dose-response curves for growth inhibition by dbcAMP that perfectly parallel their particular kinase lesion (INSEL et al. 1975). These results indicate that cytosolic protein kinase mediates G_1 growth arrest by dbcAMP.

The growth properties of a kinaseless mutant have been examined. This mutant is totally deficient in cAMP-dependent protein kinase activity. In spite of this, mutant cells have a generation time of 16.5 h compared with 18 h for the wild type (COFFINO et al. 1975). There is little difference in the cell cycle distribution between mutant and wild type cells in exponential growth. Addition of a wide range of dbcAMP concentrations to the mutant cells does not alter the growth rate. These results would appear to indicate that fluctuations in cAMP are not essential for progress of the cell cycle in S49 cells, and that the sole action of cAMP is the negative modulation of G_1 phase.

The above conclusions are strengthened further by a recent two dimensional gel analysis of changes in S49 proteins resulting from treatment of cells with analogs or inducers of cAMP (STEINBERG and COFFINO 1979). Approximately 15 proteins appeared to be phosphorylated in response to cAMP and 9 proteins showed altered rates of synthesis. None of these changes were observed in kinase mutants. Therefore, cAMP-dependent protein kinase appears to be involved in all of the changes in proteins induced by cAMP in these cells. This result is consistent with the hypothesis that there are no other receptors for cAMP which mediate its cell cycle effects in the absence of protein kinase. However, since kinase mutants are deficient in the regulatory as well as the catalytic subunit of cAMP-dependent protein kinase, effects on protein synthesis mediated by the cAMP-R complex, independent of the catalytic subunit, are not ruled out.

IX. Thymic Lymphocytes

In a series of papers, MACMANUS, WHITFIELD and co-workers have presented evidence for a stimulatory action of cAMP in proliferation of rat thymus lymphocytes (for review, see WHITFIELD et al. 1973a, 1976). The studies focus upon an actively dividing subpopulation of lymphocytes, which comprise about 10–20% of the total population. These cells are stimulated to enter DNA synthesis and divide by Ca^{++}, cAMP (10^{-7} to 10^{-5} *M*) or by either of two concentration ranges of cGMP (10^{-11} to 10^{-10} and 10^{-6} to 10^{-5}) (WHITFIELD et al. 1969, 1973b, c; MACMANUS and WHITFIELD 1969). The cells enter DNA synthesis within only an hour of stimulation, indicating that they were not previously blocked in the usual G_0 state, but rather at, or near, the G_1/S border.

In addition to the above agents, the authors defined a large number of hormones and other agents which stimulate cell division in this system. They hypothesize that the final common pathway for stimulation is an increase in cytosolic Ca^{++}. According to their idea, the divergent agents that stimulate growth either increase Ca^{++} uptake (e.g. acetylcholine, bradykinin, cortisol, growth hormone and concanavalin A) or increase the levels of cAMP (PGE_1 and epinephrine). cAMP is postulated to act to release internal Ca^{++} from mitochondrial pools (WHITFIELD et al. 1976). cGMP is postulated to act by stimulating an elevation in cellular cAMP (WHITFIELD et al. 1971).

MORGAN et al. (1977) confirmed that cAMP and cGMP are mitogenic toward thymic lymphocytes but found that both nucleotides were active over two concentration ranges. Based on this and other findings they modified the model considerably by suggesting that there are two types of mitogenic hormones. One class is calcium-dependent and is blocked by estradiol. This class is postulated to act by increasing cGMP levels secondary to elevated Ca^{++}. The second class is magnesium-dependent, blocked by testosterone and acts by increasing cAMP concentrations. The differences between this model and that of WHITFIELD et al. (1976) remain unexplained.

These investigations could be highly relevant to an understanding of the regulation cell cycle traverse. However, it remains unclear whether cyclic nucleotides mediate the action of the divalent metal ions or whether the reverse is true. Unfortunately the interpretation of the data is complicated by the fact that the proliferating cells represent a small fraction of a heterogeneous population. There could in fact be more than one proliferating subpopulation. There might also be indirect actions of agents on cell division resulting from interactions between different subpopulations.

X. Hemopoietic Stem Cells (CFU-S)

BYRON (1971–1973, 1976) has carried out a series of studies with hemopoietic stem cells from mouse bone marrow which suggest that proliferation of this tissue may be regulated in a manner similar to that of thymic lymphocytes, as just described. A complex assay is used to measure growth stimulation. Cells are removed and exposed in vitro to various drugs for 2.5 h. They are then exposed to high specific activity [^{3}H] thymidine, diluted, and injected into irradiated mice. After 9 days, spleen colonies are counted. The number of colonies is a measure of the number of viable cells in the injected population which is determined by whether cells incorporated, and were thereby killed by the [^{3}H] thymidine. Control cells are thought to have few (or slowly) cycling cells and therefore are not killed by the [^{3}H] thymidine and give rise to many colonies. Agents which stimulate cells to enter S phase result in fewer colonies. In order to be stimulated in this system, cells would have to be resting near the G_1/S border at the time of drug addition. Low doses of isoproterenol (10^{-14} *M*) stimulate about 50% of the cells to enter S phase, an effect which is inhibited by propranolol. The dose response curves with various catecholamine analogs suggest that this effect is more β_1 than β_2 in character. DNA synthesis is also stimulated by low levels of dbcAMP, which exhibits a bell-shaped concentration curve with peak stimulation at 0.01 μM and no effect at 1 μM, 5′AMP is without effect. The phosphodiesterase inhibitor RO 20–1724 also stimulates at low doses, and 4 m*M* imidazole, a presumed phosphodiesterase activator, suppresses the action of all agents. Cholinergic agents also stimulate. Carbamylcholine is effective at 10^{-12} *M* and its action is abolished by D-tubocurarine but not propranolol. Acetylcholine is active in the presence, but not the absence, of neostigmine. Finally, dbcGMP (0.01 μM) stimulates, leading to the suggestion that it mediates the action of cholinergic agents.

Like the thymic lymphocyte studies, the interpretation of these experiments is complicated by the possibility of indirect effects due to the presence of heterogeneous cell types.

XI. HeLa Cells

The involvement of cAMP in the regulation of the cell cycle of HeLa cells has been examined in our laboratory (ZEILIG et al. 1972, 1974a, b, 1976; KURZ and FRIEDMAN 1976) by determining fluctuations in cAMP content in synchronized cells and by testing the effects of experimentally altered levels of cAMP on cell cycle progress. Cells were synchronized by a double high-thymidine block to obtain data on S phase, G_2, M and early G_1. They were resynchronized by the mitotic detachment method to study M, G_1 and early S phase. The cellular cAMP concentrations were found to be at their maximum concentration at the G_1/S border and to be at a minimum in late G_2 phase and mitosis. Peaks were also observed at the 4th and 6th hours of S phase. The findings of low levels in mitosis and high levels at the G_1/S border were supported by results obtained when cells were accumulated at these points with colcemid or high levels of thymidine. Similar fluctuations in cAMP content were obtained with a hydroxyurea-amethopterin double block instead of the double thymidine block. The fall in cAMP at G_2 and M was further shown to coincide with a significant fall in the activity ratio of cAMP-dependent protein kinase (GRAY et al. 1980).

The effect of cAMP elevating agents on cell cycle progress was studied in both synchronized (ZEILIG et al. 1976) and unsynchronized (KURZ and FRIEDMAN 1976) cells. In both systems, cAMP analogs or cAMP-elevating agents, added during S phase or early G_2 caused a marked delay in G_2, but had no effect on S phase. Potentiation of the delayed progress through G_2 was observed between phosphodiesterase inhibitors and either cAMP analogs or adenyl cyclase agonists. These experiments established an inhibitory action of cAMP in G_2 phase in HeLa cells, consistent with the fall in endogenous cAMP levels at this point in the cell cycle.

In contrast with the premitotic inhibitory effect of cAMP on G_2 once cells had reached the metaphase stage of mitosis, addition of analogs or inducers of cAMP enhanced the rate at which cells completed mitosis and entered G_1 (ZEILIG et al. 1976; FRIEDMAN et al. 1976b). The physiological significance of this stimulatory effect is open to question because it does not correlate well with cell cycle changes in cAMP levels. A similar stimulation of mitosis is observed by addition of Ca^{++} or the Ca^{++} ionophore A23187. This and other evidence is consistent with the possibility that this action of cAMP is mediated by increased cytosolic Ca^{++} (FRIEDMAN et al. 1976b).

Studies on the effect of cAMP elevations on G_1 traverse were also carried out. The rationale for these experiments was that if the late G_1 peak in endogenous cAMP levels was essential for entrance into S phase, an early elevation in cAMP might induce early DNA synthesis. Though the results showed a suggestion of G_1 stimulation by elevated cAMP, the data was ambiguous due to a myriad of apparently nonspecific effects of agents used to elevate cAMP.

XII. Miscellaneous Cell Types

Alterations in cAMP and cAMP-dependent protein kinase have been determined during mitosis, G_1 and S phases in synchronized Chinese Hamster Ovary (CHO) cells by COSTA et al. (1976a). The cells were synchronized by selective detachment of mitotic cells. Similar to findings in HeLa cells (see Sect. A.XI), the levels of cAMP were minimal at mitosis, or shortly thereafter, and gradually increased 5-fold during G_1. The levels decreased as cells entered S phase. Total protein kinase levels decreased early in G_1 (2 h after mitosis), then rose to a peak in late G_1 (4–5 h after mitosis) and fell off again during S phase. The activity ratio of the kinase paralleled cAMP levels.

The possible importance of alterations in the two isozymes of protein kinase is suggested in another study by these workers (COSTA et al. 1976b, 1978). Alterations in type I and type II kinases were determined in CHO cells synchronized either by trypsinization of confluent cultures or by selective detachment of mitotic cells. Using both methods the type I enzyme was found to predominate in very early G_1. The levels of type I then decline rapidly. In mid G_1 the type II isozyme begins to increase and by the G_1/S border this form is predominant, only to decline in mid and late S phase. The authors suggest that there may be an orderly sequence of phosphorylation during the cell cycle, with different targets being phosphorylated by the different isozymes of protein kinase. Presumably this would come about through differences in subcellular distribution since the two kinases are thought to share the same catalytic subunit (P. BECHTEL et al. 1975).

In studies with peripheral blood lymphocytes the same laboratory also has shown that the type I kinase is specifically activated following growth activation by concanavalin A (BYUS et al. 1977). Addition of dbcAMP, on the other hand, inhibits mitogenesis and activates the type II isozyme. It is suggested that activation of the type I enzyme is associated with growth stimulation, whereas activation of type II is involved in inhibition of growth. However, independent evidence for this idea is lacking. Alternative explanations for the data are that differential growth regulation relates to the total amount of kinase activation or to the precise timing of kinase activation.

In addition to alterations in kinase types, the subcellular distribution of kinases during the cell cycle could be important. CHRISTENSEN et al. (1979) reported fluctuations in kinase activity in different subcellular compartments in Leydig I-10 tumor cells following synchronization by a double thymidine block. Levels of microsomal cAMP-dependent protein kinase remain constant during the cell cycle. In contrast, the activity in the mitochondria-lysosomal fraction increases in S phase, and both the cytosol and nuclear enzyme increase during G_2 and M. cAMP-independent kinases show different patterns of change. The authors suggest that the observed fluctuations could lead to selective phosphorylation at specific stages of the cell cycle.

STAMBROOK and VELEZ (1976) have examined the effect of dbcAMP on cell growth in Chinese hamster lung tumor cells (V79) with rather unusual results. Cell division is slowed by this agent (10^{-4} to 10^{-3} M) and the final cell density is reduced. After 48 h of treatment, removal of the drug leads to rapid recovery and cells proceed to grow to their normal density. The kinetics of cell division following reversal clearly indicate that cells had been blocked in G_2 phase rather than in G_1.

Table 1. Effects of elevated cAMP levels upon proliferation of normal cells

Tissue	Effect[a]	Cell Cycle stage[b]	References
Fibroblast	–	G_1	See Sect. A.I
	–	G_2	WILLINGHAM et al. (1972)
	+	G_1	WILLINGHAM et al. (1972)
Liver	+	G_1	See Sect. A.II.1
Adrenal cortex	–	(G_1)	RAMACHANDRAN and SUYAMA (1975)
Thyroid	–	ND	WESTERMARK et al. (1979)
	+	ND	WINAND and KOHN (1975)
Corpus luteum	–	ND	GOSPODAROWICZ and GOSPODAROWICZ (1975)
Sertoli cells (immature rats)	+	ND	GRISWOLD et al. (1977)
Thymic lymphocytes	+	G_1	See Sect. A.IX
Hemopoietic stem cells	+	G_1	BYRON (1971, 1972, 1973)
Schwann cells	+	ND	RAFF et al. (1978a)
Fetal chondrocytes	–	(G_1)	R. MILLER et al. (1979)
Smooth muscle (Newborn)	–	ND	CHAMLEY and CAMPBELL vas deferens (1975)
Salivary gland	–	G_2	RADLEY and HODGSON (1971, 1973)
Embryonic lens epithelium	+	ND	CREIGHTON and TREVITHICK (1974)
Chinese hamster ovary cells	–	G_1	ROZENGURT and PARDEE (1972)
	–	G_2	LEHNERT (1979)
	+	M	LEHNERT (1979)

[a] –, inhibition; +, stimulation
[b] ND, not determined; ( ), probable stage

This conclusion was confirmed using autoradiographic labeling. Though it is not uncommon for cells to be blocked in G_2 by cAMP, few studies have indicated that the blocked cells could remain viable for extended periods of time in G_2 phase.

The effect of cAMP-elevating agents has been studied on a variety of other cell types, some of which are summarized in Tables 1 and 2. In most instances, transformed cells are inhibited by cAMP (Table 2), for example, Ehrlich ascites tumor cells (KAMINSKAS et al. 1976), Walker 256 mammary carcinomas (CHO-CHUNG and GULLINO 1974; CHO-CHUNG 1974) and prostatic epithelial cells (NILES et al. 1976). In certain instances, however, the growth of tumor cells is enhanced, for example, R3230AC transplantable rat mammary tumor (KLEIN and LOIZZI 1977). Normal cells (Table 1), other than those already discussed, whose growth is inhibited include fetal rat chondrocytes in monolayer culture (R. MILLER et al. 1979), bovine luteal cells (GOSPODAROWICZ and GOSPODAROWICZ 1975) and guinea pig vas deferens smooth muscle cells (CHAMLEY and CAMPBELL 1975). In other reports normal cell growth is enhanced, as for example in young rat Sertoli cells (GRISWOLD et al. 1977), and embryonic lens epithelial cells (CREIGHTON and TREVITHICK 1974). Extensive studies have been carried out on the role of cyclic nucleotides in cell proliferation of quiescent lymphocytes and of skin. These areas are covered in other chapters of this volume and will not be reviewed here.

Table 2. Effects of elevated cAMP levels upon proliferation of transformed cells

Tissue	Effect[a]	Cell cycle stage[b]	Reference
Transformed fibroblast	−	G_2	Paul (1973) Smets (1972)
Transformed liver cultures	−	G_2	Nose and Katsuta (1975)
	−	S	Van Wijk et al. (1972, 1973)
Neuroblastoma	−	G_1	Prasad and Kumar (1974) Nomura et al. (1978)
	−	G_2	Nomura et al. (1978)
Adrenal cortical tumor	−	G_1	Weidman and Gill (1976) Gill and Weidman (1977)
	−	G_2	Weidman and Gill (1976) Gill and Weidman (1977)
Melanoma	−	ND	See Sect. A.VI
	+	ND	See Sect. A.VI
S49 Lymphoma	−	G_1	Coffino et al. (1975)
Ehrlich ascites tumor	−	ND	Kaminskas et al. (1976)
Hela cells	−	G_2	Zeilig et al. (1976)
	+	M	Zeilig et al. (1976)
Walker 256 mammary carcinoma	−	ND	Cho-Chung (1974) Cho-Chung and Gullino (1974)
R 3230AC mammary tumor	+	ND	Klein and Loizzi (1977)
V 79 lung tumor	−	G_2	Stambrook and Velez (1976)
Malignant trophoblast	−	ND	Barker and Isles (1978)
Transformed prostatic epithelium	−	ND	Niles et al. (1976)
Lymphoid cells	−	G_2	Millis et al. (1972, 1974)

[a] −, inhibition; +, stimulation
[b] ND, not determined

XIII. Generalizations on the Actions of Cyclic Nucleotides in Cell Proliferation

1. Cell Cycle Loci of cAMP Action

From a consideration of the preceeding sections, it is clear that different tissues respond to cyclic nucleotides in diverse ways. The data on cGMP is too sparse and controversial to draw conclusions at the present time. However, some general patterns emerge regarding the action of cAMP. The observations appear to segregate into 3 major actions.

a) Regulation by cAMP of the G_0–G_+ Interconversion

cAMP inhibits the growth of certain cells during the G_1 phase, inducing them to enter a G_0 state. In some cell types the question has been raised as to whether the cAMP-induced G_0 is a true G_0 state (see Sect. A.I and A.IV). In most tissues whose growth is inhibited by cAMP, there is a concomitant increase in the expression of the cell's differentiated functions.

In the case of the fibroblast, induction of quiescence by cAMP is observed only in normal cells. Following transformation, neither cAMP nor other conditions induces the transition to G_0. Cell growth is inhibited by cAMP but the block is in G_2, not G_1. The cells apparently have lost the ability to enter the G_0 state. Other malignant cell types, for example HeLa cells, also lack the ability to respond at the restriction point. However, this is not true for all malignant cell types. For example, neuroblastoma (Sect. A.III), S 49 lymphoma (Sect. A.VIII), melanoma (Sect. A.VI), and adrenal cortical cells (Sect. A.IV) can be inhibited in $G_1(G_0)$ and increase their expression of differentiated phenotypes in response to cAMP.

b) Inhibition in G_2 by cAMP

The finding that many cell types, both normal and transformed, are inhibited in G_2 by cAMP is consistent with the fall in cAMP levels in late G_2 phase and mitosis observed in a number of studies on synchronized cell populations. Inhibition in G_2 by cAMP analogs or inducers has been reported in such divergent tissues as normal and transformed fibroblasts (Sect. A.I.), cultured transformed hepatocytes (Sect. A.II), neuroblastoma cells (sect. A.III), HeLa cells (Sect. A.XI), normal intact skin (VOORHEES et al. 1974; FLAXMAN and HARPER 1975) and in certain lymphoma cell lines (MILLIS et al. 1972, 1974). G_2 inhibition is not universal, however, as it is apparently absent in S49 lymphoma cells (COFFINO et al. 1975) and Reuber hepatoma cells (VAN WIJK et al. 1973).

c) Stimulation of G_1 by cAMP

A stimulatory action of cAMP in G_1 is consistent with the general observation of a peak in cellular cAMP levels during mid or late G_1 phase of the cell cycle. Stimulation of growth by cAMP has been observed in normal hepatocytes (Sect. A.II), Schwann cells (Sect. A.VII), melanoma cells (Sect. A.VI), Sertoli cells (GRISWOLD et al. 1977), thymocytes (Sect. A.IX), hemopoietic stem cells (Sect. A.X) and 3T3 cells (Sect. A.I). It is not clear, however, that the mechanism of stimulation is the same in all of these cell types. In the case of thymocytes, homopoietic stem cells and perhaps 3T3 cells, the effect is observed late in G_1, and may be related to a Ca^{++} requirement at this stage in the cell cycle. It should be noted that, with the exception of melanoma cells, stimulatory effects of cAMP have been observed only in normal cells. BOYNTON et al. (1977) found that the Ca^{++} dependency for passage through G_1 is lost upon transformation of 3T3. They have suggested that the regulation of cell division at this cell cycle locus is lost following malignant transformation.

2. Speculations on the Physiological Role of cAMP in Growth Regulation

There are two general ways of viewing cAMP actions in cell division. First, one can postulate that fluctuations and actions of cAMP are an inherent part of the cell division cycle, i.e., cAMP is an important internal motivating force of a cell's progress through the cycle. It could act to regulate the cell cycle at a number of points and in fact could have stimulatory effects at one point and inhibitory actions at another, resulting from programmed changes in cAMP, cAMP-dependent protein kinases, and relevant protein substrates. If one assumes that the cell division cycle is a primitive eukaryotic process whose mechanism has been conserved during evolution, it follows that the cAMP fluctuations and actions should be common to all eukaryotic cells.

A second way of viewing cAMP action is to assume that it is not an inherent regulator of the cell cycle, but rather that regulation by cAMP has been superimposed upon the primitive cell cycle, just as it was apparently appended onto preexisting metabolic pathways. It might then follow that the mechanism of regulation by cAMP could vary with the requirements of a particular tissue.

The major evidence favoring the first idea is that the measured fluctuations in cAMP levels in several cell types fit into a general pattern. Levels are at their lowest during late G_2 and M, and rise to a peak in G_1 phase. Moreover, these changes are consistent with the inhibition of G_2 and stimulation of G_1 by cAMP observed in certain cells. The major arguments against such a primitive role for cAMP are the observation that different tissues respond in different ways to experimental elevations in cAMP, and the ability of "kinaseless" mutants of S49 cells (Sect. A.VIII) and other cell types to traverse the cell cycle with essentially normal kinetics.

The hypothesis that regulation by cAMP is superimposed upon the cell cycle is more flexible and is difficult to refute at the present time. Thus elevated cAMP might inhibit in early G_1 or in G_2, or stimulate in G_1 depending on the needs of a particular cell type. In fact, cyclic nucleotides could conceivably act at other points in the cell cycle as well. For example, STILES et al. (1979) have presented evidence for 3 normal regulatory sites at different temporal points in G_1. The ability of cAMP to induce the G_0 state may represent an important physiological role for hormonally regulating cell division and expression of differentiated functions. Changes in cAMP appear to be only one of a number of environmental variations that can induce this state. Regulation of G_2 may also play a physiological role in growth regulation of certain tissues. For example, a subpopulation of cells consisting of about 5% of the basal cells of mouse epidermis are normally dormant in G_2 phase (GELFANT 1963; GELFANT and CANDELAS 1972). These cells are stimulated and rapidly divide upon wounding of the skin. Subpopulations of G_2-arrested cells have also been observed in other tissues. The significance of regulation in G_2 might be that cells can undergo rapid mitosis, compared with the long lag in cells blocked at the G_1 restriction point. Finally, it is conceivable that the stimulatory effect of cAMP on cells in G_1 plays a regulatory role in certain cell types which are normally blocked just prior to DNA synthesis rather than at the more usual restriction point. Cells of this type include thymocytes, hemopoietic stem cells, and perhaps hepatocytes.

B. Cyclic Nucleotides and Cancer

I. cAMP and Properties of Transformed Fibroblasts

Transformation of cultured fibroblasts has been studied extensively as a model of malignant transformation. There is strong evidence for the participation of cAMP in this process. cAMP levels fall about 50% during transformation (e.g., ANDERSON et al. 1973b; BURSTIN et al. 1974; CARCHMAN et al. 1974; OEY et al. 1974; OTTEN et al. 1971, 1972b; SHEPPARD 1972). Transformation is accompanied by alterations in the adenylate cyclase system (see ANDERSON and JAWORSKI 1978). The fall in cAMP can account for the gross morphological changes of the transformed cell (HSIE and PUCK 1971; G. JOHNSON et al. 1971) as well as changes in motility (G. JOHNSON et al. 1972), adhesiveness (G. JOHNSON and PASTAN 1972b; SHIELDS and POLLOCK 1974), and agglutination of cells by plant lectins (HSIE et al. 1971; KURTH and BAUER 1973; SHEPPARD 1971; WILLINGHAM and PASTAN 1974). Mutant studies with CHO cells indicate that the morphological changes are mediated by cAMP-dependent protein kinase (PASTAN and WILLINGHAM 1978). Several reviews have detailed the evidence for cAMP participation in transformation and for the possible involvement of microtubules and microfilaments in its action (PASTAN et al. 1975; POLLACK and HOUGH 1974; FRIEDMAN 1976; PASTAN and WILLINGHAM 1978). However, the relationship, if any, of these altered properties to growth regulation or to the malignant state has not been elucidated. Other properties of the transformed state, such as the presence of specific cell surface antigens (KURTH and BAUER 1973) and altered membrane structure as visualized by freeze fracture (SCOTT and FURCHT 1974), appear to be unrelated to changes in cAMP. Moreover, substances other than cAMP, such as "cell surface protein" (CSP) (PASTAN and WILLINGHAM 1978) and plasminogen activator (CHRISTMAN and ACS 1974; LAUG et al. 1974; OSSOWSKI et al. 1973) are altered during transformation and have been implicated in changes of some of the same properties of transformed cells. There is as yet no convincing evidence indicating a relationship between these substances and cAMP. Treatment of transformed fibroblasts with cAMP analogs or agents which elevate cAMP leads to growth arrest in G_2 phase (PAUL 1973; SMETS 1972). Therefore, the altered cAMP metabolism does not appear to be responsible for the loss of growth control in transformed cells.

II. Cyclic Nucleotides and Tumors of Liver

Whereas the in vitro transformation of fibroblasts is accompanied by a fall in cAMP, this is not a general finding. Liver tumors are a clear example in which cAMP levels are elevated. Alterations in cAMP metabolism may become evident in livers of carcinogen treated animals even before tumors arise. For example, several changes have been observed in livers from animals treated with the carcinogen 2-acetylaminofluorene (CHRISTOFFERSON et al. 1972, 1974). The levels of cAMP gradually becomes elevated during a preneoplastic period at 4–8 weeks of treatment. A striking increase in the sensitivity of adenyl cyclase to epinephrine is also observed during this period. When tumors arise, their basal cyclase activity remains elevated severalfold though sensitivity to epinephrine diminishes. Other related carcinogens produce similar effects and their ability to increase the sensitivity of adenyl cyclase to epinephrine parallels their potency as carcinogens (CHRISTOFFERSON, 1975). Increased cAMP and adenyl cyclase have also been reported in hepatomas arising from ethionine treatment in rats (CHAYOTH et al. 1972, 1973) and in Morris hepatomas (THOMAS et al. 1973; BUTCHER et al. 1972).

MURAD and co-workers, studying transplatable Morris hepatomas, have shown that cGMP is also elevated in liver tumors (THOMAS et al. 1973). The magnitude of the cGMP elevation varies greatly, between 2 and 200-fold in different tumors, and is correlated in a general way with the growth rate of the tumor. Unexpectedly, homogenates from hepatomas have less guanylate cyclase than those from control liver. However, the tumors display a marked increase in particulate cyclase and a decrease in the soluble form of the enzyme (KIMURA and MURAD 1975). The ratio of particulate to soluble guanylate cyclase in tumors is 5- to 15-fold greater than in normal liver. In addition to an altered distribution, the tumor enzyme (both soluble and particulate) is not stimulated by sodium azide (GRISS et al. 1976), whereas the enzyme from normal liver is activated about 6-fold. DERUBERTIS and CRAVEN (1977a) have reported similar results in ethionine induced hepatomas, except that in this system both soluble and particulate guanylate cyclase were elevated relative to controls. The tumors exhibited a 2-fold increase in the ratio of particulate to soluble enzyme and, as is Morris hepatomas, the sensitivity to sodium azide was decreased.

The significance of the above results with regard to the etiology of cancer is uncertain. The results could have clinical significance, however, since it has been shown that tumor-bearing mice exhibit elevated urinary excretion of cGMP in amounts which correlate with tumor size (MURAD et al. 1975).

OLSON and RUSSELL (1979) have reported experiments which suggest that an early elevation in cAMP may be important in liver carcinogenesis possibly through its ability to induce the rate-limiting enzyme of polyamine synthesis, ornithine decarboxylase. A single carcinogenic dose of diethylnitrosamine causes a biphasic activation of cAMP-dependent protein kinase. The activity ratio (activity minus cAMP/activity plus cAMP) is elevated at one and two hours after treatment and then returns to control levels. Activity ratios increase again at 14 h and remain elevated for 7 days. The first kinase activation is followed, after several hours, by a rise in ornithine decarboxylase which remains elevated for 11 days. The conclusion that this enzyme is induced by cAMP is supported by results from a number of other systems (e.g., BYUS et al. 1976, 1978; BYUS and RUSSELL 1975). A dramatic elevation in ornithine decarboxylase activity is consistently found as an early event in growth stimulation in a variety of systems (RUSSELL and DURIE 1978).

III. Cyclic Nucleotide Levels in Tumors

The fibroblast and liver systems described above exhibit opposite effects with regard to alterations in cAMP concentration following malignant transformation. Studies on levels of cyclic nucleotides in other tumors are similarly inconsistent, as has been reviewed recently by TISDALE (1979). Various studies report elevations, no change, or decreases in cAMP content. The status of some of the studies on cyclic nucleotide levels is confused by the methods used to express the results. For example, E. BECHTEL et al. (1977), studying human mammary tissue reported markedly elevated levels of cAMP and cGMP per gram of tissue, and of cAMP-dependent protein kinase/mg protein. However, all 3 parameters were decreased significantly when expressed on a per cell basis. It is apparent that the method of expressing results is crucial to their interpretation. If one assumes the absence of compartmentalization, the most crucial consideration from a functional viewpoint is the intracellular concentration of cyclic nucleotide. Therefore, measurements are best expressed in terms of cell volume. Cell volume consistently correlates with cell protein (e.g., WEIDMAN and GILL 1976), so that it is generally valid to express results in terms of protein. Expressing results in terms of DNA content or cell number will often lead to erroneous conclusions. Since compartmentalization probably does occur (EARP and STEINER 1978), in some situations it may be useful, though not without significant pitfalls (see WALSH 1978), to measure activity ratios of cAMP-dependent protein kinase as an indication of elevated intracellular cAMP.

A number of studies have dealt with alterations in cyclic nucleotide levels or hormonal sensitivity of tissues during the preneoplastic period of carcinogen treatment. Studies of this type in liver were discussed in Sect. B.II. Topical treatment of mouse epidermis with benzo(a)pyrene increases basal cAMP levels and decreases the sensitivity of the tissue to isoproterenol (MURRAY and VERMA 1973; VERMA and MURRAY 1974). These changes are seen within 24 h of treatment with carcinogen, and are reversible. Similar effects on hormone sensitivity are observed in epidermal-dermal preparations treated with the tumor promoting phorbol esters (MUFSON et al. 1977). In this system no change in basal cAMP levels is observed. Effects of carcinogens on cGMP metabolism have been studied in a variety of tissues. Nitrosoamines, nitrosoureas, hydrazine derivatives and cigarette smoke, all highly carcinogenic, rapidly induce marked elevations in cellular cGMP and guanylate cyclase in both rat and human tissues (DERUBERTIS and CRAVEN 1976, 1977b; ARNOLD et al. 1977; VESELY et al. 1977; VESELY and LEVEY 1977a). On the other hand, other carcinogens are found to inhibit guanylate cyclase. These include the aromatic amines, polycyclic hydrocarbons, azo dyes, aflatoxins and saccharin (VESELY and LEVEY 1977b, 1978). It remains unknown whether cyclic nucleotide alterations have any relevance to the carcinogenic action of these agents.

IV. cAMP-Dependent Protein Kinase in Cancer Cells

Changes in levels of cyclic nucleotides in normal compared with malignant cells are not necessarily indicative of altered function of the cyclic nucleotide. For example, high levels of cAMP would serve no purpose if transformed cells lacked, or contained altered, cAMP-dependent protein kinase activity. Protein kinase levels, activity ratios (activity minus cAMP/activity plus cAMP) and perhaps isozyme profiles therefore are important in evaluating such a role. Even these measurements may not give a true picture of in vivo function because of the possible in vivo modulation of kinase activity by the specific protein kinase inhibitor (WALSH et al. 1971) or other undefined factors. Ultimately, it is necessary to know the phosphorylation state of specific protein substrates in normal and malignant cells to appreciate the functioning of the cyclic nucleotide system.

Studies on cAMP-dependent protein kinase levels in tumors have revealed some differences from normal cells, but there is little consistency in studies with different cell types. MASARACCHIA and WALSH (1976) reported a 2 to 4-fold increase in kinase activity in mouse lymphosarcoma cells compared with thymocytes. A two-fold increase was also observed in urethane induced lung tumors (MALKINSON et al. 1977) and very high levels relative to normal tissues have been reported in HeLa cells (GRAY et al. 1980). On the other hand, no difference in activities was observed between normal and sarcoma virus transformed bovine fibroblasts (TROY et al. 1973). Levels of kinase were also comparable in 3T3 and its SV40 transformed counterpart (WIGGLESWORTH et al. 1977; GHARRETT et al. 1976). In several rapidly growing Morris hepatomas, levels of cAMP-dependent protein kinase were reported to be decreased relative to normal liver (CRISS and MORRIS 1973).

In most tissues two separable isozymes of cAMP-dependent protein kinase are observed (CORBIN et al. 1975). Type I protein kinase elutes from DEAE cellulose between 0.05 and 0.1 *M* NaCl and type II elutes between 0.15 and 0.25 *M*. The two isozymes appear to share a common catalytic subunit but have different regulatory subunits (P. BECHTEL et al. 1975), which endow them with a number of different properties (CORBIN and KEELY 1977). The distribution of these two isozymes has been compared in several normal and transformed cell lines. GHARRETT et al. (1976) reported that mouse 3T3 cells contain only the type II kinase, whereas both types I and II are found following transformation with SV40. This result was confirmed by WIGGLESWORTH et al. (1977). However, they also showed that if S49 cells, which contain predominantly type I protein kinase, were hybridized with 3T3 cells the resulting hybrid retains the growth regulatory properties of 3T3 cells though it has both isozyme types. In other studies, WEHNER et al. (1978) showed that normal and transformed fibroblasts from other rodent species, namely, rat and vole, contained both isozyme types. WIGGLESWORTH et al. (1977) examined a number of normal and transformed cell lines and could find no consistent correlation between the isozyme distribution and cell transformation. Nine neuroblastoma and four ganglioneuroma tumors were analyzed by IMASHUKU et al. (1979) using photoaffinity labeling. Though quantitative differences were observed, all of the lines contained both isozymes and no consistent differences were observed.

To summarize, the studies on protein kinase levels and isozymes do not yield definitive patterns of change. These findings do not rule out the possibility that certain specific tumors may arise due to kinase defects. Also, kinase changes may be too subtle to detect by routine assays. For example, SIMANTOV and SACHS (1975) isolated dbcAMP resistant clones of neuroblastoma cells. The clones contained normal levels of cAMP-dependent protein kinase and the enzyme showed an unchanged K_a for cAMP. However, the enzyme was apparently defective since it exhibited a high degree of thermolability. Parenthetically, it is of interest that the resistant clones grew to higher cell densities in vitro, grew better in agar, and were considerably more tumorigenic than wild type cells.

V. Effects of Elevated cAMP Upon Tumor Growth

The possible use of cyclic nucleotide analogs or agents which elevate cyclic nucleotides in cancer chemotherapy has been considered, but a number of drawbacks are immediately apparent. First, it is clear from Sect. A and Tables 1 and 2 that some tissues are inhibited by cAMP whereas others are stimulated. While stimulatory effects in transformed cell types have been seen only rarely, no generalizations can as yet be made. It is conceivable therefore that elevations in cAMP would enhance rather than inhibit the growth of some tumors. Second, the inhibitory action of cAMP usually reverses rapidly when cAMP is removed. Third, tumor cells can readily become resistant to cAMP, through alterations in cAMP-dependent protein kinase (BOURNE et al. 1975; SIMANTOV and SACHS 1975; RAE et al. 1979; PA-

WELEK 1979). The selection of such resistant variants could result in cells with enhanced malignant properties.

cAMP-elevating agents could possibly be useful in treatment of several exceptional tumors which undergo irreversible alterations in response to cAMP. For example, some strains of neuroblastoma cells appear to be induced into a terminally differentiated, non-dividing state in response to cAMP (PRASAD and KUMAR 1974). S49 lymphoma cells are killed by high cAMP (BOURNE et al. 1975). Certain other cell types, if blocked for prolonged periods in G_2, might proceed to cell death.

The possible use of agents which elevate cAMP in combination with cytotoxic agents in treatment of neuroblastoma has been proposed by PRASAD et al. (1976) and is supported by several studies. In vitro treatment of tumor cells with dbcAMP or papavarine markedly diminishes tumorigenicity of the cells upon injection into mice (CHANG and PRASAD 1976). Treatment of the cells with combinations of the two agents completely eliminates tumorigenicity. Moreover, intraperitoneal injection of dbcAMP, papavarine and theophylline slows growth of subcutaneous neuroblastoma tumors, though after several days to weeks the cells escape and resume division. In another study with NB_4 cells (LAZO and RUDDON (1977), 3 days of treatment with PGE_1 and papaverine led to a decrease in malignancy of the cells. It required four times more cells to produce the same number of tumors in mice, and the latent period was increased for formation of a palpable tumor mass. HELSON et al. (1976) have included papaverine in a clinical treatment program, along with cyclophosphamide, vincristine and 5-trifluoromethyl-2′-deoxyuridine. Early results with 15 patients with disseminated neuroblastoma were encouraging.

ROZENGURT and PO (1976) have suggested that the ability of cAMP to induce quiescence in normal, but not transformed, fibroblasts could be used to protect normal cells against the action of agents which kill cells in S phase. They showed that hydroxyurea kills SV40 transformed 3T3 cells, but not normal 3T3 cells when cultures are pretreated with compounds that increase cAMP. PARDEE and DUBROW (1977) have presented a detailed discussion of this approach to cancer chemotherapy. They were not optimistic about the use of cAMP elevations for this purpose.

C. Concluding Remarks

The literature suggests a number of different roles for cyclic nucleotides in the regulation of cell proliferation. It is increasingly evident that growth regulation is quite complex and that cyclic nucleotides represent only one component of the process.

Our understanding of the mechanisms by which cyclic nucleotides participate in cell poliferation and cancer is still in its primitive stages. It is often assumed that initiation of the growing state is the consequence of the altered expression of a gene or battery of genes. Similarly, it is thought that progress through the cell cycle is regulated by ordered expression of genetic information. The nature of the pertinent genes in these processes in unknown, as are the mechanisms by which their expression becomes altered. A plausible approach to this problem is to begin with the interactions of regulatory molecules, e.g., cyclic nucleotides, and attempt to follow their action in a stepwise fashion to their endpoint. Such an approach is likely to lead to false starts and blind alleys, and may turn out to be a tortuous path, but ultimately should be productive. Recent approaches include studies on the effects of cyclic nucleotides upon the skeletal elements of the cells, microtubules and microfilaments (REBHUN 1977); studies on the interrelationship between cyclic nucleotides and Ca^{++} (BERRIDGE 1975; see also this volume); studies on the role of cyclic nucleotides in nuclear protein phosphorylation (JUNGMANN and RUSSELL 1977); and studies on the nuclear translocation of cAMP-binding protein complex and its interaction with chromatin (KALLOS 1977). These and other approaches should lead to important insights into growth regulation and cancer, as well as into other fundamental cellular processes.

Acknowledgements. The author wishes to thank Charlotte Boney for aid in preparing this manuscript. This work is supported by grants AM 20419 from NIH and PCM 78-08024 from NSF.

References

Abell CW, Monahan TM (1973) The role of adenosine 3′,5′-cyclic monophosphate in the regulation of mammalian cell division. J Cell Biol 59:549–558

Ahn HS, Horowitz SG, Eagle H, Makman MH (1978) Effects of cell density and cell growth alterations on cyclic nucleotide levels in cultured human diploid fibroblasts. Exp Cell Res 114:101–110

Anderson WB, Jaworski CJ (1978) Adenylate cyclase activity in normal and transformed fibroblasts in culture. Natl Cancer Inst Monogr 48:365–374

Anderson WB, Russell TR, Carchman RA, Pastan I (1973a) Interrelationship between adenylate cyclase activity, adenosine 3′,5′-cyclic monophosphate phosphodiesterase activity, adenosine 3′,5′-cyclic monophosphate levels and growth of cells in culture. Proc Natl Acad Sci USA 70:3802–3805

Anderson WB, Johnson GS, Pastan I (1973b) Transformation of chick embryo fibroblasts by wild-type and temperature-sensitive Rous sarcoma virus alters adenylate cyclase activity. Proc Natl Acad Sci USA 70:1055–1059

Armato U, Draghi E, Andreis PG, Meneghelli V (1976) Stimulation by $N^{6\prime},O^{2\prime}$-dibutyryl adenosine 3′,5′-cyclic monophosphate of RNA and DNA synthesis and of cell proliferation of rat hepatocytes in primary tissue culture. J Cell Physiol 89:157–170

Armato U, Draghi E, Andreis PG (1977) Effects of purine cyclic nucleotides on the growth of neonatal rat hepatocytes in primary tissue culture. Exp Cell Res 105:337–347

Arnold WP, Aldred R, Murad F (1977) Cigarette smoke activates guanylate cyclase and increases guanosine 3′,5′-monophosphate in tissues. Science 198:934–936

Bailey RP, Rudert WA, Short J, Lieberman I (1975) Nucleolar changes in liver before onset of deoxyribonucleic acid replication. J Biol Chem 250:4305–4309

Bannai S, Sheppard JR (1974) Cyclic AMP, ATP and cell contact. Nature 250:62–64

Barker H, Isles TE (1978) Actions of cyclic AMP, its butyryl derivates and Na butyrate on the HCG output of malignant trophoblast cells in vitro. Br J Cancer 38:158–162

Bechtel E, Kung W, Talmadge K, Almendral A, Eppenberger U (1977) Cyclic AMP, cyclic GMP and protein kinase activity in normal and neoplastic human mammary tissue. In: Folco G, Paoletti R (eds) Molecular biology and pharmacology of cyclic nucleotides. Elvisier/North-Holland Biomedical, Amsterdam Oxford New York, pp 151–154

Bechtel PJ, Beavo JA, Hofmann F, Dills WL, Krebs EG (1975) Cyclic AMP dependent protein kinase isozymes. Fed Proc 34:617

Becker H, Stanners CP (1972) Control of macromolecular synthesis in proliferating and resting Syrian hamster cells in monolayer culture. J Cell Physiol 80:51–62

Berridge MJ (1975) The interaction of cyclic nucleotides and calcium in the control of cellular activity. Adv Cyclic Nucleotide Res 6:1–98

Bombik BM, Burger MM (1973) Cyclic AMP and the cell cycle: inhibition of growth stimulation. Exp Cell Res 80:88–94

Bourne HR, Coffino P, Tomkins GM (1975) Somatic genetic analysis of cyclic AMP action: characterization of unresponsive mutants. J Cell Physiol 85:611–619

Boynton AL, Whitfield JF (1979) The cyclic AMP-dependent initiation of DNA synthesis by T51B rat liver epithelioid cells. J Cell Physiol 101:139–148
Boynton AL, Whitfield JF, Isaacs RJ, Tremblay R (1977) The control of human WI-38 cell proliferation by extracellular calcium and its elimination by SV-40 virus-induced proliferative transformation. J Cell Physiol 92:241–248
Boynton AL, Whitfield JF, Isaacs RJ, Tremblay RG (1978) An examination of the roles of cyclic nucleotides in the initiation of cell proliferation. Life Sci 22:703–710
Bucher NLR, Swaffield MN (1975) Regulation of hepatic regeneration in rats by synergistic action of insulin and glucagon. Proc Natl Acad Sci USA 72:1157–1160
Bucher NLR, Patel U, Cohen S (1978) Hormonal factors concerned with liver regeneration. Ciba Found Symp 55:95–110
Burger MM, Bombik BM, Breckenridge BMcL, Sheppard JR (1972) Growth control and cyclic alterations of cyclic AMP in the cell cycle. Nature New Biol 239:161–163
Burstin SJ, Renger HC, Basilico C (1974) Cyclic AMP levels in temperature sensitive SV40 transformed cell types. J Cell Physiol 84:69–74
Butcher FR, Scott DF, Potter VR, Morris HP (1972) Endocrine control of cyclic adenosine 3′,5′-monophosphate in several Morris hepatomas. Cancer Res 32:2135–2140
Byron JW (1971) Effect of steroids and dibutyryl cyclic AMP on the sensitivity of haemopoietic stem cells to ^{3}H-thymidine in vitro. Nature 234:39–40
Byron JW (1972) Evidence for a β-adrenergic receptor initiating DNA synthesis in haemopoietic stem cells. Exp Cell Res 71:228–232
Byron JW (1973) Drug receptors and the haemopoietic stem cell. Nature New Biol 241:152–154
Byron JW (1976) Cyclic nucleotides and the cell cycle of the haemopoietic stem cell. In: Abou-Sabé M (ed) Cyclic nucleotides and the regulation of cell growth. Dowden, Hutchinson & Ross, Stroudsburg, Pa, pp 81–93
Byus CV, Russell DH (1975) Ornithine decarboxylase activity: control by cyclic nucleotides. Science 187:650–652
Byus CV, Costa M, Sipes IG, Brodie BB, Russell DH (1976) Activation of 3′:5′-cyclic AMP-dependent protein kinase and induction of ornithine decarboxylase as early events in the induction of mixed-function oxygenases. Proc Natl Acad Sci USA 73:1241–1245
Byus CV, Klimpel GR, Lucas DO, Russell DH (1977) Type I and type II cyclic AMP-dependent protein kinase as opposite effectors of lymphocyte mitogenesis. Nature 268:63–64
Byus CV, Klimpel GR, Lucas DO, Russell DH (1978) Ornithine decarboxylase induction in mitogen-stimulated lymphocytes is related to the specific activation of type I adenosine cyclic 3′,5′-monophosphate-dependent protein kinase. Mol Pharmacol 14:431–441
Carchman RA, Johnson GS, Pastan I, Scolnick EM (1974) Studies on the levels of cyclic AMP in cells transformed by wild-type and temperature-sensitive Kirsten sarcoma virus. Cell 1:59–64
Chamley JH, Campbell GR (1975) Trophic influences of sympathetic nerves and cyclic AMP on differentiation and proliferation of isolated smooth muscle cells in culture. Cell Tissue Res 161:497–510
Chang JHT, Prasad KN (1976) Differentiation of mouse neuroblastoma cells in vitro and in vivo induced by cyclic adenosine monophosphate (cAMP). J Pediatr Surg 11:847–856
Chayoth R, Epstein S, Field JB (1972) Increased cyclic AMP levels in malignant hepatic nodules of ethionine treated rats. Biochem Biophys Res Commun 49:1663–1670
Chayoth R, Epstein SM, Field JB (1973) Glucagon and prostaglandin E_1 stimulation of cyclic adenosine 3′,5′-monophosphate levels and adenylate cyclase activity in benign hyperplastic nodules and malignant hepatomas of ethionine-treated rats. Cancer Res 33:1970–1974
Chlapowski FJ, Kelly LA, Butcher RW (1975) Cyclic nucleotides in cultured cells. Adv Cyclic Nucleotide Res 6:245–338
Chlapowski FJ, Ray KP, Butcher RW (1978) Prolonged prostaglandin E_1 stimulation of cyclic AMP production in transformed and normal WI-38 fibroblasts. In vitro 14:924–934
Cho-Chung YS (1974) In vivo inhibition of tumor growth by cyclic adenosine 3′,5′-monophosphate derivatives. Cancer Res 34:3492–3496

Cho-Chung YS, Gullino PM (1974) In vivo inhibition of growth of two hormone-dependent mammary tumors by dibutyryl cyclic AMP. Science 183:87–88
Christensen M, Schweppe JS, Jungmann RA (1979) Cyclic AMP-dependent and -independent protein phosphokinase activity in subcellular fractions of synchronously growing Leydig I-10 cells. Exp Cell Res 124:15–24
Christman JK, Acs G (1974) Purification and characterization of a cellular fibrinolytic factor associated with oncogenic transformation: the plasminogen activator from SV-40-transformed hamster cells. Biochim Biophys Acta 340:339–347
Christofferson T (1975) Effect of treatment of rats with some chemical carcinogens on the stimulatory effect of adrenaline on cyclic AMP accumulation in liver slices. Acta Pharmacol Toxicol (Copenh) 37:233–236
Christofferson T, Morland J, Osnes JB, Kjell E (1972) Hepatic adenyl cyclase: alterations in hormone response during treatment with chemical carcinogen. Biochim Biophys Acta 279:363–366
Christofferson T, Bronstad GO, Walstad P, Øye I (1974) Cyclic AMP metabolism in rat liver during 2-acetylaminofluorene carcinogenesis. Biochim Biophys Acta 372:291–303
Clark GD, Smith C (1973) The response of normal and polyoma virus transformed BHK/21 cells to exogenous purines. J Cell Physiol 81:125–132
Coffino P, Gray JW (1978) Regulation of S49 lymphoma cell growth by cyclic adenosine 3′:5′-monophosphate. Cancer Res 38:4285–4288
Coffino P, Gray JW, Tomkins GM (1975) Cyclic AMP, nonessential regulator of the cell cycle. Proc Natl Acad Sci USA 72:878–882
Coffino P, Bourne HR, Insel PA, Melmon KL, Johnson G, Vigne J (1978) Studies of cyclic AMP action using mutant tissue culture cells. In Vitro 14:140–145
Corbin JD, Keely SL (1977) Characterization and regulation of heart adenosine 3′:5′-monophosphate-dependent protein kinase isozymes. J Biol Chem 252:910–918
Corbin JD, Keely SL, Park CR (1975) The distribution and dissociation of cyclic adenosine 3′:5′-monophosphate-dependent protein kinases in adipose, cardiac and other tissues. J Biol Chem 250:218–225
Costa M, Gerner W, Russell DH (1976a) G_1 specific increases in cyclic AMP levels and protein kinase activity in Chinese hamster ovary cells. Biochim Biophys Acta 425:246–255
Costa M, Gerner EW, Russell DH (1976b) Cell cycle-specific activity of type I and type II cyclic adenosine 3′:5′-monophosphate-dependent protein kinases in Chinese hamster ovary cells. J Biol Chem 251:3313–3319
Costa M, Gerner EW, Russell DH (1978) Cyclic AMP levels and types I and II cyclic AMP-dependent protein kinase activity in synchronized cells and in quiescent cultures stimulated to proliferate. Biochim Biophys Acta 538:1–10
Creighton MO, Trevithick JR (1974) Effect of cyclic AMP, caffeine and theophylline on differentiation of lens epithelial cells. Nature 249:767–768
Criss WE, Morris HP (1973) Protein kinase activity in Morris hepatomas. Biochem Biophys Res Commun 54:380–386
Criss WE, Murad F, Kimura H, Morris HP (1976) Properties of guanylate cyclase in adult rat liver and several Morris hepatomas. Biochim Biophys Acta 445:500–508
D'Armiento M, Johnson GS, Pastan I (1973) Cyclic AMP and growth of fibroblasts: effects of environmental pH. Nature New Biol 242:78–80
Dell'Orco RT, Martin TJ, Douglas WHJ (1977) Cyclic AMP and serum arrest of the mitotic activity of human diploid fibroblasts. In Vitro 13:55–62
DeRubertis FR, Craven PA (1976) Calcium-independent modulation of cyclic GMP and activation of guanylate cyclase by nitrosamines. Science 193:897–899
De Rubertis FR, Craven P (1977a) Increased guanylate cyclase activity and guanosine 3′,5′-monophosphate content in ethionine-induced hepatomas. Cancer Res 37:15–21
DeRubertis FR, Craven PA (1977b) Activation of renal cortical and hepatic guanylate-guanosine 3′,5′-monophosphate systems by nitrosoureas. Divalent cation requirements and relationships to thiol reactivity. Biochim Biophys Acta 499:337–351
DiPasquale A, McGuire J (1977) Dibutyryl cyclic AMP arrests the growth of cultivated Cloudman melanoma cells in the late S and G_2 phases of the cell cycle. J Cell Physiol 93:395–406
Dulbecco R (1970) Topoinhibition and serum requirement of transformed and untransformed cells. Nature 227:802–806

Dulbecco R, Elkington J (1975) Induction of growth in resting fibroblastic cell cultures by Ca^{++}. Proc Natl Acad Sci USA 72:1584–1588
Dumont JE, Boeynaems JM, Decoster C et al. (1978) Biochemical mechanisms in the control of thyroid function and growth. Adv Cyclic Nucleotide Res 9:723–734
Earp HS, Steiner AL (1978) Compartmentalization of cyclic nucleotide mediated hormone action. Annu Rev Pharmacol Toxicol 18:431–459
Farese RV, Reddy WJ (1963) Observations on the interrelations between adrenal protein, RNA and DNA during prolonged ACTH administration. Biochim Biophys Acta 76:145–148
Fayet G, Lissitzky S (1970) Cyclic 3′,5′-adenosine monophosphate-mediated follicular reorganization of isolated thyroid cells in culture. FEBS Lett 11:185–188
Flaxman BA, Harper RA (1975) In vitro analysis of the control of keratinocyte proliferation in human epidermis by physiologic and pharmacologic agents. J Invest Dermatol 65:52–59
Frank W (1972) Cyclic 3′,5′-AMP and cell proliferation of embryonic rat cells. Exp Cell Res 71:238–239
Friedman DL (1976) Role of cyclic nucleotides in cell growth and differentiation. Physiol Rev 56:652–708
Friedman DL, Claus TH, Pilkis SJ, Pine GE (1981) Hormonal regulation of DNA synthesis in primary cultures of adult rat hepatocytes. Exp Cell Res 135:283–290
Friedman DL, Johnson RA, Zeilig CE (1976a) The role of cyclic nucleotides in the cell cycle. Adv Cyclic Nucleotide Res 7:69–113
Friedman DL, Johnson RA, Zeilig CE, Kurz JB, Kumar KV, Gray P (1976b) Role of cyclic AMP in the regulation of the HeLa cell cycle. In: Abou-Sabé (ed) Cyclic nucleotides and the regulation of cell growth. Dowden, Hutchinson & Ross, Stroudsburg, Pa, pp 57–80
Froehlich JE, Rachmeler M (1972) Effect of adenosine 3′,5′-cyclic monophosphate on cell proliferation. J Cell Biol 55:19–31
Froehlich JE, Rachmeler M (1974) Inhibition of cell growth in the G_1 phase by adenosine 3′,5′-cyclic monophosphate. J Cell Biol 60:249–257
Furmanski P, Silverman DJ, Lubin M (1971) Expression of differentiated functions in mouse neuroblastoma mediated by dibutyryl-cyclic adenosine monophosphates. Nature 233:413–415
Garren LD, Gill GN, Masui H, Walton GM (1971) On the mechanism of action of ACTH. Recent Prog Horm Res 27:433–474
Gelfant SA (1963) A new theory on the mechanism of cell division. In: Harris RJC (ed) Cell growth and cell division, vol 2. Academic Press, New York London, pp 229–260
Gelfant S, Candelas GC (1972) Regulation of epidermal mitosis. J Invest Dermatol 59:7–12
Gharrett A, Malkinson AM, Sheppard JR (1976) Cyclic AMP-dependent protein kinases from normal and SV40-transformed 3T3 cells. Nature 264:673–675
Gill GN, Weidman ER (1977) Hormonal regulation of initiation of DNA synthesis and of differentiated function in Y−1 adrenal cortical cells. J Cell Physiol 92:65–76
Gospodarowicz D, Gospodarowicz F (1975) The morphological transformation and inhibition of growth of bovine luteal cells in tissue culture induced by luteinizing hormone and dibutyryl cyclic AMP. Endocrinology 96:458–467
Gray JP, Johnson RA, Friedman DL (1980) Cyclic AMP dependent and independent protein kinases in HeLa cells. Arch Biochem Biophys 202:259–276
Green H (1974) Ribosome synthesis during preparation for division in the fibroblast. In: Clarkson B, Baserga R (eds) Control of proliferation in animal cells. Cold Spring Harbor Laboratory, Cold Spring Harbor, NY, pp 743–755
Griswold MD, Solari A, Tung PS, Fritz IB (1977) Stimulation by follicle-stimulating hormone of DNA synthesis and of mitosis in cultured sertoli cells prepared from testes of immature rats. Mol Cell Endocrinol 7:151–165
Gutman NS, Rae PA, Schimmer BP (1978) Altered cyclic AMP-dependent protein kinase activity in a mutant adrenocortical tumor cell line. J Cell Physiol 97:451–460
Halaban R, Lerner AB (1977) The dual effect of melanocyte-stimulating hormone (MSH) on the growth of cultured mouse melanoma cells. Exp Cell Res 108:111–117

Haslam RJ, Goldstein S (1974) Adenosine 3′:5′-monophosphate in young and senescent human fibroblasts during growth and stationary phase in vitro. Biochem J 144:253–263
Heidrick ML, Ryan WL (1971) Adenosine 3′,5′-cyclic monophosphate and contact inhibition. Cancer Res 31:1313–1315
Helson L, Helson C, Peterson RF, Das SK (1976) A rationale for the treatment of metastatic neuroblastoma. J Natl Cancer Inst 57:727–729
Hendel KB (1977) Intracellular protein degradation in growing, in density-inhibited, and serum-restricted fibroblast cultures. J Cell Physiol 92:353–364
Hibasami H, Tanaka M, Nagai J, Ikeda T (1977) Changes in ornithine decarboxylase activity and cyclic adenosine-3′-5′-monophosphate concentrations during the cell cycle of synchronized BHK cells. Aust J Exp Biol Med Sci 55:378–383
Hochman J, Insel P, Bourne H, Coffino P, Tomkins GM (1975) A structural gene mutation affecting the regulatory subunit of cyclic AMP dependent protein kinase in mouse lymphoma cells. Proc Natl Acad Sci USA 72:5051–5055
Holley RW, Kiernan J (1968) Contact inhibition of cell division in 3T3 cells. Proc Natl Acad Sci USA 60:300–304
Holley RW, Kiernan J (1974) Control of the initiation of DNA synthesis in 3T3 cells: low-molecular-weight nutrients. Proc Natl Acad Sci USA 71:2942–2945
Hovi T, Vaheri A (1973) Cyclic AMP and cyclic GMP enhance growth of chick embryo fibroblasts. Nature New Biol 245:174–177
Hsie AW, Puck TT (1971) Morphological transformation of Chinese hamster cells by dibutyryl adenosine 3′,5′-monophosphate and testosterone. Proc Natl Acad Sci USA 68:358–361
Hsie AW, Jones C, Puck TT (1971) Further changes in differentiation state accompanying the conversion of Chinese hamster cells to fibroblastic form by dibutyryl adenosine cyclic 3′:5′-monophosphate and hormones. Proc Natl Acad Sci USA 68:1648–1652
Imashuku S, Fossett MC, Green AA (1979) Characterization of adenosine cyclic 3′:5′-monophosphate-binding proteins in human neuroblastoma. Cancer Res 39:3006–3013
Imrie RC, Ramaiah TR, Antoni F, Hutchison WC (1965) The effect of adrenocorticotrophin on the nucleic acid metabolism of the rat adrenal gland. J Endocrinol 32:303–312
Insel PA, Bourne HR, Coffino P, Tomkins GM (1975) Cyclic AMP-dependent protein kinase:Pivotal role in regulation of enzyme induction and growth. Science 190:896–898
Johnson GS, Pastan I (1972a) $N^6,O^{2'}$-dibutyryl adenosine 3′,5′-monophosphate induces pigment production in melanoma cells. Nature New Biol 237:267–269
Johnson GS, Pastan I (1972b) Cyclic AMP increases the adhesion of fibroblasts to substratum. Nature New Biol 236:247–249
Johnson GS, Friedman RM, Pastan I (1971) Restoration of several morphological characteristics of normal fibroblasts in sarcoma cells treated with adenosine-3′,5′-cyclic monophosphate and its derivatives. Proc Natl Acad Sci USA 68:425–429
Johnson GS, Morgan WD, Pastan I (1972) Regulation of cell motility by cyclic AMP. Nature 235:54–56
Johnson LF, Abelson HT, Green H, Penman S (1974) Changes in RNA in relation to growth of the fibroblast. I. Amounts of mRNA, rRNA, and tRNA in resting and growing cells. Cell 1:95–100
Jungmann RA, Russell DH (1977) Cyclic AMP, cyclic AMP-dependent protein kinase, and the regulation of gene expression. Life Sci 20:1787–1798
Kallos J (1977) Photochemical attachment of cyclic AMP binding protein(s) to the nuclear genome. Nature 265:705–710
Kaminskas E, Field M, Henshaw EC (1976) Cyclic AMP and growth of Ehrlich ascites tumor cells. Lack of cyclic AMP elevation in nutritionally deprived cells and mechanism of retardation of growth by dibutyryl cyclic AMP. Biochim Biophys Acta 444:539–553
Kelly LA, Butcher RW (1974) The effects of epinephrine and prostaglandin E_1 on cyclic adenosine 3′:5′-monophosphate levels in WI-38 cells. J Biol Chem 249:3098–3102
Kimura H, Murad F (1975) Increased particulate and decreased soluble guanylate cyclase activity in regenerating liver, fetal liver and hepatoma. Proc Natl Acad Sci USA 72:1965–1969

Klein DM, Loizzi RF (1977) Enhancement of R3230AC rat mammary tumor growth and cellular differentiation by dibutyryl cyclic adenosine monophosphate. J Natl Cancer Inst 58:813–816

Knecht ME, Lipkin G (1977) Biochemical studies of a protein which restores contact inhibition of growth to malignant melanocytes. Exp Cell Res 108:15–22

Kram R, Mamont P, Tomkins GM (1973) Pleiotypic control by adenosine 3′,5′-cyclic monophosphate: a model for growth control in animal cells. Proc Natl Acad Sci USA 70:1432–1436

Kreider JW, Rosenthal M, Lengle N (1973) Cyclic adenosine 3′,5′-monophosphate in the control of melanoma cell replication and differentiation. J Natl Cancer Inst 50:555–558

Kurth R, Bauer H (1973) Influence of dibutyryl cyclic AMP and theophylline on cell surface antigens on oncornavirus transformed cells. Nature New Biol 243:243–245

Kurtz MJ, Polgar P, Taylor L, Rutenburg AM (1974) The role of adenosine 3′:5′-cyclic monophosphate in the division of WI 38 cells. The cellular response to prostaglandin E_1 and the effects of a cyclic adenosine 3′:5′-cyclic monophosphate analogue and prostaglandin E_1 on cell division. Biochem J 142:339–344

Kurz JB, Friedman DL (1976) Inhibition of G_2 phase in unsynchronized HeLa cells: synergism between adenosine 3′:5′-monophosphate analogues and phosphodiesterase inhibitors. J Cyclic Nucleotide Res 2:405–415

Landau T, Sachs L (1971) Activation of a differentiation-inducing protein by adenine and adenine-containing nucleotides. Fed Eur Biochem Soc Lett 17:339–341

Laug WE, Jones PA, Benedict WF (1974) Relationship between fibrinolysis of cultured cells and malignancy. J Natl Cancer Inst 54:173–179

Lazo JS, Ruddon RW (1977) Neurite extension and malignancy of neuroblastoma cells after treatment with prostaglandin E_1 and papaverine. J Natl Cancer Inst 59:137–143

Lehnert S (1979) Changes in morphology and cell cycle traverse induced by methyl isobutyl xanthine. Exp Cell Res 121:383–394

Levine EM, Becker Y, Boone CW, Eagle H (1965) Contact inhibition, macromolecular synthesis, and polyribosomes in cultured human diploid fibroblasts. Proc Natl Acad Sci USA 53:350–356

Lissitzky S, Fayet G, Giraud A, Verrier B, Torresani J (1971) Thyrotrophin-induced aggregation and reorganization into follicles of isolated porcine-thyroid cells. I. Mechanisms of action of thyrotrophin and metabolic properties. Eur J Biochem 24:88–99

Lotan R, Giotta G, Nork E, Nicolson GL (1978) Characterization of the inhibitory effects of retinoids on the in vitro growth of two malignant murine melanomas. J Natl Cancer Inst 60:1035–1041

MacManus JP, Whitfield JF (1969) Stimulations of DNA synthesis and mitotic activity of thymic lymphocytes by cyclic adenosine 3′,5′-monophosphate. Exp Cell Res 58:188–191

MacManus JP, Franks DJ, Youdale T, Braceland BM (1972) Increases in rat liver cyclic AMP concentrations prior to the initiation of DNA synthesis following partial hepatectomy or hormone infusion. Biochem Biophys Res Commun 49:1201–1207

MacManus JP, Braceland BM, Youdale T, Whitfield JF (1973) Adrenergic antagonists and a possible link between the increase in cyclic adenosine 3′,5′-monophosphate and DNA synthesis during liver regeneration. J Cell Physiol 82:157–164

MacPherson I, Montagnier (1964) Agar suspension culture for the selective assay of cells transformed by polyoma virus. Virology 23:291–294

Malkinson AM, Gunderson TJ, McSwigan CE (1977) Protein phosphorylation in normal and neoplastic development. Biochem J 168:319–321

Masaracchia RA, Walsh DA (1976) Protein phosphotransferase activities and cyclic nucleotide action in proliferating lymphocytes. Cancer Res 36:3227–3237

Masui H, Garren LD (1970) On the mechanism of action of adrenocorticotropic hormone. Stimulation of deoxyribonucleic acid polymerase and thymidine kinase activities in adrenal glands. J Biol Chem 245:2627–2632

Masui H, Garren LD (1971) Inhibition of replication in functional mouse adrenal tumor cells by adrenocorticotropic hormone mediated by adenosine 3′:5′-cyclic monophosphate. Proc Natl Acad Sci USA 68:3206–3210

McGowan JA, Strain AJ, Bucher NLR (1979) Glucagon and cyclic-AMP enhancement of DNA synthesis in epidermal growth factor-stimulated cultures of adult rat hepatocytes. J Cell Biol 83:7a
Miller RP, Husain M, Lohin S (1979) Long acting cAMP analogues enhance sulfate incorporation into matrix proteoglycans and suppress cell division of fetal rat chondrocytes in monolayer culture. J Cell Physiol 100:63–76
Miller Z, Lovelace E, Gallo M, Pastan I (1975) Cyclic GMP and cellular growth. Science 190:1213–1215
Millis AJT, Forest G, Pious DA (1972) Cyclic AMP in cultured human lymphoid cells: relationship to mitosis. Biochem Biophys Res Commun 49:1645–1649
Millis AJT, Forrest GA, Pious DA (1974) Cyclic AMP dependent regulation of mitosis in human lymphoid cells. Exp Cell Res 83:335–343
Minton JP, Matthews RH, Wisenbaugh TW (1976) Elevated adenosine 3′,5′-cyclic monophosphate levels in human and animal tumors in vivo. J Natl Cancer Inst 57:39–41
Moens WA, Vokaer A, Kram R (1975) Cyclic AMP and cyclic GMP concentrations in serum- and density-restricted fibroblast cultures. Proc Natl Acad Sci USA 72:1063–1067
Montagnier L (1971) Factors controlling the multiplication of untransformed and transformed BHK 21 cells under various environmental conditions. In: Wolstenholme GEW, Knight J (eds) Ciba Found. Symp Growth Control in Cell Cultures. Churchill, London p 33–44
Morgan JI, Hall AK, Perris AD (1977) The ionic dependence and steroid blockade of cyclic nucleotide-induced mitogenesis in isolated rat thymic lymphocytes. J Cyclic Nucleotide Res 3:303–314
Mufson RA, Simsiman RC, Boutwell RK (1977) The effect of the phorbol ester tumor promoters on the basal and catecholamine-stimulated levels of cyclic adenosine 3′:5′-monophosphate in mouse skin and epidermis in vivo. Cancer Res 37:665–669
Murad F, Kimura H, Hopkins HA, Looney WB, Kovacs CJ (1975) Increased urinary excretion of cyclic guanosine monophosphate in rats bearing Morris hepatoma 3924A. Science 190:58–60
Murray AW, Verma AK (1973) The adenyl cyclase system and carcinogenesis: decreased responsiveness of mouse epidermis to isoproterenol after 3,4-benzpyrene treatment. Biochem Biophys Res Commun 54:69–75
Niles RM, Makarski JS (1978) Control of melanogenesis in mouse melanoma cells of varying metastatic potential. J Natl Cancer Inst 61:523–526
Niles RM, Makarski JS, Kurz MJ, Rutenburg AM (1976) Inhibition of human prostatic epithelial cell replication by cAMP and selected analogs. Exp Cell Res 102:95–103
Nilhausin K, Green H (1965) Reversible arrest of growth in G_1 of an established fibroblast line (3T3). Exp Cell Res 40:166–168
Nomura K, Hoshino T, Knebel K, Barker M (1978) Effect of dibutyryl cAMP on cell cycle progression of rat brain tumor cells in vitro. In Vitro 14:174–179
Nose K, Katsuta H (1975) Arrest of cultured rat liver cells in G_2 phase by the treatment with dibutyryl cAMP. Biochem Biophys Res Commun 64:983–988
Oey J, Vogel A, Pollack R (1974) Intracellular cyclic AMP concentration responds specifically to growth regulation by serum. Proc Natl Acad Sci USA 71:694–698
Olson JW, Russell DH (1979) Prolonged induction of hepatic ornithine decarboxylase and its relation to cyclic adenosine 3′:5′-monophosphate-dependent protein kinase activation after a single administration of diethylnitrosamine. Cancer Res 39:3074–3079
Ossowski L, Unkeless JC, Tobia A, Quigley JP, Rifkin DB, Reich E (1973) An enzymatic function associated with transformation of fibroblasts by oncogenic viruses. II. Mammalian fibroblast cultures transformed by DNA and RNA tumor viruses. J Exp Med 137:112–126
Otten J, Johnson GS, Pastan I (1971) Cyclic AMP levels in fibroblasts: relationship to growth rate and contact inhibition of growth. Biochem Biophys Res Commun 44:1192–1198
Otten J, Johnson GS, Pastan I (1972a) Regulation of cell growth by cyclic adenosine 3′,5′-monophosphate. J Biol Chem 247:7082–7087

Otten J, Bader J, Johnson GS, Pastan I (1972b) A mutation in a Rous sarcoma virus gene that controls adenosine 3′,5′-monophosphate levels and transformation. J Biol Chem 247:1632–1633
Pardee A (1974) A restriction point for control of normal animal cell proliferation. Proc Natl Acad Sci USA 71:1286–1290
Pardee AB, Dubrow R (1977) Control of cell proliferation. Cancer 39:2747–2754
Pardee AB, Rozengurt E (1975) Role of the surface in production of new cells. In: Fox CF (ed) Biochemistry of cell walls. Technical Publishing Company, London, pp 155–185
Pastan I, Johnson GS (1974) Cyclic AMP and the transformation of fibroblasts. Adv Cancer Res 19:303–329
Pastan I, Willingham M (1978) Cellular transformation and the morphologic phenotype of transformed cells. Nature 274:645–650
Pastan I, Johnson GS, Anderson WB (1975) Role of cyclic nucleotides in growth control. Annu Rev Biochem 44:491–522
Paul D (1973) Quiescent SV40 virus transformed 3T3 cells in culture. Biochem Biophys Res Commun 53:745–753
Pawelek JM (1976) Factors regulating growth and pigmentation of melanoma cells. J Invest Dermatol 66:201–209
Pawelek J (1979) Evidence suggesting that a cyclic AMP-dependent protein kinase is a positive regulator of proliferation in Cloudman S91 melanoma cells. J Cell Physiol 98:619–626
Pawelek J, Wong G, Sansone M, Morowitz J (1973) Molecular controls in mammalian pigmentation. Yale J Biol Med 46:430–433
Pawelek J, Halaban R, Christie G (1975a) Melanoma cells which require cyclic AMP for growth. Nature 258:539–540
Pawelek J, Sansone M, Koch N et al. (1975b) Melanoma cells resistant to inhibition of growth by melanocyte stimulating hormone. Proc Natl Acad Sci USA 72:951–955
Pawlikowski M, Kunert-Radek J, Mroz-Wasilewska Z (1979) Biphasic inhibitory and stimulatory effects of thyrotropin on the mitotic activity of thyroid explants cultured in vitro. Endokrinologie 73:186–190
Pledger WJ, Gardner RM, Epstein PM, Thompson WJ, Strada SJ, Wlodyka L (1979) Cell cycle traverse and macromolecular synthesis in BHK fibroblasts are affected by insulin. Exp Cell Res 118:389–394
Pollack RE, Hough PVC (1974) The cell surface and malignant transformation. Annu Rev Med 25:431–446
Prasad KN (1972a) Cyclic AMP-induced differentiated mouse neuroblastoma cells lose tumourgenic characteristics. Cytobios 6:163–167
Prasad KN (1972b) Morphological differentiation induced by prostaglandin in mouse neuroblastoma cells in culture. Nature New Biol 236:49–52
Prasad KN (1977) Role of cyclic nucleotide in the differentiation of nerve cells. In: Fedoroff S, Hertz L (eds) Cell, tissue and organ cultures in neurobiology. Academic Press, New York London, pp 447–483
Prasad KN, Hsie AW (1971) Morphologic differentiation of mouse neuroblastoma cells induced in vitro by dibutyryl adenosine 3′:5′-cyclic monophosphate. Nature New Biol 233:141–142
Prasad KN, Kumar S (1974) Cyclic AMP and differentiation of neuroblastoma cells in culture. In: Clarkson B, Baserga R (eds) Control of proliferation in animal cells. Cold Spring Harbor Laboratory, Cold Spring Harbor, NY, pp 581–594
Prasad KN, Vernadakis A (1972) Morphological and biochemical study in X-ray- and dibutyryl cyclic AMP-induced differentiated neuroblastoma cells. Exp Cell Res 70:27–32
Prasad KN, Sahu SK, Sinha PK (1976) Cyclic nucleotides in the regulation of expression of differentiated functions in neuroblastoma cells. J Natl Cancer Inst 57:619–629
Pruss RM, Herschman HR (1979) Cholera toxin stimulates division of 3T3 cells. J Cell Physiol 98:469–474
Ramachandran J, Suyama AT (1975) Inhibition of replication of normal adrenal cortical cells in culture by adrenocorticotropin. Proc Natl Acad Sci USA 72:113–177
Radley JM, Hodgson GS (1971) Effect of isoprenaline on cells in different phases of the mitotic cycle. Exp Cell Res 69:148–160

Radley JM, Hodgson GS (1973) G_2 terminal points of action of isoprenaline, x-irradiation, cyclohexamide and actinomycin D in rat parotid gland. Exp Cell Res 80:237–244
Rae PA, Gutmann NS, Tsao J, Schimmer BP (1979) Mutations in cyclic AMP-dependent protein kinase and corticotropin(ACTH)-sensitive adenyl cyclase affect steroidogenesis. Proc Natl Acad Sci USA 76:1896–1900
Raff MC, Hornby-Smith A, Brockes JP (1978a) Cyclic AMP as a mitogenic signal for cultured rat Schwann cells. Nature 273:672–673
Raff MC, Abney E, Brockes JP, Hornby-Smith A (1978b) Schwann cell growth factors. Cell 15:813–822
Rebhun LI (1977) Cyclic nucleotides, calcium, and cell division. Int Rev Cytol 49:1–54
Rechler MM, Bruni CB, Podskalny JM, Warner W, Carchman RA (1977) Modulation of serum-stimulated DNA synthesis in cultured human fibroblasts by cAMP. Exp Cell Res 104:411–422
Richman RA, Claus TH, Pilkis SJ, Friedman DL (1976) Hormonal stimulation of DNA synthesis in primary cultures of adult rat hepatocytes. Proc Natl Acad Sci USA 73:3589–3593
Rozengurt E, Pardee AB (1972) Opposite effects of dibutyryl adenosine 3′,5′-cyclic monophosphate and serum on growth of Chinese hamster cells. J Cell Physiol 80:273–280
Rozengurt E, Po CC (1976) Selective cytotoxicity for transformed 3T3 cells. Nature 261:701–702
Rudland PS, Gospodarowicz D, Seifert W (1974a) Activation of guanyl cyclase and intracellular cyclic GMP by fibroblast growth factor. Nature 250:741–742, 773–774
Rudland PS, Seeley M, Seifert W (1974b) Cyclic GMP and cyclic AMP. Levels in normal and transformed fibroblasts. Nature 251:417–419
Russell DH, Durie BGM (1978) Polyamines as biochemical markers of normal and malignant growth. Raven, New York
Ryan WL, Heidrick ML (1974) Role of cyclic nucleotides in cancer. Adv Cyclic Nucleotide Res 4:81–116
Salas J, Gree H (1971) Proteins binding to DNA and their relation to growth in cultured mammalian cells. Nature New Biol 229:165–169
Santoro MG, Philpott GW, Jaffe BM (1977) Inhibition of B-16 melanoma growth in vivo by a synthetic analog of prostaglandin E2. Cancer Res 37:3774–3779
Schor S, Rozengurt E (1973) Enhancement by purine nucleosides and nucleotides of serum-induced DNA synthesis in quiescent 3T3 cells. J Cell Physiol 81:339–346
Scott RE, Furcht LT (1974) Effect of dibutyryl cyclic AMP and serum deprivation on the membranes of transformed mouse fibroblasts. A freeze fracture study (38304). Proc Soc Exp Biol Med 147:162–166
Seifert W, Paul D (1972) Levels of cyclic AMP in sparse and dense cultures of growing and quiescent 3T3 cells. Nature New Biol 240:281–283
Seifert WE, Rudland PS (1974a) Possible involvement of cyclic GMP in growth control of cultured mouse cells. Nature 248:138–140
Seifert WE, Rudland PS (1974b) Cyclic nucleotides and growth control in cultured mouse cells: correlation of changes in intracellular 3′:5′-cGMP concentration with a specific phase of the cell cycle. Proc Natl Acad Sci USA 71:4920–4924
Sheppard JR (1971) Restoration of contact-inhibited growth to transformed cells by dibutyryl adenosine 3′:5′-cyclic monophosphate. Proc Natl Acad Sci USA 68:1316–1320
Sheppard J (1972) Differences in the cyclic adenosine 3′,5′-monophosphate levels in normal and transformed cells. Nature New Biol 236:14–16
Sheppard JR, Hudson TH, Larson JR (1975) Adenosine 3′,5′-monophosphate analogs promote a circular morphology of cultured Schwannoma cells. Science 187:179–181
Shields R, Pollock K (1974) The adhesion of BHK and Py BHK cells to the substratum. Cell 3:31–38
Short J, Brown RF, Husakova A, Gilbertson JR, Zemel R, Lieberman I (1972) Induction of deoxyribonucleic acid synthesis in liver of the intact animal. J Biol Chem 247:1757–1766
Short J, Tsukada K, Rudert WA, Leiberman I (1975) Cyclic adenosine 3′,5′-monophosphate and the induction of deoxyribonucleic acid synthesis in liver. J Biol Chem 250:3602–3606

Simantov R, Sachs L (1975) Temperature sensitivity of cyclic adenosine 3′,5′-monophosphate-binding proteins and the regulation of growth and differentiation in neuroblastoma cells. J Biol Chem 250:3236–3242

Smets LA (1972) Contact inhibition of transformed cells incompletely restored by dibutyryl cyclic AMP. Nature New Biol 239:123–124

Smith JA, Martin L (1973) Do cells cycle? Proc Natl Acad Sci USA 70:1263–1267

Stambrook PJ, Velez C (1976) Reversible arrest of Chinese hamster V79 cells in G_2 by dibutyryl cyclic AMP. Exp Cell Res 99:57–62

Steinberg RA, Coffino P (1979) Two-dimensional gel analysis of cyclic AMP effects in cultured S49 lymphoma cells: protein modifications, inductions and repressions. Cell 18:719–733

Steiner AL, Koide Y, Earp HS, Bechtel PJ, Beavo JA (1978) Compartmentalization of cyclic nucleotide and cyclic AMP-dependent protein kinase in rat liver: immunocytochemical demonstration. Adv Cyclic Nucleotide Res 9:691–705

Stiles CD, Pledger WJ, Van Wijk JJ, Antoniades H, Scher CD (1979) Hormonal control of early events in the Balb/c-3T3 cell cycle: Commitment to DNA synthesis. Cold Spring Harbor Conf Cell Proliferation 6:425–440

Thomas EW, Murad F, Looney WB, Morris HP (1973) Adenosine 3′,5′-monophosphate and guanosine 3′,5′-monophosphate: concentrations in Moris hepatomas of different growth rates. Biochim Biophys Acta 297:564–567

Thrower S, Ord MG (1974) Hormonal control of liver regeneration. Biochem J 144:361–369

Tisdale MJ (1979) The significance of cyclic AMP and cyclic GMP in cancer treatment. Cancer Treat Rev 6:1–15

Tobey RA, Ley KD (1971) Isoleucine-mediated regulation of genome replication in various mammalian cells lines. Cancer Res 31:46–51

Todaro GJ, Green H (1963) Quantitative studies of the growth of mouse embryo cells in culture and their development into established lines. J Cell Biol 17:299–313

Todaro GJ, Green H (1964) An assay for cellular transformation by SV40. Virology 23:117–119

Todaro GJ, Lazar GK, Green H (1965) The initiation of cell division in a contact-inhibited mammalian cell line. J Cell Physiol 66:325–334

Troy FA, Vijay IK, Kawakami TG (1973) Cyclic-3′,5′-AMP-dependent and independent protein kinase levels in normal and feline sarcoma virus transformed cells. Biochem Biophys Res Commun 52:150–157

Van Wijk R, Wicks WD, Clay K (1972) Effects of derivatives of cyclic 3′,5′-adenosine monophosphate on the growth, morphology, and gene expression of hepatoma cells in culture. Cancer Res 32:1905–1911

Van Wijk R, Wicks WD, Bevers MM, Van Rijn J (1973) Rapid arrest of DNA synthesis by N^6,$O^{2'}$-dibutyryl cyclic adenosine 3′,5′-monophosphate in cultured hepatoma cells. Cancer Res 33:1331–1338

Verma AK, Murray AW (1974) The effect of benzo(a)pyrene on the basal and isoproterenol-stimulated levels of cyclic adenosine 3′,5′-monophosphate in mouse epidermis. Cancer Res 34:3408

Vesely DL, Levey GS (1977a) Enhancement of human guanylate cyclase activity by chemical carcinogens. Proc Soc Exp Biol Med 155:301–304

Vesely DL, Levey GS (1977b) Modulation of rat and human guanylate cyclase activity *in vitro* by chemical carcinogens. Clin Res 25:502A

Vesely DL, Levey GS (1978) Saccharin inhibits guanylate cyclase activity: possible relationship to carcinogenesis. Biochem Biophys Res Commun 81:1384–1389

Vesely DL, Rovere LE, Levey GS (1977) Activation of guanylate cyclase by streptozotocin and 1-methyl-1-nitrosourea. Cancer Res 37:28–31

Voorhees JJ, Duell EA, Stawiski M, Harrell ER (1974) Cyclic nucleotide metabolism in normal and proliferating epidermis. Adv Cyclic Nucleotide Res 4:117–162

Wade DR, Burkart ME (1978) The role of adenosine 3′,5′-cyclic monophosphate in the density-dependent regulation of growth and tyrosinase activity of B-16 melanoma cells. J Cell Physiol 94:265–273
Walsh DA (1978) Role of cAMP-dependent protein kinase as the transducer of cAMP action. Biochem Pharmacol 27:1801–1804
Walsh DA, Ashby CD, Gonzalez C, Calkins D, Fischer EH, Krebs EG (1971) Purification and characterization of a protein inhibitor of adenosine 3′,5′-monophosphate-dependent protein kinases. J Biol Chem 246:1977–1985
Waymire JC, Weiner N, Prasad KN (1972) Regulation of tyrosine hydroxylase activity in cultured mouse neuroblasoma cells. Elevation induced by analogs of adenosine 3′,5′-cyclic monophosphate. Proc Natl Acad Sci USA 69:2241–2245
Waymire JC, Gilmer-Waymire K, Haycock JW (1978) Cyclic-AMP-induced differentiation in neuroblastoma is independent of cell division rate. Nature 276:194–195
Wehner JM, Malkinson AM, Sheppard JR (1978) Cyclic AMP dependent protein kinases in 3T3 and other cell lines. Adv Cyclic Nucleotide Res 9:779
Weidman ER, Gill GN (1976) Differential effects of ACTH or 8-Br-cAMP on growth and replication in a functional adrenal tumor cell line. J Cell Physiol 90:91–104
Westermark B, Karlsson FA, Walinder O (1979) Thyrotropin is not a growth factor for human thyroid cells in culture. Proc Natl Acad Sci USA 76:2022–2026
White R, Hanson GC, Funan HU (1979) Tyrosinase maturation and pigment expression in B16 melanoma: relation to theophylline treatment and intracellular cyclic AMP. J Cell Physiol 99:441–450
Whitfield JF, Perris AD, Youdale T (1969) The calcium-mediated promotion of mitotic activity in rat thymocyte populations by growth hormone, neurohormones, parathyroid hormone and prolactin. J Cell Physiol 73:203–212
Whitfield JF, MacManus JP, Franks DJ, Gillan DJ, Youdale T (1971) The possible mediation by cyclic AMP of the stimulation of thymocyte proliferation by cyclic GMP. Proc Soc Exp Biol Med 137:453–457
Whitfield JF, Rixon RH, MacManus JP, Balk SD (1973 a) Calcium, cyclic adenosine 3′,5′-monophosphate, and the control of cell proliferation: a review. In Vitro 8:257–278
Whitfield JF, MacManus JP, Rixon RH, Gillan DJ (1973 b) The calcium-independent stimulation of thymic lymphoblast DNA synthesis by low cyclic GMP concentrations. Proc Soc Exp Biol Med 144:808–812
Whitfield JF, MacManus JP, Gillan DJ (1973 c) The ability of calcium to change cyclic AMP from a stimulator to an inhibitor of thymic lymphoblast proliferation. J Cell Physiol 81:241–250
Whitfield JF, MacManus JP, Rixon RH, Boynton AL, Youdale T, Swierenga S (1976)Control of cell proliferation. In Vitro 12:1
Wigglesworth NM, Mastro A, Bourne HR, Rozengurt E (1977) Cyclic AMP-binding proteins in normal and virus-transformed fibroblasts. Arch Biochem Biophys 180:258–263
Willingham MC, Pastan I (1974) Cyclic AMP mediates the concanavalin A agglutinability of mouse fibroblasts. J Cell Biol 63:288–294
Willingham MC, Johnson GS, Pastan I (1972) Control of DNA synthesis and mitosis in 3T3 cells by cyclic AMP. Biochem Biophys Res Commun 48:743–749
Winand RJ, Kohn LD (1975) Thyrotropin effects on thyroid cells in culture. Effects of trypsin on the thyrotropin receptor and on thyrotropin-mediated cyclic 3′:5′-AMP changes. J Biol Chem 250:6534–6540
Wong G, Pawelek J (1973) Control of phenotypic expression of cultured melanoma cells by melanocyte stimulating hormones. Nature New Biol 241:213–215
Wray HL, Glinos AD (1978) Cyclic nucleotides and growth regulation in suspension cultures of mammalian cells. Am J Physiol 234:C131–C138
Yasuda H, Hanai N, Kurata M, Yamada M (1978) Cyclic GMP metabolism in relation to the regulation of cell growth in Balb/3T3 cells. Exp Cell Res 114:111–116
Zeilig CE, Goldberg ND (1977) Cell-cycle-related changes of 3′:5′-cyclic GMP levels in Novikoff hepatoma cells. Proc Natl Acad Sci USA 74:1052–1056

Zeilig CE, Johnson RA, Friedman DL, Sutherland EW (1972) Cyclic AMP concentrations in synchronized HeLa cells. J Cell Biol 55:296a
Zeilig CE, Johnson RA, Friedman DL, Kumar K, Sutherland EW (1974a) Regulatory influences of cyclic AMP in synchronized HeLa cells Adv. Cyclic Nucl. Res 5:832
Zeilig CE, Johnson RA, Sutherland EW, Friedman DL (1974b) Cyclic AMP levels in synchronized HeLa cells and a dual effect on mitosis. Fed Proc 33:948a
Zeilig CE, Johnson RA, Sutherland EW, Friedman DL (1976) Adenosine 3':5'-monophosphate content and actions in the division cycle of synchronized HeLa cells. J Cell Biol 71:515–534
Zimmerman JE, Raska K (1972) Inhibition of adenovirus type 12 induced DNA synthesis in G_1-arrested BHK 21 cells by dibutyryl adenosine cyclic 3':5'-monophosphate. Nature New Biol 239:145–147

CHAPTER 19

Regulation of Development by Cyclic Nucleotides and Inorganic Ions

D. McMahon

Overview

Understanding the molecular basis of the two interlocking central problems in development, cellular position determination and gene regulation, will be an advance of great intellectual and practical importance. During the past several years, many lines of evidence have begun to accumulate which suggest that cyclic nucleotides and inorganic ions are intimately involved in this process. The present chapter reviews this evidence for three developmental systems and speculates on the molecular events which may provide the basis for cellular changes of phenotype and genotype.

A. Introduction

The fate of a cell in a developing organism is often the result of a series of decisions based upon the cell's position in the organism. The cell may divide or die; it may move to a new location; or it may assume a new morphology and/or biochemical function. The range of phenomena which are found in developing organisms are best described in textbooks of development (Ede 1978; Deuchar 1975; Kühn 1971). The experimental analysis of development decomposes into two related problems. (1) What is the molecular basis of cellular position determination during development? (2) How does a cell use information about its position to regulate the activity of its genes and their products?

Experimental analysis has revealed three types of positional specification. Two of these involve cellular interactions and one appears independent of interactions among cells.

First, during mosaic development, the cells of the embryo differentiate autonomously. If a cell is removed from the embryo, the embryo will lack those cells or tissues produced by descendants of the cell which has been removed. The isolated cell can produce these parts when cultured in vitro.

Second, developmental induction involves the interaction of two groups of cells, an inducing and an induced group of cells. If the inducing cells are removed, the inducible cells fail to differentiate. Transplanting the inducing cells to a new location in the embryo may be able to elicit differentiation of cells in an abnormal location. Recent work suggests that the molecule responsible for the primary neural induction may be smaller than 12,000 daltons (Toivonen 1979).

Third, morphogenetic fields are composed of an integrated system of cells. In contrast to induction, it is not possible to separate acting from reacting cells. If a group of cells is removed from a morphogenetic field, the remaining cells regulate to produce a population of cells which, although reduced in absolute number, produce normal proportions of differentiated cells as output.

A brief consideration of some molecular mechanisms which have been posited as the basis for positional specification is presented elsewhere (McMAHON and WEST 1976). I have proposed mechanisms for induction and morphogenetic field organization which are related to the theme of this volume. Therefore, these will be considered in detail. The reader should, however, consult other sources (EDE 1978; KÜHN 1971) for additional information.

The cell-contact model for morphogenetic field organization (McMAHON 1973) proposed that cells in a morphogenetic field determine their position using complementary contacts of plasma membrane molecules. These molecules, which can be considered as analogs of hormone receptors, were posited to control the intracellular concentration of a second messenger such as cyclic AMP (cAMP). Each of the two complementary types of molecules was postulated to have opposing actions on the intracellular concentration of cAMP. One type, when activated by contact, increased cAMP concentration. The other type was suggested to lower cAMP when activated by contact. The function of these receptors was also suggested to be under negative-feedback control by the intracellular of cAMP. Although the model may appear complex, it provides simple experimental predictions. Solution of the differential equations which model this system produce results which are congruent with knowledge of development (McMAHON 1973). A qualitative consideration of this model has been presented elsewhere (McMAHON 1981).

A variety of substances, including hormones, neurotransmitters, inorganic salts and drugs, may act as inhibitors or promoter of induction. The results of many of these studies may be rationalized if induction is considered to be a physiological process mediated by a small number of endogenous chemical messengers (McMAHON 1974). This chemical messengers hypothesis proposes that the development path of a cell is controlled by the temporal sequence of intracellular changes in cyclic nucleotides and inorganic ions. Inducing cells presumably control these changes by release of hormones or neurotransmitters or by contact-mediated interactions analogous to those described above (McMAHON and WEST 1976).

This review will not attempt to cite all publications in which the involvement of cyclic nucleotides or inorganic ions in development has been studied. Rather, it will focus on the literature (to January, 1981) of a few systems which have been intensively investigated so that the reader may gain some insight into what progress has been made and what work remains to be done.

Before considering the current status of research, it is important to re-emphasize that development is a historical process. Therefore, the timing of changes in cyclic nucleotide or inorganic ion concentration within developing cells may be critical to a chemical messenger model. Conversely, the responses of a cell and its progeny to the same first or second messenger may be expected to change during development. To physiologists and pharmacologists accustomed to dealing with stabilized tissues this may seem unusual unless it is considered that different tissues and cells, themselves, the products of a series of developmental decisions, may exhibit dramatically different responses to the same first or second chemical messenger.

B. Evidence for the Involvement of Chemical Messengers in Development

I. Maturation of the Oocyte

1. Cellular Events

In many animals, development is considered to begin with the formation of the egg from the oocyte. Both the egg and the oocyte are very differentiated cells, however. A body of work indicates very strongly that the differentiation of the oocyte into an egg cell is regulated by cAMP, Ca^{2+} and K^+. Much of this work has focused on the development of the amphibian oocyte, so this discussion will focus on this system, although the development of other oocytes will also be discussed to illustrate the widespread similarity in the pattern of control.

The mature oocyte of the african clawed toad, *Xenopus laevis*, is cell approximately 1.2 mm in diameter which is arrested at prophase of the first meiotic division. When the follicle cells surrounding the oocyte are stimulated by gonadotrophin, they secrete progesterone onto the surface of the oocyte, triggering its maturation into the egg (SCHUETZ 1972).

The cellular events which occur in formation of the egg include breakdown of the large (500 μM in diameter) nucleus; continuation of meiosis to the second meiotic metaphase; and cytokinesis which produces an egg by extrusion of a small polar body from the maturing oocyte.

2. Extracellular Messenger

Treatment with progesterone ($ED_{50} = 2\ \mu M$) induces the synthesis of an autocatalytic protein, maturation promoting factor (MPF), after 3–5 h. When MPF is transferred to other oocytes, it subsequently induces their maturation. This is indicated by germinal vesicle breakdown (GVBD) after 2–3 h in the absence of treatment with progesterone. A similar factor may regulate mitosis in many cells since extracts of HeLa cell cytoplasm extracted from cells in mitosis can cause GVBD in *Xenopus* oocytes after 1.5–2 h (SUNKARA et al. 1979). In progesterone-treated cells, GVBD occurs after 5–8 h (MASUI and MARKERT 1971; REYNHOUT and SMITH 1974).

Several lines of evidence indicate that the site of action of progesterone is the plasma membrane. Progesterone is inactive when injected into the oocyte (MASUI and MARKERT 1971; SMITH and ECKER 1971). There do not appear to be soluble intracellular progesterone receptors (BAULIEU 1978; BELLE et al. 1975; IACOBELLI et al. 1974). The most convincing evidence for an action of progesterone at a receptor on the external face of the plasma membrane is the demonstration that an analog of progesterone, 3-oxo-4-androstene-17β-carboxylic acid, can induce oocyte maturation when coupled to a polymer of polyethylene oxide with a molecular weight of 20,000 daltons. Maturation is induced when oocytes are incubated in solutions of this material ($ED_{50} = 30\ \mu M$) but injection into the oocyte of 50 pmol is ineffective (GODEAU et al. 1978).

The agonist and antagonist specificity of the progesterone effect in amphibians is quite different from that of tissues from birds and mammals which are sensitive to progesterone. Testosterone, deoxycorticosterone, and cortisol are very active agonists. Estradiol and other esterene-steroids are antagonists (Baulieu et al. 1978).

A variety of drugs will also stimulate the initiation of mitosis. These include (+) propranolol (0.5–1 m*M*) at concentrations far above those necessary to antagonize the β-adrenergic receptor; local anaesthetics such as dibucaine, lidocaine, and tetracaine (all at 0.5–1 m*M*); drugs interacting with Ca^{2+} fluxes such as verapamil (0.5 m*M*); and lanthanum (5 m*M*). All of these drugs appear to disrupt various aspects of Ca^{2+} permeability. In addition, barbiturates can cause reinitiation of meiosis. The ability of chlorpromazine (0.5 m*M*) to cause maturation suggests that calmodulin might conceivably be involved in this process (Baulieu et al. 1978), although this concentration is quite high.

3. Involvement of Cyclic Nucleotides

A number of experiments indicate that cAMP regulates the events which lead to GVBD. The content of cAMP in the *Rana pipiens* oocyte decreases from 7.5 ± 0.9 pmol/mg dry weight to 2.0 ± 0.2 pmol/mg dry weight within 4–5 h after exposure to progesterone (3.2 μ*M*) and remains at this level during GVBD until completion of the first meiotic division (Morrill et al. 1977; Speaker and Butcher 1977). Maller et al. (1979) have made a careful study of the time course of change in intracellular cAMP in *Xenopus* oocytes. They found that the internal concentration of cAMP (1–3 μ*M*) drops 60% within 15 s after exposure to progesterone (30 μ*M*) and returns to approximately basal levels by 20 min after exposure.

Speaker and Butcher (1977) have made a careful and very interesting study of the fluctuations in both cAMP and cyclic GMP (cGMP) which occur in the progesterone-stimulated oocyte of *Rana pipiens*. The concentration of these nucleotides in the unstimulated oocytes in this study was approximately 0.6 μ*M* (cAMP) and 8 μ*M* (cGMP). Within 30 min of treatment with progesterone there is a 50% decrease in cAMP content (which can be inhibited by theophylline) and a 30% decrease in cGMP (which is not prevented by theophylline). The content of cAMP rises to its initial level at the time of nuclear breakdown, drops again, and rises preceeding metaphase II of meiosis. At metaphase II the level drops by 40%. There is a complex series of fluctuations in cGMP content. The observed results are in general agreement with the idea which has been proposed that cAMP and cGMP fluctuations may produce the molecular events which produce the cellular changes which occur as cells move through mitosis (McMahon 1974).

Phosphodiesterase inhibitors block GVBD. Theophylline (10^{-4} *M*), SQ 20,006 (10^{-5} *M*) and caffeine (10^{-3} *M*) all prevent the development of the oocyte into an egg (Morrill et al. 1977). Theophylline prevents the progesterone-induced decrease in cAMP in *Rana* (Morrill et al. 1977) and *Xenopus* (Bravo et al. 1978; Maller et al. 1979) oocytes. Theophylline is ineffective if used on oocytes incubated in Ca^{2+}-free solution (Morrill et al. 1977).

Bravo et al. (1978) have studied the effects of phosphodiesterase inhibitors on progesterone-induced maturation of *Xenopus* oocytes. These studies have produced the following conclusions: Theophylline (1 m*M*) and papaverine (0.1 m*M*) can completely prevent maturation. These concentrations inhibit the activity of cAMP phosphodiesterase by 50% in vivo. Theophylline prevents the progesterone-induced decrease in cAMP in these cells. Both theophylline and papaverine appear to inhibit protein synthesis in the oocyte and both are ineffective in preventing maturation if added more than 3 h after the induction of maturation. In addition, theophylline inhibition of maturation is suppressed by increasing the concentration of Ca^{2+} in the medium to 5 m*M* (note the contrast with the results of MORRILL et al. 1979) but the action of papaverine is unaffected. Finally, both compounds inhibit the progesterone-stimulated increase in ^{45}Ca uptake by the oocyte.

Elevation of intracellular cAMP content also blocks oocyte maturation. Dibutyryl cAMP (10^{-4} to 10^{-3} *M*) effectively blocks GVBD in *Rana* oocytes induced by progesterone. There is a 60% reduction in maturation even at a concentration of 10^{-6} *M*. Butyrate (1 m*M*), 5′-AMP (1 m*M*), and cAMP (1 m*M*) have no effect. However, BRAVO et al. (1978) have reported that cAMP (1 m*M*) delays GVBD in *Xenopus* oocytes by 2 h. Dibutyryl cAMP is effective if added at any time during the first 4–5 h after exposure to progesterone. The effect of dibutyryl cAMP is reversible for at least 24 h (MORRILL et al. 1977). Maturation of *Xenopus* oocytes is also prevented by the injection of 20 pmoles of 8-thio-methyl- or 8-thio-benzyl-cAMP. Injection of 8-thio-methyl-cAMP with MPF does not allow maturation (SCHORDERET-SLATKINE et al. 1978). Finally, pretreatment of oocytes with cholera toxin increases the cell's content of cAMP and inhibits maturation. Complete inhibition of progesterone-induced maturation occurs after treatment with 10^{-11} molar cholera toxin. Injection of the A subunit of cholera toxin also prevents the effects of progesterone with a half-maximal effective concentration of 1×10^{-7} *M*. The cellular concentration of cAMP is increased 2- to 3-fold by treatment with these concentrations of cholera toxin (MALLER et al. 1979; SCHORDERET-SLATKINE 1978; MULNER et al. 1979).

The decrease in concentration of intracellular cAMP which occurs when oocytes are treated with progesterone is probably due to a decline in its synthesis. When *Xenopus* oocytes were injected with [α-^{32}P] ATP and the content of newly synthesized cAMP was measured after 1 h, there was a 30–60% decrease in the amount of newly synthesized cAMP in the presence of progesterone (1 μ*M*). This result occurred whether or not the cells were incubated in the presence of the phosphodiesterase inhibitor, 3-isobutyl-1-methyl-xanthine. A steroid which does not induce maturation, estradiol-17*β* (10 μ*M*), did not produce this effect (MULNER et al. 1979). Similar experiments with much shorter periods of labeling have shown that the inhibition of synthesis of cAMP is transitory and occurs only for several minutes after treatment with progesterone (10 μg/ml) (BALTUS et al. 1981). Two groups of investigators have shown that the activity of cAMP phosphodiesterase measured in vivo or in vitro is not affected by treatment with progesterone (MULNER et al. 1980; BALTUS et al. 1981). The phosphodiesterase from the oocyte may not be activated by calmodulin since chelation of Ca^{2+} with EGTA (1–10 m*M*); addition of calmodulin (10^{-4} *M*) or fluphenazine (10^{-5} *M*) did not affect activity in vitro (MULNER et al. 1980).

The work of MALLER and KREBS (1977) sets a standard of excellence for other studies of the importance of cyclic nucleotides in development. They found that progesterone-induced maturation of *Xenopus* oocytes could be prevented by microinjection of the catalytic subunit of cAMP-activated protein kinase from rabbit skeletal muscle ($ED_{50} = 0.1$ μ*M*) within 1 h of exposure to progesterone. Maturation was induced in the absence of progesterone by injection of regulatory subunit from the type II kinase. Microinjection of the inhibitor of cAMP-stimulated protein kinase from rabbit muscle also induced maturation. Both regulatory subunits and inhibitor were shown to inhibit the activity of the endogenous protein kinase of the oocyte. They have also shown that the injection of calmodulin (10 μM) which had been pretreated with Ca^{2+} also induced maturation. Calmodulin was not, however, able to induce maturation in oocytes which had been previously injected with the catalytic subunit of protein kinase (Maller and Krebs 1977). These results indicate that continuing phosphorylation of a protein may be necessary to freeze the oocytes in prophase 1 of meiosis.

4. Involvement of Inorganic Ions

Calcium ion is also implicated in the events which lead to the maturation of the oocyte. This is indicated by three lines of evidence: the effects of drugs which interfere with Ca^{2+} fluxes or interactions with the membrane; the action of the ionophore, A 23187; and direct measurements of changes in intracellular Ca^{2+}.

Local anesthetics, an anorexiant (fenfluramine), phenothiazine neuroleptics, verapamil and methoxyverapamil (D 600) all blocked maturation effectively. In all cases tested, these compounds also prevented the synthesis of proteins associated with maturation. This was demonstrated by comparing the spectrum of proteins synthesized by treated and untreated oocytes using SDS polyacrylamide gel electrophoresis. Many of these drugs also caused the appearance of two mitotic spindles (Schorderet-Slatkine et al. 1977; Baulieu et al. 1978).

The same workers also used the insecticide, gammexane or lindane (γ-hexachlorocyclohexane), to interfere with maturation. This substance is presumed to interfere with the metabolism of phosphatidylinositol and thereby influence interaction of Ca^{2+} with the plasma membrane (Hokin and Brown 1969). These experiments yielded several interesting results. Gammexane (10^{-4} M) inhibits progesterone (1 μM)-induced maturation. It inhibits the synthesis of maturation-induced proteins. However, it does not prevent maturation if the oocytes are injected with MPF. In addition, MPF is able to induce the synthesis of maturation-induced proteins in oocytes incubated in gammexane, and MPF can induce its own synthesis through four serial transfers in gammexane-treated oocytes. Since MPF cannot induce its own synthesis in oocytes treated with cycloheximide, this suggests that gammexane does not interfere with protein synthesis in oocytes (Schorderet-Slatkine et al. 1977).

Maturation can be induced by divalent cations in the presence of the ionophore, A 23187 (2.5 μg/ml). When $CaCl_2$ or $MgCl_2$ were added to oocytes in medium containing A 23187, optimal GVBD was obtained at 10 mM Ca^{2+} or 40 mM Mg^{2+} (Wasserman and Masui 1975). Direct injection of Ca^{2+} or Mg^{2+} into the cytoplasm does not induce maturation (Merriam 1971) but continuous iontophoresis of Ca^{2+} into the oocyte cortical cytoplasm will trigger reinitiation of meiosis (Moreau et al. 1976).

The cytoplasmic Ca^{2+} increases in oocytes which have been stimulated to mature. Using the Ca^{2+}-sensitive photoproteins, aequorin and obelin, Moreau and co-workers showed that free Ca^{2+} began to increase two hours after treatment with progesterone and reached a maximum 2–3 h before GVBD (MOREAU et al. 1980). A Ca^{2+}-sensitive microelectrode detected an increase in Ca^{2+} after ten minutes. Ca^{2+} increased from 7×10^{-7} *M* to 7×10^{-6} *M*. A variety of other agents which are able to induce maturation, including the K^+ ionophore, valinomycin, also caused an increase in cytoplasmic Ca^{2+} (MOREAU et al. 1980).

In other studies it has been shown that a Ca^{2+}-controlled Cl^- current flows between the animal and vegetal hemispheres of the *Xenopus* oocyte. This current is reduced to zero as maturation occurs (ROBINSON 1979).

Potassium ion is an inhibitor of oocyte maturation. Ouabain, an inhibitor of Na^+-K^+-ATPase, increases the rate and extent of progesterone-induced maturation (VITTO and WALLACE 1976). Valinomycin, a K^+ ionophore, improves the amount of spontaneous maturation in K^+-free medium (BALTUS et al. 1977). Finally, K^+ (>0.25 m*M*) interferes with maturation induced by progesterone and a variety of artificial inducers of maturation (KOFOLD et al. 1979).

5. Maturation of Oocytes From Starfish and Mammals

Although different external stimuli may induce maturation of oocytes from other organisms, what is known of the internal events is remarkably similar to what is known of amphibian oocyte maturation. The maturation of the starfish is induced by 1-methyladenine (2×10^{-7} *M*) which is produced by the follicle cells of the ovary (HIRAI et al. 1973) and non-germinal cells of the testis (KUBOTA et al. 1977). The production of 1-methyladenine by the follicle cells appears to be under the negative control of steroid glycosides and to be stimulated by a neuropeptide (IKEGAMI et al. 1976).

Several lines of evidence suggest that Ca^{2+} is a second messenger in starfish oocyte maturation. MOREAU et al. (1978) demonstrated this in several ways. First, increase of the external Ca^{2+} from 0–10 to 25–300 m*M* induced maturation. Second, maturation was inhibited by compounds which interfere with Ca^{2+} metabolism including D 600 (0.4 m*M*), $LaCl_3$ (10 m*M*), $MnCl_2$ (10 m*M*) and procaine·HCl (2 m*M*). In addition, 1-methyladenine (2×10^{-7} *M*) or Ca^{2+} (75 m*M*) induced a tetraphasic increase of 0.5–1 μ*M* in intracellular Ca^{2+} over a period of about 20 s, as indicated by aequorin. Finally, injection of EGTA into the egg suppressed the Ca^{2+}-stimulated emission of light by aequorin and prevented maturation. In other-studies it has been shown that procaine (2 m*M*) inhibits binding of 1-methyladenine to the surface of the oocyte (CLOUD and SCHUETZ 1979); however the balance of evidence suggests a role for Ca^{2+}.

The evidence for a potential involvement of cAMP in the maturation of starfish oocytes is modest. Theophylline (5 m*M*) inhibits maturation induced by Ca^{2+} or 1-methyladenine (MOREAU et al. 1978). Intracellular injection of dibutyryl cAMP, however, allows meiosis to be triggered by subthreshold concentrations of hormone and increases the hormone-induced surge of intracellular Ca^{2+} (MOREAU and GUERRIER 1979). This may be the result of an ability of cAMP to sensitize the membrane to 1-methyladenine. Isolated plasma membranes were treated with dibutyryl cAMP (1 n*M*), cAMP (0.1 μ*M*) or 1-methyladenine (10 n*M*). All of these released bound Ca^{2+} from the membrane. 1-methyladenine was much more effective than cAMP. The greater effectiveness of dibutyryl cAMP than cAMP may indicate that it is acting at a site within the membrane. Other nucleotides, AMP, ATP, GTP,cGMP (all at 5 m*M*) did not release Ca^{2+}. Cyclic AMP and 1-methyladenine acted synergistically since each could sensitize the membrane to the other, resulting in a more effective release of Ca^{2+} (Moreau and Guerrier 1980).

It is possible that treatment of the membrane with cAMP stimulates a greater than normal release of membrane-bound Ca^{2+} as a result of a later treatment with 1-methyladenine. The reverse may also be true. This could provide an explanation for the results of Moreau and Guerrier (1979) described above. Cyclic AMP does appear to be an obligatory intermediate in the release of Ca^{2+} caused by 1-methyladenine since it has been reported that incubation of a membrane preparation with cAMP-phosphodiesterase does not prevent 1-methyladenine effects (Moreau and Guerrier 1980). It is possible that 1-methyladenine produces its effects by regulating methylation of membrane components.

Much less is known regarding the control of maturation of the mammalian oocyte. The oocyte will mature spontaneously if dislodged from the follicle. Incubation with A 23187 (10^{-5} *M*) activates rat oocytes (Tsafriri and Bar-Ami 1978). Microinjection of Ca^{2+} (or of ions with similar physiological effects such as Sr^{2+} or Ba^{2+}) induces maturation of mouse oocytes. Mg^{2+} has been reported to be without effect (Fulton and Whittingham 1978).

6. Summary

Investigation of the maturation of oocytes from a variety of organisms strongly suggests that Ca^{2+} is a second messenger for activation. In the amphibian oocyte, it appears the cAMP is a negative regulator of maturation. Furthermore, in the amphibian, it may be possible to postulate a sequence of molecular events as follows: Progesterone first binds to a plasma membrane receptor. Next, the concentration of cAMP drops, perhaps as the result of an increase in free Ca^{2+} in the cortex caused by a change in phosphatidyl inositol metabolism of the plasma membrane. The increases in cortical Ca^{2+} may inhibit adenylate cyclase via a calmodulin-Ca^{2+} complex. The concentration of free catalytic subunit of cAMP-activated protein kinase drops as a result of the decline in cAMP, decreasing the phosphorylation of a protein(s) which keeps the oocytes in arrest. This is followed by an increase in cAMP, and free cytoplasmic Ca^{2+}, which may trigger the synthesis of MPF and other maturation related proteins.

Of course many questions remain to be answered. One of the questions which is of particular interest is whether the fluctuations in content of cAMP, cGMP and Ca^{2+} which occur following initial activation are the cause or simply the result of the complex series of intercellular events which are necessary to carry the oocyte through meiosis to metaphase II.

II. Formation of Cartilage and Muscle in the Limb

1. Developmental Events

In the chick embryo, the limbs form from outgrowths from a lateral ridge of somatic mesoderm surrounded by ectoderm. A specialized region of ectoderm called the apical embryonic ridge is found at the distal end of the limb bud. The mesoderm of the limb differentiates into four types of cells: fibroblasts, osteoblasts, chondroblasts and myoblasts. The limb bud organizes as a morphogenetic field (Kühn 1971).

Mesodermal cells become committed to become chondroblasts or myoblasts between chick embryonic stages twenty and twenty-five (Zwilling 1968; Searls 1973; Ahrens et al. 1977). Some controversy exists regarding the exact time of commitment. After this time, even when removed to culture in vitro, the cells differentiate into either chondroblasts or myoblasts depending upon the region of the embryonic limb from which they were removed. Cells removed from the core of a wing bud of a stage 23–24 embryo are more likely to be chondrogenic than peripheral cells, which are more likely to be myogenic (Ahrens et al. 1979). The third of the wing bud (stage 25) closest to the body appears to contain more myogenic cells than the most distal third. Chondrogenic cells isolated from various sections of the wing exhibit different patterns of chondrogenesis in culture. Those from the proximal third coalesce into a large chondrogenic colony; cells from the distal third from many scattered cartilaginous nodules; the cells of the middle third produce an intermediate result (Paulsen et al. 1979).

On the basis of the teratogenic action of a number of compounds, including insulin and nicotinic acid and its analogs, it has been suggested that the embryonic mesodermal cells make a developmental choice on the basis of the intracellular levels of cyclic nucleotides. High intracellular cAMP (or a high ratio of cAMP/cGMP) has been proposed to direct a cell towards becoming a chondroblast. Low intracellular cAMP (or a low ratio of cAMP/cGMP) has been suggested to steer a cell into the myoblast lineage (McMahon 1974).

2. Chondrogenesis

Solursh and Reiter (1975) have shown that when stage 24 mesodermal cells are treated with dibutyryl cAMP plus theophylline, the differentiation of chondroblasts is stimulated. This study was originally intended to determine whether agents which inhibit cell division (such as dibutyryl cAMP plus theophylline) also stimulate chondrogenesis. However, among the mitotic inhibitors tested, only dibutyryl cAMP plus theophylline stimulated the formation of chondroblasts. Therefore, the effect of cAMP was relatively specific. By plating cells from limb buds of embryos of different ages, Ahrens and co-workers showed (Ahrens et al. 1977) that cells of stages 17–19 are unable to form chondrocytes when cultured in vitro; cultures of cells from stage 20 occasionally form cartilage; cells from stages 21–24 always form cartilage. During stage 20, a period of about twelve hours, cells acquire the ability to form cartilage. Treatment of stage 19 cells with dibutyryl cyclic AMP plus theophylline induces them to become chondroblasts (Ahrens et al. 1977).

Treatment of committed (stage 25) cells with dibutyryl cAMP or 8-hydroxy cAMP stimulates the expression of the chondrogenic phenotype. The accumulation of cartilage matrix and of sulfated glycosaminoglycan are stimulated in parallel with increasing concentrations (0.5–2 m*M*) of dibutyryl cAMP. Cyclic GMP and 5′AMP do not produce these effects. Table 1 presents a sequence of events which may occur in chondrogenesis (Kosher et al. 1979).

Table 1. Hypothetical sequence of cartilage differentiation. The numbers in parentheses are embryonic stages at which these properties seem to appear. (Modified from Solursh et al. 1979)

1. Tendency of cells to aggregate (17)
2. Acquisition of ability to differentiate into chondrocytes in response to cAMP (19–20)
3. Appearance of receptors which transduce cell interactions into increased concentrations of cAMP
4. Aggregation (22)
5. Elevation in intracellular cAMP
6. Chondrocyte determination (25)
7. Chondrogenesis

The expression of differentiation (as indicated by the incorporation of SO_4^{2-} into matrix proteoglycans) of fetal rat rib-cage chondrocytes has been reported to be promoted by derivatives of cAMP (Miller et al. 1979). In these experiments dibutyryl cAMP (0.05–0.5 m*M*) and 8-bromo-cAMP (0.25 m*M*) stimulated SO_4^{2-} incorporation and inhibited cell division.

Dibutyryl cAMP also stimulated production of extracellular matrix and increased cell size. Lebovitz et al. (1976) demonstrated that dibutyryl cAMP stimulated SO_4^{2-} incorporation into chick pelvic rudiments. Dibutyryl cAMP also stimulated the incorporation of glucosamine into proteoglycans (Miller et al. 1979). Equivalent concentrations of cAMP inhibited cell division but did not affect SO_4^{2-} incorporation. Sodium butyrate (0.1–0.5 m*M*) did not produce these effects. The stimulation of SO_4^{2-} incorporation was not due to inhibition of cell division since the latter but not the former effect was produced by hydroxyurea (0.5 m*M*). Finally, labeling with ^{3}H-thymidine suggested that dibutyryl cAMP exerted its effect in the G_1 phase of the cell cycle (Miller et al. 1979).

Intracellular concentrations of cAMP have been measured under various circumstances. Caplan (personal communication) has found that, in vitro, the density at which limb cells (stage 24) are plated affects the spectrum of differentiated cells which are produced. Low density cultures produce no chondrogenic cells whereas high density cultures produce a maximum of chondrogenic cells. When cAMP content of high and low density cultures are measured as a function of time after plating, high density cells have a higher content of cAMP which varies from 2.5 times greater (day 7) to 9 times greater (day 8). In another study, cells (stage 24) were shown to increase their content of cAMP from 6.3 to 9.7 pmol/mg protein while undergoing chondrogenesis in vitro. Non-chondrogenic cultures (stage 19) contained 4.5 pmol cAMP/mg protein. The content of cAMP in intact wing buds was 4.5 pmol/mg protein during the whole course of development from stages 19–25 (Solursh et al. 1979).

Measurements of the entire wing bud do not address the changes of cAMP content which may be occurring in populations of cells which are becoming committed to different fates. It would be useful to use fluorescent-labeled antibodies to cAMP to examine whether increases in cAMP content in some cells are being masked by decreases of cAMP content in others.

If intracellular cAMP is indeed the substance which regulates the decision to become a chondroblast, the question arises as to what external factor regulates its intracellular concentration. The experiments of CAPLAN, described above, suggest that cell-cell interactions may control the concentration of cAMP.

Cell-cell interactions do appear to be important in the decision to become a chondroblast. This is indicated by studies of the effects of cell density on chondrogenesis in vitro (KARASAWA et al. 1979) and by experiments which demonstrated that addition of cells, which are non-competent to become chondrogenic cells, to cultures of chondrogenic cells inhibits chondrogenic expression (SOLURSH and REITER 1980).

The embryonic notochord and spinal chord induce the formation of vertebral cartilage by somites. Somitic chondrogenesis can also occur when somites are cultured in vitro. Chondrogenesis is inhibited in this system by dibutyryl cAMP, 8-bromocyclic AMP and theophylline. Dibutyryl cGMP, 5′-AMP, and 2′,3′-AMP do not inhibit chondrogenesis, however. Cyclic AMP derivatives and theophylline also inhibit the formation of a chondrocyte product, sulfated glycosaminoglycan (KOSHER 1976). Type I collagen stimulates chondrogenesis in this system and also lowers intracellular cAMP in cells from somites incubated on it (KOSHER and SAVAGE 1979).

Thus, cAMP cannot be considered to be a specific messenger for chondrogenesis. A more appropriate way to regard cAMP, in this context, is as an analog of a decision "flag" in a computer program. The same place in a program may be reached by different routes, even when the result of a decision made on the basis of a specific "flag" differs. Similarly, as a result of its developmental history, a cell may be directed to differentiate into the same type of product cell as the result of a high concentration of intracellular cAMP, in one case, and a low concentration of cAMP in another. Continuing research will allow us to determine these decision "trees".

3. Myogenesis

a) Myotube Formation

The formation of the skeletal muscle in limbs results from a series of processes which are individually of great biological interest. First, mesodermal cells become committed to form myoblasts. These cells proliferate and then fuse to form multinucleate myotubes. Following fusion there is an up to several-hundred fold increase in the amounts of muscle specific proteins.

Although little is known regarding the molecular events which commit a mesodermal cell to become a myoblast, much is known about the events leading to myoblast fusion, particularly because of the work of ZALIN and her collaborators. A pulsatile 10–15 fold increase in intracellular cAMP concentration (lasting for 1 h) occurs about 5–6 h before cell fusion in vitro (ZALIN and MONTAGUE 1974). In vivo, two smaller pulses of increased cAMP occur in developing muscle (ZALIN and MONTAGUE 1975). It is not clear whether two pulses rather than one occur because fusion in vivo is not completely synchronous.

Cultures of myoblasts can be induced to fuse prematurely by treating them with prostaglandin E_1 (10^{-10} to 10^{-5} *M*) which induces a premature increase in intracellular cAMP (ZALIN and LEAVER 1975; ZALIN 1977). Acetylsalicyclic acid (3×10^{-4} *M*) or indomethacin (10^{-6} *M*) prevented fusion. However, when protaglandin E_1 was added, fusion occurred after five hours (Zalin 1977). Therefore, the effect of indomethacin does not appear to be due to its ability to inhibit cAMP-dependent protein kinase (Kantor and Hampton 1978).

The termination of the pulse of cyclic AMP may result from an increase in the rate of cAMP hydrolysis. When the L6 line of rat myoblasts is treated with dibutyryl cAMP (0.1–1 m*M)* one of its three cAMP phosphodiesterases is activated within minutes by a cAMP-dependent phosphorylation. The activity of another cAMP phosphodiesterase increases apparently as a result of de novo protein synthesis (Ball et al. 1980).

Zalin (1976) has shown that two inhibitors of nucleic acid function, 5-bromodeoxyuridine (3.2×10^{-5} *M*) and 5-fluorodeoxyuridine (2×10^{-6} *M*), inhibit the pulse of cAMP and subsequent cell fusion. The pulsatile increase of cAMP occurs in the presence of EGTA (2×10^{-3} *M*) but cell fusion does not occur. If Ca^{2+} (concentration not presented) is added to these cultures, fusion occurs after 2–3 h. This suggests that cAMP has initiated a process which leads to fusion, but which requires Ca^{2+} at about its midpoint.

Both fusion and increase in myotube enzyme activities appear to depend on Ca^{2+} (Schudt et al. 1975). The increase in activity of creatine phosphokinase (CPK) which occurs after fusion does not appear to depend on the pulse of cAMP since CPK activity increases in cultures treated with 5-fluorodeoxyuridine (Zalin 1976). Experiments using added EGTA or Ca^{2+} to vary the Ca^{2+} content of the growth medium indicate that cell fusion and CPK synthesis are separately controlled by Ca^{2+} (Morris et al. 1976).

By using ^{3}H-thymidine to label cells in S phase, and examining the time course of appearance of labeled nuclei in myotubes, Zalin showed that cells are responsive to PGE_1 only during part of the G_1 phase of the cell cycle (Zalin 1979). This suggested that cells in G_1 make a decision on the basis of internal cAMP concentration whether to choose the cellular subprogram which leads to mitosis or the subprogram which leads to fusion and additional differentiation.

A controversy exists regarding the relationship between adenylate cyclase activity and fusion. The activity of this enzyme has been reported to decrease in rat myoblasts at the time of fusion (Wahrmann et al. 1973) and to increase in chick myoblasts at fusion (Zalin and Montague 1974). The intracellular concentration of cAMP rises at about the time of and after myoblast fusion. The level of cGMP drops near the time of fusion so that the ratio cAMP/cGMP increases by a factor of three and remains stable after fusion (Moriyama et al. 1976).

Analogous results have been obtained using a neurotrophic factor (apparent molecular weight, $4–5 \times 10^5$ daltons) to stimulate fusion prematurely (Festoff and Oh 1977). Although samples were not taken as frequently as in the studies of Zalin et al., the factor caused a premature increase in cellular cAMP and premature fusion. A transient (1 h) initial increase in cGMP occurred in the cultures treated with neurotrophic factor but quickly declined. The ratio, cAMP/cGMP, climbed above one more rapidly in treated than in untreated cultures and varied between three and six in the period immediately following fusion (Festoff and Oh 1977). An analogous increase in cAMP was found in the L6 line of secondary rat myoblasts. Dexamethasone (5 μg/ml) and insulin (5 μg/ml) stimulated these myoblasts to fuse prematurely and caused a premature and extended increase in cellular cAMP (Ball and Sanwal 1980).

The plasma membrane of myoblasts must change in some way which allows cells to fuse and form myotubes. L6 rat embryonic myoblast and myotube membranes contain a protein kinase which can be activated by as little as 5×10^{-7} M cAMP and which can phosphorylate histone f2b. The activity of this enzyme, using histone as a substrate, is approximately two fold greater in myoblasts then myotubes. A protein phosphatase in the plasma membrane is equally active in each cell type. Although no stimulation of the phosphorylation of endogenous membrane substrates by cAMP occurs in myotube membranes, a four-fold stimulation occurs in the membranes of myoblasts. In particular, the phosphorylation of a polypeptide with a molecular weight of 100 kilodaltons is stimulated by cAMP in myoblasts but not in myotubes (SCOTT and DOUSA 1980). It is not clear whether the change in activity of the enzyme toward endogenous substrates reflects a change in specificity of the enzyme, a change in substrates, or the possibility that endogenous membrane proteins are already fully phosphorylated. Nevertheless, these observations provide an attractive way in which the pulse of cAMP, observed by ZALIN et al. in myoblasts, could be transduced into a developmentally significant cellular change.

b) Phenotypic Transformation of Myoblasts

SCHUBERT and LACOBIERE (1976), in a very interesting paper, have examined the effect of incubation in medium containing cAMP on the phenotypic expression of cultured L6 rat myoblasts. The results which they obtained are summarized in Table 2. This table also summarizes the effects of nicotinamide analog, 6-aminonicotinamide, on the myoblasts. Chronic treatment with dibutyryl cAMP (1 mM) can cause myoblasts to assume many of the phenotypic properties of chondroblasts. This change is partially reversible. Treatment with 6-aminonicotinamide (1 mM) "converts" the myoblasts into "chondroblasts" more effectively. They do not appear to be able to revert to myoblasts.

The effects of 6-aminonicotinamide are interesting because of previous experiments which have demonstrated the teratogenic effects of nicotinamide analogs on the differentiation of skeletal muscle in vivo (LANDAUER and CLARK 1957) and in vitro (CAPLAN 1972a, b; ROSENBERG and CAPLAN 1974). CAPLAN, in particular, has advocated the hypothesis that the cellular level of NAD is an important determinant in the commitment to differentiation of mesodermal cells. Experiments such as the ones described above suggest that cAMP and NAD could both be involved in the process of commitment. A. I. CAPLAN (personal communication) has suggested that cAMP may regulate the accumulation of polyadenosinediphosphoribose (whose precursor in NAD) in the nucleus and that this may regulate gene expression. This idea will be expanded below. Interactions of metabolites and differentiation are discussed in more detail elsewhere (MCMAHON and WEST 1976).

4. Transformation by Sarcoma Viruses

Investigations of the biochemical basis of cellular transformation by avian sarcoma viruses is providing information which is very interesting to developmental biologists. When chondroblasts (PACIFICI et al. 1977) or myoblasts (FISZMAN 1978)

Table 2. Effects of 6-aminonicotinamide (6-AN) and dibutyryl cAMP (dBcAMP) on phenotypes of myoblasts summarized from Schubert and Lacorbiere (1976). The meaning of the symbol is +, an effect; −, no effect; and ±, partial effect

Property of cell treated with:	6-AN	dBcAMP
Cells become flatter and more angular	+	+
Decrease in viability	−	−
Able to fuse after 2 days exposure	−	±
Increase in secreted collagen	+	+
Increase in proline hydroxylation	+	−
Collagen exclusively α_1 chains	+	−
Increase in glycosaminoglycan synthesis	+	+
Increase in sulfation of glycosaminoglycans	+	±
Increase in chondroxtin − SO_4	+	+
Reduce NAD concentration	+	−
Increase cAMP concentration	−	+

are infected with Rous sarcoma virus (RSV), their normal program of differentiation is interrupted. Temperature-sensitive mutants of RSV which are conditionally defective in the src gene product block differentiation at a temperature which allows the src gene product to function but allow differentiation to proceed at temperatures which prevent the src product from functioning.

The src product has been identified as a protein kinase which phosphorylates tyrosine. A homologous protein kinase is the sarc (proto-src) gene in untransformed cells. Although neither kinase is dependent on cAMP both are phosphorylated by cAMP-dependent protein kinase. This may modify their activity (see Erikson et al. 1980, for review).

In this light it is interesting that dibutyryl cAMP (1 m*M*) enhances the differentiation, as indicated by cell fusion and appearance of CPK activity, of chick myoblasts which have been transformed by a murine sarcoma virus. There is no effect of 5′-AMP on these processes. The stimulatory effect of dibutyryl cAMP is most pronounced when the Ca^{2+} content of the medium is greater than 1 m*M* (Aw et al. 1973).

The src protein kinase is an integral membrane protein which is generally associated with the cytoplasmic face of the plasma membrane (Courtneidge et al. 1980) but is also a component of the nuclear membrane in at least one line transformed cells (Krueger et al. 1980). Its localization at areas of cell contact (Courtneidge et al. 1980; Krueger et al. 1980) suggests that it could play a role in cellular interaction.

5. Summary

The experimental evidence to date suggests that an increase in cellular cAMP, perhaps mediated by cell contact, triggers the determination of mesodermal cells into chondroblasts. High levels of intracellular cAMP may act to maintain the expression of macromolecules specific to chondrocytes. In the absence of high intracellular cAMP, cells may become determined as myoblasts. After this, however, the proliferating myoblasts make a decision to proliferate or to fuse into myotubes on the basis of cAMP concentrations during part of the G_1 phase of the cell cycle.

III. Pattern Formation in Dictyostelium Discoideum

1. Developmental Events

a) Pseudoplasmodial Development

The social soil amoeba, *Dictyostelium discoideum*, has become a model organism for developmental biologists. The initial stages in the development of this organism and the fundamental role which cAMP plays during aggregation in these are discussed in the chapter by VAN DRIEL. In this section, I will focus on the process of pattern formation which occurs during the pseudoplasmodium stage of development in this organism. Much of the developmental biology of *D. discoideum* has been reviewed elsewhere (BONNER 1967; LOOMIS 1975).

The pseudoplasmodium, which forms from the aggregated cells, is an integrated organism with emergent properties. The pseudoplasmodium (which may be up to 1 mm in length and composed of 10^5 cells) begins to form from the aggregate about twelve hours after the amoebae are starved under standard conditions. A theory has been proposed (CLARK and STECK 1979) which suggests propagation of waves of cAMP in circular loops of cells helps organize the pseudoplasmodium. Depending upon environmental conditions, the pseudoplasmodium may migrate for long periods or may culminate in 6–8 h and form a sorocarp, composed of a basal disk and a tapering stalk topped by a ball of spores (BONNER 1967; SUSSMAN and BRACKENBURY 1976; LOOMIS 1975). Ammonia is the messenger which regulates migration. When environmental NH_3 is high, the pseudoplasmodium will continue to migrate; when NH_3 is lowered, culmination will begin (SCHINDLER and SUSSMAN 1977b). Reciprocal grafting experiments between pseudoplasmodia composed of normal or mutant (NP 84) cells indicate that the tip controls the decision to migrate or to culminate (SMITH and WILLIAMS 1980).

Progress in development past the aggregate depends on RNA and protein synthesis. Actinomycin D and cycloheximide inhibit formation of the pseudoplasmodium and the sorocarp when the aggregate is treated with them (MIZUKAMI and IWABUCHI 1970).

Substantial changes in RNA and protein synthesis occur with formation of the pseudoplasmodium. These include the appearance of developmentally important enzymes, events which depend on normal development, since they can be prevented by inhibitors or by mutations which disrupt development (SUSSMAN and BRACKENBURY 1976; LOOMIS et al. 1978). The synthesis of approximately 400 major proteins can be detected by two-dimensional polyacrylamide gel electrophoresis in the vegetative amoeba. About 40 new proteins appear at late aggregation just prior to appearance of the pseudoplasmodium and synthesis of 10 is reduced considerably. In addition, two proteins are synthesized at much greater rate and two at a slower rate in the pseudoplasmodium. The changes in synthesis of proteins appear to result from changes in the amount of mRNA for these proteins (ALTON and LODISH 1977a).

The appearance of multicellularity appears to be the trigger for a major change in the expression of genes. Measurements of polyadenylated mRNA in the cytoplasm or on polysomes led to this conclusion. The number of poly A mRNAs in the cytoplasm of the vegetative amoeba has been estimated at 3,000–3,700 (Jacquet et al. 1981) or 5,000 (Blumberg and Lodish 1980a). At the time of organization of the pseudoplasmodium, Blumberg and Lodish (1980b) have estimated that mRNAs from approximately 3,000 previously unexpressed genes appear. Jacquet et al. (1981) have estimated that 700–900 new mRNAs appear in the pseudoplasmodium. Although the studies differ quantitatively, both reach the conclusion that a major change in gene expression occurs at the time of organization of the pseudoplasmodium. The appearance of these new mRNAs appears to result from the transcription of new genes since precursors for these RNAs were not detected in the nucleus of vegetative cells (Blumberg and Lodish 1981). Cyclic AMP (1 m*M*) can prematurely suppress the synthesis of mRNA for discoidin in vivo and in vitro and cause the premature appearance of other mRNAs (Williams et al. 1980).

b) Pattern Formation

In the pseudoplasmodium, cells determine their relative position and use that information to determine the course of their differentiation. The proportion of stalk to spore cells produced by pseudoplasmodia of different sizes is not absolutely invariant. The careful measurements of Stenhouse and Williams (1977) have shown that larger pseudoplasmodia produce proportionally more stalk cells.

A number of elegant experiments have demonstrated that cells can determine their position. One by Raper (1940) used reciprocal grafts of colored and uncolored pseudoplasmodia. If a tip from a red pseudoplasmodium was grafted to a white back, the stalk of the sorocarp was red and the spores and basal disk were white. The complementary graft gave a complementary result. In addition, Raper showed that if the front of a pseudoplasmodium was removed and forced to complete development the resulting sorocarp had an unusually high proportion of stalk. If allowed time to regulate before being forced to complete development, the sorocarp was normally proportioned. Sampson (1976) extended this work in several ways. He showed, in addition, that when rear quarters of the pseudoplasmodium were forced to differentiate, the sorocarps had disproportionately large spore heads. This result became more pronounced with increasing age of the pseudoplasmodia. Sampson's work revealed another important aspect of this process since he showed that the results of these experiments were maintained even if cells from the sections were disaggregated and therefore had to reform the multicellular pseudoplasmodium before completing development. These experiments clearly indicate that the pre-pattern of the sorocarp appears in the pseudoplasmodium.

Amoebae apparently differ in some way which prejudices them to assume different positions in the pseudoplasmodium (Takeuchi 1969; Bonner et al. 1971). Experiments such as those described above indicate that sorting of cells predisposed to become stalk or spore cells cannot be the primary determinant of pattern formation. However, it is interesting that amoebae which are predisposed to assume an anterior position in the pseudoplasmodium contain twice as much Ca^{2+}, ten times more cAMP, and are much more sensitive to cAMP than cells which assume a posterior position (MAEDA and MAEDA 1974).

The pre-pattern in the pseudoplasmodium has also been demonstrated in a convincing number of other distinct ways. Vital dyes, such as neutral red, stain the anterior zone more than the posterior (BONNER 1952). Staining sections of the pseudoplasmodium for non-starch polysaccharides with the periodic acid-Schiff's stain, stains the prespore region more intensely (BONNER et al. 1955) as does a FITC-antiserum raised against an antigen found in the spore (IKEDA and TAKEUCHI 1971).

Proteins and enzymes are also localized at this stage. ALTON and BRENNER (1979) labeled the pseudoplasmodium with ^{35}S-methionine and microdissected pseudoplasmodia into five pieces, after which the newly synthesized proteins were resolved by two-dimensional polyacrylamide gel electrophoresis. Six proteins were found exclusively in the anterior tip and 13 only in the posterior sections. Eighteen proteins were labeled more heavily in the tip and 12 were labeled more heavily in the back. Ten proteins showed a gradient of increasing or decreasing synthesis through the pseudoplasmodium. One protein appeared to be synthesized predominantly at the border between pre-stalk and pre-spore cells.

Enzymes and metabolites have also been localized in the pseudoplasmodium. Prestalk cells contain more 5′-nucleotidase and alkaline phosphatase (these are probably two different activities of the same enzyme) and more cytochrome oxidase (KRIVANEK and KRIVANEK 1958), glucose, trehalose, NH_4^+, trehalase and glycogen phosphorylase (RUTHERFORD and HARRIS 1976; WILSON and RUTHERFORD 1978; JEFFERSON and RUTHERFORD 1976), β-glucosidase and an isozyme of β-galactosidase (OOHATA and TAKEUCHI 1977) than pre-spore cells. Pre-spore cells contain more UDP galactose:polysaccharide transferase (NEWELL et al. 1969), UDP glucose pyrophosphorylase, malate dehydrogenase and citrate synthetase (MILLER et al. 1969; OOHATA and TAKEUCHI 1977) than prestalk cells.

Biological experiments demonstrated that cells apparently develop some differences on their surface at this time. This is indicated by a series of experiments begun by BONNER (1952) who grafted vitally stained cells from the anterior of a pseudoplasmodium into the rear and found that the anterior cells moved to the front of the pseudoplasmodium as it migrated. These experiments have been confirmed by YAMAMOTO (1977). In addition, if cells isolated from the rear and front are disaggregated and mixed (after one of the groups has been labeled with ^{3}H-thymidine), they sort out during pseudoplasmodium formation with a tendency to occupy their original locations (TAKEUCHI 1969). TASAKA and TAKEUCHI (1979) have shown that this sorting will also occur in spherical aggregates maintained in solution.

The difference in cell surface composition which the biological experiments suggest is circumstantially supported by other observations. GREGG and KARP (1978) demonstrated that the incorporation of ^{3}H-fucose into macromolecules is confined to the pre-spore cells with a sharp discontinuity separating them from the pre-stalk cells. This could reflect differences in synthesis of surface glycoconjugates although other explanations are possible.

It is possible to directly demonstrate position-dependent differences in the cell surface. Substantial changes in the macromolecular composition of the plasma membrane occur during development. These are most pronounced in its glycoprotein content (Hoffman and McMahon 1977; West and McMahon 1977, 1979; West et al. 1978). These changes depend on normal development since a variety of treatments which interfere with development prevent most of the changes (Hoffman and McMahon 1978). Using the fluorescent-lectin diffusion method, it was possible to show that the display of glycoconjugates on the surface of pre-stalk and pre-spore cells is different. There are a number of quantitative differences in the display of Concanavalin A receptors between the two areas. Two receptors for wheat germ agglutinin are confined to the surface of pre-stalk cells while three others are found largely on pre-spore cells. Finally, a pseudoplasmodium-specific plasma membrane antigen is confined to the pre-stalk area (West and McMahon 1979). The difference in this antigen and in the wheat-germ agglutinin receptors may be important for normal morphogenesis since treatment of dissociated pseudoplasmodial cells with the specific antibody or with wheat germ agglutinin inhibits normal morphogenesis (West and McMahon 1981).

Cells from the pre-stalk and pre-spore regions have morphological differences. Pre-stalk cells are in closer contact and have thinner plasma membranes. In addition, their nucleoli differ in morphology and the cells contain more abundant endoplasmic reticulum (Maeda and Takeuchi 1969). More distinctively, the pre-spore cells contain a vesicle, 0.6 μM in diameter (Maeda and Takeuchi 1969; Ikeda and Takeuchi 1971) whose contents are presumably emptied by exocytosis to form the coat of the spore (Maeda 1971). These pre-spore vesicles appear at late aggregation as the pseudoplasmodium is being formed (Müller and Hohl 1973; Hayashi and Takeuchi 1976; Forman and Garrod 1977a). The pre-stalk area, free of pre-spore vesicles, enlarges as the pseudoplasmodium ages (Müller and Hohl 1973) and is greater in a mutant, P4, which produces an abnormally large stalk (Forman and Garrod 1977a).

The polarity of the pseudoplasmodium might arise from an underlying cellular polarity. Individual cells in aggregates contain more 60 Å microfilaments at their anterior edge and the morphology of the plasma membrane differs between the anterior and posterior edges of the cell (Maeda and Eguchi 1977).

Pattern formation can take place in the absence of overt morphological polarization. Spherical aggregates can be incubated in liquid, and cellular differentiation will occur after 2–3 days. Stalk and spore cells are partitioned into separate regions of the resulting spherical or ellipsoid clump of cells (Sternfeld and Bonner 1977; Takeuchi et al. 1977; Garrod and Forman 1977). The process of differentiation can be accelerated by pulsing the aggregates with cAMP (Forman and Garrod 1977b). Added Ca^{2+} ($>27\ \mu M$) inhibits this process while $NH^{+}+NH_3$ ($>4\ mM$) and another factor in conditioned medium promote differentiation (Sternfeld and David 1979). Some dispute exists regarding the origin or the pattern of spores and stalk cells. This has been suggested to arise by sorting out (Garrod and Forman 1977), but the predominant evidence suggests it arises by differentiation in situ (Takeuchi et al. 1977; Sternfeld and Bonner 1977).

The experiments of Raper (1940) and Sampson (1976), described above, indicate that, in common with other morphogenetic fields, the pattern of the pseudoplasmodium can be regulated. Gregg (1965) demonstrated this process on a cellular level with fluorescent antiserum to the pre-spore antigen. More recently, Gregg and Karp (1978) have shown that within minutes of transection of a pseudoplasmodium regulation begins. They showed that incorporation of ^{3}H-fucose, a characteristic of pre-spore cells, begins to occur at the rear edge of a pre-stalk section and ceases at the leading edge of a pre-spore section.

2. Involvement of Cyclic Nucleotides and Inorganic Ions

a) In vivo

Intracellular cAMP appears to be higher in the pre-stalk than in the pre-spore area of the pseudoplasmodium. The tip of the pseudoplasmodium secretes cAMP as indicated by its ability to secrete a phosphodiesterase-sensitive substance which attracts aggregating amoebae (RUBIN 1976; MAEDA 1977). GARROD and MALKINSON (1963) showed that the tip contains about twice as much cAMP/μg DNA as was measured with the whole pseudoplasmodium (GARROD and MALKINSON 1973). BRENNER (1977) estimated the normalized amount of cAMP in the tip was 40–70% higher in the tip than in the posterior portions. PAN et al. (1974) used antiserum to cAMP which had been conjugated to fluorescin isothiocyanate to stain sections of pseudoplasmodia. They found that the early pseudoplasmodium stained uniformly but that as the pseudoplasmodium approached culmination, staining could be found only in the anterior pre-stalk section which was separated by a sharp discontinuity from the posterior pre-spore region.

Calcium ion is localized in the pre-stalk region. This has been demonstrated autoradiographically after labeling pseudoplasmodia with ^{45}Ca (MAEDA and MAEDA 1973).

b) In vitro

A number of experiments indicate that cAMP is a messenger for stalk cell differentiation. BONNER (1970) showed that cAMP (1 m*M*) induced isolated amoebae to differentiate into stalk cells. Particles of Sephadex impregnated with cAMP and inserted into pseudoplasmodia were found to induce stalk cell differentiation in 71% of the implants and spore differentiation in 30%. Control particles, infiltrated with water or 5′-AMP did not induce cell differentiation (FEIT et al. 1978).

The mutant, P4 of *D. discoideum*, produces a great excess of stalk cells. This mutant which is apparently partially deficient in cell bound cAMP-phosphodiesterase is exceptionally sensitive to cAMP-mediated induction of stalk cell differentiation (CHIA 1975).

Several workers have examined the effects of added cAMP on the differentiation of pseudoplasmodia or cells derived from them. Pseudoplasmodia exposed to cAMP (3 m*M*) produce sorocarps with accentuated stalks and few or no spores (NESTLE and SUSSMAN 1972). When pseudoplasmodia are exposed to 0.1–1 m*M* cAMP, the cells composing them leave in streams which are composed of amoebae some of which differentiate into stalk cells. Higher concentrations of cAMP disorganize the structure of the sorocarp (GEORGE 1977). If cells from the tip are treated with cAMP at concentrations of 1 m*M* (TOWN and STANFDORD 1977) or 10 m*M* (GEORGE 1977) they differentiate into stalk cells. Pre-spore cells from the rear degenerate when exposed to 10 m*M* cAMP (GEORGE 1977). Exposure to 1 m*M* cAMP can cause cells from the rear of young pseudoplasmodia to differentiate into stalk cells but these cells lose this ability when isolated from older pseudoplasmodia

(Town and Stanford 1977). Town and Stanford (1977) also showed that cells from the anterior could secrete a substance (presumably cAMP) which induced cells separated from them by cellophane to differentiate into stalk cells.

Added cAMP alters the normal pattern of developmental changes in enzyme activity. Hamilton and Chia (1975) examined the effects of cAMP (0.1 m*M*) on the synthesis of developmentally-regulated enzymes in this mutant. This treatment allows the pattern of enzyme synthesis by cells developing into "stalky" sorocarps with spores to be compared with that of cells developing into stalk cells alone. They demonstrated that cAMP-treatment increased the amount of activity produced for N-acetylglucosaminidase and alkaline phosphatase. The amount of activity of several other enzymes was reduced. These included β-glucosidase, α-mannosidase, and threonine dehydrase. Cyclic AMP strikingly reduced the activity of UDP-glucose pyrophosphorylase, UDP-galactose-4-epimerase, and trehalose-6-phosphate synthetase. As Hamilton and Chia (1975) have discussed, cAMP seems to stimulate the increase in activity of stalk cell-associated enzymes and inhibit the increase of those associated with spores. Nestle and Sussman (1972) showed that cAMP (3 m*M*) prevented developmental increases in UDP-galactose epimerase and UDP-glucose pyrophosphorylase in migrating pseudoplasmodia induced to culminate. The same concentration of cAMP added to culminating pseudoplasmodia also disrupted the developmental changes in activity of these enzymes which normally occur.

The induction of stalk cell differentiation might be the result of the continuation of some process initiated at aggregation by cAMP and continuously maintained by cAMP, or it might result from the ability of cAMP to act as a signal at an independent developmental switch. Experiments with the related species of slime mold, *Polysphondylium pallidum*, provide information on this question. *P. pallidum* produces cAMP but the nucleotide is not the chemoattractant for aggregation (Konijn et al. 1969). Hohl et al. (1977) in a thorough study have shown that cAMP (1 m*M*) can induce isolated amoebae to differentiate into stalk cells, stimulate the differentiation of stalk cells in pseudoplasmodia, and apparently convert pre-spore cells into stalk cells. A mutant of *P. pallidum*, PN 507, which produces abnormally low amounts of cAMP, produces stalks composed of undifferentiated amoebae and stalk cells. Addition of cAMP (5 m*M*) to the medium induces normal stalk cell differentiation (Francis et al. 1978).

Ammonia inhibits differentiation of *D. discoideum* and causes cellular cAMP levels to decrease (Schindler and Sussman 1977a). It has been proposed that endogenous production of NH_3 regulates the accumulation of cellular cAMP and thereby regulates cellular differentiation (Sussman and Schindler 1978; Schindler and Sussman 1979).

Maeda (1970) showed that added inorganic ions also can regulate the direction of cell differentiation. Ca^{2+} (100–200 m*M*) promotes stalk cell and inhibits spore differentiation. Li^+ (7 m*M*) produces the same effect in the presence of lower concentrations of Ca^{2+} (3 m*M*). Spore formation is stimulated by KF (15 m*M*). Although Maeda ascribes the effect of KF to the F^- ion, it may be possible that K^+ is also involved in this process, since K^+ (20 m*M*) inhibits the disappearance of pre-spore vesicles from pseudoplasmodia. This effect of K^+ is antagonized by Na^+ (Takeuchi et al. 1977).

3. Cyclic AMP-Associated Proteins in Multicellular Stages

a) Adenylate Cyclase

The adenylate cyclase in *D. discoideum* is apparently located on the inner face of the plasma membrane (FARNHAM 1975; ROSSOMANDO and CUTLER 1975; CUTLER and ROSSOMANDO 1975). The activity of the enzyme reaches a maximum at the time of aggregation and declines at a linear rate by 75% as development continues to the culmination of the sorocarp (PAHLIC and RUTHERFORD 1979). The activity of this enzyme is much higher in the developing spores than in the stalk cells of the culminating sorocarp (C. L. RUTHERFORD, personal communication).

b) cAMP-Phosphodiesterase

The membrane-bound phosphodiesterase of *D. discoideum* is a glycoprotein (CREAN and ROSSOMANDO 1977) which is located on the external face of the plasma membrane (FARNHAM 1975). The activity of the enzyme decreases from 20–40 µmol/h/gm (dry weight) to 5–10 µmol/gm in pseudoplasmodia (BROWN and RUTHERFORD 1980).

The activity of the enzyme varies with location in the pseudoplasmodium. The extreme posterior tip has the highest activity of the enzyme (16 µmol/g/h). The activity decreases at more anterior positions in the pseudoplasmodium reaching a plateau in the pre-stalk region of early pseudoplasmodia (6 µmol/h/g). The pattern of enzyme distribution in the later pseudoplasmodium is similar. The activity of the posterior tip is even greater (40 µmol/h/g) declining to 4 µmol/h/g at the border between pre-spore and pre-stalk cells. It rises to a plateau (10 µmol/h/g) in the pre-stalk region. This pattern reverses at culmination increasing greatly in the stalk cells and declining in the spores (BROWN and RUTHERFORD 1980). Although phosphodiesterase can be induced by cAMP (HAYASHI and YAMASAKI 1978), the pattern of enzyme distribution cannot be simply explained by reference to intracellular levels of cAMP.

A mutant of *D. purpureum* which forms stalks without spores has a generally similar pattern of phosphodiesterase distribution and developmental changes in activity when compared to wild type (YANAGISAWA et al. 1974).

c) cAMP-Binding Proteins

Considering the amount of work which has been devoted to understanding cAMP metabolism and function in *D. discoideum*, it is surprising that so little is known regarding possible effectors of cAMP's action in the pseudoplasmodium. TOWN (1976) suggested that there was little difference in the number of extracellular cAMP receptors between aggregating cells and cells from pre-culminating pseudoplasmodia. This conclusion has been contradicted by the work of HENDERSON (1975) who showed that specific cAMP binding to cells declined by 5- to 10-fold from early aggregation to the pseudoplasmodium stage. JULIANI and KLEIN (1981) have shown a similar decline in cAMP-binding from 0.25 pmol/4 $\times 10^6$ cells at early aggregation to 0.05 pmol/4 $\times 10^6$ cells in the pseudoplasmodium. They have also identified a polypeptide with a molecular weight of 45 kilodaltons which appears to be the cAMP receptor on the membrane of aggregating cells. This molecule is apparently absent on the cells of the pseudoplasmodium.

Garrod and Malkinson (1973) did not detect a difference in the amount of cAMP-binding protein found in cells from the back or the front of the pseudoplasmodium.

d) Calmodulin

A calmodulin-like protein has been purified from *D. discoideum*. This protein can fully activate brain cyclic nucleotide phosphodiesterase, although it is 2.5 × less active than brain calmodulin. It does not activate the extracellular phosphodiesterase from *D. discoideum* (Clarke et al. 1980). Calmodulin may play roles in growth and development of *D. discoideum* since the major tranquilizers inhibit its growth and development (Blomquist, C. and D. McMahon, unpublished work).

4. Cyclic AMP and Cell Contact

a) Substitution of cAMP for Cell Contact

Disaggregation of a pseudoplasmodium into individual cells stops and reverses overt cellular differentiation. The pre-spore vacuoles disappear from pre-spore cells within five hours of disaggregation. This can be prevented by cycloheximide (50 μg/ml), actinomycin D (125 μg/ml) or cAMP (1 m*M*) (Takeuchi and Sakai 1971), and by $(NH_4)_2SO_4$ (110 m*M*) and concanavalin A (150 μg/ml) (Takeuchi et al. 1978). Accumulation of several developmentally-regulated enzymes, UDP-glucose pyrophosphorylase, trehalose-6-phosphate synthetase, UDP-galactose epimerase and UDP-galactose:polysaccharide transferase, is inhibited by disaggregation. Upon reaggregation, a burst of new enzyme synthesis occurs. This new enzyme activity depends on RNA synthesis (Newell et al. 1972). This phenomenon is discussed in more detail elsewhere (Sussman and Newell 1972). After disaggregation, UDP-galactose polysaccharide transferase disappears with exponential kinetics ($t_{1/2}$ = 60–80 min). Cycloheximide (250 μg/ml) is only partially effective in preventing this decay (Okamoto and Takeuchi 1976). Disaggregation causes an increase in cAMP-phosphodiesterase activity, both extracellular and membrane-bound enzyme increase. The increase can be prevented by cycloheximide (250 μg/ml), emetine (2.5 m*M*), actinomycin D (125 μg/ml) and daunomycin (150 μg/ml). Therefore, the increase in activity requires protein and RNA synthesis. The protein inhibitor of cAMP phosphodiesterase is also produced after disaggregation (Okamoto 1979). The increase in activity is also inhibited by $(NH_4)_2SO_4$ (110 m*M*) and concanavalin A (150 μg/ml) (Takeuchi et al. 1978). Resolution of newly synthesized proteins by two-dimensional polyacrylamide gel electrophoresis indicates that the synthesis of many proteins which are associated with the time of pseudoplasmodium formation is shut off by disaggregation while the synthesis of some proteins characteristic of an earlier stage is reinitiated (Alton and Lodish 1977b).

Disruption of cell contact also alters RNA metabolism. Labeling of newly synthesized RNA with ^{3}H-uridine in pseudoplasmodia indicates that approximately 25–30% of the label is incorporated into poly(A)-containing RNA, whereas 45–50% of the label goes into poly(A)-containing RNA in dissociated cells and approximately 90% is found in poly(A)-containing RNA in pseudoplasmodia which have reformed from dissociated cells. Ribosomal RNA synthesis is depressed in disaggregated cells (Uchiyama et al. 1979). Since the changes in protein synthesis at the time of pseudoplasmodium formation seem to reflect changes in mRNA production, the results of UCHIYAMA et al. (1979) may reflect the substantial transcriptional changes which are occurring resulting in new mRNA production.

If normal cellular interactions are interfered with by replating dissociated pseudoplasmodial cells with purified pseudoplasmodial cell plasma membranes, cells reaggregate but cannot form pseudoplasmodia. Under these conditions, alkaline phosphatase is superinduced whereas the increase in activity of UDP-glucose pyrophosphorylase and glycogen phosphorylase are prevented (MCMAHON et al. 1975).

The effects of cell contact may be mimicked by the addition of cAMP to the disaggregated cells. Cyclic AMP (1 m*M*) completely prevents the increase in activity of cAMP phosphodiesterase which occurs on disaggregation. Note that this result would not be expected in the context of the many studies which show that cAMP can induce the phosphodiesterase. ATP, ADP, and cGMP (all 1 m*M*) had no effect on the induction in this study. Dibutyryl cAMP (1 m*M*) was less effective and 5′AMP (1 m*M*) much less effective than cAMP (TAKEMOTO et al. 1978). These workers also showed that cAMP (1 m*M*) has only a slight effect on the disaggregation-induced disappearance of UDP-galactose:polysaccharide transferase. Cyclic AMP also substitutes for cell contact in maintaining elevated levels of glycogen phosphorylase (TAKEUCHI et al. 1978). TOWN and GROSS (1978) have also examined the relationship between cell-contact stimulated processes and cyclic nucleotides. Cultures of cells were shaken in suspension at low speeds (which allow cell aggregation) or high speeds (which prevent aggregation). Fast shaking prevented the shut off of phosphodiesterase synthesis and the increases in UDP-glucose pyrophosphorylase and glycogen phosphorylase activity. Cyclic AMP (0.1 m*M*) allowed the normal developmental changes in these enzymes to occur in rapidly shaken cultures. Cyclic GMP (0.1 m*M*) had very little effect on the levels of UDP-glucose pyrophosphorylase and glycogen phosphorylase in rapidly shaken cultures. Cyclic GMP (0.1 m*M*) superinduced phosphodiesterase in fast-shaken cells although it accentuated the aggregation-induced decrease in activity which occurred in cells which were slowly shaken.

Of the 38 polypeptides whose initiation of synthesis occurs at approximately the time of pseudoplasmodium formation, four are made in disaggregated cells in the presence or absence of cAMP (7–20 μ*M*); six are inhibited by disaggregation in the presence or absence of cAMP; and 28 are made at high levels by disaggregated cells only in the presence of cAMP. The synthesis of several proteins characteristic of earlier phases of development is maintained by cAMP. Cyclic AMP can not be replaced by 5′AMP (1 m*M*) (LANDFEAR and LODISH 1980). Therefore, only 10% of the major newly synthesized proteins do not depend on continuing cell contact or cAMP for their expression. Fifteen percent require cell contact but the great majority require either cell contact or an exogenous source of cAMP.

b) Synergy Between cAMP and Cell Contact

The work of BONNER (1970) on induction of stalk cell differentiation by cAMP has been extended considerably. Cells plated on agar containing cAMP (5 m*M*) show a cooperative dependence on cell density for efficient induction of stalk cells. Low density cells may be helped to differentiate in the presence of cAMP by a layer of high density cells separated from them by a sheet of cellophane (TOWN et al. 1976).

Examination of high density cells, incubated in cAMP (1–5 m*M*), with anti-spore antibody showed that the cells express pre-spore antigen transiently before appearance of stalk cells. The induction of pre-spore cells by cAMP did not occur at low density. In contrast to the results obtained with stalk cell differentiation, helper cells separated by cellophane had little effect on the induction of pre-spore cells at low density (Kay et al. 1978). The high density cell population apparently releases a low molecular weight oligosaccharide and phosphate containing factor which acts synergistically with cAMP to induce the differentiation of stalk cells (Town and Stanford 1979). Differentiation of mature spores even in the presence of cAMP apparently has an absolute requirement for cell contact. This contact-mediated differentiation is sensitive to pronase (Kay et al. 1979). Mutants F 417 and Sci-1 have been isolated which have altered requirements for both cell contact and exogenous cAMP for the triggering of terminal cell differentiation (Town et al. 1976; Wilson and Sussman 1978).

5. Cell Contact Effects in Development

Cell contact effects in development could be mediated in a variety of ways. Contact might exert its effects by activating or inhibiting the activity of membrane molecules which control the intracellular concentrations of chemical messengers. In addition, contact may exert its effects by altering the adsorptive properties of the cytoplasmic face of the plasma membrane so that molecules such as cAMP-activated protein kinase and the src protein kinase are released into the cytoplasm. Cell density appears to affect the distribution of calmodulin in the cell in this way (Evain et al. 1979). Other examples of this process are described elsewhere (McMahon and West 1976).

6. Summary

The results of the many experiments described above indicate that cAMP and inorganic ions act as signals in directing developmentally important events in *D. discoideum*. In addition, it appears that the same substance may have different effects depending on the time and/or concentration at which it is added. The combined results from this and other systems support the ideas posited previously (McMahon 1974; McMahon and West 1976).

Cell contact is an important mediator of the events associated with pattern formation (McMahon 1973). Exogenous cAMP can substitute for cell contact in many of the events which occur. It appears that a low molecular weight oligosaccharide, in association with cAMP, can substitute for the contact-mediated interactions which lead to the differentiation of the stalk cell. It would be interesting to know whether this factor is normally associated with the plasma membrane since many surface glyproteins can be sloughed from cells of *D. discoideum* (S. Hoffman and D. McMahon, unpublished work). In addition, the question of whether cell contact is required for operation of molecular interactions between cells or for the maintenance of high concentrations of extracellular messengers must be resolved.

C. Chemical Messengers and Gene Expression in Development

As the examples discussed above illustrate, many systems in development proceed through a metastable state to a relatively stable state of differentiation. Even the relatively stable states can be perturbed, however, as the effects of transformation by sarcoma viruses indicate. It is likely that, analogously, chemical messengers exert their effects on development in ways which are metastable and others which are stable and fixed. Some ideas for possible mechanisms by which changes in chemical messengers may be remembered so that transient changes may exert continuing effects on the phenotypic properties of the cell have been suggested (McMahon and West 1976).

A full consideration of the relationship between cyclic nucleotides and the cell cycle is beyond the scope of this chapter, although clearly relevant to the cellular events which occur during maturation of the oocyte. (See the chapter by Friedman on Regulation of Cell Cycle.) For example, studies of chromatin structure in vitro (Matthews and Bradbury 1978) and of chromosome condensation in a ts cell cycle mutant (Matsumoto et al. 1980) support the idea that chromosome condensation in prophase may be regulated by phosphorylation of histone H1. Staining for type I and II regulatory subunits of protein kinase, the catalytic subunit, and cGMP protein kinase with fluorescin-conjugated antibodies shows that they are associated with the chromosomes in prophase and prometaphase (Browne et al. 1980). These workers also showed an association between type II regulatory subunits and cGMP-protein kinase and the microtubes of the mitotic spindle at metaphase in 80% of the cells examined. Calmodulin has also been localized on the mitotic spindle (Anderson et al. 1978; Welsh et al. 1975). These proteins could convert intracellular cyclic nucleotide or Ca^{2+} concentrations into movement of the mitotic spindle.

Nuclei from meiotic cells of mammals and lilies contain a DNA-binding protein, R-protein, which has been suggested to be involved in meiotic chromosome pairing or recombination. The properties of this protein are very dependent on its state of phosphorylation. The dephosphorylation of the protein abolishes the specificity for binding to single-stranded DNA as opposed to double-stranded DNA and its ability to facilitate denaturation or renaturation of DNA. A cAMP-independent protein kinase restores the native properties of the R-protein. Cyclic AMP-dependent protein kinase dependent phosphorylation abolishes the affinity of R-protein for DNA (Hotta and Stern 1979).

The few studies described above clearly indicate that cyclic nucleotide concentrations in the cell may be transduced into a variety of cellular events relevant to the operation of mitosis and meiosis.

Cyclic nucleotides and inorganic ions can potentially regulate the accessibility of genes for transcription. Previous papers have discussed this possibility (McMahon 1974; McMahon and West 1976). As described above, in *D. discoideum*, cAMP is able to both stimulate and repress the synthesis of mRNAs. Among the possible ways in which this could occur are the alteration of RNA polymerase which results in changes in initiation, rate of chain elongation, or site of termination. Phosphorylation of bacteriophage T7 polymerase alters its specificity for initiation (Zillig et al. 1975). Accessibility of genes can probably be modified via cAMP-dependent phosphorylation of histones (Fasy et al. 1979) or via changes in ionic conditions which can modify chromosome structure (Whitlock 1979; Spadafora et al. 1979; Dietrich et al. 1979). Both ionic conditions and changes in phosphorylation of chromosomal proteins can work together to change exposure of DNA (Fasy et al. 1979). By analogy with studies in prokaryotes, cAMP might also regulate production of translatable mRNAs by overcoming transcriptional polarity. Exogenous cAMP (5 m*M*) overcomes transcriptional polarity in the lactose and galactose operons of *Escherichia coli* (Ullman et al. 1979).

Changes dependent upon continued presence of the initiating stimulus (changes in cAMP, Ca^{2+}, K^{+}, etc., concentrations) would be expected to revert to their previous state in the absence of the stimulus. Several logical possibilities present themselves for maintenance of the "differentiated state." The first of these is continuation of the extracellular stimulus which has lead to an alteration in the intracellular concentration of the chemical messenger. This may occur in *D. discoideum* and may be mediated via cell contact. In addition, as discussed previously (McMahon 1974), the interpretive mechanism (e.g., protein kinases, substrates, etc.) may be modified. However, as posited (McMahon and West 1976), the messenger could cause a self-propagating change in the cell. There seem to be at least two possible biochemical mechanisms for long term development memory of an inducing stimulus. Both appear to be used in development. The first of these is activation or production of an autocatalytic protein or a protein which regulates its own synthesis, which can maintain its active state without the inducing stimulus. Phosphorylase kinase is an enzyme which can do this in vitro. Maturation-promoting factors of the oocyte appear to be another such enzyme. Alterations of the genome provide a second possible way of remembering the event.

The developmental expression of one class of proteins, the immunoglobulins, appears to be regulated via genetic alteration of the cell. The splicing of genes, variable and constant regions of immunoglobulin light and heavy chains, was predicted far in advance of its discovery by Dreyer and Bennett (1965). Such splicing has been demonstrated for the production of an active light chain gene (Hozumi and Tonegawa 1976; Rabbitts and Forster 1978) and a heavy chain gene (Davis et al. 1980). Deletion of segments of the genome similarly leads to expression of a series of immunoglobulin heavy chains (Rabbitts et al. 1980). Analogously, control of mating type in yeast apparently involves genetic rearrangement (Kushner et al. 1979).

The question of how changes in intracellular messengers might be coupled to genetic change is an intriguing one. One possible mechanism could proceed via the action of a protein such as the R-protein discussed above. Another regulatory mechanism could proceed via the enzymes and proteins which catalyze genetic recombination. At a specific time in development, a branch in the developmental tree could occur via the triggering of recombinational event by a change in concentration of a chemical messenger. This might occur in at least two different ways. First, the activity of the enzymes which catalyze recombination might be modified. The activities of the enzymes of *E. coli* recombination are very susceptible to changes in ionic conditions. The activity of the recA protein is very dependent on ionic strength (Craig and Roberts 1980), and Ca^{2+} has a dramatic effect on the pattern of activity of the recBC nuclease (Rosamond et al. 1979).

Second, chemical messengers could also change the structure of the chromatin to facilitate specific recombination. Although a variety of ways can be imagined in which chemical messengers could do this, I will discuss only one which seems very attractive to me.

Poly (adenosine diphosphoate-ribose) could be the mediator of specific recombination events. Considerable evidence, published by CAPLAN and his collaborators and discussed above, suggests that poly (ADP-ribose) is involved in some manner in cellular differentiation (CAPLAN and ROSENBERG 1975).

The synthesis and degradation of poly (ADP-ribose) is directly linked to the metabolism of the cell. This polymer is linked to histones H1, H2, and H3 in addition to other nuclear proteins (NISHIZUKA et al. 1968; YAMADA and SUGIMURA 1973; UEDA et al. 1974). The polymer is synthesized from NAD by poly (ADP-ribose) polymerase and degraded by poly (ADP-ribose) glycohydrolase (JANAKIDEVI and KOH 1974; MIWA et al. 1974, 1975). Cyclic AMP (3 m*M*) inhibits the glycohydrolase by 89% (MIWA et al. 1975) and a 39% inhibition can be produced by 0.1 m*M* cAMP. At this concentration, cGMP, 5′AMP, and ATP have no effect (MIWA et al. 1974).

A variety of evidence suggests that poly (ADP-ribose) is associated with recombination. Nuclease treatment of DNA stimulates the synthesis of poly (ADP-ribose) apparently through initiation of new chains (MILLER 1975a, b). Poly (ADP-ribose) participates in DNA excision repair (DAVIES et al. 1978; DURKACZ et al. 1980). Inhibitors of poly (ADP-ribose) polymerase induce sister chromatid exchanges (OIKAWA et al. 1980).

Therefore, it appears that poly (ADP-ribose) could participate in genotypic stabilization of differentiated phenotypes via a participation in recombinational editing of the genome. It might affect this process in several ways. Polymers of poly (ADP-ribose) bound to different chromosomal patterns might interact with each other or with the DNA duplex. In addition, since it has been demonstrated that molecules of histone H1 in the nucleus are sometimes covalently attached by poly (ADP-ribose) (STONE et al. 1977; BYRNE et al. 1978), it seems possible that recombination of areas of the chromosome might be inhibited by linking them together via poly (ADP-ribose).

How might cAMP and other second messengers participate in this process? One way is via the observed inhibition of poly (ADP-ribose) glycohydrolase. The concentration of cAMP used in the in vitro system is high, however. Therefore, it appears that another possibility for involvement of second messengers might lie in their ability to stimulate the covalent modification of chromosomal proteins. These modifications might affect the metabolism of poly (ADP-ribose) directly or might alter the ability of a chromosomal protein to be modified.

D. Conclusion

A variety of experimental protocols and experimental systems, only some of which have been discussed here, implicate cAMP and inorganic ions in morphogenesis and cellular differentiation. The most critical problem now is the mechanism by which changes in intracellular chemical messengers are coupled to gene expression.

It appears that the immediate future will provide the information which allows us to appreciate the roles which cyclic nucleotides and inorganic ions play in the drama which unfolds when amoebae of *D. discoideum* are starved or an egg is fertilized.

Acknowledgement. Preparation of this review was partially supported by NIH grant GM 29830-02.

References

Ahrens PB, Solursh M, Reiter RS (1977) Stage-related capacity for limb chondrogenesis in cell culture. Dev Biol 60:69–82

Ahrens PB, Solursh M, Reiter RS, Singley CT (1979) Position-related capacity for differentiation of limb mesenchyme in cell culture. Dev Biol 69:436–450

Alton TH, Brenner M (1979) Comparison of proteins synthesized by anterior and posterior regions of *Dictyostelium discoideum* pseudoplasmodia. Dev Biol 71:1–7

Alton TH, Lodish HF (1977a) Developmental changes in messenger RNAs and protein synthesis in *Dictyostelium discoideum.* Dev Biol 60:180–206

Alton TH, Lodish HF (1977b) Synthesis of developmentally regulated proteins in *Dictyostelium discoideum* which are dependent on continued cell-cell interactions. Dev Biol 60:201–216

Anderson B, Osborn M, Weber K (1978) Specific visualization of the distribution of the calcium dependent regulator protein of cyclic nucleotide phosphodiesterase (modulator protein) in tissue culture cells by immunofluorescence microscopy: mitosis and intracellular bridge. Cytobiologie 17:354–364

Aw EJ, Holt PG, Simons PN (1973) Myogenesis in vitro. Enhancement by dibutyryl cAMP. Exp Cell Res 83:436–438

Ball EH, Sanwal BD (1980) A synergistic effect of glucocorticoids and insulin on the differentiation of myoblasts. J Cell Physiol 102:27–36

Ball EH, Seth PK, Sanwal BD (1980) Regulatory mechanisms involved in the control of cyclic adenosine 3:5′-monophosphate phosphodiesterase in myoblasts. J Biol Chem 255:2962–2968

Baltus E, Hanocq-Quertier J, Pays AV, Brachet J (1977) Ionic requirements for induction of maturation (meiosis) in full-grown and medium-sized *Xenopus laevis* oocytes. Proc Natl Acad Sci USA 74:3461–3465

Baltus E, Hanocq-Quertier J, Guyaux M (1981) Adenylate cyclase and cyclic AMP-phosphodiesterase activities during the early phase of maturation in *Xenopus laevis* oocytes. FEBS Lett 123:37–40

Baulieu E-E (1978) Cell membrane, a target for steroid hormones. Mol Cell Endocrinol 12:247–254

Baulieu E-E, Godeau F, Schorderet M, Schorderet-Slatkine SS (1978) Steroid-induced meiotic division in *Xenopus laevis* oocytes: surface and calcium. Nature 275:593–598

Belle R, Schorderet-Slatkine S, Drury KC, Ozon R (1975) In vitro progesterone binding to *Xenopus laevis* oocytes. Gen Comp Endocrinol 25:339–345

Blumberg DD, Lodish HF (1980a) Complexity of nuclear and polysomal RNAs in growing *Dictyostelium discoideum* cells. Dev Biol 78:268–284

Blumberg DD, Lodish HF (1980b) Changes in the messenger RNA populations during differentiation of *Dictyostelium discoideum.* Dev Biol 78:285–300

Blumberg DD, Lodish HF (1981) Changes in the complexity of nuclear RNA during development of *Dictyostelium discoideum.* Dev Biol 81:74–80

Bonner JT (1952) The pattern of differentiation in amoeboid slime molds. Am Nat 86:79–89

Bonner JT (1967) The cellular slime molds. Princeton University Press, Princeton, New Jersey

Bonner JT (1970) Induction of stalk cell differentiation by cyclic AMP in the cellular slime mold *Dictyostelium discoideum.* Proc Natl Acad Sci USA 65:110–113

Bonner JT, Chiquoine AD, Kolderie MQ (1955) A histochemical study of differentiation in the cellular slime molds. J Exp Zool 130:133–158

Bonner JT, Sieja TW, Hall EM (1971) Further evidence for the sorting out of cells in the differentiation of the cellular slime mold *Dictyostelium discoideum*. J Embryol Exp Morphol 25:457–465
Bravo R, Otero C, Allende CC, Allende JE (1978) Amphibian oocyte maturation and protein synthesis: Related inhibition by cyclic AMP theophylline and papaverine. Proc Natl Acad Sci USA 75:1242–1246
Brenner M (1977) Cyclic AMP gradient in migrating pseudoplasmodia of the cellular slime mold *Dictyostelium discoideum*. J Biol Chem 252:4073–4077
Brown SS, Rutherford CL (1980) Localization of cyclic nucleotide phosphodiesterase in the multicellular stages of *Dictyostelium discoideum*. Differentiation 16:173–183
Browne CL, Lockwood AH, Su J-L, Beavo JA Steiner AL (1980) Immunofluorescent localization of cyclic nucleotide-dependent protein kinases on the mitotic apparatus of cultured cells. J Cell Biol 87:336–345
Byrne RH, Stone PR, Kidwell WR (1978) Effect of polyamines and divalent cations on histone H1-poly (adenosine diphosphate ribose) complex formation. Exp Cell Res 115:277–283
Caplan AI (1972a) Effect of a nicotinamide-sensitive teratogen 6-aminonicotinamide on chick limb cells in culture. Exp Cell Res 70:185–195
Calplan AI (1972b) The site and sequence of action of 6-aminonicotinamide in causing bone malformations of embryonic chick limb and its relationship to hormonal development. Dev Biol 28:71–83
Caplan AI, Rosenberg MJ (1975) Interrelationship between poly (ADP-ribose) synthesis, intracellular NAD levels, and muscle or cartilage differentiation from mesodermal cells of embryonic chick limb. Proc Natl Acad Sci USA 72:1852–1857
Chia WK (1975) Induction of stalk cell differentiation by cyclic AMP in a susceptible variant of *Dictyostelium discoideum*. Dev Biol 44:239–252
Clark RL, Steck TL (1979) Morphogenesis in *Dictyostelium*. an orbital hypothesis. Science 204:1163–1168
Clarke M, Basari WL, Kayman SC (1980) Isolation and properties of calmodulin from *Dictyostelium discoideum*. J Bacteriol 141:397–400
Cloud JG, Schuetz AW (1979) 1-Methyladenine induction of oocyte (starfish) maturation: inhibition by procaine and its pH dependency. J Exp Zool 210:11–16
Courtneidge SA, Levinson AD, Bishop JM (1980) The protein encoded by the transforming gene of avian sarcoma virus ($pp60^{src}$) and a homologous protein in normal cells ($pp60^{proto\ src}$) with the plasma membrane. Proc Natl Acad Sci USA 77:3783–3787
Craig NL, Roberts JW (1980) *E. coli* recA protein-directed cleavage of phage λ repressor requires poly-nucleotide. Nature 283:26–30
Crean EV, Rossomando EF (1977) Developmental changes in membrane-bound enzymes of *Dictyostelium discoideum* detected by concanavalin A sepharose affinity chromatography. Biochem Biophys Res Commun 75:488–495
Cutler LS, Rossomando EF (1975) Localization of adenylate cyclase in *Dictyostelium discoideum*. II. Cytochemical studies on whole cells and isolated plasma membrane vesicles. Exp Cell Res 95:79–87
Davies MI, Halldorsson H, Nduka N, Shall S, Skidmore CJ (1978) The involvement of poly (adenosine diphosphate-ribose) in deoxyribonucleic acid repair. Biochem Soc Trans 6:1056–1057
Davis MM, Calame K, Early PW, Livant DL, Joho R, Weissman IL, Hood L (1980) An immunoglobulin heavy-chain gene is formed by at least two recombinational events. Nature 283:733–739
Deuchar E (1975) Cellular interactions in animal development. Methuen, New York
Dietrich AE, Axel R, Cantor CR (1979) Salt-induced structural changes of nucleosome core particles. J Mol Biol 129:587–602
Dreyer WJ, Bennett JC (1965) The molecular basis of antibody formation: a paradox. Proc Natl Acad Sci USA 54:864–869
Durkacz BW, Omidiji O, Gray DA, Shall S (1980) (ADP-ribose) participates in DNA excision repair. Nature 283:593–596
Ede DA (1978) An introduction to developmental biology. John Wiley and Sons, New York Chichester

Epstein CJ, Jiminez de Asua L, Rozengurt E (1975) The role of cyclic AMP in myogenesis. J Cell Physiol 86:83–90
Erikson RL, Purchio AF, Erikson E, Collett MS, Brugge JS (1980) Molecular events in cells transformed by Rous sarcoma virus. J Cell Biol 87:319–325
Evain D, Klee C, Anderson WB (1979) Chinese hamster ovary cell population density affects intracellular concentration of calcium-dependent regulator and ability of regulator to inhibit adenylate cyclase activity. Proc Natl Acad Sci USA 76:3962–3966
Farnham CJM (1975) Cytochemical localization of adenylate cyclase and 3′,5′-nucleotide phosphodiesterase in *Dictyostelium*. Exp Cell Res 91:36–46
Fasy TM, Inoye A, Johnson EM, Allerey VG (1979) Phosphorylation of H1 and H5 histones by cyclic AMP-dependent protein kinase reduces DNA binding. Biochim Biophys Acta 564:322–334
Feit IN, Fournier GA, Needleman RD, Underwood MZ (1978) Induction of stalk and spore cell differentiation by cyclic AMP in slugs of *Dictyostelium discoideum*. Science 200:439–441
Festoff BW, Oh TH (1977) Neurotrophic control of cyclic nucleotide levels during muscle differentiation in cell culture. J Neurobiol 8:57–65
Fiszman MY (1978) Morphological and biochemical differentiation in RSV transformed chick embryo myoblasts. Cell Differ 7:89–101
Forman D, Garrod DR (1977a) Pattern formation in *Dictyostelium discoideum*. I. Development of prespore cells and its relationship to the pattern of the fruiting body. J Enbryol Exp Morphol 40:215–228
Forman D, Garrod DR (1977b) Pattern formation in *Dictyostelium discoideum*. II. Differentiation and pattern formation in non-polar aggregates. J Embryol Exp Morphol 40:229–243
Francis D, Salmon D, Moore B (1978) A mutant strain of *Polysphondylium pallidum* deficient in production of cyclic AMP. Dev Biol 67:232–236
Fulton BP, Whittingham DG (1978) Activation of mammalian oocytes by intracellular infection of calcium. Nature 273:149–151
Garrod DR, Forman D (1977) Pattern formation in the absence of polarity in *Dictyostelium discoideum*. Nature 265:144–146
Garrod DR, Malkinson AM (1973) Cyclic AMP, pattern formation, and movement in the slime mold, *Dictyostelium discoideum*. Exp Cell Res 81:492–495
George RP (1977) Disruption of multicellular organization in the cellular slime molds by cyclic AMP. Cell Differ 5:293–300
Godeau JF, Schorderet-Slatkine S, Hubert P, Baulieu E-E (1978) Induction of maturation in *Xenopus laevis* oocytes by a steroid linked to a polymer. Proc Natl Acad Sci USA 75:2353–2357
Gregg JH (1965) Regulation in the cellular slime molds. Dev Biol 12:377–393
Gregg JH, Karp GC (1978) Patterns of cell differentiation revealed by 6-[^{3}H]fucose incorporation in *Dictyostelium*. Exp Cell Res 112:31–46
Hamilton ID, Chia WK (1975) Enzyme activity changes during cyclic AMP-induced stalk cell differentiation in P4, a variant of *Dictyostelium discoideum*. J Gen Microbiol 91:295–306
Hayashi M, Takeuchi I (1976) Quantitative studies on cell differentiation during morphogenesis of the cellular slime mold *Dictyostelium discoideum*. Dev Biol 50:302–309
Hayashi H, Yamasaki F (1978) Characteristics of the induction of phosphodiesterases by cyclic adenosine 3′,5′-monophosphate in the slime mold, *Dictyostelium discoideum*. Chem Pharm Bull (Tokyo) 26:2977–2982
Hendersen EJ (1975) The cyclic 3′,5′-monophosphate receptor of *Dictyostelium discoideum*. Binding characteristics of aggregation-competent cells and variation of binding levels during the life cycle. J Biol Chem 250:4730–4736
Hirai S, Chida K, Kanatani H (1973) Role of follicle cells in maturation of starfish oocytes. Dev Growth Differ 15:21–31
Hoffman S, McMahon D (1977) The role of the plasma membrane in the development of *Dictyostelium discoideum*. II. Developmental and topographical analysis of polypeptide and glycoprotein composition. Biochim Biophys Acta 465:242–259

Hoffman S, McMahon D, (1978) The effects of inhibition of development in *Dictyostelium discoideum* on changes in plasma membrane composition and topography. Arch Biochem Biophys 187:12–24

Hohl HR, Honegger R, Traub F, Markwalder M (1977) Influence of cAMP on cell differentiation and morphogenesis in *Polysphondylium*. In: Cappuccinelli P, and Ashworth J (eds) Developments and differentiation in cellular slime molds. Elsevier, Amsterdam Oxford New York, pp 149–172

Hokin MR, Brown DF (1969) Inhibition by γ-hexachlorocyclohexane of acetylcholine-stimulated phosphatidyl-inositol synthesis in cerebral cortex slices and of phosphatic acid-inositol transferase in cerebral cortex particulate fractions. J Neurochem 16:475–483

Hotta Y, Stern H (1979) The effect of dephosphorylation on the properties of helix-destabilizing protein from meiotic cells and its partial reversal by a protein kinase. Eur J Biochem 95:31–38

Hozumi N, Tonegawa S (1976) Evidence for somatic rearrangement of immunoglobin genes coding for variable and constant regions. Proc Natl Acad Sci USA 73:3628–3632

Iacobelli S, Hanocq J, Baltus E, Brachet J (1974) Hormone-induced maturation of Xenopus laevis oocytes: effects of different steroids and study of the properties of a progesterone receptor. Differentiation 2:129–135

Ikeda T, Takeuchi I (1971) Isolation and characterization of a prespore specific structure of the cellular slime mold, *Dictyostelium discoideum*. Dev Growth Differ 13:221–229

Ikegami S, Kamiya Y, Shirai H (1976) Characterization and action of meiotic inhibitors in starfish ovary. Exp Cell Res 103:233–239

Jacquet M, Part D, Felenbok B (1981) Changes in the polyadenylated messenger RNA population during development of *Dictyostelium discoideum*. Dev Biol 81:155–166

Janakidevi K, Koh C (1974) Synthesis of polyadenosine diphosphate ribose by isolated nuclei of swine aortic tissue. Biochemistry 13:1327–1330

Jefferson BL, Rutherford CL (1976) A stalk-specific localization of trehalose activity in *Dictyostelium discoideum*. Exp Cell Res 103:127–134

Juliani MH, Klein C (1981) Photoaffinity labeling of the cell surface adenosine 3′:5′-monophosphate receptor of *Dictyostelium discoideum* and its modification in down-regulated cells. J Biol Chem 256:613–619

Kantor AS, Hampton M (1978) Indomethacin in submicromolar concentrations inhibiting cyclic-AMP-dependent protein kinase. Nature 276:841–842

Karasawa K, Kimata K, Ito K, Kato Y, Suzuki S (1979) Morphological and biochemical differentiation of limb bud cells cutures in chemically defined medium. Dev Biol 70:287–305

Kay RR, Garrod D, Tilly R (1978) Requirements for cell differentiation in *Dictyostelium discoideum*. Nature 271:58–60

Kay RR, Town CD, Gross JD (1979) Cell differentiation in *Dictyostelium discoideum*. Differentiation 13:7–14

Kofoid EC, Knauber DC, Allende JE (1979) Induction of amphibian oocyte maturation by polyvalent cations and alkaline pH in the absence of potassium ions. Dev Biol 72:374–380

Konijn TM, Chang Y-Y, Bonner JT (1969) Synthesis of cyclic AMP in *Dictyostelium discoideum* and *Polysphondylium pallidum*. Nature 224:1211–1212

Kosher RA (1976) Inhibition of "spontaneous" notochord-induced and collagen-induced somite chondrogenesis by cyclic AMP derivatives and theophylline. Dev Biol 53:265–276

Kosher RA, Savage MP (1979) The effect of collagen on the cyclic AMP content of embryonic somites. J Exp Zool 208:35–40

Kosher RA, Savage MP, Chan S-C (1979) Cyclic AMP derivatives stimulate the chondrogenic differentiation of the mesoderm subjacent to the apical ectodermal ridge of the chick limb bud. J Exp Zool 209:221–228

Krivanek JO, Krivanek RC (1958) The histochemical localization of certain biochemical intermediates and enzymes in the developing slime mold, *Dictyostelium discoideum* Raper. J Exp Zool 137:89–116

Krueger JG, Wang E, Garber EA, Goldberg AR (1980) Differences in intracellular location of $pp60^{src}$ in rat and chicken cells transformed by Rous sarcoma virus. Proc Natl Acad Sci USA 77:4142–4146
Kubota J, Nakao K, Shirai H, Kanatani H (1977) 1-Methyladenine-producing cell in starfish testis. Exp Cell Res 106:63–70
Kühn A (1971) Lectures on developmental physiology. Springer, Berlin Heidelberg New York
Landauer W, Clark E (1957) The interaction in teratogenic activity of the two niacin analogs 3-acetylpyridine and 6-aminonicotinamide. J Exp Zool 151:253–258
Landfear SM, Lodish HF (1980) A role for cyclic AMP in the expression of developmentally regulated genes in Dictyostelium discoideum. Proc Natl Acad Sci USA 77:1044–1048
Lebovitz HE, Drezner MK, Neelon FA (1976) Evidence for the role of adenosine 3′:5′ monophosphate in the growth hormone dependent serum sulfation factor (somatomedin) action on cartilage. In: Pecile A, Muller EE (eds) Growth hormone and related peptides. American Elsevier, New York, pp 202–215
Loomis WJ, Jr. (1975) Dictyostelium discoideum: A developmental system. Academic Press, New York
Loomis WF, Morrissey J, Lee M (1978) Biochemical analysis of pleiotropy in *Dictyostelium.* Dev Biol 63:243–246
MacWilliams HK, Bonner JT (1979) The prestalk-prespore pattern in cellular slime molds. Differentiation 14:1–22
Maeda Y (1970) Influence of ionic conditions on cell differentiation and morphogenesis of the cellular slime molds. Dev Growth Differ 12:217–227
Maeda Y (1971) Studies on a specific structure in differentiating slime mold cells. Mem Fac Sci Kyoto Univ Ser Biol IV:97–107
Maeda Y (1977) Role of cyclic AMP in the polarized movement of the migrating pseudoplasmodium of *Dictyostelium discoideum.* Dev Growth Differ 19:201–205
Maeda Y, Eguchi G (1977) Polarized structures of cells in the aggregating cellular slime mold *D. discoideum:* an electron microscope study. Cell Struct Funct 2:159–169
Maeda Y, Maeda M (1973) The calcium content of the cellular slime mold *Dictyostelium discoideum* during development and differentiation. Exp Cell Res 82:125–130
Maeda Y, Maeda M (1974) Heterogeneity of the cell population of the cellular slime mold *Dictyostelium discoideum* before aggregation, and its relation to the subsequent locations of the cells. Exp Cell Res 84:88–94
Maeda Y, Takeuchi I (1969) Cell differentiation and fine structures in the development of the cellular slime molds. Dev Growth Differ 11:232–245
Maller JL, Krebs EG (1977) Progesterone-stimulated meiotic cell division in *Xenopus* oocytes. Induction by regulatory subunit and inhibition by catalytic subunit of adenosine 3′:5′-monophosphate-dependent protein kinase. J Biol Chem 252:1712–1718
Maller JL, Krebs EG (1978) Intracellular cAMP levels and the initiation of meiosis in *Xenopus* oocytes. J Cell Biol 79:180a
Maller JL, Butcher FR, Krebs EG (1979) Early effect of progesterone on levels of cyclic adenosine 3′:5′-monophosphate in *Xenopus* oocytes. J Biol Chem 254:579–582
Masui Y, Markert CL (1971) Cytoplasmic control of nuclear behavior during meiotic maturation of frog oocytes. J Exp Zool 177:129–146
Matsumoto Y, Yasuda H, Mita S, Marunouchi T, Yamada M (1980) Evidence for the involvement of H1 histone phosphorylation in chromosome condensation. Nature 284:181–183
Matthews HR, Bradbury EM (1978) The role of H1 histone phosphorylation in the cell cycle. Turbidity studies of H1-DNA interaction. Exp Cell Res 111:343–351
McCurry LS, Jacobson MK (1981) Poly (ADP-ribose) synthesis following DNA damage in cells heterozygous or homozygous for the *Xeroderma pigmentosum* genotype. J Biol Chem 256:551–553
McMahon D (1973) A cell contact model for position determination in development. Proc Natl Acad Sci USA 70:2396–2400
McMahon D (1974) Chemical messengers in development: a hypothesis. Science 185:1012–1021

McMahon D (1981) Cell interactions and pattern formation in *Dictyostelium discoideum*. Recent Adv Phytochem 15:259–271

McMahon D, West C (1976) Transduction of positional information during development. In: Poste G, Nicolson GL (eds) The cell surface in animal embryogenesis and development. Elsevier, Amsterdam Oxford New York, pp 449–493

McMahon D, Hoffman S, Fry W, West CM (1975) The involvement of the plasma membrane in the development of *Dictyostelium discoideum*. In: McMahon D, Fox CF (eds) Developmental biology: pattern of formation and gene regulation. Benjamin, Menlo Park, California, pp 60–75

Merriam RW (1971) Progesterone induced maturational events in oocytes of *Xenopus laevis*. I. Continuous necessity for diffusible calcium and magnesium. Exp Cell Res 69:75–80

Miller EG (1975a) Effect of deoxyribonuclease I on the number and length of chains of poly (ADP-ribose) synthesized in vitro. Biochem Biophys Res Commun 66:280–286

Miller EG (1975b) Stimulation of nuclear poly (adenosine diphosphate-ribose) polymerase activity from HeLa cells by endonucleases. Biochim Biophys Acta 395:191–200

Miller RP, Husain M, Lohin S (1979) Long acting cAMP analogues enhance sulfate incorporation into matrix proteoglycans and suppress cell division of fetal rat chondrocytes in monolayer culture. J Cell Physiol 100:63–76

Miller ZI, Quance J, Ashworth JM (1969) Biochemical and cytological heterogeneity of the differentiating cells of the cellular slime mold *Dictyostelium discoideum*. Biochem J 114:815–818

Miwa M, Tanaka M, Matsushima T, Sugimura T (1974) Purification and properties of a glycohydrolase from calf thymus splitting ribose-ribose linkages of poly (adenosine diphosphate ribose). J Biol Chem 249:3475–3482

Miwa M, Nakatsugawa K, Hara K, Matsushima T, Sugimura T (1975) Degradation of poly (adenosine diphosphate ribose) by homogenates of various normal tissues and tumors of rats. Arch Biochem Biophys 167:54–60

Miyakawa N, Ueda K, Hayaishi O (1972) Association of poly ADP-ribose glycohydrolase with liver chromatin. Biochem Biophys Res Commun 49:239–245

Mizukami Y, Iwabuchi M (1970) Effects of actinomycin D and cycloheximide on morphogenesis and synthesis of RNA and protein in the cellular slime mold, *Dictyostelium discoideum*. Exp Cell Res 63:317–324

Moreau M, Guerrier P (1979) Free calcium changes associated with hormone action in oocytes. In: Ashley CC, Campbell AK (eds) Detection and measurement of free calcium ions in cells. North Holland, Amsterdam Oxford New York pp 219–226

Moreau M, Guerrier P (1980) In vitro interactions between membrane, hormone, and cyclic nucleotides as revealed with aequorin. Dev Biol 79:488–492

Moreau M, Doree M, Guerrier P (1976) Electrophoresis introduction of calcium ions into the cortex of *Xenopus laevis* oocytes triggers meiosis reinitiation. J Exp Zool 197:443–449

Moreau M, Guerrier P, Doree M, Ashley CC (1978) Hormone-induced release of intracellular Ca^{2+} triggers meiosis in starfish oocytes. Nature 272:251–253

Moreau M, Valain JP, Guerrier P (1980) Free calcium changes associated with hormone action in amphibian oocytes. Dev Biol 78:201–214

Moriyama Y, Hasegawa S, Murayama K (1976) cAMP and cGMP changes associated with the differentiation of cultured chick embryo muscle cells. Exp Cell Res 101:159–163

Morrill GA, Schatz F, Kostellolow AB, Poupko JM (1977) Changes in cyclic AMP levels in the amphibian ovarian follicle following progesterone induction of meiotic maturation. Differentiation 8:97–104

Morris GE, Piper M, Cole R (1976) Differential effects of calcium ion concentrations on cell fusion, cell division and creatine kinase activity in muscle cell cultures. Exp Cell Res 99:106–114

Müller U, Hohl HR (1973) Pattern formation in *Dictyostelium discoideum:* temporal and spatial distribution of prespore vacuoles. Differentiation 1:267–276

Mulner O, Huchon D, Thibier C, Ozon R (1979) Cyclic AMP synthesis in *Xenopus laevis* oocytes. Inhibition by progesterone. Biochim Biophys Acta 582:179–184

Mulner O, Cartaud A, Ozon R (1980) Cyclic AMP phosphodiesterase activities in *Xenopus laevis* oocytes. Differentiation 16:31–39
Nestle M, Sussman M (1972) The effect of cyclic AMP on morphogenesis and enzyme accumulation in *Dictyostelium discoideum*. Dev Biol 28:545–554
Newell PC, Ellingson JS, Sussman M (1969) Synchrony of enzyme accumulation in a population of differentiating slime mold cells. Biochim Biophys Acta 177:610–614
Newell PC, Franke J, Sussman M (1972) Regulation of four functionally related enzymes during shifts in the developmental program of *Dictyostelium discoideum*. J Mol Biol 63:373–382
Nishizuka Y, Ueda K, Honjo T, Hayaishi O (1968) Enzymic adenosine diphosphate ribosylation of histone and poly adenosine diphosphate ribose synthesis in rat liver nuclei. J Biol Chem 243:3765–3767
Oikawa A, Tohda H, Kawai M, Miwa M, Sugimura T (1980) Inhibitors of poly (adenosine diphosphate ribose) polymerase induce sister chromatid exchanges. Biochem Biophys Res Commun 97:1311–1316
Okamoto K (1979) Induction of cyclic AMP phosphodiesterase by disaggregation of the multicellular complexes of *Dictyostelium discoideum*. Eur J Biochem 93:221–227
Okamoto K, Takeuchi I (1976) Changes in activities of two developmentally regulated enzymes induced by disaggregation of the pseudoplasmodia of *Dictyostelium discoideum*. Biochem Biophys Res Commun 72:739–746
Oohata A, Takeuchi I (1977) Separation and biochemical characterization of the two cell types present in the pseudoplasmodium of *Dictyostelium discoideum*. J Cell Sci 24:1–9
Pacifici M, Boettinger D, Roby K, Holtzer H (1977) Transformation of chondroblasts by Rous sarcoma virus and synthesis of the sulfated proteoglycan matrix. Cell 11:891–900
Pahlic M, Rutherford CL (1979) Adenylate cyclase activity and cyclic AMP levels during the development of *Dictyostelium discoideum*. J Biol Chem 254:9703–9707
Pan P, Bonner JT, Wedner HJ, Parker CW (1974) Immunofluorescence evidence for the distribution of cyclic AMP in cells and cell masses of the cellular slime molds. Proc Natl Acad Sci USA 71:1623–1625
Paulsen DF, Parker CL, Finch RA (1979) Region-dependent capacity for limb chondrogenesis: patterns of chondrogenesis in cultures from different regions of developing chick wing. Differentiation 14:159–165
Rabbits TH, Forster A (1978) Evidence for noncontinguous variable and constant region genes in both germ line and myeloma DNA. Cell 13:319–327
Rabbitts TH, Forster A, Dunnick W, Bentley DL (1980) The role of gene deletion in the immunoglobulin heavy chain switch. Nature 283:351–356
Raper KB (1940) Pseudoplasmodium formation and organization in *Dictyostelium discoideum*. J Elisha Mitchell Sci Soc 56:241–282
Reporter M, Raveed D (1973) Plasma membranes: isolation from naturally fused and lysolecithin-treated muscle cells. Science 181:863–865
Reynhout JK, Smith LD (1974) Studies on the appearance and nature of a maturation-inducing factor in the cytoplasm of amphibian oocytes exposed to progesterone. Dev Biol 38:394–400
Robinson KR (1979) Electrical currents through full-grown and maturing *Xenopus* oocytes. Proc Natl Acad Sci USA 76:837–841
Rosamond J, Telander KM, Linn S (1979) Modulation of the action of the recBC enzyme of *Escherichia coli* K-12 by Ca^{2+}. J Biol Chem 254:8646–8652
Rosenberg MJ, Caplan AI (1974) Nicotinamide adenine dinucleotide levels in cells of developing chick limbs: possible control of muscle and cartilage development. Dev Biol 38:157–164
Rossomando EF, Cutler LS (1975) Localization of adenylate cyclase in *Dictyostelium discoideum*. I. Preparation and biochemical characterization of cell fractions and isolated plasma membrane vesicles. Exp Cell Res 95:67–78
Rubin J (1976) The signal from fruiting body and conus tips of *Dictyostelium discoideum*. J Embryol Exp Morphol 36:261–271
Rutherford CL, Harris JF (1976) Localization of glycogen phosphorylase in specific cell types during differentiation of *Dictyostelium discoideum*. Arch Biochem Biophys 175:453–462

Sampson J (1976) Cell patterning in migrating slugs of *Dictyostelium discoideum*. J Embryol Exp Morphol 36:663–668
Schindler J, Sussman M (1977a) Effect of NH_3 on cAMP associated activities and extracellular cAMP production in *Dictyostelium discoideum*. Biochem Biophys Res Commun 79:611–617
Schindler J, Sussman M (1977b) Ammonia determines the choice of morphogenetic pathways in *Dictyostelium discoideum*. J Mol Biol 116:161–169
Schindler J, Sussman M (1979) Inhibition by ammonia of intracellular cAMP accumulation in *Dictyostelium discoideum:* its significance for the regulation of morphogenesis. Dev Genet 1:13–20
Schorderet-Slatkine S, Schorderet M, Baulieu E-E (1977) Progesterone-induced meiotic reinitiation in vitro in *Xenopus laevis* oocytes. A role for the displacement of membrane-bound calcium. Differentiation 9:67–76
Schorderet-Slatkine S, Schorderet M, Boquet P, Godeau F, Baulieu E-E (1978) Progesterone-induced meiosis in *Xenopus laevis* oocytes: a role for cAMP at the "maturation-promoting factor" level. Cell 15:1269–1275
Schubert D, Lacorbiere M (1976) Phenotypic transformation of clonal myogenic cells to cells resembling chondrocytes. Proc Natl Acad Sci USA 73:1989–1993
Schudt C, Gaertner U, Dolken G, Pette D (1975) Calcium-related changes of enzyme activities in energy metabolism of cultured embryonic chick myoblasts and myotubes. Eur J Biochem 60:579–586
Schuetz AW (1972) Hormones and follicular functions. In: Biggers JD, Schuetz AW (eds) Oogenesis. University Park Press, Baltimore, Maryland, pp 479–511
Scott RE, Dousa TP (1980) Differences in the cyclic AMP-dependent phosphorylation of plasma membrane proteins of differentiated and undifferentiated L_6 myogenic cells. Differentiation 16:135–140
Searls R (1973) Chondrogenesis. In: Coward SJ (ed) Developmental regulation. aspects of cell differentiation. Academic Press, New York London, pp 219–251
Smith E, Williams KL (1980) Evidence for tip control of the "slug fruit" switch in slugs of *Dictyostelium discoideum*. J Embryol Exp Morphol 57:233–240
Smith LD, Ecker RE (1971) The interaction of steroids with *Rana pipiens* oocytes in the induction of maturation. Dev Biol 25:232–247
Solursh M, Reiter RS (1975) Determination of limb bud chondrocytes during a transient block of the cell cycle. Cell Differ 4:131–137
Solursh M, Reiter RS (1980) Evidence for histogenic interactions during in vitro limb chondrogenesis. Dev Biol 78:141–150
Solursh M, Ahrens PB, Reiter RS (1978) A tissue culture analysis of the steps in limb chondrogenesis. In Vitro 14:51–61
Solursh M, Reiter R, Ahrens PB, Pratt RM (1979) Increase of levels of cyclic AMP during avian limb chondrogenesis in vitro. Differentiation 15:183–186
Spadafora C, Oudet P, Chambon P (1979) Rearrangement of chromatin structure induced by increasing ionic strength and temperature. Eur J Biochem 100:225–235
Speaker MG, Butcher FR (1977) Cyclic nucleotide fluctuations during steroid-induced meiotic maturation of frog oocytes. Nature 267:848–850
Stenhouse FO, Williams KL (1977) Patterning in *Dictyostelium discoideum:* the proportions of the three differentiated cell types (spore, stalks and basal disk) in the fruiting body. Dev Biol 59:140–152
Sternfeld J, Bonner JT (1977) differentiation in *Dictyostelium* under submerged conditions. Proc Natl Acad Sci USA 74:268–271
Sternfeld J, David CN (1979) Ammonia plus another factor are necessary for differentiation in submerged clumps of *Dictyostelium*. J Cell Sci 38:181–191
Stone PR, Lorimer WS, Kidwell WR (1977) Properties of the complex between histone H1 and poly (ADP-ribose) synthesized in HeLa cell nuclei. Eur J Biochem 81:9–18
Sunkara PS, Wright DA, Rao PN (1979) Mitotic factors from mammalian cells induce germinal vesicle breakdown and chromosome condensation in amphibian oocytes. Proc Natl Acad Sci USA 76:2799–2802
Sussman M, Brackenbury R (1976) Biochemistry and molecular-genetic aspects of cellular slime mold development. Annu Rev Plant Physiol 27:229–265

Sussman M, Newell PC (1972) Quantal control. In: Sussman M (ed) Molecular genetics and developmental biology. Prentice-Hall, Englewood Cliffs, New Jersey, pp 275–302
Sussman M, Schindler J (1978) A possible mechanism of morphogenetic regulation in *Dictyostelium discoideum*. Differentiation 10:1–5
Takemoto S, Okamoto K, Takeuchi I (1978) The effects of cyclic AMP on disaggregation-induced changes in activities of developmentally regulated enzymes in *Dictyostelium discoideum*. Biochem Biophys Res Commun 80:858–865
Takeuchi I (1969) Establishment of polar organization during slime mold development. In: Cowdry EV, Seno S (eds) Nucleic acid metabolism, cell differentiation and cancer growth. Pergamon Oxford New York, pp 297–304
Takeuchi I, Sakai Y (1971) Dedifferentiation of the disaggregating slug cell of the cellular slime mold *Dictyostelium discoideum*. Dev Growth Differ 13:201–210
Takeuchi I, Hayashi M, Tasaka M (1977) Cell differentiation and pattern formation in *Dictyostelium*. In: Cappuccinelli P, Ashworth J (eds) Developments and differentiation in the cellular slime molds. Elsevier, Amsterdam Oxford New York, pp 1–16
Takeuchi I, Okamoto K, Tasaka M, Takemoto S (1978) Regulation of cell differentiation in slime mold development. Bot Mag Tokyo [Special Issue] 1:47–60
Tasaka M, Takeuchi I (1979) Sorting out behavior of disaggregated cells in the absence of morphogenesis in *Dictyostelium discoideum*. J Embryol Exp Morphol 49:89–102
Toivonen S (1979) Transmission problem in primary induction. Differentiation 15:177–180
Town CD (1976) Cyclic AMP receptor activity in developing cells of *Dictyostelium discoideum*. In: Bradshaw RA, Frazier WA, Merrell RC, Gottlieb DI, Hogue-Angeletti RA (eds) Surface membrane receptors. Plenum, New York, pp 443–453
Town C, Gross J (1978) The role of cyclic nucleotides and cell agglomeration in post-aggregative enzyme synthesis in *Dictyostelium discoideum*. Dev Biol 63:412–420
Town CD, Stanford E (1977) Stalk cell differentiation by cells from migrating slugs of *Dictyostelium discoideum:* special properties of tip cells. J Embryol Exp Morphol 42:105–113
Town C, Stanford E (1979) An oligosaccharide-containing factor that induces cell differentiation in *Dictyostelium discoideum*. Proc Natl Acad Sci USA 76:308–312
Town CD, Gross JD, Kay RR (1976) Cell differentiation without morphogenesis in *Dictyostelium discoideum*. Nature 262:717–719
Tsafriri A, Bar-Ami S (1978) Role of divalent cations in the resumption of meiosis of rat oocytes. J Exp Zool 205:293–300
Uchiyama S, Okamoto K, Takeuchi I (1979) Repression of rRNA synthesis induced by disaggregation in Dictyostelium discoideum. Biochim Biophys Acta 562:103–111
Ueda K, Omachi A, Kawaichi M, Hayaishi O (1974) Isolation of poly (ADP-ribosyl) histones from rat liver nuclei. In: Harris M (ed) Poly (ADP-ribose); an international symposium. National Institutes of Health, Bethesda, Maryland, pp 225–230
Ullman A, Joseph E, Danchin A (1979) Cyclic AMP as a modulator of polarity in polycistronic transcriptional units. Proc Natl Acad Sci USA 76:3194–3197
Vitto A, Wallace RA (1976) Maturation of *Xenopus* oocytes. I. Facilitation by ouabain. Exp Cell Res 97:56–62
Wahrmann JP, Winand R, Luzzati D (1973) Effect of cyclic AMP on growth and morphological differentiation of an established myogenic cell line. Nature New Biol 245:112–113
Wasserman WJ, Masui Y (1975) Initiation of meiotic maturation in *Xenopus leavis* oocytes by the combination of divalent cations and ionophore A 23187. J Exp Zool 193:369–375
Welsh MJ, Dedman JR, Brinkley BR, Means AR (1975) Calcium-dependent regulator protein localization in mitotic apparatus of eukaryotic cells. Proc Natl Acad Sci USA 75:1867–1871
West CM, McMahon D (1977) Identification of concanavalin A receptors and galactose-binding proteins in purified plasma membranes of *D. discoideum*. J Cell Biol 74:264–273
West CM, McMahon D (1979) Axial distribution of wheat germ agglutinin receptors in pseudoplasmodia of *Dictyostelium discoideum*. Exp Cell Res 124:393–401
West CM, McMahon D (1981) The involvement of a class of cell surface glycoconjugates on pseudoplasmodial morphogenesis in *Dictyostelium discoideum*. Differentiation, in press

West CM, McMahon D, Molday RS (1978) Identification of glycoproteins using lectins as probes, in plasma membranes from *Dictyostelium discoideum* and human erythrocytes. J Biol Chem 253:1716–1724
Whitlock JP (1979) The conformation of the chromatin core particle is ionic strength-dependent. J Biol Chem 254:5684–5689
Williams JG, Tsang AS, Mah-Bubani H (1980) A change in the rate of transcription of a eukaryotic gene in response to cyclic AMP. Proc Natl Acad Sci USA 77:7171–7175
Wilson DK, Sussman M (1978) Spore differentiation by isolated *Dictyostelium discoideum* cells, triggered by prior cell contact. Differentiation 11:125–131
Wilson JB, Rutherford CL (1978) ATP, trehalose, glucose and ammonium ion localization in the two cell types of *Dictyostelium discoideum*. J Cell Physiol 94:37–46
Yamamoto M (1977) Some aspects of behavior of the migrating slug of the cellular slime mold *Dictyostelium discoideum*. Dev Growth Differ 19:93–102
Yamada M, Sugimura T (1973) Effects of deoxyribonucleic acid and histone on the number and length of chains of poly (adenosine diphosphate-ribose). Biochemistry 12:3303–3308
Yanagisawa KO, Tanaka Y, Yanagisawa K (1974) Cyclic AMP phosphodiesterase in some mutants of *Dictyostelium pupureum*. Agric Biol Chem 38:1845–1849
Zalin RJ (1976) The effect of inhibitors upon intracellular cyclic AMP levels and chick myoblast differentiation. Dev Biol 53:1–9
Zalin RJ (1977) Prostaglandins and myoblast fusion. Dev Biol 59:241–248
Zalin RJ (1979) The cell cycle, myoblast differentiation and prostaglandin as a developmental signal. Dev Biol 71:274–288
Zalin RJ, Leaver R (1975) The effect of transient increase in intracellular cyclic AMP upon muscle cell fusion. FEBS Lett 53:33–36
Zalin RJ, Montague W (1974) Changes in adenylate cyclase, cyclic AMP and protein kinase levels in chick myoblasts and their relationship to differentiation. Cell 2:103–108
Zalin RJ, Montague W (1975) Changes in cyclic AMP, adenylate cyclase and protein kinase levels during the development of chick embryonic skeletal muscle. Exp Cell Res 93:55–62
Zillig W, Fujiki H, Blum W et al. (1975) In vivo and in vitro phosphorylation of DNA-dependent RNA polymerase of *Escherichia coli* by bacteriophage T7-induced protein kinase. Proc Natl Acad Sci USA 72:2506–2510
Zwilling E (1968) Morphogenetic phases in development. In: Locke M (ed) 27th symposium of the society for developmental biology. Academic Press, New York London, pp 184–207

CHAPTER 20

Regulation of Cell Secretion: The Integrated Action of Cyclic AMP and Calcium

M. J. BERRIDGE

Overview

Both cyclic AMP and calcium play a central role in stimulus-secretion coupling. As the function of cyclic AMP is described in detail elsewhere in this volume, the emphasis of this chapter is placed on calcium which often is the key second messenger in secretory cells. The first part of the review describes the mechanisms responsible for generating a calcium signal originating either from calcium entering from the outside or from calcium being released from internal reservoirs. Entry of signal calcium from the external medium is regulated either through voltage-dependent or through agonist-dependent channels.

Voltage-dependent channels are found in synaptic endings, insulin-secreting β-cells and in anterior pituitary cells. The mechanisms responsible for depolarising the membrane to open these voltage-dependent channels varies from tissue to tissue. In β-cells there is a remarkable interplay between glycolysis and a potassium channel which leads to fluctuations in membrane potential. These membrane oscillations trigger bursts of calcium-dependent action potentials which are responsible for releasing insulin. These voltage-dependent channels can be modulated by cyclic AMP which may represent an important site of interaction between these two intracellular signals. The voltage-dependent channels tend to inactivate during prolonged depolarisation and cyclic AMP may act to prevent or alleviate this process of inactivation. Another possible mechanism to avoid channel inactivation is to depolarise the membrane in short bursts which might account for the membrane oscillations which have been described in β-cells and in anterior pituitary cells.

Calcium entry across the plasma membrane can also be regulated by agonists using receptors which are quite separate from those which generate cyclic AMP. There is growing evidence for the hypothesis that the hydrolysis of phosphatidylinositol (PI) is an integral part of the receptor mechanisms responsible for opening specific calcium channels. In many systems, the PI response is apparently independent of calcium; this lends support to the idea that the hydrolysis of this phospholipid may be responsible for generating rather than being a consequence of the calcium signal.

Many secretory cells are capable of mobilizing calcium to support secretory activity when external calcium is removed from the bathing medium. The functional significance of using intracellular calcium might depend upon the fact that the diffusion of calcium in cytoplasm is exceedingly slow. In many secretory systems (mast cells, β-cells, neurosecretory and nerve terminals) the problem of low calcium diffusibility is circumvented by having the secretory process and the signal generator on the same membrane. Stimulus-secretion coupling in these cells is very dependent upon external calcium which flows into the cell to trigger secretion in the immediate vicinity of the membrane. On the other hand, secretory cells which are organised into epithelia usually have the site of signal generation on the basal membrane whereas some of the effector systems lie on the opposite side of the cell. Such systems (salivary glands and pancreas) are much less dependent upon external calcium and seem to be capable of mobilizing calcium from internal reservoirs. This release of internal calcium may represent another important site of interaction between the cyclic nucleotides and calcium because there are numerous reports suggesting that cyclic AMP may act to release calcium from these internal pools.

Further details of the way in which cyclic AMP and calcium interact with each other are provided by considering how secretion is controlled in cells which release vesicles by exocytosis (insulin-secreting β-cells, anterior pituitary, mast cells) and in cells which primarily secrete fluid (parietal cells and pancreas). These secretory cells which combine exocytosis with fluid secretion (e.g. salivary glands and pancreas) provide fascinating systems for unravelling the way in which cells can integrate the action of both cyclic AMP and calcium in order to regulate two independent processes.

A. Introduction

The integrated control networks which characterise the homeostatic mechanisms of multicellular organisms depend on the release and reception of a whole battery of chemical signals. Hormones and neurotransmitters constitute the bulk of these signals which are synthesized and released from a wide range of secretory cell types. Other secretory cells, such as the exocrine glands, form part of the reception system which responds to these external signals. When faced with such a diversity of cell types and secretory functions, it is difficult to formulate too many generalisations concerning how secretion is controlled. However, it is becoming increasingly evident that both calcium and cyclic AMP play a central role in stimulus-secretion coupling.

In many secretory cells, calcium seems to be the primary internal signal responsible for initiating cell secretion (RUBIN 1970; BERRIDGE 1975; RASMUSSEN and GOODMAN 1977). However, the action of calcium is often accompanied by that of cyclic AMP (Fig. 1). The precise action of cyclic AMP is still in doubt. In some cases, it seems to be capable of modulating the calcium signal either positively or negatively (BERRIDGE 1975; RASMUSSEN and GOODMAN 1977). In other cases, cyclic AMP may be able to activate secretion directly although unequivocal evidence for such an action is still lacking. This review will concentrate on the way in which cyclic AMP and calcium are integrated in the control of a variety of secretory processes. Before embarking on a specific description of a representative selection of secretory systems, a brief description of those features of the calcium signalling systems which are common to many secretory cells will be considered first. The general properties of the cyclic AMP signalling system, which is the main subject of this volume, will not be considered in such detail.

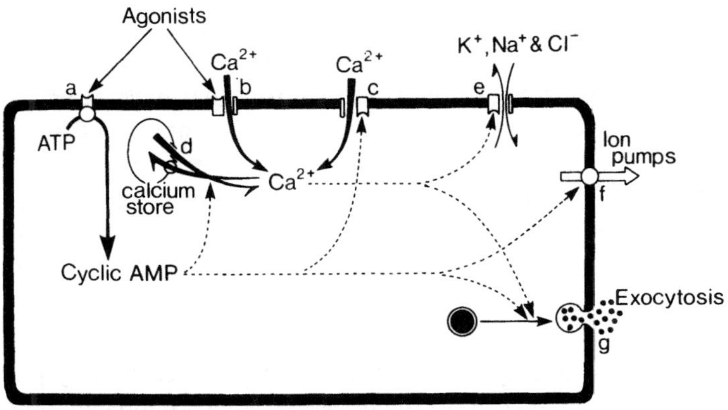

Fig. 1. A summary of the role of cyclic AMP and calcium in the control of secretion. These two intracellular signals can be increased by agonists acting through adenylate cyclase *a* or through calcium channels *b*. In addition to this agonist-dependent increase in calcium entry there are also voltage-dependent calcium channels *c* which are particularly important in excitable cells. Calcium can also be released to the cytoplasm from internal stores *d*. One important action of cyclic AMP is to modulate both the voltage-dependent calcium channels and the calcium stores. Cyclic AMP may also have direct effects on ion pumps *f* and exocytosis *g*. However, the most important intracellular regulator of secretion is calcium which controls ionic permeabilities *e*, ion pumps and exocytosis

B. The Calcium Signalling System

I. General Features

One of the major problems in analysing the role of calcium in cell activation has been to identify the source and the nature of the transducing mechanisms responsible for generating a calcium signal. One difficulty has stemmed from the fact that signal calcium can come either from outside the cell or it can be released from internal reservoirs.

In many secretory cells, an absolute requirement for extracellular calcium clearly indicates that the entry of calcium across the plasma membrane is the main transduction step during stimulus-secretion coupling. On the other hand, there are secretory cells which apparently can derive all their signal calcium form internal reservoirs at least for a short period. The possible relationship between transducing steps at the surface and the mobilisation of this internal calcium will be considered in a later section.

Plasma membranes are largely impermeable to calcium, the cell is surrounded by a barrier separating the very high external concentration of calcium from the low levels (10^{-8} to 10^{-7} *M*) maintained in the intracellular compartment. Many secretagogues act by increasing the permeability of the membrane to calcium which then floods into the cell down its enormous electrochemical gradient. The entry of calcium then raises the intracellular level sufficiently to trigger secretion. A direct demonstration for such an increase in the intracellular level of calcium during stimulation of a secretory system was obtained by injecting the photoprotein aequorin into the presynaptic terminal of the squid giant synapse (LLINÁS et al. 1972). During stimulation there was an increased light output indicating an increase in the free calcium concentration. The degree to which the intracellular calcium changes during stimulus-secretion coupling has not been established with any certainty but indirect techniques suggest that secretory mechanisms may have a calcium sensitivity similar to that of muscle. For example, cells from the adrenal medulla which have been made leaky to calcium through high-voltage electric discharges begin to release catecholamine when the calcium concentration is raised above 10^{-7} *M* (BAKER and KNIGHT 1978). A similar calcium sensitivity has been found for the fusion of secretory vesicles isolated from bovine neurohypophysis (GRATZL et al. 1977).

Another approach to this problem is to measure the intracellular level of calcium directly using calcium-sensitive microelectrodes. Preliminary measurements made on the salivary gland cells of the blowfly *Calliphora* indicate that the resting level of calcium is below 10^{-7} *M* and that the level of intracellular calcium rises to approximately 10^{-6} *M* during stimulation with 5-hydroxytryptamine (BERRIDGE 1980a). Such fluctuations in the level of calcium are certainly consistent with the observed sensitivity of the secretory mechanisms in the adrenal medulla and neurohypophysis described earlier.

The main mechanisms for generating a calcium signal are summarised on Fig. 1. Certain agonists are capable of acting on specific receptors to open calcium channels (Fig. 1 b). In certain secretory cells calcium can enter through voltage-dependent gates (Fig. 1 c). These voltage-dependent gates may be particularly important since there is a growing evidence, as described later, that they may represent one of the sites where cyclic AMP may modulate the calcium signalling system. Calcium may also be released from internal calcium stores (Fig. 1 d) which seem to be particularly important in those secreory cells which are organised into epithelia. These signalling processes will be described in greater detail in subsequent sections.

II. Voltage-Dependent Calcium Channels

Many secretory cells have channels which are sensitive to voltage in that the channels open when the membrane depolarises. In order for such channels to function as part of a calcium-signalling system, it is necessary for the primary signal to first depolarise the membrane. In excitable cells, such as nerve and muscle, this depolarisation is provided by the action potential. In other secretory cells, there are alternative and often more elaborate mechanisms for depolarising the membrane. The glucose-dependent depolarisation of β-cells, for example, results from a reduction in potassium permeability and will be discussed in more detail later (Sect. C.I). Voltage-dependent calcium channels have been extensively analysed in nerve and neurosecretory endings but they may also function in other secretory cells such as in β-cells and in cells of the anterior pituitary. However, these channels are not ubiquitous since they are not found either in exocrine pancreas or in the mammalian salivary gland. If the embryological origins of these cells is taken into consideration, the voltage-dependent channels are only found in cells of neural origin (β-cells, adrenal and anterior pituitary cells). As will be described later, many of these cells are capable of generating action potentials resulting from a phasic opening of these calcium channels which then provides the calcium signal to trigger secretion.

The voltage-dependent calcium gate in the squid giant synapse has been analysed in detail by measuring the presynaptic calcium currents induced by stepwise changes in membrane potential (LLINÁS et al. 1976). A mathematical analysis of the relationship between presynaptic depolarisation and inward calcium current suggested a model for the gate composed of 5 integral proteins. Depolarisation is thought to alter the charge distribution of each monomer such that the five monomers interact with each other to create a channel. A characteristic feature of this channel, which has not been incorporated into the model, is that the channel does not remain open during maintained depolarisation. The channel rapidly closes thus sharply curtailing further calcium entry. This inactivation phenomenon has been described in a number of secretory systems including the adrenal medulla (BAKER and RINK 1975) and the neurohypophysis (NORDMANN 1976). In some cells, such voltage-dependent calcium channels may be modulated by cyclic AMP because this cyclic nucleotide can greatly prolong the calcium-dependent action potentials in certain *Aplysia* nerve cells (KLEIN and KANDEL 1978). This ability of cyclic AMP to enhance the movement of calcium through such voltage-dependent channels might represent an important mode of action of the cyclic nucleotide in regulating the release of thyroid-stimulating hormone (TSH) from the anterior pituitary (SCHREY et al. 1978).

III. Agonist-Dependent Calcium Channels

The second method of regulating calcium entry across the plasma membrane is by way of agonist-dependent channels (Fig. 1 b). Specific agonist-receptor interactions are transduced into an increase in calcium permeability. In contrast to our growing understanding of how agonist-receptor interactions are transduced into an activation of adenylate cyclase [consult the reviews by RALL (1982) and BIRNBAUMER and IVENGAR (1982) for details], we know very little about how receptors might be coupled to calcium channels or gates. Not only are we ignorant about the nature of the transducing mechanisms but we also know very little about the amplification step which, in this case, is a change in calcium permeability. The terms "channels" or "gates" are used purely for descriptive purposes and it is important to stress that the nature of the calcium ionophore has not been established. While there is a certain predilection in assuming that the channel will be proteinaceous, as already proposed for the voltage-dependent channel, there are suggestions that they could be phospholipids such as phosphatidic acid (TYSON et al. 1976). An important reason for studying these receptors and their transducing mechanisms stems from recent observations which indicate that the activation of such receptors can seriously impair the function of those receptors which operate through adenylate cyclase. For example, the stimulation of α-adrenergic or cholinergic receptors in the mammalian salivary gland results in a marked reduction in the ability of norepinephrine to generate cyclic AMP through β-receptors (HARPER and BROOKER 1977; ORON et al. 1978 a, b). The ability of prostaglandin E_1 to increase cyclic AMP in neuroblastoma-glioma hybrid cells was also markedly reduced by activating α-adrenergic or muscarinic receptors (SABOL and NIRENBERG 1979). The receptors which generate these separate second messengers may not exist as independent avenues for passing information into the cell but they seem to interact with each other. Some of these interactions might be mediated through changes in membrane phospholipids.

Many of the agonists which stimulate calcium entry into cells induce a specific hydrolysis of phosphatidylinositol (PI). This so-called PI response was first described (HOKIN and HOKIN 1953, 1954, 1960) in the pancreas and salt gland where acetylcholine caused a specific increase in the turnover of PI without significantly altering the metabolism of the remaining phospholipids. This PI response has now been described in many different tissues (MICHELL 1975) but has remained very much a biochemical curiosity because it has proved difficult to clearly assign a function for this enhanced turnover of PI. Some of the possibilities which have been raised in the literature are of particular relevance to secretory systems. For example, on the basis of studies on the salt gland, HOKIN-NEAVERSON (1977) suggested that the change in PI metabolism in this tissue might be related the activation of tha Na-K-ATPase enzyme responsible for sodium secretion. An alternative view, suggested by MICHELL and his colleagues (MICHELL 1975; MICHELL et al. 1977a, b), is that the PI response in many tissues is connected with the mechanisms responsible for the opening of calcium gates. Yet another possibility is that the hydrolysis of PI may be responsible for triggering exocytosis (HAWTHORNE and PICKARD 1977; PICKARD and HAWTHORNE 1978). It is quite clear, therefore, that the physiological role of this PI response is still not understood. Indeed, HAWTHORNE and PICKARD (1979) have raised the question of whether there is "more than one phosphatidylinositol effect, or one effect and more than one physiological role?" For example, in the latter case one might envisage that the PI response represents a general method for altering membrane function which, in some cells, is expressed as a change in the activity of ion pumps or permeabilities whereas in another cell type it may lead to vesicle fusion. Since this PI response is potentially important for secretory cells, some of its main features will be described with particular emphasis on those aspects where crucial information is lacking.

Phosphatidylinositol (PI) is usually one of the minor plasma membrane phospholipids (of the order of 10%) and there is some evidence to suggest that it is mainly located on the inner leaflet and thus faces the cytoplasm. PI is not restricted to the plasma membrane but is also present in internal membranes. An important question concerning the PI response is whether external signals are capable of increasing the turnover of PI on these internal membranes. In the pancreas, some evidence suggests that most of the PI hydrolysed in response to acetylcholine was located in the rough endoplasmic reticulum (HOKIN-NEAVERSON 1977). However, this conclusion was based on the assumption that the subcellular fractionation technique completely separated plasma-membrane from endoplasmic reticulum. Results from such fractionation techniques are often difficult to interpret and there clearly is a need for more information on the subcellular location of the agonist-dependent hydrolysis of PI. If PI is hydrolysed at such an intracellular location, it will be necessary to invoke the existence of a second messenger to link the surface receptor to the enzymes responsible for this breakdown of PI in internal membranes (HOKIN-NEAVERSON 1977).

PI metabolism is further complicated by the fact that the inositol head group can be phosphorylated by a specific kinase to form diphosphoinositide (DPI) and triphosphoinositide (TPI) (Fig. 2). These polyphosphoinositides, particularly TPI,

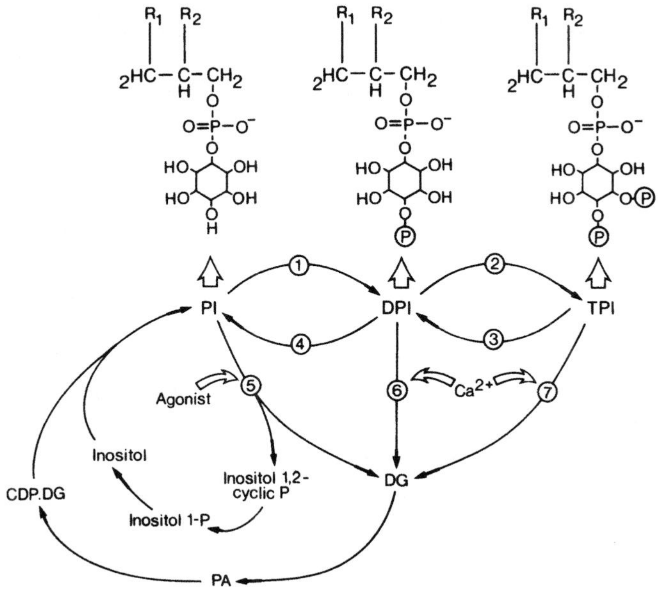

Fig. 2. The structure and metabolism of phosphatidylinositol *PI* and its two derivatives diphosphoinositide *DPI* and triphosphoinositide *TPI*. Specific kinases (enzymes *1* and *2*) are responsible for converting *PI* to *DPI* and *TPI*. These two polyphosphoinositides can be dephosphorylated back to *PI* by the phosphatase enzymes *3* and *4*. Agonists act on a phospholipase C *5* to hydrolyse *PI* to diacylglycerol *DG* which is then converted back to *PI* via phosphatidic acid *PA* and CDP diacylglycerol (CDP · DG). Calcium-dependent phospholipase C-type enzymes (*6* and *7*) hydrolyse *DPI* and *TPI* to *DG*. See text for further details

are of great importance because they bind calcium strongly. A significant proportion of membrane-bound calcium is probably associated with these phosphorylated derivatives of PI. The hydrolysis of such derivatives will thus release membrane-bound calcium leading not only to an increase in the level of intracellular calcium but may also alter the ionic permeability of the membrane as has been postulated in smooth muscle (AKHTAR and ABDEL-LATIF 1978). Since TPI and DPI may have a function separate from PI, it will be important to obtain more information on what factors determine the proportion of each derivative in the membrane. We need to know more about the equilibrium which exists between the kinases (enzymes 1 and 2 in Fig. 2) and the phosphatases (enzymes 3 and 4). TORDA (see MICHELL 1975, for references) has suggested that an interconversion between DPI and TPI might be important in generating action potentials, but this model has been criticized (MICHELL 1975). TORDA (1972) has also raised the possibility that the conversion of DPI to TPI might be sensitive to cyclic AMP; this represents one of the few instances of a proposed interaction between the cyclic nucleotides and PI metabolism. She proposes that cyclic AMP interacts with the regulatory subunit of diphosphoinositide phosphokinase (i.e. enzyme 2 in Fig. 2). It is clear that we need to know more about the factors which regulate the interconversion of these three important phosphoinositides.

The key reaction of the PI response is the hydrolysis of PI to 1,2 diacylglycerol and inositol 1,2-cyclic phosphate by phospholipase C (PI inositolphosphohydrolase or PI phosphodiesterase (Enzyme 5 in Fig. 2). Both DPI and TPI can also be cleaved to diacylglycerol liberating inositol diphosphate and inositol triphosphate respectively (Fig. 2). Unfortunately, there is still considerable uncertainty about the properties of the enzyme(s) mediating this important hydrolytic step which seems to be responsible for the changes in membrane properties mentioned earlier. For example, there is controversy concerning whether the enzyme is membrane-bound (LAPETINA and MICHELL 1973) or soluble (IRVINE and DAWSON 1978). It is also not clear whether there is a single phospholipase C enzyme mediating reaction 5, 6 and 7 (Fig. 2) as has been described for guinea pig intestine (ATHERTON and HAWTHORNE 1968) or whether there are separate enzymes. The responsiveness of this enzyme is of central important and requires clarification. While studies with the isolated enzyme seem to suggest a requirement for calcium, studies of the PI response in vivo presents a more complex picture. In attempting to determine the functional significance of the PI response, it is essential to establish whether or not the hydrolytic step is independent of an increase in the intracellular level of calcium. If calcium is omitted from the bathing medium, there is no effect on the PI response in the parotid (JONES and MICHELL 1975, 1978; ORON et al. 1975), pancreas (HOKIN 1966), adrenal medulla (TRIFARÓ 1969), smooth muscle (AKHTAR and ABDEL-LATIF 1978), hepatocytes (BILLAH and MICHELL 1978; KIRK et al. 1978), peritoneal mast cells (COCKCROFT and GOMPERTS 1979) and the insect salivary gland (FAIN and BERRIDGE 1979 a). In most of these examples, removal of external calcium inhibits cell activation presumably by preventing the intracellular level of calcium increasing sufficiently to trigger secretion. As the PI response was unaffected by this removal of calcium, it is reasonable to assume that the hydrolysis of PI can occur in the absence of a significant rise in the intracellular level of calcium. However, the enzymes which hydrolyse DPI and TPI seem to be sensitive to calcium. Another way of testing the role of calcium is to use the divalent ionophore A 23187 to increase the intracellular level of calcium independently of receptor activation. A 23187 did not induce a PI effect in the parotid (JONES and MICHELL 1975), the insect salivary gland (FAIN and Berridge 1979 a) or in synaptosomes (GRIFFIN and HAWTHORNE 1978). The latter example is particularly interesting because it suggests that there may be significant difference in the calcium sensitivity of the enzyme for hydrolysing PI as compared to those which deal with DPI and TPI. While A 23187 had no effect on the hydrolysis of PI in guinea pig synaptosomes, it did cause a rapid loss of DPI and TPI. Inositol diphosphate was a major product indicating that DPI phosphodiesterase (enzyme 6 in Fig. 2) was the most active form of the phospholipase C-type activity which is calcium-dependent (GRIFFIN and HAWTHORNE 1978). The TPI and DPI in smooth muscle shows a similar sensitivity to calcium during stimulation wich acetylcholine whereas the hydrolysis of PI was not altered by removing calcium (AKHTAR and ABDEL-LATIF 1978).

In summary, the hydrolysis of PI is insensitive to calcium; this is entirely consistent with its proposed role in calcium gating. The hydrolysis of DPI and TPI seem to require calcium; again, this is consistent with at least one of their proposed functions (i.e. exocytosis).

Under normal conditions, the two major products of phospholipase C are diacylglycerol and inositol-1,2-cyclic phosphate (Figs. 2 and 3). At one stage, the latter compound was proposed as an intracellular second messenger by analogy with cyclic AMP (MICHELL and LAPETINA 1972). There is no convincing evidence to support this idea. Some attempts to elicit a hormonal response by direct application of this cyclic derivative to anterior pituitary cells or lymphocytes were unsuccessful (FREINKEL and DAWSON 1973). Such negative results have shifted attention away from a possible second messenger role for the cyclic inositol phosphate. Diacyglycerol, the other product of PI hydrolysis, is converted back to PI through a series of intermediates. In the first step, the diacylglycerol is phosphorylated to phosphatidate which is then converted to CDP diacylglycerol by interacting with CTP. CDP-diacylglycerol represents the precursor which combines with free inositol to reform PI (Figs. 2 and 3). Although it is well established that this is the main pathway for PI synthesis, there is still some doubt concerning the cellular location for this sequence of reactions. Subcellular fractionation studies have revealed that PI synthesis is located mainly in the endoplasmic reticulum (Fig. 3) (MICHELL 1975; VAN GOLDE et al. 1974). Since it is difficult to separate out a plasma membrane fraction, which is usually mixed in with endoplasmic reticular fragments to constitute the microsomal fraction, the possibility that PI synthesis may also take place within the plasma membrane should not be excluded. If synthesis is restricted to the endoplasmic reticulum, then there must be a system of PI exchange proteins to rapidly distribute newly synthesised PI throughout the cell (Fig. 3).

A major unresolved problem concerns the nature of the calcium channel itself. Before further progress can be made in trying to unravel the way in which receptors are coupled to specific channels, it will be imperative to find out more about these channels. One interesting possibility is that the calcium ionophore might be phosphatidic acid (PA) which is formed during the PI response (Fig. 2) (PUTNEY et al. 1980; SALMON and HONEYMAN 1980). In the case of the parotid gland, it was found that PA was capable of inducing the calcium-dependent efflux of ^{86}Rb which is a characteristic action induced by activating muscarinic or α-adrenergic receptors (PUTNEY et al. 1980). It remains to be seen whether PA acts directly as an ionophore or whether it acts indirectly by combining with membrane proteins as proposed by GREEN et al. (1980). The PA formed during the PI response may also play an important role in the interaction which occurs between different receptors because it has been reported that PA results in an inhibition of adenylate cyclase (CLARK et al. 1980).

IV. Mobilization of Internal Calcium

While there has been some progress in our understanding of how calcium enters across the plasma membrane, we know relatively little about how calcium is released from internal reservoirs (Fig. 1 d). There is little doubt that most cells have internal pools of calcium stored within membrane-compartments such as the mitochondria and endoplasmic reticulum but a problem arises in trying to decide whether or not this internal calcium store is used for signaling purposes during stimulus-secretion coupling. For some secretory cells such as the adrenal medulla, mast cells and neurosecretory cells there is clear evidence that stimulation of secretion by normal agonists is almost totally dependent upon external calcium whereas in some exocrine glands, such as the salivary gland (mammalian and insect) and pancreas, normal secretion can continue for considerable periods in the absence of

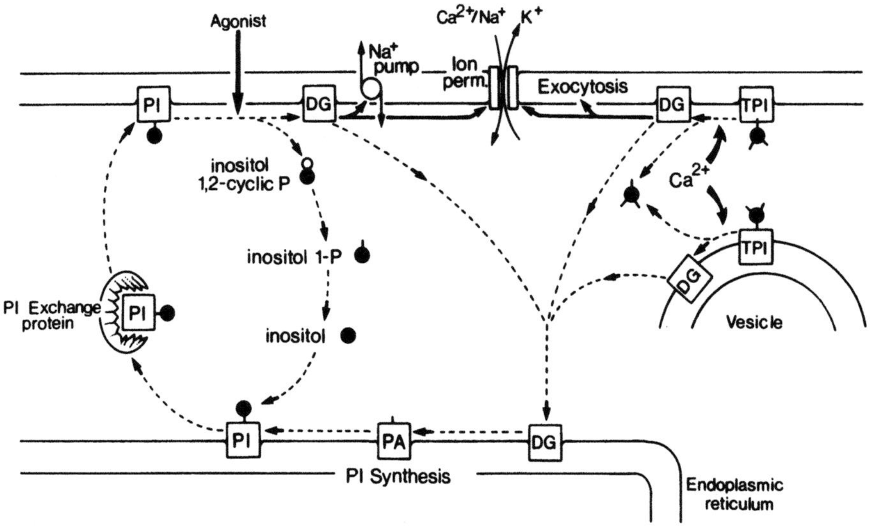

Fig. 3. Summary of the cellular location and some of the proposed functions of the *PI* response. Certain agonists stimulate the hydrolysis of phosphatidylinositol *PI* to diacylglycerol *DG* which may then increase ion permeability including the opening of calcium channels. In the case of the avian salt gland, the turnover of *PI* may be responsible for activating the sodium pump. The hydrolysis of polyphosphoinositides such as TPI depends on calcium and could play a role in mediating exocytosis or it might be responsible for altering sodium and potassium permeabilities. The *DG* formed in these reactions may be converted back into *PI* on the endoplasmic reticulum. Exchange proteins may be responsible for distributing newly-synthesized *PI* to other membranes in the cell

external calcium. This temporary independence of external calcium raises a question concerning which source of calcium is utilised under normal conditions. As yet, there is no indication as to the precise functional significance of intracellular calcium in any secretory system.

Although the "calcium-free" experiments have suggested that intracellular calcium can be mobilised, there is still some doubt concerning the identity of these internal reservoirs. In the light of their enormous capacity to sequester calcium when studied in vitro, the mitochondria are obvious candidates. However, not enough emphasis was paid to studying how much calcium was stored within mitochondria in vivo. Electron microprobe analysis of tissue sections prepared under conditions where calcium redistribution is kept to a minimum, are beginning to reveal that mitochondria within normal cells have very little calcium and certainly not enough to maintain secretion for any length of time (GUPTA and HALL 1978). Studies on smooth muscle have shown similar low values for mitochondrial calcium (SOMLYO et al. 1979). It seems that under normal conditions within the cell, mitochondria do not sequester large quantities of calcium.

This is not to deny that the mitochondria may be important in generating intracellular calcium signals. Recent studies on liver cells, for example, do suggest that there are significant changes in mitochondrial calcium fluxes during stimulation with α-adrenergic agents (BLACKMORE et al. 1979; MURPHY et al. 1980). The way in which surface stimuli alter mitochondrial function are still unknown. The other likely candidate is the endoplasmic reticulum which in skeletal muscle has been modified into a highly efficient calcium storage system which can rapidly release and reaccumulate calcium during a contraction-relaxation cycle. This specialized calcium storage system of the sarcoplasmic system may have developed from a general capacity of the endoplasmic reticulum to store calcium. High levels of calcium have been detected within the endoplasmic reticulum of β-cells (HOWELL et al. 1975) and fat cells (HALES et al. 1974). BLAUSTEIN et al. (1978) have evidence that the smooth endoplasmic reticulum of nerve cells may also store appreciable quantities of calcium. A particularly intriguing aspect of the endoplasmic reticulum which has been described in nerve cells (HENKART et al. 1976) and in fibroblasts (HENKART and NELSON 1979) is that this internal membrane system can lie very close to the plasma membrane. The two membrane system are often connected by regular strands of dense material which closely resemble the tube feet connecting the sarcoplasmic reticulum to the transverse tubular system at the triads in skeletal muscle. As in muscle, this close apposition of internal and external membrane systems might provide a mechanism for coupling surface stimuli to a release of the calcium stored within the endoplasmic reticulum (HENKART and NELSON 1979).

The uncertainty surrounding the identification of calcium stores within non-muscle cells is paralleled by an equal uncertainty concerning the intracellular signals responsible for releasing this calcium during cell activation. Some form of electrical coupling between the surface membrane and the endoplasmic reticulum, as described by HENKART and NELSON (1979) is one possibility. Another possibility is that the coupling is chemical involving some as yet unidentified second messenger. Some likely candidates include calcium itself, cyclic AMP or even inositol-1,2-cyclic phosphate. A phenomenon of calcium-induced calcium release was uncovered in studies on skinned muscle fibres where calcium was able to induce a regenerative release of calcium from the sarcoplasmic reticulum (ENDO et al. 1970; FABIATO and FABIATO 1975). This mechanism may not be restricted to muscle because a similar phenomenon occurs in medaka eggs where a local increase of calcium at the point of fertilization spreads as a wave towards the opposite pole (GILKEY et al. 1978). The possible involvement of cyclic AMP in the regulation of internal calcium has been suggested for a number of secretory systems such as the mammalian salivary gland (PUTNEY et al. 1977; KANAGASUNTHERAM and RANDLE 1976), β-cells (SEHLIN 1976), and the intestine (FRIZZELL 1977). As will be discussed later, however, much of the evidence implicating cyclic AMP as an internal regulator of calcium is indirect and there is no detailed biochemical information describing how this nucleotide might release intracellular calcium. On a more speculative note, it might be worth considering inositol-1,2-cyclic phosphate as a possible regulator of internal calcium. As noted earlier, this cyclic phosphate is formed during the PI response associated with the action of certain agonists. Since the experimental evidence used to rule out a second messenger function for this product is not entirely convincing, more effort should be made to ensure that it does not have some role to play in modulating the movement of intracellular calcium.

It may also be important to consider the possibility that phosphatidic acid, another product of the PI response formed in the plasma membrane may be transferred to the endoplasmic reticulum where it could function to gate calcium before it is converted back to PI. LIMAS (1980) has already reported that phosphatidic acid can increase the release of calcium from cardiac sarcoplasmic reticulum.

In summary, the possible role of stored calcium being used as a source of activator calcium for cell secretion remains very much an open question. This uncertainty concerning the physiological role of intracellular calcium is mirrored by the fact that we know very little about the nature of the signals which regulate this store.

V. The Role of Calcium in Stimulus-Secretion Coupling

Calcium has two main actions in secretory cells, it either triggers the release of preformed granules or vesicles by exocytosis (Fig. 1 g) or it can act on the ionic mechanisms responsible for generating fluid secretion (Fig. 1 e). The precise action of calcium has not been established but an involvement of calmodulin has been suggested for triggering exocytosis at synaptic endings (DELORENZO et al. 1979) and chloride conductance in the intestine (ILUNDAIN and NAFTALIN 1979). There is reason to believe that calcium may act by phosphorylating proteins in the membrane. During stimulus-secretion coupling in mast cells there is a calcium-dependent phosphorylation of specific membrane proteins (SIEGHART et al. 1978). However, the role of these phosphorylated proteins in exocytosis remains to be established. Cyclic AMP may also play a role in initiating secretion but again its precise function has not been established. For example, the release of amylase from the mammalian salivary gland seems to involve cyclic AMP but it is not clear whether the nucleotide stimulates exocytosis directly or whether it acts indirectly by mobilizing intracellular calcium which is then responsible for the final fusion event as proposed by PUTNEY et al. (1977). Another way that cyclic AMP may exert an indirect effect on secretion is to sensitize the secretory processes to the action of calcium.

In addition, to triggering exocytosis, calcium also regulates fluid secretion by activating the ionic mechanisms which create the osmotic gradients for water movement. So far, most information concerning this action of calcium has concentrated on its ability to alter passive permeability to either potassium, chloride or sodium (PUTNEY 1979). PUTNEY has introduced the term "stimulus – permeability coupling" to describe this ability of calcium to regulate the movement of various ions across the membrane (Fig. 1 e). This phenomenon is particularly important in secretory cells because it represents a mechanism whereby calcium controls a number of fluid secreting epithelia. For example, calcium regulates chloride fluxes in the insect salivary gland (BERRIDGE et al. 1975) and in the intestine (FRIZZELL 1977). Calcium also plays an important role in regulating the efflux of potassium and the uptake of sodium by the parotid gland (LANDIS and PUTNEY 1979). There is less information on how the pumps responsible for active transport are regulated. One again finds that cyclic AMP may also be involved in that it seems to be associated with the ability of hormones to initiate fluid secretion in the pancreas (STREWELER and ORLOFF 1977; CASE 1978), intestine (FRIZZELL 1977) parietal cell (SOLL and GROSSMAN 1978; SOLL and WALSH 1979) and the insect salivary gland (BERRIDGE and PRINCE 1972). As with exocytosis, however, it is not clear whether its role is direct or indirect. In the case of the intestine, cyclic AMP seems to act indirectly by mobilizing internal calcium (FRIZZELL 1977).

The picture which is beginning to emerge is that both cyclic AMP and calcium are intimately involved in regulating secretion. However, their precise function remains to be fully established but sufficient information is available to indicate that the relationships existing between these two intracellular signals seems to vary considerably. Such variability may have evolved to provide specialised signaling systems tailor made for the control requirements of each secretory system.

VI. Spatial and Temporal Aspects of Calcium Signalling

Spatial and temporal characteristics of calcium signalling deserve special attention because they may help us to understand some of the subtleties of the mechanisms for controlling secretory activity. The spatial aspect is largely determined by the low diffusibility of calcium in cytoplasm. An early demonstration that calcium diffuses slowly in cytoplasm was obtained using the squid axon where it was found that labelled calcium did not migrate away from its site of injection (BAKER 1976). There was a more dramatic demonstration in the giant salivary gland of an insect where the calcium injected into the cell could be visualised using the photoprotein aequorin (ROSE and LOEWENSTEIN 1975). Once again, calcium was found to spread very slowly away from the site of injection. Calcium was rapidly sequestered by the neighboring organelles which act as a buffering system to severely restrict its movement within the cytoplasmic compartment. Such experiments imply that if generation of the calcium signal is restricted to one region, it is unlikely to spread throughout the cell. This prediction has been confirmed in mast cells where an antigen was immobilised by being linked to a sepharose bead so that it made contact with the cell over a small area. Subsequent electron micrographs revealed that the release of histamine was restricted to a small area near this point of contact (LAWSON et al. 1978). The calcium which entered over a small area could stimulate secretion locally but was incapable of spreading to trigger the release of granules in neighboring parts of the cell.

The mast cell experiment highlights the problem of using calcium as an intracellular signal to transfer information over a distance. In many secretory cells, the problem is circumvented by having the secretory process and the signal generator on the same membrane (e.g. mast cells, β-cells, anterior pituitary cells, neurosecretory and nerve terminals). Stimulus-secretion coupling in these cells is very dependent upon external calcium which flows into the cell to trigger secretion in the immediate vicinity of the membrane. It has been calculated that in β-cells the calcium concentration immediately below the surface might be as high as 0.3 mM but falls away exponentially as calcium diffuses into the cytoplasmic space and is sequestered by the internal membrane systems (MATTHEWS 1975). This rapid decline in the signal as one moves away from the membrane raises the problem of how epithelial cells generate calcium signals. For example, in secretory cells which are organised into epithelia, the site of signal generation (usually the basal surface) is often separated topographically from the effector systems which are usually located on the opposite side of the cell (usually the apical surface). If the signal generator is located exclusively on one surface then calcium must run the cytoplasmic gauntlet in order to reach the opposite surface. It is of some interest, therefore, to find that many of these epithelial cells are much less dependent upon external calcium and seem to have an additional source of calcium which is mobilised from the internal reservoirs described earlier. In some of these cells, cyclic AMP may facilitate calcium diffusion by damping down the internal sequestering system which normally restricts the migration of calcium. Another device for ensuring that a calcium signal will act on the opposite surface of a cell is to reduce the diffusion path which might explain the very elaborate membrane infoldings which characterize many secretory cells (BERRIDGE and OSCHMAN 1972).

While on the subject of morphology, it is important to mention the relationship between cell size and the rate at which the intracellular level of calcium can be altered (MATTHEWS 1979). The larger the cell, the longer it will take for the calcium concentration to rise assuming that all the calcium enters from the outside. This phenomenon may restrict the use of external calcium as a signal for the larger epithelial cells which may be another reason why they seem to be more dependent upon intracellular calcium for signalling purposes as described earlier. A classical example is skeletal muscle where a well-developed sarcoplasmic reticulum surrounds each myofibril thus greatly reducing the diffusion path for calcium during excitation-contraction coupling.

In addition, to these spatial or geometric aspects, it is important to consider calcium signalling in the time domain. There are clear indications that the intracellular level of calcium may oscillate during certain forms of stimulus-secretion coupling (BERRIDGE and RAPP 1979). Although a direct demonstration for such calcium oscillations has been observed in only one system so far (*Aplysia* burster neurone), similar oscillations can be inferred on the basis of the fluctuations in membrane potential which have been described in β-cells (MEISSNER and ATWATER 1976; MATTHEWS and O'CONNOR 1979), anterior pituitary cells (KIDOKORO 1975; POULSEN and WILLIAMS 1976; TARASKEVICH and DOUGLAS 1977, 1978), *Aplysia* burster neurones (THOMAS and GORMAN 1977) and the insect salivary gland (BERRIDGE and RAPP 1979). In the burster neurons of *Aplysia*, there are trains of action potentials riding on the crests of the regular waves of depolarisation. If such neurons are filled with arsenazo III, there are periodic changes in light absorption during each burst indicating that the intracellular level of calcium is oscillating (THOMAS and GORMAN 1977). The membrane events responsible for these membrane oscillations in *Aplysia* neurons are remarkably similar to those found in β-cells (BERRIDGE and RAPP 1979) providing further indication that oscillations in intracellular calcium may be common to many secretory cells.

The functional significance of such calcium oscillations in secretory cells is not immediately apparent. One possibility is that a complex process such as exocytosis cannot proceed continuously without periods of "relaxation" during which the vesicles or membranes are primed for further release. Possibly, the intracellular motile apparatus based on the microtubule-microfilament system might play an important role in moving vesicles towards the surface. As in normal muscle, the contractile activity of these microfilaments may pass through phases of contraction and relaxation thus necessitating regular fluctuations in intracellular calcium. In some secretory systems, a continuous high level of calcium may lead to secretory tetanus.

Another possible function for membrane oscillations is to protect the signal generating system from inactivation. Many of the secretory systems which display oscillations possess voltage-dependent calcium channels which are prone to inactivation as described earlier (Sect. B.II). The regular phases of membrane hyperpolarisation interspersed between the active periods of membrane depolarisation may thus ensure that these channels continue to gate calcium. Some support for this notion comes from β-cells where glucose normally induces the membrane to oscillate with calcium-dependent action potentials riding on the crests of the waves (see Sect. C.I). However, if the membrane potential is kept depolarised with high potassium there is a phasic release of insulin after which secretion falls to a low level (HENQUIN and LAMBERT 1974). HENQUIN and LAMBERT have argued that this decline in insulin release during maintained depolarisation is due to an inactivation of the calcium channels. However, it is important to note that high levels of glucose can also induce prolonged depolarisation without inactivating the channels. The possibility that cyclic AMP may act to prevent such inactivation of the calcium channels will be discussed in the next section (C.I).

These spatial and temporal considerations stress the complexity of intracellular signalling systems. While there are often many common features, it is important to remember that these systems have diverged during evolution to suit the special requirements of each secretory system some of which are described in the following section.

VII. A Description of the Drugs Which are Used to Alter Calcium Metabolism

The role of calcium in cell secretion, as for many other processes, has often been established by studying the effects of manipulating calcium metabolism by a variety of agents. However, every possible caution must be adopted when interpreting such experiments because many of these agents may have more than one action on the cell and such side-effects can be very misleading. The safest approach is not to rely too heavily on the evidence produced from such drug experiments but to use the information as supportive evidence for a possible role of calcium. Perhaps the most useful drugs for manipulating the intracellular level of calcium are the divalent cation ionophores which can be used to bypass the normal mechanisms responsible for generating a calcium signal. The ionophore which as been used most extensively is A 23187 which is a carboxylic acid antibiotic originally introduced by REED and LARDY (1972). Another ionophore X-537A has also been used but is usually less effective. However, X-537A does seem to be capable of mobilizing calcium from internal reservoirs more effectively than A 23187 (THORN et al. 1975). These ionophores are capable of inducing a number of secretory processes such as histamine release from mast cells (FOREMAN et al. 1973; COCHRANE and DOUGLAS 1974), fluid secretion by insect salivary glands (PRINCE et al. 1973), release of potassium from the parotid gland (SELINGER et al. 1974), release of granules from blood platelets (FEINMAN and DETWILER 1974), release of vasopressin from the neurohypophysis (NAKAZATO and DOUGLAS 1974), secretion of amylase by the pancreas and parotid gland (WILLIAMS and LEE 1974; BUTCHER 1975), release of catecholamines from the adrenal medulla (GARCIA et al. 1975), insulin release from β-cells (CHARLES et al. 1975; WOLLHEIM et al. 1975), fluid secretion by the intestine (BOLTON and FIELD 1977; FRIZZELL 1977). Some caution must be exercized in using these ionophores because, as RASMUSSEN and GOODMAN (1977) have pointed out, their effects are both complex and time-dependent. They are also rather hydrophobic molecules and are best first dissolved in ethanol to provide a stock solution which is stable for several days at room temperature if kept in the dark. Immediately before use, aliquots of this stock solution can be added to physiological saline to give the concentration required taking care to add the appropriate amount of ethanol to the control saline. Other ionophores which have been used to introduce calcium into secretory cells include ionomycin (BENNETT et al. 1979; CONN et al. 1980a) and phosphatidic acid (PUTNEY et al. 1980).

Another way of investigating the possible role of calcium is to use a variety of antagonists which are thought to act by blocking the entry of calcium. Perhaps the most effective antagonists are other closely related divalent cations such as cobalt, manganese and nickel (HAGIWARA and TAKAHASHI 1967; BAKER et al. 1973; HENQUIN and LAMBERT 1975). The trivalent cation lanthanum is also an effective antagonist of Ca^{2+}-dependent physiological processes. For example, lanthanum can block the calcium response of nerve terminals (MILEDI 1971) and the release of vasopressin from the posterior pituitary (RUSSELL and THORN 1974). Experiments with lanthanum may be difficult to interpret because it acts by binding with high affinity to most calcium-binding sites and may thus exert a pleiotropic effect. In addition to blocking the entry of calcium, it may displace calcium from the membrane (CHANDLER and WILLIAMS 1974) or block its efflux from the cell (VAN BREEMEN and DE WEER 1970).

Verapamil and its methoxy derivative D 600 were introduced by KOHLHARDT et al. (1972) as selective inhibitors of "transmembrane calcium conductivity." These agents certainly are effective in blocking a number of calcium-dependent secretory processes including glucose-induced insulin secretion (MALAISSE et al. 1975), release of hormones from the pituitary (ETO et al. 1974; RUSSELL and THORN 1974; DREIFUSS et al. 1975). Once again, great care must be exercised in interpreting experiments using verapamil or D 600 because their mode of action is still uncertain. Some of the problems are described by RASMUSSEN and GOODMAN (1977) who point out that the optical isomers of D 600 may exert different effects. The (+) isomer seems to act on the fast sodium channel whereas the (−) isomer is more specific for the calcium channel. In addition to blocking such voltage-dependent ion channels, verapamil and D 600 may also interfere with agonist-dependent calcium gating. However, in this regard it is important to establish whether or not these drugs are acting as receptor blockers rather than as channel blockers.

All the agents described so far are thought to act by preventing the uptake of external calcium. However, as described earlier, many cells seem to be capable of using calcium derived from intracellular stores for signalling purposes. The drug 8(N,N-diethylamino)-octyl 3,4,5-trimethoxybenzoate-HCl (TMB-8) is a calcium antagonist which might act by inhibiting the release of calcium from some internal pool (CHARO et al. 1976). This supposed intracellular calcium antagonists has been shown to block secretion by platelets (CHARO et al. 1976; GORMAN et al. 1979) and human neutrophils (SMITH and IDEN 1979). This drug may thus provide a useful tool for distinguishing whether cells are using extracellular or intracellular calcium.

Disruption of the action of calcium at its intracellular receptor site is another potential way of interfering with the calcium signalling system. It is much more difficult to specifically inhibit events taking place inside the cell than those events occurring on the surface of the plasma membrane. Since many of the actions of calcium are mediated by calmodulin, this receptor protein is the most obvious site of action for inhibitory agents (see CHEUNG and STORM 1982). Studies in vitro have revealed that the phenothiazine antipsychotic agents can interfere with the ability of calmodulin to activate phosphodiesterase (WEISS and LEVIN 1978). Trifluoperazine (TFP) has been used extensively and was found to bind to the calcium-dependent sites of calmodulin with a K_m of 1 μM (LEVIN and WEISS 1977). While there appears to be little doubt that these phenothiazines are extremely important tools for inhibiting the action of calmodulin in vitro it is extremely dangerous to extrapolate such inhibitory effects to the in vivo situation. The main problem is that these agents also exert profound effects on the membrane which include electrical stabilization, membrane expansion and the displacement of membrane-bound calcium (WOLFF and BROSTROM 1979). These phenothiazines may also be potent receptor blockers and may thus act primarily to prevent the generation of a calcium signal. Therefore, if these drugs are found to inhibit a calcium-dependent process in the intact cell, this evidence cannot be used to implicate a functional role for calmodulin unless it can be shown that a normal calcium signal was generated.

C. The Integrated Action of Cyclic AMP and Calcium in the Control of Enzyme and Fluid Secretion

I. Insulin-Secreting *β*-Cells

The release of insulin from *β*-cells is triggered by a rise in the plasma level of glucose and is the culmination of a complicated sequence of intracellular and membrane events. When a *β*-cell is experimentally subjected to a stepwise increase in the level of glucose, insulin is released in two phases. There is an early phasic release lasting for a few minutes followed by a secondary phase which develops more slowly (Fig. 4). The electrical events associated with these two phases of release are complicated. As noted previously, the primary action of glucose is to cause the membrane to depolarise which at some critical threshold induces trains of calcium-dependent action potentials (MATTHEWS and O'CONNOR 1979). The calcium which flows in across the membrane through the voltage-dependent calcium channels provides the intracellular signal which triggers secretion (HEDESKOV 1980). Glucose-induced insulin release is inhibited by a variety of calcium antagonists such as cobalt, lanthanum and D 600 (HENQUIN and LAMBERT 1975; MALAISSE et al. 1975; MATTHEWS 1975). Under normal conditions, therefore, insulin release is very dependent upon external calcium. The possible involvement of internal calcium during certain forms of stimulation will be described later. The burst of action potentials which rides on the crest of the first wave seems to be responsible for the early phasic release of insulin (Fig. 4). After this burst of electrical activity, the membrane potential hyperpolarizes, thus switching off the action potentials; and this period of electrical quiescence corresponds to the trough in insulin release. The onset of the secondary phase of insulin release coincides with the appearance of further action potentials which once again occur on the crests of regular waves of depolarisation. These regular oscillations in membrane potential seem to be an important aspect of the signalling system because if the membrane potential is kept

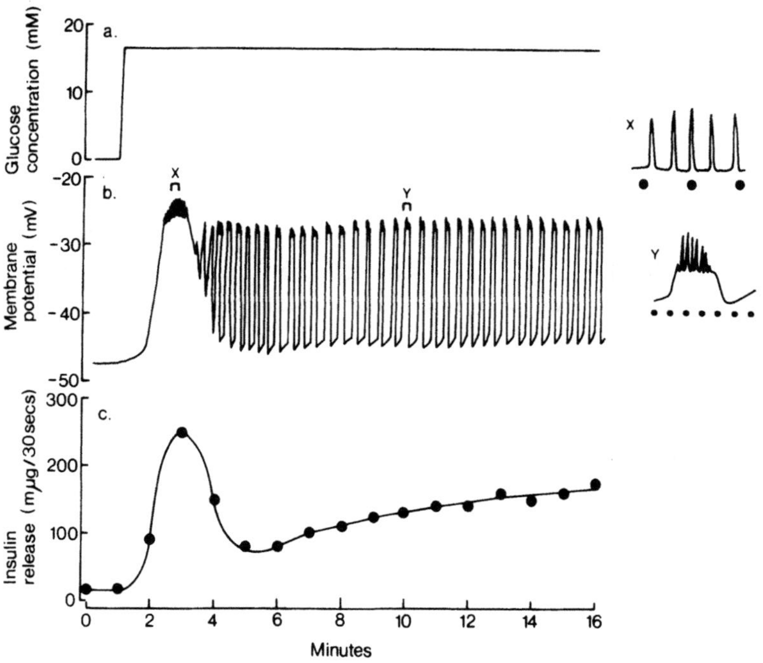

Fig. 4 a–c. The effect of increasing glucose concentration from 0–16.6 m*M* **a** on membrane potential **b** and the release of insulin **c** from β-cells. The early phase of insulin release coincides with a marked membrane depolarisation during which there are rapid calcium-dependent action potentials illustrated at a higher sweep speed in the inset *X*. After this early phasic response, insulin release gradually increases during which the membrane potential shows regular oscillations. The inset *Y* shows that there are action potentials riding on the crests of the waves (The electrical recording was redrawn from MEISSNER and ATWATER 1976; the curve showing insulin release was taken from CURRY et al. 1968)

depolarized either through prolonged treatment with high potassium or with glibenclamide, the secondary phase of insulin release is greatly reduced (MEISSNER and ATWATER 1976; HENQUIN and LAMBERT 1974). Similarly, the regular oscillations characterised by the large hyperpolarising phases are absent in the cells of diabetic mice which are also fairly insensitive to variations in the level of glucose (MEISSNER and SCHMIDT 1976). The next problem to consider, therefore, is how glucose induces these membrane fluctuations which are responsible for triggering the calcium gates.

The voltage trace obtained from these β-cells during glucose infusion is remarkably similar to that seen in burster neurones and some other membrane oscillators (BERRIDGE and RAPP 1979). It is most intriguing to find, therefore, that the unstable membrane potentials found in all these oscillatory systems is primarily caused by regular fluctuations in potassium conductance. When this potassium conductance is decreased, the membrane depolarizes; when this conductance is increased, the membrane hyperpolarizes. MATTHEWS and O'CONNOR (1979) have developed a detailed mathematical model which can account for these membrane oscillations by including this variable potassium conductance. At the troughs, where the potassium conductance is high, there is a low membrane resistance while the reverse is true at the crests (ATWATER et al. 1978). What is particularly interesting

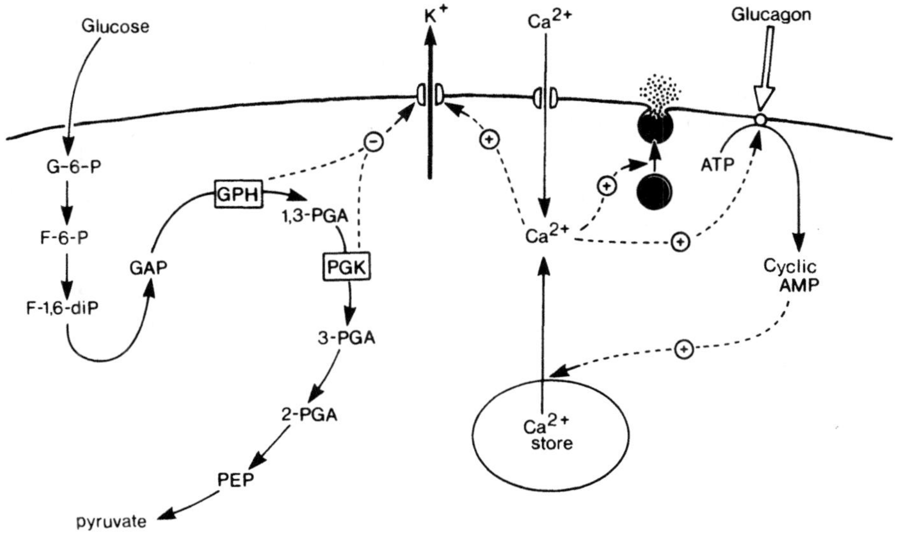

Fig. 5. A summary of the major factors responsible for regulating the release of insulin. The main calcium signal originates from the entry of this cation through voltage-dependent calcium gates. Glucose regulates whether these channels are opened or closed by adjusting the potential of the membrane by manipulating a potassium channel which is somehow sensitive to the rate at which metabolites pass through the glycolytic pathway. These potassium channels are also sensitive to calcium and these different control loops combine to generate potential oscillations (Fig. 4). See text for further details

about this conductance is its sensitivity to glucose (MALAISSE et al. 1978). Glucose must be metabolised via the glycolytic pathway in order for it to reduce potassium permeability (HENQUIN 1980a). It is the flux of intermediates through two key enzymes (glyceraldehyde phosphate dehydrogenase and phosphoglycerate kinase) which seems to be responsible for causing the membrane to depolarise by reducing potassium permeability (Fig. 5) (DEAN et al. 1975; MATTHEWS and O'CONNOR 1979). The effect of glucose on potassium permeability is rapid and reversible (HENQUIN 1978a; MALAISSE et al. 1978) which is essential if it is going to contribute to the membrane oscillations. If glucose reduces potassium conductance leading to membrane depolarisation and action potentials, the next question to consider is why the membrane hyperpolarises at the end of each burst. As in many of the membrane oscillators mentioned earlier, the potassium conductance mechanism in β-cells appears to be calcium-dependent (HENQUIN 1979; RIBALET and BEIGELMAN 1979). Therefore, during each burst of action potentials calcium will enter the cell and will function not only to trigger insulin release but also to hyperpolarise the membrane by switching on the same potassium conductance originally turned off by glucose (Fig. 5). Thus the potassium conductance acts as the focal point for the opposing actions of glucose and calcium (HENQUIN 1979). If β-cells are treated with the potassium ionophore valinomycin, which artificially increases potassium permeability, then the membrane remains hyperpolarised and insulin release is blocked (HENQUIN and MEISSNER 1978). On the other hand, tetraethylammonium (TEA) and 9-aminoacridine which acts to reduce the effectiveness of the natural glucose-sensitive potassium channels will act to potentiate the action of glucose (HENQUIN 1979; HENQUIN et al. 1979). The main factors responsible for regulating membrane potential and hence the state of the voltage-dependent calcium channels are thus becoming more and more apparent.

Even though the entry of calcium through these voltage-dependent calcium channels seems to be the main source of activator calcium, there are numerous suggestions that intracellular calcium may play an important role especially under certain conditions (HEDESKOV 1980). β-Cells are known to contain large stores of calcium (HOWELL et al. 1975; MATTHEWS 1979). While there is some evidence that this internal calcium is under physiological control (HOWELL et al. 1975; SEHLIN 1976), there are a number of uncertainties surrounding the function of intracellular calcium. Firstly, there are differing views concerning when this internal calcium is used during a normal secretory response. WOLLHEIM et al. (1978) using verapamil to block calcium entry found that the early phase is unaffected but the secondary phase is blocked. On the other hand, HENQUIN (1978b) and SIEGEL et al. (1980) consider that the early phase has an absolute requirement for calcium. Some of these differences may have arisen from different methods of pretreatment. Nevertheless, there are indications that internal calcium can be used especially during the action of methyl xanthines such as theophylline and caffeine which can overcome the inhibitory effect of removing external calcium (SOMERS et al. 1976; HENQUIN 1978b). Another area of uncertainty concerns the way in which this internal calciums is mobilised during a typical secretory response.

The ability of theophylline to overcome the lack of external calcium raises the question of a possible role for cyclic AMP in insulin release. Despite earlier reports that glucose had no effect on adenylate cyclase, subsequent studies have confirmed that, in intact β-cells, glucose does cause a significant increase in the level of cyclic AMP (ZAWALICH et al. 1975; CHARLES et al. 1975). Some confusion has arisen because glucose acts indirectly by first generating a calcium signal which then stimulates adenylate cyclase (in addition to triggering insulin release) (Fig. 5). As in several other systems, the ability of calcium to activate adenylate cyclase might be mediated through calmodulin (SUGDEN et al. 1979; VALVERDE et al. 1979). Since the level of cyclic AMP rises as a secondary consequence of the increase in calcium, it has not been easy to clearly establish a role for cyclic AMP in insulin release. Cyclic AMP also functions as the second messenger for glucagon which is another agent capable of potentiating the action of glucose (BERRIDGE 1975).

Cyclic AMP certainly does not appear to have a direct role in triggering insulin release because its level can be increased to high levels with methyl xanthines without inducing a release of insulin. CHARLES et al. (1975) have suggested that cyclic AMP may function as a "positive feed-forward" signal on the secretory process. At least two mechanisms have been proposed for this facilitatory action of cyclic AMP. Cyclic AMP may act to inhibit the uptake of calcium into the internal reservoirs thus functioning to stabilize and prolong the calcium signal (SEHLIN 1976; MATTHEWS 1979). The inability to release insulin in certain diabetic lesions could arise from a defect in the handling of internal calcium (SIEGEL et al. 1979). HEDESKOV and CAPITO (1975) have also suggested that the decreased sensitivity of the release mechanism during starvation may arise from some defect of the internal calcium system perhaps due to a failure to generate cyclic AMP. Secondly, cyclic

AMP might act by sensitizing the granule release mechanism (SIEGEL et al. 1979). SIEGEL et al. (1979) have made the interesting observation that in diabetic hamsters isobutyl methyl xanthine can greatly enhance insulin release without the concomitant increase in ^{45}Ca efflux seen in normal animals.

Another possibility worth considering is that cyclic AMP may exert some of its effects by preventing inactivation of the voltage-dependent calcium channels. Some support for such an action of cyclic AMP is certainly consistent with the observation that theophylline can overcome the inactivation which sets in during the action of tolbutamide (HENQUIN 1980b). When islets cells are stimulated with high concentrations of this sulphonylurea there is a phasic release of insulin even though this drug keeps the membrane depolarised. As noted earlier (Sect. B.II), the voltage-dependent calcium channel is prone to inactivation during prolonged depolarisation. The reduction in insulin release during tolbutamide stimulation may thus result from an inactivation of these channels (HENQUIN 1980b). The fact that theophylline can reverse this inactivation of insulin release would certainly be consistent with the idea that cyclic AMP acts to alleviate this channel inactivation. Such an action would provide a mechanism to account for its proposed role as a positive "feed forward signal."

II. Anterior Pituitary Gland

The anterior pituitary is a heterogeneous organ containing groups of cells specialised for the synthesis and release of different hormones. The secretion of these hormones is regulated by specific neurohormones from the hypothalamus and by the feedback action of hormones coming from the gonads, adrenal and thyroid. It is difficult to form any generalization concerning the mode of action of these neurohormones and it is advisable to treat each system separately. However, both cyclic AMP and calcium have been implicated as second messengers in many of these cells, thereby providing further examples of the integrated action of cyclic AMP and calcium in cell secretion. As in many other secretory cells, the role of calcium is complicated by the fact that some anterior pituitary cells can use intracellular calcium. Much of the earlier work on calcium has been reviewed by MORIARTY (1978) who draws analogies with different muscles concerning the role of either internal or external calcium. The analogy with muscle is further exemplified by the discovery that many pituitary cells have action potentials and the frequency of these action potentials can be modulated by agents which regulate secretion (KIDOKORO 1975; DAVIS and HADLEY 1976; BIALES et al. 1977; DOUGLAS and TARASKEVICH 1978; DUFY et al. 1979; TARASKEVICH and DOUGLAS 1978, 1979; OZAWA and MIYAZAKI 1979). The way in which hormone release from the pituitary is controlled will thus depend upon a careful orchestration of electrical events in the membrane with underlying biochemical processes. Some selected examples have been chosen to illustrate how second messengers regulate hormone secretion from the pituitary (see also LABRIE et al., this volume).

Adrenocorticotropic hormone (ACTH) is synthesized and released from large irregularly shaped cells comprising less than 1% of the anterior pituitary cell population. A corticotropin-releasing hormone (CRH) secreted from specific hypothalamic neurosecretory cells is responsible for stimulating the release of ACTH. CRH may act through cyclic AMP because both dibutyryl cyclic AMP and theophylline can stimulate the release of ACTH (Eto et al. 1974; Milligan and Kraicer 1974). As in many other secretory systems, the release mechanism seems also to be sensitive to calcium because depolarisation of the membrane with high potassium stimulates an uptake of calcium and triggers the release of ACTH. These cells thus have voltage-dependent calcium channels but they apparently do not function during normal release because CRH was not able to increase the uptake of calcium (ETO et al. 1974). Crude hypothalamic extracts, which presumably contained CRH, were also able to stimulate the release of ACTH in calcium-free conditions (Milligan and Kraicer 1974). CRH may thus act by first of all forming cyclic AMP which then acts on the intracellular stores to release calcium.

The release of growth hormone (GH) from purified somatotrophs may be controlled in a manner similar to that just described for ACTH. Release of GH is dependent on both cyclic AMP and calcium (Spence et al. 1980). It is proposed that the initial signal is an increase in the intracellular level of cyclic AMP which then acts to raise the level of calcium.

Thyrotropin (TSH) release from thyrotrophs is stimulated by the tripeptide thyrotropin-releasing hormone (TRH). Evidence to implicate a role for cyclic AMP in the action of TRH is summarised by Labrie et al. (1979). Somatostatin, which inhibits the release of TSH, was found to prevent this increase in cyclic AMP thus indicating that this cyclic nucleotide has a central role to play in stimulus-secretion coupling.

Calcium may also be important because the stimulatory effect of TRH required external calcium (Vale et al. 1967). Membrane depolarisation with high potassium also produced a calcium-dependent release of TSH which implies the existence of voltage-dependent calcium channels (Vale and Guillemin 1967; Eto et al. 1974). The presence of such channels may be particularly important because they may be responsible for the spontaneous action potentials which have been recorded from pituitary cells in culture (Taraskevich and Douglas 1977; Ozawa and Kimura 1979). These action potentials are insensitive to tetrodotoxin but are suppressed by D 600, lanthanum or cobalt suggesting that they are calcium spikes. Tashjian et al. (1978) have shown that the spontaneous release of TSH is inhibited by cobalt or by calcium-free solutions thus indicating that these spontaneous action potentials are functionally important for stimulus-secretion coupling. The calcium which enters during these action potentials may be responsible for initiating TSH secretion because TRH can enhance the frequency of spontaneously active cells or it can elicit action potentials in silent cells (Fig. 6). Ozawa and Kimura (1979) have suggested that TRH may act by increasing the generation of spikes. Such a positive chronotropic effect would thus be anologous to the mode of action of adrenaline on the sinoatrial node of the heart (Berridge and Rapp 1979). As in the heart, this stimulatory effect of TRH might be mediated through cyclic AMP (Wilber et al. 1969; Schrey et al. 1978).

All the evidence thus points to the fact that both cyclic AMP and calcium play an integral role in regulating the release of TSH. These two second messengers seem to exhibit a "co-operative intracellular relationship" which has been analysed by Schrey et al. (1978). They have proposed that the initial response is due to the entry of calcium probably mediated by the action potentials described earlier.

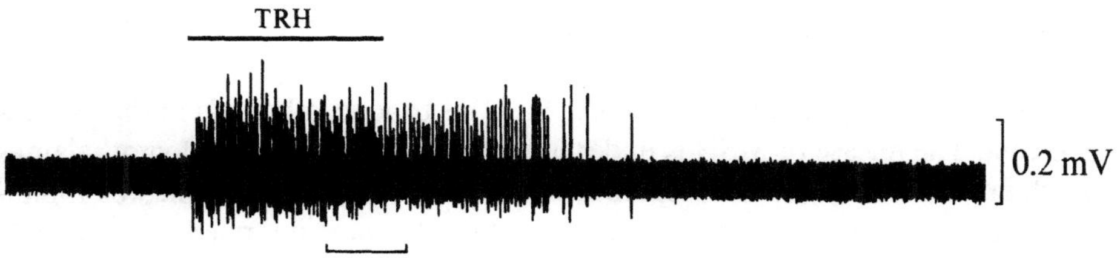

Fig. 6. A recording of the electrical activity of an adenohypophyseal cell during the application of *TRH*. The cell was initially silent but responded to TRH with bursts of action potentials. The horizontal marker represents 10 seconds (TARASKEVICH and DOUGLAS 1977)

Cyclic AMP seems to act by facilitating this calcium signalling system either by potentiating the entry of calcium across the plasma-membrane or by releasing this ion from internal stores (SCHREY et al. 1978).

Luteinizing hormone (LH) release is stimulated by the peptide luteinizing hormone-releasing hormone (LH-RH) produced in the hypothalamus. The kinetics of LH release following stimulation with LH-RH have been studied in dissociated cells (WALKER and HOPKINS 1978) and are remarkably similar to those just described for insulin release from β-cells. Immediately after applying LH-RH, there is a rapid but phasic increase in secretion which returns close to resting conditions after about 6 min. Following this phasic response there is a more gradual but longer-lasting response. Cyclic AMP, cyclic GMP and calcium have all been implicated in the action of LH-RH. During the action of LH-RH there certainly is an increase in the level of both cyclic GMP and cyclic AMP (NAOR et al. 1978; KAWAKAMI and KIMURA 1980) but these nucleotides may not be directly responsible for initiating the release of LH. Large increases in the levels of cyclic GMP can be induced by sodium nitroprusside without causing any secretion. Such observations have led NAOR and CATT (1980) to propose that the change in cyclic GMP level which occurs during the action of LH-RH is a secondary event caused by a change in calcium which is responsible for the release of LH.

The possible role of cyclic AMP in regulating the release of LH has also being questioned (RATNER et al. 1976; CONN et al. 1979). Earlier reports showing that LH-RH induced an increase in the intracellular level of cyclic AMP (BORGEAT et al. 1972) have been confirmed by one group (KAWAKAMI and KIMURA 1980) but not by another (RATNER et al. 1976). LH-RH can also bind to purified membranes without stimulating adenylate cyclase (CLAYTON et al. 1978). The role of cyclic AMP thus remains somewhat of an open question and future studies on this cyclic nucleotide must be done in relation to parallel studies on calcium which does seem to be an important regulator for LH release (CONN et al. 1980a, b). These cells seem to possess voltage-dependent calcium channels because the release of LH can be stimulated by depolarising the membrane with high potassium (SAMLI and GESCHWIND 1968; KATSUMI et al. 1969). This effect of high potassium was completely abolished by removing external calcium. On the other hand, the action of LH-RH seems to be less susceptible to the removal of external calcium (KATSUMI et al. 1969; HOPKINS and WALKER 1978). Such observations once again suggest the possible involvement of intracellular calcium. It is still not known how LH-RH act to produce a calcium signal but there are indications for an involvement of both internal and external calcium.

Melanophore-stimulating hormone (MSH) is produced by cells in the pars intermedia. The release of MSH is under inhibitory control from the hypothalamus which implies that the cells are spontaneously active and are controlled by inhibition rather than by stimulation. Secretory cells in the pars intermedia are capable of generating spontaneous action potentials which seem to play some role in this endogenous control of MSH secretion (DAVIS and HADLEY 1976; DOUGLAS and TARASKEVICH 1978; TARASKEVICH and DOUGLAS 1979). The relationship between these action potentials and the onset of secretion is still unclear. The whole subject is complicated by the fact that the ionic nature of these action potentials seems to vary from species to species. In the rat, the action potentials are predominantly due to sodium (DOUGLAS and TARASKEVICH 1978) whereas in the lizard there clearly is a significant contribution from calcium (TARASKEVICH and DOUGLAS 1979). What remains to be determined is the precise role of calcium. Experiments where calcium has been omitted from the bathing medium suggest that this ion is essential for secretion (HOPKINS 1970; BOWER and HADLEY 1972). However, this apparent requirement for calcium was based on information obtained from studies where cells were incubated in calcium-free media for long periods which makes it difficult to decide whether the decline in secretion was due to the removal of external calcium or due to a depletion of some internal pool. The precise role of calcium will have to be established before it is possible to understand how various agents modulate this secretory activity.

The adrenergic system is one important pathway for modulating the release of MSH. Cells in the intermediate lobe of rats possess both β-receptors and receptors for dopamine. What is particularly interesting is that these two adrenergic agents exert opposite effects on MSH secretion (COTE et al. 1980; MUNEMURA et al. 1980). When cells are stimulated with the β-adrenergic agent isoproterenol there is a dose-dependent increase in both intracellular cyclic AMP and in the secretion of MSH. The ability of isoproterenol to elevate the level of cyclic AMP was greatly enhanced by the addition of phosphodiesterase inhibitors such as theophylline and isobutylmethylxanthine (MUNEMURA et al. 1980). A role for cyclic AMP is also suggested by the observation that MSH secretion can be induced by the addition of dibutyryl cyclic AMP (BAKER 1974). The ability of dopamine to reduce the spontaneous release of MSH may also be mediated through cyclic AMP. Dopamine was found to greatly reduce the effects of isoproterenol on cyclic AMP accumulation and MSH secretion (MUNEMURA et al. 1980). These observations suggest that the spontaneous release can be increased or decreased simply by varying the intracellular level of cyclic AMP. It remains to be established just how such variations in cyclic AMP level interact with the electrical events to bring about changes in the rate of secretion. It is interesting to note that dopamine, which inhibits spontaneous secretion, does slow and sometimes abolishes the spontaneous action potentials in the intermediate lobe of the rat (DOUGLAS and TARASKEVICH 1978). Unfortunately, norepinephrine which presumably acts on the stimulatory β-receptors was found to act like dopamine. Such inconsistencies clearly indicate that there still is a lot to learn about the way in which cyclic nucleotides and calcium interact to regulate the release of MSH.

In addition to blocking the entry of calcium, dopamine could act at some later step as has been suggested by TAM and DANNIES (1980). They found that the dopamine agonist bromocriptine was able to inhibit the release of prolactin from pituitary cells which had been stimulated with the ionophore A 23187.

III. Mast Cells

The release of histamine from mast cells is triggered when antigens interact with immunoglobin molecules embedded in the membrane which therefore function much like conventional receptors. In addition to this immunological mechanism, a number of other chemical agents such as polymeric amines (e.g. compound 48/80), polysaccharides, and ATP will also induce the release of histamine (KAZIMIERCZAK and DIAMANT 1978). The more physiological release process induced in response to specific antigens will be considered here. This antigen-induced release of histamine seems to be mediated by an influx of external calcium (KAZIMIERCZAK and DIAMANT 1978; GOMPERTS 1976). As described earlier (Sect. B.VI), this release process can be restricted to a small part of the cell if the stimulus is applied locally by linking the antigen to a Sepharose bead (LAWSON et al. 1978). This restricted sphere of action probably implies that there are various intracellular uptake mechanisms preventing the signal from spreading through the cell. LAWSON et al. (1978) also point out that mast cells have relatively few mitochondria so there must be other mechanisms for buffering calcium to restrict its diffusion. Histamine release is thus triggered primarily by calcium entering the cell from outside.

This antigen-mediated increase in calcium permeability has much in common with the more conventional agonist-dependent calcium gating mechanisms described earlier. In particular, the action of specific antigens is associated with a large increase in the incorporation of [^{32}P] or [^{3}H]-inositol into PI (COCKCROFT and GOMPERTS 1979; KENNERLY et al. 1979). This PI response was observed even in the absence of external calcium. It is conceivable that inactivation of this transducing mechanism might be responsible for the phenomenon of desensitization which sets in rapidly during continuous treatment with antigen. FOREMAN and GARLAND (1974) have shown that this desensitization can occur in the absence of external calcium and that another acidic phospholipid, phosphatidylserine, can reduce the rate of desensitization. It is of some interest, therefore, to find that the antigen-induced PI response in mast cells was potentiated by phosphatidylserine. Both phosphatidylinositol and phosphatidylserine thus seem to be intimately involved in regulation the entry of calcium into mast cells.

Cyclic AMP has also been implicated in the control of mast cell secretion where it appears to exert an inhibitory effect (BERRIDGE 1975; GOMPERTS 1976). Before describing the mechanism which has been proposed for the inhibitory effect it is important to stress that some doubts have been expressed concerning this role of cyclic AMP (KAZIMIERCZAK and DIAMENT 1978; NORN et al. 1980). An increase in the intracellular level of cyclic AMP is not always associated with an inhibition of histamine release. Attempts to correlate total cell levels of cyclic AMP with a particular physiological response particularly one associated with the surface membrane, may not be very instructive. However, such reservations must be borne in mind in future experiments designed to test the following hypothesis concerning the mode of action of cyclic AMP. Foreman et al. (1975) have suggested that cyclic AMP may exert its inhibitory effect by acting directly on the calcium gates to reduce the entry of calcium. The calcium gates may thus represent the focal point for agents operating from the outside via the hydrolysis of PI and for the opposing effect of cyclic AMP acting from within. In fact, cyclic AMP might act by switching off the PI response (Norn et al. 1980). Such a possibility is supported by the finding that agents which elevate the level of cyclic AMP will simultaneously reduce the PI response (Kennerly et al. 1979).

IV. Exocrine Pancreas

The exocrine pancreas is a heterogenous tissue with enzymes being released from the large acinar cells whereas fluid is secreted mainly by the centro-acinar cells (Kanno and Yamamoto 1977). However, this distinction is not always so clear because, in the rat, the acinar cells are capable of considerable fluid secretion although the mechanism seems to be different to that found in the centro-acinar cells (Petersen and Ueda 1977).

Not much is known about how the secretory activity of the centro-acinar cells is regulated. The primary signal is secretin which seems to act through cyclic AMP (Streweler and Orloff 1977; Case 1978). Just how cyclic AMP acts to increase the secretion of sodium and bicarbonate has not been established. The ability of secretin to stimulate fluid secretion is apparently independent of external calcium (Kanno and Yamamoto 1977).

Much more attention has been focused on the control of enzyme release from the acinar cells which are sensitive not only to a neurotransmitter (acetylcholine) but also to a polypeptide hormone cholecystokinin-pancreozymin (CCK-PZ) (Schulz and Stolze 1980). Although these two secretagogues act on separate receptors, they seem to share a common intracellular signalling system centered primarily around calcium (Fig. 7). There have been some reports suggesting that cyclic AMP may be important, especially for the action of CCK-PZ, but the current opinion is that this cyclic nucleotide does not play a significant role in regulating the release of enzymes from the pancreas (Case 1978; Singh 1979; Schulz and Stolze 1980). Much more controversy surrounds the other nucleotide cyclic GMP. There is little doubt that its level increases rapidly in response to CCK-PZ or acetylcholine (Albano et al. 1976a; Kapoor and Krishna 1978; Case 1978; Gardner 1979). As in many other systems, this increase in the intracellular level of cyclic GMP seems to be linked to a rise in the level of calcium (Christophe et al. 1976; Lopatin and Gardner 1978; Singh 1979). The controversy concerns the functional significance of this enhanced level of cyclic GMP. Albano et al. (1976a, 1979) consider that cyclic GMP plays an important second messenger role in enzyme release whereas others consider that it has no role to play in stimulus-secretion coupling (Gunther and Jamieson 1979; Singh 1979). When the pancreas is stimulated with certain agents such as N-methyl-N′-nitro-N-nitroso guanidine (MNNG), hydroxylamine or sodium nitroprusside, the intracellular level of cyclic GMP rises to very high levels but there was no release of enzyme (Gunther and Jamieson 1979). There is thus little evidence for a direct role for either cyclic AMP or cyclic GMP

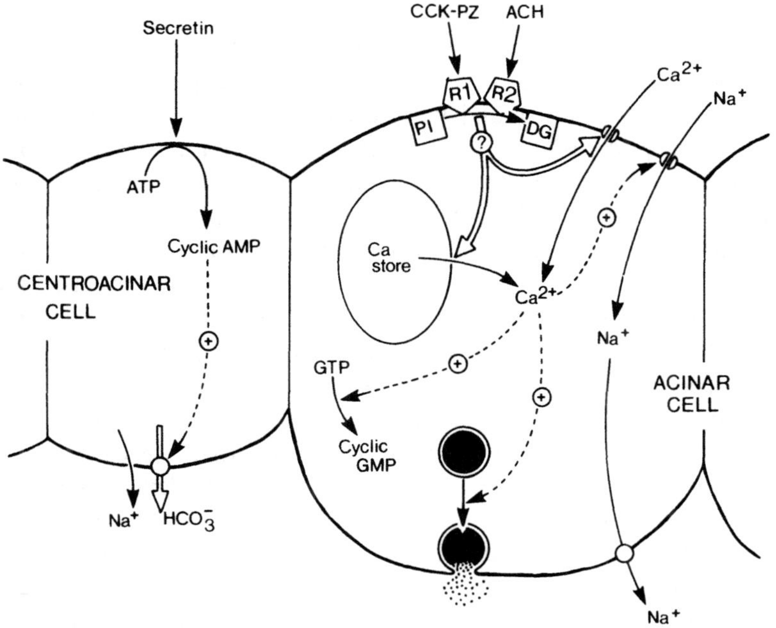

Fig. 7. Stimulus-secretion coupling in the exocrine pancreas. Secretin acts primarily on the centroacinar (duct) cells using cyclic AMP as an intermediary to stimulate bicarbonate-dependent fluid secretion. Cholecystokinin-pancreozymin *CCK-PZ* and acetylcholine *ACh*, which act on separate receptors (*R1* and *R2* respectively) on the acinar cells, are both capable of inducing the hydrolysis of phosphatidylinositol *PI* to diacylglycerol *DG*. This hydrolysis may somehow be linked to the generation of a calcium signal either by promoting the entry of external calcium or by releasing it from some internal store. The rise in internal calcium has at least three consequences, it triggers the release of enzymes, promotes the entry of sodium and stimulates the synthesis of cyclic GMP

in the control of enzyme release although they could be important in adjusting or modulating the level of calcium through various interactions (HEISLER 1976; SINGH 1979).

Even though calcium has been recognised as the primary second messenger, there is still considerable doubt about how this signal is generated. The problem arises from the observation that high levels of enzyme secretion can occur for a considerable period in the absence of external calcium. Whether this temporary independence from external calcium implies that acinar cells rely exclusively upon internal calcium under normal conditions is difficult to resolve. KANNO and NISHIMURA (1976) favour the view that an influx of calcium from the outside is the most important source of activator calcium. Studies on the effect of secretagogues on the uptake of ^{45}Ca have not resolved the problem because, while some authors have reported an increased uptake, others have seen no change (CASE 1978). RENCKENS et al. (1978) consider that many of these differences may have arisen from the use of different experimental techniques. They consider that the primary action of acetylcholine or CCK-PZ is to release calcium from some internal store which initiates secretion which is then maintained by a subsequent uptake of external calcium due to an increase in membrane permeability. PETERSEN and UEDA (1976) also consider that in order for secretion to be sustained at a high level it may be necessary to have an enhanced entry of external calcium. Such a two-stage hypothesis has also been proposed as a result of an electrophysiological study on pancreatic cells of the mouse (Laugier and Petersen 1980). The first action of cholinergic agents or the peptides is to mobilize internal calcium but this initial signal is then maintained by an influx of external calcium. A clear indication that one action of the secretagogue is to mobilize internal calcium is indicated by the large increases in ^{45}Ca efflux which preceed or accompany the onset of secretion (Case and Clausen 1973; Matthews et al. 1973). This enhanced efflux of labelled calcium can occur in the absence of external calcium and thus indicates that the secretagogues can somehow alter the distribution of internal calcium.

One aspect of stimulus-secretion coupling in pancreas is thus analogous to excitation-contraction coupling in muscle. How does a signal arriving at the surface of the cell lead to a release of calcium from some internal reservoir? This question is compounded by the fact that the nature of this internal calcium pool is uncertain. Using chlorotetracycline as a fluorescent probe, Chandler and Williams (1978) have implicated the mitochondria but it was not possible to decide whether these organelles were actually responsible for sequestering the calcium or whether they simply provided the energy for a neighbouring organelle. Electron microprobe X-ray analysis of thin sections of pancreas has implicated the endoplasmic reticulum as the calcium store because soon after the application of acetylcholine there was a large fall in the calcium content of this organelle (P. F. Heap and K. D. Bhoola, personal communication). If the endoplasmic reticulum does turn out to be an important source of calcium during stimulus-secretion coupling, then the analogy with muscle will be very close. Another possible source of activator calcium is the plasma membrane itself, calcium may be bound to the inner surface and released to the cytoplasm when secretagogues bind to external receptors (Matthews et al. 1973; Schulz and Stolze 1980). Indeed, it has been proposed that the release of this membrane bound calcium might be responsible for the increase in permeability which permits the entry of external calcium (Laugier and Petersen 1980).

The pancreatic receptors seem to be connected in some way with an internal membrane system which stores calcium. The coupling is apparently not electrical because there is no release of calcium even when the membrane is depolarised with a high potassium solution. Acetylcholine and CCK-PZ are still effective even when the membrane is in this depolarised condition. Since both agonists show a pronounced PI response, the hydrolysis of phosphatidylinositol may play some role in coupling these surface receptors to the generation of a calcium signal (Fig. 7). It was while studying the pancreas that Hokin and Hokin (1953, 1954) first discovered the PI response. The precise location of the increased turnover of PI is uncertain because there are indications that most newly synthesized PI is found in the endoplasmic reticulum (Case 1978). Whether or not this implies high breakdown at the level of the ER or simply reflects the site of synthesis is uncertain. In formulating their hypothesis concerning the role of PI hydrolysis in calcium gating, Michell and his colleagues have concentrated on effects at the plasma membrane (Michell 1975; Michell et al. 1977a, b). However, as pointed out by Gardner (1979) the hydrolysis of PI may also play a direct role in the release of internal calcium.

Another possibility is that the mobilization of internal calcium is triggered by an increase in internal sodium (CASE and CLAUSEN 1973; WILLIAMS 1975). However, electrophysiological studies have revealed that the increase in sodium permeability which accounts for the depolarisation which accompanies the action of acetylcholine or CCK-PZ seems to be mediated by calcium (IWATSUKI and PETERSEN 1977; POULSEN and WILLIAMS 1977). The injection of calcium directly into an acinar cell closely mimics the usual membrane depolarisation seen with acetylcholine. Therefore, the increased influx of sodium is not the cause but is one of the consequences of the calcium signal. The increased entry of sodium may be a part of the chain of events leading to the large increase in fluid secretion associated with the action of secretagogues on the pancreas of certain species (PETERSEN and UEDA 1976).

V. Intestine

There is a constant flux in both directions of ions and water across the intestine. The direction of net movement is normally regulated by neuronal and hormonal factors (BERRIDGE 1979; FIELD 1979; POWELL and TAPPER 1979). In pathological conditions, other factors, such as cholera toxin, switch intestinal transport processes from an absorptive to a secretory mode. Subsequent studies, which showed that cyclic AMP mediated this effect of cholera toxin, provided an important clue to the role of second messengers in the intestine (STREWELER and ORLOFF 1977). Other secretagogues, such as vasoactive intestinal peptide (VIP) and the prostaglandins, were also found to act through cyclic AMP. Further evidence that cyclic AMP plays an important role has emerged from studies using theophylline which is capable of mimicking the secretory effect of choleragen (NAFTALIN and SIMMONS 1979). On the other hand, neurotransmitters such as 5-hydroxytryptamine (5-HT) and acetylcholine can stimulate secretion without raising the intracellular level of cyclic AMP but their action is very dependent on the presence of external calcium. Further evidence for an important role of calcium has come from studies with the divalent ionophore A 23187 which can stimulate fluid secretion (BOLTON and FIELD 1977; FRIZZEL 1977). The intestine may thus have agonist-dependent calcium channels which are sensitive to either acetylcholine or 5-HT.

Activation of muscarinic and α-adrenergic receptors on rabbit ileal mucosa resulted in an increase in the level of cyclic GMP which might be linked to the action of calcium (BRASITUS et al. 1976). Cyclic GMP could play an important role in regulating ion transport because DE JONGE (1981) has identified a particulate cyclic GMP-dependent protein kinase which is localized within the microvillus. Cyclic GMP could thus act directly to modify anion channels or it might act indirectly to modify the action of calcium on these channels (DE JONGE 1981).

Like several other secretory systems, both cyclic AMP and calcium have been implicated in the control of intestinal secretion. What remains to be determined is their mode of action. It is still uncertain whether or not they both share a common site of action on the transport mechanisms themselves or whether one second messenger such as calcium is the final mediator with cyclic AMP acting indirectly. Some evidence for the latter has emerged from calcium flux studies in which cyclic AMP was found to markedly enhance the efflux of ^{45}Ca from prelabelled cells

(FRIZZELL 1977). Cyclic AMP may thus act indirectly to promote the efflux of calcium which then functions to switch the intestine from net absorption to net secretion.

VI. Parietal Cells

The mechanisms for controlling acid secretion by parietal cells has numerous similarities to those just described for regulating secretion in the intestine. In the first place, secretion can be induced by different secretagogues such as histamine, acetylcholine and gastrin. Secondly, these stimulants seem to use different second messengers. Histamine seems to act on H_2 receptors to produce a rise in the intracellular level of cyclic AMP which then activates secretion (SOLL and GROSSMAN 1978; SOLL and WALSH 1979). However, it is necessary to point out that the evidence for implicating cyclic AMP as a second messenger in gastric acid secretion is not completely convincing (JACOBSON and THOMPSON 1976; THOMPSON et al. 1977). The actions of acetylcholine and gastrin, however, are not mediated by cyclic AMP but they seem to depend on calcium, especially since the former seems to act through muscarinic receptors (SOLL 1980). Further evidence for the involvement of calcium has emerged from studies in calcium-free media which severely reduce the effect of acetylcholine but not that of histamine (BUNCE et al. 1979; BERGLINDH et al. 1980).

One of the most intriguing aspects of the control mechanisms which regulate acid secretion is that they display potentiating interactions when added in certain combinations (SOLL and GROSSMAN 1978; SOLL and WALSH 1979). For example, both acetylcholine and gastrin can potentiate the action of histamine while being incapable of potentiating each other. This phenomenon of superadditivity has some interesting implications concerning the involvement of second messengers and is certainly consistent with the fact that histamine uses a separate internal signalling system from that employed by acetylcholine and gastrin. At this stage, there is insufficient information to determine whether this potentiation occurs at the level of second messenger generation or at their site of action on the secretory system.

VII. Mammalian Salivary Gland

Control of enzyme and fluid secretion from the parotid gland has provided important insights into the role of cyclic AMP and calcium in regulating secretion. The acinar cells responsible for both enzyme and fluid secretion receive a dual innervation – a sympathetic pathway is mainly responsible for releasing enzymes whereas the parasympathetic pathway regulates fluid secretion. These two control systems are not entirely distinct in that there is some enzyme release during cholinergic stimulation and vice versa. Despite some cross-talk between these two control systems, it is remarkable that these two quite separate secretory processes can be regulated independently of each other.

The sympathetic nerves release norepinephrine which can act on either β-receptors to produce cyclic AMP or on α-receptors to gate calcium (SCHRAMM and SELINGER 1975; ALBANO et al. 1976b; LESLIE et al. 1976; PUTNEY et al. 1977; BUTCHER 1978). The parasympathetic nerves release acetylcholine which then acts on muscarinic receptors to gate calcium. The salivary gland also contains receptors for substance P which also seem to act through calcium. The activation of the three receptors which gate calcium (α-adrenergic, muscarinic and substance P) all elicit a PI response which is independent of external calcium (JONES and MICHELL 1975, 1978; KERYER and ROSSIGNOL 1978). An interesting feature of these receptors is that their affects are not additive even though they display a very specific form of refractoriness (HARPER and BROOKER 1977, 1978). This lack of additivity is displayed not only for the production of cyclic GMP but also for the stimulation of amylase secretion. A similar lack of additivity has been observed for the action of carbachol, epinephrine and substance P on potassium efflux (MARIER et al. 1978). These receptors must thus share some common component such as the calcium gate which limits such additive effects. This common component is not involved in the refractoriness which develops during continuous activation of one of other of these receptors. For example, if a parotid gland is stimulated continuously with phenylephrine there is a small increase in amylase release which fades back to basal values within 30 min. However, subsequent stimulation with carbachol will give further amylase release indicating a specific form of refractoriness (HARPER and BROOKER 1978). These receptors which gate calcium thus show a certain independence of each other but, as mentioned earlier, they do seem to be capable of modulating the β-receptors which generate cyclic AMP.

As in several other tissues, the activation of the α-adrenergic or cholinergic receptors in the rat parotid can markedly impair the generation of cyclic AMP via the β-adrenergic receptors (HARPER and BROOKER 1977; ORON et al. 1978a, b). This inhibitory effect, which seems to be exerted at the level of adenylate cyclase, is complicated by the observation that the inhibitory effect of the adrenergic system is dependent on extracellular calcium whereas that of carbamylcholine is not. This non specific refractoriness which spreads from one group of receptors to another illustrates that there are important interactions operating at the transducing mechanisms, responsible for generating cyclic AMP and calcium.

Further interactions between these second messengers may exist in their mode of action within the cell. These two second messengers are responsible for the regulation of amylase release and fluid secretion. An earlier view summarised by SCHRAMM and SELINGER (1975) considered cyclic AMP and calcium as alternative but independent second messengers which implied that exocytosis could be induced equally as well using either second messenger. An alternative view considers that calcium is the final mediator of exocytosis and that cyclic AMP works indirectly by mobilizing calcium from intracellular reservoirs (ALBANO et al. 1976b; PUTNEY et al. 1977; BUTCHER 1978). The evidence for the existence of an internal calcium reservoir is presented by PUTNEY et al. (1977) but the nature of this store and how it might be affected by cyclic AMP has not been established. PUTNEY et al. (1977) also deals with an interesting paradox raised by invoking calcium as the final mediator of the two processes of exocytosis and fluid secretion which can be regulated separately of each other. They resolve this paradox by suggesting that agents which generate a calcium signal by increasing influx may produce a distribution of intracellular free calcium which is topographically different to that resulting from the mobilization of internal calcium induced by cyclic AMP (Fig. 8). When calcium enters from the outside there will be a high concentration immediately be-

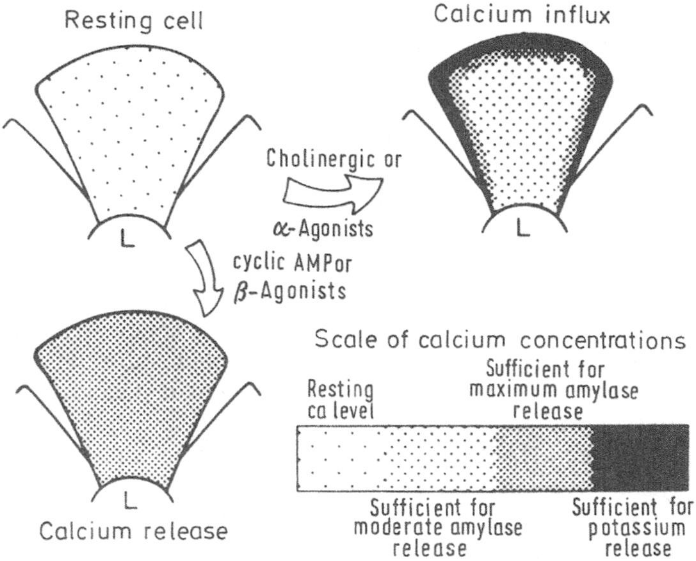

Fig. 8. A diagrammatic representation of the proposed distribution of signal calcium during stimulation of parotid acinar cells with different agonists. Cholinergic or α-adrenergic agents mainly induce an influx of external calcium which results in the calcium signal being confined to the vicinity of the baso-lateral membrane. The low diffusibility of calcium prevents the signal from spreading to the membrane facing the lumen *L* where amylase is released. Cyclic AMP or β-adrenergic agents seem to act by mobilizing internal calcium thus producing a more evenly distributed calcium signal capable of reaching the lumenal membrane to trigger the release of amylase. (PUTNEY et al. 1977)

low the surface but as calcium diffuses into the cell it will rapidly be sequestered by intracellular organelles thus reducing the concentration especially at the opposite surface of the cell where granule release occurs. The low diffusibility of calcium in cytoplasm was discussed in Sect. B.VI. The mobilization of calcium from intracellular reservoirs distributed throughout the cytoplasm may thus represent a device for overcoming this problem a calcium diffusion thus allowing a calcium signal to be transmitted from one surface of an epithelial cell to the other.

VIII. Insect Salivary Gland

The role of second messengers in regulating fluid secretion has been studied extensively in the salivary gland of the blowfly *Calliphora*. Fluid secretion is controlled by 5-hydroxytryptamine using both cyclic AMP and calcium a second messengers (BERRIDGE 1970, 1975, 1980a, b; PRINCE and BERRIDGE 1973; PRINCE et al. 1972). All the indications are that the cells have two different receptors, one linked to the formation of cyclic AMP and the other to calcium. MACDERMOT et al. (1979) have described two species of 5-HT receptors in NCB-20 neuroblastoma-brain hybrid cells. Again, one receptor was linked to adenylate cyclase whereas the other caused membrane depolarisation which might be analogous to the change in calcium permeability seen in the blowfly salivary gland.

This insect salivary gland system has provided a good model system for studying the relationship between the PI response (Sect. B.III) and calcium gating (BERRIDGE and FAIN 1979a, b; FAIN and BERRIDGE 1979a, b). One of the main advantages has stemmed from the development of a technique for continuously monitoring the permeability of the cell membrane to calcium (BERRIDGE and LIPKE 1978). Using this technique it was possible to demonstrate a close relationship between the hydrolysis of PI and the opening of calcium gates (BERRIDGE and FAIN 1979a, b; FAIN and BERRIDGE 1979a). Of particular significance was the finding that at high 5-HT concentrations not only was there an enormous increase in PI hydrolysis but there was also a parallel inhibition of PI synthesis (BERRIDGE and FAIN 1979a, b; FAIN and BERRIDGE 1979a). These two effects of 5-HT would conspire to reduce the level of PI which would result in a reduction in calcium permeability assuming, of course, that this phospholipid is intimately linked to calcium gating. This prediction was confirmed by the observation that calcium gating inactivated progressively during prolonged stimulation with high 5-HT concentrations (BERRIDGE and FAIN 1979a, b). Removing 5-HT and allowing the glands to recover in control medium for up to one hour did not restore the calcium gating system. However, if the glands were allowed to resynthesize PI by being presented with the precursor inositol, then calcium gating was completely reactivated and the cells became responsive to 5-HT (BERRIDGE AND FAIN 1979a, b; FAIN and BERRIDGE 1979b). The fact that the agonist-dependent gating of calcium can be varied by adjusting the level of PI provides strong evidence that this phospholipid plays an important role in coupling one type of 5-HT receptor to calcium gates.

These insect salivary glands resemble many other secretory systems in that both cyclic AMP and calcium have a role to play in regulating secretion. The problem of trying to work out their precise contribution in the intact cell has been tackled by studying how these internal signals affect membrane potentials. Since 5-HT stimulates water movement by first increasing the flow of ions, it is possible to learn a lot about the control of these ionic pathways by studying changes in transepithelial potential and resistance in response to 5-HT (BERRIDGE 1980b, 1981; BERRIDGE and PRINCE 1972; BERRIDGE et al. 1975). The main action of calcium is to increase the passive permeability of the membranes to chloride thus causing a large decrease in resistance with the transepithelial potential depolarising close to zero. An increase in the intracellular level of calcium by itself is not capable of eliciting a full rate of fluid secretion. For example, the calcium ionophore A 23187 at 1 μM is capable of gating the same amount of calcium as 0.05 μM 5-HT but the former can induce less than 50% of the fluid flow of 5-HT.

In order for 5-HT to stimulate these high secretion rates there appears to be a requirement for cyclic AMP to act on the potassium pump. In addition to accelerating potassium movement there is evidence from calcium efflux experiments that cyclic AMP may also be capable of mobilizing calcium from internal reservoirs (PRINCE et al. 1972; BERRIDGE and LIPKE 1978). Cyclic AMP by itself is capable of stimulating fluid secretion but its action is accompanied by no change in resistance and by a marked hyperpolarisation of the transepithelial potential in contrast to that produced by calcium. This electrophysiological picture is consistent with cyclic AMP acting in some way to speed up the transport of potassium which then creates the electrical gradient for the parallel flow of chloride which is regulated by calcium. In the insect salivary gland, therefore, there is growing evidence that these two second messengers act in concert to regulate fluid secretion.

In addition to secreting fluid, this insect salivary gland is also capable of secreting carbohydrases of which amylase and sucrase are the major components (HANSEN BAY 1978). The release of enzyme can be triggered by procedures which elevate the level of either cyclic AMP or calcium which is reminiscent of the control system found in the mammalian salivary gland described in the previous section. One particularly interesting feature of this enzyme release system in the blowfly is its sensitivity to calcium. HANSEN BAY (1978) observed that while enzyme release seemed to be stimulated by calcium, too much of this ion was inhibitory. For example, more enzyme was released from glands during 5-HT stimulation if the calcium signal was reduced either by removing external calcium or by blocking calcium entry with lanthanum. Such observations suggest that the same cell may have a number of calcium-sensitive processes which are organised in a heirarchy (HANSEN BAY 1978; BERRIDGE 1979).

D. Conclusion

The term stimulus-secretion coupling is meant to draw attention to the many similarities which exist between secretory and muscle cells. In particular, calcium seems to play a primary role as an activator in both systems. In secretory cells, most external stimuli are transduced into an increase in the intracellular level of calcium which then triggers the release of vesicles by exocytosis or activates ionic mechanisms to induce a flow of fluid. There are two main methods for regulating the flow of calcium across the plasma membrane. In some cells, secretion is initiated by membrane depolarisation which leads to an opening of voltage-dependent calcium channels. The secretion of other cells is regulated by secretagogues many of which act by opening calcium channels. The opening of these agonist-dependent calcium channels seems to depend upon the hydrolysis of phosphatidylinositol. In addition to using external calcium, many secretory cells seem to be capable of mobilizing calcium from internal reservoirs. The use of intracellular calcium seems to be associated with those secretory cells which are organised into epithelia where the calcium signal must move from one side of the cell to the other. Mobilization of calcium, from internal stores may represent a way of overcoming the problem imposed by the low diffusibility of calcium in cytoplasm.

The ubiquitous calcium signal often does not act in isolation and is either aided and abetted or sometimes even inhibited by cyclic AMP. In some systems, cyclic AMP seems to act indirectly by mobilizing calcium from intracellular reservoirs especially in those epithelia which rely to some extent on internal calcium. There are also instances where cyclic AMP may activate secretory processes directly but the precise molecular mechanisms for such an action remain to by worked out. In the light of such diverse actions and interactions it is impossible at this stage to make too many generalizations about how these two second messengers function and each secretory system must be treated separately. There is an obvious need to learn more about how these second messengers function in the intact cell.

References

Akhtar RA, Abdel-Latif AA (1978) Calcium ion requirement for acetylcholine-stimulated breakdown of triphosphoinositide in rabbit iris smooth muscle. J Pharmacol Exp Ther 204:655–668

Albano J, Bhoola KA, Harvey RF (1976a) Intracellular messenger role of cyclic GMP in exocrine pancreas. Nature 262:404–406

Albano J, Bhoola KD, Heap PF, Lemon MJC (1976b) Stimulus-secretion coupling: a role of cyclic AMP, cyclic GMP and calcium in mediating enzyme (kallikrein) secretion in the submandibular gland. J Physiol (Lond) 258:631–658

Albano J, Bhoola KD, Harvey RF (1979) The messenger role of cyclic GMP and calcium in the exocrine pancreas. J Physiol (Lond) 293:49P–50P

Atherton RS, Hawthorne JN (1968) The phosphoinositide inositolphosphohydrolase of guinea-pig intestinal mucosa. Eur J Biochem 4:68–75

Atwater I, Ribalet B, Rojas E (1978) Cyclic changes in potential and resistance of the β-cell membrane induced by glucose in islets of Langerhans from mouse. J Physiol (Lond) 278:117–139

Baker BI (1974) Effect of dibutyryl cyclic AMP on the release of melanocyte-stimulating hormone from rat neurointermediate lobe in vitro. J Endocrinol 63:533–538

Baker PF (1976) The regulation of intracellular calcium. Symp Soc Biol 30:67–88

Baker PF, Knight DE (1978) Calcium-dependent exocytosis in bovine adrenal medullary cells with leaky plasma membranes. Nature 276:620–622

Baker PF, Rink TJ (1975) Catecholamine release from bovine adrenal medulla in response to maintained depolarisation. J Physiol (Lond) 253:593–620

Baker PF, Meves H, Ridgeway EB (1973) Effects of manganese and other agents on the calcium uptake that follows depolarisation of squid axons. J Physiol (Lond) 231:511–526

Bennett JP, Cockcroft S, Gomperts BD (1979) Ionomycin stimulates mast cell histamine secretion by forming a lipid-soluble calcium complex. Nature 282:851–853

Berglindh T, Sachs G, Takeguchi N (1980) Ca^{2+}-dependent secretagogue stimulation in isolated rabbit gastric glands. Am J Physiol 239:G90–G94

Berridge M (1970) The role of 5-hydroxytryptamine and cyclic AMP in the control of fluid secretion by isolated salivary glands. J Exp Biol 53:171–186

Berridge MJ (1975) The interaction of cyclic nucleotides and calcium in the control of cellular activity. Adv Cyclic Nucleotide Res 6:1–98

Berridge MJ (1979) Relationship between calcium and the cyclic nucleotides in ion secretion. Kroc Found Ser 12:65–81

Berridge MJ (1980a) Preliminary measurements of intracellular calcium in an insect salivary gland using a calcium-sensitive microelectrode. Cell Calcium 1:217–227

Berridge MJ (1980b) The role of cyclic nucleotides and calcium in the regulation of chloride transport. Ann NY Acad Sci 341:156–169

Berridge MJ (1981) Hormone-induced changes in ion level during stimulation of fluid secretion by gland cells. In: Zeuthen T (ed) The application of ion selective microelectrodes. Elsevier/North-Holland, Amsterdam Oxford New York, pp 61–74

Berridge MJ, Fain JN (1979a) Inhibition of phosphatidylinositol synthesis and the inactivation of calcium entry after prolonged exposure of the blowfly salivary gland to 5-hydroxytryptamine. Biochem J 178:59–69

Berridge MJ, Fain JN (1979b) Phosphatidylinositol metabolism and calcium gating. Med Chem 6:117–125

Berridge MJ, Lipke H (1978) Changes in calcium transport across *Calliphora* salivary gland induced by 5-hydroxytryptamine and cyclic AMP. J Exp Biol 78:137–148

Berridge MJ, Oschman J (1972) Transporting epithelia. Academic Press, New York London

Berridge MJ, Prince WT (1972) Transepithelial potential changes during stimulation of isolated salivary glands with 5-hydroxytryptamine and cyclic AMP. J Exp Biol 56:139–153

Berridge MJ, Rapp PE (1979) A comparative survey of the function, mechanism and control of cellular oscillators. J Exp Boil 81:217–279

Berridge MJ, Lindley BD, Prince WT (1975) Membrane permeability changes during stimulation of isolated salivary glands of *Calliphora* by 5-hydroxytryptamine. J Physiol (Lond) 244:549–567

Biales B, Dichter MA, Tischler A (1977) Sodium and calcium action potentials in pituitary cells. Nature 267:172–174

Billah MM, Michell RH (1978) Stimulation of the breakdown and resynthesis of phosphatidylinositol in rat hepatocytes by angiotensin, vasopressin and adrenaline. Biochem Soc Trans 6:1033–1035

Birnbaumer L, Iyengar R (1982) Coupling of receptors to adenylate cyclases. In: Nathanson JA, Kebabian JW (eds) Cyclic nucleotides. Springer, Berlin Heidelberg New York (Handbook of experimental pharmacology, vol 58/I)

Blackmore PF, DeHaye J-P, Exton JH (1979) Studies on α-adrenergic activation of hepatic glucose output. J Biol Chem 254:6945–6950

Blaustein MP, Ratzlaff RW, Kendrick NC, Schweitzer ES (1978) Calcium buffering in presynaptic nerve terminals. I. Evidence for involvement of a nonmitochondrial Ca sequestration mechanism. J Gen Physiol 72:15–41

Bolton JE, Field M (1977) Ca ionophore-stimulated ion secretion in rabbit ileal mucosa: relation to actions of cyclic 3′,5′-AMP and carbamylcholine. J Membr Biol 35:159–173

Borgeat P, Chavancy G, Dupont A, Labrie F, Arimura A, Schally AV (1972) Stimulation of adenosine 3′,5′-cyclic monophosphate accumulation in anterior pituitary gland in vitro by synthetic luteinizing hormone-releasing hormone. Proc Natl Acad Sci USA 69:2677–2681

Bower A, Hadley ME (1972) Ionic requirements for melanophore-stimulating hormone (MSH) release. Gen Comp Endocrinol 19:147–158

Brasitus TA, Field M, Kimberg DV (1976) Intestinal mucosal cyclic AMP: regulation and relation to ion transport. Am J Physiol 231:275–282

Bunce KT, Honey AC, Parsons ME (1979) Investigation of the role of extracellular calcium in the control of acid secretion in the isolated whole stomach of the rat. Br J Pharmacol 67:123–131

Butcher FR (1975) The role of calcium and cyclic nucleotides in α-amylase release from slices of rat parotid: studies with the divalent cation ionophore A 23187. Metabolism 24:409–418

Butcher FR (1978) Calcium and cyclic nucleotides in the regulation of secretion from the rat parotid by autonomic agonists. Adv Cyclic Nucleotide Res 9:707–721

Case RM (1978) Synthesis, intracellular transport and discharge of exportable proteins in the pancreatic acinar cells and other cells. Biol Rev 53:211–354

Case RM, Clausen T (1973) The relationship between calcium exchange and enzyme secretion in the isolated rat pancreas. J Physiol (Lond) 235:75–102

Chandler DE, Wiliams JA (1974) Pancreatic acinar cells: effects of lanthanum ions on amylase release and calcium ion fluxes. J Physiol (Lond) 243:831–846

Chandler DE, Williams JA (1978) Intracellular divalent cation release in pancreatic acinar cells during stimulus-secretion coupling. II. Subcellular localization of the fluorescent probe chlorotetracycline. J Cell Biol 76:386–399

Charles MA, Lawecki J, Pictet R, Grodsky GM (1975) Insulin secretion. Interrelationships of glucose, cyclic adenosine 3′,5′-monophosphate and calcium. J Biol Chem 250:6134–6140

Charo IF, Feinman RD, Detwiller TC (1976) Inhibition of platelet secretion by an antagonist of intracellular calcium. Biochem Biophys Res Commun 72:1462–1467

Cheung WY, Storm DR (1982) Calmodulin regulation of cyclic AMP metabolism. In: Nathanson JA; Kebabian JW (eds) Cyclic nucleotides. Springer, Berlin Heidelberg New York (Handbook of experimental pharmacology, vol 58/I)

Christophe JP, Frandsen EK, Conlon TP, Krishna G, Gardner JD (1976) Action of cholecystokinin, cholinergic agents and A 23187 on accumulation of guanosine 3′,5′-monophosphate in dispersed guinea pig pancreatic acinar cells. J Biol Chem 251:4640–4645

Clark RB, Salmon DM, Honeyman TW (1980) Phosphatidic acid inhibition of PGE_1-stimulated cAMP accumulation in WI-38 fibroblasts: similarities with carbachol inhibition. J Cyclic Nucleotide Res 6:37–49

Clayton RN, Shakespear RA, Marshall JC (1978) LH-RH binding to purified pituitary plasma membranes: absence of adenylate cyclase activation. Mol Cell Endocrinol 11:63–78

Cochrane DE, Douglas WW (1974) Calcium-induced extrusion of secretory granules (exocytosis) in mast cells exposed to 48/80 or the ionophores A 23187 and X-537A. Proc Natl Acad Sci USA 71:408–412
Cockcroft S, Gomperts BD (1979) Evidence for a role of phosphatidylinositol turnover in stimulus-secretion coupling. Studies with rat peritoneal mast cells. Biochem J 178:681–687
Conn PM, Rogers DC, Sandhu FS (1979) Alteration of the intracellular calcium level stimulates gonadotropin release from cultured rat anterior pituitary cells. Endocrinology 105:1112–1127
Conn PM, Kilpatrick D, Kirshner N (1980a) Ionophoretic Ca^{2+} mobilization in rat gonadotropes and bovine adrenomedullary cells. Cell Calcium 1:129–133
Conn PM, Marian J, McMillian M, Rogers D (1980b) Evidence for calcium mediation of gonadotropin releasing hormone action in the pituitary. Cell Calcium 1:7–20
Cote T, Munemura M, Eskay RL, Kebabian JW (1980) Biochemical identification of the β-adrenoreceptor and evidence for the involvement of an adenosine 3′,5′-monophosphate system in the β-adrenergically-induced release of α-melanocyte stimulating hormone in the intermediate lobe of the rat pituitary gland. Endocrinology 107:108–116
Curry DL, Bennett LL, Grodsky EM (1968) Dynamics of insulin secretion by the perfused rat pancreas. Endocrinolgoy 83:572–584
Davis MD, Hadley ME (1976) Spontaneous electrical potentials and pituitary hormone (MSH) secretion. Nature 261:422–423
Dean PM, Matthews EK, Sakamoto Y (1975) Pancreatic islet cells: effects of monosacharides, glycolytic intermediates and metabolic inhibitors on membrane potential and electrical activity. J Physiol (Lond) 246:459–478
De Jonge HR (1981) Cyclic GMP-dependent protein kinase in intestinal brushborders. Adv Cyclic Nucleotide Res 14:315–333
DeLorenzo RJ, Freedman SD, Yohe WB, Maurer SC (1979) Stimulation of Ca^{2+}-dependent neurotransmitter release and presynaptic nerve protein phosphorylation by calmodulin and a calmodulin-like protein isolated from synaptic vesicles. Proc Natl Acad Sci USA 76:1838–1842
Douglas WW, Taraskevich PS (1978) Action potentials in gland cells of rat pituitary pars intermedia: inhibition by dopamine, an inhibitor of MSH secretion. J Physiol (Lond) 285:171-184
Dreifuss JJ, Grau JD, Nordmann JJ (1975) Calcium movements related to neurohypophysial hormone secretion. In: Carafoli E, Clementi F, Drabikowski W, Margreth A (eds) Calcium transport in contraction and secretion. North-Holland, Amsterdam Oxford New York, pp 271–279
Dufy B, Vincent J-D, Fleury H, Du Pasquier P, Gourdji D, Tixier-Vidal A (1979) Dopamine inhibition of action potentials in a prolactin secreting cell line is modulated by oestrogen. Nature 282:855–857
Endo M, Tanaka M, Ogawa Y (1970) Calcium induced release of calcium from the sarcoplasmic reticulum of skinned skeletal muscle fibres. Nature 228:34–36
Eto S, Wood JM, Hutchins M, Fleischer N (1974) Pituitary $^{45}Ca^{++}$ uptake and release of ACTH, GH and TSH: effect of verapamil. Am J Physiol 226:1315–1320
Fabiato A, Fabiato F (1975) Contractions induced by a calcium-triggered release of calcium from the sarcoplasmic reticulum of single skinned cardiac cells. J Physiol (Lond) 249:469–495
Fain JN, Berridge MJ (1979a) Relationship between hormonal activation of phosphatidylinositol hydrolysis, fluid secretion and calcium flux in the blowfly salivary gland. Biochem J 178:45–58
Fain JN, Berridge MJ (1979b) Relationship between phosphatidylinositol synthesis and recovery of 5-hydroxytryptamine -responsive Ca^{2+} flux in blowfly salivary glands. Biochem J 180:655–661
Feinman RD, Detwiler TC (1974) Platelet secretion induced by divalent cation ionophores. Nature 249:172–173
Field M (1979) Intracellular mediators of secretion in the small intestine. Kroc Found Ser 12:83–91

Foreman JC, Garland LG (1974) Desensitization in the process of histamine secretion induced by antigen and dextran. J Physiol (Lond) 239:381–391
Foreman JC, Mongar JL, Gomperts BD (1973) Calcium ionophores and movement of calcium ions following the physiological stimulus to a secretory process. Nature 245:249–251
Foreman JC, Garland LG, Mongar JL (1975) The role of calcium in secretory processes: model studies in mast cells. Symp Soc Exp Biol 30:193–218
Freinkel N, Dawson RMC (1973) Role of inositol cyclic phosphate in stimulated tissues. Nature 243:535–536
Frizzell RA (1977) Active chloride secretion by rabbit colon: calcium-dependent stimulation by ionophore A 23187. J Membr Biol 35:175–187
Garcia AG, Kirpekar SM, Prat JC (1975) A calcium ionophore stimulating the secretion of catecholamines from the cat adrenal. J Physiol (Lond) 244:253–262
Gardner JD (1979) Regulation of pancreatic exocrine function in vitro: initial steps in the actions of secretagogues. Ann Rev Physiol 41:55–66
Gilkey JC, Jaffe LF, Ridgeway LB, Reynolds GT (1978) A free calcium wave traverses the activating egg of the medaka, *Oryzias latipes*. J Cell Biol 76:448–466
Gomperts BD (1976) Calcium and cell activation. In: Cuatrecasas P, Greaves MF (eds) Receptors and recognition, Serie A, vol 2. Chapman & Hall, London, pp 43–102
Gorman RR, Wierenga W, Miller OV (1979) Independence of the cyclic AMP-lowering activity of thromboxane A_2 from the platelet release reaction. Biochim Biophys Acta 572:95–104
Gratzl M, Dahl G, Russel JT, Thorn NA (1977) Fusion of neurohypophyseal membranes in vitro. Biochim Biophys Acta 470:45–57
Green DE, Fry M, Blondin GA (1980) Phospholipids as the molecular instruments of ion and solute transport in biological membranes. Proc Natl Acad Sci USA 77:257–261
Griffin HD, Hawthorne JN (1978) Calcium-activated hydrolysis of phosphatidyl-*myo*-inositol 4-phosphate and phosphatidyl-*myo*-inositol 4,5-bisphosphate in guinea pig synaptosomes. Biochem J 176:541–552
Gunther GR, Jamieson JD (1979) Increased intracellular cyclic GMP does not correlate with protein discharge from pancreatic acinar cells. Nature 280:318–320
Gupta BL, Hall TA (1978) Electron microprobe X-ray analysis of calcium. Ann NY Acad Sci 307:28–51
Hagiwara S, Takahashi K (1967) Surface density of calcium ions and calcium spikes in the barnacle muscle fiber membrane. J Gen Physiol 50:583–601
Hales CN, Luzio JP, Chandler JA, Herman L (1974) Localization of calcium in the smooth endoplasmic reticulum of rat isolated fat cells. J Cell Sci 15:1–15
Hansen Bay CM, (1978) The control of enzyme secretion from fly salivary glands. J Physiol (Lond) 274:421–435
Harper JF, Brooker G (1977) Refractoriness to muscarinic and adrenergic agonists in the rat parotid: responses of adenosine and guanosine cyclic 3′,5′-monophosphate. Mol Pharmacol 12:1048–1059
Harper JF, Brooker G (1978) Amylase secretion from the rat parotid: refractoriness to muscarinic and adrenergic agonists. Mol Pharmacol 14:1031–1045
Hawthorne JN, Pickard MR (1977) Metabolism of phosphatidic acid and phosphatidylinositol in relation to transmitter release from synaptosomes. Adv Exp Med Biol 83:419–427
Hawthorne JN, Pickard MR (1979) Phospholipids in synaptic function. J Neurochem 32:5–14
Hedeskov CJ (1980) Mechanism of glucose-induced insulin secretion. Physiol Rev 60:442–509
Hedeskov CJ, Capito K (1975) The restoring effect of caffeine on the decreased sensitivity of the insulin secretory mechanism in mouse pancreatic islets during starvation. Horm Metab Res 7:1–5
Heisler S (1976) Effects of an ATP analogue (α,β-methylene-adenosine-5-triphosphate) on cyclic AMP and cyclic GMP levels, ^{45}Ca efflux, and protein secretion from rat pancreas. Can J Physiol Pharmacol 54:692–697
Henkart M, Nelson PG (1979) Evidence for an intracellular calcium store releasable by surface stimuli in fibroblast (L cells). J Gen Physiol 73:655–673

Henkart M, Landis DMD, Reese TS (1976) Similarity of junctions between plasma membranes and endoplasmic reticulum in muscle and neurons. J Cell Biol 70:338–347
Henquin J-C (1978 a) D-Glucose inhibits potassium efflux from pancreatic islet cells. Nature 271:271–273
Henquin J-C (1978 b) Relative importance of extracellular and intracellular calcium for the two phases of glucose-stimulated insulin release: studies with theophylline. Endocrinology 102:723–730
Henquin J-C (1978) Opposite effects of intracellular Ca^{2+} and glucose on K^+ permeabilitiy of pancreatic islets cells. Nature 280:66–68
Henquin J-C (1980 a) Metabolic control of the potassium permeability in pancreatic islet cells. Biochem J 186:541–550
Henquin J-C (1980 b) Tolbutamine stimulation and inhibition of insulin release; studies of the underlying ionic mechanisms in isolated rat islets. Diabetologia 18: 151–160
Henquin J-C, Lambert AE (1974) Cationic environment and dynamics of insulin secretion. II. Effect of a high concentration of potassium. Diabetes 23:933–942
Henquin J-C, Lambert AE (1975) Cobalt inhibition of insulin secretion and calcium uptake by isolated rat islets. Am J Physiol 228:1669–1677
Henquin J-C, Meissner HP (1978) Valinomycin inhibition of insulin release and alteration of the electrical properties of pancreatic B-cells. Biochim Biophys Acta 543:455–464
Henquin J-C, Meissner HP, Preissler M (1979) 9-Aminoacridine- and tetraethylammonium-induced reduction of the potassium permeability in pancreatic B-cells. Biochim Biophys Acta 586:579–592
Hokin LE (1966) Effects of calcium omission on acetylcholine-stimulated amylase secretion and phospholipid synthesis in pigeon pancreas slices. Biochim Biophys Acta 115:219–221
Hokin LE, Hokin MR (1960) Studies of the carrier function of phosphatidic acid in sodium transport. I. The turnover of phosphatidic acid and phosphoinositide in the avian salt gland on stimulation of secretion. J gen Physiol 44:61–85
Hokin MR, Hokin LE (1953) Enzyme secretion and the incorporation of ^{32}P into phospholipids of pancreas slices. J Biol Chem 203:967–977
Hokin MR, Hokin LE (1954) Effects of acetylcholine on phospholipids in the pancreas. J Biol Chem 209:549–558
Hokin-Neaverson M (1977) Metabolism and role of phosphatidylinositol in acetylcholine-stimulated membrane function. Adv Exp Med Biol 83:429–445
Hopkins CR (1970) Studies on secretory activity in the pars intermedia of *Xenopus laevis.* Tissue Cell 2:83–98
Hopkins CR, Walker AM (1978) Calcium as a second messenger in the stimulation of luteinizing hormone secretion. Mol Cell Endocrinol 12:189–208
Howell SL, Montague W, Tyhurst M (1975) Calcium distribution in Islets of Langerhans: a study of calcium concentrations and of calcium accumulation in B cell organelles. J Cell Sci 19:395–409
Ilundain A, Naftalin RJ (1979) Role of Ca^{2+}-dependent regulator protein in intestinal secretion. Nature 279:446–448
Irvine RF, Dawson RMC (1978) The distribution of calcium-dependent phosphodiesterase in rat brain. J Neurochem 31:1427–1434
Iwatsuki N, Petersen OH (1977) Acetylcholine-like effects of intracellular calcium application in pancreatic cells. Nature 268:147–149
Jacobson ED, Thompson WJ (1976) Cyclic AMP and gastric secretion: the illusive second messenger. Adv Cyclic Nucleotide Res 7:199–224
Jones LM, Michell RH (1975) The relationship of calcium to receptor-controlled stimulation of phosphatidylinositol turnover. Biochem J 148:479–485
Jones LM, Michell RH (1978) Enhanced phosphatidylinositol breakdown as a calcium independent response of rat parotid fragments to substance P. Biochem Soc Trans 6:1035–1037
Kanagasuntheram P, Randle PJ (1976) Calcium metabolism and amylase release in rat parotid acinar cells. Biochem J 160:547–564
Kanno T, Nishimura O (1976) Stimulus-secretion coupling in pancreatic acinar cells: inhibitory effects of calcium removal and manganese addition on pancreozymin-induced amylase release. J Physiol (Lond) 257:309–324

Kanno T, Yamamoto M (1977) Differentiation between the calcium-dependent effects of cholecystokinin-pancreozymin and the bicarbonate dependent effects of secretin in exocrine secretion of the rat pancreas. J Physiol (Lond) 264:787–799
Kapoor C, Krishna G (1978) A possible role for guanosine 3′,5′-monophosphate in the stimulus-secretion coupling in exocrine pancreas. Biochim Biophys Acta 544:102–112
Katsumi W, Kamberi IA, McCann SM (1979) In vitro response of the rat pituitary to gonadotropin-releasing factors and to ions. Endocrinology 85:1046–1056
Kawakami M, Kimura F (1980) Stimulation of guanosine 3′,5′-monophosphate accumulation in anterior pituitary glands in vivo by synthetic luteinizing hormone-releasing hormone. Endocrinology 106:626–630
Kazimierczak W, Diamant B (1978) Mechanisms of histamine release in anaphylactic and anaphylactoid reactions. Prog Allergy 24:295–365
Kennerly DA, Sullivan TJ, Parker CW (1979) Activation of phospholipid metabolism during mediator release from stimulated rat mast cells. J Immunol 122:152–159
Keryer G, Rossignol B (1978) Lanthanum as a tool to study the role of phosphatidylinositol in the calcium transport in rat parotid glands upon cholinergic stimulation. Eur J Biochem 85:77–83
Kidokoro Y (1975) Spontaneous calcium action potentials in a clonal pituitary cell line and their relationship to prolactin secretion. Nature 258:741–742
Kirk CJ, Verrinder TR, Hems DA (1978) The influence of extracellular calcium concentration on the vasopressin-stimulated incorporation of inorganic phosphate into phosphatidylinositol in hepatocyte suspensions. Biochem Soc Trans 6:1031–1033
Klein M, Kandel ER (1978) Presynaptic modulation of voltage-dependent Ca^{2+} current: mechanisms for behavioural sensitization in *Aplysia californica*. Proc Natl Acad Sci USA 75:3512–3516
Kohlhardt M, Bauer B, Krause H, Fleckenstein A (1972) New selective inhibitors of the transmembrane Ca conductivity in mammalian myocardial fibres. Studies with the voltage clamp technique. Experientia 28:288–289
Labrie F, Borgeat P, Drouin J, Beaulieu M, Legacé L, Ferland L, Raymond V (1979) Mechanism of action of hypothalamic hormones in the adenohypophysis. Annu Rev Physiol 41:555–569
Landis CA, Putney JW (1979) Calcium and receptor regulation of radiosodium uptake by dispersed rat parotid acinar cells. J Physiol (Lond) 297:369–377
Lapetina EG, Michell RH (1973) A membrane-bound activity catalysing phosphatidylinositol breakdown to 1,2 diacylglycerol, D-*myo*-inositol 1,2-cyclic phosphate and D-*myo*-inositol-1-phosphate. Biochem J 131:433–442
Laugier R, Petersen OH (1980) Pancreatic acinar cells: electrophysiological evidence for stimulant-evoked increase in membrane calcium permeability in the mouse. J Physiol (Lond) 303:61–72
Lawson D, Fewtrell C, Raff MC (1978) Localized mast cell degranulation induced by concanavalin A-sepharose beads. J Cell Biol 79:394–400
Leslie BA, Putney JW, Sherman JM (1976) α-Adrenergic, β-adrenergic and cholinergic mechanisms for amylase secretion by rat parotid gland in vitro. J Physiol (Lond) 260:351–370
Levin RM, Weiss B (1977) Binding of trifluoperazine to the calcium-dependent activator of cyclic nucleotide phosphodiesterase. Mol Pharmacol 13:690–697
Limas CJ (1980) Phosphatidate releases calcium from cardiac sarcoplasmic reticulum Biochem Biophys Res Commun 95:541–546
Llinás R, Blinks JR, Nicholson C (1972) Calcium transient in presynaptic terminal of squid giant synapse: detection with aequorin. Science 176:1127–1129
Llinás R, Steinberg IZ, Walton K (1976) Presynaptic calcium currents and their relation to synaptic transmission: voltage clamp study in squid giant synapse and theoretical model for the calcium gate. Proc Natl Acad Sci USA 73:2918–2922
Lopatin RN, Gardner JD (1978) Effects of calcium and chelating agents on the ability of various agonists to increase cyclic GMP in pancreatic acinar cells. Biochim Biophys Acta 543:465–475
MacDermot J, Higashida H, Wilson SP, Matsuzawa H, Minna J, Nirenberg M (1979) Adenylate cyclase and acetylcholine release regulated by separate serotonin receptors of somatic cell Hybrids. Proc Natl Acad Sci USA 76:1135–1139

Malaisse WJ, Herchuelz A, Levy J et al. (1975) Insulin release and the movements of calcium in pancreatic islets. In Carafoli E, Clementi F, Drabikowski W, Margreth A (eds) Calcium transport in contraction and secretion. North Holland, Amsterdam Oxford, pp 211–326
Malaisse WJ, Boschero AC, Kawazu S, Hutton JC (1978) The stimulus secretion coupling of glucose-induced insulin release. XXVII. Effect of glucose on K^+ fluxes in isolated islets. Pfluegers Arch 373:237–242
Marier SH, Putney JW, Van De Walle CM (1978) Control of calcium channels by membrane receptors in the rat parotid gland. J Physiol (Lond) 279:141–151
Matthews EK (1975) Calcium and stimulus-secretion coupling in pancreatic islets cells. In: Carafoli E, Clementi F, Drabikowski W, Margreth A (eds) Calcium transport in contraction and secretion. North Holland, Amsterdam Oxford New York, pp 203–210
Matthews EK (1979) Calcium translocation and control mechanisms for endocrine secretion. Soc Exp Biol Symp 33:225–249
Matthews EK, O'Connor MDL (1979) Dynamic oscillations in the membrane potential of pancreatic islet cells. J Exp Biol 81:75–91
Matthews EK, Petersen OH, Wiliams JA (1973) Pancreatic acinar cells; acetylcholine-induced membrane depolarization, calcium efflux and amylase release. J Physiol (Lond) 234:689–701
Meissner HP, Atwater I (1976) The kinetics of electrical activity of Beta cells in response to a "square wave" stimulation with glucose or glibenclamide. Horm Metab Res 8:11–16
Meissner HP, Schmidt H (1976) The electrical activity of pancreatic β-cells of diabetic mice. FEBS Lett 67:371–374
Michell RH (1975) Inositol phospholipids and cell surface receptor function. Biochim Biophys Acta 415:81–147
Michell RH, Lapetina EG (1972) Production of cyclic inositol phosphate in stimulated tissues. Nature New Biol 240:258–260
Michell RH, Jafferji SS, Jones LM (1977a) The possible involvement phosphatidylinositol breakdown in the mechanism of stimulus-response coupling at receptors which control cell-surface calcium gating. Adv Exp Med Biol 83:447–464
Michell RH, Jones LM, Jafferji SS (1977b) A possible role for phosphatidylinositol breakdown in muscarinic cholinergic stimulus-response coupling. Biochem Soc Trans 5:77–81
Miledi R (1971) Lanthanum ions abolish the "calcium response" of nerve terminals. Nature 229:410–411
Milligan JV, Kraicer J (1974) Physical characteristics of the Ca^{++} compartments associated with in vitro ACTH release. Endocrinology 94:435–443
Moriarty CM (1978) Role of calcium in the regulation of adenohypophysial hormone release. Life Sci 23:185–194
Munemura M, Eskay RL, Kebabian JW (1980) Release of alpha-melanocyte stimulating hormone from dispersed cells of the intermediate lobe of the rat pituitary gland: involvement of catecholamines and adenosine 3',5'-monophosphate. Endocrinology 106:1795–1803
Murphy L, Coll K, Rich TL, Wiliamson JR (1980) Hormonal effects on calcium homeostasis in isolated hepatocytes. J Biol Chem 255:6600–6608
Nakazato Y, Douglas WW (1974) Vasopressin release from the isolated neurohypophysis induced by a calcium ionophore, X-537 A. Nature 249:479–481
Naftalin RJ, Simmons NL (1979) The effects of theophylline and choleragen on sodium and chloride ion movements within isolated rabbit ileum. J Physiol (Lond) 290:331–350
Naor Z, Catt KJ (1980) Independent action of gonadotropin releasing hormone upon cyclic GMP production and luteinizing hormone release. J Biol Chem 255:342–344
Naor Z, Fawcett CP, McCann SM (1978) Involvement of cGMP in LHRH-stimulated gonadotropin release. Am J Physiol 235:E586–E590
Nordmann JJ (1976) Evidence for calcium inactivation during hormone release in the rat neurohypophysis. J Exp Biol 65:669–683
Norn S, Stahl Skov P, Geisler A, Klysner R (1980) Cyclic nucleotides and allergic-inflammatory reactions. Prog Pharmacol 4:101–108
Oron Y, Löwe M, Selinger Z (1975) Incorporation of inorganic (^{32}P) phosphate into rat parotid phosphatidylinositol. Mol Pharmacol 11:79–86

Oron Y, Kellog J, Larner J (1978 a) Stable cholinergic-muscarinic inhibition of rat parotid adenylate cyclase. FEBS Lett 94:331–334

Oron Y, Kellog J, Larner J (1978 b) *Alpha* adrenergic and cholinergic-muscarinic regulation of adenosine cyclic 3′,5′-monophosphate levels in the rat parotid. Mol Pharmacol 14:1018–1030

Ozawa S, Kimura N (1979) Membrane potential changes caused by thyrotropin-releasing hormone in the clonal GH_3 cell and their relationship to secretion of pituitary hormone. Proc Natl Acad Sci USA 76:6017–6020

Ozawa S, Miyazaki S (1979) Electrical excitability in the rat clonal pituitary cell and its relation to hormone secretion. Jpn J Physiol 29:411–426

Petersen OH, Ueda N (1976) Pancreatic acinar cells: the role of calcium in stimulus-secretion coupling. J Physiol (Lond) 254:583–606

Petersen OH, Ueda N (1977) Secretion of fluid and amylase in the perfused rat pancreas. J Physiol (Lond) 264:819–835

Pickard MR, Hawthorne JN (1978) The labelling of nerve ending phospholipids in guinea pig brain in vivo and the effect of electrical stimulation on phosphatidylinositol metabolism in prelabelled synaptosomes. J Neurochem 30:145–155

Poulsen JH, Williams JA (1976) Spontaneous repetitive hyperpolarizations from cells in the rat adenohypophysis. Nature 263:156–158

Poulsen JH, Williams JA (1977) Effects of the calcium ionophore A 23187 on pancreatic acinar cell membrane potentials and amylase release. J Physiol (Lond) 264: 323–339

Powell DW, Tapper EJ (1979) Intestinal ion transport: cholinergic-adrenergic interactions. Kroc Found Ser 12:175–192

Prince WT, Berridge MJ (1973) The role of calcium in the action of 5-hydroxytryptamine and cyclic AMP on salivary glands. J Exp Biol 58:367–384

Prince WT, Berridge MJ, Rasmussen H (1972) Role of calcium and adenosine-3′,5′-cyclic monophosphate in controlling fly salivary gland secretion. Proc Natl Acad Sci USA 69:553–557

Prince WT, Rasmussen H, Berridge MJ (1973) The role of calcium in fly salivary gland secretion analysed with the ionophore A 23187. Biochim Biophys Acta 329:98–107

Putney JW (1979) Stimulus-permeability coupling: role of calcium in the receptor regulation of membrane permeability. Pharmacol Rev 30:209–245

Putney JW, Weiss SJ, Leslie BA, Marier SH (1977) Is calcium the final mediator of exocytosis in the rat parotid gland? J Pharmacol Exp Ther 203:144–155

Putney JW, Weiss SJ, Van de Walle CM, Haddas RA (1980) Is phosphatidic acid a calcium ionophore under neurohumoral control? Nature 284:345–347

Rall TW (1982) Formation and degradation of cyclic nucleotides: an overview. In: Nathanson JA; Kebabian JW (eds) Cyclic nucleotides. Springer, Berlin Heidelberg New York (Handbook of experimental pharmacology, vol 58/I)

Ratner A, Wilson MC, Srivastava L, Peake GT (1976) Dissociation between LH release and pituitary cyclic nucleotide accumulation in response to synthetic LH-releasing hormone in vivo. Neuroendocrinology 20:35–42

Rasmussen H, Goodman DBP (1977) Relationships between calcium and cyclic nucleotides in cell activation. Physiol Rev 57:421–509

Reed PW, Lardy HA (1972) A 23187: a divalent cation ionophore. J Biol Chem 247:6970–6977

Renckens BAM, Schrijen JJ, Swart HGP, De Pont JJHHM, Bonting SL (1978) Role of calcium in exocrine pancreatic secretion. IV. Calcium movements in isolated acinar cells of rabbit pancreas. Biochim Biophys Acta 544:338–350

Ribalet B, Beigelman PM (1979) Cyclic variation of K^+ conductance in pancreatic B-cells: Ca^{2+} and voltage dependence. Am J Physiol 237:C137–C146

Rose B, Loewenstein WR (1975) Calcium ion distribution in cytoplasm visualized by aequorin: diffusion in cytosol restricted by energised sequestering. Science 190:1204–1206

Rubin RP (1970) The role of calcium in the release of neurotransmitter substances and hormones. Pharmacol Rev 22:389–428

Russell JT, Thorn NA (1974) Calcium and stimulus-secretion coupling in the neurohypophysis. Acta Endocrinol (Copenh) 76:471–487

Sabol SL, Nirenberg M (1979) Regulation of adenylate cyclase of neuroblastoma x glioma hybrid cells by α-adrenergic receptors. I. Inhibition of adenylate cyclase mediated by α-receptors. J Biol Chem 254:1913–1920
Salmon DM, Honeyman TW (1980) Proposed mechanism of cholinergic action in smooth muscle. Nature 284:344–345
Samli MH, Geschwind II (1968) Some effects of energy-transfer inhibitors and of Ca^{2+} free or K^+ enhanced media on the release of luteinizing hormone (LH) from the rat pituitary gland in vitro. Endocrinology 82:225–231
Schramm M, Selinger Z (1975) The functions of cyclic AMP and calcium as alternative second messengers in parotid gland and pancreas. J Cyclic Nucleotide Res 1:181–192
Schrey MP, Brown BL, Ekins RP (1978) Studies on the role of calcium and cyclic nucleotides in the control of TSH secretion. Mol Cell Endocrinol 11:249–264
Schulz I, Stolze HH (1980) The exocrine pancreas: the role of secretagogues, cyclic nucleotides, and calcium in enzyme secretion. Annu Rev Physiol 42:127–156
Sehlin J (1976) Calcium uptake by subcellular fractions of pancreatic islets. Biochem J 156:63–69
Selinger Z, Eimerl S, Schramm M (1974) A calcium ionophore simulating the action of epinephrine on the α-adrenergic receptor. Proc Natl Acad Sci USA 71:128–131
Siegel EG, Wollheim CB, Sharp GWG, Herberg L, Renold AE (1979) Defective calcium handling and insulin release in islets from diabetic Chinese hamsters. Biochem J 180:233–236
Siegel EG, Wollheim CB, Sharp GWG (1980) Glucose-induced first phase insulin release in the absence of extracellular Ca^{2+} in rat islets. FEBS Lett 109:213–215
Sieghart W, Theoharides TC, Alper SL, Douglas WW, Greengard P (1978) Calcium-dependent protein phosphorylation during secretion by exocytosis in the mast cell. Nature 275:329–331
Singh M (1979) Calcium and cyclic nucleotide interaction in secretion of amylase from pancreas in vivo. J Physiol (Lond) 296:159–176
Smith RJ, Iden SS (1979) Phorbol myristate acetate-induced release of granule enzymes from human neutrophils: inhibition by the calcium antagonist 8-(N,N-diethylamino)-octyl 3,4,5-trimethoxybenzoate hydrochloride. Biochem Biophys Res Commun 91:262–271
Soll AH (1979) Secretagogue stimulation of [^{14}C]-aminopyrine accumulation by isolated canine parietal cells. Am J Physiol 238:G366–G375
Soll AH, Grossman MI (1978) Cellular mechanisms in acid secretion. Annu Rev Med 29:495–507
Soll AH, Walsh JH (1979) Regulation of gastric acid secretion. Annu Rev Physiol 41:35–53
Somers G, Devis G, Van Obberghen E, Malaisse WJ (1976) Calcium antagonists and islet function. II. Interaction of theophylline and verapamil. Endocrinology 99:114–124
Somlyo AP, Somylo AV, Shuman H (1979) Electron probe analysis of vascular smooth muscle. J Cell Biol 81:316–335
Spence JW, Sheppard MS, Kraicer J (1980) Release of growth hormone from purified somatotrophs: interrelation between Ca^{2+} and adenosine 3′,5′-monophosphate. Endocrinology 106:764–769
Streweler GJ, Orloff J (1977) Role of cyclic nucleotides in the transport of water and electrolytes. Adv Cyclic Nucleotide Res 8:311–361
Sugden MC, Christie MR, Ashcroft SJH (1979) Presence and possible role of calcium-dependent regulator (calmodulin) in rat islets of Langerhans. FEBS Lett 105:95–100
Tam SW, Dannies PS (1980) Dopaminergic inhibition of ionophore A 23187-stimulated release of prolactin from rat anterior pituitary cells. J Biol Chem 255:6595–6599
Taraskevich PS, Douglas WW (1977) Action potentials occur in cells of the normal anterior pituitary gland and are stimulated by the hypophysiotropic peptide thyrotropin-releasing hormone. Proc Natl Acad Sci USA 74:4064–4067
Taraskevich PS, Douglas WW (1978) Catecholamines of supposed inhibitory hypophysiotropic function suppress action potentials in prolactin cells. Nature 276:832–834
Taraskevich PS, Douglas WW (1979) Stimulant effect of 5-hydroxytryptamine on action potential activity in pars intermedia cells of the lizard *Apolis carolinensis:* contrasting effects in pars intermedia of rat and rostral pars distalis of fish *(Alosa pseudoharengus)*. Brain Res 178:584–588

Tashjian AH, Lomedico ME, Maina D (1978) Role of calcium in the thyrotropin-releasing hormone-stimulated release of prolactin from pituitary cells in culture. Biochem Biophys Res Commun 81:798–806
Thomas MV, Gorman ALF (1977) Internal calcium changes in bursting pacemaker neuron measured with Arsenazo III. Science 196:531–533
Thompson WJ, Rosenfeld GC, Jacobson ED (1977) Adenylyl cyclase and gastric acid secretion. Fed Proc 36:1938–1941
Thorn NA, Russell JT, Robinson ICAF (1975) Factors affecting intracellular concentration of free calcium ions in neurosecretory nerve endings. In: Carafoli E, Clementi F, Drabikowski W, Margreth A (eds) Calcium transport in contraction and secretion. North Holland, Amsterdam Oxford New York, pp 261–269
Torda C (1972) Cyclic AMP-dependent diphosphoinositide kinase. Biochim Biophys Acta 286:389–395
Trifaró JM (1969) The effect of Ca^{++} omission on the secretion of catecholamine and the incorporation of orthophosphate-^{32}P into nucleotides and phospholipids of bovine adrenal medulla during acetylcholine stimulation. Mol Pharmacol 5:420–431
Tyson CA, Vande Zande H, Green DE (1976) Phospholipids as ionophores. J Biol Chem 251:1326–1332
Vale W, Guillemin R (1967) Potassium-induced stimulation of thyrotropin release in vitro. Requirement for presence of calcium and inhibition by thyroxine. Experientia 23:855–857
Vale W, Burgess R, Guillemin R (1967) Presence of calcium ions as a requisite for the in vitro stimulation of TSH-release by hypothalamic TRF. Experientia 23:853–855
Valverde I, Vandermeers A, Anjaneyulu R, Malaisse WJ (1979) Calmodulin activation of adenylate cyclase in pancreatic islets. Science 206:225–227
Van Breemen C, De Weer P (1970) Lanthanum inhibition of ^{45}Ca efflux from the squid giant axon. Nature 226:760–761
Van Golde LMG, Raben J, Batenburg JJ, Fleischer B, Zambrano F, Fleischer S (1974) Biosynthesis of lipids in golgi complex and other subcellular fractions from rat liver. Biochim Biophys Acta 360:179–192
Walker AM, Hopkins CR (1978) Dissociation of the porcine anterior pituitary: the kinetics of luteinizing hormone release in response to luteinizing hormone-releasing hormone. Mol Cell Endocrinol 12:177–187
Weiss B, Levin RM (1978) Mechanism for selectively inhibiting the activation of cyclic nucleotide phosphatidiesterase and adenylate cyclase by antipsychotic agents. Adv Cyclic Nucleotide Res 9:285–303
Wilber JF, Peake GT, Utiger RD, (1969) Thyrotropin release in vitro: stimulation by cyclic 3′,5′ adenosine monophosphate. Endocrinology 84:758–760
Williams JA (1975) Na^{+} dependence of in vitro pancreatic amylase release. Am J Physiol 229:1023–1026
Williams JA, Lee M (1974) Pancreatic acinar cells: use of a Ca^{2+} ionophore to separate enzyme release from the earlier steps in stimulus-secretion coupling. Biochem Biophys Res Commun 60:542–548
Wolff DJ, Brostrom CO (1979) Properties and functions of the calcium-dependent regulator protein. Adv Cyclic Nucleotide Res 11:27–88
Wollheim CB, Blondel B, Trueheart PA, Renold AE, Sharp GWG (1975) Calcium-induced insulin release in monolayer culture of the endocrine pancreas. J Biol Chem 250:1354–1360
Wollheim CB, Kikuchi M, Reynold AG (1978) The roles of intracellular and extracellular Ca^{++} in glucose-stimulated biphasic insulin release by rat islets. J Clin Invest 62:451–458
Zawalich WS, Karl RC, Ferrendelli J, Matschinsky FM (1975) Effects of glucose, Ca^{++} and an ionophore on cyclic-3′,5′-AMP (cAMP) and insulin release in isolated pancreatic islets. Diabetes 23:337

CHAPTER 21

Regulation of Water and Electrolyte Movement by Vasopressin and Cyclic Nucleotides in Kidney

D. A. AUSIELLO and J. ORLOFF

Overview

A direct effect of cyclic AMP (cAMP) on water and electrolyte transport was first reported in 1962 (ORLOFF and HANDLER 1962). The authors noted that the nucleotide mimicked vasopressin (ADH) in the urinary bladder of the toad *Bufo marinus* in that it increased both osmotic water flow and net sodium transport across the tissue. Since then a large body of data has accumulated implicating cAMP as the biochemical messenger for hormones that influence transport in kidney and other epithelial target tissues (for recent review, see STREWLER and ORLOFF 1977; DOUSA 1979).

ADH action is initiated when the hormone binds to its receptor at the basolateral surface of target epithelial cells and stimulates adenylyl cyclase. Hormone-receptor-enzyme interactions can be modulated in many ways. ADH induces a decrease in the affinity of its receptor and an associated uncoupling of the hormone-receptor complex from adenylyl cyclase. The change in receptor affinity is prevented by hypertonic NaCl. It is conceivable that the degree of hypertonicity of the renal medulla in vivo may regulate ADH binding.

Prostaglandins inhibit ADH-stimulation of water flow in toad bladder and renal collecting duct, presumably by inhibiting an ADH-sensitive adenylyl cyclase, perhaps through an effect on the action of Ca^{++} and calmodulin. ADH stimulates prostaglandin synthesis in toad bladder and kidney, and may thereby influence its own effects on transport.

Consistent with the current view that most, if not all, responses to cAMP are mediated by cAMP-dependent protein kinases, several studies have demonstrated that ADH is capable of stimulating protein phosphorylation and dephosphorylation. The 50,000 dalton protein dephosphorylated in toad bladder in response to ADH is very likely the regulatory unit of type II cAMP-dependent protein kinase. It is therefore unlikely that this phosphoprotein is the final mediator of hormone action. It is possible that such a cAMP-dependent protein phosphorylation is the initial event in a sequence of reactions that lead to a physiological response. Alternatively, a specific apical membrane protein or proteins phosphorylated by a cAMP-dependent kinase may be directly responsible for increased water or NaCl transport in ADH-responsive tissue.

During the last decade a role for cytosolic calcium as a mediator of ADH-induced sodium and water transport has been proposed. In most studies, manipulations of the cell environment leading to increases in cytosolic calcium have blunted the effects of vasopressin on water flow and sodium transport.

There is still much to be learned about the interactions of cAMP and calcium in the production of these responses but effects of these mediators on microtubule and microfilament assembly may be involved.

Although this chapter focuses on the biochemical events associated with ADH action in kidney, toad bladder and cultured renal epithelial cells, it is probable that many of these also play a role in cellular responses to other agonists, e.g., PTH, calcitonin, and β-adrenergic agents. In all cases, however, the mechanism of hormone-mediated transport itself remains to be defined.

A. Vasopressin Action in Kidney and Toad Bladder

The ability of the mammalian kidney to excrete a concentrated urine is dependent on its responsiveness to vasopressin (ADH). The hormone increases the water permeability of the renal collecting tubules and medullary collecting duct (HANDLER and ORLOFF 1973) and has minor effects on sodium reabsorption in collecting tubules (GANOTE et al. 1968; SCHAFER and ANDREOLI 1972). It also increases active chloride transport in the medullary thick ascending limb of Henle's loop in the mouse (HALL and VARNEY 1980; SASAKI and IMAI 1980).

The urinary bladder of the toad has been used extensively as a model system for examining the effects of ADH on transport since in many respects the effects of the hormone are analogous to those in the renal collecting tubule. The bladder responds to ADH by increasing: a) the active transport of sodium from the mucosal (urinary) to the serosal (blood) surface; b) the rate of water flow along an osmotic gradient; and c) the permeability to urea and other small solutes. The physical-chemical changes in the membrane responsible for the alterations in permeability are not fully understood. The subject is beyond the scope of this review but is dealt with in detail elsewhere (SCHAFER and ANDREOLI 1977, 1978; ANDREOLI and SCHAFER 1976). Certain features will be noted briefly for purposes of orientation. Thus, although ADH is known to interact with its receptor at the serosal surface of the pertinent epithelial cell, it alters the permeability of a limiting barrier at the luminal surface of the cell (HAYS and LEAF 1962) via the intermediacy of cAMP (ORLOFF and HANDLER 1962). Cells of the renal collecting tubule bathed in isotonic fluid and perfused through its lumen with hypotonic fluid swell in consequence of osmotic uptake of water from lumen to cell only if ADH is added to the medium bathing the serosal surface. This effect of ADH is associated with an increase in apical membrane deformability (GRANTHAM 1970). DIBONA (1979) has extended these observations to toad bladder granular cells and has concluded that an increase in apical membrane compliance is a primary feature of the swelling response to ADH-induced water flow.

Although it was originally proposed that ADH increased osmotic flow across responsive anuran and mammalian epithelial membranes by increasing the size of pores in the structure (KOEFOED-JOHNSON and USSING 1953), this view was discarded in favor of one that ascribed the effect to an alteration in the luminal membrane that permitted more rapid diffusion rather than bulk flow of water across the structure (ANDREOLI and SCHAEFER 1976 for review of subject). More recently, FINKELSTEIN (1976a, b) has pointed out that the 100-fold increase in the ratio of water permeability to the permeability of certain solutes produced in toad bladder by ADH is inconsistent with a simple diffusion model, but compatible with the view that water flows through aqueous channels in the apical membrane. His view differs in detail from that of KOEFOED-JOHNSON and USSING (1953) in that he ascribes the effect of vasopressin to an increase in the size or number of small aqueous channels through which water moves by single file diffusion.

Direct evidence for ADH induction of aqueous channels is derived from studies by GLUCK and AL-AWQATI (1980) who measured the proton permeability of toad bladder. They reason that protons would not be able to cross lipid bilayers easily, since even fluid lipids have a very low dielectric constant. On the other hand, protons would traverse aqueous channels since, unlike other ions, they could jump from one water molecule in the bulk solution onto another at the mouth of the channel. This would lead to proton transfer through the chain of water molecules in the channel. Their results support this hypothesis. Hydrogen ion permeability across the toad bladder correlated with increased water permeability in response to ADH, but not with changes in sodium or urea permeability.

The results of several other studies have been interpreted to support the pore or aqueous channel thesis. Thus ADH and cAMP have been shown to induce the appearance of intramembranous particle aggregates in the apical membrane of granular cells in frog and toad bladder (CHEVALIER et al. 1974; BOURGUET et al. 1976; KACHADORIAN et al. 1975). The number of aggregates and the cumulative area of toad bladder epithelial cell membrane occupied by aggregates are related directly to the magnitude of ADH-induced changes in water permeability in toad bladder under a variety of circumstances (KACHADORIAN et al. 1977a, b; WADE 1980). It has been proposed that particle aggregation sites may behave as pores (KACHADORIAN et al. 1979a; MULLER et al. 1980).

The particle aggregates seen in the apical membrane after ADH stimulation appear to be transferred preformed by fusion of membranes of cytoplasmic vacuoles with the apical membrane (MULLER et al. 1980). Initiation of the fusion may be dependent on intact microtubules. Microfilaments seem not to be involved in the process of membrane fusion, but once fusion has occurred, may play a role in the movement of aggregates from the intracellular membranes to apical membranes (see below).

B. Cell Culture Models

In the last few years, several laboratories have utilized cultured cells to study a number of renal cell functions, including transepithelial transport and hormone action. Cultured cells offer the advantage of homogeneity, relatively large quantities of material, and the ability to control the cells' growth media and environment. These conditions are rarely met in intact organs, even in simple epithelia such as toad bladder.

Four types of cultured cell systems that respond to ADH and/or cAMP have recently been described. Two are established cell lines (MDCK and LLC-PK$_1$ cells) and two are derived from primary cultures. The characteristics of the effects of ADH on these cells will be briefly described. Detailed reviews of studies with these cell lines have been published recently (CEREIJIDO et al. 1978; TAUB and SAIER 1979a; HANDLER et al. 1980).

I. MDCK Cell Line

The Maden Darby canine kidney cell line (MDCK) was derived from the kidney of a normal male cocker spaniel in 1958. Morphologically, these cells exhibit a structural polarity characteristic of transporting epithelia (LEIGHTON et al. 1969; MISFELDT et al 1976). The monolayer formed by MDCK cells transports approximately 10 μl $cm^{-2} \cdot h^{-2}$ of fluid toward the basolateral surface (MISFELDT et al. 1976). The cells contain an adenylyl cyclase system sensitive to ADH, glucagon, prostaglandin E_2 (PGE_2) and isoproterenol (RINDLER et al. 1979; HANDLER et al. 1980). Analogues of cAMP stimulate the formation of cyst-like structures called "hemicysts" or "domes" (VALENTICH et al. 1976). These domes result from the accumulation of reabsorbed components of the medium between the cell surface and the culture dish (LEIGHTON et al. 1969). Hemicyst formation is thus ascribed to and correlates with transepithelial transport of fluid from bathing medium to the basolateral surface of the cells attached to the culture dish. This cell line has served as a useful model for study of the regulation of epithelial cell growth and Na^+ uptake (TAUB and SAIER 1979a, b).

II. LLC-PK_1 Cells

These cells, originally derived from male Hampshire pig kidney by HULL et al. (1976), also form monolayers of polar epithelial cells in culture. Their functional polarity was demonstrated by the ability of the cells to bind [^{3}H]-ouabain only to their basolateral cell surfaces (MILLS et al. 1979). Monolayers of the cells exhibit sodium-dependent, phlorizin-inhibitable hexose transport with characteristics similar to those observed in kidney (RABITO and AUSIELLO 1980). Active transport of α-methyl glucopyranoside (αMGP), a non-metabolized sugar, was inhibited both by omitting Na^+ from the medium or by ouabain. Kinetic analysis of the effect of Na^+ on the uptake of αMGP indicates that Na^+-sugar co-transport occurs via a system in which binding of either sugar or Na^+ to the carrier increases the affinity for the ligand without affecting the V_{max}.

Whereas the transport characteristics of the LLC-PK_1 cells so far observed are generally analogous to those found in the proximal tubules of kidney, the hormone sensitivity of these cells is not, but rather reflects that of the distal nephron. GOLDRING et al. (1978) observed that ADH or calcitonin increased cAMP content of LLC-PK_1 cells 30-fold in 10 min in the absence of phosphodiesterase inhibitors. Parathyroid hormone, epinephrine or PGE_2 did not affect cAMP content, nor did PGE_2 inhibit the ADH or calcitonin response. Further studies have demonstrated that the specificity of the ADH receptor for analogues of ADH is identical to that of the ADH receptor in pig medullary membranes (ROY and AUSIELLO 1981a).

To demonstrate the usefulness of these cells as a model system in which to investigate the biochemical events of ADH action distal to cAMP production, the activation of cAMP-dependent protein kinase (cAMP·PK) was examined

(AUSIELLO et al. 1980a). As will be discussed below, phosphorylation of membrane and/or cytosolic proteins, catalyzed by cAMP · PK, may be the essential final step in the action of ADH and other hormones that affect transport in responsive epithelial structures. Both ADH and calcitonin activated cAMP · PK. This effect was most pronounced on soluble cAMP · PK which accounted for 80% of the total cell protein kinase activity. DEAE-cellulose chromatography demonstrated a predominance of the type II cAMP · PK isoenzyme in LLC-PK_1 cells and in rat and guinea pig renal medulla. Thus the LLC-PK_1 cell line may serve both as a model for the study of hormonal modulation of protein kinase and as a source of the endogenous substrates for isolation and/or identification.

III. Primary Culture of Toad Bladder Epithelial Cells

HANDLER et al. (1979) have established five lines of epithelial cells derived from the urinary bladder of the toad. Unlike the permanent cell lines described above, these cells when grown on filters form more than one layer. Cells of the apical layer contain microvilli, junctional complexes and, in some cases, granules. The latter resemble those found in the granular cells of the toad bladder which are presumed responsible for vasopressin-stimulated sodium and water flow (DIBONA et al. 1969a, b). The transport properties of a cell line TB-M have been studied. These cells develop a shortcircuit current (I_{SC}) of 8 μA · cm^{-2} (about half that of the intact bladder). I_{SC} is the equivalent of net mucosa-to-serosa Na^+ transport (HANDLER et al. 1980). Although both aldosterone and cAMP stimulate active Na^+ transport in these cell lines, the cells do not respond to ADH, apparently the result of the absence of ADH receptors (JOHNSON et al. 1979). Exogenous cAMP also alters urea permeability, but not osmotic water flow. These cells represent the first cultured epithelial cell line that maintain the characteristics of "tight" epithelia and thus offer the opportunity to study basal and hormone stimulated transepithelial Na^+ transport.

IV. Primary Culture of Glomerular Mesangial Cells

KREISBERG and KARNOVSKY (to be published) have been able to isolate and maintain in tissue culture three clones of cells from rat glomeruli. One contains numerous microfilaments and is morphologically similar to a mesangial cell. To identify the physiological role of glomerular mesangial (MS) cells, their responses to ADH, angiotensin II (AG II), PGE_2 and parathyroid hormone were investigated (AUSIELLO et al. 1980b). ADH (0.1 n*M*) and AG II (1 n*M*) induced contraction of MS cells as observed by phase contrast and electron microscopy. [^{3}H] (8-lysine) vasopressin bound to these cells with an apparent affinity of 10 n*M*. ADH at low concentrations did not induce cAMP production although PGE_2 increased cell cAMP content as much as six-fold; neither agent altered cGMP content. These observations provide no evidence for a relationship between cAMP and contraction. It might be inferred that the ADH effect was mediated by interaction with the putative "pressor" receptor similar to that described in smooth muscle (ALTURA 1970) and hepatocytes (CHEN et al. 1978; CANTAU et al. 1980). Both AG II and ADH decrease the glomerular ultrafiltration coefficient, K_f, which is a reflection of glomerular permeability and capillary surface area (BLANTZ et al. 1976; ICHIKAWA and BRENNER 1977). A decrease in glomerular surface area might conceivably be achieved by the hormone-induced contraction of mesangial cells.

The "pressor" response to ADH is correlated with alterations in Ca^{++} efflux from hepatocytes (CHEN et al. 1978; EXTON 1980) whereas the antidiuretic response to the hormone in responsive epithelial cells is mediated by an increase in cAMP content which may be associated with changes in cytosolic Ca^{++} (see discussion below). Further studies with cultured cells should help to define the similarities and differences in the biochemical events associated with these two physiological responses to ADH.

C. Role of Cyclic AMP in ADH Action – Cellular Mechanisms

It is now established that cAMP is the mediator of the effects of ADH on transport. Following the initial observations that cAMP and theophylline, a phosphodiesterase inhibitor, reproduced the effects of ADH on water, urea permeability, and active sodium transport in toad urinary bladder (ORLOFF and HANDLER 1962) it was demonstrated that the cAMP content of toad bladder epithelial cells increased in response to ADH (HANDLER et al. 1965). Succeeding experiments demonstrated that cAMP mimics ADH in the kidney in that it increases the permeability of the isolated cortical collecting tubule of the rabbit to water (GRANTHAM and BURG 1966).

ADH increased adenylyl cyclase activity in isolated segments of rabbit cortical collecting tubules 26-fold; a 15-fold increase was noted in medullary collecting tubules, and a 9-fold increase in the thick ascending limb of Henle (IMBERT et al. 1975). Similar results were obtained in renal collecting tubules from mouse, rat, and man. In contrast, the medullary thick ascending limb of the loop of Henle is highly responsive to ADH in rat and mouse, less responsive in rabbit and insensitive in man (MOREL et al. 1978; CHABARDÈS et al. 1980). These data are consistent with the view that the ADH-induced changes in transport in renal collecting ducts result from the hormone's ability to increase cAMP production. The precise physiologic role for ADH and cAMP in the medullary thick ascending limb remains to be established.

I. ADH Receptors and Adenylyl Cyclase

The initial event in the response of a target organ to ADH is the interaction between the hormone and its receptor that results in a train of events leading to activation of adenylyl cyclase and acceleration of the synthesis of cAMP. The enzyme system is complex and the mode by which the occupied hormone receptor increases its activity is unknown. Hormone receptors and adenylyl cyclase activation have been considered in detail in earlier Chaps. (see Chapters 3 and 4 in Vol. 58/I on Biochemistry of Cyclic Nucleotides). In this discussion we shall focus specifically on the activation of adenylyl cyclase by ADH.

1. ADH Receptor Occupancy and Coupling to Adenylyl Cyclase

Detailed studies of ADH interaction with its receptor have been conducted by SERGE JARD and his colleagues at the Collège de France. They have been successful in preparing [^{3}H] labeled vasopressin, the only suitable radiolabeled ligand for binding studies. Their results have been summarized elsewhere (JARD et al. 1977). The more readily available ^{125}I-labeled hormone has no ADH-like activity as assessed by binding or activation of adenylyl cyclase (FLOURET et al. 1977).

BOCKAERT et al. (1973) demonstrated specific binding of [^{3}H] (8-lysine) vasopressin (LVP) to pig kidney medullary plasma membranes. The preparation proved to be particularly useful for studying the properties of the receptor-adenylyl cyclase system, especially in its ability to discriminate between structurally related ADH analogues (ROY et al. 1975 a, b). Of particular interest were the observations on receptor occupancy and coupling to adenylyl cyclase. Significant activation of adenylyl cyclase occurred with very low fractional occupancy of receptors. When relative adenylyl cyclase stimulation was plotted as a function of relative receptor occupancy, a non-linear relationship was observed, i.e., as total receptor occupancy increased, a given increment in receptor occupancy resulted in a smaller increase in adenylyl cyclase activity. This raised the possibility of heterogenous populations of receptors, only some of which were coupled efficiently to adenylyl cyclase. Kinetic analysis of [^{3}H] LVP binding, however, was consistent with a single population of receptors ($K_m = 20$ nM). Similar observations were made in bovine renal medullary membranes (see BERGMAN and HECHTER 1978). However, in recent studies with the porcine renal cell line, LLC-PK$_1$, kinetic analysis of [^{3}H] LVP binding to monolayers of intact cultured cells was consistent with the existence of receptors with high and low affinities (ROY and AUSIELLO 1981 a). Several lines of evidence favored a transition of high (R) to low (R′) affinity receptors with increasing hormonal receptor occupancy, rather than two independent populations of binding sites. Equation (1) illustrates this "receptor transition" model. The ADH receptors are assumed to exist as dimers, since site-site interaction between receptors likely requires receptor clustering or aggregation.

$$H + RR \underset{(1)}{\overset{K_1}{\rightleftharpoons}} HRR \underset{(2)}{\rightleftharpoons} HRR' \underset{(3)}{\overset{K_2\ \ H}{\rightleftharpoons}} HRR'H \qquad (1)$$

Prior to hormonal (H) binding, both units (R) of the dimer have a high affinity, K_1. With the binding of hormone to one unit of the dimer, the affinity of the other unoccupied site (R′) is lowered to K_2. The change in affinity from K_1 to K_2 occurs only in those dimers which previously bound H. This transition in receptor affinity is associated with uncoupling of the hormone receptor complex from adenylyl cyclase (ROY et al. 1981): at low hormone concentrations with bound H predominately present as HRR or HRR′ (reaction 1 and 2) a linear relationship was observed between receptor occupancy and cAMP production in intact cells; when with increasing hormone concentration, HRR′H increased (reaction 3), non-linear coupling to adenylyl cyclase was observed.

Further support for the concept that HR′ is poorly coupled to adenylyl cyclase was obtained from the following experiments: intact LLC-PK$_1$ cells were exposed for four minutes to a concentration of ADH which would occupy all receptor sites and thus maximize conversion of R to R′. Cells were washed and membranes prepared for the in vitro assay of adenylyl cyclase. Despite the fact that enzyme activity had returned to basal levels, less than 60% of the maximum ADH activation of adenylyl cyclase was achieved on restimulation with hormone. If the incubation medium bathing intact cells was modified to prevent the transition of R to R′, then maximal ADH-activation of adenylyl cyclase was preserved. These data support the view that receptor transition is necessary for uncoupling of the hormone receptor enzyme complex.

It has been proposed that a single ADH receptor, upon binding hormone, has the ability to activate several adenylyl cyclase molecules within a limited interaction field (BERGMAN and HECHTER 1978). Since only a small fraction of total receptors are occupied at physiological concentrations of ADH (~0.01 n*M*), it would seem advantageous to a target cell if each hormone molecule binds to a receptor that is capable of coupling to adenylyl cyclase. Receptor transition may serve the cell in this capacity: the large population of spare receptors enhances the probability of a hormone molecule interacting with its target (receptor). Once this interaction has been achieved, within the framework of the model described above, a rapid decrease in the affinity of those receptors within the same interaction field will insure that each hormone molecule binds to a receptor capable of eliciting a physiological response.

2. Effects of NaCl

The ADH receptor is constantly exposed to 200–500 m*M* NaCl in the renal medulla of a normal intact kidney (MORGAN 1977). It is therefore not surprising that hypertonic NaCl results in large modifications in ADH-sensitive adenylyl cyclase in vitro. When 250 m*M* NaCl was added to the incubation medium with pig kidney medullary membranes, an 8- to 30-fold increase in ADH-stimulated adenylyl cyclase was observed (ROY et al. 1977). These changes in maximal enzyme stimulation occurred with only minimal modification in the catalytic activity of adenylyl cyclase measured under basal conditions. No ^{3}H-binding studies were conducted to determine if NaCl induced changes in ADH receptor number, affinity, or coupling to enzyme.

MORGAN (1977) demonstrated that the isolated rat renal papilla exposed to a medium containing 300 m*M* NaCl has an intracellular NaCl concentration of 200 m*M*. Thus in vivo, the ADH receptor on the outer surface of the plasma membrane and cytalytic unit of adenylyl cyclase situated at the interior of the plasma membrane are likely to be exposed to different NaCl concentrations. Since in isolated membranes it is not possible to reproduce the physiological assymetry of NaCl concentrations bathing the ADH receptor and adenylyl cyclase, the effect of hypertonic NaCl on [^{3}H] LVP binding and ADH-stimulated adenylyl cyclase in the intact LLC-PK$_1$ cells was examined (ROY et al. 1981; ROY and AUSIELLO 1981 b). Increasing medium NaCl concentration from 150 m*M* to 450 m*M* led to a progressive increase in the binding of 10 n*M* [^{3}H] LVP (3-fold maximal increase) as well as increased adenylyl cyclase activation and cAMP production.

It remains to be established whether the effects of NaCl observed in isolated membranes and intact cultured cells occur in vivo in hypertonic renal medullary cells exposed to only 1–10 p*M* ADH. Results obtained in Brattleboro rats with hypothalamic diabetes insipidus (DI) however, are consistent with this hypothesis. In these rats, the sensitivity of the medullo-papillary adenylyl cyclase to ADH is reduced (DOUSA et al. 1975; RAJERISON et al. 1977). Chronic administration of physiological concentrations of ADH in vivo induced a 30% increase in the responsiveness of the enzyme to ADH in vitro (RAJERISON et al. 1977). In this study, the reduction of ADH secretion in normal rats during induced water diuresis was associated with a 30% reduction of maximal adenylyl cyclase activation by ADH in vitro. Hormone-sensitive enzyme activity was restored to maximal levels following chronic administration of ADH as it was in DI rats. These results were interpreted to indicate that the number of specific ADH-receptor sites present on target cells is normally regulated by the concentration of the hormone in body fluids. The ADH receptor-adenylyl cyclase interaction could be controlled by the chemical composition of the renal medullary interstitial fluid, as in LLC-PK_1 cells. The inability of the DI rats to maximally concentrate urine (VALTIN and SCHROEDER 1964) presumably as a consequence of minimal stimulation of adenylyl cyclase may be due to the subnormal solute concentration prevailing in the renal medulla. This hypothesis is consistent with the observation that prolonged treatment of DI rats with ADH, which gradually increases medullary osmolality, restores the concentrating ability of the kidney to normal (HARRINGTON and VALTIN 1968).

Recent studies by IMBERT-TEBOUL et al. (1978) utilizing microdissected segments of renal tubules from Brattleboro rats (DI), support this view. They have demonstrated that the impaired response of adenylyl cyclase to ADH was limited to the medullary thick ascending limb of Henle's loop (MAL). This is the segment of the nephron chiefly responsible for solute accumulation in the medullary interstitial fluid (BURG and GREEN 1973). Thus a causal relationship may exist between the solute environment and decreased ADH-sensitive adenylyl cyclase activity in the MAL of DI rats, as well as the impairment of their ability to produce a concentrated urine.

3. Effects of Glucocorticoid Hormones

In the rat (RAJERISON et al. 1974), adrenalectomy reduced the responsiveness of kidney medullary adenylyl cyclase to ADH. ADH stimulation was specifically affected; basal and parathyroid hormone- and fluoride-stimulated activities were unaffected. Adrenalectomy (with mineralocorticoid replacement) reduced the efficiency of the ADH receptor-enzyme coupling process; both the number and affinity of ADH receptors remained unchanged, and their specificity towards ADH structural analogues was preserved. In vivo treatment of glucocorticoid deficient rats with dexamethasone restored the efficiency of receptor-enzyme coupling, whereas the in vitro addition of the glucocorticoid to the adenylyl cyclase assay was without effect. It is possible that glucocorticoids control the synthesis of a protein responsible for the coupling of the hormone-receptor complex to adenylyl cyclase.

A small reduction in ADH binding capacity was observed in adrenalectomized rats deficient in both mineralocorticoids and glucocorticoids. Although receptor number was returned to normal by treatment with either aldosterone or dexamethasone (a glucocorticoid), only the glucocorticoid restored the receptor-enzyme coupling defect described above.

4. Interactions with Prostaglandins

a) Effects of ADH on Prostaglandin Synthesis

Experiments in one of our laboratories in the 1960's first demonstrated the inhibition of ADH-induced water flow by prostaglandins (PG). PGE_1 and PGE_2 inhibited the effects of ADH and theophylline on the water permeability of the isolated toad urinary bladder, but did not inhibit the response to exogenous cAMP (ORLOFF et al. 1965; URAKABE et al. 1975). Similar results were obtained from studies in the isolated rabbit renal collecting tubule, an analogous ADH-responsive epithelium (GRANTHAM and ORLOFF 1968). On the basis of these observations, GRANTHAM and ORLOFF suggested that endogenous PG modulates the water permeability response to ADH. Support for this hypothesis has been obtained in studies in isolated toad bladder where ADH stimulation of PGE_2 synthesis has been measured directly (ZUSMAN et al. 1977a). ADH, theophylline, and cAMP each increased the water permeability of this tissue, but only ADH stimulated PGE_2 synthesis. The latter was dependent on activation of a hormone-sensitive phospholipase. Inhibition of PGE_2 biosynthesis resulted in augmented ADH- and theophylline-stimulated water flow but had no effect on cAMP-stimulated water flow. The authors interpreted these results to indicate that endogenous PGE_2 inhibited basal and ADH-stimulated adenylyl cyclase activity (see below).

Further studies have provided a unifying mechanism for the modulation of ADH action by chlorpropamide, an oral hypoglycemic sulfonylurea, and steroid hormones (ZUSMAN et al. 1977b, 1978; ORLOFF and ZUSMAN 1978). Chlorpropamide enhances the hydroosmotic effect of ADH in toad bladder (MENDOZA and BROWN 1974) by inhibiting the conversion of arachidonic acid to PGE_2 (ZUSMAN et al. 1977b). Adrenal steroid hormones known to enhance ADH-induced water flow in toad bladder (HANDLER et al. 1969) and renal collecting tubule (M. SCHWARTZ and KOKKO 1980) also inhibit ADH-stimulated PGE_2 in toad bladder by decreasing arachidonic acid release from the phospholipid storage pool (ZUSMAN et al. 1978). Their inhibitory effect on cAMP phosphodiesterase also contribute to the permissive effect of the steroid on ADH-induced water flow (STOFF et al. 1973) (v.i.).

Indirect evaluation of the relationship between ADH action and endogenous PG synthesis have been performed in studies in mammalian kidney. Indomethacin, an inhibitor of PG biosynthesis, enhances the antidiuretic effect of ADH in man (BERL et al. 1977), rat (LUM et al. 1977), and dog (ANDERSON et al. 1975). Furthermore, in rats (WALKER et al. 1978) and rabbits (LIFSCHITZ and STEIN 1977), ADH administration increases urinary PG excretion.

In intact kidney, there appear to be four different regions capable of PG biosynthesis: (1) the glomerulus (HASSID et al. 1979), particularly the glomerular mesangial cells (SRAER et al. 1979; AUSIELLO et al. 1980b); (2) the renal vasculature (SMITH and BELL 1978); (3) medullary and cortical collecting ducts (SMITH and BELL 1978); and (4) medullary interstitial cells (ZUSMAN and KEISER 1977). In rabbit renomedullary interstitial cells in tissue culture (ZUSMAN and KEISER 1977), stimulation of PG biosynthesis by ADH has been demonstrated directly. This effect is due to an increase in the rate of arachidonic acid released from a storage pool following activation of a hormone-sensitive phospholipase. ADH presumably mediated this effect via its pressor receptor since DDAVP (1-desamino-8-D-arginine vasopressin), a synthetic analog with antidiuretic activity but no pressor activity, had no effect on PGE_2 biosynthesis by the cells in culture (BECK et al. 1980). It has not been demonstrated however, that the increase in urinary PG excretion described in studies referred to above is a consequence of ADH stimulation of PG synthesis in medullary interstitial cells in vivo. It is possible that this effect of ADH could be mediated by "pressor" receptors in glomerular mesangial cells (AUSIELLO et al. 1980b) and renal vasculature (ALTURA 1970), and/or „antidiuretic" receptors in renal collecting tubules (ROY et al. 1975a, b). Indirect evidence supports such a role for the renal antidiuretic receptors. DDAVP, the non-pressor analogue of ADH, has been shown to increase the urinary excretion of PG in rats with hereditary pituitary diabetes insipidus (DI) (DUNN et al. 1978). In further studies, it was demonstrated that the urinary osmolality in DI rats was inversely related to the ratio of PG excretion and the ingested dose of DDAVP (DUNN et al. 1979). Indomethacin potentiated the effect of DDAVP on urine osmolality. Thus, the effects of ADH on urine concentration in vivo reflect a balance between the cAMP-mediated effects of the hormone on the collecting tubule and the antagonistic actions of renal PG. Studies with isolated collecting tubules will be required to determine whether ADH directly stimulates PG biosynthesis in these cells.

It also has been demonstrated that derivatives of arachidonic acid other than prostaglandins affect the hydroosmotic response to ADH. The toad urinary bladder synthesizes thromboxane B_2 (the metabolite of thromboxane A_2). Its synthesis is stimulated by ADH during the period of the water permeability response to the hormone (BURCH et al. 1979, 1980). cAMP did not affect thromboxane synthesis. A thromboxane antagonist, 13-azaprostonoic acid (13 APA), inhibited ADH-stimulated water flow in a dose dependent fashion. An inhibitor of thromboxane biosynthesis, 7-(l-Imidazolyl)-heptanoic acid, inhibited both the hydroosmotic effect of ADH and thromboxane B_2 synthesis, but did not affect synthesis of PGE_1 or PGE_2. Neither of these agents affected the water flow response to cAMP.

An effect of exogenous thromboxanes on water flow in toad bladder has been reported (BURCH and HALUSHKA 1979). These agents increased the water permeability of the bladder, and the effect was blocked by the thromboxane antagonist, 13 APA. The data are consistent with the hypothesis that an increase in thromboxane A_2 synthesis in response to ADH enhances the effect of the hormone on water flow (BURCH et al. 1980).

Several studies have demonstrated a role for Ca^{++} in stimulating prostaglandin and thromboxane biosynthesis in renal medulla (KNAPP et al. 1977; ZENSER and DAVIS 1978; CRAVEN et al. 1980). As discussed below, the interaction of ADH with its receptors may result in an increase in cytosolic Ca^{++} in the region of the basolateral surface of hormone-sensitive cells which is responsible, in part, for the stimulation of adenylyl cyclase. It is possible that this Ca^{++} signal is also the stimulus for ADH-induced prostaglandin synthesis.

b) Effects of PG on ADH-Sensitive Adenylyl Cyclase

In the toad bladder, an increase in the Ca^{++} concentration of the serosal medium impairs the hydroosmotic response but not the active Na^+ transport response to

Table 1. The effects of PGE_1 on cAMP production and Na^+ and H_2O transport in toad bladder

PGE_1 (M)	Cell cAMP content	H_2O flow		Na^+ transport
		Theophylline	ADH [a]	
10^{-8}	↔	↓	↓	+
10^{-7}	↑	↓↓	↓↓	+
10^{-6}	↑↑	↑	↓	++
10^{-5}	↑↑↑	↑↑	↔	+++

[a] 25 mU/ml

submaximal concentrations of ADH (PETERSEN and EDELMAN 1964). These findings prompted the authors to propose that ADH activates two adenylyl cyclase systems, one of which is Ca^{++}-sensitive and coupled to the regulation of osmotic water flow. Results of studies in intact toad bladder cells may indicate that PG inhibits this same Ca^{++}-sensitive enzyme (OMACHI et al. 1974).

Table 1 includes data extrapolated from studies of OMACHI et al. (1974), FLORES et al. (1975) and LIPSON et al. (1971). Increasing concentrations of PGE_1 (10^{-7} to 10^{-5} M) progressively enhance cAMP production and Na^+ transport, but have no effect on basal water flow. Over this same concentration range PGE_1 has a biphasic effect on both theophylline- and ADH-stimulated water flow. Maximal inhibition by PGE_1 is observed with 10^{-7} M as a result of inhibition of theophylline- and ADH-stimulated cAMP production (data not shown). As cell cAMP content increases with higher concentrations of PGE_1, a progressive enhancement of theophylline-stimulated water flow is seen and inhibition of the hydroosmotic effect of ADH is no longer observed. This is not due to a partial agonist effect of 10^{-5} M PGE_1 since this concentration of PGE_1 is still inhibitory when a submaximal concentration of ADH is used. Rather, the response may be a consequence of an increase in total cell cAMP content. The inhibitory effects of PGE_1 were not observed with concentrations of PGE_1 alone, or of PGE_1 plus ADH, that raised the level of intracellular cAMP to 30 pmol/mg protein or higher. Thus, it may be that while the ADH-sensitive adenylyl cyclase "responsible" for water flow is inhibited by PGE_1, PGE_1 and ADH stimulate the second adenylyl cyclase and the cAMP generated by it may spill over into the "water flow" compartment with the resultant physiological effect. This also explains the lack of an inhibitory effect of PGE_1 on the water flow response to exogenous cAMP which, at mM concentrations, presumably increases cell cAMP content in all compartments.

Since it is likely that the water flow and sodium transport stimulated by ADH and PGE_1 occurs in the same type of cell, i.e., the granular cell of the toad bladder (DIBONA et al. 1969a, b), the activation of two adenylyl cyclases controlling these transport events must be independently regulated. The existence of two forms of adenylyl cyclase has been demonstrated in brain (BROSTROM et al. 1978) and other tissues (WOLFF and BROSTROM 1979). One enzyme is independent of μM Ca^{++} for activity, and moderately inhibited at higher Ca^{++} concentrations. The second enzyme demonstrates a biphasic response to Ca^{++} with activation observed at μM Ca^{++} concentrations and inhibition at higher concentrations. Both activation and inhibition of this enzyme by Ca^{++} are mediated by calmodulin (BROSTROM et al. 1978). It is possible that toad bladder contains a similar Ca^{++}-calmodulin-sensitive adenylyl cyclase responsible for water flow and inhibited by PGE_1. Recent in vivo studies in dog have demonstrated that cellular Ca^{++} uptake is involved in the hydroosmotic effect of ADH and that prostaglandins attenuate the action of ADH primarily by blocking cellular Ca^{++} transport (BERL et al. 1980). Similar inhibitory effects may be produced by norepinephrine (HANDLER et al. 1968; OMACHI et al. 1974), general anesthetics (LEVINE et al. 1976, 1979), and verapamil (HUMES et al. 1980). These agents selectively inhibit ADH-stimulated water flow by decreasing the hormones ability to increase cAMP production. PGE_1 (RAMWELL and SHAW 1970), norepinephrine (CHEN et al. 1978), general anesthetics (ENDO 1977) and verapamil (HUMES et al. 1980) each can alter Ca^{++} fluxes across cell membranes, a possible common mechanism of action of these agents.

Although the data from studies with intact toad bladders are consistent with an effect of PG on ADH-stimulated adenylyl cyclase(s), PGE_1 has been reported to produce only barely detectable inhibition of the response to ADH (LIPSON et al. 1971) or no inhibition at all (BAR et al. 1970) of adenylyl cyclase activity in homogenates of toad bladder. These results are consistent with an indirect effect of PG via an alteration in cellular calcium flux as proposed above. However, the adenylyl cyclase system is complex. At least three components of the system have been characterized in part (RODBELL 1980): (1) receptors for agonists and antagonists; (2) guanine nucleotide binding subunit(s), and (3) the catalytic subunit which generates cAMP from ATP. In addition, calmodulin may play an important role in toad bladder and other tissues as described above. In assays of toad bladder adenylyl cyclase inappropriate concentrations of substrates or cofactors such as ATP, GTP, Mg^{++}, Ca^{++}, etc. or absence of one or more of the above components may have prevented demonstration of the effect of PG on cAMP production. Support for this hypothesis has been obtained by KATHER and SIMON (1979). They demonstrated that adenylyl cyclase from human fat cells exhibited a biphasic response to PGE_2, with inhibition occurring at submicromolar concentrations and stimulation at higher concentrations of the hormone. The inhibitory component of PGE_2 became apparent only at GTP concentrations exceeding 10^{-6} *M*. Thus, appropriate alterations in nucleotide, cation, and calmodulin concentrations e.g., in toad bladder adenylyl cyclase assays might permit demonstration of an effect of PG on stimulation of the enzyme by ADH.

II. Activation of Protein Kinase and Protein Phosphorylation

In ADH-sensitive epithelia, the hormone binds to the basolateral membrane and activates adenylyl cyclase (I. SCHWARTZ et al. 1974). The cAMP that is generated is responsible for eliciting the physiological response at the apical membrane of the polar epithelial cell. As indicated in earlier chapters (see Chaps. 10 and 11 of Vol. 58/I on Biochemistry of Cyclic Nucleotides) evidence has accumulated in the last decade that the physiological effects of cAMP are mediated predominately, if not solely, via cAMP-dependent protein kinases (cAMP-PK). These enzymes consist of regulatory (R) and catalytic (C) units (see Eq. 2) (NIMMO and COHEN 1977). Two isoenzymes, type I and II, exist in mammalian tissues; these differ solely in the characteristics of their regulatory units. The tetrameric holoenzyme is inactive;

dissociation of the subunits following the binding of cAMP to R liberates catalytically active C which can phosphorylate protein substrates in the cell.

$$R_2C_2 + 2\ \text{cAMP} \rightleftharpoons R_2\ (\text{cAMP})_2 + 2C \qquad (2)$$

In ADH-responsive tissue, cAMP-dependent protein phosphorylation may be only the initial event in a sequence of reactions that leads to a physiological response. Alternatively, a specific apical membrane protein or proteins phosphorylated by a cAMP dependent kinase may be directly responsible for increased water or NaCl transport.

ADH can activate cAMP-PK in intact cells from kidney medulla (DOUSA and BARNES 1977), toad bladder (SCHLONDROFF and FRANKI 1978), and in cultured LLC-PK_1 cells (AUSIELLO et al. 1980a). These enzymes are found predominantly (>80%) in a 20–40,000 g supernatant fraction. Soluble cAMP-PK from bovine renal medulla is capable of phosphorylating proteins in a plasma membrane fraction from the same tissue (DOUSA et al. 1972). In other studies DOUSA and BARNES (1977) demonstrated increased cAMP-PK activity in particulate fractions of bovine kidney medulla following exposure to ADH. These authors postulated that ADH stimulation resulted in activation of cytosolic cAMP-PK. The free catalytic unit was then "translocated" to the apical membrane where phosphorylation of protein substrates occurred. Since tissue homogenization and fractionation were required to assess translocation, its relationship to hormone action in the intact cell remains uncertain. When LLC-PK_1 cells were fractionated in the presence of 150 m*M* KCl, no ADH induced translocation of protein kinase activity from the supernatant to pellet fraction was detected, i.e., increased cAMP-PK was found only in the supernant (AUSIELLO et al. 1980a). Omission of KCl during fractionation resulted in recovery of over 30% of the hormone-activated cAMP-PK in the pellet fraction. It has been demonstrated that the soluble catalytic unit of cAMP-PK in rat kidney cortex will bind non-specifically to particulate elements during cell fractionation (DERUBERTIS and CRAVEN 1976). Precise evaluation of the role of translocation of cytosolic cAMP-PK in the action of ADH will require direct measurement of enzyme activity and localization in intact cells.

Studies by I. SCHWARTZ et al. (1974) support the hypothesis that membrane phosphorylation is important in ADH action. These investigators purified apical plasma membranes from bovine renal papilla using free-flow electrophoresis. The membranes contained cAMP-PK which was capable of phosphorylating endogenous membrane protein, although no specific membrane substrates were identified. The addition of cytosolic cAMP-PK to the apical membranes did not result in a further increase in phosphorylation. The authors concluded that the data were indicative of the presence of a unique cAMP-PK in the apical membranes. However, recent data suggest that the type II isoenzyme is the predominant cAMP-PK in both soluble and particulate fractions from several ADH-sensitive tissues (DERUBERTIS and CRAVEN 1979; AUSIELLO et al. 1980a). A detailed study of protein kinases in bovine cerebral cortex (RUBIN et al. 1979) has demonstrated that membrane-derived and cytosolic type II cAMP-PK exhibit nearly identical immunological, physiological, and structural properties. Similar studies will be necessary in ADH-target tissues before specific phosphoprotein substrates in the biochemical pathway of ADH action can be defined.

The predominance of the type II cAMP-PK isoenzyme in kidney medulla has particular importance for ADH action. In subcellular preparations of several tissues, the type II isoenzyme is resistant to activation by 0.5 *M* NaCl in the absence of cAMP (CORBIN et al. 1975), whereas a high salt concentration makes the enzyme more sensitive to cAMP-stimulated activation (CORBIN et al. 1973). It is difficult to extrapolate from studies with isolated enzymes to the effects of intracellular NaCl on cAMP-PK in intact cells. However, as discussed above, the renal medulla of kidney is unique among mammalian tissues in that its cells are bathed at their basolateral surfaces by fluid containing high concentrations of NaCl and urea. This extracellular environment results in an increased cell content of these same constituents (MORGAN 1977). Therefore, based on the characteristics of the type II isoenzyme in vitro, it can be inferred cAMP-PK in the renal medulla must be resistant to direct dissociation (activation) by the high concentrations of solutes normally encountered. Moreover, it might be anticipated that ADH activation of cAMP-PK in renal medullary cells would be enhanced by high solute concentration in the bathing medium. Data consistent with this hypothesis have been provided by DERUBERTIS and CRAVEN (1978, 1979). They exposed rat kidney medullary slices to media of different osmolalities from 305–1650 mOsm attained by adding urea and NaCl to standard Krebs-Ringer bicarbonate buffer. ADH-stimulation of cAMP-PK in tissue slices exposed to 1650 mOsm buffer was 40% greater than in tissue incubated in 750 mOsm buffer. Thus, the osmotic changes that occur in renal medulla in vivo may conceivably influence the activation of cAMP-PK by ADH.

III. Protein Dephosphorylation

Greengard's group in the early 70's incubated intact toad bladders with ^{32}P-labeled inorganic phosphate to incorporate radioactivity into cell ATP and phosphoproteins and then exposed them to concentrations of ADH (200 mU/ml) or monobutyryl cAMP (2 m*M*) sufficient to induce effects on water permeability and short circuit current. On subsequent analysis of total tissue proteins by sodium dodecyl sulfate polyacrylamide gel electrophoresis, a 50,000 dalton protein was found to be the richest in ^{32}P but, surprisingly, a net decrease in the phosphorylation of this protein was observed in bladders exposed to ADH and cAMP (DELORENZO et al. 1973; DELORENZO and GREENGARD 1973). This 50,000 dalton phosphoprotein was initially called protein D but, subsequently, the acronym SCARP (LIU and GREENGARD 1976), for steroid- and cAMP-regulated phosphoprotein, was chosen.

DELORENZO et al. (1973) utilized broken cell preparations of toad bladder cells in an attempt to define the location of SCARP and the regulation of its phosphorylation by cAMP. They found most of ^{32}P-SCARP in cell sap fractions; however, cAMP-induced dephosphorylation of SCARP was most pronounced in crude membrane preparations. To distinguish between a decrease in the phosphorylation of SCARP and an increase in the dephosphorylation induced by cAMP, the investigators repeated the phosphorylation studies in toad bladder homogenates in the presence of inhibitors of protein kinase (adenosine; EDTA) and/or protein phosphatase ($ZnCl_2$) (DELORENZO and GREENGARD 1973). After the phosphorylation of SCARP was maximal, cAMP significantly increased the rate of removal of ^{32}P from SCARP. This effect of the nucleotide was inhibited by the simultaneous addition of $ZnCl_2$, but unaltered by protein kinase inhibitors. The authors concluded that cAMP was responsible for the activation of membrane-bound SCARP phosphatase. It was not determined whether this was a direct effect of cAMP on phosphatase activity since other endogenous or exogenous phosphoprotein substrates for the enzyme were not evaluated. As the authors noted, the possibility remained that cAMP made SCARP more available to a protein phosphatase and thus increased the dephosphorylation of this protein (DELORENZO and GREENGARD 1973).

WALTON et al. (1975) studied the effects of several agents, including ADH, cAMP, PGE_1, $MnCl_2$, and $ZnCl_2$, in an attempt to correlate changes in the phosphorylation of SCARP with the transport of salt and water in intact toad bladder. They concluded that the regulation of SCARP dephosphorylation correlated with the ability of these agents to stimulate sodium transport. Their hypothesis was supported by the results of studies with aldosterone (LIU and GREENGARD 1974), a steroid hormone known to increase sodium transport, but not water flow, to toad bladder. A several-fold increase in the rate of SCARP dephosphorylation was observed in cell homogenates obtained from intact bladders exposed to aldosterone. FERGUSON and TWITE (1974), however, did not agree. They observed that ADH at a concentration of 10 mU/ml produced maximal effects on sodium transport but had no effect on the dephosphorylation of SCARP, whereas ADH at 50 mU/ml produced maximal effects on sodium and water transport as well as significant dephosphorylation of the protein. It should be noted that in the studies from both laboratories there was no attempt to correlate changes in the cell cAMP content or the activity of cAMP-PK with the dephosphorylation of SCARP.

The data presented to this point have implicated the metabolism of SCARP in the action of hormones that stimulate salt and water transport in toad bladder. However, Greengard's laboratory has found SCARP in a wide variety of vertebrate tissues in which its phosphorylation is regulated by cAMP and steroid hormones: LIU and GREENGARD (1976) found that the effects of several steroid hormones on their respective target tissues resembled the effect of aldosterone in toad bladder on the dephosphorylation of SCARP. The effects of testosterone on seminal vesicles and prostate, of estradiol on the uterus, and of cortisol on liver were evaluated utilizing control and steroid-deprived animals. In cell fractions of tissues exposed to steroid, there was a marked decrease in SCARP phosphorylation as well as an enhanced dephosphorylation of this protein by an endogenous protein phosphatase. These effects were blocked by inhibitors of protein synthesis. The dephosphorylation of SCARP was stimulated by cAMP in all tissue fractions studied. It thus appears that steroids and cAMP can regulate the rate of dephosphorylation of SCARP, while, in addition, steroid hormones regulate either the amount of SCARP or its ability to become phosphorylated. On the basis of these data, LIU and GREENHARD (1976) proposed that the SCARP system may be the link in the synergism between the biological actions of steroid hormones and those hormones whose effects are mediated through cAMP.

1. Relationship of SCARP to Type II cAMP-PK

MALKINSON et al. (1975) demonstrated the cAMP-induced dephosphorylation of SCARP in both soluble and microsomal fractions from fifteen vertebrate tissues.

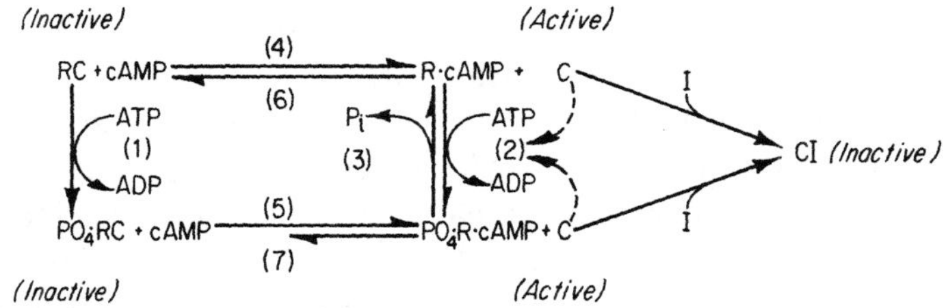

Fig. 1. Activation of type II cAMP-dependent protein kinase. See text for description of reactions. *Abbreviations: R*, regulatory unit; *C*, catalytic unit; *I*, inhibitor protein; *RC*, holoenzyme; *PO_4 · RC*, phosphorylated holoenzyme

These investigators suggested that this ubiquitous protein might be the regulatory unit of type II cAMP-PK, which is a 50,000 dalton phosphoprotein (see NIMMO and COHEN 1977). They used a photoaffinity analogue of cAMP to label covalently the cytosolic cAMP-binding protein and found in several tissues, including kidney and toad bladder, that covalently bound cAMP comigrated with phospho-SCARP during sodium dodecyl sulfate polyacrylamide electrophoresis. Although these experiments do not prove unequivocally the identify of SCARP and the type II regulatory units this conclusion is attractive.

As indicated earlier, cAMP-PK exist as holoenzymes consisting of regulatory (R) and catalytic (C) subunits (see Eq. 2). The holoenzyme is probably a tetramer (R_2C_2), but for convenience it is depicted as RC in Fig. 1 which summarizes the known reactions involved in activation and deactivation of type II cAMP-PK. In attempting to identify SCARP as R, the following characteristics of the equilibrium reactions in Fig. 1 must be considered: (1) R can be phosphorylated by C, either by an intramolecular phosphorylation of the holoenzyme (reaction 1), or by an intermolecular phosphorylation of dissociated R catalyzed by free C (reaction 2) (RANGEL-ALDAO and ROSEN 1976). The intramolecular reaction occurs at concentrations of ATP (Km = 0.4 μ*M*) several orders of magnitude below the cellular levels of ATP and thus the holoenzyme exists predominantly in the phosphorylated inactive form in vivo (RANGEL-ALDAO et al. 1979); (2) the dissociated phospho-R at the right of the figure, but not the phospho-R residing in the holoenzyme (left), can be dephosphorylated by the action of phosphoprotein phosphatase (reaction 3) (CHOU et al. 1977), or by the reversal of the phosphotransferase reaction (2) in the presence of ADP and Mg^{++} (ROSEN and ERLICHMAN 1975); (3) although both-phospho- and dephospho-holoenzymes can be completely dissociated by cAMP (reactions 4 and 5), the dephospho-R reassociates with C to regenerate the inactive holoenzyme (reaction 6) more readily than does the phosphorylated R (reaction 7).

Based on these observations, the data on the effects of ADH and cAMP on SCARP may be interpreted as an effect on phospho R. ADH stimulates cAMP production in the intact cell which in turn activates the phosphoholoenzyme by dissociation into phospho R and C (reaction 5). The phosphorylated R is converted to dephospho R by a protein phosphatase (reaction 3). The effect of cAMP is thus indirectly to enhance dephosphorylation of R while activating C. As long as cAMP levels remain elevated, the subunits are dissociated and the free catalytic unit C catalyzes the phosphorylation of the appropriate substrate(s). The latter is or are likely involved in effects of ADH on transport.

Support for this scheme has recently been obtained by I. SCHWARTZ et al. (1979). They have demonstrated the cAMP-dependent dephosphorylation of a 50,000 dalton protein from the microsomal fraction of canine renal inner medulla. This protein has several characteristics of the regulatory unit of type II kinase: It has the expected mol wt; it suppresses the activity of the catalytic subunit of cAMP-PK; it binds ^{3}H-cAMP, and it undergoes autophosphorylation. Furthermore, cAMP had no direct effect on protein phosphatase activity in this tissue when phosphohistone and phosphocasein were used as substrates.

2. Effects of Steroids on SCARP: A Hypothesis

An attempt to explain the effects of steroid hormones on SCARP in terms of the events associated with the phosphorylation of the type II cAMP-PK regulatory unit is at best speculative. Since protein synthesis is involved in the effects of these hormones, an increase in the synthesis of protein phosphatase is possible. An estrogen-induced phosphatase has been reported (VOKAER et al. 1974). However, since the holoenzyme is not dephosphorylated (v.s.) an increase in phosphatase activity would only enhance the dephosphorylation of R if steroid hormones induced dissociation of the kinase. Similarly, phosphatase-induction would not explain the observed decrease in the phosphorylation of SCARP in the presence of a phosphatase inhibitor (LIU and GREENGARD 1976).

A second possibility is that steroid-hormones decrease the synthesis of the type II isoenzyme. Again this would explain a decrease in the phosphorylation of R, but not an increase in its dephosphorylation. In fact, steroid-hormones have been shown to increase type I cAMP-PK in steroid-depleted animals with no effect on the type II enzyme (FULLER et al. 1978).

A third possibility which allows us to explain most of the available data is that steroid hormones induce the synthesis of a protein inhibitor of the catalytic subunit, perhaps similar to the one described by ASHBY and WALSH (1972). This is described on the right side of Fig. 1. Catalytic inhibitor protein (I) interacts only with the free catalytic unit (ASHBY and WALSH, 1972, 1973) forming the inactive complex, CI. The intramolecular phosphorylation of R (reaction 1) in the holoenzyme state is not impeded. The presence of I decreases the amount of free C and thereby increases the dissociation of the holoenzyme even at low basal concentrations of cAMP (reactions 4 and 5). The free phospho-R (as in reaction 5) is then available as a substrate for protein phosphatase (reaction 3). Thus the sequence of events may be as follows: steroid hormones induce I which converts C to inactive CI. This leads to a decrease in phosphoholoenzyme. Since in the absence of free C only intramolecular phosphorylation can occur in the in vitro assay, there will be a decrease in the amount of R phosphorylated as is observed. In the dephosphorylation assay, more phospho-R is available as the dissociated subunit and thus more dephosphorylation should also occur.

Within the framework of this hypothesis, although ADH and steroid hormones have similar effects on the dephosphorylation of the regulatory subunit (SCARP?), they could have opposing effects on cAMP-PK activity. This seems incompatible with the known permissive effects of these hormones, i.e., aldosterone-treated toad bladders (HANDLER et al. 1969) and rabbit renal collecting tubule (M. SCHWARTZ and KOKKO 1980) have an enhanced water flow response to vasopressin. However, BEAVO et al. (1974) has pointed out that the role of the protein kinase inhibitor may be most important at basal cAMP levels. Under these conditions as much as 20% of cell cAMP-PK is dissociated, but its activity can be rendered almost completely inactive by the inhibitor. It is of interest that the kidney has very low levels of inhibitor protein in comparison in other tissues (ASHBY and WALSH 1972), and it may be important to steroid-hormone action to increase the tissue concentration of inhibitor. This would be expected to alter the level of cAMP necessary to allow protein kinase activity to be expressed. However, a several-fold increase in tissue cAMP levels in the toad bladder is achieved by incubation with ADH in the presence of steroid hormone in comparison to ADH alone. This large increase in cAMP would likely overcome the effect of inhibitor protein and result in the augmentation of ADH-stimulated water permeability (HANDLER et al. 1969). This steroid effect reflects at least two actions of the hormone: adrenal steroids inhibit ADH-stimulated PGE_2 synthesis (ZUSMAN et al. 1978; see discussion above) thus reducing the inhibitory effects of PGE_2 on ADH-sensitive adenylyl cyclase (vida infra); 2) steroids decrease phosphodiesterase activity (STOFF et al. 1973). This effect may also be a result of steroid-induced inhibitor synthesis. A protein has been purified from rat testes (BEALE et al. 1977) which inhibits cAMP-PK and phosphodiesterase and its synthesis is enhanced by follicle-stimulating hormone (TASH et al. 1979).

This discussion has raised several points which need further verification. It would appear, however, that the dephosphorylation of SCARP reflects one of several complex regulatory steps in the activation and inhibition of cAMP-PK. Furthermore, it is unlikely that SCARP is "the" phosphoprotein responsible for the membrane permeability changes induced by ADH.

IV. ADH Action and Calcium

In many systems in which cAMP has been implicated as the second messenger in the activation of a cellular process, there is evidence for an equally important role of calcium ion either as a direct messenger or as a modulator of nucleotide related responses in association with calmodulin, a calcium-binding protein (RASMUSSEN and GOODMAN 1977; CHEUNG 1980; MEANS and DEDMAN 1980). For example, both the hydroosmotic and sodium-transport effects of ADH in anuran bladder can be modulated by altering the extracellular and presumably cytosolic Ca^{++} content.

1. Effect of Ca^{++} on Sodium Transport in Toad Bladder

The Ca^{++}-ionophores, A 23187 and X 537A, have been employed to increase the Ca^{++} content of toad bladder cells in a number of studies (WIESMANN et al. 1977; TAYLOR et al. 1979). The effects of these ionophores on sodium transport were shown to be dependent on the extracellular (serosal) calcium concentration. Thus in the presence of 2.5 mM Ca^{++}, basal sodium transport was inhibited whereas at lower concentrations of Ca^{++} minimal inhibition was observed.

On the basis of these and other findings TAYLOR and WINDHAGER (1979) have proposed that changes in cytosolic calcium modulate net Na^+ transport across responsive epithelial cells. Their thesis is discussed elsewhere (TAYLOR and WINDHAGER 1980) in which the appropriate experimental details of their own studies and those of others are cited. A brief summary will suffice for the purpose of this review.

It is generally accepted that net transcellular transport of Na^+ from urine to blood (mucosal to serosal solution) in epithelia of anuran bladder, skin, and certain segments of the renal tubule is effected by a series of steps only one of which is rate-limiting. Na^+ from the mucosal solution crosses the luminal membrane by a carrier mediated process along a favorable (down-hill) electrochemical gradient. The sodium is then transported out of the cell by an active process energized by a Na^+-K^+ exchanger in the basolateral membrane. The entry step at the luminal surface is rate-limiting. CURRAN and GILL (1962) had demonstrated some years ago that a rise in the calcium concentration of the external medium decreased transepithelial sodium transport across frog skin. They proposed that an elevation of Ca^{++} in the mucosal solution resulted in a decrease in the permeability to Na^+ of the luminal membrane. This view has been adopted and extended by TAYLOR and colleagues and incorporated into a model that explains some of the effects of the calcium ionophores, ADH and cyclic nucleotides on sodium (and water movement, see below) (TAYLOR and WINDHAGER 1979).

In their model both Ca^{++} and Na^+ cross the luminal membrane along their respective electrochemical gradients. Na^+ is extruded by the exchange pump at the basolateral surface. Calcium, however, exists from the cell via a process involving a Na^+-Ca^{++} exchanger (as well as an active calcium pump). It is the former which is of importance to their thesis since it requires that passive Na^+ influx back into cell from the serosal solution energizes coupled extrusion of calcium.

Na^+-Ca^{++} exchange across plasma membranes has been demonstrated in excitable tissues (BLAUSTEIN 1974; BAKER 1976). Direct evidence for Na^+-Ca^{++} exchange in renal tubular epithelium has been reported by KINNE et al. (1978) and indirect evidence for such a system in toad bladder (TAYLOR et al. 1979; TAYLOR and WINDHAGER 1980) and frog skin (GRINSTEIN and ERLIJ 1978) has been obtained in experiments involving manipulation of the electrochemical gradient for Na^+ entry into the epithelial cells across their basolateral surfaces. As implied above, one would predict that a decrease in the rate of basolateral sodium entry would raise cytosolic calcium levels, and thus mimic the effects of the ionophores described above. Indeed, decreasing sodium backflux by lowering the sodium concentration at the basolateral surface of bladder inhibited basal sodium transport; the degree of inhibition being dependent on the calcium concentration: as Ca^{++} was lowered, the extent of the inhibition was reduced (TAYLOR et al. 1979). This has led TAYLOR and WINDHAGER (1979) to propose a role for cytosolic Ca^{++} in the regulation of the apical membrane permeability to sodium, P_{Na}, (e.g., an increase in Ca^{++} reduces apical P_{Na}). This effect would constitute a negative feedback mechanism whereby the rate of apical Na^+ entry is kept in step with the rate of sodium extrusion across the basolateral cell surface. CHASE and AL-AWQATI (1979) have recently provided direct evidence for this model in toad bladder.

A 23187 also inhibits ADH-stimulated Na^+ transport in toad bladder (WIESMANN et al. 1977). This effect is probably a consequence of inhibition of hormone-stimulated cAMP production, since it was not observed when DBcAMP was added to the medium. ADH also reverses the inhibition of basal Na^+ transport induced by a low serosal Na^+ concentration (TAYLOR et al. 1979). Since the increased transepithelial transport of Na^+ following exposure to ADH (or cAMP) is the result of an increase in the apical membrane permeability to this ion (MACKNIGHT et al. 1980), TAYLOR et al. (1979) have proposed that the hormone effect results from transient lowering of the level of ionized Ca^{++} in epithelial cell cytosol by an unknown mechanism. The resultant increase in cell sodium concentration would decrease the downhill backflux of this ion across the basolateral membrane and ultimately via the Ca^+-Na^+ exchanger restrict calcium efflux with a resultant elevation in cell calcium. This would complete a negative feedback mechanism whereby Ca^{++} would block ADH-induced increases in cAMP production and apical membrane permeability to sodium. This series of events may explain, in part, the transient nature of the increase in sodium transport in response to ADH (TAYLOR et al. 1979).

2. Effect of Ca^{++} on Water Flow in Toad Bladder

The Ca^{++} ionophores A 23187 and X 537A inhibit the hydroosmotic response to ADH and exogenous cAMP in toad urinary bladder (TAYLOR et al. 1979). The inhibitory effect is variable (40–90% maximum inhibition), independent of external calcium or ADH concentrations, and fully reversible. These findings differ in part from those reported by HARDY (1978) in frog urinary bladder. The latter noted that the effect of a supramaximal dose of ADH was diminished in bladders pretreated with A 23187, while the hydroosmotic effect of a submaximal dose was enhanced when the ionophore was added together with the hormone. The reason for these differences in results is unclear.

Experiments designed to evaluate the effects of the proposed Na^+-Ca^{++} exchange mechanism on water flow in toad bladder have been conducted in a manner similar to that described in the preceding section (TAYLOR et al. 1979). When potassium was removed from the serosal bathing medium of toad bladder, a maneuver that results in inhibition of the sodium pump, or sodium backflux was reduced by lowering the sodium concentration of the serosal medium the hydroosmotic effects of ADH and cAMP were diminished. The degree of inhibition was dependent on the serosal calcium concentration; as calcium was lowered, the degree of inhibition was reduced.

3. Conclusions

The above data are consistent with the hypothesis that maximal effects of ADH and cAMP on salt and water transport require the maintenance of low cytosolic calcium levels. They do not, however, provide evidence that a primary event in ADH action is to lower cytosolic calcium. An answer to this question is hampered not only by our inability to directly determine changes in cytosolic calcium, but by the complex distribution and regulation of the calcium content of cells (see DEDMAN et al. 1979). The response of cells to changes in intracellular calcium content is best stated by the term "private line intracellular communication by Ca^{++}" introduced by LOEWENSTEIN and ROSE (1978). Increases in cytosolic calcium can be restricted to a very small volume because the sequestering capacity of the Ca^{++} "sinks" (mitochondria and endoplasmic reticulum) exceeds the diffusion rate of free hydrated calcium (KRETSINGER 1979). Hence the volume within which free Ca^{++} concentration is raised (or lowered) is so restricted that several such domains could serve opposing messenger functions and coexist within the cytosol of a single cell. The asymmetric distribution of intracellular organelles in polar epithelial cells may further serve to segregate cellular calcium domains. cAMP has been demonstrated to alter both the intracellular distribution of calcium and the efflux of cellular calcium in several cell types (see reviews by RASMUSSEN and GOODMAN 1977; WOLFF and BROSTROM 1979; DEDMAN et al. 1979). It is likely that similar events occur in ADH-sensitive tissue (I. SCHWARTZ and WALTER 1969; CUTHBERT and WONG 1974).

A working hypothesis for the role of Ca^{++} in ADH action can be developed as follows: ADH interacts with its receptor at the basolateral membrane of its target cells and activates two distinct adenylyl cyclases. One of the two enzymes requires an increase in the Ca^{++} concentration within the physiological range (μM) for activation (see earlier discussion). Larger increases in cytosolic Ca^{++} lead to inhibition of ADH-sensitive adenylyl cyclases. In contrast to an increase in cytosolic Ca^{++} in the region of the basolateral membrane after exposure to ADH, the increase in cAMP production induced by the hormone leads to a decrease in cytosolic Ca^{++} in the area of the apical membrane, facilitating the increase in permeability to salt and water. Proof of this hypothesis will require the definition of the biochemical mechanisms involved in these transport processes. For cAMP action, this involves the study of protein phosphorylation. The messenger function of Ca^{++} is intimately associated with its interaction with calmodulin. The Ca^{++}-calmodulin complex modulates many enzyme activities, including protein kinases (WOLFF and BROSTROM 1979). It is thus important to define the physiological substrates for Ca^{++}-calmodulin- and cAMP-dependent protein kinases, and to establish whether their respective substrates are functionally independent, complementary, or antagonistic.

V. Role of Microtubules and Microfilaments in ADH Action

1. Physiological Studies

In recent years, several investigators have focused on the involvement of microtubules and microfilaments in the hydroosmotic action of ADH (see reviews by TAYLOR et al. 1979; TAYLOR 1977). Colchicine, podophyllotoxin, and vinblastine, which disrupt microtubules by binding to tubulin, irreversibly inhibit ADH- and cAMP- induced water flow across the toad bladder without altering basal or ADH-stimulated sodium transport or urea flux (TAYLOR et al. 1978). The ability of these agents to inhibit the response to ADH closely parallels the interactions of colchicine and podophyllotoxin with tubulin (WILSON and TAYLOR 1978). Morphologically, these effects were expressed as a reduction in assembled microtubules in the granular cells of toad bladder with no effect on the mitochondrial-rich cells (REAVEN et al. 1978). These data are consistent with the cellular specificity for ADH in this tissue (DIBONA et al. 1969a) since it is presumed that only the granular cells respond to ADH. In freeze fracture electron microscopic studies, KACHADORIAN et al. (1979b) and CHEVALIER et al. (1977) have shown that colchicine prevents the appearance of apical membrane particle aggregates (see section A) in granular cells of toad and frog bladder, in parallel with its effect on ADH-induced water movement.

Cytochalasin B has been found to inhibit both ADH-induced water movement and the appearance of membrane particle aggregates in toad bladder (TAYLOR et al. 1973, 1979; KACHADORIAN et al. 1979b). The effects of cytochalasin B occurred at concentrations of the drug known to interfere with actin-related functions in other cell systems (TAYLOR 1977), presumably by binding to actin (HARTWIG and STOSSEL 1979; BRENNER and KORN 1979) and disrupting microfilament organization. PEARL and TAYLOR (1979) purified a protein from toad bladder epithelial cells which comigrated with rabbit actin on SDS polyacrylamide gels and, in the polymerized form, demonstrated 50–70 A filaments. Similar filaments seen in the apical and lateral subplasmalemmal region of granular cells were identified as actin by their ability to be decorated by heavy meromyosin (PEARL and TAYLOR 1979).

KACHADORIAN et al. (1979b) have demonstrated that although addition of either colchicine or cytochalasin B prior to ADH will inhibit the hydroosmotic effect of the hormone, only cytochalasin B alters the hormone response when added thirty minutes after ADH. These data are consistent with the suggestion (MULLER et al. 1980) that intact microtubules normally function to promote the fusion of cytoplasmic structures with the luminal membrane and that this is one of the initiating events that leads to the appearance of apical membrane particle aggregates. Once fusion has occurred, however, microtubules do not seem necessary to sustain the hormone response. In contrast, these authors propose (MULLER et al. 1980) that the maintenance of the hydroosmotic effect of ADH is mediated by microfilament-induced movement of particle aggregates from the intracellular membranes to the luminal membrane.

2. Control of Microfilament and Microtubule Organization – A Working Hypothesis for ADH Action

The above results are consistent with the view that the integrity of microfilament and microtubule organization is necessary for the hydroosmotic effect of ADH to occur. It appears that ADH induces an alteration in either the assembly or functional activity of these structures which results in the appearance of apical membrane particle aggregates, the presumed transmembrane channels for water passage (KACHADORIAN et al. 1979a; MULLER et al. 1980). How this effect of the hormone is achieved remains to be defined.

We have proposed that ADH interaction with its target cells results in an increase in cAMP content and a decrease in cytosolic Ca^{++} in the region of the apical membrane. Figure 2 illustrates the possible consequences of these effects of the hormone on microtubule and microfilament organization. The figure is drawn

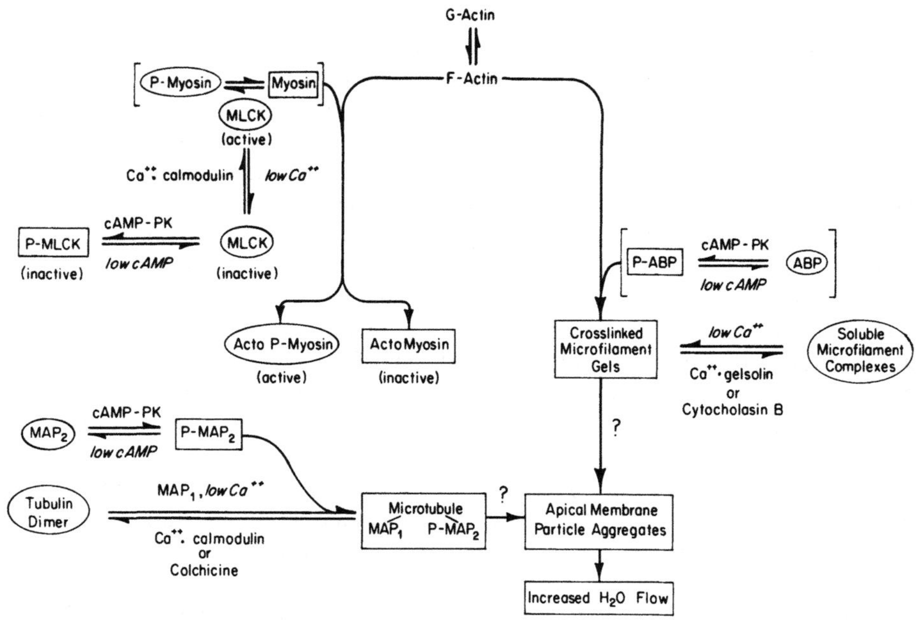

Fig. 2. Possible regulation of functional complexes of microfilaments and microtubules by cAMP and Ca^{++}. Products within rectangles are forms favored by high cAMP and/or low Ca^{++}. Products within ellipses are forms favored by low cAMP and/or high Ca^{++}. F-Actin can interact with either P-myosin or myosin (bracketed reaction) to form inactive or active actomyosin. It is uncertain whether P-ABP interacts more readily than non-phosphorylated ABP with F-Actin. Therefore this reaction appears within brackets. The association between crosslinked microfilament gels, polymerized microtubules and apical membrane particles is a hypothesis as indicated by the question marks. *Abbreviations: P-*, phosphorylated; *MLCK*, myosin light chain kinase; MAP_1 and MAP_2, microtubule-associated proteins; *ABP*, actin-binding protein; *cAMP-PK*, cAMP-dependent protein kinase

from a composite of data obtained from studies with proteins purified from a variety of different smooth muscle and non-muscle cells; no single cell has been shown to contain all of the proteins (KORN 1978; DEDMAN et al. 1979; YIN and STOSSEL 1979; ADELSTEIN 1980). Toad bladder cells contain actin (PEARL and TAYLOR 1979), myosin, actin-binding protein, and gelsolin (AUSIELLO and HARTWIG 1980; unpublished work). Furthermore, none of the reactions in Fig. 2 has yet been shown to occur in ADH target cells.

a) Formation of Crosslinked Microfilament Gels

The state of actin polymerization (monomer-polymer) is regulated by the cell but is not known to be affected by Ca^{++} or cAMP. Polymerized actin (F-actin) has the capacity to interact with actin binding proteins (collectively referred to as ABP in text and Fig. 2), including the high molecular weight filamin (WANG et al. 1975). cAMP-dependent phosphorylation of filamin has been demonstrated (WALLACH et al. 1978). It is possible that phosphorylated ABPs differ from non-phosphorylated ABPs in their interaction with F-actin in epithelial cells. Crosslinked actin gels can be disrupted into soluble complexes by the action of a Ca^{++}-dependent protein, gelsolin (YIN and STOSSEL 1979), or by cytochalasin B which binds to filament ends and which may lead to a reduction in average filament length (BRENNER and KORN 1979; HARTWIG and STOSSEL 1979).

Thus, one might suggest that low Ca^{++} (and more speculatively high cAMP) would favor crosslinked gels and ADH-induced water flow. High Ca^{++}, possibly low cAMP, or cytochalasin B would solubilize gels and inhibit ADH action. If cAMP lowers cytosolic Ca^{++}, it could have its effect on actin gels in this way.

b) Formation of Non-Functional Actomyosin

Enzymatically active actomyosin from non-muscle and smooth muscle cells requires that the 20,000 dalton myosin light chains be phosphorylated by a Ca^{++}-calmodulin-dependent myosin light chain kinase (MLCK). MLCK can be phosphorylated by a cAMP-dependent protein kinase. This appears to weaken the affinity of the enzyme for calmodulin and hence results in a decrease in MLCK activity (ADELSTEIN 1980). Thus high cAMP and/or low Ca^{++} would favor the formation of the enzymatically inactive actomyosin resulting in a decrease in cell tension. This would be consistent with the observations that ADH increases the apical membrane surface deformability in renal collecting duct cells (GRANTHAM 1970) and the granular cells of the toad bladder (DIBONA 1979).

c) Microtubule Polymerization

Several lines of evidence (see DEDMAN et al. 1979) have implicated a functional role for Ca^{++}-calmodulin and cAMP in microtubule assembly. Tubulin dimers polymerize to microtubules only when the Ca-calmodulin activity is very low (MARCUM et al. 1978) and in the presence of the microtubule-associated proteins (MAP), MAP_1 and phosphorylated MAP_2. MAP_2 is phosphorylated by cAMP-dependent protein kinase. Thus, low Ca^{++} and high cAMP would favor microtubule assembly, and high Ca^{++}, low cAMP, and colchicine (which forms a complex with tubulin dimer) would favor depolymerization and inhibition of ADH-induced water flow.

The biochemical reactions illustrated in Fig. 2 can be tested for in ADH target tissues. Such studies should provide a definition of the role of cAMP and Ca^{++} in ADH action.

D. Conclusion

In a recent review (DOUSA 1979), no fewer than sixteen hormones are reported to alter the cellular levels of cAMP in kidney. In this chapter we have used ADH as a model to describe the observed or probable pathways between adenylyl cyclase activation and the physiological response of a hormone. It is likely that many if not all of these events occur in response to other hormones (see STREWLER and ORLOFF 1977). At what point the functional specificity in the action of a hormone becomes manifest remains unclear. The cellular components necessary for cAMP generation and protein phosphorylation are ubiquitous. It is also evident that Ca^{++}-calmodulin is intimately associated with cAMP production, degradation and action. In each case of a hormone-mediated transport event, we can expect the biological response to closely correlate with the level of phosphorylation of a specific protein(s) rather than the level of the messenger, such as cAMP or Ca^{++}. We need to isolate and identify these phosphoproteins to establish their roles, integral or modulatory, in effecting the transport of water, electrolytes and other solutes.

Acknowledgements. The authors would like to thank Drs. MARTHA VAUGHAN and EDWARD KORN of the National Heart, Lung, and Blood Institute for their helpful discussions during the preparation of this manuscript.

References

Adelstein RS (1980) Phosphorylation of muscle contractile proteins. Fed Proc 39:1544–1545

Altura BM (1970) Significance of amino acid residues in vasopressin on contraction in vascular muscle. Am J Physiol 219:222–229

Anderson RJ, Berl T, McDonald KM, Schrier RW (1975) Evidence for an in vivo antagonism between vasopressin and prostaglandin in the mammalian kidney. J Clin Invest 56:420–426

Andreoli TE, Schafer JA (1976) Mass transport across membranes: the effects of antidiuretic hormone on water and solute flows in epithelia. Annu Rev Physiol 39:451–500

Ashby CD, Walsh DA (1972) Characterization of the interaction of a protein inhibitor with adenosine 3′,5′-monophosphate-dependent protein kinases. J Biol Chem 247:6637–6642

Ashby CD, Walsh DA (1973) Characterization of the interaction of a protein inhibitor with adenosine 3′,5′-monophosphate-dependent protein kinase. J Biol Chem 248:1255–1261

Ausiello DA, Hartwig JH (1980) Evidence for actin-binding protein and gelsolin activity in vasopressin-sensitive epithelia. Kidney Int 19:230

Ausiello DA, Hall DH, Dayer JM (1980a) Modulation of cyclic AMP-dependent protein kinase by vasopressin and calcitonin in cultured porcine renal LLC-PK_1 cells. Biochem J 186:773–780

Ausiello DA, Kreisberg JI, Roy C, Karnovsky MJ (1980b) Contraction of cultured rat glomerular cells of apparent mesangial origin after stimulation with angiotensin II and arginine vasopressin. J Clin Invest 65:754–760

Baker PF (1976) Regulation of intracellular Ca and Mg in squid axons. Fed Proc 35:2589–2595

Bar HP, Hechter O, Schwartz IL, Walter R (1970) Neurohypophyseal hormone-sensitive adenylyl cyclase of toad urinary bladder. Proc Natl Acad Sci USA 67:7–12

Beale EG, Dedman JR, Means AR (1977) Isolation and characterization of a protein from rat testis which inhibits cyclic AMP-dependent protein kinase and phosphodiesterase. J Biol Chem 252:6322–6327

Beavo JA, Bechtel PJ, Krebs EG (1974) Activation of protein kinase by physiological concentrations of cyclic AMP. Proc Natl Acad Sci USA 71:3580–3583

Beck TR, Hassid A, Dunn MJ (1980) The effect of arginine vasopressin and its analogs on the synthesis of prostaglandin E_2 by rat renal medullary interstitial cells in culture. J Pharmacol Exp Ther 215:15–19

Bergman RN, Hechter O (1978) Neurohypophyseal hormone-responsive renal adenylate cyclase. J Biol Chem 253:3238–3250

Berl T, Raz A, Wald H, Horowitz J, Czaczkes W (1977) Prostaglandin synthesis inhibition and the action of vasopressin studies in man and rat. Am J Physiol 232:F529–F537

Berl T, Erickson AL, Schrier RW (1980) In vivo evidence for a role of cellular calcium uptake in the hydroosmotic response to vasopressin. Clin Res 437A

Blantz RC, Ronnen KS, Tucker BJ (1976) Angiotensin UU effects upon the glomerular microcirculation and ultrafiltration coefficient of the rat. J Clin Invest 56:419–434

Blaustein MP (1974) The interrelationship between sodium and calcium fluxes across cell membranes. Rev Physiol Biochem Pharmacol 70:33–82

Bockaert J, Roy C, Rajerison R, Jard S (1973) Specific binding of [^{3}H] lysine-vasopressin to pig kidney plasma membranes. Relationship of receptor occupancy to adenylate cyclase activators. J Biol Chem 248:5922–5931

Bourget J, Chevalier J, Hugon JS (1976) Alterations in membrane-associated particle distribution during antidiuretic challenge in frog urinary bladder epithelium. Biophys J 16:627:639

Brenner SL, Korn ED (1979) Substoichiometric concentrations of cytochalasin B inhibit actin polymerization. J Biol Chem 254:9982–9985

Brostrom MA, Brostrom CO, Breckenridge BMcL, Wolff DJ (1978) Calcium-dependent regulation of brain adenylate cyclase. Adv Cyclic Nucleotide Res 9:85–99

Burch RM, Halushka PV (1979) Thromboxane is a positive modulator of vasopressin-stimulated water flow in the toad urinary bladder. Kidney Int 16:869A

Burch RM, Knapp DR, Halushka PV (1979) Vasopressin stimulates thromboxane synthesis in the toad urinary bladder: effects of imidazole. J Pharmacol Exp Ther 210:344–348

Burch RM, Knapp DR, Halushka PV (1980) Vasopressin-stimulated water flow is decreased by thromboxane synthesis inhibition or antagonism. Am J Physiol 239:F160–F166

Burg MB, Green N (1973) Function of the thick ascending limb of Henle's loop. Am J Physiol 224:659–668

Cantau B, Keppens S, DeWulf H, Jard S (1980) [^{3}H]-vasopressin binding to isolated rat hepatocytes and liver membranes: regulation by GTP and relation to glycogen phosphorylase activation. J Receptor Res 1:137–158

Cereijido M, Rotunno CA, Robbins ES, Sabatini DD (1978) Polarized epithelial membranes produced in vitro. In: Hoffman JF (ed) Membrane transport processes. Raven, New York, pp 433–461

Chabardes D, Gagnan-Brunette M, Imbert-Teboul M, Bontcharevskaa O, Montegut M, Clique A, Morel F (1980) Adenylate cyclase responsiveness to hormones in various portions of the human nephron. J Clin Invest 65:439–448

Chase HS, Al-Awqati Q (1979) Regulation of Na permeability of luminal border of toad bladder by intracellular Na^+ and Ca^{++}. Kidney Int 16:809A

Chen JLJ, Babcock DF, Lardy HA (1978) Norepinephrine, vasopressin, glucagon, and A 23187 induce efflux of calcium from an exchangeable pool in isolated rat hepatocytes. Proc Natl Acad Sci USA 75:2234–2238

Cheung WY (1980) Calmodulin plays a picotal role in cellular regulation. Science 207:19–27

Chevalier J, Bourguet J, Hugon JS (1974) Membrane associated particles: distribution in frog urinary bladder epithelium at rest and after oxytocin treatment. Cell Tissue Res 152:129–140

Chevalier J, Bourguet J, Hugon JS (1977) Actions compinées de la colchicine et de la cytochalasine B. sur la perméabilité à l'eau et la distribution des particules intramembranaires de la vessie de grenouille. Proc Int Union Physiol Sci 13:135

Chou CK, Alfano J, Rosen OM (1977) Purification of phosphoprotein phosphatase from bovine cardiac muscle that catalyzes dephosphorylation of cyclic AMP-binding protein component of protein kinase. J Biol Chem 252:2855–2859

Corbin JD, Soderling TR, Park CR (1973) Regulation of adenosine 3′,5′-monophosphate-dependent protein kinase. J Biol Chem 248:1813–1821

Corbin JD, Keely SL, Park CR (1975) The distribution and dissociation of cyclic adenosine 3′:5′-monophosphate-dependent protein kinases in adipose, cardiac, and other tissues. J Biol Chem 250:218–225

Craven PA, Briggs R, DeRubertis FR (1980) Calcium-dependent action of osmolality on adenosine 3′,5′-monophosphate accumulation in rat renal inner medulla. J Clin Invest 65:529–542

Curran PF, Gill JR Jr (1962) The effect of calcium on sodium transport by frog skin. J Gen Physiol 45:625–641

Cuthbert AW, Wong PYD (1974) Calcium release in relation to permeability changes in toad bladder epithelium following antidiuretic hormone. J Physiol (Lond) 241:407–422

Dedman JR, Brinkley BR, Means AR (1979) Regulation of microfilaments and microtubules by calcium and cyclic AMP. Adv Cyclic Nucleotide Res 11:131–174

Delorenzo RJ, Greengard P (1973) Activation by adenosine 3′.5′-monophosphate of a membrane-bound phosphoprotein phosphatase of toad bladder. Proc Natl Acad Sci USA 70:1831–1835

Delorenzo RJ, Walton KG, Curran PF, Greengard P (1973) Regulation of phosphorylation of a specific protein in toad-bladder membrane by antidiuretic hormone and cyclic AMP, and its possible relationship to membrane permeability changes. Proc Natl Acad Sci USA 70:880–884
DeRubertis FR, Craven PA (1976) Hormonal modulation of cyclic adenosine 3′,5′-monophosphate-dependent protein kinase activity in rat renal cortex. Specificity of enzyme translocation. J Clin Invest 57:1142–1450
DeRubertis FR, Craven PA (1978) Effects of osmolality and oxygen availability on soluble cyclic AMP-dependent protein kinase activity of rat renal inner medulla. J Clin Invest 62:1210–1221
DeRubertis FR, Craven PA (1979) Properties of soluble cyclic AMP-dependent protein kinase activity of renal inner medulla. Biochim Biophys Acta 585:499–511
DiBona DR (1979) Direct visualization of ADH-mediated transepithelial osmotic flow. In: Bourguet J, Chevalier J, Parisi M, Ripoche P (eds) Hormonal control of epithelial transport. INSERM, Paris, pp 195–206
DiBona DR, Civan MM, Leaf A (1969a) The cellular specificity of the effect of vasopressin on toad urinary bladder. J Membr Biol 1:79–91
DiBona DR, Civan MM, Leaf A (1969b) The anatomic site of the transepithelial permeability barriers of toad bladder. J Cell Biol 40:1–7
Dousa TP (1979) Cyclic nucleotides in renal pathophysiology. In: Brenner BM, Stein JH (eds) Hormonal function and the kidney, Churchill Livingstone, Edinburgh London New York, pp 251–285
Dousa TP, Barnes LD (1977) Regulation of protein kinase by vasopressin in renal medulla in situ. Am J Physiol 232:F50–F57
Dousa TP, Sands H, Hechter O (1972) Cyclic AMP-dependent reversible phosphorylation of renal medullary plasma membrane protein. Endocrinology 91:757–763
Dousa TP, Hui YFS, Barnes LD (1975) Renal medullary adenylate cyclase in rats with hypothalamic diabetes insipidus. Endocrinology 97:802–807
Dunn MJ, Greely HP, Valtin H, Kinter LB, Beeuwkes R III (1978) Renal excretion of prostaglandins E_2 and F_{2a} in diabetes insipidus rats. Am J Physiol 235:E624–E627
Dunn MJ, Kinter LB, Shier O Beeuwkes R III (1979) The interaction of vasopressin and renal prostaglandins in the homozygous diabetes insipidus rat. Clin Res 27:496A
Endo M (1977) Calcium release from sarcoplasmic reticulum. Physiol Rev 57:71–108
Exton JH (1980) Mechanisms involved in α-adrenergic phenomena: role of calcium ions in actions of catecholamines in liver and other tissues. Am J Physiol 253:E3–E12
Ferguson DR, Twite BR (1974) Effects of vasopressin on toad bladder membrane proteins: relationship to transport of sodium and water. J Endocrinol 61:501–507
Finkelstein A (1976a) Water and nonelectrolyte permeability of lipid bilayer membranes. J Gen Physiol 68:127–135
Finkelstein A (1976b) Nature of the water permeability increase induced by antidiuretic hormone (ADH) in toad urinary bladder and related tissues. J Gen Physiol 68:137–143
Flores J, Witkum PA, Beckman B, Sharp GWG (1975) Stimulation of osmotic water flow in toad bladder by prostaglandin E_1. J Clin Invest 56:256–267
Flouret G, Terada S, Nakagawa SH, Nakahara T, Hechter O (1977) Iodinated neurohypophyseal hormones as potential ligands for receptor binding and intermediates in synthesis of tritiated hormone. Biochemistry 16:2119–2124
Fuller DJM, Byus CV, Russell DH (1978) Specific regulation by steroid hormones of the amount of type I cyclic AMP-dependent protein kinase holoenzyme. Proc Natl Acad Sci USA 75:223–227
Ganote CE, Grantham JJ, Moses HL, Burg MG, Orloff J (1968) Ultrastructural studies of vasopressin effect on isolated perfused renal collecting tubules of the rabbit. J Cell Biol 36:355–367
Gluck S, Al-Awqati Q (1980) Vasopressin induces aqueous channels in luminal membrane of toad bladder. Nature 284:531–532
Goldring SR, Dayer JM, Ausiello DA, Krane SM (1978) A cell strain cultured from porcine kidney increases cyclic AMP content upon exposure to calcitonin or vasopressin. Biochem Biophys Res Commun 83:434–440

Grantham JJ (1970) Vasopressin: effect on deformability of urinary surface collecting duct cells. Science 168:1093–1095
Grantham JJ, Burg MB (1966) Effect of vasopressin and cyclic AMP on permeability of isolated collecting tubules. Am J Physiol 211:255–259
Grantham JJ, Orloff J (1968) Effect of prostaglandin E_1 on the permeability response of the isolated collecting tubule to vasopressin, adenosine 3′,5′-monophosphate, and theophylline. J Clin Invest 47:1154–1161
Grinstein S, Erlij D (1978) Intracellular calcium and the regulation of sodium transport in the frog skin. Proc R Soc Lond [Biol] 202:353–360
Hall DA, Varney DM (1980) Effect of vasopressin on electrical potential difference and chloride transport in mouse medullary thick ascending limb of Henle's loop. J Clin Invest 66:792–802
Handler JS, Orloff J (1973) The mechanism of action of antidiurectic hormone. In: Orloff J, Berliner RW (eds) Renal physiology. American Physiological Society, Washington, DC (Handbook of physiology, sect 8, pp 791–814)
Handler JS, Butcher RW, Sutherland EW, Orloff J (1965) The effect of vasopressin and of theophylline on the concentration of adenosine-3′,5′-phosphate in the urinary bladder of the toad. J Biol Chem 240:4524–4526
Handler JS, Bensinger R, Orloff J (1968) Effect of adrenergic agents on toad bladder response to ADH, 3′,5′-AMP and theophylline. Am J Physiol 215:1024–1031
Handler JS, Preston AS, Orloff J (1969) Effect of adrenal steroid hormones on the response of the toad's urinary bladder to vasopressin. J Clin Invest 48:823–833
Handler JS, Steele RE, Sahib M, Wade JB, Preston AS, Lawson N, Johnson JP (1979) Toad urinary bladder epithelial cells in culture: maintenance of epithelial structure, sodium transport and response to hormones. Proc Natl Acad Sci USA 76:4151–4155
Handler JS, Perkins FM, Johnson JP (1980) Studies of renal cell function using cell culture techniques. Am J Physiol 238:F1–F9
Hardy MA (1978) Intracellular calcium as a modulator of transepithelial permeability to water in frog urinary bladder. J Cell Biol 76:787–791
Harrington AR, Valtin H (1968) Impaired urinary concentration after vasopressin and its gradual correction in hypothalamic diabetes insipidus. J Clin Invest 47:502–510
Hartwig JH, Stossel TP (1979) Cytochalasin B and the structure of actin gels. J Mol Biol 134:539–553
Hassid A, Konieczkowski M, Dunn MJ (1979) Prostaglandin synthesis in isolated rat kidney glomeruli. Proc Natl Acad Sci USA 76:1155–1159
Hays RM, Leaf A (1962) Studies on the movement of water through the isolated toad bladder and its modification by vasopressin. J Gen Physiol 45:905–919
Hull RN, Cherry WR, Weaver GW (1976) The origin and characteristics of a pig kidney cell strain LLC-PK_1. In vitro 12:670–677
Humes HD, Simmons CF Jr, Brenner BM (1980) Effect of verapamil on the hydroosmotic response to antidiuretic hormone in toad urinary bladder. Am J Physiol 8:F250–F257
Ichikawa I, Brenner BM (1977) Evidence for glomerular actions of ADH and dibutyryl cyclic AMP in the rat. Am J Physiol 233:F102–F117
Imbert M, Chabardes D, Montegut M, Clique A, Morel F (1975) Vasopressin dependent adenylate cyclase in single segments of rabbit kidney cortex. Pfluegers Arch 357:173–186
Imbert-Teboul M, Chabardes D, Montegut M, Clique A, Morel F (1978) Impaired response to vasopressin of adenylate cyclase of the thick ascending limb of Henle's loop in Brattleboro rats with diabetes insipidus. Renal Physiol (Basel) 1:3–10
Jard S, Butlen D, Rajerison R, Roy C (1977) The vasopressin-sensitive adenylate cyclase from mammalian kidney: Mechanisms of activation and regulation of hormonal responsiveness. In: Dumont JE, Nunez J (eds) First European symposium on hormones and cell regulation. Elsevier/North-Holland Biomedical, Amsterdam Oxford New York, pp 15–30
Johnson J, Perkins F, Roy C, Butkus D, Preston A, Handler J (1979) Cyclic-AMP stimulates sodium transport and urea permeability without changing water permeability in epithelial cells in culture. Kidney Int 16:822A

Kachadorian WA, Wade JB, DiScala VA (1975) Vasopressin – induced structural change in toad bladder luminal membrane. Science 190:67–69
Kachadorian WA, Wade JB, Uiterwyk CC, DiScala VA (1977a) Membrane structural and functional responses to vasopressin in toad bladder. J Membr Biol 30:381–401
Kachadorian WA, Levine SD, Wade JB, DiScala VA, Hays RM (1977b) Relationship of aggregated intramembranous particles to water permeability in vasopressin-treated toad urinary bladder. J Clin Invest 59:576–581
Kachadorian WA, Muller J, Rudich SW, DiScala VA (1979a) Temperature dependence of ADH-induced water flow and intramembranous particle aggregates in toad bladder. Science 205:910–912
Kachadorian WA, Ellis SJ, Muller J (1979b) Possible roles for microtubules and microfilaments in ADH action on toad urinary bladder. Am J Physiol 236:F14–F20
Kather H, Simon B (1979) Biphasic effects of prostaglandin E_2 on the human fat cell adenylate cyclase. J Clin Invest 64:609–612
Kinne R, Keljo D, Gmaj P, Murer H (1978) The energy source of glucose and calcium transport in the renal proximal tubule. In: Vogel HG, Ullrich KJ (eds) New aspects of renal function. Excerpta Medica, Amsterdam London New York, pp 41–47
Knapp HR, Oelz O, Roberts J, Sweetman BJ, Oates JA, Reed PW (1977) Ionophores stimulate prostaglandin and thromboxane biosynthesis. Proc Natl Acad Sci USA 74:4251–4255
Koefoed-Johnson V, Ussing HH (1953) The contribution of diffusion and flow to the passage of D_2O through living membranes: effect of neurohypophyseal hormone on isolated anuran skin. Acta Phys Scand 28:60–76
Korn ED (1978) Biochemistry of actomyosin-dependent cell motility (a review). Proc Natl Acad Sci USA 75:588–599
Kreisberg JI, Karnovsky MJ (to be published) Characterization of rat glomerular cells in vitro. In: Michael A, Cummings N (eds) Immune mechanisms in renal disease. Plenum, New York
Kretsinger RH (1979) The informational role of calcium in the cytosol. Adv Cyclic Nucleotide Res 11:1–26
Leighton J, Brada Z, Estes LW, Justh G (1969) Secretory activity and oncogenicity of a cell line (MDCK) derived from canine kidney. Science 163:472–473
Levine SD, Levine RD, Worthington RE, Hays RM (1976) Selective inhibition of osmotic water flow by general anesthetics in toad urinary bladder. J Clin Invest 58:980–988
Levine SD, Weber H, Schlondorff D (1979) Inhibition of adenylate cyclase by general anesthetics in toad urinary bladder. Am J Physiol 237:F372–F378
Lifschitz M, Stein JH (1977) Antidiuretic hormone stimulates renal postaglandin E (PGE) synthesis in the rabbit. Clin Res 25:440A
Lipson L, Hynie S, Sharp GWG (1971) Effect of prostaglandin E_1 on osmotic water flow and sodium transport in the toad bladder. Ann NY Acad Sci 180: 261–277
Liu AYC, Greengard P (1974) Aldosterone-induced increase in protein phosphatase activity of toad bladder. Proc Natl Acad Sci USA 71:3869–3873
Liu AYC, Greengard P (1976) Regulation by steroid hormones of phosphorylation of specific protein common to several target organs. Proc Natl Acad Sci USA 73:568–572
Loewenstein WR, Rose B (1978) Calcium in (junctional) intercellular communication and a thought on its behavior in intracellular communication. Ann NY Acad Sci 307:285–305
Lum GM, Aisenbrey GA, Dunn MJ, Berl T, Schrier RW, McDonald KM (1977) In vivo effect of indomethacin to potentiate the renal medullary cyclic AMP response to vasopressin. J Clin Invest 59:8–13
MacKnight ADC, DiBona DR, Leaf A (1980) Sodium transport across toad urinary bladder: A model "tight" epithelium. Physiol Rev 60:615–715
Malkinson AM, Krueger BK, Rudolph SA, Casnellie JE, Haley BE, Greengard P (1975) Widespread occurrence of a specific protein in vertebrate tissues and regulation by cyclic AMP of its endogenous phosphorylation and dephosphorylation. Metabolism 24:331–341
Marcum JM, Dedman JR, Brinkley BR, Means AR (1978) Control of microtubule assembly-disassembly by calcium-dependent regulator protein. Proc Natl Acad Sci USA 75:3771–3775

Means AR, Dedman JR (1980) Calmodulin – an intracellular calcium receptor. Nature 285:73–77
Mendoza SA, Brown CF Jr (1974) Effect of chlorpropamide on osmotic water flow across toad bladder and the response to vasopressin, theophylline, and cyclic AMP. J Clin Endocrinol Metab 38:883–889
Mills JW, Macknight ADC, Dayer JM, Ausiello DA (1979) Localization of [^{3}H] ouabain-sensitive Na^+ pump sites in cultured pig kidney cells. Am J Physiol 236:C157–C162
Misfeldt DS, Hamamoto ST, Pitelka DR (1976) Transepithelial transport in culture. Proc Natl Acad Sci USA 73:1212–1216
Morel F, Chabardes D, Imbert-Teboul M (1978) Heterogeneity of hormonal control in the distal nephron. In: Proceedings of the VIIth international congress of nephrology, Montreal. Karger, New York, pp 209–216
Morgan T (1977) Effect of NaCl on composition and volume of cells of the rat papilla. Am J Physiol 232:F117–F122
Muller J, Kachadorian WA, DiScala VA (1980) Evidence that ADH-stimulated intramembrane particle aggregates are transferred from cytoplasmic to luminal membranes in toad bladder epithelial cells. J Cell Biol 85:83–95
Nimmo HG, Cohen P (1977) Hormonal control of protein phosphorylation. Adv Cyclic Nucleotide Res 8:145–226
Omachi RS, Robbie DE, Handler JS, Orloff J (1974) Effects of ADH and other agents on cyclic AMP accumulation in toad bladder epithelium. Am J Physiol 226:1152–1157
Orloff J, Handler JS (1962) The similarity of effects of vasopressin, adenosine-3′,5′-monophosphate (cyclic AMP) and theophylline on the toad bladder. J Clin Invest 41:702–709
Orloff J, Zusman R (1978) Role of prostaglandin E (PGE) in the modulation of the action of vasopressin on water flow in the urinary bladder of the toad and mammalian kidney. J Membr Biol (Special Issue) 40:297–304
Orloff J, Handler JS, Bergstrom S (1965) Effect of prostaglandin (PGE_1) on the permeability response to toad bladder to vasopressin, theophylline and adenosine 3′,5′-monophosphate. Nature 205:314–315
Pearl M, Taylor A (1979) Isolation and localization of actin-like protein from toad bladder epithelium. Fed Proc 38:1241A
Petersen MJ, Edelman IS (1964) Calcium inhibition of the action of vasopressin on the urinary bladder of the toad. J Clin Invest 43:583–594
Rabito CA, Ausiello DA (1980) Na^+-dependent sugar transport in a cultured epithelial cell line from pig kidney. J Membr Biol 54:31–38
Rajerison R, Marchetti J, Roy C, Bockaert J, Jard S (1974) The vasopressin-sensitive adenylate cyclase of the rat kidney. J Biol Chem 249:6390–6400
Rajerison RM, Butlen D, Jard S (1977) Effects of in vivo treatment with vasopressin and analogues on renal adenylate cyclase responsiveness to vasopressin stimulation in vitro. Endocrinology 101:1–12
Ramwell PW, Shaw JE (1970) Biological significance of the prostaglandins. Recent Prog Horm Res 26:149
Rangel-Aldao R, Rosen OM (1976) Mechanism of self-phosphorylation of adenosine 3′:5′-monophosphate-dependent protein kinase from bovine cardiac muscle. J Biol Chem 251:7526–7529
Rangel-Aldao R, Kupiec JW, Rosen OM (1979) Resolution of the phosphorylated and dephosphorylated cAMP-binding proteins of bovine cardiac muscle by affinity labeling and two-dimensional electrophoresis. J Biol Chem 254:2499–2508
Rasmussen H, Goodman DBP (1977) Relationships between calcium and cyclic nucleotides in cell activation. Physiol Rev 57:421–509
Reaven E, Maffly R, Taylor A (1978) Evidence for involvement of microtubules in the action of vasopressin in toad urinary bladder. III. Morphological studies on the content and distribution of microtubules in bladder epithelial cells. J Membr Biol 40:251–267
Rindler MJ, Chuman LM, Shaffer L, Saier MH (1979) Retention of differentiated properties in an established dog kidney epithelial cell line (MDCK). J Cell Biol 81:635–648
Rodbell M (1980) The role of hormone receptors and GTP-regulatory proteins in membrane transduction. Nature 284:17–22
Rosen OM, Erlichman J (1975) Reversible autophosphorylation of a cyclic 3′,5′-AMP-dependent protein kinase from bovine cardiac muscle. J Biol Chem 250:7788–7794

Roy C, Ausiello DA (1981 a) Characterization of (8-lysine) vasopressin binding sites on a pig kidney cell line (LLC-PK_1): Evidence for hormone-induced receptor transition. J Biol Chem 256:3415–3422
Roy C, Ausiello DA (1981 b) Regulation of vasopressin binding to intact cells. Ann NY Acad Sci 372:92–105
Roy C, Barth T, Jard S (1975 a) Vasopressin-sensitive kidney adenylate cyclase. Structural requirements for attachment to the receptor and enzyme activation: studies with vasopressin analogues. J Biol Chem 250:3149–3156
Roy C, Barth T, Jard S (1975 b) Vasopressin-sensitive kidney adenylate cyclase. Structural requirements for attachment to the receptor and enzyme activation: studies with oxytoxin analogues. J Biol Chem 250:3157–3168
Roy C, Lebars NC, Jard S (1977) Vasopressin-sensitive kidney adenylate cyclase. Differential effects of monovalent ions on stimulation by fluoride, vasopressin and guanylyl 5′-imidodiphosphate. Eur J Biochem 78:325–332
Roy C, Hall D, Karish M, Ausiello DA (1981) Relationship of (8-lysine) vasopressin receptor transition to receptor functional properties in a pig kidney cell line (LLC-PK_1). J Biol Chem 256:3423–3427
Rubin CS, Rangel-Aldao R, Sarkar D, Erlichman J, Fleischer N (1979) Characterization and comparison of membrane-associated and cytosolic cAMP-dependent protein kinases. J Biol Chem 254:3797–3805
Sasaki S, Imai M (1980) Effects of vasopressin on water and NaCl transport across the in vitro perfused medullary thick ascending limb of Henle's loop of mouse, rat, and rabbit kidneys. Pfluegers Arch 383:215–221
Schafer JA, Andreoli TE (1972) Cellular restraints to diffusion: The effect of antidiuretic hormone on water flows in isolated mammalian collecting tubules. J Clin Invest 51:1264–1278
Schafer JA, Andreoli TE (1977) Action of antidiuretic hormone on water and nonelectrolyte transport processes in mammalian collecting tubules. In: Andreoli TE, Grantham JJ, Rector FC Jr (eds) Disturbances in body fluid osmolality. American Physiological Society, Bethesda, Maryland, pp 57–83
Schafer JA, Andreoli TE (1978) The collecting duct. In: Andreoli TE, Hoffman JF, Fanestil DD (eds) Physiology of membrane disorders. Plenum, New York, pp 707–737
Schlondorff D, Franki N (1978) Activation through dissociation of cAMP-Protein kinase in vasopressin-treated toad bladder. Kidney Int 14:779A
Schwartz IL, Walter R (1969) Neurohypophyseal hormone-calcium interrelationships in the toad bladder. In: Margoulies M (ed) Protein and polypeptide hormones. Excerpta Medica, Amsterdam London New York, pp 264–269
Schwartz IL, Shlatz L, Kinne-Saffron E, Kinne R (1974) Target cell polarity and membrane phosphorylation in relation to the mechanism of action of antidiuretic hormone. Proc Natl Acad Sci USA 71:2595–2599
Schwartz IL, Huang CJ, Reisman L et al. (1979) Cyclic AMP mediated dephosphorylation in renal collecting duct epithelial cell plasma membrane: a substrate level phenomenon. In: Bourguet J, Chevalier J, Parisi M, Ripoche P (eds) Hormonal control of epithelial transport. INSERM, Paris, pp 71–84
Schwartz MJ, Kokko JP (1980) Urinary concentrating defect of adrenal insufficiency. Permissive role of adrenal steroids on the hydroosmotic response across the rabbit cortical-collecting tubule. J Clin Invest 66:234–242
Smith WL, Bell TG (1978) Immunohistochemical localization of the prostaglandin-forming cyclooxygenase in renal cortex. Am J Physiol 235:F451–F457
Sraer J, Foidart J, Chansel D, Mahieu P, Kouznetzova B, Ardaillou R (1979) Prostaglandin synthesis by mesangial and epithelial glomerular cultured cells. FEBS Lett 104:420–424
Stoff JS, Handler JS, Preston AS, Orloff J (1973) The effect of aldosterone on cyclic nucleotide phosphodiesterase activity in toad urinary bladder. Life Sci 13:545–552
Strewler GJ, Orloff J (1977) Role of cyclic nucleotides in the transport of water and electrolytes. Adv Cyclic Nucleotide Res 8:311–361
Tash JS, Dedman JR, Means AR (1979) Protein kinase inhibitor in Sertoli cell-enriched rat testis. Specific regulation by follicle-stimulating hormone. J Biol Chem 254:1241–1247
Taub M, Saier MH Jr (1979 a) An established but differentiated kidney epithelial cell line (MDCK). Methods Enzymol LVIII:552–560

Taub M, Saier MH Jr (1979 b) Regulation of $^{22}Na^+$ transport by calcium in an established kidney epithelial cell line. J Biol Chem 254:11440–11444
Taylor A (1977) Role of microtubules and microfilaments in the action of vasopressin. In: Andreoli T, Grantham JJ, Rector FC Jr (eds) Disturbances in body fluid osmolatily. American Physiological Society, Bethesda, Maryland, pp 97–124
Taylor A, Windhager EE (1979) Possible role of cytosolic calcium and Na-Ca exchange in regulation of transepithelial sodium transport. Am J Physiol 236:F505–F512
Taylor A, Windhager EE (1980) Effects of sodium-calcium interaction on sodium transport by epithelia. In: Leaf A, Giebisch G, Bolis L, Gorini S (eds) Renal pathophysiology – recent advances. Raven, New York, pp 129–138
Taylor A, Mamelak M, Reaven E, Maffly R (1973) Vasopressin: possible role of microtubules and microfilaments in its action. Science 181:347–350
Taylor A, Mamelak M, Golbetz H, Maffly R (1978) Evidence for involvement of microtubules in the action of vasopressin to toad urinary bladder. I. Functional studies on the effects of antimitotic agents on the response to vasopressin. J Membr Biol 40:213–235
Taylor A, Eich E, Pearl M, Brem A (1979) Role of cytosolic Ca^{++} and Na-Ca exchange in the action of vasopressin. In: Bourguet J, Chevalier J, Parisi M, Ripoche P (eds) Hormonal control of epithelial transport. INSERM, Paris, pp 167–174
Urakabe S, Takamitsu Y, Shirai D, Yuasa S, Kimura A, Orita Y, Abe H (1975) Effect of different prostaglandins on the permeability of the toad urinary bladder. Comp Biochem Physiol 52:1–4
Valentich JD, Tchao R, Leighton J (1976) Functional control of transporting epithelia by cAMP and divalent cations. J Cell Biol 70:330A
Valtin H, Schroeder HA (1964) Familial hypothalamic diabates insipidus in rats (Brattleboro strain). Am J Physiol 206:425–430
Vokaer A, Iacobelli S, Kram R (1974) Phosphoprotein phosphatase activity associated with estrogen-induced protein in rat uterus. Proc Natl Acad Sci USA 71:4482–4486
Wade JB (1980) Hormonal modulation of epithelial structure. Curr Top Membr Transp 13:123–147
Walker L, Whorton R, Smigel M, France R, Frolich JC (1978) Antidiuretic hormone increases renal prostaglandin synthesis in vivo. Am J Physiol 235:F180–185
Wallach D, Davies PJA, Pastan I (1978) Cyclic AMP-dependent phosphorylation of filamin in mammalian smooth muscle. J Biol Chem 253:4739–4745
Walton KG, Delorenzo RJ, Curran PF, Greengard P (1975) Regulation of protein phosphorylation and sodium transport in toad bladder. J Gen Physiol 65:153–177
Wang K, Ash JF, Singer SJ (1975) Filamin, a new high-molecular weight protein found in smooth and non-muscle cells. Proc Natl Acad USA 72:4483–4486
Wiesmann WJ, Sinha S, Klahr S (1977) Effects of ionophore A 23187 on base-line and vasopressin-stimulated sodium transport in the toad bladder. J Clin Invest 59:418–425
Wilson L, Taylor A (1978) Evidence for involvement of microtubules in the action of vasopressin in toad urinary bladder. II. Colchicine binding properties of toad bladder epithelial cell tubulin. J Membrane Biol 40:237–250
Wolff DJ, Brostrom CO (1979) Properties and functions of the calcium-dependent regulator protein. Adv Cyclic Nucleotide Res 11:27–88
Yin HL, Stossel TP (1979) Control of cytoplasmic actin gel-sol transformation by gelsolin, a calcium-dependent regulatory protein. Nature 281:583–586
Zenser TV, Davis BB (1978) Effects of calcium on prostaglandin E_2 synthesis by rat inner medullary slices. Am J Physiol 235:F213–F218
Zusman RM, Keiser HR (1977) Prostaglandin biosynthesis by rabbit renomedullary interstitial cells in tissue culture: stimulation by vasoactive peptides. J Clin Invest 60:215–223
Zusman RM, Keiser HR, Handler JS (1977 a) Vasopressin-stimulated prostaglandin E biosynthesis in the toad urinary bladder. Effect on water flow. J Clin Invest 60:1339–1347
Zusman RM, Keiser HR, Handler JS (1977 b) Inhibition of vasopressin-stimulated prostaglandin E biosynthesis by chlorpropamide in the toad urinary bladder. Mechanism of enhancement of vasopressin-stimulated water flow. J Clin Invest 60:1348–1353
Zusman RM, Keiser HR, Handler JS (1978) Effect of adrenal steroids on vasopressin stimulated PGE synthesis and water flow. Am J Physiol 234:F532–540

CHAPTER 22

Regulation of Cellular Excitability by Cyclic Nucleotides

G. R. SIGGINS

Overview

Considerable research indicates that cyclic nucleotides serve as second messengers in excitable cells for a variety of hormones and neurotransmitters. However, attempts to demonstrate exact mimicry of humoral responses by cyclic nucleotides are frustrated by impediments to adequate measures of excitability and to proper drug delivery. In most cases the cell type under study displays properties (e.g., small size, inaccessability) requiring more expedient technologies. Nonetheless, a survey of the research to date across a wide variety of species and cell types indicates that cyclic AMP and cyclic GMP may evoke a distinctive repertoire of responses. Hence, in most cell types cyclic AMP either (1) hyperpolarizes cells and/or inhibits spontaneous discharges, usually with no change or a decrease in ionic conductance, (2) enhances certain synaptic potentials, or (3) alters the voltage-dependent (usually Ca^{++}) conductances generally associated with generation or prolongation of action potentials. Responses to cyclic GMP remain more covert, although in many cell types depolarization is the predominant response. It is speculated that cyclic AMP in many cases may be a second messenger for direct transmission of humoral or synaptic information. The mechanism of the hyperpolarizing responses may involve reduced conductance to sodium ions or activation of electrogenic pumps; either mechanism may involve phosphorylation of membrane constituents. The alteration of voltage-dependent calcium conductances may have important consequences for the many slower cellular processes (e.g., cell growth, movement, secretion) which utilize calcium ions. Indeed, many of the electrophysiological effects of the cyclic nucleotides could serve to bring about ionic conditions in the cell favorable for initiation of such slower phenomena.

A. Introduction

Research over the last two decades has demonstrated that excitable tissue constitutes a major store of cyclic nucleotides (SUTHERLAND et al. 1962; KLAINER et al. 1962; N. GOLDBERG et al. 1969). The resulting question of possible physiological roles for these nucleotides has presented a great avenue of experimentation. The first step along this route was the observation that several mammalian hormones and neurotransmitters were capable of stimulating cyclic AMP (cAMP) production (see KLAINER et al. 1962; ROBISON et al. 1971).

Since the best known function of neurotransmitters is the modulation of the electrical activity of neurons and muscle, a next logical step in determining the role of cyclic nucleotides was to assess the effects of the nucleotide on the excitability of these cells. To establish that the action of a particular hormone or transmitter is mediated by a cyclic nucleotide four major criteria need to be satisfied (see BLOOM 1975; SIGGINS 1978a): (1) The exogenous neurotransmitter or hormone, as well as activation of the synaptic pathway utilizing that transmitter, must both regulate intracellular levels of cyclic nucleotide in the postsynaptic cell. (2) The change in intracellular cyclic nucleotide content observed should precede the biological event triggered by the hormone, transmitter or nerve pathway. (3) Responses to the hormone, transmitter or nerve pathway should be altered in the same manner by drugs that specifically interact with the nucleotide cyclase or that inhibit the appropriate phosphodiesterase. (4) Exogenous cyclic nucleotides (and analogues which activate cAMP dependent protein kinase) should elicit the biological event caused by the hormone, transmitter or nerve pathway.

This chapter is devoted primarily to an analysis of criterion 4, with regard to the electrophysiological effects of cyclic nucleotides and their putative (neuro)hormones or first messengers on excitable tissue. Little attempt will be made to cite all the literature pointing to a role for cyclic nucleotides in a given function since this subject has been recently surveyed by many authors (DALY 1975; BLOOM 1975) as well as by other authors in this volume. Nor will methodology be explored in detail. Rather, I will pursue significant implications of second messenger mediation of humoral, synaptic or junctional events, especially within the nervous system. Methodology will be discussed only where variations lead to artifacts or controversies. However, a simplified introduction on what bioelectrical events might be measured and what methods may be used to administer first and second messengers will greatly facilitate the subsequent discussion of the electrophysiologically effects of these messengers.

B. Measures of Excitability

I. Transmembrane Properties Using Intracellular Recording

The most direct measure of cell excitability is obtained by recording the potential difference across the intact cell membrane, usually by penetrating the cell with a glass ultramicroelectrode filled with electrolyte (see LING and GERARD 1949; KATZ 1966). Changes in cell excitability are generally reflected by changes in the resting transmembrane potential (RMP), with increased intracellular potentials (hyperpolarization) usually indicating reduced excitability and moderately diminished potentials (depolarization), increased excitability. Moderate depolarization tends to increase the probability of the abrupt regenerative reversals of potential known as action potentials or spikes, while hyperpolarization usually reduces the likelihood of action potentials by shifting the membrane potential away from the threshold for spike generation (KATZ 1966).

Intracellular recording offers an added powerful advantage because appropriate intracellular stimulation with current can be used to assess the relative permeability (conductance) of the membrane to ions (the inverse of electrical resistance).

Since changes in membrane ionic conductance (e.g., induced by neurotransmitters) are usually the cause of changes in membrane potential and excitability, measurement of conductance provides information about ionic mechanisms of the excitability change; manipulation of the intra- or extracellular concentrations of various ions then allows evaluation of the specific ion or ions responsible for the change in excitability. Determination of the ionic basis of excitatory and inhibitory postsynaptic potentials (PSPs) is a classic example of the use of measurements of membrane conductance (see J. ECCLES 1964; KATZ 1966).

The most conventional mechanism of hormone or transmitter action on cell excitability involves binding to a specific receptor, resulting in a change in the transmembrane permeabilities to one or more ions. The influence on membrane potential depends upon the ionic permeability changes. Each ionic species is in unequal concentration on either side of the membrane due to the relative membrane impermeability to some ions and to the activity of ion pumps; thus there is a driving force, determined by the concentration gradient, for each ionic species. An equilibrium potential, E_x, can be defined for each ion (X), at which the electrical gradient is exactly equal to the chemical gradient for that ion by the Nernst equation:

$$E_x = \frac{RT}{ZF} \cdot \ln \frac{[X]_o}{[X]_i},$$

where R is the universal gas constant, T is absolute temperature, F is the Faraday constant, Z is the ionic valence, and the subscripts i and o indicate inside and outside concentrations of the ion.

Figure 1 is a schematic representation of the types of ionic channels likely to generate the equilibrium potentials for the major ionic species involved in determining RMP, action potentials and receptor-mediated potential shifts in excitable cells. The approximate range of ionic equilibrium potentials involved in determining membrane potentials for most excitable cells are: Ca^{++}, +20 to +50 mV; Na^+, +20 to +40 mV, Cl^-, −10 to −80 mV; K^+, −40 to −80 mV. The resting membrane potential usually can be approximated by the sum of the contributions of Na^+, K^+, and Cl^-; thus most excitable cells display RMPs in the range of 40–100 mV, internally negative. Under resting conditions, K^+ permeability usually predominates and RMP is relatively near but slightly positive to E_{K^+}. When a hormone, neurotransmitter or second messenger *increases* permeability to a single ion, the potential will approach the equilibrium potential for that ion. If such an agent causes a *decrease* in the permeability to one ionic species, the potential will move away from the equilibrium potential for that ion toward that of the ion with the dominant permeability. Thus, an increase in K^+ permeability will generally hyperpolarize, whereas an increase in Na^+ permeability will depolarize an excitable cell. In most brain neurons, E_{Cl^-} is more negative than RMP; here permeability increases to Cl^- are hyperpolarizing. In the vertebrate neuromuscular junction and many synapses mediating fast excitation the transmitter opens a channel allowing movement of both Na^+ and K^+, pushing the potential at the neuromuscular junction to about −15 mV, approximately midway between E_{K^+} and E_{Na^+}.

However, it is not clear what changes in ionic conductance, if any, would appear if ionic pumps were the cause of excitability changes (THOMAS 1972). Such electrogenic pumps are thought by some to account for certain slow synaptic po-

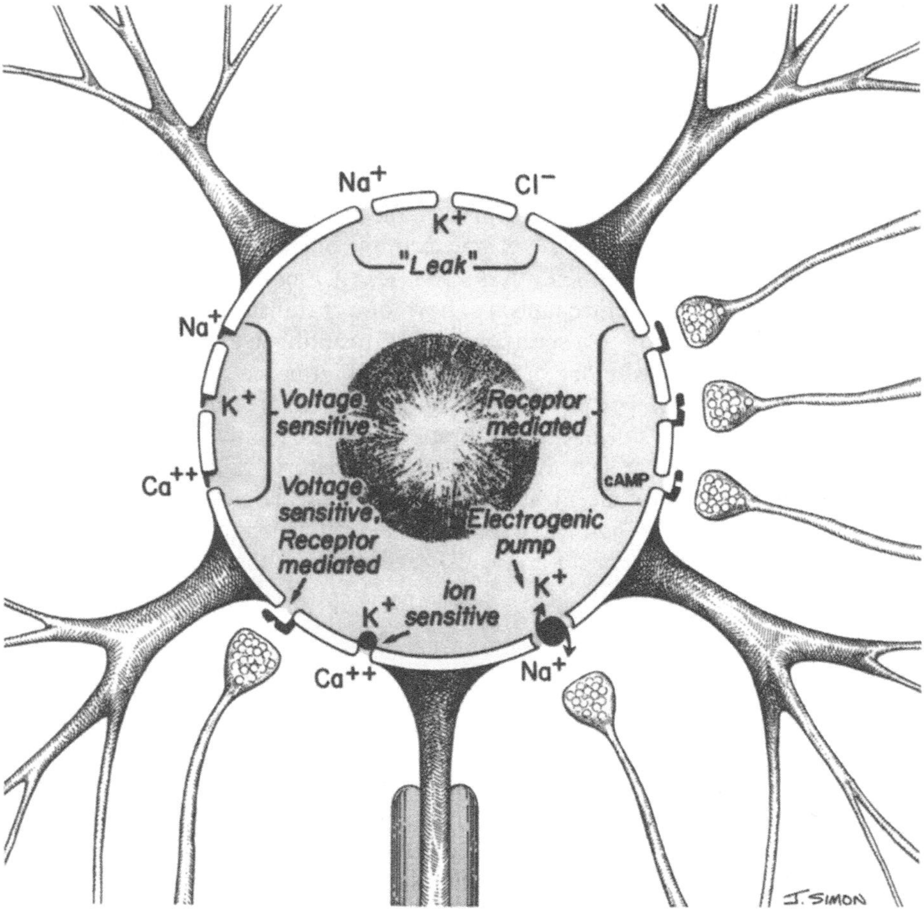

Fig. 1. Schematic of several types of ion channels and related processes contributing to the electrical activity of excitable cells. Most electrical activity is generated by the flow of ions through such conductance channels. Those which are always open (top of figure) are termed *"leak" conductances;* these, especially those for potassium and sodium ions, contribute largely to the resting membrane potential. The *receptor-mediated channels* are depicted on the right. These are activated or inactivated by chemicals (most hormones or neurotransmitters) and are thought to account for the conventional non-voltage-dependent or passive responses to activation of synaptic pathways. The traditional *voltage-dependent channels* (left) are those which are open only at certain membrane potentials; these contribute to the generation of an action potential, after the membrane potential is brought to a threshold (trigger) level of depolarization by injected current or chemical activation of passive conductances. One result of a voltage-sensitive conductance is shown at the bottom left, wherein the entry of calcium during the action potential triggers the efflux of potassium ions, resulting in membrane repolarization (and sometimes the hyperpolarizing afterpotential) at the conclusion of the action potential. Such *ion sensitive channels* are opened only when a particular ion (e.g. calcium) is present. A relatively new concept is the existence of *voltage sensitive, receptor-mediated ion channels (lower left);* as with conventional synapses, such channels may be opened or closed by neurotransmitters, but only at certain membrane potentials. Since most voltage-dependent conductances are associated with action potential mechanisms, activation of such receptors would be expected to alter properties of the spike (see text). Activation or inhibition of *electrogenic ion pumps (lower right)* could also contribute to receptor- or non-receptor-coupled changes in membrane potential. Generation of *cyclic nucleotides* by nucleotide cyclases, possibly through activation of transmitter receptors (see text) could open or close ion channels directly (or perhaps via protein phosphorylation) or alter voltage sensitive conductances or membrane pumps, thus significantly altering neuronal excitability

tentials in sympathetic ganglia (see NISHI and KOKETSU 1967). Moreover, electrophysiological studies of vertebrate and invertebrate neurons suggest that some neurotransmitters can alter excitability without directly changing membrane potential. For example, in some neurons where E_{Cl^-} is very near RMP, transmitter-increased permeability to Cl^- would produce no potential change, but any other synaptic inputs would be reduced in effectiveness because of the "shunting" effect of the reduced resistance. Conversely, a neurotransmitter which reduces ionic permeabilities (increasing resistance and therefore the "voltage drop" for a given second synaptic current) would increase the responsiveness of neurons to other synaptic inputs.

Another recently described phenomenon of some importance is the voltage-dependent action of some hormones and neurotransmitters. Here, concentrations of the agonists often below those normally producing potential changes are capable of altering ionic permeabilities which are usually not active at the RMP. For example, alteration of spike threshold have been seen with GABA and opioid peptides in some cultured spinal neurons (BARKER et al. 1980). Since spikes or action potentials involve membrane conductances which are activated by changes in membrane voltage (the so-called voltage-dependent conductances) and these actions are blocked by specific receptor antagonists, such a novel phenomenon can be ascribed to a receptor-mediated voltage-sensitive conductance change (Fig. 1). Receptor-mediated changes in voltage-dependent calcium channels are of even greater interest because calcium has so many regulatory functions upon a variety of cellular activities, e.g., secretion, calcitonin activation. Examples of this phenomenon are the decreases in the late (calcium) plateau component of the spike in mammalian dorsal root nerves produced by GABA, norepinephrine, serotonin and enkephalin (DUNLAP and FISCHBACH 1978, MUDGE et al. 1979) and in rat sympathetic nerves by norepinephrine (HORN and MCAFEE 1979). Activation or prolongation of voltage sensitive Ca^{++} channels by serotonin has been observed in aplysia neurons (M. KLEIN and KANDEL 1978; PELLMAR and CARPENTER 1979).

Furthermore, BROWN and ADAMS (1980) report a muscarinic cholinergic action (sometimes depolarizing) of neurons of sympathetic ganglia which arises from inactivation of a voltage-dependent K^+ channel. This latter action is similar to one action of catecholamines on cardiac Purkinje fibers, where the slow inactivation of a voltage-dependent K^+ conductance is responsible in part for a depolarizing pacemaker potential (see below). By speeding the inactivation of this channel, norepinephrine increases the frequency of firing. In addition, norepinephrine (and cyclic AMP as well) appears to enhance the slow inward current (mostly calcium) of the cardiac action potential and the outward K^+ current responsible for repolarization (see below); both of these affects involve voltage-sensitive conductances.

Although pharmacological agents (e.g. tetrodotoxin, TEA and divalent cations) are useful, the voltage clamp technique is the method of choice for critical analysis of such voltage-sensitive conductances. This method is capable of determining effects of hormones and transmitters on ionic currents which are active only at certain membrane potentials, and is enormously helpful in revealing covert actions of agonists which do not involve changes in RMP. However, to date this method has been rarely used for analysis of cyclic AMP actions (other than in cardiac cells, photoreceptors, and invertebrate neurons... see below), mostly because of the technical difficulties in applying this method to small cells. Nonetheless, because of the many recent reports of voltage-dependent actions of hormones and transmitters, future research on the role of 2nd messengers in these systems will need to develop the use of voltage clamp methods for analysis of the effects of cyclic nucleotides.

II. Summed Potentials of Cell Populations

Intracellular recording with micropipettes is convenient for large, easily isolated cells which are relatively uninjured by the impaling electrode. However, many excitable cells are too small to withstand electrode penetration and require less direct measures of excitability. One such approach is the sucrose gap method of recording either single large fibers or the summed activity of a large number of longitudinally arrayed and electrically isolated cells (see STÄMPFLI 1954). In this technique, one measures the potential difference between one end of the fiber or cellular array placed in Ringer's solution and the other end bathed in concentrated KCl and consequently depolarized; electrical shunting between the two ends along extracellular pathways is minimized by bathing the mid-section of the tissue in a non-conducting sucrose solution. The potential measured is essentially "intracellular." Although changes in ionic conductance and absolute RMP cannot be determined by this method (except with single large fibers), changes in the summed membrane potentials of the population of cells can be followed. This technique has proved useful in studies on isolated axon trunks, smooth muscle arrays, myocardial bundles, autonomic ganglia, and nerve trunks from spinal cords.

A more recently-popularized means of extracellular recording from aggregates of nerve cells is the method of "field potentials," which takes advantage of the stereotyped laminar arrangement of some arrays of neurons in mammalian brain (e.g., in the cerebellar cortex or the hippocampal formation). So-called source/sink relationships of populations of cells with well-oriented dendritic processes, upon which are found specific afferent nerve terminations, can be used to generate large fields of synchronous synaptic potentials from many cells or dendrites following afferent stimulation. Although population spikes can also be recorded, resting potentials or ionic conductance cannot be inferred from such potentials. Still, the synaptic and spike fields can afford a valuable parameter for the study of drug actions, such as those on the role of cyclic nucleotides (see DUNNWIDDIE and HOFFER, this volume). Field potentials can be studied either in vivo or in in vitro preparations such as the hippocampal slice; in vitro slice preparations have the added advantage of ease of drug administration (see below).

III. Extracellular Action Potentials of Single Units

A disadvantage of the sucrose gap or any gross recording method is the requirement for the existence of a large number of nearly homogenous cell types, preferably arranged in a longitudinal or laminar array; this is difficult for most mammalian central neurons. However, we may take advantage of the frequent spontaneous action potentials seen in many central neurons. Recording these action potentials extracellularly with appropriate glass or metal microelectrodes offers another indirect index of cell excitability, assuming that a high rate of discharge reflects membrane depolarization and a reduced rate of firing, hyperpolarization. If the neuron under study does not fire spontaneously it can often be activated to generate evoked spikes by stimulating excitatory inputs to the cell. Changes in excitability will then be reflected in changes in the response to the excitatory input. If specific excitatory inputs cannot be activated, then an alternate means of making the cell discharge artificially is to apply an excitatory agent (e.g. glutamate) directly to the cell by iontophoresis.

Three major caveats are required for analysis of extracellular recordings. First, extracellular activity is not a sure reflection of membrane potential: for example, excessive depolarization can result in an actual cessation of discharge. For this reason artificial excitation of neurons with agents such as glutamate can be hazardous because the subsequent addition of a second excitatory agent may further depolarize the cell to the extent of total blockade of discharge; extracellular recording would then only reveal an apparent inhibition. Second, in order to satisfy criterion four above for cyclic nucleotide mediation, one needs to compare effects of agonists (e.g. catecholamines) to evaluate identity of action (mimicry) with that of the cyclic nucleotide; since only two qualitative changes in firing rate are possible, many agents will show a false mimicry by extracellular recording. In extracellular recording, complicated studies of interaction of agonists with antagonists and synergists are required to substantiate agonist mimicry (criterion 3). Third, agonists can modify pre-junctional release of neurotransmitters as well as elicit post-junctional responses; thus, extracellular recording of responses will not distinguish between these two effects.

C. Problems of Drug Administration

I. Perfusion and Superfusion

With those tissues which can be safely isolated and which are largely composed of homogeneous cell types, in vitro perfusion or superfusion of agents may be the method of choice. Artifacts here are mostly the minor correctible ones of tissue or ion movement (due to fluid flow), temperature and pH. However, perfusion, whether through an intact vascular system or in a bath, is often used in studies of isolated populations of heterogeneous cell types (e.g. brain slices). Here controls for the different cell types involved and their possible interconnections must be used, since drug effects may be exerted at a site (cell type) remote from the actual cell under study. For example, inhibition of neuronal activity (hyperpolarization) could arise from the excitation by perfused drug of a remote (inter)neuron which sends inhibitory terminals to the cell under study; the conclusion that the agent was inhibitory would constitute an interpretive error. The use of drugs or ions (e.g., Mg^{++}) which block synaptic transmission can control for such artifacts.

Superfusion of drugs (that is, topical application) to in situ structures such as surfaces of cerebral or cerebellar cortex, or brain tissue transplanted in oculo (HOFFER et al. 1977) require similar controls. In addition, the intact vascular supply, which may carry the drug to remote but connected brain areas, constitutes an additional source of error in these studies. Experimental removal of major afferent pathways to the cell under study, as for example by surgery (HOFFER et al. 1977) or X-irradiation (WOODWARD et al. 1974), genetic mutations (SIGGINS et al. 1976 b) or chemical denervation (HOFFER et al. 1971 b) can often surmount these problems.

II. Microiontophoresis

The most widely-used method of drug administration for mammalian central neurons in the last two decades has been the local application of drug in the immediate environment of the recorded cell by iontophoresis (CURTIS 1964). The reasons for the popularity of this technique are several-fold: (1) the area of brain, and numbers of cell and cell types, affected by the drug are substantially reduced: therefore single neurons may be studied in intact brain with little remote action on other neurons; (2) drugs may be applied directly to a cell in quantities insufficient to reach the systemic circulation to cause cardiovascular changes and subsequent mechanical or metablic alterations in neuronal firing; (3) drugs that do not penetrate pial surfaces or the blood brain barrier can be studied even in deep brain structures.

The method of iontophoresis can be adapted for recording either extracellular neuronal activity, or, for larger cells, transmembrane potentials. The review by HOFFER and SIGGINS (1975) provides details of the construction and use of the most common types of microiontophoretic electrodes, the most widely used of which – for extracellular recording – contain 5 to 7 pipettes fused together and pulled to a fine open tip (4–10 μm overall tip diameter). The center barrel of this array is usually filled with 3 *M* NaCl and is used for recording neuronal discharge. Another barrel is also usually filled with electrolyte and is used as a current control or for current neutralization (see SALMOIRAGHI and WEIGHT 1967). The remaining barrels are filled with concentrated solutions of ionized drugs. Current of the same polarity as the drug ion is applied to these barrels to eject the drugs into tissue. Since the glass pipettes are fused together in close proximity, drugs can be applied at the exact site of the neuronal recording and drug-evoked changes in neuronal discharge can be assessed. However, many problems are encountered with this technique, especially regarding negative results and current effects; the interested reader should consult the review of methodology by BLOOM (1974).

It is apparent that the best method of electrophysiological recording is obtained by intracellular electrodes. Methods are available for recording cells intracellularly while applying drugs extracellularly by iontophoresis (Fig. 2; see HOFFER and SIGGINS 1975). However, since cyclic nucleotides are only sparingly permeable across cell membranes, and their presumed site of action is intracellular (KUO and GREENGARD 1969) the best approach is to administer the cyclic nucleotides intracellularly. Although this has been accomplished for some large non-neuronal and invertebrate neuronal cells, it is a formidable task to inject nucleotides into the smaller mammalian central neurons without injuring them. Only a few studies of this type have been reported for vertebrate neurons (SWARTZ and WOODY 1979, GALLAGHER and SHINNICK-GALLAGHER 1977; KRNJEVÍC and VAN METER 1976).

III. Micropressure Application

Recently the common technique of pressure ejection has been modified for use with fine drug-filled micropipettes – often glued or fastened to recording microelectrodes – such that they may be used in studies of drug effects on single central neurons

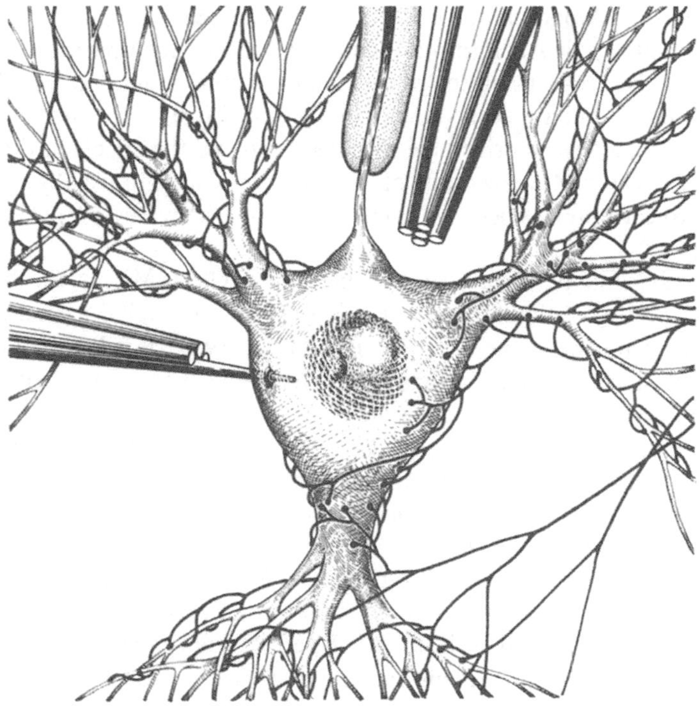

Fig. 2. Diagrammatic representation of two types of assemblies for iontophoresis or micropressure drug delivery and unit recording, drawn to approximate scale for comparison to a mammalian brain neuron. The extracellular assembly on the top has 5 barrels, one for recording neuronal discharge, one for current controls (see text) and 3 for ejection of drugs by pressure or current. The assembly on the left has an intracellular ultra-microelectrode glued with its tip in advance of a multiple-barreled iontophoresis or pressure pipette; the optimum assembly in this system may be obtained with two or three extracellular pipettes, one or two containing ionized drug for ejection and one for current "neutralization." Also depicted are many synaptic boutons constituting possible sources of indirect drug actions in iontophoresis experiments

(McCaman et al. 1977; M. Sakai et al. 1979), much in the same way that iontophoresis electrodes are used. Indeed, the more sophisticated methods allow the use of pressure application and iontophoresis from the same micropipette barrel; thus, the results obtained with the two methods may be compared to minimize the artifacts inherent in each technique alone. Among other advantages, the micropressure methods has the ability to eject drugs that are poorly ionized or weakly soluble. This method will likely prove very useful in studies of cyclic AMP because of the poor releasing properties of cyclic AMP passed from pipettes by iontophoresis (Shoemaker et al. 1975; Hill-Smith and Purves 1978).

D. Effect of Cyclic Nucleotides and Related First Messengers on Excitable Cells

Of all the neurotransmitters and humoral substances known to elevate levels of cyclic nucleotides in excitable tissues, the catecholamines (specifically, epinephrine, norepinephrine, dopamine and isoproterenol) seem the most universal in their ability to stimulate cyclic AMP formation in vertebrates. The β-receptor is most often involved in such actions, although dopamine receptors and occasionally α-receptors may also stimulate cyclic AMP production. Most of the vertebrate electrophysiological studies described below have compared the effects of β-receptor agonists and cyclic AMP. Accounts of invertebrate work will usually provide comparisons to serotonin, since this agent must often activates adenylate cyclase in lower phyla.

While the link between acetylcholine and cyclic GMP as the mediator of muscarinic receptor stimulation in vertebrates has been well documented recently for certain peripheral tissues (N. GOLDBERG et al. 1973), it is less well understood in the CNS, since acetylcholine has such diverse effects in many areas of the CNS and because so many non-cholinergic agonists elevate cyclic GMP levels (FERRENDELLI et al. 1974; MAO et al. 1974a, b). Moreover, relatively few studies have appeared on the electrophysiological effects of cyclic GMP. Another potential neurotransmitter, ATP, and its metabolite adenosine, have provoked some interest due to the ability of adenosine to stimulate adenylate cyclase in the CNS. Therefore, the following survey of cell types highlights primarily the comparisons between catecholamines (serotonin in invertebrates), adenosine and cyclic AMP and between acetylcholine and cyclic GMP. An effort will be made to provide data on the effects of these agents on membrane conductance and ionic permeability, where those parameters have been studied.

I. Liver

Although not usually categorized as an excitable tissue, liver cells exhibit substantial resting membrane potentials and respond to catecholamines and glucagon with increases in cyclic AMP levels (see ROBISON et al. 1971). Furthermore, hyperpolarization of liver cells has been reported with administration of catecholamines and glucagon in perfused rat liver (FRIEDMAN et al. 1971), with catecholamines in superfused guinea pig liver slices (HAYLETT and JENKINSON 1969) and with iontophoresis of catecholamines in short-term tissue cultures of guinea pig liver parenchymal cells (GREEN et al. 1972). Therefore, it is of some interest that both cyclic AMP and cyclic GMP hyperpolarize perfused rat liver cells; these hyperpolarizations are preceded by an increase in calcium efflux, paralleled by an increase in K^+ efflux, and are blocked by tetracaine (FRIEDMAN et al. 1971). The similarity of action of glucagon, isoproterenol and cyclic AMP greatly supports the hypothesis that cyclic AMP is the second messenger in a variety of hormonal effects produced by catecholamines and glucagon in liver (see ROBISON et al. 1971).

II. Fat Cells

Fat cells represent another tissue thought to utilize cyclic AMP as a second messenger for a variety of hormone effects (ROBISON et al. 1971; FAIN, this volume). Intracellular recording of brown fat cells has revealed that norepinephrine (NE), whether superfused in vitro, perfused in situ or released by stimulation of the sympathetic nerves, depolarizes the membrane (GIRARDIER et al. 1968; B. HOROWITZ et al. 1969; KRISHNA et al. 1970). This depolarization is accompanied by a decrease in membrane resistance (J. HOROWITZ et al. 1971) and is blocked by the antilipolytics insulin and propranolol (a β-receptor antagonist).

Although early reports indicated that cyclic nucleotides had no effect on membrane potentials of brown fat cells (GIRARDIER et al. 1968; B. HOROWITZ et al. 1969; KRISHNA et al. 1970), a later study by WILLIAMS and MATHEWS (1974a, b) showed pronounced depolarization of 11–28 mV with dibutyryl cyclic AMP (2 mM) or theophylline. It was suggested that the earlier negative finding might have resulted from poor intracellular penetration of the nucleotide. The ionic mechanism behind these depolarizations is unclear, although Na^+ and Cl^- may be involved. Moreover, WILLIAMS and MATHEWS (1974a, b) point out that it has not yet been determined if the depolarizing effect of catecholamines and cyclic AMP result from a direct or indirect action on the membrane, since the fatty acid octanoate (perhaps released by these agents) will also depolarize fat cells.

III. Glandular Tissue

1. Invertebrate Salivary Glands

There is pharmacological evidence that cyclic AMP mediates at least part of the secretory response of blowfly (Calliphora) salivary glands to 5-hydroxytryptamine (5-HT) (BERRIDGE and PRINCE 1971, 1972; see BERRIDGE, this volume). However, when the transepithelial (extracellular) potential is measured via a liquid paraffin-gap technique, the electrical responses to 5-HT and cyclic AMP are completely different: 5-HT causes a negative luminal potential (with respect to the bathing medium) while cyclic AMP (or theophylline) makes the lumen more positive (BERRIDGE and PRINCE 1972). However, when 5-HT is administered in the presence of theophylline or in a chloride-free medium, luminal positivity results. BERRIDGE and PRINCE (1972) therefore conclude that 5-HT has two actions: (1) elevation of anion transport (perhaps mediated by Ca^{++} fluxes) and (2) stimulation of cyclic AMP production which results in enhanced cation transport.

RAPP and BERRIDGE (1977) present an interesting theoretical model of a calcium-cyclic AMP control loop to account for the sustained oscillations in the transepithelial potential produced by treatment with cyclic AMP or low concentrations of 5-HT. This model depends on a feedback loop in which cyclic AMP (generated by 5-HT) increases free cytoplasmic calcium, which in turn inhibits adenylate cyclase. RAPP and BERRIDGE extend their cyclic AMP-calcium loop hypothesis to other secretory tissues, such as pancreatic β-cells, the adrenal cortex and the anterior pituitary, all of which also generate oscillatory membrane potentals. However, confirmation of the hypothesis for these latter tissues must await investigation of the direct effects of cyclic nucleotides on membrane potential.

Recent work by HAX et al. (1974) suggests that cyclic AMP might have yet another function in isolated salivary glands of the larvae of Drosophila hydie. Cyclic AMP and its dibutyryl derivative hyperpolarize these cells with a decrease in ionic permeability of non-junctional membranes and increased permeability of the specialized low-resistance junctions between cells. These responses are mimicked by theophylline or ecdysterone (a hydroxylated derivative of the insect molting hormone ecdysone) both of which elevate intracellular cyclic AMP levels. HAX et al. (1974) propose that cyclic AMP thus plays a role in passive electrical communication between cells.

2. Parotid Acinar Cells

Both acetylcholine and epinephrine hyperpolarize acinar cells in conjunction with an increase in membrane conductance (probably to K^+ ions). The epinephrine effect appears to be mediated by an α-adrenergic receptor, while the β-receptor agonist isoproterenol stimulates adenylate cyclase in this tissue. Dibutyryl cyclic AMP also hyperpolarizes, but isoproterenol depolarizes, acinar cells, thus casting doubt on the role of cyclic AMP in the electrophysiological response of this tissue to β-receptor activation (PETERSEN 1975). Unfortunately, it is difficult to determine if cyclic AMP might mediate the α-receptor-induced hyperpolarization, since the effect of cyclic AMP on membrane conductance was not reported.

3. Pineal Gland

A more definitive role for cyclic AMP is found in pineal gland for the conversion of serotonin to N-acetyl serotonin, by induction of the enzyme serotonin N-acetyltransferase (see D. KLEIN et al. 1970; ZATZ, this volume). Since it is well known that norepinephrine stimulates cyclic AMP production in the pineal (see e.g. WEISS and COSTA 1968), it is of some interest that K. SAKAI and MARKS (1972) and KAKIUCHI and MARKS (1972), using intracellular microelectrode recording, found that norepinephrine and isoproterenol evoked a rapid hyperpolarization of pinealocytes. More recently, PARFITT et al. (1975) noted that cyclic AMP or dibutyryl cyclic AMP, as well as norepinephrine, induced a small but significant hyperpolarization of rat pinealocytes. Furthermore, ouabain or a high extracellular K^+ concentration blocks the hyperpolarizing effects of norepinephrine and cyclic AMP. Since ouabain does not prevent the stimulation of cyclic AMP generation by norepinephrine, but does block the induction of the N-acetyl-transferase enzyme, KLEIN and PARFITT (1975) proposed that hyperpolarization of the pineal cell may serve to establish an intracellular ionic environment more conductive for the cyclic AMP induction of the N-acetyltransferase. However, since membrane conductance was not measured it is difficult to determine which ions might be involved in this process and which produce the hyperpolarizations. Indeed, the involvement of an electrogenic pump as the source of the hyperpolarization is not ruled out.

IV. Epithelial Electrolyte Transporting Tissue

Changes in the potential difference (extracellular), and an associated "short-circuit current," are measured across certain arrays of cells (e.g., amphibian skin, toad bladder, gastric mucosa) during changes in transport of cations (e.g., sodium) and water (see ORLOFF and AUSIELLO, this volume). Such changes are dramatically evoked by application of epinephrine, vasopressin, oxytocin and angiotensin II, all of which also appear to stimulate the production of cyclic AMP (see OMACHI et al. 1974; HYNIE and SHARP 1971; SCHORDERET et al. 1975; COVIELLO et al. 1978). Since exogenous cyclic AMP produces similar ion transport and electrical events (see for example, WIESMANN et al. 1977), it is thought that cyclic AMP mediates the action of epinephrine and the peptides in these tissues. However, strict proof of this hypothesis will require intracellular recording of the transporting cells to show exact mimicry by cyclic AMP of the hormonal response, in terms of transmembrane electrical parameters.

Similar reasoning applies to the case of the proximal convoluted tubule, where both parathyroid hormone and cyclic AMP can inhibit volume reabsorption. Interestingly, the 8-[p-chloro-phenylthio] analogue of cyclic AMP produces a significant decrease in the lumen negative transepithelial potential difference and in net fluid reabsorption in the superficial proximal convoluted tubule of the rabbit, perfused in vitro (JACOBSON 1979).

V. Muscle

1. Skeletal Muscle

In spite of early studies showing elevation of cyclic AMP levels in skeletal muscle by β-adrenergic receptor stimulation (KLAINER et al. 1962), little is known of the functional role of either catecholamines or cyclic AMP in this tissue. In a variety of types of vertebrate and invertebrate skeletal muscle examined to date, β-adrenergic receptor stimulation has been reported to result in hyperpolarization, usually associated with decreased membrane conductance (BOWMAN and RAPER 1965; A.P. SOMLYO and SOMLYO 1969; HIDAKA and KURIYAMA 1969; KUBA 1970; KUBA and TOMITA 1971; ITO et al. 1971; TASHIRO 1973; EVANS and SMITH 1973; J. SMITH and THESLEFF 1976; BRAY et al. 1976). Both isoproterenol (a selective β-receptor agonist) and cyclic AMP were reported to hyperpolarize the "slow" or tonic skeletal muscle fibers of the pigeon (A.P. SOMLYO and SOMLYO 1969). More recently dibutyryl cyclic AMP applied together with theophylline has been found to mimic β-receptor activation, hyperpolarizing rat diaphragm (BRAY et al. 1976) and soleus (CLAUSEN and FLATMAN 1977) muscle fibers, probably via an electrogenic Na^+/K^+ pump (CLAUSEN and FLATMAN 1977).

Also consistent with cyclic AMP-induced hyperpolarization in skeletal muscle are reports of increased calcium efflux (CHENG and CHEN 1975) and sodium efflux (BITTAR and WALKOWIAK 1975; CLAUSEN and FLATMAN 1977) in barnacle and rat diaphragm muscle following treatment with analogues of cyclic AMP. Cyclic AMP analogues are also capable of enhancing excitation-contraction coupling in invertebrate muscles, possibly without changing membrane potential (KUPFERMAN et al. 1979).

The role of cyclic GMP in skeletal muscle has not been well elucidated. However, stimuli which elicit muscle contraction in general (nerve stimulation, nicotinic agents, direct electrical stimulation) are capable of doubling muscle cyclic GMP levels, perhaps through an increase in the intracellular concentration of free calcium (BEAM et al. 1977; NESTLER et al. 1978).

Catecholamines also affect motor nerve terminals of some of these preparations, but generally such effects have been characterized pharmacologically as α-adrenergic. Stimulation of these receptors restores junctional transmission after fatigue (BRECKENRIDGE et al. 1967) and facilitates the frequency of miniature end-plate potentials, which provide an index of excitability of motor nerve terminals (JENKINSON et al. 1968; A. GOLDBERG and SINGER 1969, KUBA 1970; KUBA and TOMITA 1971). In several of these studies the presynaptic effects of exogenous cyclic AMP were similar to those of the catecholamines (A. GOLDBERG and SINGER 1969; TAKAMORI et al. 1973). WILSON (1974) reported that the quantum size of end-plate potentials, mobilization rate and probability of transmitter release evoked by nerve stimulation in the rat diaphragm were increased by dibutyryl cyclic AMP or theophylline. Recently, SKIRBOLL et al. (1977) found evidence for a cyclic AMP-mediated calcium influx in motor nerve terminals, thus accounting for catecholamine or cyclic AMP-induced facilitation of transmission. Voltage-dependent conductances could provide the mechanism for this action (see Sect. G below) although this is difficult to study in nerve terminals on skeletal muscle.

2. Cardiac Muscle

The action of catecholamines and cyclic nucleotides in the heart is complex, in part because the heart is composed of heterogenous cells: some regulate the speed of beating (chronotropy) while others are responsible for the force of contraction (inotropy). The sino-atrial nodal cells are the primary pacemakers of the heart, and ventricular and atrial fibers are the major contractile elements; Purkinje fibers also possess properties of pacemakers.

In both sino-atrial nodal cells and Purkinje fibers catecholamines act primarily at β-adrenergic receptors, leading to a more rapid pacemaker depolarization. An elegant series of voltage clamp studies by TSIEN and colleagues (TSIEN et al. 1972; TSIEN 1973) showed that this chronotropic action was brought about by hastening the rate of decay of a slow potassium current (which is responsible for maintaining RMP). Qualitatively identical chronotropic effects on the pacemaker potential of sino-atrial nodal cells (YAMASAKI et al. 1974) and Purkinje fibers (TSIEN et al. 1972; TSIEN 1973; REUTER 1974) have been seen with external application of theophylline, cyclic AMP with theophylline, or butyrylated derivatives of cyclic AMP.

The action potential in Purkinje and ventricular fibers displays an initial spike followed by a prolonged plateau of depolarization thought to arise from a slow inward calcium (and possibly sodium) current. The function of this calcium current may to be load the fiber with calcium for excitation-contraction coupling. Both the slow inward calcium current and the following outward potassium current (which repolarizes the membrane) are voltage-dependent phenomena. It is thus of some interest that β-adrenergic receptor agonists, theophylline and cyclic adenosine nucleotides alter these two currents in Purkinje fibers, leading to enhanced plateau amplitude and either shortening (TSIEN et al. 1972; TSIEN 1973) or lengthening of its duration (REUTER 1974). In either case the likely result would be increased intracellular calcium, possibly accounting for the inotropic effects of these agents (KUKOVETZ and PÖCH 1970; see KATZ, this volume). Similar electrophysiological effects of cyclic AMP and theophylline are also seen in invertebrate heart muscle (see S-ROZSA and KISS 1976), although here the first messenger is not adrenaline but probably serotonin or dopamine.

The proposition that cyclic AMP produced intracellularly mediates the physiological action of the catecholamines (see KRAUSE et al. 1970; KUKOVETZ and PÖCH

1970; ROBISON et al. 1971) is strengthened by the finding that cyclic AMP has a more potent action in mimicking the electrophysiological action of catecholamines when injected directly into myocardial cells by iontophoresis (TSIEN 1973), while catecholamines injected into the cell are less effective than when applied externally (TSIEN 1973; REUTER 1974; YAMASAKI et al. 1974). On the negative side, the studies of BENFY (1971) and DANILO et al. (1978) indicate that the increases in cyclic AMP and automaticity produced by epinephrine in Purkinje fibers can be dissociated under certain conditions. Moreover, cyclic AMP and its analogues can evoke *negative* inotropic and chronotropic effects when applied extracellularly (JAMES 1965; CHIBA et al. 1972), possibly by stimulation of extracellular inhibitory adenosine receptors (BERTELLI et al. 1972).

While cyclic GMP has been strongly implicated in acetylcholine-induced tachycardia (N. GOLDBERG et al. 1973; GEORGE et al. 1970), to my knowledge no studies of the electrophysiological effects of cyclic GMP in heart have been published to date.

3. Smooth Muscle

The actions of catecholamines on membrane properties of smooth muscle is complicated by the presence of varying ratios of α- and β-receptors. For example, BULBRING and TOMITA (1969) found that noradrenaline (a mixed receptor agonist) hyperpolarized the intestinal smooth muscle of guinea pig taenia coli by increasing conductance mainly to K^+, whereas isoproterenol (a β-receptor agonist) hyperpolarized the membrane without changing the membrane conductance. Isoproterenol also hyperpolarizes myometrial fibers (DIAMOND and MARSHALL 1969; KROEGER and MARSHALL 1973). In support of a role for cyclic AMP in these β-responses (TRINER et al. 1970) are the findings that dibutyryl cyclic AMP and aminophylline hyperpolarize smooth muscle cells of the taenia coli (TAKAGI et al. 1971) and uterus (KROEGER and MARSHALL 1973; MARSHALL 1977; GROSSET and MICRONNEAU 1977). It is interesting that while dibutyryl cyclic AMP relaxes and hyperpolarizes uterine smooth muscle with an elevation in evoked action potential threshold, once triggered, the spikes can evoke larger contractions than without DB cAMP (GROSSET and MICRONNEAU 1977).

In vascular smooth muscle, isoproterenol has been shown to produce hyperpolarization of the membrane accompanied by muscular relaxation (A. P. SOMLYO and SOMLYO 1969; VON LOH 1971), although JOHANSSON et al. (1967) reported depolarizations with high concentrations of isoproterenol, possibly a result of using media with fairly high K^+ concentrations (A. P. SOMLYO and SOMLYO 1969). The mechanism of the relaxation of smooth muscle produced by isoproterenol is still debated (see review of MARSHALL 1977). Indeed, relaxation can result without significant potential change (DANIEL et al. 1970). Some authors suggest that an electrogenic sodium pump may be involved (A. P. SOMLYO and SOMLYO 1969) while others (e.g. ANDERSSON and MOHME-LUNDHOLM 1969; MARSHALL 1977) speculate that a Ca^{++} pump or Ca^{++} sequestration into sarcoplasmic reticulum, which reduces intracellular free Ca^{++} levels, (thus causing relaxation) may be involved (MAGARIBUCHI and KURIYAMA 1972).

Cyclic AMP has also been suggested to play a role in β-receptor-mediated vasodilation (ROBISON et al. 1971; NAMM, this volume). Indeed, it has been reported that cyclic AMP in the presence of cAMP-dependent protein kinase increases the uptake of calcium into subcellular fractions of vascular smooth muscle (WEBB and BHALLA 1976). However, few studies have appeared on the effects of cyclic AMP on vascular smooth muscle electrophysiology. A. P. SOMLYO and SOMLYO (1969) AND A. V. SOMLYO et al. (1970) report dibutyryl cyclic AMP induced-hyperpolarization of the smooth muscle of the rabbit main pulmonary vein which is inversely dependent on extracellular potassium levels, as are hyperpolarizing responses to isoproterenol. The fact that the hyperpolarizing responses to both agents are potentiated by theophylline further supports a second messenger role for cyclic AMP in this isoproterenol effect.

VI. Photoreceptors

Cyclic nucleotides have been implicated in the role of modulation of photoreceptors (see reviews by BITENSKY et al. 1973; FARBER, this volume). Although early studies suggested the presence in frog retinal rod outer segments (ROS) of a light inactivated adenylate cyclase (BITENSKY et al. 1971), later studies by this group (MIKI et al. 1973) and others (CHADER et al. 1974; GORIDIS et al. 1973; GORIDIS and VIRMAUX 1974) indicated that the phosphodiesterase (PDE) of ROS in vertebrates is stimulated by light while the cyclase is unaffected. Moreover, the PDE is more specific for cyclic GMP than for cyclic AMP (GORIDIS and VIRMAUX 1974). The implication therefore is that the most important nucleotide in photoreception is cyclic GMP, although the associated protein kinase is more sensitive to cyclic AMP (FARBER and LOLLEY 1979).

However, prior to the discovery that cyclic GMP might be the relevant nucleotide in ROS of vertebrate, several studies were conducted on the effects of cyclic AMP on the electrophysiology of photoreceptors. At this point it should be pointed out that light depolarizes invertebrate photoreceptors but hyperpolarizes those of vertebrates. The limulus lateral eye retinular cell has been chosen as a model because it is sufficiently large to impale by intracellular microelectrode. W. MILLER et al. (1971) reported that cyclic AMP, theophylline and aminophylline (all in high concentrations) all depolarized limulus retinular cells. WULFF (1971, 1973) noted that extracellular application of cyclic AMP decreased: retinular cell membrane potentials, the effective input resistance, the receptor potential magnitude and the reversal potential of the receptor potential; the duration of the latent period to the receptor potential was increased. However, extracellular 5′AMP mimicked the effects of cyclic AMP (WULFF 1973). In contrast to the results of W. MILLER et al. (1971), WULFF (1973) found that low concentrations of aminophylline (2 m*M* or less) hyperpolarized the retinular cells, elevated input resistance and receptor potentials, and shortened the latency to receptor potentials. WULFF (1973) interpreted these results as indicating that the effects of extracellular cyclic AMP (and 5′AMP) may not reflect the effects of increased intracellular cyclic AMP; the enhancement of the receptor potential by aminophylline was taken to suggest a role for cyclic AMP (modulated by Ca^{++}) in the genesis of the receptor potential in the retinular cell.

However, as noted above, recent developments indicate that cyclic GMP and not cyclic AMP may be the relevant nucleotide in retinal tissue (GORIDIS and VIRMAUX 1974). Moreover, the fast primary response to light is likely to involve a more rapidly generated mediator such as Ca^{++} rather than cyclic nucleotides. Unfortunately, to date only one preliminary report has appeared on the electrophysiological effects of cyclic GMP on photoreceptors (W. MILLER 1973). Although the results of this study are described as inconsistent, it is interesting that intracellular injection of both cyclic AMP and cyclic GMP in several experiments produced large increases in membrane potential and receptor potentials. However, the exact role of cyclic nucleotides in photoreception still remains unclear, although studies with cyclic nucleotide-dependent phosphorylation of a 30,000-dalton protein in vertebrate ROS suggest that reduction of cyclic GMP may be involved in light adaptation, providing a means of amplifying the visual response (FARBER and LOLLEY 1979).

Recently, a detailed voltage-clamp study on the type B photoreceptor of the nudibranch *Hermissenda* has been reported (ALKON 1979). In this invertebrate receptor, light induces a long-lasting depolarization (LLD) thought to derive in part from a voltage-dependent calcium current. Interestingly, intracellular iontophoresis of cyclic AMP reduces the amplitude of this calcium current without directly affecting RMP or membrane resistance. This covert action of cyclic AMP reinforces the appeal for applying voltage-clamp methodologies to cyclic nucleotide effects.

VII. Invertebrate Neurons

Prior to 1976 there was scant information in the literature on a putative electrophysiological role of cyclic AMP in invertebrate neurons, even though several neurotransmitter candidates (dopamine, octopamine, serotonin) were known to elevate cyclic AMP in invertebrate nervous tissue (see LINGLE, MARDER and NATHANSON, this volume). This situation arose partly because of the fact that cyclic AMP had no apparent effect on the resting electrical membrane properties of many invertebrate neurons (see, e.g., GAINER and BARKER 1975; GERSHENFELD, personal communication). The most extensive paper on this subject prior to 1976 (TAKEUCHI et al. 1975) reported that neither cyclic AMP nor cyclic GMP had any effect on two types of DA-sensitive neurons in the subesophageal ganglion of the African giant snail.

Research since 1976 has provided more positive data with regard to several electrophysiological actions of cyclic AMP in invertebrate neurons, and has helped suggest several reasons for the previous reports of negative findings with the nucleotides. For example, work by KACZMAREK et al. (1978) has shown that phosphodiesterase-resistant derivatives of cyclic AMP (8-benzylthio- and 8-methylthiocyclic AMP) are capable of initating after-discharges in neurites of *Aplysia* bag cells, similar to the actions of dopamine and phosphodiesterase inhibitors, while cyclic AMP and even its dibutyryl derivative were inactive.

The series of studies on *Aplysia* neurons (R15 and others) by LEVITAN, TREISTMAN and co-workers provides an interesting on-going story on the interactions of derivatives of cyclic AMP and cyclic GMP, phosphodiesterase inhibitors and phosphodiesterase. Early studies showed that 8-substituted benzylthio- and parachlorophenylthio-derivatives of cyclic AMP (but not intracellular injection of cyclic AMP or cyclic GMP) modified the bursting behavior of cells R15 and F-1 after a 20–45 min lag, often with enhancement of the interburst hyperpolarizations (TREISTMAN and LEVITAN 1976a). The PDE inhibitor IBMX produced variable results ranging from induction of bursts in silent cells to enhanced hyperpolarization in bursting cells (TREISTMAN and DRAKE 1979). However, TREISTMAN and LEVITAN (1976b) also reported that intracellular injection of guanylylimidodiphosphate (GMP-PNP), which stimulates adenylate cyclase in *Aplysia*, induces long-lasting hyperpolarization and decreases in bursting activity in R15 and other cells.

Later, combined electrophysiological and biochemical studies by LEVITAN and NORMAN (1980) help to clarify the meaning of the changes in bursting and the variability in response: lower doses of the two 8-substituted cyclic AMP derivatives (5 μ*M* to 0.3 m*M*) than used previously primarily enhance the interburst hyperpolarizations and in some cells bursting was completely inhibited; in contrast, 8-parachlorophenylthio-cyclic GMP leads to some depolarization and enhanced bursts, with little effect on the inter-burst phase. Biochemical assays of the differential interactions of these agents with the cyclic AMP- and cyclic GMP-related phosphodiesterases and protein kinases (showing that the high concentrations of cyclic AMP derivatives previously used can inhibit *both* cyclic AMP and cyclic GMP PDEs) lead these authors to conclude that the variability of earlier results may have been due to combined effects of elevated intracellular cyclic AMP and cyclic GMP (LEVITAN and NORMAN 1980). Thus a case may be presented for cyclic AMP-induced hyperpolarization, and cyclic GMP-induced depolarization in this preparation. Although the first messenger for these responses is not known, one or more peptide factors are suspected (TREISTMAN and LEVITAN 1976a).

The elegant pharmacological studies of KANDEL and colleagues, also on Aplysia neurons, represent another instance of the frequently covert action of cyclic AMP. These workers have shown that serotonin, which pre-synaptically enhances synaptic transmission between a sensory neuron and a motor neuron responsible for gill withdrawal, also generates cyclic AMP in this ganglion; the EPSPs responsible for this transmission are also enhanced by extracellular dibutyryl cyclic AMP or by intracellularly injected cyclic AMP (BRUNELLI et al. 1976), with little or no change in resting potential (M. KLEIN and KANDEL 1978). Subsequent studies (M. KLEIN and KANDEL 1978) indicate that either cyclic AMP, PDE inhibitors, serotonin, or stimulation of the sensitizing pathway exert their facilitatory effect by prolonging a voltage-sensitive calcium current (seen during the action potential) in the presynaptic terminal, probably by delaying the late outward potassium current. Essentially similar conclusions have been reported by SHIMAHARA and TAUC (1977). This cyclic AMP effect may not only prolong the action potential in the terminal but the enhanced entrance of calcium is likely to account for the release of larger amounts of neurotransmitter.

Thus, interpretation of negative results in these invertebrate preparations would have been initially hazardous, for several reasons: (1) in many cases proof was (or is) needed that the neurotransmitter candidate (first messenger) studied is actually a neurotransmitter for the cell being recorded; (2) stimulation of cyclic AMP generation by the first messenger should be shown for the specific cells studied electrophysiologically; (3) some proof is needed that exogenous nucleotide reaches intracellular "receptors" in significant amounts, penetrating membrane barriers and/or escaping degradation by PDEs; (4) opposing interactions of cyclic AMP and cyclic GMP systems should be considered; (5) cyclic nucleotides should be studied for effects on voltage-dependent conductances as well as on resting properties.

VIII. Vertebrate Nervous Tissue

By far the greatest proportion of literature on the electrophysiology of cyclic nucleotides concerns vertebrate nervous tissue. The primary reason for this is the well-documented effect of neurotransmitter candidates on cyclic AMP or cyclic GMP levels in vertebrate brain (seen reviews by DALY 1975; BLOOM 1975; NATHANSON 1977; DUNWIDDIE and HOFFER, this volume). Most of the early reports described a post-synaptic action of the nucleotides. Although recent studies have shown pre-synaptic effects of ATP and adenosine; it is not yet clear whether this effect involves cyclic nucleotides. Therefore, the following account is concerned primarily with the effect of cyclic nucleotides (and their presumed first messengers) at the post-synaptic level of integration.

1. Peripheral Nervous System

a) Autonomic Ganglia

The vertebrate sympathetic ganglia would seem a favorable model for the study of cyclic nucleotide electrophysiology, since: (1) the principle neurons are large enough to impale with microelectrodes; (2) the tissue is easily isolated and suitable for sucrose gap recording; (3) at one time the synaptic circuitry was thought to be fairly simple, (4) repetitive stimulation of the inputs produces a unique "slow inhibitory postsynaptic potential" (sIPSP) and a "slow excitatory postsynaptic potential" (sEPSP) (R. ECCLES and LIBET 1961; NISHI and KOKETSU 1967) while elevating the levels both of cyclic AMP and cyclic GMP (MCAFEE et al. 1971; WEIGHT et al. 1974); (5) superfused catecholamines evoke increases in ganglionic cyclic AMP (KEBABIAN and GREENGARD 1971; CRAMER et al. 1973); (6) immunohistochemistry shows increases in cyclic AMP and cyclic GMP in response to superfused dopamine (DA) and acetylcholine (ACh), respectively, appearing predominantly in the post-ganglionic neurons (KEBABIAN et al. 1975).

These and other data (see reviews of DALY 1975; BLOOM 1975) have implicated cyclic AMP as the intracellular postsynaptic mediator of the sIPSP, and cyclic GMP for the sEPSP; the 1st messengers for these systems in mammals are thought to be DA or NE for the sIPSP (but see WEIGHT and PADJEN 1973a, for evidence implicating ACh in amphibia) and ACh (muscarinic) for the sEPSP. The source of the DA or NE in mammals is thought to be the small intensely fluorescent (SIF) cell, suggested to function as an interneuron interposed between the input fibers and the principal ganglio-neurons. However, recent data has also implicated certain neuropeptides (e.g. LH-RH, substance P) in these slow potentials (JAN et al. 1979). On intracellular recording, the sIPSP and sEPSP are both often accompanied by an increase in membrane (input) resistance (decrease in ionic conductance). Controversy has centered on whether the sIPSP and sEPSP arise as a result of activation of electrogenic pumps (NISHI and KOKETSU 1967; KOBAYASHI and LIBET 1968) or from a decreased membrane conductance to Na^+ or K^+, respectively (WEIGHT and VOTAVA 1970; WEIGHT and PADJEN 1973b). However, the elegant voltage clamp studies of B. BROWN and ADAMS (1980) now indicate that the cholinergic sEPSP may result from muscarinic attenuation of a slow voltage-sensitive K^+ current (outward).

The first electrophysiological studies of cyclic nucleotides in sympathetic ganglia, using the sucrose gap, indicated that both cyclic AMP and dopamine hyperpolarized, while cyclic GMP mainly depolarized, ganglion neurons (McAFEE and GREENGARD 1972); theophylline potentiated the dopamine response. These data were taken as evidence that cyclic AMP post-synaptically mediates the sIPSP.

Recent research from a number of laboratories casts some doubt whether cyclic nucleotides actually mimic the RMP changes of the sPSPs (e.g., see AKASU and KOKETSU 1977; DUN and KARCZMAR 1977; DUN et al. 1977; HSU and McISAC 1978; GALLAGHER and SHINNICK-GALLAGHER 1977; KOBAYASHI et al. 1978; WEIGHT et al. 1978; BUSIS et al. 1978; P. SMITH et al. 1979; LINDL 1978; D. BROWN et al. 1979). Most of these investigators (but see D. BROWN et al. 1979) report difficulty in evoking hyperpolarization with cyclic AMP or its dibutyryl derivatives when bath-applied extracellularly, Although responses to extracellular cyclic GMP and its derivatives have been nearly as inconclusive, several groups do report depolarizations with these nucleotides extracellularly applied or intracellularly injected; these responses are associated either with a decrease (GALLAGHER and SHINNICK-GALLAGHER 1977) or no change in membrane resistance (HASHIGUCHI et al. 1978).

However, in general the research reports on the effects of the nucleotides in sympathetic ganglia are strewn with inconsistencies. For example, the same preparation (rat sympathetic ganglia) can yield either depolarization or no change (GALLAGHER and SHINNICK-GALLAGHER 1977; HSU and McISAAC 1978), or frank hyperpolarization (D. BROWN et al. 1979), with administration of cyclic AMP or adenosine. Similarly, rat and rabbit ganglion cells show depolarizations with cyclic guanosine nucleotides (GALLAGHER and SHINNICK-GALLAGHER 1977; HASHIGUCHI et al. 1978) while bullfrog ganglion neurons generally do not respond to a variety of nucleotides (WEIGHT et al. 1978). Moreover, while dibutyryl cyclic AMP or cyclic GMP is reported to have no effect on the spike after-hyperpolarization in bullfrog ganglia (P. SMITH et al. 1979), dibutyryl cyclic AMP enhances this afterhyperpolarization in hamster submandibular ganglion cells (SUZUKI and KUSANO 1978).

It thus seems possible that many of the reservations concerning interpretations of negative results with cyclic nucleotides on the electrophysiology of invertebrate neurons (see Sect. VIII) may also apply to the autonomic ganglia. In particular only a few studies have utilized intracellular injection of cyclic AMP or dibutyryl cyclic AMP into sympathetic ganglion cells, and none has employed intracellular or extracellular administration of the 8-substituted cyclic AMP derivates known to be more resistant to PDE hydrolysis and more potent in activating protein kinase (LEVITAN and NORMAN 1980; MEYER and MILLER 1974; SIGGINS and HENRIKSEN 1975). Antagonistic actions of cyclic AMP and cyclic GMP, due to unspecific PDE inhibition, may be another factor. Recent studies on cultured bullfrog sympathetic neurons support the idea that inconsistent or negative responses to extracellularly-applied cyclic adenosine nucleotides may still arise from technical problems such as poor penetration through the plasmolemma or hydrolysis by PDE: while extracellular application of cyclic AMP, monobutyryl cyclic AMP or 8-benzylthio cyclic AMP give only weak or unreproducible responses, intracellular iontophoresis of N^6 monobutyryl cyclic AMP produces more pronounced and repeatable hyperpolarizations (GRUOL et al. 1981).

Nonetheless, several recent reports (LIBET et al. 1975; LIBET 1981; KOBAYASHI et al. 1978) suggest a function for the cyclic nucleotides beyond direct effects on resting membrane properties: with both gross and intracellular recording methods, application of DA or cyclic AMP to the sympathetic ganglion causes long-term enhancement of the sEPSP or the slow depolarizing response to methacholine; addition of cyclic GMP to the bath abolishes this effect. It is thus proposed that the cyclic AMP could function to produce a "memory trace" in the ganglion which is "disrupted" by cyclic GMP. However, understanding the mechanisms behind these and other nucleotide effects may require analysis of voltage-dependent conductances (see e.g. HORN and MCAFEE 1979; B. BROWN and ADAMS 1980).

b) Sciatic Nerve

An early study on frog sciatic nerve indicated that cyclic AMP, dibutyryl cyclic AMP and theophylline could decrease the spike amplitude and raise the firing threshold for the evoked compound action potential (VANDE BERG 1974). However, a more recent report by HORN and MCAFEE (1977) on the same preparation could not verify this finding. Thus, while isoproterenol caused an increase in cyclic AMP and carbachol evoked an increase in cyclic GMP (both nucleotides were elevated by theophylline), neither isoproterenol, carbachol, theophylline, cyclic AMP, cyclic GMP nor their dibutyryl derivatives affected the magnitude of the resting or compound action potential of the frog sciatic nerve. These authors conclude that cyclic nucleotide metabolism in peripheral nerve is unrelated to control of axonal excitability.

2. Central Nervous System

a) Spinal Cord

The electrophysiological effects of cyclic nucleotides have been studied in several CNS regions, including, more recently, spinal cord neurons. As in other central regions, the first messenger most likely to generate cyclic AMP in the spinal cord is norepinephrine, which has been reported to hyperpolarize spinal motorneurons with an increase in input resistance (ENGBERG and MARSHALL 1971). It is suggested that these effects are due to a reduced conductance to sodium ions (K. MARSHALL and ENGBERG 1979).

In accord with this mechanism, intracellular injection of cyclic AMP by means of "push-pull" iontophoresis often induced a rise in resistance and membrane hyperpolarization (KRNJEVÍC and VAN METER 1976), although the most striking effect was acceleration of the rising and falling phases of the action potential and enhancement of the after-hyperpolarization. Intracellular cyclic GMP most often generated a diminished resistance and occasional depolarizations, and also accelerated the action potential (KRNJEVÍC et al. 1976), yet, surprisingly, combined injection of both nucleotides enhanced the ability of cyclic AMP to increase input resistance (KRNJEVÍC and VAN METER 1976). Cyclic AMP tended to enhance EPSPs (KRNJEVÍC and VAN METER 1976) while cyclic GMP diminished EPSPs (KRNJEVÍC et al. 1976), as might be predicted from their occasional effects on membrane potential and resistance. Unfortunately, no derivatives of cyclic AMP or cyclic GMP were tested in these studies.

A variety of nucleosides and nucleotides have been tested recently on the isolated, hemisected toad spinal cord perfused in vitro (PHILLIS and KIRKPATRICK 1978). In this preparation most of the adenine and adenosine nucleotides had pronounced presynaptic inhibitory actions and occasional excitatory actions on dorsal and ventral root potentials (gross recording of many cells), but it is not clear whether these effects involve generation of cyclic nucleotides as in the mammalian brain. Perfusion of cyclic AMP and cyclic GMP at concentrations up to 10 m*M* had no effect on polarization levels or the evoked dorsal and ventral root potentials of this preparation (PHILLIS and KIRKPATRICK 1978). However, again no derivatives of these cyclic nucleotides were tested.

b) Cerebellum

Positive results which cyclic nucleotides on neuronal electrophysiology were first reported for the cerebellum of the rat, in which a concordance of data favors a role for cyclic AMP in synaptic transmission. Furthermore, the modularity of the neuronal architecture and "circuitry" of this region facilitates electrophysiological identification of the only output cell of this structure, the Purkinje cell (J. ECCLES et al. 1967). The biochemical, pharmacological and histochemical data implicating a role for cyclic AMP in noradrenergic transmission to the Purkinje cells have been reviewed elsewhere (BLOOM 1975; SIGGINS 1978a). However, a major line of evidence linking cyclic AMP to this system is derived from electrophysiological studies. With extracellular recording of the spontaneous action potentials of identified Purkinje cells of many species, iontophoresis of cyclic AMP and several more potent derivatives produce a reduction of firing rate in most Purkinje cells similar to that produced by NE and stimulation of the locus coeruleus (LC), the source of cerebellar norepinephrine fibers (SIGGINS et al. 1969, 1971a, b, c, d; BLOOM et al. 1975; SIGGINS and HENRIKSEN 1975; HOFFER et al. 1971a, 1973). Moreover, with intracellular recording, stimulation of the LC or extracellular application of cyclic AMP, dibutyryl cyclic AMP or NE all hyperpolarize Purkinje cells in association with no change or an increase in the input resistance (SIGGINS et al. 1971b, d; HOFFER et al. 1973). The latter effect is unique since most inhibitory neurotransmitters and pathways generally reduce membrane resistance. Thus, there appears to be an exact mimicry between the 1st messenger and the presumed 2nd messenger. Interestingly, iontophoresis of adenosine (also known to elevate cerebellar cyclic AMP levels) also inhibits Purkinje cell firing, although this effect, unlike that of cyclic AMP, is blocked by theophylline (BLOOM et al. 1975).

Nonetheless, other laboratories have reported difficulty in obtaining inhibitory responses to cyclic AMP in extracellular recording of Purkinje cells (GODFRAIND and PUMAIN 1971; LAKE and JORDAN 1974). Although many factors may account for their negative findings (SIGGINS et al. 1971c; BLOOM et al. 1974; BLOOM 1974) probably the single most important factor may be the variability with which iontophoresis pipettes pass cyclic AMP (SHOEMAKER et al. 1975). Since, as with other tissues, much larger amounts of cyclic AMP are needed to produce an effect compared to the 1st messenger, this variability in release from pipettes is a critical factor in obtaining positive responses to cyclic AMP. As suggested above for invertebrate and vertebrate autonomic neurons, cautious interpretation of negative results is required, especially in iontophoresis experiments. The observation of reproducible inhibitory responses of cultured Purkinje cells to superfusion of high concentrations of cyclic AMP (GÄHWILER 1976; see below) reinforces the assumption that the method of drug administration is critical and that cyclic AMP mimics NE effects. The latter point is further supported by the finding that iontophoresis of certain derivatives of cyclic AMP possessing a greater ability to activate protein kinase (the intracellular "receptor" for cyclic AMP) inhibits 80–92% of Purkinje cells compared to 60–65% with cyclic AMP itself (SIGGINS and HENRIKSEN 1975).

More recent work from the laboratory of PHILLIS indicates that more frequent inhibitory responses of Purkinje cells to cyclic AMP are now obtained (KOSTOPOULOS et al. 1975). Moreover, this group also finds very potent and reproducible inhibitory responses of Purkinje cells to several adenine derivatives such as adenosine, 5′AMP, ADP and ATP, which they ascribe in cerebral cortex to the activation of a "purinergic" or adenosine receptor, with the resultant postsynaptic generation of cyclic AMP (see Sect. D.VIII., 2.d below; PHILLIS et al. 1975; PHILLIS and KOSTOPOULOS 1975). The implication here is that the effect of intracellular cyclic AMP therefore must be also inhibitory if it is to mediate the potent inhibitions produced by the other adenine derivatives.

Thus, the preponderance of evidence indicates a mediator role for cyclic AMP in the noradrenergic and "purinergic" inhibitions of the spontaneous activity of cerebellar Purkinje cells. However, it should be noted that cyclic AMP, like NE, can *enhance* synaptically evoked activity such as that produced by the climbing fiber input to Purkinje cells, as shown by the enlargement of climbing fiber EPSPs with cyclic AMP, NE and LC activation (SIGGINS et al. 1971 b, d; HOFFER et al. 1973). In this respect the end effect of cyclic AMP bears resemblance to that reported for sympathetic ganglia (see LIBET 1980), although the mechanism may be different in the two cases.

The role of cyclic GMP in the cerebellum remains more covert, even though several putative neurotransmitters (e.g. acetylcholine, glutamate) are reported to elevate cyclic GMP levels (FERRENDELLI et al. 1970, 1974; MAO et al. 1974 a, b). Certain pharmacological data are thought to suggest that cyclic GMP may be the intracellular mediator for the unique depolarizing response of Purkinje cells to activation of climbing fiber inputs (MAO et al. 1974 a, b). Glutamate might be a candidate for the climbing fiber neurotransmitter. However, all of these biochemical studies on cyclic GMP in cerebellum have utilized slices of cerebellum treated with very high concentrations of agonists, or intact animals injected systemically; the results of these studies are therefore difficult to interpret because of the multiple sites of possible indirect actions of the agonists (see Sect. C.I.A). Moreover, early iontophoresis studies in rat cerebellum showed mostly inhibitory responses of Purkinje cells to cyclic GMP (HOFFER et al. 1971 a), although a more recent study of normal and mutant (weaver) mouse cerebellum gave a predominance of excitatory (presumed depolarizing) responses (SIGGINS et al. 1976b). Glutamate but not acetylcholine also excites normal mouse Purkinje cells; this is more consistent with a role in mouse for glutamate as a first messenger than for acetylcholine. However, weaver Purkinje neurons showed more (40%) excitations to acetylcholine. Obviously many more criteria of 2nd messenger mediation need to be satisfied before a synaptic role for cyclic GMP can be verified in cerebellum.

c) Hippocampus

The locus coeruleus sends noradrenergic fibers to several other cortical areas as well as cerebellum. Recent pharmacological and electrophysiological studies of the rat hippocampus, whose granule and pyramidal cells receive a noradrenergic input, suggest that this input is similar, but not identical, to that in cerebellum (SEGAL and BLOOM 1974a, b; see DUNWIDDIE and HOFFER, this volume). The reader should refer to the reviews by BLOOM (1975) and DUNWIDDIE and HOFFER (this volume) for a more detailed account of data suggesting cyclic nucleotide mediation of synaptic events. In brief, electrical stimulation of the LC and iontophoresis of NE inhibit the spontaneous activity (recorded extracellularly) of hippocampal pyramidal cells probably via a β-receptor, and PDE inhibitors potentiate both of these inhibitions. A major link between cyclic AMP and NE-evoked inhibition of pyramidal cells has been derived from electrophysiological studies showing that extracellular iontophoresis of cyclic AMP acts like NE and stimulation of LC in inhibiting a majority (57%) of pyramidal cells (SEGAL and BLOOM 1974a). More exact mimicry of responses to NE and cyclic AMP was seen in the intracellular in vivo studies of OLIVER and SEGAL (1974): cyclic AMP (but not ATP or 5′AMP) injected inside pyramidal cells by intracellular iontophoresis, and LC stimulation or NE applied outside the cell, evoked hyperpolarization accompanied by no change or an increase in membrane input resistance.

However, recent extracellular and intracellular studies on the in vitro hippocampal slice preparation reveal a more complicated picture of NE and cyclic AMP-mediated events. For example, a preliminary intracellular report by SEGAL (1980) suggests that NE may hyperpolarize pyramidal cells in association with a *decrease* in input resistance. In parallel with this finding, perfusion of monobutyryl cyclic AMP (50–100 μM) also hyperpolarizes pyramidal neurons, often with a decrease in input resistance (SIGGINS and SCHUBERT 1981). However, care must be exercised in interpreting these results, since hippocampal pyramidal cells possess both α- and β-adrenergic receptors (see DUNWIDDIE and HOFFER, this volume) and NE can activate either receptor type. Furthermore, it has been shown that extracellularly-applied cyclic AMP activates adenosine receptors in the hippocampal slice, producing some inhibitory actions which may not involve generation of intracellular cyclic AMP (see DUNWIDDIE and HOFFER, this volume). Therefore, in order to completely verify a link between NE effects and cyclic AMP, intracellular studies should be repeated using a range of α- and β-adrenergic drugs, and using theophylline to block the adenosine receptor-mediated actions of cyclic AMP. Since it is likely that at least some of the inhibitory actions of adenosine are mediated by cyclic AMP, the reader is referred to the chapter by DUNWIDDIE and HOFFER where this topic is covered in detail.

A possible electrophysiological role for cyclic GMP in rat hippocampus is also emerging, owing to the studies of HOFFER et al. (1977) on explants of hippocampus transplanted to the anterior chambers of adult rat eyes. As with brain slices in vitro, this preparation allows the use of superfusion techniques as well as iontophoresis and permits better evaluation of the indirect effects of the two techniques of drug delivery (see Sect. C). In this preparation both ACh and cyclic GMP (or its derivatives) evoke reproducible increases in the spontaneous firing rate of all pyramidal cells, often to the point of epileptiform activity (HOFFER er al. 1977). Certain phosphodiesterase inhibitors potentiate the excitations to ACh. These results thus predict a postsynaptic role for cyclic GMP in mediating the excitatory responses to ACh, a physiologically relevant concept in view of evidence showing a large cholinergic input to the hippocampus via the septum (LEWIS and SHUTE 1967).

d) Cerebral Cortex

Although the cerebral cortex of several species responds well to catecholamines by generating cyclic AMP in vitro (KAKIUCHI and RALL 1968a; CHASIN et al. 1971), electrophysiological studies linking cyclic AMP to the effects of catecholamines are inconclusive. One problem has been the inability to determine exactly which type(s) of cortical neuron(s) receive input from the locus coeruleus. The importance of identifying cell types in obtaining positive responses to cyclic AMP has been described for cerebellum (SIGGINS et al. 1971c; SIGGINS and HENRIKSEN 1975). Indeed, the early inability of LAKE et al. (1972, 1973) and JORDAN et al. (1972) to correlate extracellular unit responses to iontophoretically applied cyclic AMP with those to NE appears to have been a result of studying unidentified cortical neurons; later studies by STONE et al. (1975), STONE and TAYLOR (1977) and PHILLIS et al. (1975) showed good correlations between cyclic AMP and NE responses in electrophysiologically identified pyramidal tract cells. In general, both NE and cyclic AMP depress the spontaneous or glutamate-evoked discharge of these neurons, with cyclic AMP inhibiting about 70% of the cells. The potentiation of NE responses by the phosphodiesterase inhibitor papaverine (STONE et al. 1975) and a clear distinction between the inhibitory actions produced by cyclic AMP and those produced by adenosine (TAYLOR and STONE 1977, 1980), adds further evidence that cyclic AMP may be the 2nd messenger for NE in cerebral cortex.

An interesting development is the possibility that adenosine (or some other non-cyclic adenine derivative) may be, among other things, a first messenger for cyclic AMP in cerebral cortex (see DUNWIDDIE and HOFFER, this volume). It is pertinent that PHILLIS et al. (1975) and PHILLIS and KOSTOPOULOS (1975) have shown that the iontophoresis of adenosine and a variety of adenine derivatives inhibit the spontaneous extracellular electrical activity of almost all pyramidal tract and other unidentified cortical neurons. The proposition that this effect is mediated through an adenosine receptor is strengthened by the finding that iontophoresis of methyl xanthines antagonizes the inhibitions produced by adenosine (PHILLIS and KOSTOPOULOS 1975). Similar findings have recently been reported for slices of olfactory cortex maintained in vitro: adenosine, 5′-AMP, ATP and ADP (at concentrations of 5×10^{-6} to $5 \times 10^{-3} M$) all depressed the orthodromically-evoked field potential (N-wave) indicative of a population of EPSPs, and enhanced the formation of cyclic AMP (OKADA and KURODA 1975; KURODA and KOBAYASHI 1975; SCHOL-

FIELD 1978). Theophylline inhibited both these effects of the adenine derivatives (KURODA and KOBAYASHI 1975). Cyclic AMP itself also has an inhibitory effect on the N-wave (OKADA and KURODA 1975; SCHOLFIELD 1978). However, the implication that intracellular cyclic AMP mediates the inhibitory effect of adenosine in this preparation is clouded by the weak correlation between adenosine-induced electrical and biochemical actions across slice preparations from several brain areas (OKADA and SAITO 1979), and by the finding that dibutyryl cyclic AMP and drugs that increase intracellular cyclic AMP do not have inhibitory actions (SCHOLFIELD 1978).

The iontophoretic studies of STONE et al. (1975) suggest a possible role for cyclic GMP in rat cerebral cortex. In contrast to an earlier report by PHILLIS et al. (1974), STONE et al. (1975) find a strong correlation in identified pyramidal tract neurons in situ between excitations of extracellular discharge produced by acetylcholine and cyclic GMP. Roughly 75% of these cells are excited by cyclic GMP (STONE et al. 1975). An even stronger correlation has recently been communicated by SWARTZ and WOODY (1979), who compared the effects of intracellular iontophoresis of cyclic GMP with those of extracellular iontophoresis of ACh during intracellular recording of cortical pyramidal cells in the awake cat. In brief, these workers found that 57% of neurons tested with ACh showed an increase in input resistance and 50% displayed an increase in firing rate; 65% of cells tested with cyclic CMP developed an increase in input resistance and 60%, an increase in firing rate. All cells tested with both ACh and cyclic GMP and which developed increases in resistance to ACh also showed comparable responses to cyclic GMP. However, because of the interference of the iontophoretic currents used it was not possible to measure the effects of these two agents on membrane potential.

Thus the above findings suggest that cyclic AMP and cyclic GMP could function as reciprocal intracellular second messengers in cerebral cortex for NE and acetylcholine, respectively, as first proposed in the "yin-yang" hypothesis of N. GOLDBERG et al. (1973) for peripheral systems.

e) Caudate Nucleus

Although catecholamines are known to stimulate cyclic AMP formation in the caudate nucleus (KEBABIAN et al. 1972; WALKER and WALKER 1973; R. MILLER et al. 1974), the adenylate cyclase system in this brain structure more closely resembles that of sympathetic ganglia than of the brain cortices. The endogenous catecholamine is predominantly dopamine (DA), not NE, derived from cell bodies in the substantia nigra. Furthermore the DA receptor, as assayed either biochemically or electrophysiologically is antagonized by neuroleptic agents such as haloperidol, chlorpromazine and fluphenazine, rather than β-adrenergic blockers.

In spite of these differences, over 90% of unidentified caudate neurons respond like cerebral and cerebellar cortical neurons to iontophoresis of cyclic AMP, monobutyryl cyclic AMP and DA, with a reduction in spontaneous or amino acid-evoked discharge rate (SIGGINS et al. 1974, 1976a). It must be admitted that a controversy still abounds as to whether DA is an inhibitory or excitatory transmitter in the caudate, although it seems likely than the reported excitatory effects arise as artifacts of iontophoresis currents (SIGGINS 1978b). In contrast, it seems clear that the inhibitory actions of DA or cyclic AMP are not due to current artifacts, since these agents are still potent inhibitory agents when applied to caudate neurons by the micropressure technique (G. SIGGINS and ZIEGLGÄNSBERGER, unpublished work). Furthermore, the enhancement of dopamine and cyclic AMP-induced inhibitions by PDE inhibitors such as papaverine and isobutyl methylxanthine (SIGGINS et al. 1974) further strengthens the link between DA and cyclic AMP in caudate neurons at the electrophysiological level.

Adenosine may also play a role in caudate. The biochemical studies of WILKENING and MAKMAN (1975) show that 2-chloroadenosine stimulates cyclic AMP in caudate. This derivative of adenosine does not enter the pool of precursors for ATP and cyclic AMP (STURGILL et al. 1975); thus it may function primarily as an agonist for an "adenosine" receptor. The formation of cyclic AMP in response to 2-chloroadenosine is blocked by the methyl xanthines (WILKENING and MAKMAN 1975). Recent electrophysiological studies reinforce these biochemical findings; iontophoresis of adenosine and 2-chloroadenosine inhibits the spontaneous firing of nearly all caudate neurons studied (SIGGINS et al. 1976a). Unlike the inhibitory response to cyclic AMP and dopamine, responses to adenosine are blocked by methyl xanthines such as aminophylline or isobutyl methylxanthine. Hence, an inhibitory adenosine/adenylate cyclase system distinct from the dopamine/adenylate cyclase system may exist in rat caudate as well as cerebral cortex. However, it still remains to be determined whether these systems are located on pre- or post-synaptic elements.

f) Other Dopamine-Rich Areas

Dopamine containing fibers, with cells of origin in areas A9 (substantia nigra) or A10, densely innervate several other areas besides the caudate nucleus. Principal among these are the limbic structures such as olfactory tubercle, amygdala and limbic cortex, and the nucleus accumbens. It is therefore of interest that iontophoretically applied DA or cyclic AMP inhibits the spontaneous activity of about 90% of unidentified cells in the nucleus accumbens and the olfactory tubercle (BUNNEY and AGHAJANIAN 1973). Furthermore, OBATA and YOSHIDA (1973) note that iontophoresis of both DA and cyclic AMP predominantly inhibits neuronal firing of neurons in the entopeduncular nucleus, another region rich in DA. Biochemical studies have shown that DA can stimulate adenylate cyclase in the nucleus accumbens and olfactory tubercle (CLEMENT-CORMIER et al. 1974). However, proof of the intermediation of the inhibitory dopamine responses in these structures by cyclic AMP awaits further electrophysiological tests with agents (e.g. PDE inhibitors) known to influence biochemically the dopamine/cyclic AMP system.

g) Brain Stem

An effort has also been made to find a relationship between responses to NE, histamine and cyclic AMP in unidentified neurons in the cat brain stem (ANDERSON et al. 1973). Here, iontophoresis of cyclic AMP depressed about 80% of all neurons studied, including 95% of those units inhibited by NE and about 90% of those depressed by histamine. Responses to NE were blocked by nicotinate. However, only 3 of 11 cells showed potentiation of the monoamine effects by the PDE inhibitors theophylline and aminophylline, and prostaglandin E_1 blocked 50% of the NE-induced depressions. As a result, ANDERSON et al. (1973) were reluctant to conclude that cyclic AMP might mediate monoamine depressions. However, in view of the lack of histochemical data on the percentage of the test cells showing the presence of NE or histamine synapses, and the likelihood of diverse isozymes of PDE in this brain region (see, e.g. SIGGINS et al. 1974), the data of ANDERSON et al. (1973) do not rule out a link between cyclic AMP and the depressant responses to NE and histamine in brain stem.

h) Cultured Neurons

A few attempts have been made to study electrophysiological responses of cultured neurons to cyclic nucleotides. In general, these studies have not always produced positive results. Indeed it has often proved difficult to evoke responses even to the presumed first messengers NE and DA, as for example in intracellularly recorded, cultured superior cervical ganglion neurons of the rat (OBATA 1974). Secondly, responses to the presumed 2nd messengers are not often reproducible with extracellular application, as for example in cultured frog sympathetic ganglion neurons recorded intracellularly (GRUOL et al. 1981); in this preparation high extracellular concentrations (2–5 m*M*) of catecholamines or intracellular iontophoresis of monobutyryl cyclic AMP hyperpolarizes the principal neurons more consistently. It is possible that the culture system itself modifies monoamine receptor or enzymes of the cyclic AMP system.

Several studies have noted modulation by cyclic AMP of on-going excitability of cultured neurons. Thus, CRAIN and POLLACK (1973) showed that cyclic AMP or dibutyryl cyclic AMP restores the excitability of neurons of fetal explant cultures of mouse cerebral cortex and spinal cord after Ca^{++} deprivation. Likewise, CHALAZONITIS and GREEN (1974) reported larger RMPs and a greater excitability of neuroblastoma cell lines cultured for long periods in media with high cyclic AMP levels. A similar elevation of excitability was seen with superfusion of dibutyryl cyclic AMP onto exposed kitten cerebral cortex in situ (PURPURA and SHOFER 1972). However, these studies do not show that cyclic AMP excites these neurons directly, but that cyclic AMP so alters the membrane that it is easier to excite by other means (e.g. by intracellular injections of current). Such increase in excitability could be produced by changes in voltage-dependent conductances or by slight hyperpolarizing actions (in somewhat depolarized cells) accompanied by increased membrane resistance, wherein a constant amount of stimulating or synaptic current would produce a larger potential deflection across the greater membrane resistance. The latter action would permit the evoked potential to more closely approach or exceed the threshold for spike generation, while spontaneous firing (arising from pacemaker potentials) would be depressed by the hyperpolarization.

A recent study by GÄHWILER (1976) on explants of rat cerebellar cortex reinforces the notion that cyclic AMP mediates the inhibitory effects of NE on Purkinje cells. In this study perfusion of the culture chamber with NE at greater than 10^{-5} *M* decreased spontaneous firing of Purkinje cells. While cyclic AMP at 10^{-4} *M* had no effect, 10^{-3} *M* slowed the firing of 44% of the cells. Phosphodiesterase inhibitors alone also depressed Purkinje cell firing, but in doses subthreshold for this effect they also strongly potentiated the inhibitions produced by either cyclic

AMP or NE. GÄHWILER (1976) concludes that this data supports the cyclic AMP-mediation hypothesis for the depressant action of noradrenergic neurotransmission in Purkinje cells.

The role of cyclic GMP has been little studied in cultured neurons. However, the biochemical and pharmacological investigations of STUDY et al. (1978) on neuroblastoma cultures seem to indicate that cyclic GMP can be elevated by two distinct mechanisms: (1) by depolarization with veratridine or high potassium concentrations, probably resulting from the opening of voltage-sensitive calcium channels; (2) by activation of muscarinic receptors with carbachol, arising from the opening of voltage-insensitive calcium channels.

3. Glia

Few studies have been performed on the physiology of cyclic AMP in glial cells, in part because of the difficulty in recording from such cells: because they do not fire action potentials they must be recorded intracellularly. However, in view of the large increases in cyclic AMP produced by catecholamines and prostaglandins in glial cell lines (GILMAN and NURENBERG 1971), this area is of some importance. It is therefore noteworthy that iontophoresis of cyclic AMP into presumed glial cells of the cat spinal cord produces hyperpolarization associated with an increase in membrane conductance, probably to potassium ions (KRNJEVÍC and VAN METER 1976). Similarly, ARLOCK and KANJE (1977) have shown that cultured human glioma cells (and particularly stellate cells) incubated in the presence of dibutyryl cyclic AMP exhibit significantly greater resting potentials than do those without cyclic AMP in the medium. However, this effect appears to require a two hour incubation before an effect is seen.

E. Conclusions and Speculations

Although it is still premature to suggest that cyclic AMP has a specific or universal electrophysiologic effect across a variety tissue types, it is tempting to survey the data for possible equivalencies in response to cyclic AMP (see Table 1). Such a survey shows that with a few exceptions (e.g. heart and lipocytes), and barring negative results, cyclic AMP predominantly hyperpolarizes or inhibits firing of most cell types studied; cyclic GMP when active usually depolarizes cells. These cell types include smooth muscle, skeletal muscle, hepatocytes, salivary cells, pineal cells, possibly retinulocytes, glia and many types of vertebrate and invertebrate neurons. Those studies utilizing extracellular recording of evoked or spontaneously firing neurons strongly imply hyperpolarizing effects. Responses of the two tissues representing exceptions to the above generality, lipocytes, are in question because of the possibility that released lipid may in fact be responsible for the depolarizations observed with NE or cyclic AMP. Myocardial cells may represent a special case because of the complexity of the cells and of the response (depolarizing and repolarizing) to NE and cyclic AMP.

However, a second theme seems to emerge from this survey, namely the significant action of cyclic AMP, and possibly cyclic GMP as well, on voltage-sensitive conductances, especially those involving or affecting inward calcium currents.

Table 1. Summary of effects of cyclic AMP and related substances on membrane electrical properties

Cell or tissue	MP	R_m	Comments; Other effects
Hepatocytes	↑	–	↑ K^+ efflux, tetracaine blocks effects
Lipocytes	↓	↓	
Blowfly salivary gland	–	–	↑ Luminal positivity, ↑ cation transport
Drosophila larvae salivary gland	↑	↑↓[a]	↓ Junction R_m, ↑ non-junctional R_m; theophylline mimics[a]
Parotid acinar cells	↑	–	
Pinealocytes	↑	–	Ouabain or high K_0^+ blocks hyperpolarization
Epithelial tissues	–	–	Alters ion transport and short circuit current
Convoluted tubule	–	–	↓ Lumen neg. transepithelial potential and fluid absorption
Skeletal muscle	↑[a]	↑	[a]DBcAMP and theophylline hyperpolarize, ↑ Na^+, Ca^{++} efflux and K^+ influx; all effects antagonized by ouabain
Cardiac sinoatrial and Purkinje fibers	[a]	–	[a]↑ Decay of slow K^+ current, ↑ inward Ca^{++} current, ↑ or ↓ late K^+ current
Smooth muscle of:			
Taenia coli	↑[a]	↑ or 0	DBcAMP and aminophylline hyperpolarize[a]
Uterus	↑[a]	↑ or 0	DBcAMP and aminophylline hyperpolarize[a]
Blood vessels	↑[a]	–	Inversely dependent on K_0, potentiated by theophylline[a]
Photoreceptors:			
Limulus retinular	↓	↓	↓ Receptor potential and its reversal potential; ↑ latency
Limulus retinular	↑[a]	↑	[a]Aminophylline in low concentration; ↑ receptor potential and ↓ latency
Limulus retinular	↑	–	Intracellular injection of cAMP; ↑ receptor potential
Hermissenda B cells	0	0	Intracellular injection of cAMP; ↓ voltage-dependent Ca^{++} current
Invertebrate neurons:			
Aplysia R15 and others	↑[a]		[a]GMP-PNP, 8-substituted cAMPs; 8-sub'd cGMP depolarizes
Aplysia sensory neuron	↓[a] or 0	↑	[a]Slight. Slows late outward K^+ current prolongs slow inward Ca^{++} current
Vertebrate neurons:			
Autonomic	↑[a] or 0	– or 0	[a]Not verified by several groups; potentiation of sEPSP; cGMP may depolarize
Spinal cord	↑[a]	↑[a]	[a]Occasional; acceleration of rising and falling phase of spike; ↑ of afterhypolarization and EPSP; cGMP depolarizes, accelerates spike phases, ↓ R_m and EPSPs
Cerebellar Purkinje cell	↑	↑	↓ Spontaneous firing (potentiated by PDE inhibitors), ↑ EPSPs. cGMP has mixed effects
Hippocampus	↑	↑↓[a]	[a]Effect depends on preparation ↓ spontaneous firing

Table 1 (continued)

Cell or tissue	MP	R_m	Comments; Other effects
Cerebral cortex	–	–	↓ Spontaneous firing, enhanced by PDE inhibitors; cGMP ↑ R_m, ↑ firing
Caudate n.	–	–	↓ Spontaneous firing, enhanced by PDE inhibitors
N. accumbens and olfactory tub.	–	–	↓ Spontaneous firing
Entopeduncular n.	–	–	↓ Spontaneous firing
Brain stem	–	–	↓ Spontaneous firing
Cultured neurons:			
Cortex and spinal cord	–	–	Restores excitability
Neuroblastoma	–	–	↑ Excitability
Cerebellum	–	–	↓ Spontaneous activity, potentiated by PDE inhibitors
Neuroglia:			
Spinal cord	↑	↓	
Cultured stellate glia	↑[a]	–	Requires time[a]

MP = membrane potential; R_m = membrane or input resistance (inverse of ionic conductance); ↑ = increases; ↓ = decreases; 0 = no effect; – = not tested or reported; DBcAMP = dibutyryl cAMP.
Several instances of a lack of effect were omitted if other cell properties also were not changed. See text for details and references.
[a] Comment refers to the effect listed under MP or R_m which is also marked with [a]

Such effects are exemplified by responses of myocardial cells, certain photoreceptors and certain invertebrate neurons, and they could prove prevalent in other excitable tissues (e.g. vertebrate autonomic ganglia), following completion of voltage-clamp and other relevant tests, at concentrations of cyclic nucleotides lower than those reported to affect resting membrane properties. The effect of such actions of cyclic nucleotides could be highly significant, especially with respect to calcium conductances, since calcium is known to play a role not only in transmitter and hormone release, but also in such vital processes as cyclic nucleotide synthesis and degradation (perhaps via calmodulin; see CHEUNG, this volume), cyclic nucleotide dependent and independent protein phosphorylation (see WALTER and GREENGARD, this volume), cell motility (PORTER 1976), genome expression (RODAN et al. 1978) and cell growth and development (LLINAS and SUGIMORI 1979). Moreover, in mammalian CNS it is now well-known that calcium can carry the current responsible for generation of the action potentials in the dendrites of a number of neuron types (see LLINAS and SUGIMORI 1979).

Tissues like heart, bursting neurons and salivary glands which exhibit pacemaker activity or oscillations in electrical events may represent a special case for the interactions between calcium and cyclic nucleotides. RAPP and BERRIDGE (1977) present an appealing hypothesis suggesting that such potentials shifts may arise from oscillations of a control loop involving intracellular calcium and cyclic AMP. The type of control loop may be unique for each tissue type, depending upon whether calcium stimulates or inhibits cyclic AMP formation, and whether cyclic AMP reduces or elevates cytoplasmic calcium levels.

However, determination of the ionic mechanism underlying responses of excitable cells to cyclic AMP will obviously require further tests, since many studies reported to date neither measured membrane resistance, nor changed ionic concentrations during recording of membrane properties, nor evaluated effects on voltage-sensitive conductances. As a result, several mechanisms of action have not been eliminated as candidates. These include decreases or increases in resting or active conductance to several ions (K^+, Na^+, Ca^{++}, Cl^-), and activation of electrogenic pumps. The latter mechanism is a strong candidate in skeletal muscle, smooth muscle and adipocytes, where active extrusion of ions or activation of $Na+/K+$ ATPase by catecholamines or cyclic AMP has been observed (HAYS et al. 1974; BRESSLER et al. 1975; B. HOROWITZ and EATON 1975). It is speculated that there will be little if any change in membrane resistance with activation of an electrogenic pump (THOMAS 1972).

The molecular events whereby cyclic nucleotides might evoke these ionic or membrane changes is another avenue of investigation. It is thought that protein kinase activation may be involved as the intracellular (or perhaps intra-membranous) receptor for many actions of the nucleotides or calcium (KUO and GREENGARD 1969; see WALTER and GREENGARD, this volume). Electrophysiologically, this theory is supported for central neurons by the finding that derivatives of cyclic AMP inhibit Purkinje cell firing in direct correlation with their ability to activate protein kinase (SIGGINS and HENRIKSEN 1975). There is evidence that the protein kinase activated by cyclic AMP, cyclic GMP or calcium may catalyze the phosphorylation of some membrane-bound protein or activate membrane phosphatases (see WALTER and GREENGARD; BEVO; KUO; SCHULMAN, this volume), and that these alterations in the phosphate content of membrane components might result in the observed electrical changes in membrane properties (GREENGARD and KEBABIAN 1974).

However, the production by cyclic nucleotides of electrophysiologically detectable events in a given cell type does not rule out other cyclic nucleotide-dependent physiological events in that cell that might escape detection. Such covert epiphenomena may be much slower in time-course than the electrical events and may involve induction or activation of enzymes, cell growth, differentiation and mitogenesis (see MCMAHON, this volume). Indeed, further investigation could show that the electrophysiological changes in some cells are superfluous or perhaps ontogenic vestiges. A more likely possibility is that these changes serve to bring about ionic conditions in the cell or its membrane that are favorable for initiation of these later, slower phenomena, as suggested by D. KLEIN and PARFITT (1975). In this regard, neurons could represent a special case wherein the slow cyclic AMP-evoked hyperpolarizations are utilized both for tonic modulations of electrical excitability and for optimization of conditions necessary for long-term changes in proteins and enzymes. The hyperpolarizations in some muscle cells may bring about conditions favorable for sequestion of calcium (TADA et al. 1974; ANDERSSON and MOHME-LUNDHOLM 1970). In the final analysis, each excitable cell type may be unique in its ultimate use of the cyclic nucleotides.

Acknowledgements. I thank my colleagues, Drs. FLOYD BLOOM, BARRY HOFFER, DONNA GRUOL, JAMES NATHANSON, QUENTIN PITTMAN and JESSE SCHULMAN for helpful discussions and reading of the manuscript. Particular thanks go to NANCY CALLAHAN for typing the manuscript and preparing the bibliography.

References

Akasu T, Koketsu K (1977) Effects of dibutyryl cyclic adenosine 3′,5′-monophosphate and theophylline on the bullfrog sympathetic ganglion. Br J Pharmacol 60:331–336

Alkon DL (1979) Voltage-dependent calcium and potassium ion conductances: a contingency mechanism for an associative learning model. Science 205:810–816

Arlock P, Kanje M (1977) Effects of db-cAMP on the transmembrane potentials of cultured human glioma cells. Exp Cell Res 109:105–109

Anderson EG, Haas H, Hösli L (1973) Comparison of effects of noradrenaline and histamine with cyclic AMP on brain stem neurones. Brain Res 49:471–475

Andersson R, Mohme-Lundholm E (1969) Metabolic actions in intestinal smooth muscle associated with relaxation by adrenergic α and β-receptors. Acta Physiol Scand 79:244–261

Barker JL, Gruol DL, Huang LyM, MacDonald JF, Smith TG Jr (1980) Peptide receptor functions on cultured spinal neurons. In: Costa E, Trabucchi M (eds) Neural peptides and neural communication. Raven, New York, pp 409–423

Beam KG, Nestler EJ, Greengard P (1977) Increased cyclic GMP levels associated with concentration in muscle fibers of the giant barnacle. Nature 267:534–536

Benfy BG (1971) Lack of relationship between myocardial cyclic AMP concentration and inotropic effects of sympathomimetic amines. Br J Pharmacol 43:757–763

Berridge MJ, Prince WT (1971) The electrical response of isolated salivary glands during stimulation with 5-hydroxytryptamine and cyclic AMP. Philos Trans R Soc Lond [Biol] 262:111–120

Berridge MJ, Prince WT (1972) Transepithelial potential changes during stimulation of isolated salivary glands with 5-hydroxytryptamine and cyclic AMP. J Exp Biol 56:139–153

Bertelli A, Bianchi C, Beani L (1972) Effects of AMP and cyclic AMP on the mechanical and electrical activity of isolated mammalian atria. Eur J Pharmacol 19:130–133

Bitenski MW, Gorman RE, Miller WH (1971) Adenyl cyclase as a link between photon capture and changes in membrane permeability of frog photoreceptors. Proc Natl Acad Sci USA 68:561–562

Bitensky MW, Miki N, Marcus FR, Keirns JU (1973) The role of cyclic nucleotides in visual excitation. Life Sci 13:1451–1472

Bittar EE, Walkowiak H (1975) Stimulation by 5′-methylene cyclic phosphonate analogue of cAMP of sodium efflux in barnacle muscle fibres. Gen Pharmacol 6:271–274

Bloom FE (1974) To spritz or not to spritz: the doubtful value of aimless iontophoresis. Life Sci 14:1819–1834

Bloom FE (1975) The role of cyclic nucleotides in central synaptic function. Rev Physiol Biochem Pharmacol 74:1–103

Bloom FE, Siggins GR, Hoffer BJ (1974) Interpreting the failures to confirm the depression of cerebellar Purkinje cells by cyclic AMP. Science 185:627–629

Bloom FE, Siggins GR, Hoffer BJ, Segal M, Oliver AP (1975) The role of cyclic nucleotides in the central synaptic actions of catecholamines. Adv Cyclic Nucleotide Res 5:603–618

Bowman WC, Raper C (1965) The effects of sympathomimetic amines on chronically denervated skeletal muscles. Br J Pharmacol 24:98–109

Bray JJ, Hawken MJ, Hubbardt JI, Pockett S, Wilson L (1976) The membrane potential of rat diaphragm muscle fibres and the effect of denervation. J Physiol (Lond) 255:651–667

Breckenridge BM, Burn JH, Matschinsky FM (1967) Theophylline, epinephrine, and neostigmine facilitation of neuromuscular transmission. Proc Natl Acad Sci USA 57:1893–1897

Bressler BH, Phillis JW, Kozachuk W (1975) Noradrenaline stimulation of a membrane pump in frog skeletal muscle. Eur J Pharmacol 33:201–204

Brown DA, Adams PR (1980) Muscarinic suppression of a novel voltage-sensitive K^+ current in a vertebrate neurone. Nature 283:673–676

Brown DA, Caulfield MP, Kirby PJ (1979) Relation between catecholamine-induced cyclic AMP changes and hyperpolarization in isolated rat sympathetic ganglia. J Physiol (Lond) 290:441–451

Brunelli M, Vastellucci V, Kandel ER (1976) Synaptic facilitation and behavioral sensitization in Aplysia: possible role of serotonin and cyclic AMP. Science 194:1178–1181
Bulbring E, Tomita T (1969) Increase of membrane conductance by adrenaline in the smooth muscle of guinea-pig taenia coli. Proc R Soc Lond [Biol] 172:89–102
Bunney BS, Aghajanian GK (1973) Electrophysiological effects of amphetamine in dopaminergic neurons. In: Usdin E, Snyder S (eds) Frontiers in catecholamine research. Pergamon, Oxford, New York, pp 957–962
Busis NA, Weight FF, Smith PA (1978) Synaptic potentials in sympathetic ganglia: are they mediated by cyclic nucleotides? Science 200:1079–1081
Chader GJ, Herz LR, Fletcher T (1974) Light-activation of PDE activity in ROS. Biochim Biophys Acta 347:491–493
Chalazonitis A, Greene LA (1974) Enhancement in excitability properties of mouse neuroblastoma cells cultured in the presence of dibutyryl cyclic AMP. Brain Res 72:340–345
Chasin M, Rivkin I, Mamrak F, Samaniego G, Hess SM (1971) α- and β-adrenergic receptors as mediators of accumulation of cyclic adenosine 3′,5′-monophosphate in specific areas of guinea pig brain. J Biol Chem 246:3037–3041
Cheng SC, Chen SC (1975) Stimulation by cyclic nucleotides of calcium efflux in barnacle muscle fibers. Life Sci 16:1711–1716
Chiba S, Kuboto K, Hashimoto K (1972) Absence of chronotropic effects of dibutyryl cyclic adenosine 3′,5′-monophosphate on the dog S-A node. Tohoku J Exp Med 197:103–104
Clausen T, Flatman JA (1977) The effect of catecholamines on NA-K transport and membrane potential in rat soleus muscle. J Physiol (Lond) 270:383–414
Clement-Cormier YC, Kebabian JW, Petzold GI, Greengard P (1974) Dopamine-sensitive adenylate cyclase in mammalian brain: a possible site of action of antipsychotic drugs. Proc Natl Acad Sci USA 71:1113–1171
Coviello A, Raisman R, Elso G, Orce G (1978) Role of cyclic AMP and angiotensin III in the response of toad skin to angiotensin II. Biochem Pharmacol 27:611–612
Crain SM, Pollack ED (1973) Restorative effects of cyclic AMP on complex bioelectric activities of cultured fetal rodent CNS tissues after acute Ca^{++} deprivation. J Neurobiol 4:321–342
Cramer H, Johnson DG, Hanbauer I, Silberstein SD, Kopin IJ (1973) Accumulation of adenosine 3′,5′-monophosphate induced by catecholamines in the rat superior cervical ganglion in vitro. Brain Res 53:97–104
Curtis DR (1964) Microelectrophoresis. In: Nastuk WL (ed) Physical techniques in biological research, vol 5. Academic Press, New York London, pp 144–190
Daly J (1975) The role of cyclic nucleotides in the nervous system. In: Iversen LL, Iversen SD, Snyder SH (eds) Handbook of psychopharmacology, vol 5. Plenum, New York, pp 47–128
Daniel DE, Paton DM, Taylor GS, Hodgson BJ (1970) Adrenergic receptors for catecholamine effects on tissue electrolytes. Fed Proc 29:1410–1425
Danilo P, Vulliemoz Y, Verosky M, Rosen MR (1978) Epinephrine-induced automaticity of canine cardiac purkinje fibers and its relationship to the adenylate cyclase-adenosine 3′,5′-monophosphate system. J Pharmacol Exp Ther 205:175–182
Diamond J, Marshall JM (1969) Smooth muscle relaxants: dissociation between resting membrane potential and resting tension in rat myometrium. J Pharmacol Exp Ther 168:13–20
Dun NJ, Karczmar AG (1977) A comparison of the effect of theophylline and cyclic adenosine 3′:5′-monophosphate on the superior cervical ganglion of the rabbit by means of the sucrose-gap method. J Pharmacol Exp Ther 202:89–96
Dun JN, Kaibara K, Karczmar AG (1977) Dopamine and adenosine 3′,5′-monophosphate responses of single mammalian sympathetic neurons. Science 197:778–788
Dunlap K, Fischbach GD (1978) Neurotransmitters decrease the calcium component of sensory neurone action potentials. Nature 276:837–839
Eccles JC (1964) The physiology of synapses. Academic Press, New York London
Eccles JC, Ito M, Szentagothai J (1967) The cerebellum as a neuronal machine. Springer, Berlin Heidelberg New York
Eccles R, Libet B (1961) Origin and blockade of the synaptic responses of curarized sympathetic ganglia. J Physiol (Lond) 157–484

Engberg I, Marshall KC (1971) Mechanism of noradrenaline hyperpolarization in spinal cord motor neurons of the cat. Acta Physiol Scand 83:142–144
Evans RH, Smith JW (1973) Mode of action of catecholamines on skeletal muscle. J Physiol (Lond) 232:81–82P
Farber DB, Lolley RN (1979) Phosphoproteins as proposed modulators of visual function. In: Ehrlich YH, Volvaka J, Davis LG, Brunngraber EG (eds) Modulators, mediators, and specifiers in brain function. Plenum, New York, pp 103–115
Ferrendelli JA, Steiner AL, McDougal DB, Kipnis DM (1970) The effect of oxotremorine and atropine on cGMP and cAMP levels in mouse cerebral cortex and cerebellum. Biochem Biophys Res Commun 41:1061–1067
Ferrendelli JA, Chang MM, Kinscherf DA (1974) Elevation of cyclic GMP levels in central nervous system by excitatory and inhibitory amino acids. J Neurochem 22:535–540
Friedman N, Somlyo AV, Somlyo AP (1971) Cyclic adenosine and guanosine monophosphate and glucagon: effect on liver membrane potentials. Science 171:400–402
Gähwiler BH (1976) Inhibitory action of noradrenaline and cyclic adenosine monophosphate in explants of rat cerebellum. Nature 259:483–484
Gainer H, Barker J (1975) Selective modulation and turnover of proteins in identified neurons of Aplysia. J Comp Biochem Physiol 51B:221–227
Gallagher JP, Shinnick-Gallagher P (1977) Cyclic nucleotides injected intracellularly into rat superior cervical ganglion cells. Science 198:851–852
George WJ, Polson JB, O'Toole AG, Goldberg ND (1970) Elevation of guanosine 3′,5′-cyclic phosphate in rat heart after perfusion with acetylcholine. Proc Natl Acad Sci USA 66:398–403
Gilman AG, Nurenberg M (1971) Effect of catecholamines on the adenosine 3′,5′-cyclic monophosphate concentrations of clonal satellite cells of neurons. Proc Natl Acad Sci USA 68:2165–2168
Girardier L, Seydoux J, Clausen T (1968) Membrane potential of brown adipose tissue. A suggested mechanism for the regulation of thermogenesis. J Gen Physiol 52:925–940
Godfraind JM, Pumain R (1971) Cyclic adenosine monophosphate and norepinephrine: effect on Purkinje cells in rat cerebellar cortex. Science 174–1257
Goldberg AL, Singer JJ (1969) Evidence for a role of cyclic AMP in neuromuscular transmission. Proc Natl Acad Sci USA 64:134–141
Goldberg ND, Dietz SB, O'Toole AG (1969) Cyclic guanosine 3′,5′-monophosphate in mammalian tissues and urine. J Biol Chem 244:4458–4466
Goldberg ND, O'Dea RF, Haddox MK (1973) Cyclic GMP. Adv Cyclic Nucleotide Res 3:155–223
Goridis C, Virmaux N (1974) Light regulated guanosine 3′,5′-monophosphate phosphodiesterase of bovine retina. Nature 248:57–58
Goridis C, Virmaux N, Urban PF, Mandel P (1973) Guanyl cyclase in a mammalian photoreceptor. FEBS Lett 30:163–166
Green RD, Dale MM, Haylett DG (1972) Effect of adrenergic amines on the membrane potential of guinea pig liver parenchymal cells in short term tissue culture. Experientia 28:1073–1074
Greengard P, Kebabian JW (1974) Role of cyclic AMP in synaptic transmission in the mammalian peripheral nervous system. Fed Proc 33:1059–1068
Grosset A, Micronneau J (1977) An analysis of the actions of prostaglandin E_1 on membrane currents and contraction in uterine smooth muscle. J Physiol (Lond) 270:765–784
Gruol DL, Siggins GR, Padjen AL, Forman DS (1981) Explant cultures of adult amphibian Sympathetic ganglia: electrophysiological and pharmacological investigation of neurotransmitter and nucleotide action. Brain Res 223:81–106
Hashiguchi T, Ushiyama NW, Kobayashi H, Libet B (1978) Does cyclic GMP mediate the slow excitatory synaptic potential in sympathetic ganglia? Nature 271:267–268
Hax WMA, Van Venroolj GEPM, Vossenberg JBJ (1974) Cell communication: a cyclic AMP mediated phenomenon. J Membr Biol 19:253–266
Haylett DG, Jenkinson DH (1969) Effects of noradrenaline on the membrane potential and ionic permeability of parenchymal cells in the liver of the guinea-pig. Nature 224:80–81
Hays ET, Dwyer TM, Horowitz P, Swift JF (1974) Epinephrine action on sodium fluxes in frog striated muscle. Am J Physiol 227:1340–1347

Hidaka T, Kuriyama H (1969) Effects of catecholamines on the cholinergic neuromuscular transmission in fish red muscle. J Physiol (Lond) 201:61–71
Hill-Smith I, Purves RD (1978) Synaptic delay in the heart: an iontophoretic study. J Physiol (Lond) 279:31–54
Hoffer B, Siggins GR (1975) Electrophysiological techniques for the study of hormone action in the central nervous system. Methods Enzymol 39:429–442
Hoffer BJ, Siggins GR, Oliver AP, Bloom FE (1971 a) Cyclic AMP mediation of norepinephrine inhibition in rat cerebellar cortex: A unique class of synaptic responses. Ann NY Acad Sci 185:531–549
Hoffer BJ, Siggins GR, Woodward DJ, Bloom FE (1971 b) Spontaneous discharge of Purkinje neurons after destruction of catecholamine-containing afferents by 6-hydroxydopamine. Brain Res 30:425–430
Hoffer BJ, Siggins GR, Oliver AP, Bloom FE (1973) Activation of the pathway from locus coeruleus to rat cerebellar Purkinje neurons: pharmacological evidence of noradrenergic central inhibition. J Pharmacol Exp Ther 184:553–569
Hoffer B, Seiger A, Freedman R, Olson L, Taylor D (1977) Electrophysiology and cytology of hippocampal formation transplants in the anterior chamber of the eye. II. cholinergic mechanism. Brain Res 119:107–132
Horn JP, McAfee DA (1977) Modulation of cyclic nucleotide levels in peripheral nerve without effect on resting or compound action potentials. J Physiol (Lond) 269:753–766
Horn JP, McAfee DA (1979) Norepinephrine inhibits calcium-dependent potentials in rat sympathetic neurons. Science 204:1233–1235
Horowitz BA, Eaton M (1975) The effect of adrenergic agonists and cyclic AMP on the Na^+/Ka^+-ATPase activity of brown adipose tissue. Eur J Pharmacol 34:241–245
Horowitz BA, Horowitz JM, Smith RE (1969) Norepinephrine-induced depolarization of brown fat cells. Proc Natl Acad Sci 64:113
Horowitz JM, Horowitz BA, Smith RE (1971) Effect in vivo of norepinephrine on the membrane resistance of brown fat cells. Experientia 27:1419
Hsu SY, McIsaac RJ (1978) Effects of theophylline and N^6,O^2-dibutyryl adenosine 3′:5′-monophosphate on sympathetic ganglionic transmission in rats. J Pharmacol Exp Ther 205:91–103
Hynie S, Sharp GWG (1971) Adenyl cyclase in the toad bladder. Biochim Biophys Acta 230:40–43
Ito Y, Kuriyama H, Tashiro N (1971) Effects of catecholamines on the neuromuscular junction of the somatic muscle of the earthworm pheretima communissima. J Exp Biol 54:167–186
Jacobson HR (1979) Altered permeability in the proximal tubule response to cyclic AMP. Am J Physiol 236:F81–F79
James TN (1965) The chronotropic action of ATP and related compounds studied by direct perfusion of the sinus node. J Pharmacol Exp Ther 149:233–247
Jenkinson DH, Stamenovic BA, Whitaker BDL (1968) The effect of noradrenaline on the end-plate potential in twitch fibres of the frog. J Physiol (Lond) 195:743–754
Johansson B, Jonsson O, Axelsson J, Wahlstrom B (1967) Electrical and mechanical characteristics of vascular smooth muscle response to norepinephrine and isoproterenol. Circ Res 21:19–633
Jordan LM, Lake N, Phillis JW (1972) Mechanism of noradrenaline depression of cortical neurones: a species comparison. Eur J Pharmacol 20:381–384
Kaczmarek LK, Jennings K, Strumwasser F (1978) Neurotransmitter modulation, phosphodiesterase inhibitor effects, and cyclic AMP correlates of afterdischarge in peptidergic neurites. Proc Natl Acad Sci USA 75:5200–5204
Kakiuchi KS, Marks BH (1972) Adrenergic effects on pineal cell membrane potential. Life Sci 11:285–291
Kakiuchi S, Rall TW (1968) Studies on adenosine 3′,5′-phosphate in rabbit cerebral cortex. Mol Pharmacol 4:379–388
Katz B (1966) Nerve, muscle and synapse. McGraw-Hill, New York
Kebabian JW, Greengard P (1971) Dopamine-sensitive adenyl cyclase: possible role in synaptic transmission. Science 174:1346–1349

Kebabian JW, Petzold GL, Greengard P (1972) Dopamine-sensitive adenylate cyclase in caudate nucleus of rat brain and its similarities to the dopamine receptor. Proc Natl Acad Sci USA 69:2145–2150
Kebabian JW, Bloom FE, Steiner AL, Greengard B (1975) Neurotransmitter induced increases in cyclic nucleotides of postganglionic neurons in mammalian sympathetic ganglia: immunocytochemical demonstration. Science 190:157–160
Klainer LM, Chi Y-M, Friedberg SL, Rall TW, Sutherland E (1962) Adenyl cyclase. IV. The effects of neurohormones on the formation of adenosine 3′–5′ phosphate by preparations from brain and other tissues. J Biol Chem 237:1239–1243
Klein DC, Parfitt A (1975) Ouabain blocks the adrenergic-cyclic AMP stimulation of pineal N-acetyltransferase activity. In: Weiss B (ed) Cyclic nucleotides in disease. University Park Press, Baltimore, pp 257–265
Klein DC, Berg GR, Weller J (1970) Melatonin synthesis. Adenosine 3′,5′-monophosphate and norepinephrine stimulate N-acetyltransferase. Science 168:979–980
Klein M, Kandel ER (1978) Presynaptic modulation of voltage-dependent Ca^{+2} current: mechanism for behavioral sensitization in Aplysia californica. Proc Natl Acad Sci USA 75:3512–3516
Kobayashi H, Libet B (1968) Generation of slow postsynaptic potentials without increases in ionic conductance. Proc Natl Acad Sci 60:1304–1311
Kobayashi H, Hashiguchi T, Ushiyama NS (1978) Postsynaptic modulation of excitatory process in sympathetic ganglia by cyclic AMP. Nature 271:268–270
Kostopoulos GK, Limacher JJ, Phillis JW (1975) Action of various adenine derivatives on cerebellar Purkinje cells. Brain Res 88:162–165
Krishna G, Moskowitz J, Dempsey P, Brodie BB (1970) The effect of norepinephrine and insulin on brown fat cell membrane potentials. Life Sci 9:1353–1361
Krnjevíc K, Van Meter WG (1976) Cyclic nucleotides in spinal cells. Can J Physiol Pharmacol 54:416–420
Krnjevíc K, Puil E, Werman R (1976) Is cyclic guanosine monophosphate the internal "second messenger" for cholinergic actions on central neurons? Can J Physiol Pharmacol 54:172–176
Kroeger EA, Marshall JM (1973) Beta-adrenergic effects on rat myometrium: mechanism of membrane hyperpolarization. Am J Physiol 225:1339–1345
Krause EG, Halle W, Kallabis E, Wollenberger A (1970) Positive chronotropic response of cultured rat heart cells to N^6-2-O-dibutyryl-3′-5′-adenosine monophosphate. J Mol Cell Cardiol 1:1–10
Kuba K (1970) Effects of catecholamines on the neuromuscular junction in the rat diaphragm. J Physiol (Lond) 211:551–570
Kuba K, Tomita T (1971) Noradrenaline action on nerve terminal in the rat diaphragm. J Physiol (Lond) 217:19–31
Kukovetz WR, Pöch G (1970) Cardiostimulatory effects of cyclic 3′,5′-adenosine monophosphate and its acylated derivatives. Naunyn Schmiedebergs Arch Pharmacol 266:236–254
Kuo JF, Greengard P (1969) Cyclic nucleotide-dependent protein kinases. IV. Widespread occurrence of adenosine 3′,5′monophosphate dependent protein kinase in various tissues and phyla of the animal kingdom. Proc Natl Acad Sci USA 64:1359–1355
Kupfermann I, Cohen JL, Mandelbaum DE, Schonberg M, Susswein AJ, Weiss KR (1979) Functional role of serotonergic neuromodulation in Aplysia. Fed Prod 38:2095–2102
Kuroda Y, Kobayashi K (1975) Effects of adenosine and adenine nucleotides on the postsynaptic potential and on the formation of cyclic adenosine 3′,5′-monophosphate from radioactive adenosine triphosphate in guinea pig olfactory cortex slices. Proc Jpn Acad 51:495–500
Lake N, Jordan LM (1974) Failure to confirm cyclic AMP as second messenger for norepinephrine in rat cerebellum. Science 183:663–664
Lake N, Jordan LM, Phillis JW (1972) Mechanism of noradrenaline actions in cat cerebral cortex. Nature 240:249–250
Lake N, Jordan LM, Phillis JW (1973) Evidence against cyclic adenosine 3′,5′-monophosphate (AMP) mediation of noradrenaline depression of cerebral cortical neurones. Brain Res 60:411–421

Levitan IB, Norman J (1980) Different effects of cAMP and cGMP derivatives on the activity of an identified neuron: biochemical and electrophysiological analysis. Brain Res 187:415–429
Lewis PR, Schute CD (1967) The cholinergic limbic system: projection to hippocampal formation, medial cortex, nuclei of the ascending cholinergic reticular system and the subfornical organ and supra-optic crest. Brain 90:521–540
Libet B (1981) Long-lasting modulation of slow-excitatory-postsynaptic potential (s-EPSP), by catecholamines. Adv Physiol Sci 4:305–309
Libet B, Kobayashi H, Tanaka T (1975) Synaptic coupling into the production and storage of a neuronal memory trace. Nature 258:155–157
Lindl T (1978) Cyclic AMP and its relation to ganglionic transmission. A combined biochemical and electrophysiological study of the rat superior cervical ganglion in vitro. Neuropharmacology 18:227–235
Ling G, Gerard RW (1949) Normal membrane potential of frog sartorius fibers. J Cell Comp Physiol 34:383–394
Llinas R, Sugimori M (1979) Calcium conductances in purkinje cell dendrites: their role in development and integration. Prog Brain Res 51:323–334
Magaribuchi M, Kuriyama H (1972) Effects of noradrenaline and isoprenaline on the electrical and mechanical activities of guinea pig depolarized taenia coli. Jpn J Physiol 22:253–270
Mao CC, Guidotti A, Costa E (1974a) Inhibition by diazepam of the tremor and the increase of cerebellar cGMP content elicited by harmaline. Brain Res 83:526–529
Mao CC, Guidotti A, Costa E (1974b) The regulation of cyclic guanosine monophosphate in rat cerebellum: possible involvement of putative amino acid neurotransmitters. Brain Res 79:510–514
Marshall KC, Engberg I (1979) Reversal potential for noradrenaline-induced hyperpolarization of spinal motoneurons. Science 205:422–424
Marshall JM (1977) Modulation of smooth muscle activity by catecholamines. Fed Proc 36:2450–2455
McAfee DA, Greengard P (1972) Adenosine 3′,5′-monophosphate: electrophysiological evidence for a role in synaptic transmission. Science 178:310–312
McAfee DA, Schorderet M, Greengard P (1971) Adenosine 3′,5′-monophosphate in nervous tissue: increase associated with synaptic transmission. Science 171:1156–1158
McCaman RE, McKenna DG, Ono JK (1977) A pressure system for intracellular and extracellular ejections of picoliter volumes. Brain Res 136:141–147
Meyer RB, Miller JP (1974) Analogs of cyclic AMP and cyclic GMP: general methods of synthesis and the relationship of structure to enzymic activity. Life Sci 14:1019–1040
Miki N, Keirns JJ, Markus FR, Freeman J, Bitensky MW (1973) Regulation of cyclic nucleotide concentrations in photoreceptors: an ATP-dependent stimulation of cyclic nucleotide phosphodiesterase by light. Proc Natl. Acad Sci USA 70:3820–3824
Miller WH (1973) Cyclic nucleotides and photoreception. Exp Eye Res 16:357–363
Miller WH, Gorman RE, Bitensky MW (1971) Cyclic adenosine monophosphate: function in photoreceptors: Science 174:295–297
Miller RJ, Horn AS, Iversen LL (1974) The action of neuroleptic drugs on dopamine-stimulated adenosine cyclic 3′,5′-monophosphate production in rat neostriatum and limbic forebrain. Mol Pharmacol 10:759–766
Mudge AW, Leeman SE, Fischbach GD (1979) Enkephalin inhibits release of substance P from sensory neurons in culture and decreases action potential duration. Proc Natl Acad Sci USA 76:526–530
Nathanson J (1977) Cyclic nucleotides in nervous system function. Physiol Rev 57:157–256
Nestler EJ, Beam KG, Greengard P (1978) Nicotinic cholinergic stimulation increases cyclic GMP levels in vertebrate skeletal muscle. Natur 275:451–453
Nishi S, Koketsu K (1967) Origin of ganglionic inhibitory postsynaptic potentials. Life Sci 6:2049–2055
Obata K 81974) Transmitter sensitivities of some nerve and muscle cells in culture. Brain Res 73:71–88
Obata K, Yoshida M (1973) Caudate-evoked inhibition and actions of GABA and other substances on cat pallidal neurons. Brain Res 64:455–459

Okada Y, Kuroda Y (1975) Inhibitory action of adenosine and adenine nucleotides on the postsynaptic potential of olfactory cortex slices of the guinea pig. Proc Jpn Acad 51:491–494
Okada Y, Saito M (1979) Inhibitory action of adenosine, 5-HT (serotonin) and GABA (γ-aminobutyric acid) on the postsynaptic potential (PSP) of slices from olfactory cortex and superior colliculus in correlation to the level of cyclic AMP. Brain Res 160:368–371
Oliver AP, Segal M (1974) Transmembrane changes in hippocampal neurons: hyperpolarizing actions of norepinephrine, cyclic AMP, and locus coeruleus (Abstr) Soc Neurosci 4th Annual Meeting, p 361
Omachi RS, Robbie DE, Handler JS, Orloff J (1974) Effects of ADH and other agents on cyclic AMP accumulation in toad bladder epithelium. Am J Physiol 226:1152–1157
Parfitt A, Weller JL, Klein DC, Sakai KK, Marks BH (1975) Blockade by ouabain or elevated potassium ion concentration of the adrenergic and adenosine cyclic 3′,5′-monophosphate-induced stimulation of pineal serotonin N-acetyltransferase activity. Mol Pharmacol 11:241–245
Pellmar TC, Carpenter DO (1979) Voltage-dependent calcium current induced by serotonin. Nature 277:483–484
Petersen OH (1975) Increase in membrane conductance by adrenaline in parotid acinar cells. Experientia 32:471–472
Phillis JW, Kirkpatrick JR (1978) The actions of adenosine and various nucleosides and nucleotides on the isolated toad spinal cord. Gen Pharmacol 9:239–247
Phillis JW, Kostopoulos GK (1975) Adenosine as a putative transmitter in the cerebral cortex. Studies with potentiators and antagonists. Life Sci 17:1085–1094
Phillis JW, Kostopoulos GK, Limacher JJ (1974) Depression of corticospinal cells by various purines and pyrimidines. Can J Physiol Pharmacol 52:1227–1229
Phillis JW, Kostopoulos GK, Limacher JJ (1975) A potent depressant action of adenine derivatives on cerebral cortical neurons. Eur J Pharmacol 30:125–129
Porter KR (1976) Motility in cells. Cold Spring Harbor Conf Cell Proliferation 3:1–28
Purpura DP, Shofer RJ (1972) Excitatory action of dibutyryl cyclic adenosine monophosphate on immature cerebral cortex. Brain Res 38:179–181
Rapp PE, Berridge MJ (1977) Oscillations in calcium-cycle AMP control loops form the basis of pacemaker activity and other high frequency biological rhythms. J Theor Biol 66:497–525
Reuter H (1974) Localization of beta adrenergic receptors, and effects of noradrenaline and cyclic nucleotides on action potentials, ionic currents and tension in mammalian cardiac muscle. J Physiol (Lond) 242:429–452
Robison GA, Butcher RW, Sutherland EW (1971) Cyclic AMP. Academic Press, New York London
Rodan GA, Bourret LA, Norton LA (1978) DNA synthesis in cartilage cells is stimulated by oscillating electric fields. Science 199:690–692
Sakai K, Marks B (1972) Adrenergic effects on pineal cell membrane potential. Life Sci 11:285–291
Sakai M, Swartz BE, Woody CD (1979) Controlled micro-release of pharmacological agents: measurements of volumes ejected in vitro through fine-tipped glass microelectrodes by pressure. Neuropharmacology 18:209–213
Salmoiraghi GC, Weight F (1967) Micromethods in neuropharmacology: an approach to the study of anesthetics. Anesthesiology 28:54–64
Scholfield CN (1978) Depression of evoked potentials in brain slices by adenosine compounds. Br J Pharmacol 63:239–244
Schorderet M, Grosso A, de Sousa RC (1975) Intracellular cAMP: hormone-induced changes in frog skin epithelium. Experientia 31:732
Segal M (1980) The noradrenergic innervation of the hippocampus. In: Hobson JA, Brazier MAB (eds) The reticular formation revisited. Raven, New York, pp 415–425
Segal M, Bloom FE (1974a) The action of norepinephrine in the rat hippocampus. I. Iontophoretic studies. Brain Res 72:79–97
Segal M, Bloom FE (1974b) The action of norepinephrine in the rat hippocampus. II. Activation of the input pathway. Brain Res 72:99–114

Shimahara T, Tauc L (1977) Cyclic AMP induced by serotonin modulates the activity of an identified synapse in Aplysia by facilitating the permeability to calcium. Brain Res 127:168–172

Shoemaker WJ, Balentine LT, Siggins GR, Hoffer BJ, Henriksen SJ, Bloom FE (1975) Characteristics of the release of cyclic adenosine 3′,5′-monophosphate from micropipets by microiontophoresis. J Cyclic Nucleotide Res 1:97–106

Shute CCD, Lewis PR (1974) The ascending cholinergic reticular system: neocortical, olfactory, and subcortical projections. Brain 90:497–520

Siggins GR (1978 a) Electrophysiological assessment of mononucleotides and nucleosides as first and second messengers in the nervous system. In: Karlin A, Tennyson VM, Vogel HJ (eds) Neuronal information transfer. Academic Press, New York, p 339

Siggins GR (1978 b) The electrophysiological role of dopamine in striatum. Excitatory or inhibitory? In: Lipton MA, DiMascio A, Killam KF (eds) Proc Am Coll Neuropsychopharmacol. Raven, New York, pp 143–157

Siggins GR, Henriksen SJ (1975) Inhibition of rat Purkinje neurons by analogues of cyclic adenosine monophosphate: correlation with protein kinase activation. Science 189:559–561

Siggins GR, Hoffer BJ , Bloom FE (1969) Cyclic 3′,5′-adenosine monophosphate: possible mediator for the response of cerebellar Purkinje cells to microelectrophoresis of norepinephrine. Science 165:1018–1020

Siggins GR, Hoffer BJ, Bloom FE (1971 a) Studies on norepinephrine-containing afferents to Purkinje cells of rat cerebellum. III. Evidence for mediation of norepinephrine effects by cyclic 3′,5′-adenosine monophosphate. Brain Res 25:535–553

Siggins GR, Hoffer BJ, Oliver AP, Bloom FE (1971 b) Activation of a central noradrenergic projection to cerebellum. Nature 233:481–483

Siggins GR, Hoffer BJ, Bloom FE (1971 c) Cyclic adenosine monophosphate and norepinephrine: effect on purkinje cells in rat cerebellar cortex. Science 174:1258–1259

Siggins GR, Oliver AP, Hoffer BJ, Bloom FE (1971 d) Cyclic adenosine monophosphate and norepinephrine: effects on transmembrane properties of cerebellar Purkinje cells. Sience 171:192–194

Siggins GR, Hoffer BJ, Ungerstedt U (1974) Electrophysiological evidence for involvement of cyclic adenosine monophosphate in dopamine responses of caudate neurons. Life Sci 15:779–792

Siggins GR, Hoffer B, Bloom F, Ungerstedt U (1976 a) Cytochemical and electrophysiological studies of dopamine in the caudate nucleus. In: Yahr M (ed) The basal ganglia. Raven, New York, pp 227–248

Siggins GR, Henriksen SJ, Landis SC (1976 b) Electrophysiology of Purkinje neurons in the weaver mouse: iontophoresis of neurotransmitters and cyclic nucleotides, and stimulation of the nucleus locus coeruleus. Brain Res 114:53–65

Siggins GR, Schubert P (1981) Adenosine depression of hippocampal neurons in vitro: an intracellular study of dose-dependent actions on synaptic and membrane potentials. Neurosci Lett 23:55–60

Skelton CL, Levey GS, Epstein SE (1970) Positive inotropic effects of dibutyryl cyclic adenosine 3′,5′-monophosphate. Circ Res. 26:35–43

Skirboll LR, Baizer L, Dretchen KL (1977) Evidence for a cyclic nucleotide-mediated calcium flux in motor nerve terminals. Nature 268:352–354

Smith JW, Thesleff S (1976) Spontaneous activity in denervated mouse diaphragm muscle. J Physiol (Lond) 257:171–186

Smith PA, Weight FF, Lehne RA (1979) Potentiation of Ca^{++}-dependent K^+ activation by theophylline is independent of cyclic nucleotide elevation. Nature 280:400–402

Somlyo AP, Somlyo AV (1969) Pharmacology of excitation-contraction coupling in vascular smooth muscle and in avian slow muscle. Fed Proc 28:1634–1642

Somlyo AV, Haeusler G, Somlyo AP (1970) Cyclic adenosine monophosphate: potassium-dependent action on vascular smooth muscle membrane potential. Science 169:490–491

S-Rozsa K, Kiss T (1976) Role of cyclic nucleotides in the effect of transmitters on the heart of helix pomatia L. Comp Biochem Physiol 53C:13–16

Stämpfli R (1954) A new method for measuring membrane potentials with external electrodes. Experientia 10:508–509

Stone TW, Taylor DA (1977) Microiontophoretic study of the effects of cyclic nucleotides on excitability of neurones in the rat cerebral cortex. J Physiol (Lond) 266:523–543
Stone TW, Taylor DA, Bloom FE (1915) Cyclic AMP and cyclic GMP may mediate opposite neuronal responses in the rat cerebral cortex. Science 187:845–847
Study RE, Breakefield XO, Bartfa T, Greengard P (1978) Voltage-sensitive calcium channels regulate guanosine 3′,5′-cyclic monophosphate levels in neuroblastoma cells. Proc Natl Acad Sci USA 75:6295–6299
Sturgill TW, Schrier BK, Gilman AG (1975) Stimulation of cyclic AMP accumulation by 2-chloroadenosine: lack of incorporation of nucleoside into cyclic nucleotides. J Cyclic Nucleotide Res 1:21–30
Sutherland EW, Rall TW, Menon T (1962) Adenyl cyclase. I. Distribution, preparation and properties. J Biol Chem 237:1220–1227
Swartz BE, Woody CD (1979) Correlated effects of acetylcholine and cyclic guanosine monophosphate on membrane properties of mammalian neocortical neurons. J Neurobiol 10:465–488
Suzuki T, Kusano K (1978) Hyperpolarizing potentials induced by Ca^{++}-mediated K^+ conductance increase in hamster submandibular ganglion cells. J Neurobiol 9:367–392
Tada M, Kirchberger MA, Repke DI, Katz AM (1974) The stimulation of calcium transport in cardiac sarcoplasmic reticulum by adenosine 3′,5′-monophosphate dependent protein kinase. J Biol Chem 249:6174–6180
Takagi K, Takayanagi I, Tomiyama A (1971) Action of dibutyryl cyclic adenosine monophosphate on the intestinal smooth muscle. Jpn J Pharmacol 21:271–273
Takamori M, Ishii N, Mori M (1973) The role of cyclic 3′,5′-adenosine monophosphate in neuromuscular transmission. Arch Neurol 29:420–424
Takeuchi H, Yokoi I, Mori A, Kohsaka M (1975) Effects of nucleic acid components and their relatives on the excitability of dopamine sensitive giant neurones, identified in subesophageal ganglia of the african giant snail (Achatina Fulica Ferussac). Gen Pharmacol 6:77–85
Tashiro N (1973) Effects of isoprenaline on contractions of directly stimulated fast and slow skeletal muscles of the guinea pig. Br J Pharmacol 48:113–122
Taylor DA, Stone TW (1977) Neuronal responses to extracellularly applied cyclic AMP: role of the adenosine receptor. Experientia 34:481–482
Taylor DA, Stone TW (1980) The action of adenosine on noradrenergic neuronal inhibition induced by stimulation of locus coeruleus. Brain Res 183:367–376
Thomas RC (1972) Electrogenic sodium pump in nerve and muscle cells. Physiol Rev 52:563–594
Treistman SN, Drake PF (1979) The effects of cyclic nucleotide agents on neurons in Aplysia. Brain Res 168:643–647
Treistman SN, Levitan IB (1976a) Alteration of electrical activity in molluscan neurones by cyclic nucleotides and peptide factors. Nature 261:62–64
Treistman SN, Levitan IB (1976b) Intraneuronal guanylylimidodiphosphate injection mimics long-term synaptic hyperpolarization in Aplysia. Proc Natl Acad Sci 73:4689–4692
Triner L, Overweg NIA, Nahas GG (1970) Cyclic 3′,5′-AMP and uterine contractility. Nature 225:282–283
Tsien RW (1973) Adrenaline-like effects of intracellular iontophoresis of cyclic AMP in cardiac Purkinje fibres. Nature 245:120–122
Tsien RW, Giles W, Greengard P (1972) Cyclic AMP mediates the effects of adrenaline on cardiac Purkinje fibers. Nature 240:181–183
Vande Berg JS (1974) Inhibitory effects of dibutyryl and cyclic AMP on the compound action potential in the frog (rana pipiens) sciatic nerve. Experientia 30:1025–1027
Von Loh D (1971) The effect of adrenergic drugs on spontaneously active vascular smooth muscle studied by long-term intracellular recording of membrane potential. Angiologia 8:144–155
Walker JB, Walker JP (1973) Neurohumoral regulation of adenylate cyclase activity in rat striatum. Brain Res 54:386–390
Webb RC, Bhalla RC (1976) Calcium sequestration by subcellular fractions isolated from vascular smooth muscles: effects of cyclic nucleotides and prostaglandins. J Mol Cell Cardiol 8:145–157

Weight FF, Padjen A (1973a) Acetylcholine and slow synaptic inhibition in frog sympathetic ganglion cells. Brain Res 55:225–228
Weight FF, Padjen A (1973b) Slow synaptic inhibition: evidence for synaptic inactivation of sodium conductance in sympathetic ganglion cells. Brain Res 55:219–224
Weight FF, Votava J (1970) Slow synaptic excitation in sympathetic ganglion cells: evidence for synaptic activation of potassium conductance. Science 170:755–758
Weight FF, Petzold G, Greengard P (1974) Guanosine 3′,5′-monophosphate in sympathetic ganglia: increase associated with synaptic transmission. Science 186:942–944
Weight FF, Smith PA, Schulman JA (1978) Postsynaptic potential generation appears independent of synaptic elevation of cyclic nucleotides in sympathetic neurons. Brain Res 158:197–202
Weiss B, Costa E (1968) Regional and subcellular distribution of adenyl cyclase and 3′,5′-cyclic nucleotide phosphodiesterase in brain and pineal gland. Biochem Pharmacol 17:2107–2116
Wiesmann WP, Sinha S, Klahr S (1977) Effects of insulin, ADH, and cyclic AMP on sodium transport in the toad bladder. Am J Physiol 232(4):F307–F314
Wilkening D, Makman MH (1975) 2-chloroadenosine-dependent elevation of adenosine 3′,5′-cyclic monophosphate levels in rat caudate nucleus slices. Brain Res 92:522–528
Williams JA, Mathews EK (1974a) Effects of ions and metabolic inhibitors on membrane potential of brown adipose tissue. Am J Physiol 277:981–986
Williams JA, Mathews EK (1974b) Membrane depolarization, cyclic AMP, glycerol release by brown adipose tissue. Am J Physiol 227:987–992
Wilson DF (1974) The effects of dibutyryl cyclic adenosine 3′,5′-monophosphate, theophylline and aminophylline on neuromuscular transmission in the rat. J Pharmacol Exp Ther 188:447–452
Woodward DJ, Hoffer BJ, Altman J (1974) Physiological and pharmacological properties of Purkinje cells in rat cerebellum degranulated by postnatal X-irradiation. J Neurobiol 5:283–304
Wulff VJ (1971) The effect of cyclic AMP on limulus lateral eye retinular cells. Vision Res 11:1493–1495
Wulff VJ (1973) The effect of cyclic AMP and aminophylline on limulus lateral eye retinular cells. Vision Res 13:2335–2344
Yamasaki Y, Fujiwara M, Toda N (1974) Effects of catecholamines injected into sinoatrial nodal cells on their electrical activity. Jpn J Pharmacol 24:383–391

CHAPTER 23

Regulation of Cardiac Contractile Activity by Cyclic Nucleotides *

A. M. Katz

Overview

The electrical, mechanical, and metabolic properties of the heart are influenced by changing levels of Ca^{2+} and cyclic AMP within the myocardial cell. In general, Ca^{2+} serves as an effector, or signal, that initiates key functional responses in heart muscle when it is bound to various Ca^{2+}-binding proteins. Cyclic AMP, in contrast, serves primarily to regulate myocardial function.

Active and passive Ca^{2+} movements across the sarcolemmal and sarcoplasmic reticulum membranes of the myocardium appear to be controlled in part by cyclic AMP. Ca^{2+} entry into the myocardium via the slow channel, which is partly responsible for depolarization of the myocardial cell and may contribute to intracellular Ca^{2+} stores used to activate the contractile proteins, is enhanced by cyclic AMP. The mechanism responsible for this effect has not been elucidated, but may involve phosphorylation of the sarcolemma by a cyclic AMP-dependent protein kinase. Cyclic AMP, by stimulating a cyclic AMP-dependent protein kinase, appears also to increase active Ca^{2+} transport into the sarcoplasmic reticulum and Ca^{2+} efflux from this intracellular membrane structure. Both of these effects are related to phosphorylation of phospholamban, a 22,000 dalton protein in the membranes of the sarcoplasmic reticulum that is distinct from the 100,000 dalton ATPase protein. The phosphorylation of phospholamban influences several properties of the Ca^{2+} pump ATPase, including an increase in the Ca^{2+}-sensitivity of the Ca^{2+} pump, an apparent change in the cooperatively between the two Ca^{2+}-binding sites of the Ca^{2+} pump ATPase, and an increased turnover rate of this protein. Some of these effects may also be involved in the promotion of Ca^{2+} efflux from the sarcoplasmic reticulum during excitation.

Troponin I, one component of the regulatory protein complex of the thin filament of cardiac muscle, can be phosphorylated by cyclic AMP-dependent protein kinase. Although the functional consequences of this phosphorylation reaction remain in dispute, recent data indicate that troponin I phosphorylation reduces the Ca^{2+}-sensitivity of the cardiac contractile proteins. The resulting increase in the Ca^{2+} requirement for contractile protein activation would have a relaxing effect in the intact myocardium.

The significance of the apparent opposite shifts in Ca^{2+}-sensitivities of the Ca^{2+} pump of the cardiac sarcoplasmic reticulum and of the cardiac con-

* Supported by Research Grants HL-21812 and HL-22135 from the U.S. Public Health Service, and a Grant-in-Aid from the American Heart Association

tractile proteins may be related to the inherent slowness of the Ca^{2+} fluxes during muscle relaxation, compared to the more rapid intrinsic rates of the Ca^{2+} fluxes that initiate contraction. While the latter are the result of "downhill" Ca^{2+} fluxes that are limited only by the rate of diffusion, relaxation is effected by an ATP-dependent calcium pump. The increased Ca^{2+}-sensitivity of the cardiac sarcoplasmic reticulum coupled with a decreased Ca^{2+}-sensitivity of the contractile proteins, by accelerating relaxation of cardiac muscle, would facilitate filling of the heart when it comes under the influence to catecholamines, which markedly increase heart rate.

A "negative feedback" may exist between intracellular Ca^{2+} levels and those of cyclic AMP such that cyclic AMP accumulation is inhibited by high levels of Ca^{2+} within the myocardial cells. Several studies indicate that high levels of intracellular Ca^{2+} activate phosphodiesterase and inhibit cardiac sarcolemmal adenylate cyclase. Thus, under conditions where intramyocardial Ca^{2+} reaches high levels, the ability of the myocardium to accumulate cyclic AMP would be reduced.

A. Introduction

The performance of the heart is regulated by variations in the cellular processes that control the contractile performance of the individual myocardial cells. This means of contractile regulation differs from that in most skeletal muscles, the cells of which respond in an essentially stereotypical manner to nerve stimulation. Thus, the contractile performance of a skeletal muscle is controlled by variations in the number of muscle cells that are electrically stimulated. These variations in the number of active motor units are integrated by, and conveyed to the skeletal muscle from the central nervous system. By virtue of the cellular basis for the physiological control of muscle function in the heart, this tissue provides an excellent model in which to examine the interplay between Ca^{2+} and cyclic AMP in regulating physiological behavior (KATZ 1977).

Cardiac muscle exhibits a complex array of electrical, mechanical and metabolic properties, many of which respond directly or indirectly to messages transmitted within the cell by changing levels of Ca^{2+} and cyclic AMP. The present review examines several aspects of these responses of the heart. Emphasis is directed to a number of known points of interaction between these two important intracellular messengers as they affect the energy-consuming reactions associated with the electrical and mechanical behavior of the myocardium.

It appears reasonable to assign somewhat different general functions to Ca^{2+} and cyclic AMP within the myocardial cell. Calcium ion acts mainly as an effector, or signal, that directly initiates specific aspects of myocardial cell function, whereas cyclic AMP serves primarily a regulatory role in the heart. For example, the intensity of the mechanical response of the heart appears to be directly proportional to the amount of Ca^{2+} made available for binding to troponin C, the Ca^{2+}-receptor protein of thecontractile apparatus. While Ca^{2+} plays a role in regulating the fluxes of ions into and out of the heart, this cation itself contributes directly to changes in membrane potential by serving as a carrier for electric charge. Inward Ca^{2+}

movements, by carrying current into most cells of the mammalian heart, make a major contribution to the characteristic contour of the cardiac action potential (TSIEN 1977). In the case of cyclic AMP, important regulatory effects are exerted on the energy-producing reactions of intermediary metabolism (LARNER and VILLAR-PALASI 1971; FISHER et al. 1971; NEELY and MORGAN 1974; NIMMO and COHEN 1977). In addition, cyclic AMP influences a number of ion fluxes across the sarcolemma. These regulated processes, which are mediated by specific ion channels, include those responsible for trans-sarcolemmal Ca^{2+} fluxes (TADA et al. 1978). Cyclic AMP also regulates the Ca^{2+} fluxes within the myocardium that are responsible for the initiation and termination of cardiac contraction, and may modify the interaction between Ca^{2+} and the troponin complex. These latter effects of cyclic AMP constitute the major subject of this review.

Like any generalization, the assignment of an "effector function" to Ca^{2+} and a "regulatory function" to cyclic AMP is of limited validity. Especially in the case of Ca^{2+}, which can regulate a number of intracellular reactions–probably including the formation and breakdown of cyclic AMP, this generalization is unwarranted. Yet from a didatic point of view, this distinction is probably useful in facilitating an understanding of the way in which Ca^{2+} and cyclic AMP interact to regulate cardiac function.

B. Effector Role of Ca^{2+}

The direct actions of Ca^{2+} that initiate specific steps in the cardiac process can be most easily understood by examination of the role of Ca^{2+} in effecting communications between three regions of the heart (Table 1). Communications between the extracellular and intracellular spaces are mediated by the sarcolemmal (plasma) membrane; those between the interior of the sarcoplasmic reticulum and the cytosol are affected by the membranes of the sarcoplasmic reticulum; while the influence of cytosolic Ca^{2+} upon the contractile proteins is governed by the Ca^{2+}-affinity of the troponin complex. The list of Ca^{2+}-regulated process in Table 1 is incomplete; for example, Ca^{2+} also may act via the Ca^{2+}-dependent protein kinases to control specific aspects of cardiac function. Thus, extrapolations from what is known in other contractile tissues (CHACKO et al. 1977; HARTSHORNE et al. 1977; DABROWSKA et al. 1978) suggest that phosphorylation of some of the structures listed in Table 1 by Ca^{2+}-dependent protein kinases may play an important, but as yet poorly understood role in the control of cardiac function.

The ability of Ca^{2+} to effect communications between different regions of the myocardium results from fluxes of this ion between different membrane-delimited spaces and between Ca^{2+}-binding sites and the surrounding fluids. To understand the way in which these Ca^{2+} fluxes are controlled it is essential to have some idea of the Ca^{2+} concentrations (or, more precisely, the Ca^{2+} activities) in each of the "pools" or sites listed in Table 1. In the extracellular space, Ca^{2+} concentrations are in the *millimolar* range, while those in the cytosol of the heart probably fluctuate between approximately 0.1 and up to 10 *micromolar* during diastole and systole, respectively. The Ca^{2+} concentration within the sarcoplasmic reticulum is not known with precision; it is higher than in the cytosol and probably 100 μM or

Table 1. Role of Ca^{2+} in effecting communication between different regions of the heart

Communication Between:	Major Control Exerted by:
Extracellular *and* Intracellular Spaces	Sarcolemma
Sarcoplasmic Reticulum *and* Cytosol	Sarcoplasmic Reticulum
Cytosol *and* Contractile Proteins	Troponin Complex

more. The amount of cytosolic Ca^{2+} bound to troponin during cardiac systole is determined in part by the cytosolic Ca^{2+} concentration and partly by the Ca^{2+}-affinity of the troponin complex, which has a dissociation constant for Ca^{2+} of approximately 1–3 μM (EBASHI and ENDO 1968; KATZ 1970).

Changing distributions of Ca^{2+} between the regions of the myocardium listed in Table 1 depend on the activities of sarcolemmal and sarcoplasmic reticulum Ca^{2+} transport systems, on the Ca^{2+} permeabilities of the sarcolemma and sarcoplasmic reticulum, and on the Ca^{2+}-affinity of the troponin complex. As discussed below, many aspects of these Ca^{2+} regulatory systems appear to be controlled by cyclic AMP.

C. Regulatory Effects of Cyclic AMP on Ca^{2+} Fluxes in the Heart

I. Calcium Fluxes Across the Sarcolemma

It is now well established that catecholamines increase Ca^{2+} influx across the sarcolemma into the cardiac cell (REUTER 1974a; TSIEN 1977). This effect has been attributed to increased Ca^{2+} flux through a Ca^{2+}-selective ionic channel that allows inward current to flow across the sarcolemma. This depolarizing current, which is activated during cardiac systole, has been designated the *slow inward current* because of the relative slowness of its kinetics compared to those of the *fast inward current*. The fast inward current, which carries Na^+ into the cells, is responsible for the initial rapid upstroke of the action potential in the contractile cells of the atria and ventricles, and in rapidly conducting cells of the His-Purkinje system. In contrast, the slow inward current prolongs depolarization in these cardiac cell types and thus generates the "plateau" which typifies the cardiac action potential in these cells. In other regions of the heart, notably the S-A and A-V nodes where a well-developed fast inward current is absent, a current analogous to the slow inward current constitutes the major, and possibly the only, depolarizing current.

The electrogenic Ca^{2+} fluxes that are responsible for the slow inward current are "downhill", as Ca^{2+} moves from a region of high activity in the extracellular space to one of lower activity within the cell. The mechanism by which catecholamines promote the slow inward current in the ventricular myocardium has been shown by REUTER and SCHOLZ (1977) to be due to an increase in the number of active slow channels, and not a modulation of either their kinetics or size. These investigators observed no change in either the rates of opening or closing of the slow channels, nor in ion selectivity such as might be expected to occur if the channel increased in size. These findings might be explained if catecholamines led to the phosphorylation of a site which in the dephospho-state inactivated the slow channel. Direct evidence for this hypothesis, however, is lacking.

Although the mechanism by which the catecholamine-induced changes in the Ca^{2+}-permeability of the sarcolemma are brought about has not been defined at a biochemical level, many, if not all, of these permeability changes appear to be mediated by cyclic AMP. Thus, several aspects of the response of the cardiac sarcolemma to catecholamines can be induced by cyclic AMP analogues or by intracellular injection of this nucleotide (TSIEN et al. 1972; TSIEN 1973, 1977; REUTER 1974b). An intracellular receptor for the catecholamines appears to have been excluded by the failure of epinephrine injection into the cardiac cell to produce a typical catecholamine response (REUTER 1974b).

Several investigators have attempted to define the biochemical basis for effects of cyclic AMP on Ca^{2+} fluxes across the cardiac sarcolemma using sarcolemmal vesicles purified from the cardiac microsomal fraction. Evidence has been obtained that cyclic AMP-dependent phosphorylation of a Ca^{2+}-binding system in these membranes could explain some of these effects (WOLLENBERGER 1975; SULAKHE et al. 1976; WALSH et al. 1979; JONES et al. 1979), but further work is needed before any final conclusions as to the physiological significance of these observations can be drawn in terms of the control of sarcolemmal Ca^{2+} fluxes.

No clear data have been obtained to define cyclic AMP effects on Ca^{2+} efflux from the myocardial cell. This "uphill" movement of Ca^{2+}, which appears to be effected mainly by an exchange with Na^{+} present at higher concentrations in the extracellular space (REUTER 1974a), could be subject to control by cyclic AMP, but as yet no definitive studies of such a regulatory mechanism have appeared.

II. Calcium Fluxes Across the Sarcoplasmic Reticulum

An enhancement by cyclic AMP of Ca^{2+} fluxes across the sarcoplasmic reticulum can be deduced from the mechanical response of the heart to agents that increase cellular levels of the nucleotide (Fig. 1). The increased tension developed in response to catecholamines implies that more Ca^{2+} becomes bound to the troponin complex. This could result, in part, from the increased Ca^{2+} influx across the sarcolemma described above. However, this Ca^{2+} influx alone is insufficient to account for activation of the contractile proteins in the adult myocardium, (BASSINGTHWAITE and REUTER 1972) so that a role for cyclic AMP to increase Ca^{2+} release from stores within the sarcoplasmic reticulum also appears likely. A stimulatory effect of cyclic AMP on Ca^{2+} release from the cardiac sarcoplasmic reticulum is suggested by the finding that catecholamines and cyclic AMP analogues accelerate the rate of tension development in the heart (Fig. 1), which probably reflects an increase in the rate at which Ca^{2+} becomes available for binding to troponin. A third effect of catecholamines, to increase the rate of cardiac muscle relaxation (Fig. 1), appears to result from direct stimulation of calcium transport into the sarcoplasmic reticulum because shortening of systole by the catecholamines is independent of effects on the duration of the action potential (REUTER 1974b; MORAD and ROLETT 1972). This latter effect, which can be attributed to an increased rate of dissociation of Ca^{2+} from the troponin complex, could result from a reduction in the Ca^{2+}-affinity of the cardiac troponin complex as well as an accelerated rate of Ca^{2+} transport into the sarcoplasmic reticulum (see below).

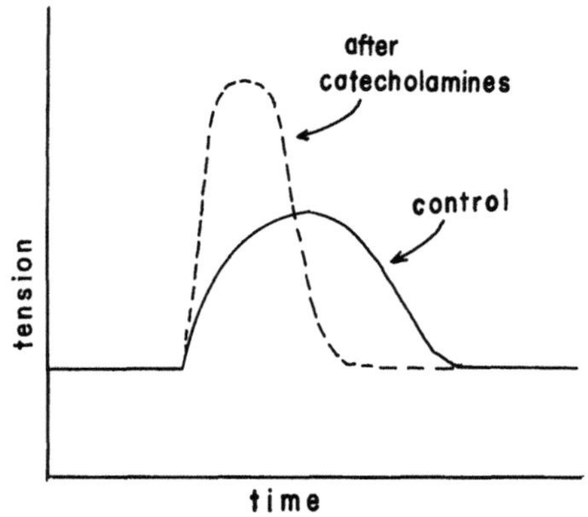

Fig. 1. Schematic representation of the effects of catecholamines on the mechanical response of cardiac muscle. Catecholamines increase maximal tension, the rate of tension rise, and the rate of tension fall. As a result, the duration of mechanical systole is shortened

All three aspects of the mechanical response of the myocardium to catecholamines described above, and shown diagrammatically in Fig. 1, can be evoked by application of cyclic AMP to mechanically "skinned" cardiac fibers (Fabiato and Fabiato 1975). This finding provides further evidence that all three aspects of the mechanical response to catecholamines are due to effects of cyclic AMP that are at least partly independent of actions on the sarcolemma.

Membrane vesicles derived from the cardiac sarcoplasmic reticulum represent an extremely useful preparation in which to study both active and passive Ca^{2+} fluxes across a biological membrane. Extensive study of the active uptake of Ca^{2+} into these vesicles has demonstrated that this active process is effected by an ATP-dependent Ca^{2+} pump that transports 2 moles of this cation per mole of ATP hydrolyzed in both skeletal (Hasselbach and Makinose 1963; Weber et al. 1965) and cardiac (Tada et al. 1974) sarcoplasmic reticulum vesicles. A number of proteins have been identified in cardiac sarcoplasmic reticulum preparations (Suko and Hasselbach 1976; Louis and Katz 1977). The Ca^{2+} pump itself is a 100,000 dalton protein that forms a phosphorylated ATPase intermediate (Suko and Hasselbach 1976; Fanburg and Matsushita 1973). The resulting acyl phosphoprotein (EP) represents an intermediate in the Ca^{2+} pump reaction as EP formation by both skeletal (MacLenan and Holland 1975; Tada et al. 1977) and cardiac (Shigekawa et al. 1976) sarcoplasmic reticulum vesicles requires Ca^{2+}, and the Ca^{2+}-sensitivity of this EP formation closely parallels that of the Ca^{2+} pump. Additionally, slight differences in the Ca^{2+} sensitivity of the Ca^{2+} pumps of cardiac and skeletal sarcoplasmic reticulum are paralleled by similar differences in the Ca^{2+}-sensitivity of EP formation in these two membranes (Shigekawa et al. 1976).

III. Phosphorylation of the Cardiac Sarcoplasmic Reticulum by Cyclic AMP-Dependent Protein Kinases and Catecholamine-Induced Acceleration of Cardiac Relaxation

The possibility that acceleration of the Ca^{2+} pump of the cardiac sarcoplasmic reticulum is responsible for the more rapid relaxation of the heart in the presence of catecholamines led several groups to attempt to define the biochemical mechanism underlying this response by examining the effects of epinephrine and cyclic AMP on Ca^{2+} uptake by cardiac sarcoplasmic reticulum vesicles (HESS et al. 1968; ENTMAN et al. 1969; SHINEBOURNE and WHITE 1970). Results from these early studies were conflicting. We (KATZ and REPKE 1973) were unable to identify effects of physiological concentrations of either epinephrine or cyclic AMP on the initial rate of Ca^{2+} uptake in cardiac sarcoplasmic reticulum.

The explanation for these discrepant results was provided by the discovery that intracellular effects of cyclic AMP could be mediated by cyclic AMP-dependent protein kinases (WALSH et al. 1968; MIYAMOTO et al. 1969) which commonly contaminate cardiac sarcoplasmic reticulum preparations. Four groups independently studied the effects of cyclic AMP-dependent protein kinases on cardiac sarcoplasmic reticulum vesicles in an attempt to define the biochemical mechanism responsible for the ability of catecholamines to accelerate relaxation in the myocardium. WOLLENBERGER (1972), WRAY et al. (1973), and LARAIA and MORKIN (1974) demonstrated that cardiac sarcoplasmic reticulum was a substrate for this enzyme. The resulting phosphoester is chemically distinct from the acyl phosphoprotein formed as a intermediate by the Ca^{2+}-pump ATPase. Our group, which was actively studying the control of the cardiac sarcoplasmic reticulum Ca^{2+} pump, first demonstrated that Ca^{2+} uptake rate could be increased 2–3 fold after pre-incubation with cyclic AMP and a cyclic AMP-dependent protein kinase (KIRCHBERGER et al. 1972). Our subsequent findings summarized below have provided evidence that phosphorylation of the cardiac sarcoplasmic reticulum causes stimulation of Ca^{2+} transport, and that this reaction is responsible for the accelerated relaxation of the heart response to catecholamines.

A causal relationship between protein kinase-catalyzed phosphoester formation and stimulation of Ca^{2+} transport is suggested by the finding that the extent to which Ca^{2+} uptake is stimulated correlates closely with the amount of phosphorylation (KIRCHBERGER et al. 1974). The relationship is the same when cyclic AMP-dependent protein kinases from sources other than cardiac muscle are used. The maximal amount of cyclic AMP-stimulated phosphoester formed in cardiac sarcoplasmic reticulum vesicles, slightly less than 2 nmoles/mg protein (KIRCHBERGER et al. 1974) is similar to the maximal amount of EP formed by the Ca^{2+} pump ATPase in these vesicles (SHIGEKAWA et al. 1976). This relationship suggests that there is a 1:1 stoichiometry between EP and phosphoester phosphoprotein, and that each mole of the latter affects one mole of the Ca^{2+} pump. Additional evidence that cyclic AMP-dependent protein kinase-catalyzed phosphorylation of the sarcoplasmic reticulum is causally related to stimulation of Ca^{2+} transport was obtained by studies of the effects of controlled tryptic digestion of cardiac sarcoplasmic reticulum. Very mild trypsinization, which minimally inhibited the Ca^{2+} transport process, was found to abolish the ability of the cyclic AMP-dependent protein kinase both to phosphorylate these membranes and to stimulate Ca^{2+} transport (TADA et al. 1975 a). A protein kinase modulator was also able to inhibit both phosphorylation and stimulation of Ca^{2+} transport (TADA et al. 1977). Perhaps the most convincing demonstration of a causal relationship between phosphorylation of the cardiac sarcoplasmic reticulum and stimulation of Ca^{2+} transport was provided by the finding that dephosphorylation of the phosphoester formed by the protein kinase was paralleled by loss of the stimulation of Ca^{2+} transport, and that rephosphorylation of the membranes was accompanied by a renewed stimulation of Ca^{2+} uptake (Kirchberger and Raffo 1977). This study also confirmed earlier reports (Tada et al. 1975b) that phosphoprotein phosphatases provide a potential physiological mechanism by which the cyclic AMP-induced stimulation of Ca^{2+} transport could be reversed.

The substrate for cyclic AMP-dependent protein kinase-catalyzed phosphorylation is not the 100,000 dalton ATPase of the sarcoplasmic reticulum, but a smaller 22,000 dalton protein named *phospholamban* (Katz et al. 1975) which is readily separated from the ATPase protein on SDS-polyacrylamide gels (LaRaia and Morkin 1974; Tada et al. 1975a). The amount of phospholamban relative to the ATPase protein has not been determined directly, but the approximately 1:1 ratio between acyl phosphate formation by the ATPase protein and phosphoester phosphorylation of phospholamban (see above), suggests that there is one mole of phospholamban per mole of the ATPase protein in cardiac sarcoplasmic reticulum.

A physiological role for the cyclic AMP-dependent protein kinase catalyzed phosphorylation of phospholamban and the associated stimulation of Ca^{2+} transport is suggested by our studies of different muscle types. In these studies, we compared cardiac sarcoplasmic reticulum vesicles with similar preparations from fast skeletal muscles in which relaxation is not stimulated by catecholamines (Goffart and Ritchie 1952; Bowman and Raper 1967). The absence of a substrate for cyclic AMP-protein kinase-catalyzed phosphorylation in skeletal muscle sarcoplasmic reticulum, and the failure of protein kinases purified from either cardiac or fast skeletal muscles to stimulate Ca^{2+} transport in the skeletal sarcoplasmic reticulum (Katz et al. 1975; Kirchberger and Tada 1976) are in accord with the view that enhancement of Ca^{2+} transport by phospholamban phosphorylation represents, at least in part, a component of the biochemical mechanism responsible for catecholamine-induced acceleration of relaxation in the heart.

The conclusions reached in our studies of the mechanism of catecholamine-induced acceleration of cardiac relaxation have been challenged by Schwartz et al. (1976). While these investigators, and others (Nayler and Berry 1975; Will et al. 1976; Wray and Gray 1977) have subsequently confirmed our essential findings regarding the reactions in cardiac sarcoplasmic reticulum, Schwartz et al. (1976) and Bornet et al. (1977) reported that cyclic AMP-dependent protein kinases can also stimulate Ca^{2+} transport in sarcoplasmic reticulum vesicles prepared from fast skeletal muscle. We regard these latter findings as being of uncertain significance as both our own group and Schwartz et al. (1976) have failed to demonstrate a substrate for the cyclic AMP-dependent protein kinase in fast skeletal sarcoplasmic reticulum. Furthermore, the stimulation of Ca^{2+} transport described by Schwartz et al. in fast skeletal sarcoplasmic reticulum vesicles was obtained at high ($>10\ \mu M$) Ca^{2+} concentrations by the use of an optical method that depends on changes in the absorbance of the Ca^{2+}-sensitive dye murexide. Blayney et al. (1977) have questioned the accuracy of the murexide method, which in any case is unsuitable for Ca^{2+} uptake studies in the physiological, micromolar, range of Ca^{2+} concentration. Furthermore, we have found that phospholamban phosphorylation maximally stimulates Ca^{2+} transport by the cardiac sarcoplasmic reticulum at Ca^{2+} concentrations well below $10\ \mu M$ (Tada et al. 1974; Hicks et al. 1979), so that the physiological significance of the findings of Schwartz et al. (1976) and Bornet et al. (1977) that the cyclic AMP-dependent protein kinase stimulates Ca^{2+} transport by fast skeletal sarcoplasmic reticulum in the range of Ca^{2+} concentration above 10 μM can be questioned. The significance of Ca^{2+} transport stimulation in skeletal sarcoplasmic reticulum remains uncertain in view of the report that cyclic AMP can cause the relaxation of tension in mechanically skinned fast skeletal fibers of the cat (FABIATO and FABIATO 1978).

Stimulation of Ca^{2+} transport in cardiac sarcoplasmic reticulum as a consequence of phospholamban phosphorylation appears to result from an effect of this phosphoprotein on the interactions between the two Ca^{2+}-binding sites on each molecule of the ATPase protein of the cardiac sarcoplasmic reticulum (HICKS et al. 1979). Although there appears to be a significant positive cooperativity between the two Ca^{2+}-binding sites of skeletal sarcoplasmic reticulum during the initial interactions between Ca^{2+} and the ATPase protein (KANAZAWA et al. 1971), once Ca^{2+} uptake has begun, the kinetic properties of the reaction indicate that these interact independently in skeletal sarcoplasmic reticulum. Thus, in these preparations, no cooperativity has been found during the Ca^{2+}-dependent ATPase reaction (YAMAMOTO and TONOMURA 1976) and during oxalate- (LI et al. 1974) or phosphate-supported Ca^{2+} uptake (HICKS et al. 1979). In cardiac sarcoplasmic reticulum, on the other hand kinetic studies of the Ca^{2+}-dependence of phosphate-supported Ca^{2+} uptake by cardiac sarcoplasmic reticulum suggest a high degree of positive cooperativity between the two Ca^{2+} binding sites on each molecule of the ATPase protein (HICKS et al. 1979). This positive cooperativity is significantly decreased by exposure to a cardiac cyclic AMP-dependent protein kinase (HICKS et al. 1979) suggesting that phospholamban phosphorylation reduces an interaction between the two Ca^{2+} binding sites on the ATPase protein. At the same time, phospholamban phosphorylation reduces the level of Ca^{2+} at which the Ca^{2+}-transport reaction achieves half-maximal velocity. Phosphorylation of phospholamban has also been found to increase the velocity of the Ca^{2+} transport ATPase without increasing the amount of EP (TADA et al. 1979). This effect, which represents accelerated turnover of the Ca^{2+} pump, is associated with an increased rate of EP decomposition (TADA et al. 1979). As these studies indicate that phospholamban phosphorylation influences a number of different aspects of the Ca^{2+} transport reaction, it appears likely that the interaction between phospholamban and the Ca^{2+} pump ATPase in the membrane of the cardiac sarcoplasmic reticulum is relatively non-specific.

A tentative mechanism that can explain the effects of phospholamban phosphorylation on the cardiac sarcoplasmic reticulum is shown in Fig. 2. While evidence for this mechanism is incomplete, it is consistent with our current knowledge of the effects of the cyclic AMP-dependent protein kinase on these membranes. As shown in Fig. 2A, phospholamban in its dephospho-form interacts with the ATPase protein in a manner that inhibits Ca^{2+} binding and confers positive cooperativity upon the two Ca^{2+}-binding sites of the ATPase. Phosphorylation of phospholamban reduces the extent of these interactions and increases the Ca^{2+}-sensitivity of the Ca^{2+} pump, thereby increasing its rate at low Ca^{2+} concentrations (Fig. 2B). The finding that the Ca^{2+}-sensitivity of ATP hydrolysis by the purified cardiac sarcoplasmic reticulum ATPase protein is similar to that of the corresponding protein from fast skeletal muscle (LEVITSKY et al. 1976) and does not show the lower Ca^{2+} sensitivity seen in native cardiac sarcoplasmic reticulum vesicles (SHI-

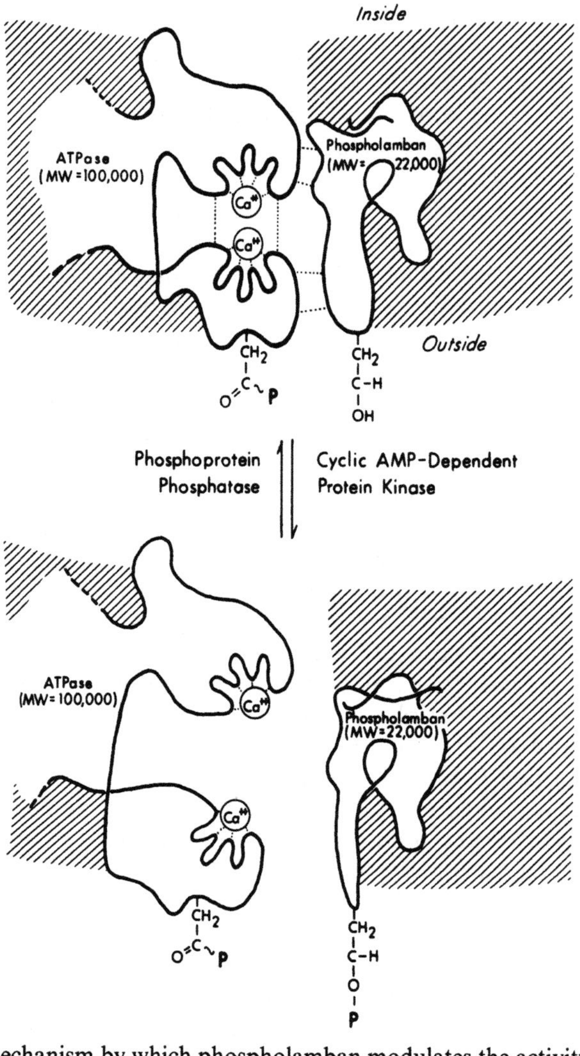

Fig. 2. Possible mechanism by which phospholamban modulates the activity of the calcium pump of the cardiac sarcoplasmic reticulum. *Upper*, Dephospho-phospholamban interacts with the calcium pump ATPase in the membrane *(shaded)*, conferring positive cooperatively on the two Ca^{2+} binding sites and lowering the Ca^{2+} sensitivity of the ATPase. *Lower*, Phosphorylation of phospholamban reduces its interaction with the calcium pump ATPase, increasing the Ca^{2+} sensitivity of calcium uptake and allowing the Ca^{2+} binding sites of the calcium pump to interact independent with Ca^{2+}. These effects increase calcium transport rate at low Ca^{2+} concentrations. (HICKS et al. 1979, by permission of the American Heart Association, Inc.)

GEKAWA et al. 1976) is in accord with this view that the dephospho-form of phospholamban is at least partly responsible for the high degree of positive cooperativity and lesser Ca^{2+} affinity of the cardiac sarcoplasmic reticulum Ca^{2+} pump. More direct evidence for this proposed mechanism is needed, however, and may stem from current efforts to purify phospholamban and to incorporate the dephospho- and phospho-forms into reconstituted sarcoplasmic reticulum vesicles.

IV. Phosphorylation of the Cardiac Sarcoplasmic Reticulum and the Catecholamine-Induced Increases in Tension Development and Rate of Tension Rise in the Heart

Phosphorylation of the cardiac sarcoplasmic reticulum may directly mediate the action of catecholamines to increase tension development and the rate of tension rise in the heart (Fig. 1). This is suggested by the observations that cyclic AMP applied to skinned cardiac fibers can induce these same effects of catecholamines as in the intact heart (FABIATO and FABIATO 1975). KATZ et al. (1975) reported that the rate of Ca^{2+} release from Ca^{2+}-filled cardiac sarcoplasmic reticulum vesicles could be increased after exposure to a cyclic AMP-dependent protein kinase and proposed that phosphorylation of the cardiac sarcoplasmic reticulum might explain this catecholamine effect.

It has been suggested that a "Ca^{2+}-triggered Ca^{2+} release" from stores in the sarcoplasmic reticulum is responsible for initiating cardiac contraction (FABIATO and FABIATO 1977). Such a mechanism would allow the inward movement of a small of Ca^{2+} across the sarcolemma to trigger a much larger Ca^{2+} release from the sarcoplasmic reticulum, much like the explosion of a small powder change in the firing pan of an old flintlock musket explodes the larger charge of powder within the barrel. Recently we have obtained evidence that the rate of Ca^{2+} efflux from sarcoplasmic reticulum vesicles is increased by elevation of the Ca^{2+} concentration in the medium surrounding the vesicles and that this Ca^{2+}-dependent efflux may be mediated by the Ca^{2+} pump of the sarcoplasmic reticulum (KATZ et al. 1977a, b, c). Thus, the ability of increased Ca^{2+} concentrations at the external surface of cardiac sarcoplasmic reticulum vesicles to increase Ca^{2+} efflux rate (DUNNETT and NAYLER 1978) might be promoted by cyclic AMP-catalyzed phosphorylation of phospholamban (KATZ et al. 1975). If these phenomena involving Ca^{2+} efflux from the sarcoplasmic reticulum play a physiological role in the initiation of cardiac contraction, the apparent ability of phospholamban phosphorylation to stimulate Ca^{2+} efflux from the sarcoplasmic reticulum (KATZ et al. 1975) may partly explain the ability of catecholamines to increase both total tension and the rate of tension rise in the myocardium.

V. Calcium Fluxes Between the Cytosol and Troponin: Phosphorylation of the Troponin Complex

The possibility that phosphorylation of the troponin complex by a cyclic AMP-dependent protein kinase could play a role in regulation of myocardial contractility was suggested by early studies which demonstrated phosphorylation of the contractile proteins isolated from fast skeletal muscle (BAILEY and VILLAR-PALASI 1971; STULL et al. 1972; PRATJE and HEILMEYER 1972). Subsequent studies, however, failed to demonstrate significant functional changes in the skeletal muscle contractile proteins after this phosphorylation, and exposure of skeletal muscle to isoproterenol in vivo did not lead to phosphorylation of the troponin complex (STULL 1975). Furthermore, troponin I in the intact skeletal troponin complex was found to be a poor substrate for this enzyme, and its phosphorylation was inhibited when troponin I was bound to troponin C (COLE and PERRY 1975). BYLUND and

KREBS (1975) presented evidence suggesting that the phosphorylation of skeletal troponin was an artifact arising from partial denaturation of the protein. The apparent inability of native skeletal troponin I to serve as a substrate for cyclic AMP-dependent protein kinase is in accord with the observation that agents which increase cellular levels of cyclic AMP do not modify greatly the contractile response of this type of muscle, which is much less regulated by catecholamines than is cardiac muscle (GOFFART and RITCHIE 1952; BOWMAN and RAPER 1967). In view of the much more important role of changing cellular function in mediating the regulation of cardiac performance, the findings that cyclic AMP-induced phosphorylation of skeletal troponin I does not change the Ca^{2+}-sensitivity of skeletal actomyosin do not preclude a physiological role for such an effect in the cardiac contractile proteins.

In contrast to the findings in skeletal muscle, cardiac troponin I can be phosphorylated in vivo by agents that increase cyclic AMP (ENGLAND 1975), and in vitro by cyclic AMP-dependent protein kinases (SOLARO et al. 1976; REDDY and WYBORNY 1976; STULL and BUSS 1977; BAILIN 1979). The phosphorylation of cardiac troponin I by cyclic AMP-dependent protein kinase does not require its prior dissociation from the troponin complex, and this protein is readily phosphorylated even when bound to F-actin in a structure similar to that of the thin filament of muscle (BAILIN 1979).

The functional significance of the phosphorylation of cardiac troponin I, however, remains in dispute. An early study of the effects of phosphorylation of cardiac troponin I suggested that the troponin complex containing this phosphorylated protein had an increased Ca^{2+}-sensitivity in that the Ca^{2+} levels needed to activate actomyosin ATPase were lowered afer phosphorylation (RUBIO et al. 1975). Such an effect, which in the intact muscle would increase the amount of troponin-bound Ca^{2+} at low levels of cytosolic Ca^{2+}, could contribute to the increased tension developed by the heart under the influence of catecholamines (Fig. 1). The determinations of Ca^{2+}-sensitivity in this initial study appeared to suffer from methodologic deficiencies, however, and a number of more recent studies have failed to document an increased Ca^{2+}-sensitivity of cardiac actomyosin ATPase after phosphorylation of the cardiac troponin complex. While STULL and BUSS (1977) reported that no significant change in Ca^{2+} sensitivity occurred after cyclic AMP-dependent protein kinase catalyzed phosphorylation of cardiac troponin I, other laboratories (SOLARO et al. 1976; REDDY and WYBORNY 1976; BAILIN 1979) have documented a decrease in the Ca^{2+}-sensitivity of cardiac actomyosin ATPase activity after troponin I phosphorylation. The latter effect, while tending to reduce the myocardial contractile response to a given amount of Ca^{2+} released into the cell during excitation-contraction coupling, would promote relaxation. This latter effect would result from a reduction in the Ca^{2+} affinity of the troponin complex, as this change would facilitate the dissociation of activator Ca^{2+} from the contractile proteins while cytosolic Ca^{2+} was taken up by the sarcoplasmic reticulum.

A lowering of the Ca^{2+}-sensitivity of the cardiac contractile proteins following phosphorylation by cyclic AMP-dependent protein kinase, as suggested by several recent studies, would be opposite in direction from the apparent increase in the Ca^{2+}-sensitivity of the cardiac sarcoplasmic reticulum brought about by phospholamban phosphorylation (see above). It is of some interest that both of these reported changes in Ca^{2+} sensitivity appear to result not from phosphorylation of the Ca^{2+}-binding proteins of the sarcoplasmic reticulum (the Ca^{2+} pump ATPase) or the contractile proteins (troponin C), but from a changing cooperative interaction between the cyclic AMP-dependent protein kinase substrates (phospholamban and troponin I) and the Ca^{2+}-binding proteins themselves.

IV. Significance of Phosphorylation of Cardiac Phospholamban and Troponin

Should the finding of a decrease in the Ca^{2+}-sensitivity of the cardiac troponin complex after cyclic AMP-induced phosphorylation be confirmed, it might be asked why the cardiac cell has chosen to respond to catecholamines by favoring Ca^{2+}-dissociation during relaxation instead of Ca^{2+}-binding during contraction. One explanation for this apparent favoring of reactions that promote relaxation was suggested by P. GREENGARD (personal communication), who noted that Ca^{2+}-binding to troponin results from an energy-independent "downhill" Ca^{2+} flux that is initiated by permeability changes in the sarcoplasmic reticulum, and possibly the sarcolemma, whereas Ca^{2+} removal from troponin requires the action of an energy-linked ion pump. The rates of the activating, downhill, Ca^{2+} fluxes are limited only by that of diffusion, which is several orders of magnitude more rapid than of the ATP-dependent Ca^{2+} pump of the sarcoplasmic reticulum, which ultimately initiates cardiac relaxation by causing Ca^{2+} to be dissociated from the contractile proteins. In view of the major physiological effect of catecholamines to increase heart rate (see above), and the fact that tachycardia causes diastole to shorten to a much greater extent than systole in the intact heart, it becomes mandatory that relaxation be accelerated when the heart comes under the influence of the catecholamines. Failure of the catecholamine-stimulated heart to accelerate its rate of relaxation would impair diastolic filling so that, at rapid heart rates, the output of the heart would be reduced. This physiological fact may underlie the increase in the Ca^{2+}-sensitivity of the cardiac sarcoplasmic reticulum that would accelerate the rate of Ca^{2+} uptake at low Ca^{2+} concentrations. At the time, an opposite shift that decreases the Ca^{2+}-sensitivity of the cardiac troponin complex would facilitate the dissociation of Ca^{2+} from the contractile proteins at low levels of cytosolic Ca^{2}. This combination of effects would allow catecholamines to cause the contractile proteins of the heart to relax at higher levels of cytosolic Ca^{2+} at the same time that the Ca^{2+} pump of the sarcoplasmic reticulum would be operating at a more rapid rate. Even though this reduction in the Ca^{2+} sensitivity of the troponin complex would require that an increased amount of Ca^{2+} be delivered to initiate contraction, the rate of this Ca^{2+} delivery process would probably not be limiting in view of the ability of catecholamines to increase Ca^{2+} influx across the sarcolemma and efflux from the sarcoplasmic reticulum, the virtually inexhaustible supply of extracellular Ca^{2+}, and the inherent rapidity of the diffusion processes that mediate the downhill fluxes of Ca^{2+} to the contractile proteins.

An additional advantage to the catecholamine-stimulated heart of the opposite shifts in the Ca^{2+}-sensitivity of the sarcoplasmic reticulum Ca^{2+} pump and the troponin complex described above would arise from the reported decrease in the efficiency of the Ca^{2+} pump at low Ca^{2+} concentrations (MAKINOSE and THE (1965).

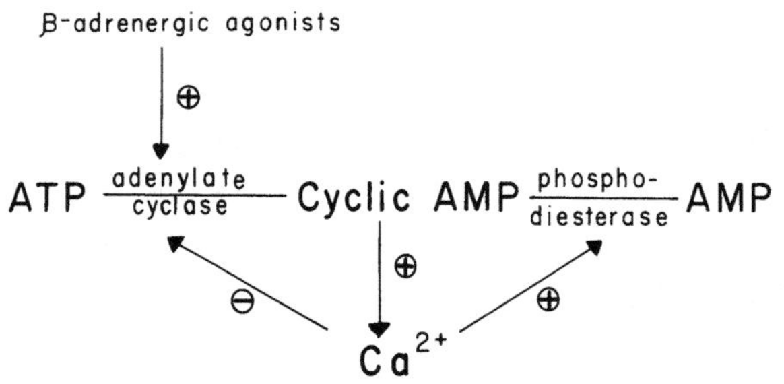

Fig. 3. Proposed interrelationships between Ca^{2+} and cyclic AMP in the myocardium. (TADA et al. 1975c, by permission of the American Heart Association, Inc.)

An effect of cyclic AMP to facilitate Ca^{2+} dissociation from the contractile proteins might, by allowing the heart to relax at higher levels of cytosolic Ca^{2+}, have an energy-sparing effect under conditions where catecholamines profoundly increase the work of the heart.

D. Regulatory Effect of Ca^{2+} on Cyclic AMP Levels

Up to this point, this article has focused on the effector role of Ca^{2+} both as a carrier of electrical change across the sarcolemma and as the signal that initiates the contractile process. There is also evidence that changing Ca^{2+} concentration in the micromolar range can regulate the production and degradation of cyclic AMP in the heart. These effects, which appear to be mediated by a Ca^{2+}-dependent regulator protein (calmodulin) that is evolutionarily related to troponin C, allow increased cytosolic Ca^{2+} concentrations to reduce cyclic AMP levels in the heart.

There is now abundant evidence that phosphodiesterase activity is enhanced by Ca^{2+} (KAKIUCHI et al. 1973; WANG et al. 1975), so that increased Ca^{2+} levels in the heart could, by activating this enzyme, accelerate cyclic AMP breakdown. In addition to promoting cyclic AMP breakdown, we have found that micromolar levels of Ca^{2+} inhibit cardiac sarcolemmal adenylate cyclase (TADA et al. 1975c), thereby reducing cyclic AMP production. A more complex response of cerebral cortex adenylate cyclase to Ca^{2+} has been attributed to an effect of a Ca^{2+}-dependent regulatory protein (BROSTROM et al. 1978). These findings suggest that when elevated cardiac cytosolic cyclic AMP levels increase intracellular Ca^{2+} concentration (see above), a "negative feedback" mechanism is initiated that, in turn, tends to reduce cyclic AMP levels (Fig. 3). This inhibitory effect of Ca^{2+} on adenylate cyclase was less when the enzyme was activated by catecholamines (TADA et al. 1975c).

A physiological role for the "negative feedback" mechanisms described above is not clear. The apparent ability of Ca^{2+} to reduce cyclic AMP levels may reflect a "fine tuning" mechanism that controls cyclic AMP and Ca^{2+} concentrations in the heart under basal conditions. The observation that catecholamine-stimulated adenylate cyclase activity is less sensitive to the inhibitory effects of Ca^{2+} than is the basal activity (TADA et al. 1975c) suggests that this balance is reset to allow both higher cyclic AMP and Ca^{2+} levels in the myocardium when it is stimulated by catecholamines.

References

Bailey C, Villar-Palasi C (1971) Cyclic AMP dependent phosphorylation of troponin (Abstr). Fed Proc 30:1147

Bailin G (1979) Phosphorylation of a bovine cardiac actin complex. Am J Physiol 236:C41–C46

Bassingthwaite JB, Reuter H (1972) Calcium movements and excitation-contraction coupling in cardiac cells. In: DeMello WC (ed) Electrical phenomena in the heart. Academic Press, New York London, pp 353–395

Blayney LM, Thomas H, Muir J, Henderson A (1977) Critical reevaluation of the murexide technique in the measurement of calcium transport by cardiac sarcoplasmic reticulum. Biochim Biophys Acta 470:128–133

Bornet EP, Entman ML, van Winkle WB, Schwartz A, Lehotay DC, Levey GS (1977) Cyclic AMP modulation of calcium accumulation by sarcoplasmic reticulum from fast skeletal muscle. Biochim Biophys Acta 468:188–193

Bowman WC, Raper C (1967) Adrenotropic receptors in skeletal muscle. Ann NY Acad Sci 139:741–753

Brostrom MA, Brostrom CO, Breckenridge B McL, Wolff DJ (1978) Calcium-dependent regulation of brain adenylate cyclase. Adv Cyclic Nucleotide Res 9:85–99

Bylund DB, Krebs EG (1975) Effect of denaturation on the susceptibility of enzyme proteins to enzymic phosphorylation. J Biol Chem 250:6355–6361

Chacko S, Blose SH, Adelstein RS (1977) Phosphorylation and Ca^{2+} regulation of actin-activated ATPase activity of myosin isolated from cultured aortic and vas deferens smooth muscle cells. In: Casteels R, Godfraind T, Ruegg JC (eds) Excitation-contraction coupling in smooth muscle. Elsevier/North-Holland, Amsterdam Oxford New York

Cole HA, Perry SV (1975) The phosphorylation of troponin I from cardiac muscle. J Biochem (Tokyo) 149:525–533

Dabrowska R, Sherry JMF, Aromatorio DK, Hartshorne DJ (1978) Modulator protein as a component of the myosin light chain kinase in chicken gizzard. Biochemistry 17:253–258

Dunnett J, Nayler WG (1978) Calcium efflux from cardiac sarcoplasmic reticulum: effects of calcium and magnesium. J Mol Cell Cardiol 10:487–498

Ebashi S, Endo M (1968) Calcium ion and muscular contraction. Prog Biophys Mol Biol 18:123–183

England PJ (1975) Correlation between contractions and phosphorylation of the inhibitory subunit of troponin in perfused rat heart. FEBS Lett 50:57–60

Entman ML, Levey GS, Epstein SE (1969) Mechanism of action of epinephrine and glucagon on the canine heart. Evidence for increase in sarcotubular calcium stores mediated by cyclic 3′,5′-AMP. Circ Res 25:429–438

Fabiato A, Fabiato F (1975) Relaxing and inotropic effects of cyclic AMP in skinned cardiac cells. Nature 253:556–558

Fabiato A, Fabiato F (1977) Calcium release from the sarcoplasmic reticulum. Circ Res 40:119–129

Fabiato A, Fabiato F (1978) Cyclic AMP-induced enhancement of calcium accumulation by the sarcoplasmic reticulum with no modification of the sensitivity of the myofilaments to calcium in skinned fibres from a fast skeletal muscle. Biochim Biophys Acta 539:253–260

Fanburg BL, Matsushita S (1973) Phosphorylated intermediate of ATPase of isolated cardiac sarcoplasmic reticulum. J Mol Cell Cardiol 5:111–115

Fisher EH, Heilmeyer LMG Jr, Hascke RA (1971) Phosphorylase and the control of glycogen degradation. Curr Top Cell Regul 4:211–251

Goffart M, Ritchie JM (1952) The effect of adrenaline on the contration of mammalian skeletal muscle. J Physiol (Lond) 116:357–371

Hartshorne DJ, Gorecka A, Aksoy MO (1977) Aspects of the regulatory mechanism is smooth muscle. In: Casteels R, Godfraind T, Ruegg JC (eds) Excitation-contraction coupling in smooth muscle. Elsevier/North-Holland, Amsterdam Oxford New York

Hasselbach W, Makinose M (1963) Über den Mechanismus des Calciumtransportes durch die Membranen des sarkoplasmatischen Reticulum. Biochem Z 339:94–111
Hess ML, Briggs FN, Shinebourne E, White R (1968) Effect of adrenergic blocking agents on the calcium pump of the fragmented cardiac sarcoplasmic reticulum. Nature 220:79–80
Hicks M, Shigekawa M, Katz AM (1979) Mechanism by which cyclic AMP-dependent protein kinase stimulates calcium transport in cardiac sarcoplasmic reticulum. Circ Res 44:384–391
Jones LR, Besch HR Jr, Fleming JW, McConnaughey MM, Watanabe AM (1979) Separation of vesicles of cardiac sarcolemma from vesicles of cardiac sarcoplasmic reticulum. Comparative biochemical analyses of component activities. J Biol Chem 254:530–539
Kakiuchi S, Yamazaki R, Teshima Y, Venishi K (1973) Regulation of nucleotide cyclic 3′,5′-monophosphate phosphodiesterase activity from rat brain by a modulator and Ca^{2+}. Proc Natl Acad Sci USA 70:3526–3530
Kanazawa T, Yamada S, Yamamoto T, Tonomura Y (1971) Reaction mechanism of the Ca^{2+}-dependent ATPase of sarcoplasmic reticulum from skeletal muscle V. Vectorial requirements for calcium and magnesium ions of three partial reactions of ATPase: formation and decomposition of a phosphorylated intermediate and ATP-formation from ADP and the intermediate. J Biochem (Tokyo) 70:95–123
Katz AM (1970) Contractile proteins of the heart. Physiol Rev 50:63–158
Katz AM (1977) Physiology of the heart. Raven, New York
Katz AM, Repke DI (1973) Calcium-membrane interactions in the myocardium: effects of ouabain, epinephrine and 3′,5′-cyclic adenosine monophosphate. Am J Cardiol 31:193–201
Katz AM, Tada M, Kirchberger MA (1975) Control of calcium transport in the myocardium by the cyclic AMP-protein kinase system. Adv Cyclic Nucleotide Res 5:453–472
Katz AM, Repke DI, Fudyma G, Shigekawa M (1977a) Control of calcium efflux from sarcoplasmic reticulum vesicles by external calcium. J. Biol. Chem. 252:4210–4214
Katz AM, Repke DI, Fudyma G, Shigekawa M (1977b) Calcium efflux from sarcoplasmic reticulum vesicles. In: Wasserman RH et al. (eds) Calcium-binding proteins and calcium function. Elsevier/North-Holland, Amsterdam Oxford New York, pp 147–154
Katz AM, Repke DI, Dunnett J, Hasselbach W (1977c) Dependence of calcium permeability of sarcoplasmic reticulum vesicles on external and internal calcium ion concentrations. J Biol Chem 252:1950–1956
Kirchberger MA, Raffo A (1977) Decrease in calcium transport associated with phosphoprotein phosphatase-catalyzed dephosphorylation of cardiac sarcoplasmic reticulum. J Cyclic Nucleotide Res 3:45–53
Kirchberger MA, Tada M (1976) Effects of adenosine 3′,5′-monophosphate dependent protein kinase on sarcoplasmic reticulum isolated from cardiac and slow and fast contracting skeletal muscles. J Biol Chem 251:725–729
Kirchberger MA, Tada M, Repke DI, Katz AM (1972) Cyclic adenosine 3′,5′-monophosphate-dependent protein kinase stimulation of calcium uptake by canine cardiac microsomes. J Mol Cell Cardiol 4:673–680
Kirchberger MA, Tada M, Katz AM (1974) Adenosine 3′,5′monophosphate-dependent protein kinase-catalyzed phosphorylation reaction and its relationship to calcium transport in cardiac sarcoplasmic reticulum. J Biol Chem 249:6166–6173
Larner J, Villar-Palasi C (1971) Glycogen synthase and its control. Curr Top Cell Regul 3:195–236
LaRaia PJ, Morkin E (1974) Adenosine 3′,5′-monophosphate dependent membrane phosphorylation; a possible mechanism for the control of microsomal calcium transport in heart muscle. Circ Res 25:298–306
Levitsky DO, Aliev MK, Kuzmin AL, Levchenko TS, Smirnov VN, Chazov EI (1976) Isolation of calcium pump system and purification of calcium ion-dependent ATPase from heart muscle. Biochim Biophys Acta 443:468–484
Li H-C, Katz AM, Repke DI, Failor A (1974) Oxalate dependence of calcium uptake kinetics of rabbit skeletal muscle microsomes (fragmented sarcoplasmic reticulum). Biochim Biophys Acta 367:385–389

Louis CF, Katz AM (1977) Lactoperoxidase coupled iodination of cardiac sarcoplasmic reticulum proteins. Biochim Biophys Acta 494:255–265
MacLennan DH, Holland PC (1975) Calcium transport in sarcoplasmic reticulum. Annu Rev Biophys Bioeng 4:377–404
Makinose M, The R (1965) Calcium-Akkumulation und Nucleosidtriphosphatspaltung durch die Vesikel des sarkoplasmatischen Reticulum. Biochem Z 343:383–393
Miyamoto E, Kuo JF, Greengard P (1969) Adenosine 3',5'-monophosphate dependent protein kinase from brain. Science 165:63–65
Morad M, Rolett EL (1972) Relaxing effects of catecholamines on mammalian heart. J Physiol (Lond) 224:537–558
Nayler WG, Berry D (1975) Effect of drugs on the cyclic adenosine 3',5'-monophosphate-dependent protein kinase-induced stimulation of calcium uptake by cardiac microsomal fractions. J Mol Cell Cardiol 7:387–395
Neely JR, Morgan HE (1974) Relationship between carbohydrate and lipid metabolism and the energy balance of heart muscle. Annu Rev Physiol 31:413–459
Nimmo HG, Cohen P (1977) Hormonal control of protein phosphorylation. Adv Cyclic Nucleotide Res. 8:145–266
Perry SV, Cole HA (1973) Phosphorylation of the "37,000 component" of the troponin complex (Troponin-T). Biochem J 131:425–428
Pratje E, Heilmeyer LMG (1972) Phosphorylation of rabbit muscle troponin and actin by a 3',5'-cAMP-dependent protein kinase. FEBS Lett 27:89–93
Reddy YS, Wyborny LE (1976) Phosphorylation of guinea pig actomyosin and its effect on ATPase activity. Biochem Biophys Res Commun 73:703–709
Reuter H (1974a) Exchange of calcium ions in the mammalian myocardium: mechanisms and physiological significance. Circ Res 34:599–605
Reuter H (1974b) Localization of *beta* adrenergic receptors and effects of noradrenaline and cyclic nucleotides on action potentials, ionic currents and tension in mammalian cardiac muscle. J Physiol (Lond) 242:429–451
Reuter H, Scholz H (1977) The regulation of the calcium conductance of cardiac muscle by adrenaline. J Physiol (Lond) 264:49–62
Rubio R, Bailey C, Villar-Palasi C (1975) Effects of cyclic AMP dependent protein kinase on cardiac actomyosin: increase in Ca^{2+} sensitivity and possible phosphorylation of troponin I. J Cyclic Nucleotide Res 1:143–150
Schwartz A, Entman ML, Kaniike K, Lane LK, van Winkle WB, Bornet EP (1976) The rate of calcium uptake in sarcoplasmic reticulum of cardiac muscle and skeletal muscle. Effects of cyclic AMP-dependent protein kinase and phosphorylase b kinase. Biochim Biophys Acta 426:57–72
Shigekawa M, Finegan JAM, Katz AM (1976) Calcium transport ATPase of canine cardiac sarcoplasmic reticulum: a comparison with that of rabbit fast skeletal muscle sarcoplasmic reticulum. J Biol Chem 251:6894–6900
Shinebourne E, White R (1970) Cyclic AMP and calcium uptake of the sarcoplasmic reticulum in relation to increased rate of relaxation under the influence of catecholamines. Cardiovasc Res 4:194–200
Solaro RJ, Moir AJG, Perry SV (1976) Phosphorylation of the inhibitory component of troponin and the inotropic effect of adrenaline in perfused rabbit heart. Nature 262:615–616
Stull JT (1975) Phosphorylation of skeletal muscle troponin in vivo. Pharmacologist: 234
Stull JR, Russ JE (1977) Phosphorylation of cardiac troponin by cyclic adenosine 3',5'-monophosphate-dependent protein kinase. J Biol Chem 252:851–857
Stull JR, Brostrom CV, Krebs EG (1972) Phosphorylation of the inhibitor component of troponin by phosphorylase kinase. J Biol Chem 247:5272–5274
Suko J, Hasselbach W (1976) Characterization of cardiac sarcoplasmic reticulum ATP-ADP phosphate exchange and phosphorylation of the calcium transport adenosine triphosphatase. Eur J Biochem 64:123–130
Sulakhe PV, Leung NL-K, St Louis P (1976) Stimulation of calcium accumulation in cardiac sarcolemma by protein kinase. Can J Biochem 54:438–445

Tada M, Kirchberger MA, Repke DI, Katz AM (1974) Stimulation of calcium transport in cardiac sarcoplasmic reticulum by adenosine 3′:5′-monophosphate-dependent protein kinase. J Biol Chem 249:6174–6180

Tada M, Kirchberger MA, Katz AM (1975a) Phosphorylation of a 22,000-dalton component of the cardiac sarcoplasmic reticulum by adenosine 3′,5′-monophosphate dependent protein kinase. J Biol Chem 250:2640–2647

Tada M, Kirchberger MA, Li H-C (1975b) Phosphoprotein phosphatase catalyzed dephosphorylation of the 22,000 dalton phosphoprotein of cardiac sarcoplasmic reticulum. J Cyclic Nucleotide Res 1:329–338

Tada M, Kirchberger MA, Iorio J-AM, Katz AM (1975c) Control of cardiac sarcolemmal adenylate cyclase and sodium, potassium-activated adenosine triphosphatase activities. Circ Res 36:8–17

Tada M, Ohmori F, Nimura Y, Abe H (1977) Effect of myocardial protein kinase modulator on adenosine 3′,5′-monophosphate-dependent protein kinase-induced stimulation of calcium transport by cardiac sarcoplasmic reticulum. J Biochem (Tokyo) 82:885–892

Tada M, Yamamoto Y, Tonomura Y (1978) Molecular mechanism of active calcium transport by sarcoplasmic reticulum. Physiol Rev 58:1–79

Tada M, Ohmori F, Yamada M, Abe H (1979) Mechanism of the stimulation of Ca^{2+}-dependent ATPase of cardiac sarcoplasmic reticulum by adenosine 3′:5;-monophosphate-dependent protein kinase. J Biol Chem 254:319–326

Tsien RW (1973) Adrenaline-like effects of intracellular iontophoresis of cyclic AMP in cardiac Purkinje fibers. Nature New Biol 245:120–122

Tsien RW (1977) Cyclic AMP and contractile activity in heart. Adv Cyclic Nucleotide Res 8:363–420

Tsien RW, Giles W, Greengard P (1972) Cyclic AMP mediates the effects of adrenaline on cardiac Purkinje fibers. Nature New Biol 240:181–183

Walsh DA, Perkins JP, Krebs EG (1968) An adenosine 3′,5′-monophosphate dependent protein kinase from rabbit skeletal muscle. J Biol Chem 243:3763–3765

Walsh DA, Clippinger MA, Sivaramakrishnan S, McCullough TE (1979) Cyclic adenosine monophosphate dependent and independent phosphorylation of sarcolemma membrane proteins in perfused rat heart. Biochemistry 18:871–877

Wang JH, Teo TS, Ho HC, Stevens FC (1975) Bovine heart protein activator of cyclic nucleotide phosphodiesterase. Adv Cyclic Nucleotide Res 5:179–194

Weber A, Herz R, Reiss I (1965) Study of the kinetics of calcium transport by isolated fragmented sarcoplasmic reticulum. Biochem Z 333:518–528

Will H, Blanck J, Smettar G, Wollenberger A (1976) A quench-flow kinetic investigation of calcium ion accumulation by isolated cardiac sarcoplasmic reticulum. Dependence of initial velocity of free calcium ion concentrations and influence of preincubation with a protein kinase, MgATP and cyclic AMP. Biochim Biophys Acta 449:297–303

Wollenberger A (1972) Cyclic nucleotides and the regulation of heart beat. Abstr Fifth Int Congr Pharmacol, pp 231–233

Wollenberger A (1975) The role of cyclic AMP in the adrenergic control of the heart. In: Nayler WG (ed) Contraction and relaxation in the myocardium. Academic Press, New York London, pp 113–190

Wray HL, Gray RR (1977) Cyclic AMP stimulation of membrane phosphorylation and Ca^{2+}-activated, Mg^{2+}-dependent ATPase in cardiac sarcoplasmic reticulum. Biochem Biophys Acta 461:441–459

Wray HL, Gray RR, Olsson RA (1973) Cyclic adenosine 3′,5′-monophosphate-stimulated protein kinase and a substrate associated with cardiac sarcoplasmic reticulum. J Biol Chem 248:1496–1498

Yamamoto T, Tonomura Y (1976) Reaction mechanism of the Ca^{2+}-dependent ATPase of sarcoplasmic reticulum from skeletal muscle. I. Kinetic studies. J Biochem (Tokyo) 62:558–575

CHAPTER 24

Cyclic Nucleotides as First Messengers

R. VAN DRIEL

Overview

Do cyclic nucleotides play a role in *inter*cellular communication in addition to their well-established function as *intra*cellular second messengers? Only for certain cellular slime molds can this question be answered affirmatively. Slime molds live as single amoebae in the soil as long as sufficient food is available. Upon starvation, the amoebae start to secrete pulses of adenosine-3′,5′-cyclic-monophosphate (cAMP) into the surrounding medium. These signals are received by neighboring, which respond chemotactically. In this way, the cells are able to find each other and aggregate into a multi-cellular organism, a process that is part of their life cycle (shown in Fig. 2). Furthermore, the cAMP signals play an important role in the control of cell development and possibly cell differentiation.

Is such a first messenger role of extracellular cAMP unique to slime molds? There is suggestive evidence that a similar type of intercellular communication occurs during early development of the chick embryo (see Sect. E). One wonders whether the same is true for other embryonic organisms. It is conceivable that the slime molds constitute a special example of a more generally used communication mechanism occurring during early development. Because the distance between the slime mold cells during cell aggregation is much greater than that between cells in an embryo, the signals in the latter case can be expected to be weaker than those observed for *Dictyostelium*. Therefore they may be more difficult to measure in a multi-cellular organism, particularly because there is a relatively high background of intracellular cyclic nucleotides.

This chapter will almost exclusively deal with cAMP-mediated communication between *Dictyostelium* cells, which is the only well-studied case of cyclic nucleotides acting as a first messenger. Attention will be paid particularly to the molecular aspects of the *Dictyostelium* system, which can be dissected in to the following steps: a) generation of the cAMP signal, involving a transient activation of the enzyme adenylate cyclase; b) reception of the signal by cell surface receptors that are specific for cAMP; c) transfer of information from the cell membrane to various intracellular systems that are responsible for (i) chemotaxis, (ii) cAMP production and secretion, and (iii) cell development (these processes probably involve cyclic nucleotides as second messengers); and d) signal destruction by extracellular and cell surface bound cyclic nucleotide phosphodiesterase. It is hoped that this review which covers the literature through August, 1979, will stimulate workers using other organisms to investigate whether cyclic nucleotides are used more commonly as first messengers in other developmental systems.

A. Intercellular Communication by cAMP Signals

I. Cyclic Nucleotides and the Cellular Slime Molds

Cyclic nucleotides are thought to play a central role in the control of cellular processes. This volume gives ample evidence for this. In almost all cases studied so far, the action of these small molecules is confined to the intracellular space. It is well established that cyclic nucleotides function as secondary messengers, transmitting into cells signals that are received by the cell surface. However, as we will see in this chapter, cAMP can also play a role in *inter*cellular communication, acting as a primary messenger. The cAMP secreted by certain cells, diffuses to others, is recognized by specific receptors, and elicits response in the recipient cells.

Although there are indications that extracellular cAMP plays such a role in other organisms (see Sect. E), a first messenger function is well-established only in certain cellular slime molds, particularly *Dictyostelium discoideum*. Most of this review will therefore be concerned with this organism. Recent research in this field has strongly emphasized the regulatory role of cyclic nucleotides in chemotaxis, cell development, and cell differentiation (see, also, the chapter by McMAHON on Cyclic Nucleotides in Development).

Cellular slime molds are relatively simple, eukaryotic organisms. The single amoeboid cells live in the soil. They show a fascinating behavioural pattern and are able to aggregate into a multicellular organism in a highly controlled way. This process is to a large extent governed by fluctuating extra- and intracellular cyclic nucleotide levels. A comprehensive introduction into the field has been written by LOOMIS (1975).

Micrographs of *Dictyostelium discoideum* in the single cell stage and during aggregation are shown in Fig. 1. The life cycle of *D. discoideum* is depicted in Fig. 2. During periods when sufficient nutrients, mainly bacteria, are available, the cells live and divide as independent, single cell units (Fig. 1 a). A most remarkable change in behavior occurs after food resources have been used up and the cells begin to starve. Within a few hours, aggregation centers are formed that attract surrounding cells (Fig. 1 b, c). The aggregation territories are large and can be over 2 cm in diameter. A single aggregate, called a pseudo-plasmodium, can contain up to 10^5 cells. In the multicellular state, the behaviour of the amoebae becomes more social, as is shown by their coordinated response (as a pseudo-plasmodium) to external stimuli like temperature, light, and chemoattractants. At a later developmental stage, the initially identical cells differentiate into stalk cells and spores. The former build the stalk of the slender fruiting body, the head of which carries the spores. Spores are resistant to fairly harsh environmental conditions and are able to germinate if favourable conditions are encountered, giving rise to single amoeboid cells (Fig. 2).

These at first sight peculiar properties have attracted attention because they involve several fundamental aspects of cell behavior, including (i) intercellular communication, (ii) chemotaxis, (iii) cell development, (iv) formation of specific cell-cell contacts, and (v) pattern formation. Because the cellular slime mold is a relatively simple organism and can be cultured relatively easely in the laboratory, it is an attractive object for studying these basic phenomena. Slime mold control mechanisms involve cyclic nucleotide signals both outside and inside the cell. Although

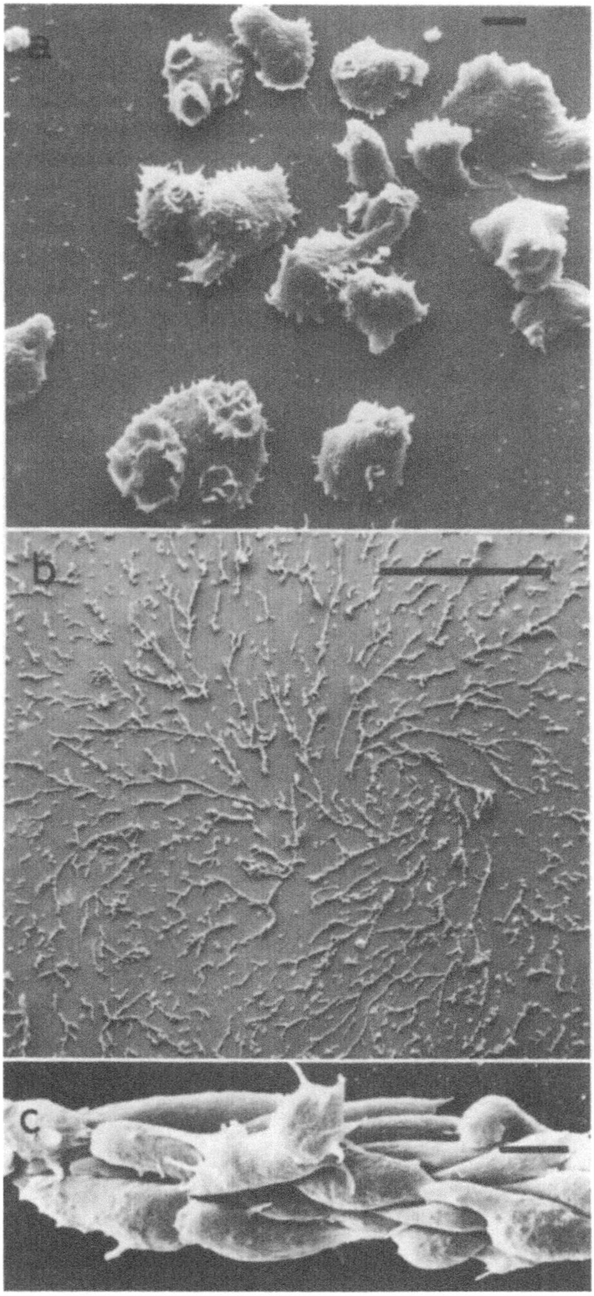

Fig. 1 a–c. Scanning electron micrographs of *Dictyostelium discoideum* cells: **a** vegetative cells; **b, c** starving cells that are beginning to aggregate. Note that the cells move in streams to an aggregation center which is located about in the middle of micrograph b. In **c**, part of such a stream of cells is shown at higher magnification. The scale bars represent 1 μm in **a** and **c**, and 100 μm in **b**. (The micrographs were kindly provided by Dr. G. GERISCH)

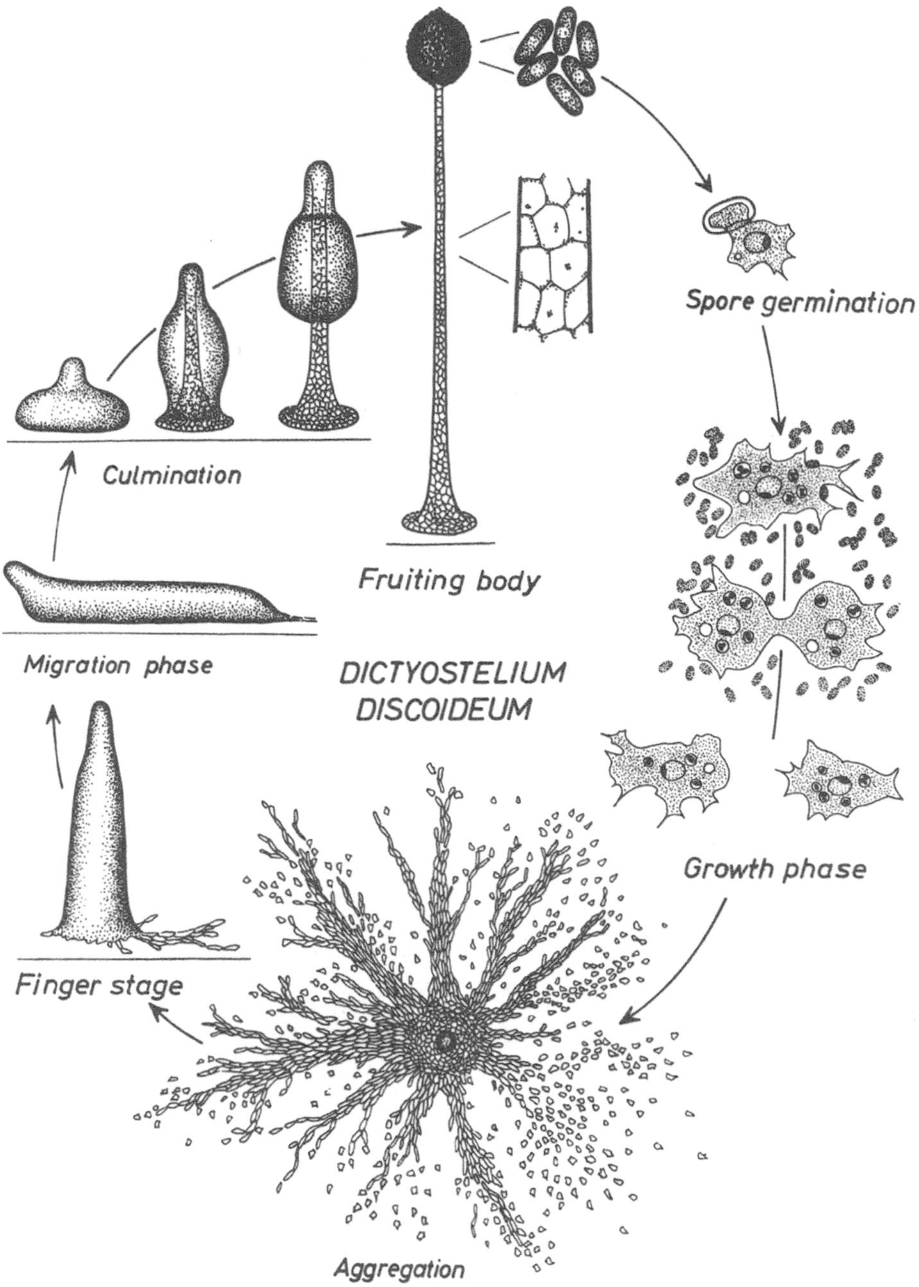

Fig. 2. Schematic representation of the life cycle of *Dictyostelium discoideum*. After growth has stopped, due to the lack of nutrients, the cells start to aggregate and form a pseudo-plasmodium that contains up to 10^5 cells. The aggregate is subsequently transformed into a fruiting body that is 1–2 mm high and produces about 7×10^4 spores. The spores can germinate and give rise to single amoeboid cells. (GERISCH 1980)

Table 1. Recent reviews concerning cellular slime molds

Topic	Reference
Regulation of enzyme activity during differentiation	KILLICH and WRIGHT (1974)
General introduction	LOOMIS (1975)
Biochemical and molecular aspects of development	SUSSMAN and BRACKENBURY (1976)
cAMP and the control of cell aggregation	GERISCH and MALCHOW (1976)
Cell adhesion	ROSEN and BARONDES (1978)
Genetics of cellular slime molds	JACOBSON and LODISH (1975); NEWELL (1978)
Cell aggregation and development	DARMON and BRACHET (1978); LOOMIS (1979); NEWELL (1979)
Pattern formation in the pseudoplasmodium	MACWILLIAMS and BONNER (1979)

this review will stress the role of extracellular cAMP, one has to keep in mind that primary and secondary messenger functions are intimately related and often tightly coupled. Several recent reviews that deal with various aspects of the slime mold systems are listed in Table 1.

II. cAMP Signals Elicit a Chemotactic Response, Can be Relayed and are Involved in Cell Development

In this section we will present a brief overview of the cell aggregation process and show that pulsatile cAMP signals are involved in chemotaxis and development. In this first few hours after the onset of starvation, which triggers developmental changes, cells remain single and continue their non-oriented, random movement (POTEL and MACKAY 1979). Aggregation centers are then formed, and these centers attract surrounding cells by emitting a diffusable chemotactic factor, originally called acrasin. The aggregation centers consist of cells that have acquired the developmentally controlled ability to autonomously release attractant into the medium. KONIJN et al. (1967, 1969) found that cAMP in the nanomolar range acts as an efficient chemoattractant for *Dictyostelium discoideum* amoebae. ROBERTSON et al. (1972) showed that the function of an aggregation center can be mimicked by electrophoretically released cAMP. This suggests that the naturally emitted attractant is cAMP.

Cells are attracted towards the aggregation center over distances of more than 1 cm. It is very unlikely that cAMP itself can diffuse over such distances, because the molecule is hydrolyzed by cyclic nucleotide phosphodiesterases that are present in the extra-cellular medium (see Sect. B IV). To overcome this problem certain slime mold species have developed a fascinating cell communication system which does not require physical contact between the amoebae. Cells on a solid substrate move towards an aggregation center in a pulsatile way (ARNDT 1937; BONNER 1944; ALCANTARA and MONK 1974). SHAFFER (1957) first suggested that this periodic behaviour could be due to the emission of pulses of attractant by the aggregation center, combined with a relay of the signal by surrounding cells. Later work has justified this hypothesis. ROBERTSON et al. (1972) showed that electrophoretically re-

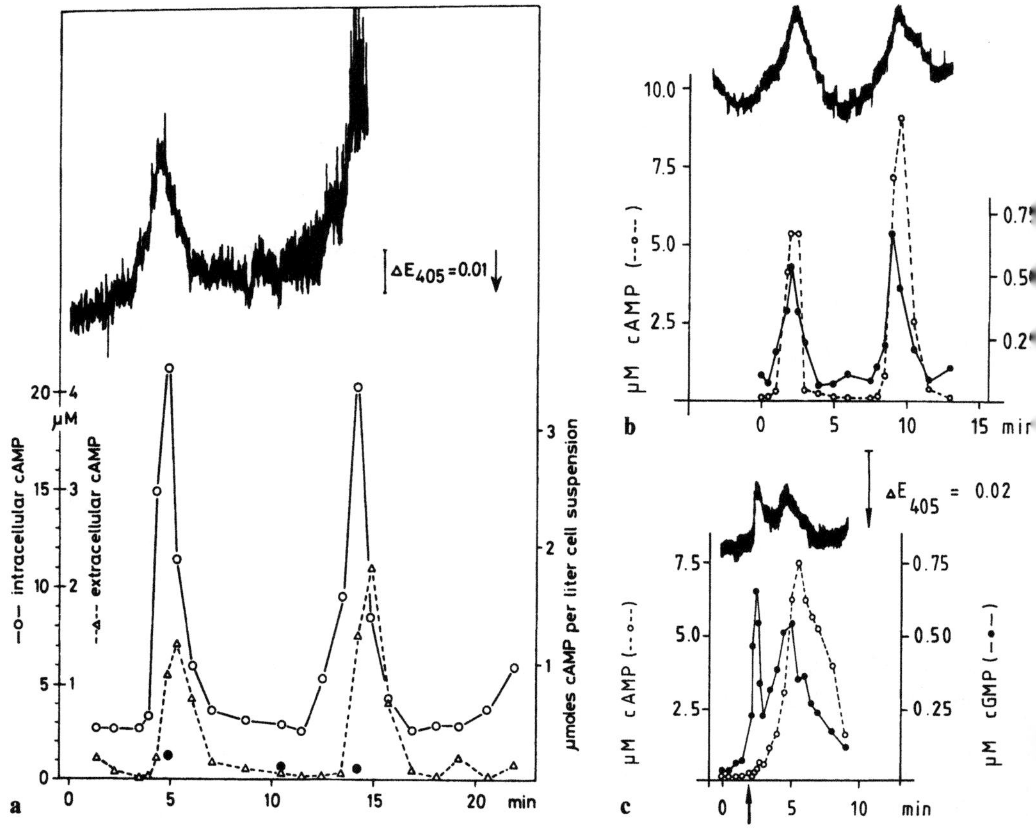

Fig. 3 a–c. Periodic changes in light scattering, measured at 405 nm, and oscillations of cAMP and cGMP concentrations in a suspension of starving *Dictyostelium discoideum* cells. **a** Spontaneous oscillation of intracellular and extracellular cAMP (GERISCH and WICK 1975). **b** Spontaneous oscillations of cAMP and cGMP, both in phase with changes in optical density (WURSTER et al. 1977). **c** A transient change in (i) optical density, (ii) cAMP, and (iii) cGMP is induced by a pulse of exogenous cAMP (5 n*M* final concentration), added at the time indicated by the arrow (WURSTER et al. 1977). Cyclic nucleotide concentrations are given in micromoles per liter cell sediment, except on the right ordinate in **a**

leased pulses of cAMP in a field of aggregating cells give rise to the same pattern of periodic cell movement as found around a natural aggregation center. This observation suggests that the aggregation center also emits pulsatile cAMP signals. The period of the signals is on the order of 4 to 10 min.

The cells in the aggregation territory relay the cAMP signal; in other words, a cell that is stimulated by a pulse of cAMP responds by emitting its own cAMP pulse. By this means, the cell amplifies the received signal and stimulates cells farther away from the aggregation center. These cells, in turn, relay the signal still farther. In this way, signals can travel through the aggregation territory.

ALCANTARA and MONK (1974) showed that the effective range of an emitted cAMP pulse is about 60 µm. At larger distances the pulse becomes ineffective because the cAMP is detroyed by extracellular phosphodiesterase. Because a cell emits a signal about 10 s after it has been stimulated, the rate of signal propagation is about 360 µm min^{-1} (ALCANTARA and MONK 1974). Thus roughly 30 min are required for the repeatedly relayed signal to travel from an aggregation center to the edge of an aggregation territory with a radius of 1 cm. The signal is transmitted exclusively outward. This appears to be due to a short refractory period, which occurs immediately after stimulation, during which the cell is insensitive to a second stimulus. This mechanism ensures a chemotactic movement in the direction of the aggregation center only.

So far we have described the cAMP-controlled aggregation behaviour of cells on a solid support. A molecular approach towards understanding this mechanism has been greatly facilitated by the observation of GERISCH and HESS (1974) that stirred cell suspensions develop the ability to produce regulator oscillations in optical density a few hours after the beginning of starvation (Fig. 3 b). The period is about 8 min, which is similar to that of aggregation centers on a solid support. Moreover, GERISCH and WICK (1975) found peaks of intra- and extracellular cAMP associated with the periodic optical density changes (Fig. 3 a). This is direct evidence that cells are able to emit periodic cAMP signals into the extracellular medium. In addition, starving cells, that are not yet able to pulse autonomously, respond to the addition of exogenous cAMP (nanomolar range) with an often biphasic, transient change in optical density and the secretion of a pulse of cAMP, as shown in Fig. 3 c (ROOS et al. 1975; WURSTER et al. 1977).

The biochemical equipment that the cells need for the generation and relay of cAMP signals is developmentally controlled. After initiation of development by starvation, the cAMP pulses, themselves, stimulate and speed up the expression of the gene products that are required for signal relay (Fig. 4; see Sect. D). In this respect, the system acts in an autocatalytic way. cAMP pulses also stimulate the developmentally controlled appearance of certain intercellular contact sites (contact sites A) (GERISCH et al. 1975a; MÜLLER et al. 1979). These are important for the formation of the multicellular organism. All this together constitutes a remarkably efficient aggregation system that enables the cells to form an organism in which up to 10^5 cells can respond in a coordinated way to external stimuli, differentiate into stalk cells and spores, and form a fruiting body.

B. Biochemical Aspects of the cAMP Signal Generating System

I. Introduction

In the previous section we have seen that pulses of extracellular cAMP play an important role in cell aggregation by acting as a chemoattractant and a stimulant for developmental processes. Signals can be propagated over long distances by a relay system that: (i) perceives the signal by cell surface cAMP receptors, (ii) responds by synthesizing and secreting a pulse of cAMP, and (iii) destroys extracellular cAMP to reduce the signal-to-noise ratio. Bits and pieces of the interwined networks that are responsible for chemotaxis, signal relay and development are now emerging from experiments at the molecular level. In this section we will discuss biochemical aspects of the relay system. Several of the elements that are discussed here may also act in chemotaxis and developmental control.

II. Cell Surface Receptors for cAMP

Extracellular cAMP signals are received by highly specific receptors. The following evidence indicates that the receptors are located on the outer cell surface and that cAMP does not have to pass through the plasma membrane for cell stimulation: (i) intact cells have saturable high affinity cAMP binding sites (see below); (ii) the cell membrane appears to be impermeable to cAMP (MOENS and KONIJN 1974); (iii) cell bound, labeled cAMP is rapidly displaced by an excess of unlabeled nucleotide (MULLENS and NEWELL 1978), and (iv) dibutyryl-cAMP, which is supposed to pass more easily through the cytoplasmic membrane because it is more lipophylic than cAMP, is a poor attractant (KONIJN 1972). The ultimate proof for the existence of a cell surface receptor will be the isolation of a polypeptide which specifically binds cAMP and is exposed on the cell surface.

The chemotactic receptor is highly specific for cAMP. KONIJN (1972, 1973) and KONIJN and JASTORFF (1973) showed that any substitution in the base or the ribose moiety reduces chemotactic activity dramatically. For instance, cyclic GMP (cGMP) and cyclic IMP (cIMP) are 10^3 to 10^4 times less active than cAMP. (Only substitutions of the 5′C-linked oxygen of the ribose by nitrogen or carbon are tolerated.) Based on the relative chemotactic activity of about 50 cAMP-analogues, MATO et al. (1978a) proposed a model for the cAMP-receptor interaction in which specificity is thought to be due to five specific contacts between cAMP and the receptor. Several groups have studied the binding of cAMP to intact cells (MALCHOW and GERISCH 1973, 1974; GREEN and NEWELL 1975; HENDERSON 1975; MATO and KONIJN 1975; MULLENS and NEWELL 1978). A major technical problem with which these studies have had to contend with is the presence of cyclic nucleotide phosphodiesterases on the cell surface and in the extracellular medium (see Sect. B IV.).

The appearance of cell surface cAMP receptors is developmentally controlled (Fig. 4b). A maximum of between 10^5 and 5×10^5 binding sites per cell has been found in aggregating cells, whereas vegetative cells bind very little or no cAMP (MALCHOW and GERISCH 1973, 1974; GREEN and NEWELL 1975; HENDERSON 1975). The binding studies of GREEN and NEWELL (1975) and MULLENS and NEWELL (1978) indicate a marked heterogeneity of binding sites; Scatchard plots suggest the existence of 0.1 to 0.2×10^5 high affinity sites ($K_D = 9$ n*M*) and roughly 2×10^5 low affinity sites ($K_D = 200$ n*M*), as shown in Fig. 5. MALCHOW and GERISCH (1974) found about 4×10^5 binding sites with a K_D of 150–200 n*M*. This study probably did not detect the high affinity sites because it was conducted in the presence of high concentrations of cGMP to suppress phosphodiesterase activity.

Are these binding activities identical to the cAMP receptors involved in chemotaxis, signal relay and the stimulation of development? cAMP acts as an attractant at concentrations less than 1 n*M* (KONIJN 1972). Concentrations as low as 0.1 n*M* cAMP elicit a cAMP secretory response (DEVREOTES and STECK 1979), and 1 n*M* cAMP pulses stimulate development (YEH et al. 1978). This suggests that the high affinity sites ($K_D = 9$ n*M*) are involved in chemotaxis, signal relay and developmental control. However, because the cells can be stimulated over a wide cAMP concentration range, up to 10^{-5} *M* (DEVREOTES and STECK 1979), the low affinity binding sites ($K_D = 100$–200 n*M*) probably play a role too. Both the low and the high affinity sites are specific for cAMP (GREEN and NEWELL 1975). An-

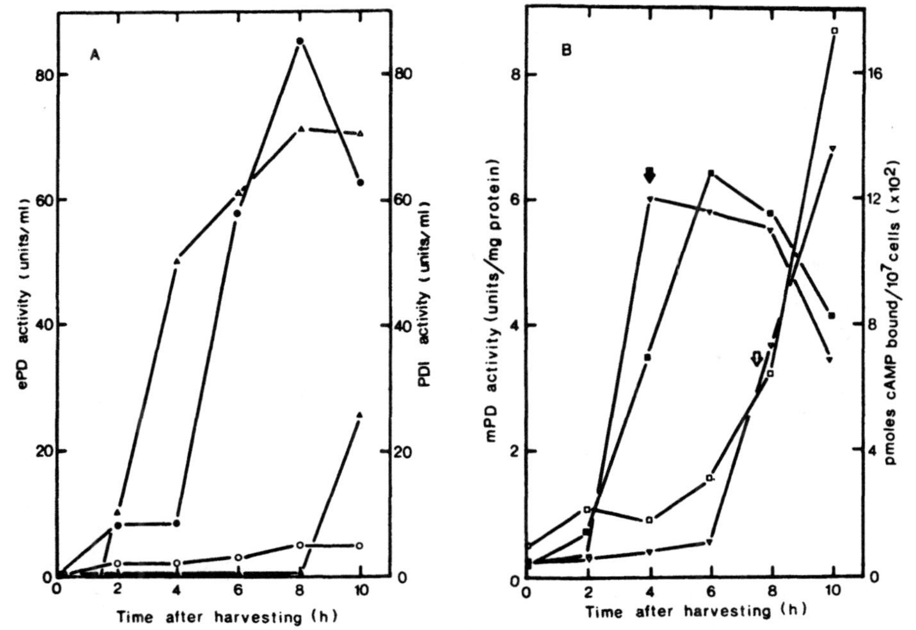

Fig. 4. Exogenous pulses of cAMP stimulate the expression of the developmentally controlled activities of extracellular phosphodiesterase (○, ●), membrane bound phosphodiesterase (▽, ▼) and cell surface cAMP binding sites (□, ■). At the same time the expression of the inhibitor of extracellular phosphodiesterase is suppressed (△, ▲). (*Open symbols* refer to untreated cells, *filled symbols* to cells that received a 100 m*M* cAMP pulse each 5 min) The time after the onset of starvation of the *Dictyostelium discoideum* cells is indicated on the horizontal axis. (YEH et al. 1978)

other argument that the same set of cAMP receptors is involved in signal relay and the control of cell development is that the number of cell surface binding sites is developmentally controlled and reaches a maximum value during the period of full aggregation competence, i.e. when the signal relay system works optimally (Fig. 4b). In conclusion, it seems that chemotaxis, signal relay, and development are all controlled via very similar if not identical cell surface receptors for cAMP.

KLEIN and JULIANI (1977) demonstrated that the number of cAMP binding sites decreased following incubation with relatively high cAMP concentrations (10^{-6} to 10^{-3} *M*). This treatment did not appear to change the receptor affinity. After removal of cAMP, the binding activity reappeared. This reversible effect was not inhibited by cycloheximide, suggesting that protein synthesis was not involved. Such desensitization or down-regulation has been observed for several hormone receptors in mammalian cells. However, considering the high, nonphysiological cAMP concentrations that are required in the slime mold, it remains doubtful whether desensitization is a useful control mechanism in *Dictyostelium*.

III. Synthesis and Secretion of cAMP

The enzyme adenylate cyclase, which catalyzes the conversion of ATP into cAMP and pyrophosphate, is a key element in the cAMP signal relay mechanism. Its basal

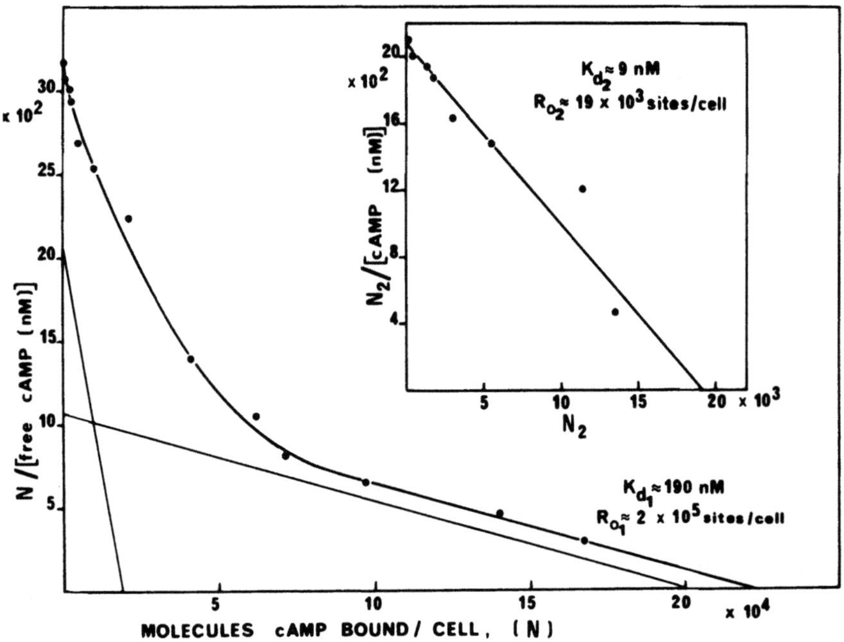

Fig. 5. Scatchard plot of cAMP binding activity of intact *Dictyostelium discoideum* cells, 9.5 h after the onset of starvation. The results indicate that there are per cell about 0.2×10^5 high affinity sites ($K_D = 9 \times 10^{-9}$ *M*) and 2×10^5 low affinity sites ($K_D = 190 \times 10^{-9}$ *M*). The inset shows a scatchard plot which results when the experimental points at low cAMP concentrations (less than 30 n*M*) are corrected for the contribution of the low affinity sites. (GREEN and NEWELL 1975)

activity increases during development (KLEIN 1976; ROOS et al. 1977b). Furthermore, the enzyme is rapidly activated about 10-fold when aggregating cells are stimulated by a cAMP pulse (ROOS et al. 1977b). Activation is transient and lasts 2–4 min (Fig. 6b). A similar, periodic increase in enzyme activity is observed in cells that autonomously produce cAMP pulses (ROOS et al. 1977a), as shown in Fig. 6a.

Theoretical, allosteric models have been forwarded to explain the relationship between enzyme activation during relay and autonomous pulsations (COHEN 1977, 1978; GOLDBETER and SEGEL 1977). Discussion of these models is, however, beyond the scope of this review.

There is cytochemical evidence that adenylate cyclase is located on the inner surface of the plasma membrane (FARNHAM 1975; ROSSOMANDO and CUTLER 1975; CUTLER and ROSSOMANDO 1975). This location makes a direct interaction between receptor and enzyme in the plane of the membrane possible, analogous to what is found for other systems (see, for a recent review, FAIN 1978). However, because there is often a lag of about 30–60 s between cell stimulation and cAMP synthesis (e.g. see Fig. 3c), it may also be that second messengers or protein modification are involved. In Sect. C, fast cellular responses to cAMP stimulation that precede cAMP production will be discussed. KLEIN (1976) and LOOMIS et al. (1978) showed that *Dictyostelium* adenylate cyclase is inhibited by Ca^{++} ions at concentrations in the millimolar range. In other cell types, Ca^{++} ions are known to activate the en-

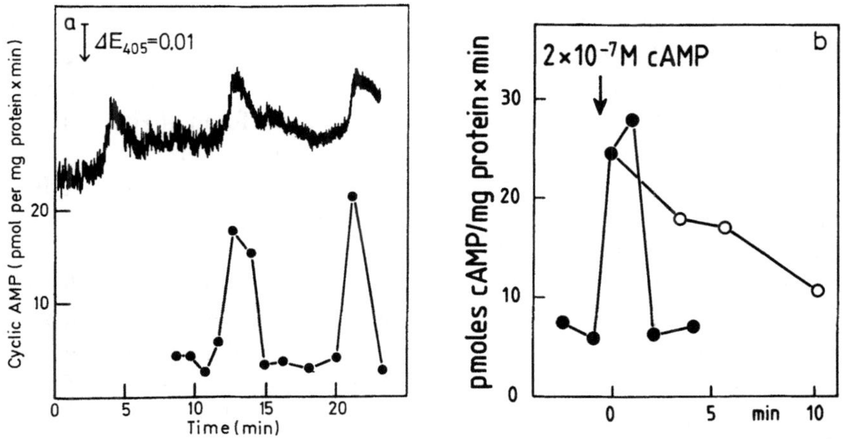

Fig. 6 a, b. A transient activation of adenylate cyclase in starving *Dictyostelium discoideum* cells can occur spontaneously and periodically **a** or can be induced by a pulse of exogenous cAMP **b**. Immediately after taking a sample from the cell suspension, the cells are lysed and the enzyme activity is measured *(Filled circles)*. If the lysate is stored at 0 °C, the enzyme activity decays rapidly (*open circles* in **b**). (Roos et al. 1977 a, b)

zyme at low concentrations while higher concentrations sometimes inhibit [see Rasmussen and Goodman (1977) for a review]. Activation may involve the calcium-dependent regulator (calmodulin) (Brostrom et al. 1975), a protein that mediates Ca^{++} sensitivity to several other enzymes. Such a protein has also been found in *Dictyostelium* cells (Clarke et al. 1980). Thus it is conceivable that Ca^{++}ions are involved in the control of adenylate cyclase activity in *Dictyostelium*. It may also be that inactivation by Ca^{++}ions is responsible for the instability of the activated state of adenylate cyclase in lysates, as was observed by Roos et al. (1977 a, b) and is illustrated in Fig. 5b. Loomis et al. (1978) showed that millimolar concentrations of Mn^{++}ions overcome the inhibitory effect of Ca^{++}ions. This finding may make possible an investigation of the molecular mechanisms that switch this key enzyme on and off.

Recently, Devreotes et al. (1979) and Devreotes and Steck (1979), in a very careful study, showed that the magnitude of the relay response depends on the magnitude of the stimulus. The stimulated state requires the persistent presence of the stimulant cAMP, but is limited to a maximum of about 4 min. Although this conclusion is based on measurement of cAMP secretion rather than adenylate cyclase activity, these observations may tell us that the enzyme is in the activated state only as long as the receptor is occupied. The number of activated enzyme molecules, assuming one low and one high activity state, apparently depends on the number of cAMP-receptor complexes. The simplest explanation for this correlation would be a direct receptor-adenylate cyclase interaction. This control mechanism is overridden by an adaptation process that reduces the sensitivity of the cell to external cAMP stimuli. The rate of adaptation then determines the maximum response time which seems to be independent of the magnitude of the stimulus. Adaptation explains why the cell responds only to an increase of cAMP concentration and not to constant stimulant levels. In bacterial cells, adaptation is tightly linked to carboxy-0-methylation of certain cell proteins (for a review see SPRINGER et al. 1979). Nuske has shown that cAMP stimulation triggers a very rapid, transient methylation of *Dictyostelium* macromolecules (personal communication). Such a rapid time course, however, supports a role for methylation in the signal transduction process in the cell rather than in adaptation.

What is the mechanism of cAMP secretion? The localization of adenylate cyclase on the inner side of the plasma membrane (FARNHAM 1975; CUTLER and ROSSOMANDO 1975) suggests that the enzyme reaction may be vectorial in the sense that substrate (ATP) is taken up on the inside and cAMP is released at the outside of the cell. Two pieces of evidence speak against this. Firstly, measurement of the time dependence of intra- and extracellular cAMP levels of autonomously oscillating cells shows that a peak of intracellular cAMP slightly precedes that of extracellular cAMP (Fig. 3a) (GERISCH and WICK 1975). This indicates an accumulation in the cell before secretion. Secondly, ultrastructural studies of MAEDA and GERISCH (1977) indicate a transient increase in cytoplasmic vesicles that parallels cAMP production. This result suggests a mechanism by which newly synthesized cAMP is first accumulated in vesicles and then secreted by exocytosis. In some ways this is analogous with the cholinergic synapse, in which the transmitter acetylcholine is stored in presynaptic vesicles and is secreted by exocytosis. An important difference is, however, that under most conditions the synaptic vesicles store acetylcholine over long periods, whereas in *Dictyostelium* cAMP is synthesized immediately before secretion. Such a secretory mechanism appears, cyclase on the inside of the plasma membrane.

IV. Destruction of the cAMP Signal

In the previous sections, we have seen that pulses of extracellular cAMP control cell aggregation by affecting both chemotaxis and development. Because the cells respond to a relative increase in extracellular cAMP level rather than to an absolute one (DEVREOTES and STECK 1979), it is important for *Dictyostelium* to keep the background low. This is achieved by producing extracellular cyclic nucleotide phosphodiesterase (PDE). Cell populations are able to control the average extracellular cAMP level using feedback loops in which an increased extracellular nucleotide concentration leads to an increase in extracellular PDE activity. It is clear that the activity must not become too high, otherwise the cAMP signal itself would be destroyed. For this reason, a complex, highly controlled system has evolved. Elements of this system are: (i) membrane bound phosphodiesterase (mPDE) (PANNBACKER and BRAVARD 1972; MALCHOW et al. 1972) located at the outer cell surface (FARNHAM 1975); (ii) soluble, extracellular phosphodiesterase (ePDE) (PANNBACKER and BRAVARD 1972); and (iii) an extracellular, soluble phosphodiesterase inhibitor (RIEDEL et al. 1972).

The role of the mPDE may be to steepen the local cAMP gradient near the cell surface (MALCHOW et al. 1975; NANJUNDIAH and MALCHOW 1976). The ePDE is probably important for keeping the background cAMP level low. Mutants that are unable to hydrolyze extracellular cAMP are unable to aggregate. This block can be overcome by adding PDE to the medium (DARMON et al. 1978). Thus ePDE, rather than mPDE, may participate in aggregation. The inhibitor acts on the ePDE; the mPDE is not affected (RIEDEL et al. 1972). The latter, however, becomes sensitive upon detergent solubilization (MALCHOW et al. 1975). Both enzymes show similarly low K_m values in the micromolar range, and have the same substrate specificity. They hydrolize cAMP and cGMP about equally well (MALCHOW et al. 1973). This raises the question about the relationship between mPDE and ePDE. Both activities are controlled differently during development, suggesting that the enzymes are products of two different genes. In developing cells, mPDE and ePDE are induced by pulses of cAMP, as are the cAMP receptors (Fig. 4). Constant, elevated cAMP levels are inhibitory for mPDE expression (YEH et al. 1978), but stimulate ePDE activity as cAMP pulses do (KLEIN 1975; KLEIN and DARMON 1977; YEH et al. 1978; C. ROSSIER and G. GERISCH, unpublished work). The cAMP-induced increase in ePDE activity is due either to repression of ePDE-inhibitor synthesis or release and de novo synthesis of ePDE (TSANG and COUKELL 1977, 1979a, b). This dual regulatory mechanism enables the cell to fine-control ePDE activity and maintain a high signal to noise ratio. Induction of PDE activities and inhibitor suppression do not require cAMP hydrolysis. A slowly hydrolyzed cAMP-analogue is a good inducer as well (ROSSIER et al. 1978; C. ROSSIER and G. GERISCH, unpublished work). Therefore, the feedback loops most probably involve the cell-surface cAMP receptor described in Sect. B II.

In contrast to the very limited information we have about the mPDE molecule, quite a lot is known about ePDE (Table 2). TSANG and COUKELL (1979a, b) have isolated ePDE and its inhibitor from *Dictyostelium purpureum*. Two enzymes were found, one is produced during vegatative growth, another appears early during development. Since the enzymes have different peptide maps, they are probably not related. The former enzyme has a molecular weight of 60,000, the latter of about 50,000. Their isoelectric points are 8.5 and 7.5, respectively. Both have broad pH optima and show K_m values around 5 μM. Such K_m's have been found by most other investigators for *Dictyostelium* ePDE's (Table 2). This K_m-value is remarkably low compared to the classical beef heart enzyme that has a K_m of about 100 μM (BUTCHER and SUTHERLAND 1962). Activity measurements of ePDE are often somewhat difficult because of the presence of inhibitor. The inhibitor usually causes curved Lineweaver-Burk plots (RIEDEL et al. 1972), because the K_m of the enzyme-inhibitor complex is in the millimolar range (KESSIN et al. 1979). The inhibitor of *Dictyostelium purpureum* ePDE is an acidic protein (pI about 4) with a molecular weight of 50,000 (TSANG and COUKELL 1979b). DICOU and BRACHET (1979) found, in supernatant fluids of *Dictyostelium discoideum* cultures that had been starved for very long times (36 h), there ePDE activities with isoelectric points (pI) of 4.6, 6.5, and 8.3. The first two may occur in at least two aggregation states. It seems likely that the two with the highest pI's correspond to those found in *Dictyostelium purpureum*. A puzzling observation was made by KESSIN et al. (1979), who found that ePDE's induced by starvation in the absence and in the presence of cAMP have largely different isoelectric points (Table 2).

It remains to be seen to what extent the multiple enzyme activities found by DICOU and BRACHET (1979) and KESSIN et al. (1979) are real or reflect preparation artifacts. It may be, for instance, that complexes between the enzyme and its very acidic inhibitor are responsible for some forms with low isoelectric points. The relatively high sedimentation constants (Table 2), compared to the monomeric molecular weight of 50 to 60 $\times 10^3$ suggests that the enzyme occurs in one or more oligomeric forms which may be an additional source of heterogeneity.

Table 2. Properties of purified extracellular cyclic nucleotide phosphodiesterase and its inhibitor

Organism	Protein	Molecular weight	Sedimentation constant (S)	Iso-electric point	K_m for cAMP (μM)	Isolated after	Reference
D. purpureum	ePDE	60,000	–	8.5	10	Late exponential phase	TSANG and COUKELL (1979b)
		50,000	–	7.5	10		
	Inhibitor	50,000	–	4.0	–	12 h starvation	TSANG and COUKELL (1979b)
D. discoideum	ePDE	–	5.4	8.3	–	36 h starvation	DICOU and BRACHET (1979)
		–	5.4/9.7	6.5	–		
		–	5.4/9.7	4.6	–		
		–	–	–	4	4 h starvation	RIEDEL et al. (1972)
		–	6	8.5	10	12 h starvation (+exogenous cAMP pulses)	KESSIN et al. (1979)
		–	6	4.2	10	12 h starvation (no cAMP addition)	
	Inhibitor	50,000	3	–	–	12 h starvation	
	ePDE-inhibitor complex	–	6.7	–	1,300	–	

C. Transduction of cAMP Signals in the Cell

I. Introduction

Extracellular cAMP signals are transduced in the *Dictyostelium* cell to at least three intracellular systems: (i) the signal relay system, where an increase in receptor occupancy results in a transient activation of adenylate cyclase and cAMP secretion (Sect. B. III), (ii) the chemotactic system, implying a connection between receptor and the acto-myosin system, and (ii) the nucleus, where developmental processes are presumably controlled. Because the stimulatory cAMP signal does not seem to cross the plasma membrane, second messengers may transfer information from the receptor to these systems. It is for the moment unclear to what extent the three pathways overlap. This section will summarize some evidence that cyclic nucleotides and Ca^{++}ions are involved. RASMUSSEN and GOODMAN (1977) have discussed possible relationships between these two substances in signal transduction pathways in cell types other than cellular slime molds.

II. Cyclic Nucleotides as Possible Second Messengers

In many cells the role of cAMP as a second messenger is well established. Although most cAMP that is synthesized upon cAMP stimulation of *Dictyostelium* cells is secreted for signal relay, it is quite possible that some of this nucleotide plays an intracellular role (probably in another cell compartment than the bulk of the cAMP). Supporting such a view is the observation that the basal level of intracellular cAMP increases during development (MALKINSON and ASHWORTH 1973; KLEIN and BRACHET 1975; BRENNER 1978); arguments that this cAMP is required for developmentally controlled gene expression will be summarized in Sect. D. I. In addition, several soluble cAMP binding activities have been found in *Dictyostelium* cells (SAMPSON 1977; RAHMSDORF and GERISCH 1978). Photoaffinity labeling with ^{32}P-labeled 8-azido-cAMP (HALEY 1975) reveals at least two cAMP binding proteins in whole cell lysates (R. VAN DRIEL, unpublished work), and SAMPSON (1977) found two cAMP-dependent protein kinase activities in developing cells. This latter result could not, however, be reproduced by others (RAHMSDORF and GERISCH 1978; RAHMSDORF and PAI 1979).

Cyclic GMP may also play an important messenger in *Dictyostelium*. After stimulation by cAMP, there is an immediate, short burst of cGMP, followed, about 3 min later, by a second broader cGMP peak, as shown in Fig. 3c (MATO et al. 1977; WURSTER et al. 1977, 1978). In spontaneously oscillating cell suspensions, cGMP is transiently synthesized in phase with cAMP production (Fig. 3b; WURSTER et al. 1977). Unlike cAMP, cGMP is not secreted. The fast cGMP response is also induced by exposure of cells to other chemo-attractants, like folic acid (WURSTER et al. 1977, 1978); thereby suggesting a role for cGMP in chemotaxis. A terminal step in this signal transduction pathway may be the rapid phosphorylation of the myosin heavy chain upon cell stimulation, as found by RAHMSDORF et al. (1978). No cGMP stimulated protein kinase activity has been found, however (MATO et al. 1978b; RAHMSDORF and PAI 1979), suggesting that additional components may be involved in signal transduction. On the other hand, the kinase may be myosin-specific and may have remained undetected because histone and casein were used as exogenous sustrates.

Cyclic AMP stimulated cGMP synthesis is due to a transient activation of the guanylate cyclase enzyme (Mato and Malchow 1978). As has been found for adenylate cyclase, the activated state decays rapidly after homogenization, and guanylate cyclase cannot be activated in vitro (Mato and Malchow 1978). Mato (1979) showed that ATP (0.1–2 m*M*) stimulates the enzyme by lowering the K_M for GTP from 1.0–0.2 m*M*. Nonhydrolyzable ATP-analogues had no effect. Because these experiments were carried out with crude extracts, it is unclear whether ATP interacts directly with guanylate cyclase. The very rapid activation of guanylate cyclase upon stimulation of the intact cell with cAMP precedes adenylate cyclase activation (see Fig. 3c) and suggests a very close linkage, possibly a physical contact, between receptor and enzyme.

III. Ca^{++} Ions as a Second Messenger

Ca^{++}ions have been implicated in almost all of the processes discussed in the previous sections. However, published results are often contradictory with respect to the effects of Ca^{++}ions. The only direct measurements have been made by Wick et al. (1978). These authors showed that cell stimulation by cAMP leads to a rapid, transient influx of Ca^{++}ions during the first minute after stimulation. However, extracellular Ca^{++} is not required for signal relay because the Ca^{++} chelating agent, EGTA, does not inhibit cAMP-stimulated cAMP production (Gerisch et al. 1975b). As suggested by Darmon and Brachet (1978), it may be that a primary effect of cAMP stimulation is a rapid translocation of Ca^{++}ions between different intracellular pools. A subsequent, possibly passive, filling of a depleted pool by extracellular Ca^{++} may be what has been measured by Wick et al. (1978). Such an explanation is attractive in the light of recent work of Loomis et al. (1978), showing that adenylate cyclase is reversibly inhibited by Ca^{++}ions.

D. Extracellular cAMP Controlled Developmental Changes

I. Changes During Cell Aggregation

Starvation is the primary event that initiates development and differentiation in slime mold cells (Marin 1976; Darmon and Klein 1978). Although early developmental effects are certainly speeded up by pulses of cAMP, it is hard to prove that development absolutely requires cAMP-mediated cell communication. One wonders whether pulses per se are necessary for communication or whether a continuous increase in receptor occupancy by a positive temporal gradient may work as well. Devreotes and Steck (1979) showed that the latter is true for cAMP-dependent cAMP production. They found that cells adapt within a few minutes to a constant stimulant level and become insensitive to it. The available data suggest that a similar adaptation is also true for cAMP stimulation of development, i.e., constant levels of cAMP do not increase the number of cell surface receptors, the activity of membrane-bound phosphodiesterase, or the number of cell contact sites. cAMP pulses may, however, have another important role, i.e., synchronizing the development of cells within an aggregation territory so that they enter the multicellular aggregate in about the same developmental state. This synchronization may be a prerequisite for the formation of a pseudoplasmodium in which cells act in a coördinated way.

There is evidence that elevated intracellular cAMP levels are required for the development of *Dictyostelium* cells. First, the intracellular cAMP concentration has been shown to increase during cell development (MALKINSON and ASHWORTH 1973; KLEIN and BRACHET 1975; BRENNER 1978). Normally, this increase is probably due to an increase in basal adenylate cyclase activity. Second, stimulation of development can be mimicked by incubation of cells in medium that contains an extremely high cAMP concentration (millimolar range) as has been shown by SAMPSON et al. (1978) and KAY et al. (1979). Under these non-physiological conditions, cAMP may leak directly into the cell and increase the intracellular level of the nucleotide.

Other evidence that cyclic nucleotides may be involved in the control of nuclear processes comes from PAN et al. (1974) and PAN and WEDNER (1979), who detected, using immunofluorescence, bound cAMP and cGMP in the nuclear region of various cellular slime molds.

II. Differentiation into Spore and Stalk Cells

As the cells enter the multicellular stage and form the pseudoplasmodium, they are able to respond in a coordinated way to external stimuli such as chemotaxis towards cAMP (MAEDA 1977), phototaxis (LOOMIS 1975), and thermotaxis (LOOMIS 1975). Two other types of cell behaviour observed in the pseudoplasmodium are typical for a multicellular organism: cell differentiation and pattern formation. The posterior part of the slug differentiates into prespore cells which later form spores, and the anterior cells become prestalk cells that later form the stalk of the fruiting body. Prespore and prestalk cells can be discriminated morphologically or by using vital stains (LOOMIS 1975; DURSTON and VORK 1979).

Cell communication mediated by extracellular cAMP is probably important in the multicellular stage, too. The extreme anterior tip of the slug (not to be confused with the prestalk region) is known to direct slug movement. If extra tips are grafted on to the slug, the organism splits up so that each tip leads its own fragment (RUBIN and ROBERTSON 1975). The tip is known to emit cAMP because it can act as an aggregation center in a field of starving cells (MAEDA 1977). Furthermore, pseudoplasmodial cells are attracted by cAMP (MAEDA 1977). This suggests that movement of the slug is directed by cAMP produced by the tip. Recently, DURSTON and VORK (1979) presented that, in the pseudoplasmodial stage, sorting out of prestalk and prespore cells occurs. The prestalk cells are attracted by cAMP and move to the anterior side. Recently MACWILLIAMS and BONNER (1979) published a thorough discussion of three possible mechanisms that could provide the differentiating cells with positional information in the pseudoplasmodium. In this context, it is possible that cAMP acts as a morphogen stimulating cells, located at the side of the cAMP producing tip, to become stalk cells. BRENNER (1977) showed that a front to back cAMP gradient really exists in the slug, although it remains to be seen whether this is a prerequisite for pattern formation, or a consequence of it. The idea that cAMP is a stalk cell morphogen is supported by the observation that high cAMP concentrations induce stalk cell formation (BONNER 1970). However differentiation seems to proceed via a morphologically prespore cell-like state (KAY et al. 1978), suggesting that additional factors are involved.

E. Are There Other Systems That Use cAMP as a Primary Messenger?

Cyclic nucleotide mediated intercellular communication may occur in organisms other than the cellular slime molds. It has been found in the slime mold system probably because the cAMP signals are strong and give rise to periodic cell movements. In tissues where the cells are close together, the signals may be much weaker and, consequently, the concentration of extracellular cyclic AMP may be much lower.

ROBERTSON et al. (1978) have presented evidence that dissociated chick embryo cells rapidly produce cAMP in response to cAMP stimulation, in the concentration range of 10^{-8} to 10^{-6} *M*. Another parallel between early chick embryo and slime mold cells was observed by GINGLE (1977), who showed that reaggregation of plated embryo cells is enhanced by cAMP. Furthermore, ROBERTSON and GINGLE (1977) showed that electrophoretically released exogenous cAMP can bend the developmental longitudinal axis of early chick embryos. The effect is specific for cAMP and may involve chemotaxis. Although there are still many uncertainties, these results point to a role of cAMP in intracellular communication during development of higher organisms.

Acknowledgement. The author is indebted to Drs. R. BERNSTEIN, G. GERISCH, J. NUSKE, C. ROSSIER and C. SUND for critical comments.

References

Alcantara F, Monk M (1974) Signal propagation during aggregation in the slime mold *Dictyostelium discoideum.* J Gen Microbiol 85:321–334

Arndt A (1937) Untersuchungen über *Dictyostelium mucoroides Brefeld.* Wilhelm Roux Arch Entwicklungsmech Org 136:681–774

Bonner JT (1944) A descriptive study of the development of the slime mold *Dictyostelium discoideum.* Am J Bot 31:175–182

Bonner JT (1970) Induction of stalk cell differentiation by cyclic AMP in the cellular slime mold *Dictyostelium discoideum.* Proc Natl Acad Sci USA 65:110–113

Brenner M (1977) Cyclic AMP gradients in migrating pseudoplasmodia of the cellular slime mold *Dictyostelium discoideum.* J Biol Chem 252:4073–4077

Brenner M (1978) Cyclic AMP levels and turnover during development of the cellular slime mold *Dictyostelium discoideum.* Dev Biol 64:210–223

Brostrom CO, Huang YC, Breckenridge B, Wolf DJ (1975) Identification of a calcium-binding protein as a calcium dependent regulator of brain adenylate cyclase. Proc Natl Acad Sci USA 72:64–68

Butcher RW, Sutherland EW (1962) Adenosine 3′,5′ phosphate in biological material. I. Purification and properties of cyclic 3′,5′ nucleotide phosphodiesterase and use of this enzyme to characterize adenosine 3′,5′phosphate in human urine. J Biol Chem 237:1244–1250

Clarke M, Bazari WL, Kayman SC (1980) Isolation and properties of calmodulin from *Dictyostelium discoideum.* J Bacteriol 141:397–400

Cohen MS (1977) The cyclic AMP control system in the development of *Dictyostelium discoideum*. I. Cellular dynamics. J Theor Biol 69:57–85

Cohen MS (1978) The cyclic AMP control system in the development of *Dictyostelium discoideum*. II. An allosteric model. J Theor Biol 72:231–255

Cutler LS, Rossomando EF (1975) Localization of adenylate cyclase in *Dictyostelium discoideum*. II. Cytochemical studies on whole cells and isolated plasma membrane vesicles. Exp Cell Res 95:79–87

Darmon M, Brachet P (1978) Chemotaxis and differentiation during aggregation of *Dictyostelium discoideum* amoebae. Receptors Recognition B5:103–139

Darmon M, Klein C (1978) Effects of amino acids and glucose on adenylate cyclase and cell differentiation of *Dictyostelium discoideum*. Dev Biol 63:377–389

Darmon M, Barra J, Brachet P (1978) The role of phosphodiesterase in aggregation of *Dictyostelium discoideum*. J Cell Sci 31:233–243

Devreotes PN, Steck TL (1979) Cyclic 3′,′ AMP relay in *Dictyostelium discoideum*. II. Requirements for the initiation and termination of the response. J Cell Biol 80:300–309

Devreotes PN, Destine PL, Steck TL (1979) Cyclic 3′,5′ AMP relay in *Dictyostelium discoideum*. I. A technique to monitor responses in controlled stimuli. J Cell Biol 80:291–299

Dicou EL, Brachet P (1979) Multiple forms of an extracellular cyclic AMP phosphodiesterase from *Dictyostelium discoideum*. Biochim Biophys Acta 578:232–242

Durston AJ, Vork F (1979) A cinematographical study of the development of vitally stained *Dictyostelium discoideum*. J Cell Sci 36:261–279

Fain JN (1978) Hormones, membranes and cyclic nucleotides. Receptors Recognition 6A:3–61

Farnham CJM (1975) Cytochemical localization of adenylate cyclase and 3′,5′ nucleotide phosphodiesterase in *Dictyostelium*. Exp Cell Res 91:36–46

Gerisch G (1980) Univalent antibody fragments as tools for the analysis of cell interactions in *Dictyostelium*. Curr Top Dev Biol 14:243–270

Gerisch G, Hess B (1974) Cyclic-AMP controlled oscillations in suspended *Dictyostelium discoideum*. Their relation to morphogenetic cell interactions. Proc Natl Acad Sci USA 71:2118–2127

Gerisch G, Malchow D (1976) Cyclic AMP receptors and the control of cell aggregation in *Dictyostelium*. Adv Cyclic Nucleotide Res 7:49–68

Gerisch G, Wick U (1975) Intracellular oscillations and release of cyclic AMP from *Dictyostelium* cells. Biochem Biophys Res Commun 65:364–370

Gerisch G, Fromm H, Huesgen A, Wick U (1975a) Control of cell-contact sites by cyclic AMP pulses in differentiating *Dictyostelium* cells. Nature 255:547–549

Gerisch G, Malchow D, Huesgen A, Nanjundiah V, Roos W, Wick U (1975b) Cyclic-AMP reception and cell recognition in *Dictyostelium discoideum*. ICN-UCLA Symp Mol Cell Biol 2:76–88

Gingle AR (1977) cAMP enhanced aggregation of cells from early chick embryos. Dev Biol 58:394–401

Goldbeter A, Segel LA (1977) Unified mechanism for relay and oscillation of cyclic AMP in *Dictyostelium discoideum*. Proc Natl Acad Sci USA 74:1543–1547

Green AA, Newell PC (1975) Evidence for the existence of two types of cAMP binding sites in aggregating cells of *Dictyostelium discoideum*. Cell 6:129–136

Haley BE (1975) Photoaffinity labeling of adenosine 3′,5′-cyclic monophosphate binding sites of human red cell membranes. Biochemistry 14:3852–3857

Henderson EJ (1975) The cyclic adenosine 3′:5′-monophosphate receptor of *Dictyostelium discoideum*. J Biol Chem 250:4730–4736

Jacobson A, Lodish HF (1975) Genetic control of development of the cellular slime mold *Dictyostelium discoideum*. Annu Rev Genet 9:145–185

Kay RR, Garrod D, Tilly R (1978) Requirements for cell differentiation in *Dictyostelium discoideum*. Nature 271:58–60

Kay RR, Town CD, Gross JD (1979) Cell differentiation in *Dictyostelium discoideum*. Differentiation 13:7–14

Kessin RH, Orlow SJ, Shapiro RI, Franke J (1979) Binding of inhibitor alters the kinetic and physical properties of the extracellular cyclic AMP phosphodiesterase from *Dictyostelium discoideum.* Proc Natl Acad Sci USA 76:5450–5454
Killich KA, Wright BE (1974) Regulation of enzyme activity during differentiation in *Dictyostelium discoideum.* Annu Rev Microbiol 28:139–166
Klein C (1975) Induction of phosphodiesterase by cyclic adenosine 3′:5′ monophosphate in differentiating *Dictyostelium discoideum* amoebae. J Biol Chem 250:7134–7138
Klein C (1976) Adenylate cyclase activity in *Dictyostelium discoideum* amoebae and its changes during differentiation. FEBS Lett 68:125–128
Klein C, Brachet P (1975) Effects of progesterone and EDTA on cyclic AMP and phosphodiesterase in *Dictyostelium discoideum.* Nature 254:432–434
Klein C, Darmon M (1977) Effects of cyclic AMP pulses on adenylate cyclase and the phosphodiesterase inhibitor of *D. discoideum.* Nature 268:76–78
Klein C, Juliani MH (1977) cAMP-induced changes in cAMP-binding sites on *D. discoideum* amoebae. Cell 10:329–335
Konijn TM (1972) Cyclic AMP and cell aggregation in the cellular slime molds. Acta Protozool 11:137–143
Konijn TM (1973) The chemotactic effect of cyclic nucleotides with substitutions in the base ring. FEBS Lett 34:263–266
Konijn TM, Jastorff B (1973) The chemotactic effect of 5′-amido-analogues of adenosine cyclic 3′,5′-monophosphate in the cellular slime molds. Biochim Biophys Acta 304: 774–780
Konijn TM, Van der Meene JGC, Bonner JT, Barkley DS (1967) The acrasin activity of adenosine-3′,5′-cyclic phosphate. Proc Natl Acad Sci USA 58:1152–1154
Konijn TM, Van der Meene JGC, Chang Y-Y, Barkley DS, Bonner JT (1969) Identification of adenosine-3′,5′-monophosphate as the bacterial attractant for myxamoebae of *Dictyostelium discoideum.* J Bacteriol 99:510–512
Loomis WF (1975) *Dictyostelium discoideum.* A developmental system. Academic Press, New York London
Loomis WF (1979) Biochemistry of aggregation in *Dictyostelium.* Dev Biol 70:1–12
Loomis WF, Klein C, Brachet P (1978) The effect of divalent cations on aggregation of *Dictyostelium discoideum.* Differentiation 12:83–89
MacWilliams HK, Bonner JT (1979) The prestalk-prespore pattern in cellular slime molds. Differentiation 14:1–22
Maeda Y (1977) Role of cyclic AMP in the polarized movement of the migrating pseudoplasmodium of *Dictyostelium discoideum.* Dev Growth Differ 19:201–205
Maeda Y, Gerisch G (1977) Vesicle formation in *Dictyostelium discoideum* cells during oscillations of cAMP synthesis and release. Exp Cell Res 110:119–126
Malchow D, Gerisch G (1973) Cyclic AMP binding to living cells of *Dictyostelium discoideum* in the presence of excess of cyclic AMP. Biochem Biophys Res Commun 55:200–204
Malchow D, Gerisch G (1974) Short-term binding and hydrolysis of cyclic 3′:5′-adenosine monophosphate by aggregating *Dictyostelium* cells. Proc Natl Acad Sci USA 71:2423–2427
Malchow D, Nägele B, Schwarz H, Gerisch G (1972) Membrane bound cyclic AMP phosphodiesterase in chemotactically responding cells of *Dictyostelium discoideum.* Eur J Biochem 28:136–142
Malchow D, Fuchila J, Jastorff B (1973) Correlation of substrate specificity of cAMP phosphodiesterase in *Dictyostelium discoideum* with chemotactic activity of cAMP analogues. FEBS Lett 34:5–9
Malchow D, Fuchila J, Nanjundiah V (1975) A plausible role for a membrane-bound cyclic AMP phosphodiesterase in cellular slime mold chemotaxis. Biochim Biophys Acta 385:421–428
Malkinson AM, Ashworth JM (1973) Adenosine 3′-5′-cyclic monophosphate concentrations and phosphodiesterase activities during axenic growth and differentiation of cells in the cellular slime mould *Dictyostelium discoideum.* Biochem J 134:311–319
Marin FT (1976) Regulation of development in *Dictyostelium discoideum.* Initiation of the growth to development transition by amino acid starvation. Dev Biol 48:110–117

Mato JM (1979) Activation of *Dictyostelium discoideum* guanylate cyclase by ATP. Biochem Res Commun 88:569–574

Mato JM, Konijn TM (1975) Chemotaxis and binding of cyclic AMP in cellular slime molds. Biochim Biophys Acta 385:173–179

Mato JM, Malchow D (1978) Guanylate cyclase activation in response to chemotactic stimulation in *Dictyostelium discoideum*. FEBS Lett 90:119–122

Mato JM, Krens FA, Van Haastert PJM, Konijn TM (1977) 3′:5′-cyclic AMP-dependent 3′:5′-cyclic GMP accumulation in *Dictyostelium discoideum*. Proc Natl Acad Sci USA 74:2348–2351

Mato JM, Jastorff B, Morr M, Konijn TM (1978) A model for cyclic AMP-chemoreceptor interaction in *Dictyostelium discoideum*. Biochim Biophys Acta 544:309–314

Mato JM, Woelders H, Haastert PJM, Konijn TM (1978b) Cyclic GMP binding activity in *Dictyostelium discoideum*. FEBS Lett 90:261–264

Moens PB, Konijn TM (1974) Cyclic AMP as a cell surface activating agent in *Dictyostelium discoideum*. FEBS Lett 45:44–46

Müller K, Gerisch G, Fromme J, Mayer H, Tsugita A (1979) A membrane glycoprotein of aggregating *Dictyostelium* cells with the properties of contact sites. Eur J Biochem 99:419–426

Mullens JA, Newell PC (1978) cAMP binding to cell surface receptors in *Dictyostelium*. Differentiation 10:171–176

Nanjundiah V, Malchow D (1976) A theoretical study of the effects of cyclic AMP phosphodiesterases during aggregation in *Dictyostelium*. J Cell Sci 22:49–58

Newell PC (1977) Aggregation and cell surface receptors in cellular slime molds. Receptors Recognition B3:1–58

Newell PC (1978) Genetics of the cellular slime molds. Annu Rev Genet 12:69–93

Pan P, Wedner HJ (1979) Immunohistochemical localization of cyclic GMP in aggregating *Polysphondylium violaceum*. Differentiation 14:113–118

Pan P, Bonner JT, Wedner HJ, Parker CM (1974) Immunofluorescence evidence for the distribution of cyclic AMP in cells and cell masses of the cellular slime molds. Proc Natl Acad Sci USA 71:1623–1625

Pannbacker RG, Bravard LJ (1972) Phosphodiesterase in *Dictyostelium discoideum* and the chemotactic response to cyclic adenosine monophosphate. Science 175:1014–1015

Potel MJ, MacKay SA (1979) Preaggregative cell motion in *Dictyostelium*. J Cell Sci 36:281–309

Rahmsdorf HJ, Gerisch G (1978) Specific binding proteins for cyclic AMP and cyclic GMP in *Dictyostelium discoideum*. Cell Differentiation 7:249–257

Rahmsdorf HJ, Pai S-H (1979) The protein kinases of *Dictyostelium discoideum*, strain AX-2. Biochim Biophys Acta 567:339–346

Rahmsdorf HJ, Malchow D, Gerisch G (1978) Cyclic AMP-induced phosphorylation in *Dictyostelium* of a polypeptide comigrating with myosin heavy chains. FEBS Lett 88:322–326

Rasmussen H, Goodman DBP (1977) Relationships between calcium and cyclic nucleotides in cell activation. Physiol Rev 57:421–509

Riedel V, Malchow D, Gerisch C, Nägele B (1972) Cyclic AMP phosphodiesterase interaction with its inhibitor of the slime mold, *Dictyostelium discoideum*. Biochem Biophys Res Commun 46:279–287

Robertson A, Gingle AR (1977) Axial bending in the early chick embryo by a cyclic adenosine monophosphate source. Science 197:1078–1079

Robertson A, Drage DJ, Cohen MH (1972) Control of aggregation in *Dictyostelium discoideum* by an external periodic pulse of cyclic adenosine monophosphate. Science 175:333–334

Robertson A, Grutch JF, Gingle AR (1978) Cyclic ȧdenosine monophosphate production by embryonic chick cells. Science 199:990–991

Roos W, Nanjundiah V, Malchow D, Gerisch G (1975) Amplification of cyclic-AMP signals in aggregating cells of *Dictyostelium discoideum*. FEBS Lett 53:139–142

Roos W, Scheidegger C, Gerisch G (1977a) Adenylate cyclase activity oscillations as signals for cell aggregation in *Dictyostelium discoideum*. Nature 266:259–261

Roos W, Malchow D, Gerisch G (1977 b) Adenylyl cyclase and the control of cell differentiation in *Dictyostelium discoideum*. Cell Differentiation 6:229–239

Rosen SD, Barondes SH (1978) Cell adhesion in the cellular slime molds. Receptors Recognition B4: 235–264

Rossier C, Gerisch G, Malchow D, Eckstein F (1978) Action of a slowly hydrolysable cyclic AMP analogue on developing cells of *Dictyostelium discoideum*. J Cell Sci 35:321–338

Rossomando EF, Cutler LS (1975) Localization of adenylate cyclase in *Dictyostelium discoideum*. I. Preparation and biochemical characterization of cell fractions and isolated plasma membrane vesicles. Exp Cell Res 95:67–78

Rubin J, Robertson A (1975) The tip of the *Dictyostelium discoideum* pseudoplasmodium is an organizer. J Embryol Exp Morphol 33:227–241

Sampson J (1977) Developmentally regulated cyclic AMP-dependent protein kinases in *Dictyostelium discoideum*. Cell 11:173–180

Sampson J, Town C, Gross J (1978) Cyclic AMP and the control of aggregative phase gene expression in *Dictyostelium discoideum*. Dev Biol 67:54–64

Shaffer BM (1957) Aspects of aggregation in cellular slime molds. I. Orientation and chemotaxis. Am Nat 91:19–35

Springer MS, Goy MF, Adler J (1979) Protein methylation in behavioural control mechanisms and in signal transduction. Nature 280:279–284

Sussman M, Brackenbury R (1976) Biochemical and molecular-genetic aspects of cellular slime mold development, Annu Rev Plant Physiol 27:229–265

Tsang AS, Coukell MB (1977) The regulation of cyclic AMP-phosphodiesterase and its specific inhibitor by cyclic AMP in *Dictyostelium*. Cell Differentiation 6:75–84

Tsang AS, Coukell MB (1979 a) Biochemical and genetic evidence for two extracellular adenosine 3′:5′-monophosphate phosphodiesterases in *Dictyostelium discoideum*. Eur J Biochem 95:407–417

Tsang AS, Coukell MB (1979 b) Direct evidence for extracellular adenosine 3′:5′-monophosphate phosphodiesterase induction and phosphodiesterase inhibitor repression by exogenous adenosine 3′:5′-monophosphate in *Dictyostelium purpureum*. Eur J Biochem 95:419–429

Wick U, Malchow D, Gerisch G (1978) Cyclic-AMP stimulated calcium influx into aggregating cells of *Dictyostelium discoideum*. Cell Biol Int Rep 2:71–79

Wurster B, Schubiger K, Wick U, Gerisch G (1977) Cyclic GMP in *Dictyostelium discoideum* oscillations and pulses in response to folic acid and cyclic AMP signals. FEBS Lett 76:141–144

Wurster B, Bozzaro S, Gerisch G (1978) Cyclic GMP regulation and responses of *Polysphondylium violaceum* to chemoattractants. Cell Biol Int Rep 2:61–69

Yeh RP, Chan FK, Coukell MB (1978) Independent regulation of the extracellular cyclic AMP phosphodiesterase-inhibitor system and membrane differentiation by exogenous cyclic AMP in *Dictyostelium discoideum*. Dev Biol 66:361–374

Section IV: Physiology and Pharmacology of Organ Systems

CHAPTER 25

The Role of Cyclic Nucleotides in the Nervous System

T. V. DUNWIDDIE and B. J. HOFFER

Overview

A wide variety of roles have been suggested for cyclic nucleotides in both the central and peripheral nervous systems. Cyclic AMP has been hypothesized to be the intracellular second messenger for a variety of inhibitory transmitters, most notably norepinephrine, dopamine, and serotonin. In addition, cyclic GMP has been suggested to mediate the effects of acetylcholine and glutamate. While this "second messenger" role of cyclic nucleotides is perhaps most well known, there are indications that they serve a variety of other functions as well. Cyclic AMP appears to be involved in the modulation of the postsynaptic responsiveness of several transmitter systems; adenosine, which can raise cyclic AMP levels by itself, appears implicated in many of these effects. Cyclic nucleotides have also been suggested as being either directly involved in exocytosis, or affecting the release of transmitter indirectly via a regulatory action on release processes. Cyclic nucleotides appear to act by activating a class of cyclic AMP and cyclic GMP-dependent protein kinases. While the functions of some of the endogenous substrates for these kinases, and the effect of phosphorylation are largely unknown, in some cases (e.g., phosphorylation of tyrosine hydroxylase) the physiological significance of the phosphorylated and dephosphorylated states of the protein are quite clear. In the case of tyrosine hydroxylase, cyclic AMP certainly does not appear to be functioning as a second messenger to mediate the physiological effects of a neurotransmitter, but instead to be mediating a more complex type of regulatory effect. Glial cells also have cyclic nucleotide generating systems; while their functions is somewhat unclear, there are indications that changes in cyclic AMP in glial cells may influence intermediary metabolism in the brain. In terms of behavior, it is difficult to summarize the interrelationships between cyclic nucleotides and behavioral responses, particularly in animals with well-developed and therefore complex nervous systems. It would appear that cyclic nucleotide levels are affected under certain conditions, such as during epileptic activity or possibly in affective disorders. However, it is not clear whether the alterations in cyclic nucleotides are directly involved in the etiology of these conditions, or vice versa.

In spite of the fact that some of these putâtive roles of the cyclic nucleotides have been under investigation for well over a decade, it has not been possible to unequivocally establish a role for cyclic AMP or cyclic GMP in any of these specific aspects of nervous system function. Nevertheless, the importance of cyclic nucleotides to nervous system function seems apparent. Virtually any treatment which affects the general function of the nervous system affects the levels of cyclic AMP, cyclic GMP, or both. Conversely, both nucleotides have profound effects on electrophysiological as well as biochemical processes.

The primary difficulty in so far as characterizing the functional role of cyclic nucleotides is concerned is to demonstrate the causal relationship between biochemical events and physiological responses. The general lack of information about the dynamics of cyclic nucleotide synthesis and degradation at the cellular level is a serious hindrance to establishing such causal links. The most informative types of physiological experiments (at least as far as cellular mechanisms are concerned) generally utilize measurements made on single neurons with time resolutions in the sub-millisecond range. Most biochemical studies of cyclic nucleotides have neither the spatial nor the temporal resolution of these electrophysiological experiments, hence it is difficult to establish whether cyclic nucleotide changes precede physiological events. Since rapid changes in cyclic AMP levels occur in other systems (BROOKER 1975; DRUMMOND et al. 1966), rapid regulation of cyclic nucleotide levels in the nervous system is at least possible. If cyclic nucleotides are involved in extremely rapid processes (e.g., exocytosis), rather sophisticated technical developments will have to be made before these types of changes can be quantified.

Attempts to link slower phenomena, such as changes in transmitter synthesis, slow synaptic potentials, or epileptiform activity, have met with greater success than those involving faster activity. In some cases, where the endpoint of cyclic nucleotide action can be quantified in cell-free systems, and occurs slowly enough to be resolved with conventional biochemical methods, it has been possible to establish a close correspondence between cyclic nucleotides and particular biochemical or physiological changes. For example, tyrosine hydroxylase, the rate-limiting step in catecholamine biosynthesis, is phosphorylated in a cyclic AMP-dependent fashion, and the incorporation of phosphate into the molecule is directly reflected in increased enzymatic activity. In this case, the link between cyclic nucleotides and the response (enzyme activation) is particularly strong.

As just described, the lack of appropriate information concerning the dynamics of cyclic nucleotide formation makes the interpretation of physiological experiments somewhat difficult. On the other hand, there is a wealth of information concerning the biochemical effects of cyclic nucleotides, particularly in regard to protein phosphorylation, but the relationship of these changes to physiological processes remains obscure. Many nervous system proteins are substrates for cyclic nucleotide-dependent phosphorylation, but the physiological role played by the phosphorylated and dephosphorylated forms of these proteins in cellular function is unclear. The fact that large changes in the phosphorylation state of proteins may occur within seconds simply compounds the problems associated with the rapid dynamics of cyclic nucleotide changes discussed above.

Another major problem regarding cyclic nucleotide action concerns the regulation of cyclic nucleotide levels. The list of putative transmitters and/or neuromodulators that can alter cyclic nucleotide levels is much longer than that of agents which are known to activate adenylate or guanylate cyclase in cell-free systems. Much more needs to be known about which of these have direct effects on cyclases, which have indirect effects mediated via other transmitters, and which might affect cyclic nucleotide levels indirectly by means of more complex interactions with other cellular regulators manifesting actions either on the cyclase, or at other sites (e.g., phosphodiesterase).

A convincing demonstration that cyclic nucleotides are involved in a given physiological process rests upon satisfactory characterization of a variety of biochemical and physiological processes (see Introduction). At present, most biochemical and physiological studies of cyclic nucleotides are carried out in totally different preparations; a more suitable marriage of these techniques applied to simple systems (e.g., homogenous cell populations in tissue culture, brain slices, peripheral ganglia, and invertebrate nervous systems) is required before many of the more stringent criteria concerning cyclic nucleotide action can be met.

The past decade has witnessed a remarkable development in terms of what is known concerning cyclic nucleotides in the nervous system. In general, most of this knowledge is fragmentary and has quite naturally led to the development of a larger number of hypotheses concerning the roles played by cyclic nucleotides. What remains is to extend these hypotheses to the point where complete pictures of cyclic nucleotide action can be described.

A. Introduction

I. Cyclic Nucleotides as Second Messengers

The need to transmit information about changes in the extracellular environment to the interior of cells is a fundamental requirement of nearly all types of cells. In many cases, the cells must respond to the external stimulus in a very specific manner; hence, a functional link is required between cell membrane receptors and intracellular biochemical processes. The evidence is now fairly compelling that cyclic adenosine 3′,5′-monophosphate (cylic AMP) provides this essential link, acting as a "second messenger" in the intracellular compartment to convey information about extracellular "first messengers" and their interactions with receptor sites on the exterior cell surface.

The second messenger role of cyclic AMP has been studied extensively in various hormonal target tissues. The need for individual cell function within a given

Abbreviations

cyclic AMP: cyclic adenosine 3′,5′-monophosphate
cyclic GMP: cyclic guanosine 3′,5′-monophosphate
ATP: adenosine triphosphate
GABA: γ-amino butyric acid
NE: norepinephrine
E: epinephrine
DA: dopamine
5-HT: 5-hydroxytryptamine, serotonin
ACh: acetylcholine
5′AMP: adenosine 5′-monophosphate
IBMX: 3-isobutyl-1-methylxanthine
H: histamine
CNS: central nervous system
NMJ: neuromuscular junction
Li: lithium
Ca^{+2}: calcium
Mg^{+2}: magnesium
P-cells: Purkinje cells
LC: locus coeruleus
3AP: 3-acetylpyridine

tissue to be coordinated with the activities of other cells in that organ, as well as the physiological state of the organism, has been resolved in many cases by systems in which extracellularly circulating hormones regulate the intracellular processes of large groups of cells via interactions with extracellular receptors. In the liver, exposure to either epinephrine (a catecholamine) or the peptide hormone glucagon results in increased glycogenolysis, and in both cases, the change in the extracellular milieu (i.e., the arrival of the hormone) is signaled to the intracellular environment by the catalytic hydrolysis of ATP to cyclic AMP by the enzyme adenylate cyclase. This enzyme is located in the membranes of receptive cells and is apparently activated in most cases via an interaction with other membrane proteins, particularly receptor molecules. The essential role of cyclic AMP in the activation of specific enzymes and the elaboration of the appropriate physiological response to circulating hormones has been well-characterized in a variety of systems (see other chapters, this volume).

The nervous system has a unique requirement for mechanisms for the selective transfer of information when compared with other tissues such as the liver. Whereas a single hormonal signal can be used to alter the physiological state of the entire liver, the brain does not usually function as such a unit; instead, systems are required whereby specific information can be transferred from individual neuron to neuron.

By and large, the means by which this is accomplished is fairly well known. Transmitters released by terminal elements of presynaptic neurons diffuse across synaptic clefts where they interact with receptors located upon the postsynaptic cells. The binding of the transmitter molecule to the receptor is usually associated with the opening of specific channels in the membrane, and the subsequent passage of ions in or out of the neuron exerts an influence upon electrophysiological activity of that particular cell (see KRNJEVIĆ 1974, for a review). While the ionic mechanisms of transmitter action are known in a few cases (e.g., GABA appears to act by opening conductance channels to potassium and chloride ions), there still exists a wide variety of transmitters for which it is difficult to establish such a simple mechanism. Catecholamines, such as norepinephrine (NE) and epinephrine (E), dopamine (DA), serotonin (5HT), acetylcholine (ACh), and a variety of other putative neurotransmitters clearly affect electrophysiological activity of the central nervous system, but in many cases, it has not been possible to demonstrate unequivocally that the primary consequence of receptor occupancy is the opening of an ion channel. In some cases, such as with NE, changes in membrane potential occasionally appear with *no* change in membrane resistance (HOFFER et al. 1973; SIGGINS et al. 1971b; OLIVER and SEGAL 1974; PHILLIS 1977) suggesting that no ion channels have opened. In such cases, the suggestion has frequently been made that a particular transmitter may produce its postsynaptic effects in a more complex fashion, specifically by means of a "second messenger", which translates an extracellular event (binding of agonists to receptors) into an intracellular signal that can be used to modify the functioning of a target neuron. Both calcium and cyclic nucleotides have frequently been suggested as second messengers in the central nervous system, but only the latter will be discussed at any length in this review.

The importance of cyclic nucleotides, both cyclic AMP as well as guanosine cyclic 3′,5′-monophosphate (cyclic GMP) in central nervous function derives support from several sources. The brain maintains levels of cyclic AMP and GMP which are generally higher than any other tissue (KLAINER et al. 1962; GOLDBERG et al. 1969). In addition, a wide variety of treatments which affect nervous activity will influence the levels of one or both of these nucleotides.

The cyclic nucleotide second messenger hypothesis is also one which is experimentally testable. The mechanisms by which hormones (and by inference, neurotransmitters) influence cyclic nucleotide levels and, more specifically, the way in which changes in cyclic nucleotide levels are translated into intracellular events is fairly well known, particularly in some hormonal systems. For example, in the liver, the sequence of events involving cyclic nucleotides as second messengers has been well-established (see SUTHERLAND et al. 1965) and it appears that the effects of cyclic nucleotides in the central nervous system occur via similar mechanisms (GREENGARD 1976, 1978a, b, 1979). Briefly, this is thought to occur as shown in Fig. 1. The first step is the binding of a transmitter to a specific receptor molecule in the cell membrane. This transmitter-receptor complex can then interact (perhaps via intermediates) with a membrane-bound adenylate cyclase, which catalyzes the hydrolysis of ATP to cyclic AMP. Cyclic AMP is thought to affect intracellular events by binding to the regulatory subunit of a cyclic AMP-dependent protein kinase(s). The subsequent dissociation of the complex releases free catalytic subunit which then transfers the terminal phosphate group of ATP to substrate proteins in the target cell. The termination of this process is thought to involve the breakdown of cyclic AMP to adenosine 5′-monophosphate (5′-AMP) by phosphodiesterases, and the removal of the phosphate group from the substrate protein by a phosphatase. This process has been outlined in greatly oversimplified form, and there exist numerous other points in this system besides the adenylate cyclase at which regulatory control may be exerted (see other chapters, this volume).

The complexity of the responses mediated by this system derives from the variety of substrates which may be phosphorylated; the number of different substrates which have been shown to be phosphorylated in a cyclic AMP-dependent fashion probably number over a hundred. Phosphorylation itself provides a means by which enzymes can be activated (e.g., phosphorylase b to phosphorylase a) or deactivated (glycogen synthetase I to D). Phosphorylation could likewise change the properties of nearly any protein which has sites which can be phosphorylated by cyclic AMP-dependent protein kinases; structural proteins, receptor molecules, ionophores and histones all reflect sites at which cyclic AMP could produce changes in cellular function. At least ten different substrates for cyclic AMP-dependent protein kinases have been shown in the synaptic membranes (DE BLAS et al. 1979; REDDINGTON and MEHL 1979; EHRLICH 1979); more probably exist in smaller concentrations or in forms which are not detectable by current assay techniques. Some of the ways in which cyclic nucleotide accumulation in the nervous system can be stimulated, and the physiological effects of such changes, are shown in Table 1.

As far as cyclic GMP is concerned, it is generally thought to have a similar mode of action. Cyclic GMP would be formed by guanylate cyclase from GTP, and increased levels of this nucleotide would activate cyclic GMP-dependent kinase(s), which would then phosphorylate other types of substrates. However, there are several important differences between cyclic AMP and cyclic GMP systems. In particular, guanylate cyclase, the enzyme responsible for the formation of cyclic GMP,

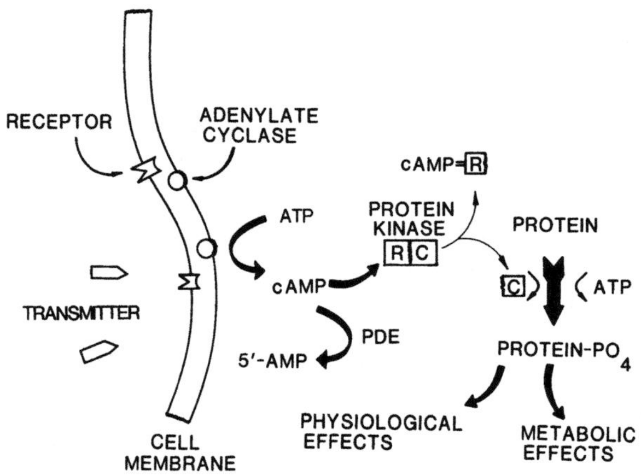

Fig. 1. This figure schematizes the basic hypothesis concerning cyclic AMP as a second messenger in the central and peripheral nervous systems. Transmitters and neuromodulators (see Table 1) are thought to interact with membrane receptors in such a way that the receptor can activate adenylate cyclase molecules located in the membrane. Activation of the adenylate cyclase leads to the formation of cyclic AMP, which can subsequently be degraded to 5′-AMP via the action of phosphodiesterase *(PDE)*, which is largely present in the soluble cell fraction. Cyclic AMP itself binds to the regulatory subunit *R* of protein kinase, which then separates from the catalytic subunit *C* of the kinase. Since the action of the regulatory subunit is inhibitory, the free catalytic subunit then catalyzes the transfer of terminal phosphate molecules from ATP to cellular proteins. Phosphorylation of cellular proteins can result in a variety of effects on cellular function (Table 1). Activation of adenylate cyclase by transmitters is not the only way in which this system is regulated; virtually every aspect of this system from the receptor to the endpoints of cyclic nucleotide action is controlled in a variety of ways. Other intracellular messengers, such as calcium, can interact with cyclic nucleotide systems as well. There are also regulatory agents (e.g., protein kinase inhibitors) not shown in this model which can also influence individual aspects of cyclic AMP-mediated effects. Cyclic GMP is thought to act as a second messenger in a manner quite similar to that shown for cyclic AMP. However, guanylate cyclase is a primarily soluble enzyme, so the initial steps in its activation may be somewhat different

is found primarily in the soluble fraction of homogenates (GORIDIS and MORGAN 1973), suggesting an intracellular location, and apparently depends upon Ca^{+2} influx for its activation. Hence, it would appear, at least superficially, that cyclic GMP would be of less value as a second messenger, since guanylate cyclase is generally not found in locations where it would be sensitive to extracellular events. In addition, it has been extremely difficult to isolate endogenous substrates of cyclic GMP-dependent protein kinases in the nervous system. Even though cyclic GMP-dependent protein kinases have been known to exist for some time in cerebellum (GREENGARD and KUO 1970; HOFMANN and SOLD 1972; TAKAI et al. 1975), the existence of endogenous substrates for this kinase were unknown until SCHLICHTER et al. (1978) were able to demonstrate a 23,000 protein in cerebellum (but not hippocampus, cortex, or striatum), which was phosphorylated in a cyclic GMP-dependent fashion.

This is the basic outline of the sequence of events by which the interaction of a transmitter at an extracellular site is thought to influence intracellular events using cyclic nucleotides as intermediaries. However, it should be pointed out that

Table 1. This is a partial listing of some of the putative transmitters which have been shown to alter cyclic nucleotide levels in nervous tissue from mammals (i.e., first messengers), and some of the types of physiological events which have been hypothesized to result from cyclic nucleotide-mediated events. More detailed information on cyclic nucleotide accumulation in nervous tissue, and the physiological responses which result, can be found in any of several reviews (BLOOM 1975; NATHANSON 1977; DALY 1975, 1977a, b)

Factors which release first messengers	Possible first (i.e. extracellular) messengers	Possible second messengers	Physiological responses
Electrical stimulation	NE } catecholamines	Cyclic AMP	1) Fast permeability changes
Endogenous activity	E } catecholamines	Cyclic GMP	2) Slow permeability changes
High potassium	DA } catecholamines	(Calcium)	3) Modulation of other synaptic inputs
Veratridine	ACh		4) Effects on microtubules
Ouabain	Serotonin		5) Transmitter synthesis
Glutamate	Peptides (VIP, substance P, enkephalins)		6) Protein synthesis
	Amino acids (glutamate, aspartate, GABA, glycine)		7) Receptor density regulation
	Adenosine		8) Metabolic effects
	Histamine		9) Transmitter release
			10) Others?

there are several problems associated with this model, in so far as the nervous system is concerned. It is probably safe to say that in the nervous system, it has not been possible to demonstrate this complete sequence of events occurring in response to any single transmitter. There are many examples of independent steps in this sequence, but as of yet, it has not been possible to demonstrate the causal relationship between the appropriate biochemical and physiological events.

As an example, it was mentioned above that there are a variety of substrates for cyclic AMP-dependent kinase in the central nervous system. One such substrate is Protein I, which has been extensively characterized by Greengard's group (UEDA et al. 1973; UEDA and GREENGARD 1977; FORN and GREENGARD 1978). Protein I, which actually consists of two proteins, Proteins I a and I b, is found exclusively in neurons, and is apparently associated with synaptic regions, both pre- and postsynaptically. In vivo, CNS depressants tend to reduce the fraction of Protein I in the phosphorylated state, while convulsants increase the proportion of phosphorylated Protein I (STRÖMBOM et al. 1979). Its conversion to the phosphorylated form in vitro is increased by cyclic AMP and its analogs, as well as the phosphodiesterase inhibitor isobutylmethyxanthine (IBMX), and by depolarization of tissue slices by high K^+ or veratridine. Nonetheless, no putative transmitters have been found which appear to change the phosphorylated state of this protein; catecholamines, carbachol, serotonin, excitatory and inhibitory amino acids, histamine and adenosine, all have no apparent effect on phosphorylation of Protein I (FORN and

GREENGARD 1978). Phosphorylation of this protein, as well as most other substrates associated with synaptic membranes, is quite rapid, usually maximal within 15–30 s. What is lacking in these studies is any kind of understanding of either the events which lead to phosphorylation in vivo, i.e., the "first" messengers which increase cyclic AMP levels, or of the physiological consequences of a shift from the unphosphorylated to the phosphorylated form of the protein.

Numerous examples of this kind of fragmentary knowledge of cyclic AMP actions could be described. Dopamine has been shown to stimulate adenylate cyclase to form cyclic AMP; dopamine also exerts a primarily inhibitory influence on spontaneous cell firing. Thus, unlike the situation with protein I, this represents a situation where the first messenger (dopamine) is known, as well as its ultimate effect (inhibition of cell firing), but the intermediate steps (i.e., cyclic AMP-dependent phosphorylation of a substrate protein) is unknown. In still other cases, proteins of known function, such as tyrosine hydroxylase, phosphorylase B, glycogen synthetase I, microtubular protein, and the regulatory subunit of cyclic AMP-dependent protein kinase are phosphorylated by cyclic AMP-dependent kinases. For each of these proteins, some aspect of the process is unknown; either the events which lead to in vivo phosphorylation, the role of cyclic AMP, or the physiological relevance of the phosphorylated form of the protein are unresolved. Thus, one of the major directions which this research is likely to take is to begin to link up various individual steps to provide more complete pictures concerning cyclic nucleotide actions.

The other major thrust in terms of research in this field will be to gain better understanding of the complex regulation of these types of processes. These events are not simple on-off types of events, where proteins are either phosphorylated or not phosphorylated. Levels of cyclic AMP represent a dynamic balance between the activity of adenylate cyclase and phosphodiesterase, both of which are sensitive to a variety of factors, including intracellular calcium. Certain protein kinases are highly activated by cyclic nucleotides, but, in addition, can be inhibited by specific endogenous kinase inhibitors (SZYMIGIELSKI et al. 1977; WALSH et al. 1971), which can affect the activity of cyclic AMP- or cyclic GMP-dependent kinases. The regulatory unit of cyclic AMP-dependent protein kinase represents one of the major substrates of endogenous phosphorylation (MAENO et al. 1974; termed Protein II of UEDA et al. 1973; Protein E of EHRLICH 1979). The significance of this phosphorylation is not entirely clear, but it may be related to the manner in which the catalytic and regulatory subunits of the kinase bind (EHRLICHMAN et al. 1974). Thus, there are complex ways in which nearly every aspect of cyclic nucleotide formation and subsequent phosphorylation can be regulated, but the physiological events which influence these regulatory factors are largely unknown.

A final problem with this entire model is that it has not been established that phosphorylation represents the only way in which cyclic nucleotides can exert their effects. The regulatory subunit of cyclic AMP-dependent protein kinase is not the only protein which can bind cyclic AMP (WALSH 1978); this certainly suggests that this nucleotide might be able to regulate the activity of other enzymes, and hence cellular processes, by an entirely different mechanism.

In summary, at least 3 factors conspire to make the role of cyclic nucleotides in the nervous system somewhat unclear. First, for various reasons, it has not been possible to describe in detail the entire sequence of events from activation of cyclase to physiological response, although individual steps in the process may be quite well characterized. Secondly, the regulation of cyclic nucleotide-dependent effects is extremely complex, and it is quite clear that the complete spectrum of physiological events which can influence various aspects of cyclic AMP formation and degradation, and the corresponding physiological and biochemical responses, is just beginning to be known. Finally, cyclic nucleotides may exert effects which have nothing to do with protein phosphorylation; if they do, then there might be other categories of biochemical effects which also occur in a cyclic AMP-dependent fashion.

What we have briefly described is the way in which cyclic nucleotides have been thought to exert their effects as second messengers, and some of the problems encountered in trying to extend this model to the nervous system. At the most basic level, any model of cyclic nucleotide action would be expected to answer at least four questions: a) What is the signal, i.e., the extracellular event which is to be transmitted? b) How are the cyclic nucleotide levels regulated by extracellular events? c) What types of biochemical events are regulated by cyclic nucleotides? d) What is the physiological endpoint of these processes?

A complete discussion of all of the physiological processes which are thought to involve cyclic nucleotides would require far more space than is available here, and in spite of the current progress being made in many individual areas, would yield few, if any, complete "answers" to the questions outlined above. In addition, extensive reviews have been published in recent years which have been extremely useful in organizing an already massive literature (BLOOM 1975; NATHANSON 1977; DALY 1975, 1976, 1977a, b; PHILLIS 1977; SIGGINS 1977, 1979; KEBABIAN 1977; FERRENDELLI 1978). The reader is referred to these reviews if more complete information is desired concerning specific areas not covered by this review.

The primary concern of this review will be with the first and last questions discussed above, viz., what extracellular events influence cyclic nucleotide levels, and the physiological events which result from changes in nucleotide levels.

The primary problem with attempting to review the literature in such an area concerns the fact that there are relatively few strong cases for cyclic nucleotide-mediated responses, but many cases in which the preponderance of evidence would seem to suggest an involvement of cyclic nucleotides. What will be attempted here will be to discuss at some length several "prototypic" models of cyclic nucleotide action, i.e., examples in which cyclic nucleotides have been suggested to regulate some particular aspect of the physiology of the target cell, to suggest criteria by which such models can be evaluated, and to discuss the problems which are typically encountered in these types of experiments. Related systems will generally by mentioned but not discussed at any length. An effort has also been made to select subjects which have developed more recently, since much of the older work has been reviewed extensively elsewhere. Finally, the examples chosen for this review are intended to be somewhat provocative, and display a wide variation in the probability that cyclic nucleotides are involved. Thus, consideration is made of some cases where cyclic nucleotides are probably not involved, and examples in which quite speculative (or completely unknown) modes of action of cyclic nucleotides are suggested or discussed as well.

The review of the literature contained in this chapter (ending December 1979) is by no means exhaustive. Many studies not described herein were omitted merely because of space considerations, in order to give fuller treatment to a few selected topics. Others were excluded because the effort expended in attempting to infer a physiological role for substances administered in grossly unphysiological amounts is rarely justified.

II. Criteria for Evaluating Cyclic Nucleotide Mediation of Physiological Responses

A problem frequently encountered in physiological experiments is to demonstrate that a particular physiological response to a drug or transmitter is mediated by cyclic nucleotides when the intervening steps leading to a response are unknown. For example, norepinephrine is known to inhibit the firing of cerebellar Purkinje neurons; norepinephrine frequently increases cyclic AMP levels in brain as well. This has led to the suggestion that norepinephrine inhibits Purkinje cell firing as a direct result of its effects on cyclic AMP levels. The problem is that the intermediate steps are unknown, so that if cyclic AMP is involved, the way in which it slows firing is unclear. What are needed are criteria which can be used to evaluate such a hypothesis without having to describe the complete set of intervening events. Obviously, the latter approach is preferable, but is often not possible, particularly in the nervous system.

For this reason, a set of criteria have been developed which should ideally be met if an extracellular messenger uses cyclic nucleotides as intracellular messenger to achieve physiological response. Various criteria have been suggested and discussed numerous times (SUTHERLAND et al. 1968; ROBISON et al. 1971, BLOOM 1975; PHILLIS 1977). Basically, these criteria in somewhat modified form are as follows:

(1) *The extracellular messenger should be able to stimulate the activity of the appropriate cyclase in broken cell preparations, and to increase cyclic nucleotide levels in target cells which manifest the physiological response being considered. Inactive transmitters should have no effect, nor should increases in cyclic nucleotides be observed in cases where an antagonist blocks the appropriate receptor.* In general, this criterion has been met only in a few unusual circumstances. The problems with applying this criterion to the central nervous system are numerous. In the first place, as discussed above, it is often difficult to obtain activation of cyclases in homogenates. Thus, when an agent which increases cyclic AMP in slices (e.g., glutamate) fails to activate cyclase, it is not clear whether it is because there is no glutamate-stimulated cyclase, or because some aspect of the assay conditions prevents the activation of the cyclase. Secondly, the nervous system is a very heterogenous tissue; with a few exceptions, it has not been possible to show that the changes in cyclic nucleotides which are observed are localized to the "target cells", which show the physiological response. Experiments with cultured cells relieve this problem to some extent, but only immunohistochemical methods (which have problems of their own) can localize cyclic nucleotide changes with sufficient resolution to establish where the changes are occurring, both with regard to cell type and cellular location (e.g., pre- versus post-synaptic).

(2) *The changes in cyclic nucleotides must occur prior to the elaboration of the physiological response.* Again, this is an extremely difficult criterion to meet. In cases where cyclic nucleotides lead to phosphorylation of nuclear histone proteins and subsequent *de novo* protein synthesis, this criterion may be practicable. However, when the physiological response is a rapid electrical one, such as the inhibition of Purkinje cell firing induced by NE or locus coeruleus stimulation (which occurs in less than 100 msec), fairly elaborate procedures would have to be used to determine whether cyclic nucleotide changes precede physiological response. Such experiments have not been done.

(3) *The effects of a hormone or transmitter on cyclic nucleotide levels should be apparent at the lowest concentrations required to elicit a physiological response.* This criterion, while perhaps not as important as the others, deserves some mention. One possible complication is that in some systems in which a second messenger role for cyclic nucleotides is quite firmly established, the dose response curve for cyclic nucleotide accumulation is shifted to the right by as much as two orders of magnitudes when compared to the physiological response which it elicits (RODBARD 1974; BEALL and SAYERS 1972; MACKIE et al. 1972). The explanation for this is not clear; one possibility is that cyclic nucleotide "accumulation" is basically an unphysiological process, one that represents the spilling over of cyclic nucleotide from some small physiologically relevant compartment where it has reached high concentrations into the rest of the cell. Thus, this criterion might have to be accepted in somewhat modified form. At the very least, the converse of this criterion must be true, i.e., if detectable changes in cyclic nucleotide levels are observed, then there must be a physiological response. One suggestion which might also be made in this regard concerns the concentrations of agents which are used in biochemical and electrophysiological experiments. In general, the results of such experiments can be most easily interpreted if these concentrations lie in a physiological range. As an example the K_D of l-norepinephrine at the β-receptor in brain, the EC_{50} for electrophysiological responses to NE in brain slices, and the EC_{50} for cyclic AMP increases in brain slices all range between 0.5–5 μM (SPORN and MOLINOFF 1976; MAGUIRE et al. 1976; DUNWIDDIE and MUELLER, unpublished observations; KRISHNA et al. 1970; RALL and SATTIN 1970; SCHMIDT et al. 1970; SHIMIZU et al. 1970). However, when the effects of NE concentrations over an order of magnitude higher are measured (SATTIN and RALL 1970; SCHULTZ and DALY 1973), it is difficult to relate these effects back to responses observed at perhaps more physiological levels. This problem is complicated by the fact that even maximal electrical stimulation of the locus coeruleus produces only 30% increases in cyclic AMP (KORF and SEBENS 1979), compared to the 260–2,000% increases observed both in vivo (BURKARD 1972) and in vitro (cf. DALY 1977a). This suggests that even the effects produced by less than maximal concentrations of NE may be totally out of the physiological range. Thus, in both electrophysiological and biochemical experiments, interpretive problems can be minimized if the concentrations of drugs investigated are as conservative as possible, preferably at levels substantially below those which produce maximal biochemical responses.

(4) *Potentiation of the physiological response should be observed in situations where the cyclic nucleotide response is potentiated.* Classically, it has been suggested that phosphodiesterase inhibitors might be used to potentiate cyclic nucleotide ac-

cumulation as well as physiological responses. In the nervous system this approach, with a few exceptions, is generally a difficult strategy to employ. In a tissue containing many different cell types, each of which may utilize cyclic nucleotides as both pre- and postsynaptic second messengers, and which contain phosphodiesterases of several types with varying sensitivities to different phosphodiesterase inhibitors, it is impossible to be certain of the site of phosphodiesterase activity which is of physiological interest. Furthermore, many of the common phosphodiesterase inhibitors (particularly the methyl xanthines) have a wide variety of actions on the nervous system which are completely unrelated to phosphodiesterase inhibition. Perhaps a slightly more productive approach would to be combine these types of studies with others using other drugs which can potentiate cyclic nucleotide increases by different mechanisms (e.g., adenosine-norepinephrine combinations; see STONE and TAYLOR 1978).

(5) *Exogenous cyclic nucleotide should produce the same effect as the hormone or transmitter.* The same criticism applied to the use of phosphodiesterase inhibitors, i.e., a lack of specificity in terms of the locus of the effect, may be applied to this criterion. In addition, this requirement has been the source of considerable controversy in this field, largely because various adenine nucleotides including cyclic AMP can interact with extracellular adenosine receptors. Thus, extracellular cyclic AMP can produce both the increases in intracellular cyclic AMP (CHASIN et al. 1974; HUANG et al. 1973; MAH and DALY 1976; SATTIN and RALL 1970) as well as the physiological effects (see PHILLIS 1977; DUNWIDDIE and HOFFER 1980) produced by adenosine. A partial solution to this problem is to demonstrate that the potency of cyclic nucleotide derivatives corresponds to their ability to cross the cell membrane, their ability to stimulate protein kinases (e.g., SIGGINS and HENRIKSEN 1975), and to compare their effects in the presence and absence of blockers of adenosine receptors (TAYLOR and STONE 1978; DUNWIDDIE and HOFFER 1980). The ideal solution in many ways is to use intracellular injection of cyclic nucleotides, but this has proven possible in but a few cases (KRNJEVIĆ et al. 1976; KRNJEVIĆ and VAN METER 1976; SWARTZ and WOODY 1979).

It is not known if guanine nucleotides, and cyclic GMP in particular, can interact with unknown extracellular sites in an analogous fashion. In general, the GTP binding site which influences adenylate cyclase activity is thought to be intracellularly directed and relatively insensitive to cyclic GMP (RODBELL 1980), so that it would not be expected to introduce complications.

(6) *The physiological effects of the transmitter or hormone are preceded by or occur in conjunction with changes in the state of phosphorylation of a relevant protein.* This criterion, which has been suggested by various groups (KUO and GREENGARD 1969 a, b; BLOOM 1975), presupposes that all cyclic nucleotide-dependent events involve phosphotransferase reactions; while there is not evidence to the contrary, there are indications that other mechanisms may be involved as well (see WALSH 1978). Nevertheless, in view of the ubiquity of cyclic nucleotide-dependent phosphorylation, this criterion is not unreasonable. The problems with this are similar to those with criterion 2), discussed above; basically, biochemical measures cannot achieve the temporal resolution of electrophysiological ones, and hence, the types of processes involving phosphorylation which can be studied are those in which phosphorylation occurs slowly, or persists for some time following a given event.

As can be seen, the strict application of these six criteria to processes in the central nervous system is virtually impossible, primarily for methodological reasons. Nevertheless, they are useful for several reasons. First, they indicate the types of techniques which will have to be developed before it will be possible to rigorously demonstrate that cyclic nucleotides act as second messengers in any given event. Secondly, they represent criteria by which current hypotheses of cyclic nucleotide action may be judged. Finally, their consideration will make apparent what types of information will be needed to complete our knowledge of cyclic nucleotide mediation of specific responses. In the succeeding sections, as the various examples of cyclic nucleotide action are discussed, reference will be made to these criteria in order to establish a framework within which the experimental data may be considered.

B. Cyclic AMP

I. The Role of Cyclic AMP as a Postsynaptic Second Messenger

In the nervous system, the physiological role for cyclic AMP which has received probably the greatest amount of attention is that of a second messenger for the catecholamine neurotransmitters, NE and DA. Cyclic GMP has been suggested for an analogous role, most notably in the muscarinic cholinergic system. However, the study of the role of cyclic GMP presents some unique problems and hence is considered separately in another section (see Sect. C).

According to the second messenger hypothesis, the binding of a neurotransmitter to an extracellular receptor results in the activation of a membrane-bound adenylate cyclase and the formation of cyclic AMP. Subsequent cyclic AMP-dependent events in the target cell (most probably phosphorylation of membrane and cytosolic proteins) constitutes an essential element in the physiological response to that transmitter (e.g., GREENGARD 1976). Thus, the formation of cyclic AMP is a necessary step which precedes the physiological response to a neurotransmitter. In the central nervous system, this second messenger role of cyclic AMP has been suggested for a variety of transmitters (primarily NE, DA, 5-HT, histamine and adenosine) in many different parts of the brain as well as in the peripheral nervous system. Basically, every substance listed in Table 1 which increases cyclic AMP constitutes a possible transmitter which could use cyclic AMP as an intracellular messenger. Perhaps the more well-known cases in which cyclic AMP is thought to act are in the β-adrenergic depression of Purkinje cell firing (SIGGINS et al. 1969; HOFFER et al. 1970), in inhibitory dopaminergic responses in the striatum (SIGGINS et al. 1974), and in synaptic responses in peripheral ganglia (McAFEE and GREENGARD 1972; McAFEE et al. 1971; GREENGARD and KEBABIAN 1974).

Space precludes a discussion of more than a few of the possible synapses at which cyclic AMP is thought to be important. What will be considered here will be two different types of cases where cyclic AMP has been implicated as a second messenger. In the discussion of these examples, an attempt will be made to illustrate the types of problems and pitfalls frequently encountered in these types of electrophysiological experiments. The particular examples to be considered are the actions of norepinephrine on the Purkinje (P) cells of the cerebellum, and the effects of adenosine and related adenine nucleotide on neuronal activity.

1. Is Cyclic AMP the Second Messenger for NE in the Cerebellum?

The evidence implicating cyclic AMP as a second messenger for NE in the cerebellum has been reviewed in considerable detail. The converging biochemical, electrophysiological and histochemical evidence supporting this hypothesis is described in detail elsewhere in this volume (see SIGGINS, this volume). Briefly, NE increases cyclic AMP levels in cerebellum via activation of a β-receptor. Both NE and cyclic AMP depress cerebellar Purkinje (P) cell spontaneous discharge via a hyperpolarization of the P cell with increases in membrane resistance. Responses to NE are blocked by substances like lanthanum and lithium, which reduce adenylate cyclase activity. Moreover, phosphodiesterase inhibitors, which reduce cyclic AMP breakdown, augment responses to both NE and cyclic AMP. Finally, activation of the noradrenergic input to the P cell, either pharmacologically or physiologically, increases cyclic AMP immunoreactivity of these neurons.

A number of the technical problems encountered in studies of the electrophysiological actions of cyclic AMP are detailed in the chapter by SIGGINS (this volume). Other problems concerning the relationship of extracellular adenosine receptors and "purinergic transmission" to the effects of exogenously applied cyclic AMP are discussed below.

2. Does Cyclic AMP Mediate the Central Effects of Adenosine and Adenine Nucleotides?

Adenosine, as well as other adenine nucleotides, represent another class of compounds with a variety of electrophysiological effects upon the central nervous system for which cyclic AMP has been suggested as a second messenger. ATP has been suggested as a putative transmitter in the periphery (BURNSTOCK 1972, 1978, 1979), but this receptor appears to be somewhat different from the "adenosine" receptor which is observed in brain slices, and apparently does not involve cyclic AMP synthesis.

a) Biochemical Effects of Adenosine

The first indication that adenosine might affect brain levels of cyclic AMP is the report of Sattin and Rall (1967), who found large increases in cyclic AMP produced by brain extracts; the active constituent of these extracts was later shown to be adenosine and/or adenine nucleotides (SHIMIZU et al. 1969; SATTIN and RALL 1970). Increases in cyclic AMP produced by adenosine are antagonized by methylxanthines such as theophylline or isobutylmethylxanthine (SATTIN and RALL 1970; HUANG and DALY 1972; MAH and DALY 1976). Adenosine is released from brain slices by electrical or chemical stimulation in a calcium-dependent fashion (MCILWAIN 1972, PULL and MCILWAIN 1973; KURODA and MCILWAIN 1974), and electrical stimulation elicits increases in cyclic AMP which can be antagonized by theophylline, suggesting mediation by released adenosine. However, the cyclic AMP increases in response to electrical stimulation are not affected, or are actually facilitated in calcium-free medium (KAKIUCHI et al. 1969; ZANELLA and RALL 1973), suggesting that perhaps a more complex interaction of factors is involved.

A variety of experimental approaches suggest that adenosine increases cyclic AMP levels via an interaction with an extracellular receptor. As mentioned above, such increases can be competitively antagonized by a variety of drugs, most notably methyl xanthine derivatives (SATTIN and RALL 1970; HUANG and DALY 1972; KURODA et al. 1976; MAH and DALY 1976; SMELLIE et al. 1979b); increases in cyclic AMP are potentiated by treatments which prevent uptake or metabolic degradation of adenosine (HUANG and DALY 1974). The case for an adenylate cyclase-coupled adenosine receptor has been strengthened by the direct demonstration of adenosine-stimulated cyclase activity in rat striatal homogenates (PREMONT et al. 1977; BOCKAERT 1978). However, while adenosine has been shown to raise cyclic AMP levels in every brain region that has been studied (see DALY 1979), the adenosine-stimulated cyclase is not ubiquitous (PREMONT et al. 1979) and is notably absent in some brain regions which show excellent cyclic AMP responses to exogenously applied adenosine. The literature concerning cyclic AMP accumulations in brain slice preparations in different species elicited by adenosine has been reviewed in detail elsewhere (Daly 1979).

b) Electrophysiological Effects of Adenosine

Because of the ability of adenosine to increase cyclic AMP in many brain regions just discussed, cyclic AMP might be a likely candidate for a second messenger for purinergic transmitters. The electrophysiological evidence that this is the case is primarily correlative. Iontophoretically applied adenosine has been shown to be a potent depressant of spontaneous neuronal activity in most brain regions which have been studied (PHILLIS et al. 1974, 1975; KOSTOPOULOS et al. 1975; PHILLIS and KOSTOPOULOS 1975; STONE and TAYLOR 1978; see PHILLIS et al. 1979b for a recent review). Adenosine, adenine nucleotides such as 5′-AMP, ADP and ATP, and various non-metabolized purine derivatives, such as 2-chloroadenosine and 2′-deoxyadenosine, all have generally depressant effects on single unit firing. Furthermore, the relative potencies of these purinergic agonists in depressing single unit activity correlates fairly well with their ability to stimulate cyclic AMP formation in brain slice preparation (PHILLIS and KOSTOPOULOS 1975; PHILLIS and EDSTROM 1976). Drugs which antagonize cyclic AMP accumulation, such as methyl xanthines, are also relatively potent blockers of the electrophysiological response to adenosine (PHILLIS and KOSTOPOULOS 1975; KURODA et al. 1976; SCHOLFIELD 1978; STONE and TAYLOR 1977). Cyclic AMP accumulations in brain slices can be potentiated either by blocking the reuptake of adenosine, or by blocking its metabolic breakdown to inosine by inhibiting adenosine deaminase (HUANG and DALY 1974; MAH and DALY 1976; SKOLNICK et al. 1978). Both adenosine reuptake blockers and adenosine deaminase inhibitors have generally depressant effects in cortical unit activity (PHILLIS and EDSTROM 1976; PHILLIS et al. 1979a), suggesting an endogenous release of adenosine.

Nevertheless, there is also some conflicting evidence in which the effects of drugs upon cyclic AMP generating systems and physiological activity do not show parallels. Two purine derivatives, 2′- and 3′-deoxyadenosine, antagonize adenosine-mediated cyclic AMP formation (MAH and DALY 1976), but appear to have depressant properties when applied iontophoretically (EDSTROM and PHILLIS 1976). Direct approaches to the problem, such as iontophoresis of cyclic AMP or its derivatives have been somewhat difficult to interpret. Because cyclic AMP is an adenine nucleotide, it probably, via metabolism to adenosine, shares with adenosine the ability to increase intracellular cyclic AMP formation via an interaction with extracellular site viz. the adenosine receptor (CHASIN et al. 1974; MAH and DALY 1976). Electrophysiological experiments disagree as to the extent by which the effects of exogenous cyclic AMP can be blocked by adenosine antagonists (PHILLIS 1977; STONE and TAYLOR 1977). This, in addition to the fact that most phosphodiesterase blockers are either adenosine antagonists (e.g., theophylline; SATTIN and RALL 1970) or reuptake blockers (e.g., papaverine, dipyridamole; MAH and DALY 1976), has made it extremely difficult to test electrophysiologically whether cyclic AMP is involved in the postsynaptic actions of adenosine. These two problems, the effects of cyclic AMP and related compounds on the extracellular adenosine receptor, and the effects of phosphodiesterase inhibitors on other adenosine-related processes, are serious obstacles to the electrophysiological demonstration that cyclic AMP is involved in the postsynaptic action of any transmitter, be it NE, dopamine, adenosine or any other agent which is known to raise cyclic AMP levels.

Regarding adenosine, there is no compelling electrophysiological evidence to suggest that adenosine exerts its depressant effects at a postsynaptic site; in fact, the preponderance of the data would seem to suggest that most such effects stem from an action at a presynaptic site (see LEKIĆ 1977; PHILLIS et al. 1979b; EDSTROM and PHILLIS 1976; see Sect. 2.b).

To summarize, the evidence appears to be fairly strong that adenosine can produce increases in cyclic AMP via an interaction with an extra-cellular adenosine receptor. However, these effects of adenosine and related compounds on cyclic AMP formation do not *always* correlate well with the electrophysiological effects of adenosine, and the pre- or postsynaptic localization of these adenosine receptors is largely unknown. Thus, in contrast to the situation with norepinephrine, the evidence that adenosine uses cyclic AMP as a postsynaptic second messenger is weak. Until more evidence in support of this role becomes available, this hypothesis should remain highly tentative.

II. Cyclic AMP as a Modulator of Synaptic Responses

In the examples just discussed, it was hypothesized that cyclic AMP acted directly upon some aspect of the postsynaptic neuron to alter its electrophysiological activity. Two of the most readily apparent ways in which it might do so would be to directly affect conductance channels in the postsynaptic cell, or to activate membrane pumps which would effect a redistribution of ions, primarily Na^+ and K^+. In either case, such an action would be readily apparent, and could be measured with an intracellular electrode in terms of changes in membrane resistance and/or resting potential.

Another possibility is that cyclic AMP is involved in the modulation of synaptic responses; by modulation, we refer to processes which affect some aspect of neurotransmission, but which do not directly affect measurable electrophysiological parameters of the postsynaptic cell. These types of effects would not be detectable under most circumstances with an intracellular electrode, but would become apparent when responses along a "modulated" pathway are tested. One type of modulation could be presynaptic; changes in transmitter synthesis or release could occur as a result of interaction of a transmitter with its own terminals ("autoreceptors"), or with terminals which release another transmitter. Modulation could also be postsynaptic, perhaps through some type of influence on the postsynaptic processes by which another transmitter produces its electrophysiological effects. An example might help to clarify what is meant by this; the acetylcholine receptor of *Torpedo* is apparently a substrate for an endogenous protein kinase (GORDON et al. 1977). Although the physiological significance of phosphorylation of the ACh receptor is unclear, this represents a way in which cyclic AMP produced in a postsynaptic neuron by one neurotransmitter, could modulate transmission in other transmitter systems. Phosphorylation of the ACh receptor does not occur in a cyclic AMP-dependent fashion, so it is unlikely that this occurs in *Torpedo*, but other receptors in the CNS might be regulated by cyclic AMP-dependent phosphorylation.

Perhaps more germane is the suggestion that adenylate cyclase itself is a substrate for endogenous kinases (RICHARDS and SWISLOCKI 1979). This could provide a very basic mechanism by which the increases in cyclic AMP produced by a modulator (e.g., adenosine) could influence responses to other agents which activate adenylate cyclase in the same cells.

1. Cyclic AMP as a Postsynaptic Modulator

There are a large number of factors which can influence cyclic AMP-mediated effects in postsynaptic neurons. Modulators could interact with cyclases, phosphodiesterases, or even with cyclic nucleotide-dependent kinases to modify physiological responsiveness of the entire system. RODBELL (1980) discusses a wide variety of factors which can influence adenylate cyclase activation. Calmodulin (CHEUNG 1980; see also CHEUNG, Volume I) imparts a calcium sensitivity not only to the adenylate cyclase, but to phosphodiesterase as well. In addition, the endogenous inhibitory factors which regulate cyclic AMP-dependent protein kinase activity are affected by neuronal activity as well (SZMIGIELSKI and GUIDOTTI 1979). Thus, the possibilities for regulation of the cyclic AMP system by modulators are numerous.

In this section, we will discuss two specific types of experiments which suggest that functional modulation can take place at the postsynaptic side of the synapse. First, there is evidence that adenosine can modulate the biochemical responsiveness of brain slices to a variety of other putative transmitters. Secondly, there is considerable evidence from electrophysiological experiments which indicates that NE can modulate the effects of other transmitters in the cerebellum; however, there is as of yet little evidence either for or against an involvement of cyclic AMP in either of these two examples.

a) Adenosine-Modulation of the Responsiveness of Cyclic AMP Generating Systems

The earliest report of adenosine-mediated increases in cyclic AMP formation noted that combinations of either NE or histamine with adenosine would produce increases in cyclic AMP accumulation which were greater than the sum of the individual responses (SATTIN and RALL 1970; HUANG et al. 1971). These types of synergistic responses are observed both at low drug concentrations, and at levels sufficient to elicit maximal cyclic AMP accumulations as well. The biochemical evidence for these types of synergistic interactions has been reviewed and discussed (DALY 1977a; RALL 1979).

Nevertheless, the physiological significance of these results is not at all clear. In the first place, such effects are apparently observed only in tissue slices. A variety of different types of cultured cells have been examined, and the cyclic AMP responses to various amines measured; combinations of amines never produce more than additive accumulations of cyclic AMP (CLARK et al. 1974; SCHULTZ and HAMPRECHT 1973; PERKINS et al. 1975; MCCARTHY and DE VELLIS 1978; SCHULTZ et al. 1972). In primary glial cultures and clonal cell lines, NE actually inhibits adenosine-mediated cyclic AMP accumulation through an interaction with an α_2-receptor site (MCCARTHY and DE VELLIS 1978; SABOL and NIRENBERG 1979). In homogenates, adenylate cyclase activation by dopamine, adenosine and NE are all additive (PREMONT et al. 1977, 1979). All this might lead one to question whether potentiative interactions between putative transmitters occur within the same cell population. It would appear more likely that they involve different types of cells, neurons and/or glial, and perhaps involve the release of other neurohumoral substances. This latter possibility is also supported by the finding that the removal of calcium from the medium in which slices are maintained changes NE-adenosine synergism to a purely additive effect (SCHWABE and DALY 1977).

The synergism between NE and adenosine in rat cortex (SCHWABE and DALY 1977; PERKINS et al. 1975) and in guinea pig cortex (SATTIN et al. 1975) has been attributed to activation of α-receptor sites by NE. It has been suggested by RALL (1979) that this effect might occur via a direct influx of Ca^{+2} following stimulation of α-receptors, which would potentiate the increases in cyclic AMP stimulated by adenosine. However, if increased calcium influx facilitates adenylate cyclase activation, it is not clear why removal of extracellular Ca^{+2} enhances, rather than diminishes adenosine-mediated increases in cyclic AMP in the absence of NE (SCHWABE and DALY 1977; SCHULTZ 1975).

A more recent paper from this group (SCHWABE et al. 1978) suggests that the interaction between calcium and adenosine is even more complex. Treatment of slices with adenosine deaminase, which breaks down adenosine in the extracellular space, significantly alters the types of responses to other transmitters in both rat and guinea pig cortical slices, suggesting that the slices themselves release enough adenosine to modulate the responsiveness of the slices to other putative transmitters. In the presence of adenosine deaminase and calcium, histamine, NE, and N^6-phenylisopropyl adenosine (a non-metabolizable adenosine analog) all increase cyclic AMP levels. With adenosine deaminase and no calcium, NE and histamine have no effect. Thus, accumulations of cyclic AMP in response to both NE and histamine in guinea pig cortex apparently require either calcium or adenosine to be present in the extracellular space; in the absence of both, no increases in cyclic AMP can be seen (see Table 2).

In addition to exerting a kind or permissive influence over NE-mediated cyclic AMP accumulations, adenosine also appears to change the basic agonist/antagonist properties of some adrenergic drugs. Specifically, methoxamine is not able to

Table 2. Effects of various drugs on cyclic AMP accumulation guinea pig cerebral cortex

Calcium Adenosine	Normal Basal	Normal 0	0 (2 m*M* EGTA) Basal	0 (2 m*M* EGTA) 0
Basal levels of cAMP	8.9 pg/mg protein	7.2	17.9	10.4
Histamine (100 μ*M*)	X 3.9	X 3.0	X 2.0	X 0.9
Norepinephrine (100 μ*M*)	X 3.8	X 1.8	X 3.9	X 1.0
N6PA[a] (100 μ*M*)	X 15	X 22	X 14	X 22
Histamine + N6PA[a]	X 4.1	X 2.9	X 1.8	X 1.1

[a] N6PA = N^6-phenyl isopropyl adenosine

This table shows the effects of histamine, norepinephrine, and N^6-phenyl-isopropyl adenosine on the accumulation of cyclic AMP in slices from guinea pig cortex. Slices were maintained either in Krebs-Ringer bicarbonate buffered medium (normal calcium), or medium to which 2 m*M* EGTA had been added, effectively reducing the extracellular calcium concentration to almost 0. Some slices had small amounts of adenosine in the extracellular space from endogenously released adenosine ("basal"); others were treated with adenosine deaminase to eliminate extracellular adenosine. Increases in tissue cyclic AMP are shown for histamine, norepinephrine, and N6PA as fold increases above basal cyclic AMP levels in the different media. For the last row, the increases produced by histamine-N6PA combinations were synergistic; therefore, the increases are shown as the fold increase over what would have been expected had the two been merely additive in their effects. Note that while strongly synergistic effects are observed in normal medium, the responses in EGTA-adenosine deaminase medium were apparently additive (only 1.1 X of what would have been expected based upon individual responses) (Data adapted from SCHWABE et al. 1978)

increase cyclic AMP levels by itself, and antagonizes NE-mediated increases. However, in the presence of exogenously applied adenosine, methoxamine increases cyclic AMP levels, and no longer antagonizes NE-mediated increases (SCHULTZ and KLEEFELD 1979).

Without belaboring the point, the conclusions which may be derived from this admittedly superficial coverage of the literature are clear. Adenosine has the capability to radically alter the responsiveness of cyclic AMP generating systems to various other putative transmitters. While the way in which it produces these effects defies simple explanation at this point, the possible involvement of calcium as an intermediary has been suggested.

So far, we have discussed the ability of adenosine to stimulate cyclic AMP formation directly and to influence the types of changes produced by other putative transmitters. In addition, adenosine has been shown to have direct inhibitory effects on adenylate cyclase in the brain and elsewhere (MCKENZIE and BÄR 1973; LONDOS and WOLFF 1977), and to antagonize β-adrenergically mediated increases in cyclic AMP in mouse brain cultures (VAN CALKER et al. 1978). This has led to the proposal that there are two distinct types of adenosine-sensitive sites on the receptor-cyclase complex which can be distinguished pharmacologically (LONDOS and WOLFF 1977; LONDOS et al. 1979). One site (the "R" site) is thought to be externally directed and antagonized by methylxanthines, while the second ("P") site, which inhibits cyclase activity, is internally directed and not antagonized by xanthine derivatives. Thus, adenosine can a) directly stimulate cyclase activity, b) potentiate cyclic AMP increases elicited by other putative transmitters, and c) inhibit adenylate cyclase directly.

While the data which has just been discussed may be somewhat complex and not readily amenable to the development of testable theories of neuronal interaction, the message of such experiments in terms of physiological function is clear. Classical electrophysiology would hold that the effects of several transmitters applied to the same neuron would be readily predictable in terms of the individual conductance changes produced by each transmitter. The locus of interaction, as it were, is the cell membrane; the factors to be considered are the conductance changes and the electrochemical gradients involved. Biochemical experiments with adenosine would suggest another mode of interaction, via changes in cyclic nucleotide systems in the postsynaptic neuron. In such situations, the electrophysiological response to simultaneous application of two or more transmitters could not be predicted from summation of their known electrophysiological effects. Furthermore, it appears quite likely that transmitter substances exist (defined here as one type of neuromodulator) which produce no direct effects on membrane conductances, but whose primary effect is at this second locus of interaction, intracellular biochemical effects.

The electrophysiological evidence that such modulatory interactions can take place is exceedingly scant. As far as adenosine is concerned, it has been reported that the duration of the depression of single cell firing in rat cortex elicited by iontophoretically applied NE is enhanced by the concurrent application of adenosine (STONE and TAYLOR 1978); however, the specificity of this interaction is unclear, since changes of nearly comparable magnitude were observed in serotonin-mediated depressions. More recently, TAYLOR and STONE (1980) have reported that iontophoretic application of adenosine has multiple effects on NE released by stimulation of the locus coeruleus (LC). If the adenosine is applied prior to LC stimulation, the response to LC stimulation is diminished, whereas concurrent iontophoresis of adenosine potentiates the effects of LC stimulation. These authors suggest that adenosine may act presynaptically to inhibit NE release, and postsynaptically to facilitate the β-adrenergic depression of cell firing. Attempts to produce physiological interactions between exogenously applied adenosine and NE in the hippocampus in vitro have, to this point, been unsuccessful (DUNWIDDIE, unpublished observations).

b) Norepinephrine: Modulation of Responsiveness to Other Transmitters

Recent studies have expanded our concept of the functional interaction of NE with neuronal circuitry beyond that of the early work in this area, in which NE was thought to be primarily an inhibitory neurotransmitter. Based upon the interactions of NE with a variety of neurotransmitters, primarily ACh, GABA, and glutamate, it would appear that the ability of NE to modulate responsiveness to other transmitters is at least as important as its ability to directly affect neuronal activity.

Much of the work implicating NE as a neuromodulator comes from work in the cerebellum, where the functional role of the adrenergic pathway from the locus coeruleus has been well-established (SIGGINS et al. 1971c; HOFFER et al. 1973; SIGGINS, this volume). In addition to a direct depressant action on Purkinje (P) cell activity, NE produces a relative or absolute potentiation of either excitatory or inhibitory synaptic inputs to the P cell. As seen in Fig. 2 and 3, microiontophoreti-

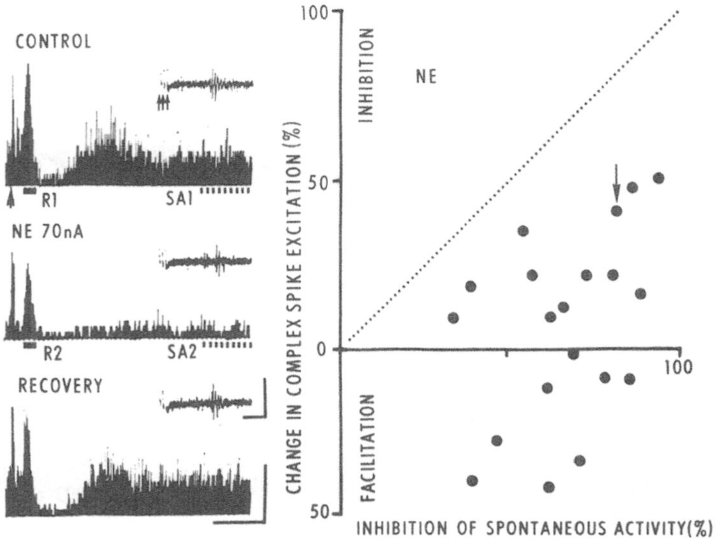

Fig. 2. Changes in evoked complex spikes and spontaneous activity induced by norepinephrine *(NE)* iontophoresis. Oscillograph and poststimulus-time histogram records *(left)* show the complex spike response of a cerebellar Purkinje cell from stimulation of the cerebral cortex. Responses during the control, NE iontophoresis, and recovery periods are shown. Spontaneous activity (broken bars beneath histograms) was inhibited 80% by NE from 49.0 spikes/s *SA1* to 10.0 spikes/s *SA2*. The evoked activity *(solid bars)* was inhibited only 46% from 2.13 spikes/stimulus *R1* to 1.15 spikes per stimulus *R2*. Each histogram contains 100 sweeps. The graph at right summarizes results from similar experiments with 20 Purkinje cells. The point corresponding to the data from the cell shown at left is marked by the arrow. Note that eight of the cells show an apparent potentiation of evoked activity. Calibrations: Histograms-vertical, 10 counts per address; horizontal, 100 ms. Specimen record-vertical, 1 mV; horizontal, 10 ms (Taken from FREEDMAN et al. 1977)

cally applied NE, or NE released via stimulation of LC, enhances responses to stimulation of excitatory cerebellar afferents, as well as potentiating GABAergic inhibition of P cell firing (MOISES et al. 1979; MOISES and WOODWARD 1980). No enhancement of glycine-induced depressions are seen; this accords well with other evidence suggesting that glycine is not an endogenous transmitter in cerebellum. In addition, dopamine, which is found in very low concentrations in cerebellum, is not able to mimic the effects of NE. The ability of NE to potentiate both inhibitory or excitatory responses in cerebellum is occasionally observed with amounts of NE insufficient to produce any detectable changes in the spontaneous firing rate; thus, it would appear that the cerebellar P cells are, if anything, more sensitive to the modulatory influences of NE than they are to its direct effects of cell firing rate.

The work in cerebellum presents by far the most compelling evidence for NE modulation of synaptic responses. Nevertheless, there is evidence for modulatory actions of NE not only in cerebellum, but in cerebral cortex (FOOTE et al. 1975; WATERHOUSE et al. 1979; WATERHOUSE and WOODWARD 1980), hippocampus (SEGAL and BLOOM 1976), and other brain areas. If the function of NE is primarily to induce a bias that augments responsiveness to conventional excitatory and inhibitory synaptic input, is such as bias mediated via cyclic AMP? There have been no systematic tests of this hypothesis, although examples of increased synaptic po-

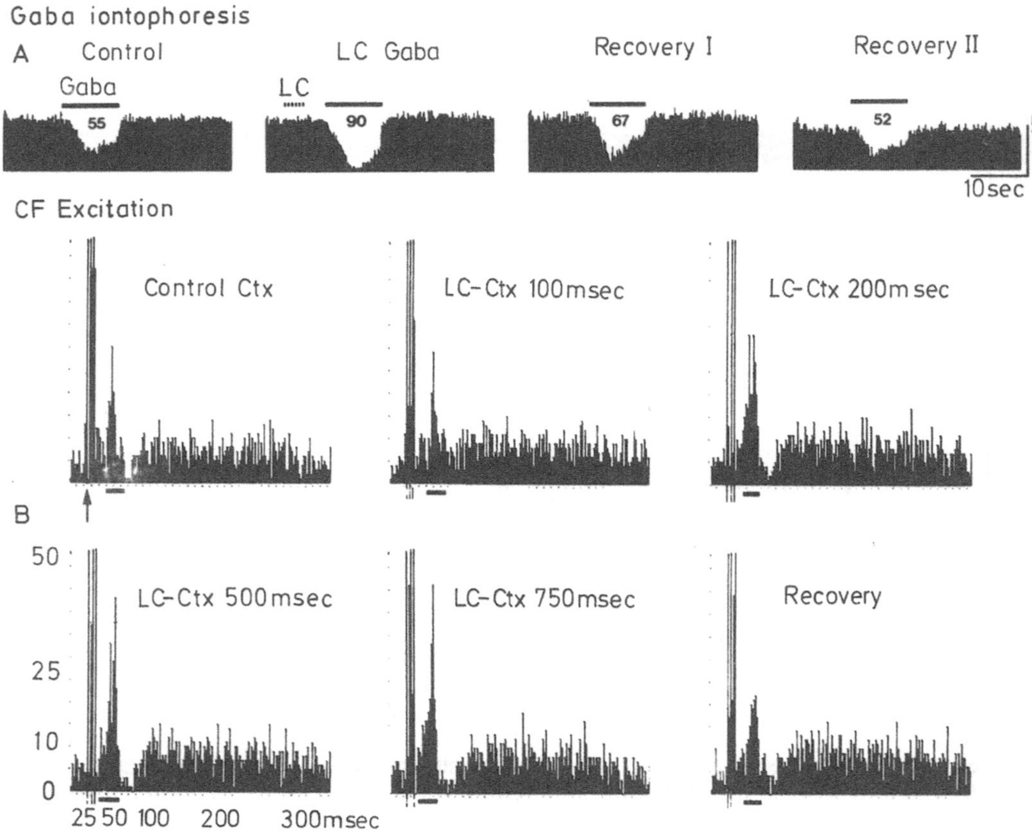

Fig. 3 A, B. Drug response histograms in **A** show the response of a cerebellar Purkinje cell to microiontophoretic pulses of GABA *(solid bar)* applied before, in conjunction with, and long after preconditioning stimulation of the locus coeruleus *(LC; dotted line)*. Stimulation of the LC for 3.5 s at 10 Hz, initiated 6.0 s prior to the onset of drug iontophoresis, greatly enhanced the inhibitory effect of GABA. Numbers beneath the horizontal bars in all histograms indicate the percent inhibition of background firing produced by GABA. Note that LC stimulation was subthreshold for directly affecting spontaneous discharge of the cell. All histograms contain 8 sweeps. Poststimulus time histograms in **B** show the effect of LC preconditioning stimulation on the climbing fiber excitation of a Purkinje cell evoked by sensorimotor cortex stimulation (*triple vertical bars* in histogram). Stimulation of LC (3 shocks at 100 Hz) at currents subthreshold for directly affecting spontaneous discharge of this cell greatly enhanced activity evoked by the climbing fiber input *(solid bar histograms)*. Facilitation of the evoked responses was observed when LC stimulation was delivered 200–750 msec prior to the cortical test stimulus. Note that at 500 and 750 msec intervals, post-climbing fiber inhibition was also increased by LC conditioning. All histograms contain 100 sweeps. (Taken from WOODWARD et al. 1979)

tentials after application of cyclic AMP have been reported (SIGGINS et al. 1971 a; HOFFER et al. 1973; SIGGINS, this volume).

Thus, it would appear, on the basis of electrophysiological experiments, that NE has not only the direct depressant effects discussed earlier (Sect. B.I.1), but that it has effects consistent with our definition of a neuromodulator as well. The precise role played by cyclic AMP in these phenomena remains to be determined.

2. Cyclic AMP as a Presynaptic Modulator

Another basic way in which modulation can take place is via a regulatory influence on the amount of transmitter which is released by a single nerve impulse. One way in which this might occur is if cyclic AMP can directly influence the synthesis of transmitter. This appears to be the case in the activation of tyrosine hydroxylase, which is the rate-limiting enzyme in catecholamine biosynthesis. Since the involvement of cyclic AMP has been studied in rather extensive detail, it will be considered at length in the following section (Sect. II.2.a). The phosphorylation and consequent activation of tyrosine hydroxylase represents the type of process by which cyclic AMP could regulate synthesis of other transmitters as well, but at this point, the generality of this mechanism in unknown.

A second possibility for a presynaptic action of cyclic AMP is in the process of transmitter release. Cyclic AMP has been proposed to either by directly involved in transmitter release, or to exert a modulatory influence on release, perhaps by controlling the availability of intracellular calcium for the process of exocytosis. This possibility is discussed in Sect. B.II.2.b.

a) Regulation of Transmitter Synthesis: Cyclic AMP-Dependent Phosphorylation of Tyrosine Hydroxylase

Although it has been possible to demonstrate the cyclic AMP-dependent phosphorylation of a variety of protein substrates in the nervous system, their functions are largely unknown. However, one such protein which does have a well-known function is tyrosine hydroxylase, the rate-limiting enzyme in the synthesis of catecholamines (WEINER 1975). Two features make this system somewhat unique. First, because it is an enzyme, its activity can be measured quantitatively in a purified preparation, and detailed comparisons made between the properties of the phosphorylated and de-phosphorylated forms. Secondly, it is clearly located presynaptically, and provides perhaps the strongest evidence that cyclic AMP systems can affect physiological activity in pre- as well as postsynaptic compartments in the nervous system.

The evidence that tyrosine hydroxylase (TH) can be activated in an apparently cyclic AMP-dependent manner has been demonstrated in a variety of systems, i.e., in vivo, in vitro, and in purified membrane preparations, and has been reviewed at some length in various reports (DALY 1977a; WEINER et al. 1977; WEINER 1979b). In vivo, a wide variety of treatments which result in enhanced release of catecholamines increase TH activity, although release per se is not essential to the activation.

Stimulation of peripheral nerves (WEINER et al. 1978) as well as central catecholaminergic pathways (ROTH et al. 1975; SALZMAN and ROTH 1978) result in relatively rapid increases in enzyme activity. Both the speed (maximal within 30–60 sec in peripheral nerve; WEINER et al. 1977) as well as the magnitude of the changes (300% increase; WEINER et al. 1977; SALZMAN and ROTH 1978) which are observed suggest that these types of changes may be of significant importance in the short-term regulation of transmitter concentrations. The problem with these types of experiments is that, although treatments that increase cyclic AMP levels elicit parallel changes in TH activity (ZIVKOVIC et al. 1975, 1976; SALZMAN and

ROTH 1978) and administration of exogenous cyclic AMP derivatives produces increases in TH activity (SALZMAN and ROTH 1978; WEINER et al. 1978; GOLDSTEIN et al. 1973; ANAGNOSTE et al. 1974; TANEDA et al. 1974; MACKAY and IVERSEN 1972), it is not possible to show in these types of preparations that there is a strict cause and effect relationship between cyclic AMP-dependent phosphorylation and the increases in TH activity.

Evidence from experiments using broken-cell preparations (either homogenates or partially purified enzyme preparations) supports the basic hypothesis that phosphorylation is involved in TH activation (LOVENBERG and BRUCKWICK 1974; EBSTEIN et al. 1974; MORGENROTH et al. 1975; HARRIS et al. 1974; LOVENBERG et al. 1975; LLOYD and KAUFMAN 1975; HOELDTKE and KAUFMAN 1977; DRUMMOND et al. 1978). When such preparations are subjected to phosphorylating conditions, subsequent measurements reveal an increase in TH activity. This activation appears to be due primarily to a decrease in the K_m for the pterin cofactor and an increase in the K_i for inhibitory catechols, although changes in the K_m for tyrosine and in the V_{max} have been reported as well. In general, the activation appears to demonstrate an absolute requirement for Mg^{+2}, ATP and cyclic AMP in order for the conversion to the activated state to occur.

Following some early attempts to demonstrate direct phosphorylation of TH, there was some question as to whether TH itself, or perhaps some regulatory protein, was phosphorylated in order to activate TH. LOVENBERG et al. (1975) and LLOYD and KAUFMAN (1975) both showed that phosphorylating conditions produced decreases in the K_m for the tetrahydropteridine cofactor and consequent increases in enzymatic activity, but were unable to demonstrate enhanced incorporation of ^{32}P into immunprecipitable TH.

Subsequently, at least five groups have been able to show direct incorporation of ^{32}P into purified TH with subsequent increases in activity (LETENDRE et al. 1977; EDELMAN et al. 1978; JOH et al. 1978; YAMAUCHI and FUJISAWA 1979; VULLIET et al. 1980). In general, the activation, as with the in vitro systems, appears to correspond to a decrease in K_m for the pterin cofactor, although changes in V_{max} have been reported as well (JOH et al. 1978). The interpretation of changes in V_{max} are somewhat difficult since several minor contaminants (possibly regulatory subunits) were observed in the purified enzyme preparation following acrylamide gel electrophoresis. However, JOH et al. (1978) did observe the phosphorylation to occur in what was apparently the same ~60,000 dalton subunit of TH seen by others.

In spite of these discrepancies, it seems apparent in highly purified preparations that phosphorylation of TH occurs in the presence of Mg^{+2}, ATP and purified catalytic subunit of cyclic AMP-dependent protein kinase. When TH is extracted from tissue and purified, is usually is found to be approximately 20–40% in the phosphorylated form, and demonstrates non-linear kinetics indicating two forms of the enzyme with different K_m values for the pterin cofactor. When maximally activated, approximately 0.7 mole of additional phosphate is incorporated per mole of TH, indicating the probable existence of one phosphorylated site per enzyme molecule; in this form, the enzyme demonstrates linear kinetics with regards to pterin cofactor, indicating a single form of the enzyme. Finally, the degree and time course of activation of the purified TH preparation corresponds nearly exactly with incorporation of ^{32}P into the enzyme (YAMAUCHI and FUJISAWA 1979; VUL-

LIET et al. 1980). In addition, it does not appear to make a difference whether purified TH is derived from peripheral tissues, cultured cells, or brain tissue. In all cases, the phosphorylation of the enzyme results in increases in enzymatic activity.

These elegant experiments demonstrate directly that activation of tyrosine hydroxylase proceeds via the incorporation of phosphate into the enzyme molecule with consequent alteration in its kinetic properties. However, the physiological significance of this type of phosphorylation has been questioned by others (BUSTOS and ROTH 1979). Difficulties have arisen particularly in trying to find in vivo conditions under which TH is activated in a cyclic AMP-dependent fashion.

There are a variety of in vivo treatments which can induce short-term activation of the enzyme, such as nerve stimulation (MORGENROTH et al. 1974; WEINER et al. 1978), decapitation (MASSERANO and WEINER 1979) and treatment of slices with high potassium, phospholipids and cyclic AMP analogs (RAESE et al. 1976; BUSTOS and ROTH 1979; MASSERANO and WEINER, unpublished observations). In many cases, the in vivo activation is not additive with that produced by subsequent exposure of the purified TH to phoshorylating conditions. This nonadditivity would suggest that the same site is phosphorylated during endogenous activation of the TH molecule, and in vitro in the presence of cyclic AMP.

However, there are also a variety of ways in which TH may be activated in intact tissue such that the increases in activity *are* additive with those produced by subsequent phosphorylation. BUSTOS and ROTH (1979) reported that stimulation of striatal slices with either high K^+ or dBcAMP resulted in an activation of TH when subsequently assayed in a crude supernatant fraction prepared from the slices. However, when this supernatant was incubated with Mg^{+2}, ATP and cyclic AMP (i.e., phosphorylating conditions), increases in TH activity were observed which were actually greatest in the slices which had previously been treated with dBcAMP. If the original treatment with dBcAMP activated TH by a phosphorylation of the TH molecule, then subsequent exposure to phosphorylating conditions should have had little if any effect of enzymatic activity.

What implications does this have for the postulated mechanism of short-term TH activation via cyclic AMP-dependent phosphorylation? First, it suggests that there are other noncyclic AMP-dependent mechanisms by which TH is activated (e.g., by calcium as was suggested by BUSTOS and ROTH). Secondly, in vivo and in crude cytosolic fractions, there may be various cyclic AMP-dependent regulators of TH activity which contribute to the activation of TH, but which, of course, are lost in purified enzyme preparations. Furthermore, in a crude preparation, activated TH molecules may be exposed to the action of endogenous phosphatases, which might reverse any changes in the phosphorylated state of the protein by the time the in vitro assay is carried out. The phosphorylated state of some proteins appears to be quite labile unless particular precautions are taken to block the action of phosphatases (e.g., FORN and GREENGARD 1978). In view of the extremely rapid phosphorylation of TH in some preparations, the action of similarly active phosphatases cannot be discounted. The failure of initial attempts to demonstrate phosphate incorporation into TH (LLOYD and KAUFMAN 1975; LOVENBERG et al. 1975) may have been the result of this type of dephosphorylation. Finally, there are indications that the active phosphorylated form of the TH molecule may be somewhat unstable (Vulliet et al. 1980), and hence, might not persist long enough to be manifested in a subsequent in vitro assay.

In short, these experiments do not suggest that phosphorylation is unrelated to the regulation of TH activity, but indicate as well a) that other mechanisms besides cyclic AMP-dependent phosphorylation exist which may alter the activity of TH, and b) that a test of the physiological significance of endogenous phosphorylation of TH may await the development of techniques for extracting phosphorylated proteins from tissue without affecting their state of phosphorylation.

b) Regulation of Transmitter Release

There are at least two ways in which cyclic AMP might influence the release of synaptic transmitters. First, it might be directly involved as an essential step in the process of exocytosis. This suggestion has been made by Rasmussen (1970; see also Rasmussen et al. 1975; Berridge, this volume), and might provide an explanation for the apparent release of various substances following treatment with cyclic AMP derivatives and phosphodiesterase inhibitors in the adrenal medulla (Peach 1972; Poisner 1973), and in peripheral nerves (Wooten et al. 1973; Standaert et al. 1976b). Another possibility is that cyclic nucleotides can affect some variable associated with transmission (e.g., intracellular levels of calcium); in this case, cyclic nucleotides might regulate transmission even though they are not directly involved in the transmission process per se. The current status of these two hypotheses is somewhat difficult to evaluate; basically, it is not feasible at this point to measure cyclic nucleotide levels in nerve terminals with anything near the temporal resolution necessary to correlate cyclic nucleotide changes with various aspects of the release process. The alternative is to characterize the effects of drugs which affect cyclic nucleotide levels, and relate them to their effects on synaptic transmission. While these techniques might provide suggestive evidence concerning cyclic nucleotide involvement in transmitter release, they are insufficient to distinguish between the two alternatives just discussed.

If cyclic nucleotides do act to modulate neurotransmission, how do changes in presynaptic nucleotide levels come about? The assumption has been that presynaptic receptors activate adenylate or guanylate cyclase to regulate cyclic nucleotide levels in the presynaptic compartment. Here, the actions of cyclic nucleotides as second messengers would be comparable to their postsynaptic actions, except that in terminals, the intracellular "message" concerns the subsequent release of transmitter. The question then becomes what type of first (i.e., extracellular) messengers might use cyclic nucleotides as a means of influencing transmitter release.

Many transmitters can apparently influence transmitter release from their own terminals. Probably the best known example of this mechanism is at noradrenergic synapses, where NE itself appears to act on presynaptic α-receptors, termed "autoreceptors", whose physiological role is generally to inhibit subsequent NE release. At other synapses, it would appear that substances besides the neurotransmitter are released and that these substances can exert a feedback influence upon the presynaptic element. For example, ATP has been shown to be stored in cholinergic vesicles (Meunier et al. 1975) and apparently can be released by synaptic stimulation (Silinsky 1975). It has also been suggested that coenzyme A might be released simultaneously with ACh (Cook et al. 1978, 1979). Since both of these purine derivatives have inhibitory effects upon synaptic transmission, the release of these putative modulators may be physiologically significant; a negative feedback role for purine derivatives in neurotransmission has frequently been discussed (e.g., RIBEIRO 1979). Finally, many putative transmitters appear to affect transmitter release at synapses where other substances are the primary transmitter. For example, not only noradrenergic autoreceptors regulate release of NE, but putative presynaptic receptors for epinephrine, dopamine, prostaglandins, nicotinic and muscarinic cholinergic compounds, and opiates have all been postulated to control the release of NE (see WEINER 1979a). Although not all of these are likely to be operative in the same system, they suggest that heterosynaptic regulation of transmission may be fairly ubiquitous. The fact that almost all of these substances can affect cyclic nucleotide levels raises the issue of whether they exert their effects via cyclic nucleotides. In general, while the experimental evidence presents no unequivocal case for cyclic AMP (or cyclic GMP) modulating transmitter release, there is much evidence suggesting such a role.

In the following sections, we will consider several examples in which presynaptic modulatory effects on transmitter release are thought to occur; two cases in which autoreceptors are involved (dopaminergic D_1 and β-noradrenergic), one in which the modulator may be released along with the normal transmitter (adenosine), and the neuromuscular junction, where modulation of several different types appears to occur.

α) Autoreceptors: Norepinephrine. The existence of presynaptic α-receptors which inhibit the release of NE from peripheral terminals has been known for some time (see LANGER 1977 for a review). In addition, there appears to be a β-mediated positive feedback system by which NE release is facilitated (ADLER-GRASCHINSKY and LANGER 1975; STJÄRNE and BRUNDIN 1975). The proposal has been made that the β-response (viz. facilitation of release) is observed at low levels of transmitter release while the α-inhibition occurs at higher levels.

The physiological events which occur in the terminal to alter release are unclear. A likely hypothesis is that the α-inhibition of release is mediated via a decreased availability of intracellular Ca^{+2}, since the inhibitory effects of most α-agonists can be reversed by increased levels of Ca^{+2} (STJÄRNE 1973; DISMUKES et al. 1977; WESTFALL 1977). A similar calcium dependency was observed in release of ^{3}H-NE from synaptosomes (DE LANGEN and MULDER 1980), where the basal release of NE is apparently insufficient to stimulate the α-receptors. The apparent calcium-dependency of α-modulation of NE release does not necessarily rule out an involvement of cyclic AMP. For example, if changes in the levels of cyclic AMP restricted calcium fluxes into the terminal, higher concentrations of calcium might override this type of inhibition. However, there is little evidence to suggest that this is the case. Moreover, the existence of β-receptors at some of the same synapses, and the effect of exogenous cyclic nucleotides on transmitter release (see below) make it unlikely that cyclic AMP is involved in the inhibition of NE release by presynaptic noradrenergic autoreceptors.

As mentioned above, β-receptor activation has been shown to increase NE release from peripheral nerve terminals. Because β-receptors are frequently if not universally coupled to adenylate cyclases (PERKINS 1973), it has been proposed that the β-adrenergic facilitation of NE release involves increases in cyclic AMP levels

(SERCK-HANNSSEN 1974). However, it has not been shown directly that cyclic AMP increases in peripheral nerve terminals in response to β-agonists, nor has a loss of β-receptor binding or β-stimulated cyclase been described following lesions of the noradrenergic fibers.

The evidence in favor of a cyclic AMP involvement comes from experiments of a more indirect sort, using perfusion with dBcAMP or with phosphodiesterase inhibitors. These drugs have been shown to have effects somewhat similar to those of β-receptor agonists, in that they affect spontaneous release of NE from the adrenal (PEACH 1972; POISNER 1973) and from sympathetic nerves (WOOTEN et al. 1973; but see CUBEDDU et al. 1975), and facilitate release in response to nerve stimulation as well (CUBEDDU et al. 1974, 1975; LANGER et al. 1975; LANGER 1976).

The way in which β-agonists, cyclic AMP derivatives and phosphodiesterase inhibitors affect release is not known, nor is there any certainty that they do so by the same mechanism. One possibility is that nerve stimulation causes activation of presynaptic β-receptors, increases in cyclic AMP, and consequent activation of tyrosine hydroxylase (see Sect. B.II.2.a). Activation of TH would result in higher rates of synthesis for NE, and hence a greater pool of transmitter available for release. However, it has not been possible to link cyclic AMP-dependent increases in TH activity directly with increases in NE release. As of yet, there has also been no unequivocal demonstration of central presynaptic β-receptors. However, since the α-mediated control of NE release demonstrated for the periphery appears to be exerted on central NE terminals as well (e.g., DISMUKES et al. 1977; MULDER et al. 1978), an analogous role for β-receptors in the periphery and in the CNS might also be expected.

β) Autoreceptors: Dopamine. Receptors for dopamine appear to be of several types (see KEBABIAN and CALNE 1979; for a review). These receptors differ in their pharmacological specificity, their cellular localization, and in whether or not they are able to increase adenylate cyclase activity. Dopamine-sensitive adenylate cyclase activity is maintained in homogenates, and for that reason, it has been possible to compare the binding of radioactive dopaminergic ligands with DA-sensitive cyclase activity in essentially the same preparation. The lack of a complete correlation between binding and cyclase activation has led to the conclusion that some, but not all dopaminergic receptors are functionally coupled to adenylate cyclase.

To be more specific, kainate lesions of the striatum (which destroy cell bodies while sparing presynaptic fibers and glial cells), virtually eliminate the DA-sensitive cyclase in this region while only 50% of specific ^{3}H-spiroperidol binding is lost (MINNEMAN et al. 1978b). Thus, postsynaptic DA receptors (referred to as D-1 receptors; KEBABIAN and CALNE 1979) appear to be linked with the cyclase. Lesions of the cortical afferents to the striatum (SCHWARCZ et al. 1978), or of the nigral afferents to the striatum (KRUEGER et al. 1976) do not alter DA-sensitive cyclase activity, but there are significant decreases in spiroperidol or haloperidol binding (SCHWARCZ et al. 1978; CREESE et al. 1977; MURRIN et al. 1979). Thus, in the striatum, presynaptic dopaminergic autoreceptors (on the nigral fibers) and on the possibly glutamatergic cortical afferents (SPENCER 1976) are not coupled to adenylate cyclases. Thus it would appear unlikely that the physiological response to stimulation of D-2 (presynaptic) dopaminergic autoreceptors involves cyclic AMP. The physiological response to stimulation of autoreceptors in striatum appears to be decrease in tyrosine hydroxylase activity (GOLDSTEIN et al. 1970, KAROBATH 1971; PATRICK and BARCHAS 1974; IVERSEN et al. 1976), rather than a direct influence on transmitter release.

In addition to dopaminergic autoreceptors, there are presynaptic dopamine receptors on the terminals of non-dopaminergic neurons as well. As just discussed, presynaptic receptors on the cortico-striate pathway are apparently not coupled to adenylate cyclase. However, there now is good evidence that there is an adenylate cyclase-coupled presynaptic dopaminergic receptor in the substantia nigra on the terminals of striato-nigral fibers. Lesions of dopaminergic neurons in the nigra do not result in a decrease in DA-sensitive cyclase activity (KEBABIAN and SAAVEDRA 1976), while intra-striatal kainate lesions cause a large reduction in nigral cyclase activity (MCGEER et al. 1976; PHILLIPSON et al. 1977; SCHWARCZ and COYLE 1977; QUIK et al. 1979). Thus, there does appear to be a mechanism whereby dopamine can alter cyclic AMP levels in the terminals of the non-dopaminergic neurons of the striato-nigral projections.

The physiological evidence for a cyclic AMP link in the modulation of dopaminergic transmission is relatively scanty. It has been demonstrated in striatal slices that dBcAMP facilitates the release of (^{3}H)-dopamine (WESTFALL et al. 1976). Because the dopaminergic autoreceptor in the striatum is not coupled to adenylate cyclase, it would appear unlikely that DA is involved in these effects. The obvious alternative is that some other transmitter is able to modulate DA release. One possibility is that the β-receptors in the striatum, which are not located on striatal neurons (MINNEMAN et al. 1978 a, b; ZAHNISER et al. 1979) are presynaptic, and facilitate dopaminergic transmission via an interaction at this site.

γ) Adenosine as a Modulator of Transmitter Release. The role of cyclic AMP as second messenger for a putative purinergic transmitter was discussed previously (see Sect. B.I.2). It was concluded that the receptor which mediates the depressant effects of adenosine on single cell firing, and the receptor which is responsible for cyclic AMP accumulations in response to adenosine show considerable similarities in terms of their pharmacological specifities. Nonetheless, there is little direct evidence that would suggest either that cyclic AMP serves as a second messenger for adenosine or that adenosine can act postsynaptically in a neurotransmitter-type role.

A frequently discussed alternative concerns the presynaptic actions of adenosine; adenosine (or perhaps adenine nucleotides such as ATP) are known to inhibit the release of transmitter in a variety of systems, and to depress synaptic transmission in brain slices probably via a similar mechanism. In this section, we will consider these two cases, and the evidence for a presynaptic role for cyclic AMP in these types of processes.

One way in which to establish a presynaptic effect for adenosine has been to directly measure the release of transmitter in the presence of adenosine or related nucleotides. In the noradrenergic system, ATP has been shown to inhibit release of ^{3}H-NE in blood vessels (SU 1978; ENEROZ and SAIDMAN 1977; HEDQVIST and FREDHOLM 1976), vas deferens (CLANACHAN et al. 1977; HEDQVIST and FREDHOLM 1976), and rat cerebral cortex (HARMS et al. 1978). Indirect evidence suggesting an inhibition of release comes from experiments in which adenosine diminishes a physiological response to nerve stimulation, while responsivity to exogenously applied NE is unaffected (CLANACHAN et al. 1977; SU 1978; VERHAEGE et al. 1977). On the other hand, increased efflux of ^{3}H-NE has been reported to result from adenosine perfusion of the spleen (MUELLER et al. 1979). In all these cases, theophylline appears to be able to at least partially antagonize adenosine-mediated changes in either release of physiological responsiveness. Where it has been examined, the pharmacological properties of the putative adenosine receptor responsible for these effects correspond well to those of the receptor which mediates cyclic AMP accumulations in other tissues (PATON et al. 1978). However, exceptions have been found; PATON et al. (1978) reported that adenosine arabinoriboside, adenine xylofuranoside, and 2′-deoxyadenosine were not able to block physiological effects of adenosine; in fact, 2′deoxyadenosine potentiated the adenosine-mediated inhibition of a neurally evoked response. Since these compounds generally act as adenosine antagonists in cyclic AMP generating systems (HUANG et al. 1972; LONDOS and WOLFF 1977; MAH and DALY 1976), this would argue against an involvement of cyclic AMP in the physiological response. What is needed in this case is some way of determining whether or not changes in cyclic AMP occur with adenosine concentrations sufficient to modify NE release, and to establish whether such changes are pre- or postsynaptic. The use of exogenous cyclic AMP derivatives or phosphodiesterase inhibitors at these types of synapses would be problematic, primarily because of complications with possible presynaptic β-receptors which might also affect cyclic AMP levels.

There is evidence that adenosine may mediate a similar inhibition of transmitter release at cholinergic nerve terminals as well. Adenosine depresses release of ACh in the periphery (GINSBORG and HIRST 1972; RIBEIRO and WALKER 1973; HAYASHI et al. 1978; VIZI and KNOLL 1976), and probably in the central nervous system as well (JHAMANDAS and SAWYNOK 1976; VIZI and KNOLL 1976). The endogenous source of the adenosine (or perhaps ATP) mediating these effects could be either presynaptic (e.g., SILINKSY 1975) or postsynaptic, as appears to be the case with Torpedo electroplaque (ISRAEL et al. 1977). As far as the central nervous system is concerned, Schubert and co-workers have demonstrated that adenosine can be transported by neurons to their terminals and released, in the rat central nervous system. This release is enhanced by electrical stimulation (SCHUBERT et al. 1976). In the septo-hippocampal pathway, the adenosine release occurs from what are presumably cholinergic nerve terminals (ROSE and SCHUBERT 1977; SCHUBERT et al. 1979). This suggests that in the CNS, the presynaptic terminal may be an important source of adenosine. Thus, adenosine can decrease the release of at least two transmitters, NE and ACh, at both central and peripheral sites. However, the evidence that cyclic AMP is involved in either of these effects is scanty.

In addition to the direct measures of transmitter release, there is also considerable electrophysiological evidence which suggests that adenosine has depressant effects on synaptic transmission, most probably via a reduction in the release of transmitter. Intracellular recordings indicate that adenosine appears to hyperpolarize neurons and to diminish the amplitude of both spontaneous and evoked synaptic potentials (EDSTROM and PHILLIS 1976; SCHOLFIELD 1978, PHILLIS et al. 1979b; SIGGINS, SCHUBERT, ZIEGLGÄNSBERGER and HERZ, unpublished results). Because of the failure to find consistent changes in membrane resistance, and because of a reduction of spontaneous synaptic potentials, PHILLIS et al. (1979b) have suggested that adenosine acts by blocking the release of excitatory transmitters. It should be pointed out that a reduction in membrane resistance in dendritic regions could also produce an apparent loss of synaptic activity; if the conductance increases were sufficiently remote, such changes might not be detectable with intrasomatic recordings, even though their shunting action on synaptic potentials generated in the same dendritic region would be readily apparent. In addition, intracellular experiments do not distinguish between a presynaptic inhibition of transmitter release on the one hand and a reduction in sensitivity of the postsynaptic neuron on the other; either type of change could produce the type of effects which were observed. SIGGINS et al. (unpublished work) reported consistent changes in membrane resistance which they interpreted as being a direct postsynaptic effect, suggesting that adenosine may have mixed pre- and postsynaptic effects.

Using extracellular recording techniques, LEKIĆ (1977) has shown that the depressant effect of 5′-AMP on the Renshaw cell firing is primarily due to a reduction in the responsiveness of that neuron to synaptic input; excitations induced by the iontophoresis of ACh or excitatory amino acids were unaffected. In the rat cortex, adenine nucleotides also appear to be more potent in depressing spontaneous activity as compared with ACh- or particularly glutamate-evoked activity (PHILLIS et al. 1979b), although the differences here are not as striking as in the spinal cord. This selective antagonism of synaptically driven cell firing would seem to indicate that adenosine can diminish the release of excitatory neurotransmitters, while the partial antagonism of responses to iontophoretically applied excitatory agents in cortex again suggests a mixed pre- as well as postsynaptic action.

The role of cyclic AMP in these effects of adenosine has not been directly studied in these preparations. However, adenosine has been shown to antagonize excitatory synaptic responses in several types of in vitro slice preparations, and in these cases, direct tests have been made for an involvement of cyclic AMP in these effects.

Using in vitro preparations from olfactory cortex and hippocampus, adenosine and adenine nucleotides have been shown to depress the amplitude of synaptic responses (KURODA and KOBAYASHI 1975; KURODA et al. 1976; SCHOLFIELD 1978; SMELLIE et al. 1979a; OKADA and SAITO 1979; SCHUBERT and MITZDORF 1979; DUNWIDDIE and HOFFER 1980; see also Fig. 4). The decreases in field EPSP's occur with no change in the presynaptic fiber potential (OKADA and KURODA 1975; SCHOLFIELD 1978; SCHUBERT and MITZDORF 1979; DUNWIDDIE and HOFFER 1980). Thus, the decreases in synaptic responses must reflect either a decrease in the release of transmitter, or a diminished postsynaptic sensitivity to the transmitter which is released. Although some of the initial reports indicated that the cyclic AMP increases paralleled the decreases in postsynaptic potentials (KURODA et al. 1976), there is now evidence that the two types of changes may not be closely linked. Adenosine increased cyclic AMP levels in both olfactory cortex and superior colliculus slices, but depressed synaptic responses only in the former (OKADA and KURODA 1975; OKADA and SAITO 1979). The conclusion from these experiments was that the depressant effects of adenosine on synaptic transmission were not related to changes in cyclic AMP levels. An alternative possibility is that adenosine modifies release only in certain pathways, and that the excitatory re-

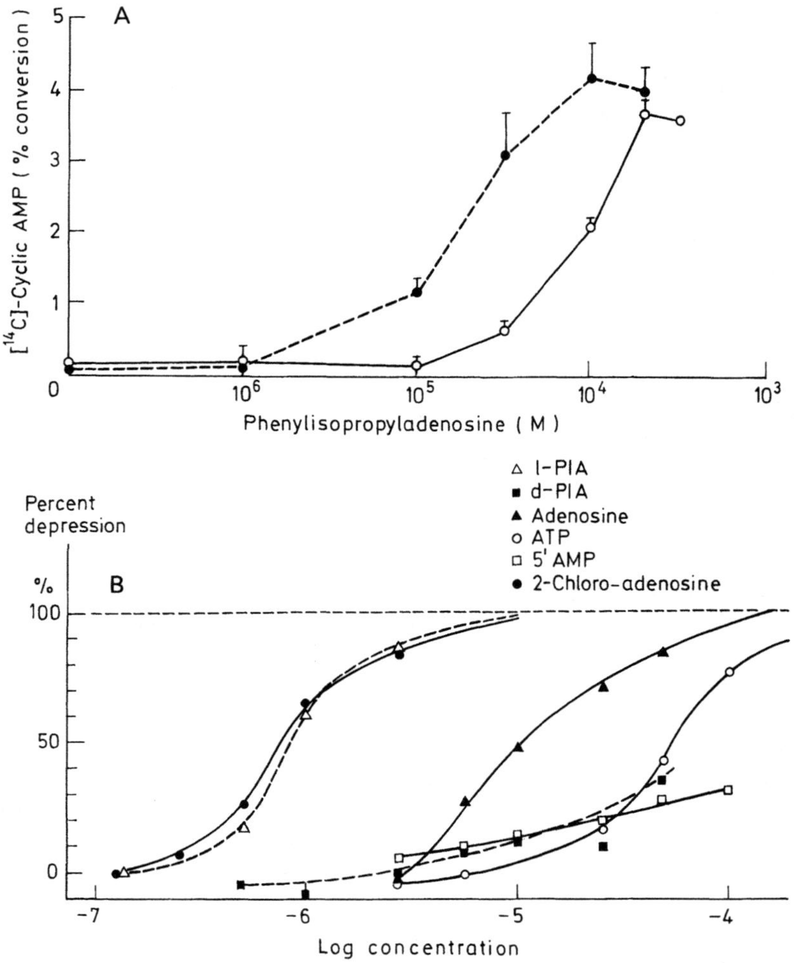

Fig. 4. A Accumulation of radioactive cyclic AMP in guinea pig cerebral cortical slices: Effect of levo (●---●) and dextro (o——o) rotatory isomers of N^6-phenylisopropyladenosine (PIA). Slices were labelled with (^{14}C)adenine for 40 min, washed, post-incubated and then stimulated with various concentrations of phenylisopropyladenosine for 15 min. Values are means +/− S.E.M. ($N=3$). (Taken from Smellie et al. 1979 a) **B** Dose response curves showing the depression of synaptically mediated responses in the in vitro hippocampal slice preparation with adenosine and various adenosine analogs. Dose-response curves are shown for several different adenine nucleotides, as well as the two stereoisomeric derivatives for which biochemical data on cyclic AMP accumulation is shown (part **A**). The values used in this figure were obtained from 67 individual determinations of the effects of various concentrations of these drugs; individual points represent the results of 1–5 experiments. (Taken from Dunwiddie and Hoffer 1980)

sponses evoked from the superior colliculus involved a pathway which was not affected by adenosine. The experiments of Kostopoulos and Phillis (1977) which showed depressant effects of adenosine on spontaneous cell firing in superior colliculus indicate that adenosine is certainly not without effect in this region.

In experiments with two stereoisomeric derivatives of adenosine, Dunwiddie and Hoffer (1980) found l-phenylisopropyl adenosine ($IC_{50} \sim 7\ \mu M$) to be ~100

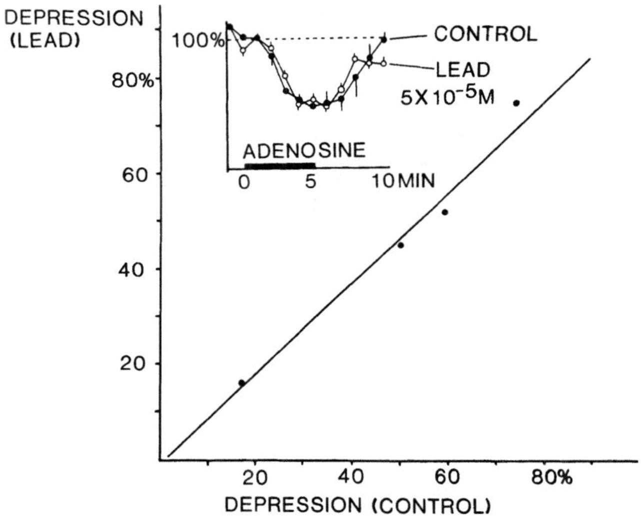

Fig. 5. The effects of lead pretreatment on adenosine-mediated depressions of synaptic responses in rat hippocampus in vitro are illustrated. Slices were tested with varying concentrations of adenosine (5–20 μ*M*), then perfused with medium containing 50 μ*M* lead, and subsequently perfused with the same concentration of adenosine. The magnitude of the adenosine-induced depressions in control medium *(abscissa)* are unaffected by lead treatment *(ordinate)*. The inset shows responses from a single slice which was tested several times with 5 μ*M* adenosine either with or without lead. Individual responses evoked at one minute intervals are displayed as a percentage of the pre-drug control amplitude. Neither the time course nor the amplitude of adenosine depression of these synaptic responses is affected by lead. Adenine arabinofuranoside, which has also been reported to inhibit the activation of adenylate cyclase, was also ineffective in inhibiting physiological responses to adenosine (DUNWIDDIE, unpublished observations)

times more potent in inhibiting excitatory postsynaptic potential in rat hippocampus in vitro than was the d-isomer. On the other hand, biochemical data from the same preparation (SMELLIE et al. 1979a) show only a 4- to 5-fold difference in potency in increasing cyclic AMP levels (see Fig. 4). Furthermore, much lower concentrations of both isomers were required for threshold electrophysiological responses than for increases in cyclic AMP.

Moreover, treatments which potentiate the cyclic AMP increases produced by adenosine, such as perfusion with adenosine in conjunction with phosphodiesterase inhibitors or with other biogenic amines, do not influence the adenosine-mediated decreases in synaptic responses in the hippocampal slice preparations. Conversely, agents which can antagonize adenylate cyclase activity, such as lead or adenine arabinofuranoside (NATHANSON and BLOOM 1975; LONDOS and WOLFF 1977) have no effect on depressant responses to adenosine although they can at least partially antagonize increases in cyclic AMP (DUNWIDDIE, unpublished observations; see Fig. 5). Finally, the primary effect of exogenously applied cyclic AMP analogs in the hippocampus in vitro was to increase rather than decrease synaptic responses (Fig. 6).

The effects of cyclic AMP and cyclic AMP analogs are particularly interesting and illustrate a common problem when cyclic nucleotides are administered extracellularly. Perfusion of hippocampal slices with cyclic AMP or dibutyryl cyclic

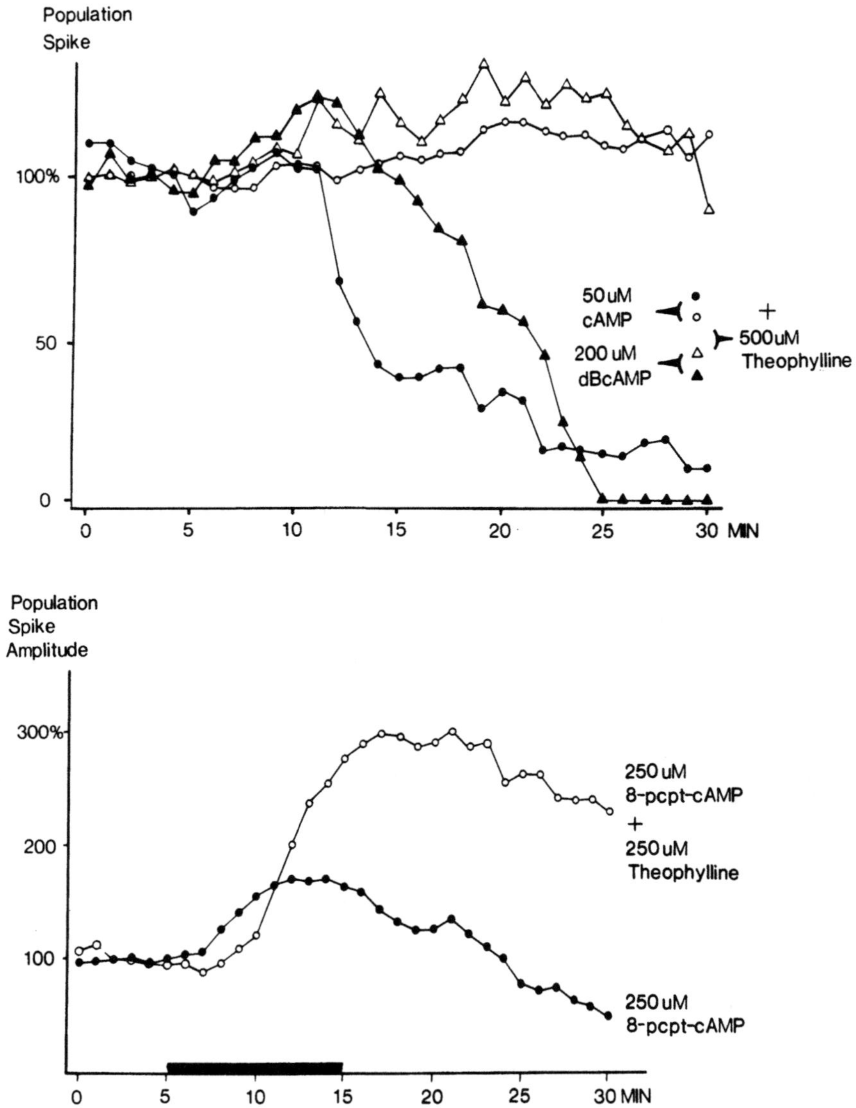

Fig. 6. Effects of cyclic AMP, dibutyryl cyclic AMP (dBcAMP), and 8-p-chlorophenylthio-cyclic AMP (8-pcpt-cAMP) on the amplitude of synaptically evoked responses *(population spikes)* recorded from the rat hippocampus in vitro. Both cyclic AMP and dibutyryl cyclic AMP produced potent depressant effects on the amplitude of population spike responses *(upper)*. However, when slices were pretreated with theophylline, the depressant effects were abolished, suggesting that the effects were due largely to an interaction at an extracellular site with the adenosine receptor. In each case, the original response to the drug and the subsequent test in the presence of theophylline were conducted in the same slice. In the *lower half* of the figure, the effect of 8-pcpt-cyclic AMP is seen with and without pretreatment with 250 μM theophylline. In both cases, increases rather than decreases in population spike amplitude were initially observed, and with this analog, theophylline was seen to potentiate rather than antagonize the observed response. The indicated figure represent the means from 9 experiments; both increases were significally different from control values ($p < 0.05$). (Taken from DUNWIDDIE and HOFFER 1980)

AMP (dBcAMP) depressed synaptic responses, and these effects were completely antagonized by theophylline. Thus, it would appear that this depressant effect represents the action of these drugs at the extracellular adenosine receptor, rather than at an intracellular site. Another cyclic AMP derivative, 8-para-chlorophenylthio cyclic AMP had modest excitatory effects which were potentiated by theophylline. These excitatory effects mirrored those produced by β-agonists in this tissue; hence it would appear that, apart from their actions at adenosine receptors, the physiological effects produced by application of cyclic AMP analogs correspond more nearly to those of β-agonists rather than to the effects of adenosine. Similar increases in synaptic potentials in response to exogenous cyclic nucleotide derivatives have been reported in olfactory cortex as well (SCHOLFIELD 1978).

The problem which remains is to determine the significance of the adenosine-elicited increases in cyclic AMP which *do* occur. The biochemical literature indicates that adenosine is probably the putative transmitter with the most widespread and uniform effects on cyclic AMP. Although it has been suggested that this may reflect a glial localization of adenosine-sensitive adenylate cyclase, this would appear unlikely. Kainate lesions of the striatum induce a loss of adenosine-stimulated cyclase activity (PREMONT et al. 1979) and adenosine-stimulated accumulations of cyclic AMP are reported in cultured neuronal cells (BLUME and FOSTER 1975; PENIT et al. 1976). Although some glial cell lines show increases in cyclic AMP in response to adenosine (BLUME 1979; CLARK et al. 1975), others which appear to be primarily glioblasts actually show an inhibition of cyclic AMP in the presence of low concentrations ($IC_{50} \sim 0.5\ \mu M$) of adenosine (VAN CALKER et al. 1978). This would indicate that the changes in cyclic AMP which are observed in brain slices may occur primarily in neuronal rather than glial elements.

If the changes in cyclic AMP levels are neuronally located, how can this be reconciled with the apparent lack of correlation between such changes and electrophysiological effects? One possibility is that there are multiple adenosine receptors, only some of which are coupled to adenylate cyclase (as appears to be the case with dopamine receptors). These multiple adenosine receptors might also be differentially distributed, i.e., they may be pre- or postsynaptic, or located upon some cell types and not others. The largely unsuccessful attempts to develop a ligand to measure specific binding at an adenosine receptor have precluded direct measurements of adenosine receptors and hence, localization of possible sites of adenosine action.[1]

When attempting to physiologically differentiate between a possible pre- versus postsynaptic action of adenosine, it would appear likely that, during a treatment with cyclic nucleotide analogs, intracellular concentrations of these agents would be expected to reach diffusional equilibrium much more rapidly in nerve terminals than in cell bodies, since the latter have much less membrane surface area in relation to their intracellular volume. Therefore, it would be expected that, all other factors being equal, the pre- rather than postsynaptic effects of exogenously ap-

1 *Added in proof:* This speculation now appears to have been largely confirmed. Adenosine can mediate both inhibition as well stimulation of adenylate cyclase activity via interactions with extracellular receptors (LONDOS et al., Proc. Natl. Acad. Sci. 77:2551, 1980; see DALY et al., Life Sci. 28:2083, 1981, for a brief review), adding still more complexities to the relationship between adenosine and cyclic AMP levels

plied cyclic nucleotides would be more apparent. It might also be pointed out that the apparently preferential accumulation of ^{3}H-adenosine in presynaptic elements of cerebral cortex (SHIMIZU 1979) might simply reflect the type of diffusional process just described for cyclic AMP. Be that as it may, there is at least suggestive evidence for both pre- and postsynaptic effects of adenosine, and it may be that only one of these is mediated via cyclic AMP.

Another possibility is that occupation of the adenosine receptor can simultaneously activate several processes (e.g., increase conductance to certain ions, activate adenylate cyclase) in parallel in the same cellular element, but that these processes are relatively independent. If this were the case, the electrophysiological effects (depression of cell firing and synaptic transmission) might reflect one effect of adenosine, while the increase in cyclic AMP could be responsible for more complex (and as of yet unknown) physiological action of adenosine. Modulation of responsiveness of other cyclic AMP generating systems (see Sect. B.II.1.a) is one such possibility, and the development of long-term synaptic plasticity is another (DUNWIDDIE and HOFFER 1980). In these types of situations, a close correspondence would be expected between the pharmacological properties of the "biochemical" and "electrophysiological" receptors, even though the biochemical and electrophysiological endpoints would be unrelated.

In summary, there is not yet enough evidence to either establish or eliminate a role for cyclic AMP in the electrophysiological effects of adenosine, either at a pre- or postsynaptic site. The complexity of the interactions of adenosine with other putative transmitters on cyclic AMP generating systems suggests that adenosine plays a fairly significant role in the regulation of some yet unknown aspect of nervous activity. The problems just described which are encountered in trying to establish such a role for cyclic AMP in terms of the physiological effects of adenosine clearly illustrate the problems that are encountered in any such study.

c) Cyclic AMP and Neuromuscular Transmission

No discussion of the presynaptic modulatory role of cyclic nucleotides would be complete without some discussion of their possible involvement at peripheral neuromuscular junctions. The major problem in so far as these studies are concerned is that it has not been possible to measure the changes in cyclic nucleotides in presynaptic terminals. Thus, the types of experiments which have been done are largely electrophysiological and pharmacological, and the presumed actions of drugs on cyclic AMP generating systems have been extrapolated from their known effects primarily in brain slices. Thus, where discrepancies or disagreements have arisen, these can largely be attributed to a fundamental ignorance of the effects of these treatments on cyclic nucleotides in the motor nerve terminal.

The suggestion that cyclic AMP may be involved in transmitter release originated with experiments which demonstrated that a variety of treatments which would be expected to increase cyclic AMP levels elevate release of acetylcholine (ACh). These treatments include perfusion with dibutyryl cyclic AMP (dBcAMP), epinephrine, and phosphodiesterase inhibitors (BRECKENRIDGE et al. 1967; GOLDBERG and SINGER 1969; WILSON 1974; JACOBS and MCNIECE 1977; TAKAMORI et al. 1973). In general, there appears to be agreement that these treatments increase both the amount of transmitter released (measured as either quantal content in preparations in high Mg^{+2}/low Ca^{+2}, or as end-plate potential amplitude in curare-paralyzed preparations) as well as the frequency of miniature end-plate potentials. Others have shown repetitive firing of the presynaptic terminal in response to similar treatments (STANDAERT et al. 1976a, b; STANDAERT and DRETCHEN 1979). The conduction of nerve impulses along the axon appears to be unaffected by changes in cyclic nucleotides (HORN and MCAFEE 1977).

Two basic problems have arisen in this area, and they largely hinge around differences in interpretation. First, it has been suggested by some workers (STANDAERT et al. 1976b; STANDAERT and DRETCHEN 1979) that cyclic nucleotides mediate an *essential* step in transmitter release; depolarization of the terminal element results in an activation of adenylate cyclase, which subsequently leads to a phosphorylation of membrane proteins, which in turn permits the influx of calcium and subsequent release of transmitter. Not all evidence would seem to support this, however. MIYAMOTO and BRECKENRIDGE (1974) found that NE, epinephrine and dBcAMP had no effect on transmission at the phrenic nerve-diaphragm synapse under normal conditions. In a depolarized (i.e., "fatigued") preparation, all of these treatments were able to increase both spontaneous and evoked release. This would suggest that cyclic nucleotides might subserve a type of metabolic role in cases of excessive transmitter release. Further support for this hypothesis comes from the experiments of WILSON (1974) who also used the isolated rat diaphragm. Both dBcAMP and theophylline were found to increase quantal content, mobilization rate and the releasable pool of transmitter, but not the probability of release. This latter parameter would seem to be the one most likely to change if cyclic AMP were directly involved in exocytosis. The changes in mobilization would appear to support a metabolic role for cyclic nucleotides rather than a direct control over the release process.

The other major problem which has arisen concerns the interpretation of the effects of various agents which are thought to increase cyclic AMP levels. For example, sodium fluoride produces effects on the neuromuscular junction (NMJ) which appear similar to those produced by repetitive stimulation or dBcAMP. However, while it is well known that fluoride can activate adenylate cyclase in broken cells, there appears to be no evidence that it can do so in whole cells (cf. DALY 1977a). Thus, it would appear that this action at the neuromuscular synapse represents another action of fluoride unrelated to cyclic AMP, probably at an extracellular site.

Similar problems have arisen with the effects of other drugs, such as adenosine and theophylline, on the neuromuscular junction. Adenosine depresses transmitter release, theophylline facilitates release, and the effects of both are mutually antagonistic. It has been suggested that adenosine's effects are due to the inhibition of protein kinase activity (e.g., MIYAMOTO et al. 1969), and that theophylline is working via its known actions as a phosphodiesterase inhibitor (e.g., BUTCHER and SUTHERLAND 1962). There are several problems with this. First, the potency of adenosine as a kinase inhibitor ($IC_{50} > 50$ μM; MIYAMOTO et al. 1969) is more than an order of magnitude less than its potency in depressing release of ACh ($IC_{50} < 0.7$ μM; HAYASHI et al. 1978). Moreover, the effect of adenosine on ACh release is due to the interaction of adenosine with an extracellular site, since the potency of adenosine is increased by uptake blockers. If adenosine were inhibiting release because of effects on protein kinases, reuptake blockers would be expected to antagonize, not potentiate this effect. Thus, it would appear extremely unlikely that adenosine inhibits transmission via an inhibition of kinases. It is also somewhat unlikely that either theophylline or SQ 20009, which potentiate synaptic transmission, do so via an inhibition of phosphodiesterases. In general, theophylline has been found to be a relatively weak inhibitor of various phosphodiesterases (IC_{50} 200–500 μM; BUTCHER and SUTHERLAND 1962; UZUNOV et al. 1974; LEVIN and WEISS 1976; CHASIN et al. 1972) and has little or no effect on cyclic AMP accumulations in brain slices (cf. DALY 1977a, p. 127). SQ 20009, which is a relatively potent inhibitor of phosphodiesterase in brain homogenates ($IC_{50} < 6\ \mu M$; CHASIN et al. 1972) also is relatively ineffective in potentiating cyclic AMP increases, while other inhibitors such as diazepam and RO 20-1724 do potentiate such increases (cf. DALY 1977a, p. 128).

While theophylline may be a relatively poor phosphodiesterase inhibitor, it does share a variety of actions with other methylxanthines. Methylxanthines are antagonists of 5′-nucleotidase activity (TSUZUKI and NEWBURGH 1975) and adenosine antagonists (SATTIN and RALL 1970; HUANG and DALY 1972; MAH and DALY 1976). They can alter Ca^{+2} distribution and fluxes (WEBER and HERZ 1968; JOHNSON and INESI 1969; CHAPMAN and MILLER 1974; BLINKS et al. 1972), and can facilitate the binding of cyclic AMP to the regulatory subunit of cyclic AMP-dependent protein kinase (MIECH et al. 1979). Of these possibilities, it would appear most likely that the actions of theophylline at the NMJ reflect the antagonism of the extracellular effects of endogenously released ATP or adenosine. The depressant effects of adenosine on cholinergic transmission are well known and competitively antagonized by theophylline (VIZI and KNOLL 1976; HAYASHI et al. 1978; RIBEIRO and WALKER 1973; GINSBORG and HIRST 1972). There is also evidence for the endogenous release of adenine nucleotides; ATP is released along with ACh by nerve stimulation (SILINSKY 1975), and has been estimated to reach sufficient amounts following a single impulse (80 μM) to affect physiological activity. Perhaps if experiments were conducted comparing the effects of adenosine deaminase to those of theophylline on neuromuscular transmission, a better understanding might be gained of the physiological significance of this release.

What remains unknown is whether cyclic AMP mediates the effects of adenosine on the terminal element. As has already been discussed, it would appear that cyclic AMP is *not* involved in adenosine-mediated depressions of synaptic transmission in the brain. Without direct measures of changes in cyclic AMP levels during neuromuscular transmission, its possible involvement at this synapse must remain on open question. However, since the effects of dBcAMP on neuromuscular transmission appear to be facilitory, this would suggest that the depressant effects of adenosine on transmission do not involve cyclic AMP.

Thus, the evidence that cyclic nucleotides are involved in neuromuscular cholinergic transmission is fairly strong. A wide variety of treatments which would be expected to alter cyclic nucleotide levels all have fairly consistent effects upon both transmission per se (i.e., ACh release, amplitude of the end-plate potential), as well as on electrophysiological events in the presynaptic element (STANDAERT and DRETCHEN 1979). The primary disagreements concern a) whether these treatments actually do affect cyclic AMP levels in the way in which they are hypothesized to act; b) whether cyclic AMP is directly involved in the secretory process; c) whether it regulates a facilitatory presynaptic process prior to exocytosis (i.e., that it serves as a type of second messenger for NE and E); and d) whether it might inhibit transmitter release (by acting as a second messenger for adenosine). The resolution of these differences will probably depend at least partially upon the development of techniques for direct measurement of cyclic nucleotides in presynaptic terminals.

In general, the evidence seems to suggest that not only at the neuromuscular junction, but in a variety of central and peripheral systems, cyclic AMP is involved in *augmenting* synaptic responses, although clearly not by the same mechanism in all cases. In noradrenergic pathways, cyclic AMP appears involved in increased synthesis of transmitter via activation of TH; in hippocampal slices and at the NMJ, postsynaptic responses are augmented by cyclic nucleotide derivatives. In both the cerebellum (SIGGINS et al. 1969) and in the hippocampus (SEGAL and BLOOM 1974), cyclic AMP appears to inhibit spontaneous cell firing. However, in both of these regions, NE appears to facilitate excitatory synaptic responses (see Sect. B.II.1.b). While it has not been directly tested, if NE produces its effects via cyclic AMP, then cyclic AMP should produce a similar facilitation of synaptic responses. Here again, this would be consistent with a cyclic AMP facilitation of transmitter release. Using direct tests, transmitter release can be shown to be augmented by either β-receptor agonists, by dBcAMP, or by phosphodiesterase inhibitors at both peripheral and central synapses. Whether this general pattern of apparent facilitation of neurotransmission by cyclic AMP will continue to hold up is unclear, but at least for the present, it would appear that putative transmitters which antagonize transmission (e.g., adenosine) are unlikely to do so via a cyclic AMP-dependent mechanism.

III. Cyclic AMP and Intermediary Metabolism

In general, cyclic AMP has been thought to act as a second messenger for various neurotransmitters in the central nervous system, in which case the end result is generally thought to be a change in cell firing. Another possible role for cyclic AMP which has been suggested is as a regulator of cellular metabolic processes. In this respect, its action would be somewhat analogous to the function of cyclic AMP in the liver, where epinephrine acts at extracellular receptors to produce increases in cyclic AMP which subsequently activated the glycogenolytic response of liver cells (RALL and SUTHERLAND 1958, 1961). There is considerable evidence to suggest that changes in cyclic AMP may similarly be involved in glycogenolysis in the central nervous system. The specific question which we would like to discuss in this section is whether cellular metabolism in the central nervous system is regulated by cyclic AMP, and if so, what types of extracellular events can elicit the cyclic AMP increases, and in what types of cells these changes take place.

1. Increases in Cyclic AMP and Metabolic Changes

A formidable obstacle which complicates determining a physiological role for cyclic nucleotides in the nervous system is the heterogeneity of cell types. It would seem likely that cyclic nucleotides may have multiple roles, with the function depending primarily upon the cell type being considered. In terms of changes in intermediary metabolism, two types of problems are encountered. First, any physiological manipulation which is sufficient to elicit metabolic changes probably involves changes in the release of other substances which can by themselves increase cyclic AMP levels. Hence, the first problem is to establish the specificity of the response, i.e., to show that cyclic AMP changes are essential for the change in metabolic state, and are not simply a process which occurs in parallel with metabolic change. Secondly, it is important to demonstrate that the changes in cyclic AMP are not simply a result of the altered state. Ideally, one would like to show that some agent acts at an extracellular site to increase cyclic AMP levels, and that this increase leads to the subsequent phosphorylation and activation of enzymes involved in metabolic regulation.

In spite of the difficulties outlined above, the evidence that cyclic AMP is involved in the mobilization of cerebral glycogen stores is fairly strong. In vivo, it has been shown that activation of β-adrenergic and histamine H_2 receptors induce cAMP formation in the cerebral hemispheres of the chick, and there is a concomitant increase in the percentage of phosphorylase a (the active form), and a decrease in glycogen (EDWARDS et al. 1974; NAHORSKI et al. 1975). The increases in brain phosphorylase a observed after decapitation (BRECKENRIDGE and NORMAN 1962; LUST and PASSONNEAU 1976), trauma (WATANABE and PASSONNEAU 1974, 1975), electroconvulsive shock (LUST and PASSONEAU 1976), and spreading depression (Křivánek 1977) may reflect activation of these types of receptors. The difficulty with these kinds of approaches is in establishing the causal involvement of cyclic nucleotides in the glycogenolytic process; at best, correlation between cAMP levels and measures such as phosphorylase a can be obtained which might simply reflect changes in some underlying variable. It is not even certain whether the changes from phosphorylase b to a and the changes in cyclic AMP occur in the same cells.

The problem of the heterogeneity of cell types in intact tissue has been attacked by the use of cultured cells. Primary glial cultures and glioma cells often show very large increases (as much as 200-fold) in cyclic AMP upon exposure to various agonists, including β-adrenegeric agonists (CLARK and PERKINS 1971; GILMAN and NIRENBERG 1971; MCCARTHY and DE VELLIS 1978) and prostaglandins (CLARK et al. 1975; PERKINS et al. 1975). In addition, exposure of these cells to adrenergic agonists or cyclic AMP analogs has been shown to increase conversion of phosphorylase b to phosphorylase a, and to reduce the glycogen content of these cultures (BROWNING et al. 1974; OPLER and MAKMAN 1972; NEWBURGH and ROSENBERG 1972; PASSONNEAU and CRITES 1976). Treatments which increase cyclic AMP in astrocytoma cells (NE, IBMX) and in neuroblastoma cells (PGE_1 and IBMX), all reduced cellular glycogen concentrations and increased phosphorylase a. This suggests that in both types of cells, glycogenolysis may be regulated by cyclic AMP-dependent mechanisms (PASSONNEAU and CRITES 1976). In the last study, changes in glycogen metabolism were also observed following changes in the glucose content of the medium, but, under these conditions, were not accompanied by changes in cyclic AMP levels.

2. Striatal β-Receptors

The hypothesis that has developed is that the cells in the central nervous system, and glial cells in particular, may respond to various stimuli with increases in glycogenolysis via cyclic AMP-dependent mechanisms. One source of indirect support for this hypothesis comes from experiments on striatal β-receptors. The existence of β-adrenoreceptors in the striatum is somewhat surprising, insofar as noradrenergic input to this region is almost nonexistent (UNGERSTED 1971). Furthermore, the fact that NE-mediated increases in cyclic AMP content of striatal slices are considerably greater than those elicited by dopamine (MINNEMAN et al. 1978b), which is found in the striatum, would seem inconsistent if cyclic AMP functions as a second messenger only for neurotransmitters.

One possible resolution to this somewhat anomalous situation is that the β-receptors are located upon glial cells, and are sensitive to circulating NE and E. This hypothesis is supported by experiments using local kainate lesions of the striatum. These lesions produce decreases in basal adenylate cyclase activity, almost a complete loss of dopamine-stimulated adenylate cyclase activity, no changes in basal cyclic AMP levels, and an increase in cyclic AMP accumulation in slices elicited by β-adrenergic stimulation (MCGEER et al. 1976; MINNEMAN et al. 1978a, b; ZAHNISER et al. 1979). Since kainate lesions destroy primarily neuronal elements, while sparing fibers of passage and glial cells (of which the latter generally show hypertrophy subsequent to kainate lesions), the interpretation which has been given to these results is that striatal dopamine-sensitive adenylate cyclase is located upon striatal neurons, while the β-receptors are found upon glia. Because PGE_1-stimulated increases in cyclic AMP were unchanged by kainate lesions, this would suggest that other receptors may have a primarily glial localization as well. Another possibility is that the striatal β-receptors are located on microvessels; these receptors would also be unaffected by kainate lesions, and would receive noradrenergic input from the sympathetic innervation of the brain vasculature (HARTMAN et al. 1972). However, these vascular receptors appear to be primarily β_2 in character (NATHANSON 1980), and β_2-receptors comprise only 20–25% of the total β-receptor complement of the striatum (MINNEMAN et al. 1979b). Thus, a substantial proportion of β-receptors in the striatum would appear to be localized to non-vascular cellular elements which are not destroyed by kainate lesions.

As mentioned above, absolute increases in β-stimulated cyclic AMP formation are observed following kainate lesions; however, there appears to be no change in β-receptor number, either in the β_1 or β_2 receptor subtypes (ZAHNISER et al. 1979). Other work has not been entirely confirmatory, in that NAHORSKI et al. (1979) found decreases in β-receptor binding sites following kainate lesions of the striatum, with the decrease a loss of primarily β_1 binding; these authors did not measure changes in cyclic AMP response subsequent to the kainate lesion. These results present an interesting problem. In spite of the fact that β-receptor number in unchanged, or perhaps even decreases, stimulation of β-receptors produces a 2- to 4-fold greater increase in cyclic AMP. Two possible explanations for this finding might be advanced. First, there might be a compensatory change in the dynamics of cyclic AMP formation/degradation, which permits larger accumulations of cyclic AMP. This is supported by the fact that reductions in phosphodiesterase activity following this type of lesion (up to 84%; MINNEMAN et al. 1978a) are considerably larger than the changes in basal adenylate cyclase activity (up to 50%). This might indicate that compensatory decreases in phosphodiesterase activity occurred following the lesion which could result in considerably larger accumulations of cyclic AMP with no change (or even a reduction) in the formation of cyclic AMP.

An alternative explanation, suggested by MINNEMAN et al. (1978b) is that phosphodiesterase is preferentially located in the neurons destroyed by the kainate lesion. This is an intriguing suggestion, since it suggests that some pools of cyclic AMP in tissue (neuronal pools) might be turning over at an appreciably faster rate, and that these cells contribute relatively little to either the basal or stimulated cyclic AMP levels which are measured. A primarily neuronal localization of phosphodiesterase is not unreasonable; if cyclic AMP does serve as a second messenger in the dopaminergic nigro-striatal pathway as has been suggested, the time courses of such responses would be likely to be faster than any metabolic changes associated with glial cells in the same region. Hence, the enzyme responsible for lowering cyclic AMP levels and shutting off the response should be somewhat higher.

If this hypothesis is correct, it might be expected that there should be a relatively uniform distribution of glia-associated receptors throughout the brain. The β_2-receptor, which is relatively unaffected by kainate lesions (NAHORSKI et al. 1979; ZAHNISER et al. 1979) does, in fact, show a nearly uniform distribution in all brain regions except cerebellum, while the β_1-receptor can show as much as 20-fold differences in receptor density in different areas (MINNEMAN et al. 1979b). Secondly, it would seem that kainate lesions in other brain regions should have similar effects, i.e., there should be relatively little change or even an increase in β_2-stimulated adenylate cyclase activity. The caudate appears to be the only region in which this has been studied, and a mentioned previously, total adenylate cyclase levels go down (SCHWARCZ and COYLE 1977, MINNEMAN et al. 1978a), while β-stimulated cyclic AMP accumulations are increased. In the cerebellum, kainate lesions actually increase basal adenylate cyclase by approximately 300%, but it is not known how these changes relate to β-stimulated adenylate cyclase (BIGGIO et al. 1978c). Cerebellar cyclic GMP and guanylate cyclase are nearly abolished by such lesions, suggesting a neuronal localization for cyclic GMP systems.

The evidence which has just been described suggests a glial and partially vascular localization for β-receptors in the striatum. Is there any evidence that these β-receptors are involved in the type of metabolic changes discussed previously? WILKENING and MAKMAN (1976, 1977, 1979) have shown that β-agonists induce glycogenolysis in rat striatal slices, and that changes in glycogen content correlate well with increases in cyclic AMP as well as with the conversion of phosphorylase b to a. The general spectrum of changes which is observed (increased glycogenolysis, conversion of phosphorylase b to the a form, decreases in hexose uptake, and increased lactic acid production) all tend to suggest a change from oxidative to glycolytic metabolism. Dibutyryl cyclic AMP and IBMX produced similar effects, but dopamine, which also increases cyclic AMP levels, could not induce these types of metabolic changes. This would again suggest that the β-adrenergic and dopaminergic receptors are located on different cell types, and the increases in cyclic AMP which they stimulate have functionally different consequences. A potent adenosine analog, 2-chloro-adenosine, produced some but not all of the metabolic changes described above. However, its effects were not blocked by methyl xanthines, which antagonized cyclic AMP increases; this would seem to suggest that metabolic changes are under the control of cyclic AMP-independent as well as -dependent mechanisms.

3. Electrophysiological Experiments

In terms of electrophysiological responses, there is little to draw upon, since glial cells are not usually recorded from. However, some mention should be made of the work of KRNJEVIĆ and others (KRNJEVIĆ and VAN METER 1976), who recorded intracellularly from both neurons and presumptive glial cells in the spinal cord, and injected cyclic AMP and GMP intracellularly. The experiments with neurons were somewhat inconclusive, in that no consistent changes were observed either in resting membrane potential or in membrane resistance. There were changes in spike shape and height, but these were produced by both cyclic AMP and cyclic GMP. On the other hand, injections into glial cells (identified by stable resting potentials, absence of spiking and no synaptic potentials) produced consistent hyperpolarizations, accompanied by as much as 10-fold decreases in membrane resistance. Membrane depolarizations were never observed with either cyclic AMP or cyclic GMP (KRNJEVIĆ and VAN METER 1976).

The interpretation of these results is somewhat difficult, in that it is unclear what significance such hyperpolarizations might have in functional terms for glial cells, and possibly for the surrounding neurons as well. Nevertheless, the consistency which was observed in terms of electrophysiological responses would seem to suggest that cyclic nucleotides are more closely linked to membrane conductance changes in glial cells than in spinal cord neurons. Alternatively, cyclic nucleotide actions in neurons may be so complex that intracellular injections of cyclic nucleotides are unable to mimic the effects of cyclic AMP produced at the appropriate intracellular loci.

The conclusions which may be drawn from the preceding discussion are twofold. First, it is apparent that glial cells in culture and in the brain possess adenylate cyclase functionally coupled to a variety of receptors. The physiological function of cyclic AMP in glial cells is unclear, but one possible role is the initiation of glycolysis consequent to activation of a β-adrenergic receptor. Whether neurons demonstrate similar responses is unclear, although there are suggestions that they do. Since the role of glial cells in relation to neuronal function is poorly understood, the ramifications of changes in glial metabolism are unclear. However, changes in ion-transport systems or membrane conductance in glial cells may influence the external milieu in such a way as to affect the function of nearby neurons.

What is also unclear is the source of the stimuli which might provoke such changes; in the case of β-activation of glycolysis, such receptors might be stimulated by "overflow" from nearby noradrenergic afferents. In some regions where the blood-brain barrier appears to be fairly permeable, such as in circumventricular organs, area postrema, or in locus coeruleus, activation may depend upon systemic circulating hormones such as epinephrine. However, this would not appear to be particularly likely in areas such as the striatum, where the blood-brain barrier is relatively impermeable to circulating hormones such as epinephrine.

The second point which might be made from these studies is more of a caveat than a conclusion. Clearly, not all cyclic nucleotides in the nervous system are neuronal in origin. If, as suggested by MINNEMAN et al. (1978b), neuronal pools of cyclic AMP are turning over more rapidly than the glial, then the predominant effects which are observed in in vivo or in vitro studies of cyclic nucleotide synthesis may be derived from those tissue compartments which exhibit relatively slow changes in cyclic nucleotide levels. In fact, there might be some pools of cyclic nucleotides which contribute virtually nothing to measureable basal and stimulated cyclic AMP levels. This might provide a partial explanation for why central nervous system dose-response curves in slices for various drugs in terms of cyclic nucleotides accumulation often appear shifted to the right when compared to the dose-response curves in terms of physiological responses, or in terms of radioligand receptor binding. In the absence of effective inhibitors of phosphodiesterase, a much higher degree of activation of adenylate cyclase will be required to achieve a given amount of total cyclic AMP accumulation in a fast-turnover system than in a slower one, even though the concentrations of cyclic AMP at a physiologically relevant site (e.g., near the cyclic AMP-dependent kinase) may be much higher in cells associated with rapidly turning over nucleotides.

In any case, the implications for physiological experiments are fairly clear. In the absence of any information as to a) the types of cells in which cyclic nucleotide changes are occurring, and b) as to whether there might be changes in more rapidly turning over pools of nucleotides which are obscured by others with less rapid turnover, extrapolation from experiments involving measurement of cyclic nucleotide accumulation to physiological effects will be somewhat difficult.

C. Physiological Role of Cyclic GMP

The biochemical characterization of cyclic AMP generating systems has been extremely useful in establishing functional roles for cyclic AMP in the nervous system. Hormone-stimulated adenylate cyclases have been characterized in homogenates, cyclic AMP formation has been extensively studied in brain slice preparations, cyclic AMP-dependent kinase and its regulatory subunit have been investigated, and it has been possible to measure the phosphorylated state of various substrate proteins of cyclic AMP-dependent kinase in vivo and in vitro. On the other hand, much less is known regarding the cyclic GMP system. For various reasons, certain aspects of the biochemical events involved in cyclic GMP formation and the subsequent physiological events are very poorly understood. For this reason, it has been much more difficult to use biochemical data to infer a physiological role for this nucleotide.

A primary problem in studying guanylate cyclase is that it displays virtually no hormone-stimulated activity in broken cell preparations (cf. MURAD et al. 1979). The reason for this is not clear, but it probably reflects some requirement for activation which is not met under in vitro conditions. In brain slices, stimulation of guanylate cyclase appears to be almost universally dependent upon the presence of extracellular calcium (SCHULTZ et al. 1973; CLYMAN et al. 1975). Because almost 70% of guanylate cyclase exists in a soluble form inside cells, it has been suggested that the primary activation of cyclase is not by extracellularly-acting agents (e.g., hormones or neurotransmitters), but depends instead upon an influx of calcium. Thus, activation of guanylate cyclase by transmitters may be an indirect effect, in that such activation occurs as a result of calcium fluxes generated by transmitter action or related physiological events. Thus, the failure to observe guanylate cyclase activation by transmitters in broken cell preparations may reflect the fact that transmitters can no longer generate calcium fluxes when the normal ionic gradients across cell membranes are lost.

If cyclic GMP is formed only in response to influx of calcium, its importance as a second messenger per se would appear somewhat diminished. However, this does not in any way reduce its significance for neuronal activity in other possible roles. Most indications are that guanylate cyclase is a predominantly neuronal enzyme; in cultures from the nervous system of the chick, it is found only in those containing neurons (GORIDIS et al. 1974). In addition, kainate lesions of the cerebellum result in a nearly complete loss of basal guanylate cyclase activity (BIGGIO et al. 1978c). This primarily neuronal localization would suggest that it has particular significance in so far as nervous activity is concerned, even though it may not necessarily function as a second messenger.

In spite of the fact that guanylate cyclase is a predominantly soluble enzyme, there is a significant percentage of cyclase activity in the membrane-bound form; this fraction ranges from 16% in the striatum to 45% in the hippocampus. Furthermore, although the hippocampus has the lowest overall guanylate cyclase activity (when compared to cortex, cerebellum and striatum), it has the highest level of absolute activity in the particulate fraction (GREENBERG et al. 1978). This membrane-bound fraction may represent a transmitter-sensitive type of guanylate cyclase for which the appropriate conditions for enzymatic assay are not known. In any case, the failure to observe stimulated guanylate cyclase activity in membrane preparations has presented a formidable stumbling block to establishing a physiological role for cyclic GMP, because the primary events responsible for cyclic GMP formation remain unknown.

It has been suggested that cyclic GMP affects physiological processes by the same mechanism invoked for cyclic AMP, via the activation of a cyclic nucleotide-dependent protein kinase and subsequent phosphorylation of substrate proteins (GREENGARD and KUO 1970). Although this role has not been firmly established as the only mode of action even for cyclic AMP (WALSH 1978), the existence of cyclic GMP-dependent protein kinases (KUO and GREENGARD 1970; CASNELLIE and GREENGARD 1974; KUO 1974; TAKAI et al. 1975; HOFMANN and SOLD 1972) suggests that this may be the primary way in which cyclic GMP regulates cellular activity as well. The level of cyclic GMP-dependent protein kinase appears to be particularly high in the cerebellum (BANDLE and GUIDOTTI 1978, 1979), and to be associated with intact Purkinje cells and functional innervation by inhibitory pathways. In addition, probably the only well characterized endogenous substrate for cyclic GMP-dependent kinase in mammalian brain has also been found in cerebellum, but not in hippocampus, caudate or cortex (SCHLICHTER et al. 1978; see also MALKINSON 1975). Thus, it appears that the biochemical machinery for cyclic GMP-dependent phosphorylation exists in the brain, and particularly in the cerebellum. However, the physiological significance of these cyclic GMP-dependent biochemical events remains unknown.

Despite these handicaps arising from a lack of direct information concerning cyclic GMP-dependent processes, there have been numerous attempts to establish a functional physiological role for this nucleotide. Generally, the approach that has been used has been to characterize electrophysiologically and behaviorally a wide variety of treatments which have been observed to increase tissue cyclic GMP levels, both in vivo and in vitro (cf. DALY 1977a; FERRENDELLI 1976; FERRENDELLI et al. 1972, 1975; GOLDBERG and HADDOX 1977). Although it is difficult to provide generalizations which accurately reflect all the experimental data, it would appear that treatments in vivo which increase behavioral excitability (i.e., motor activity) or electrophysiological activity (e.g., seizures) lead to increases in cyclic GMP levels, while treatments which have the opposite effects (e.g., sedatives and anesthetics, membrane stabilizers) reduce cyclic GMP levels (FERRENDELLI 1978). In vitro, treatment of brain slices with various putative transmitters has widely varying effects, depending upon the species and brain region being considered; only the excitatory amino acids and norepinephrine are relatively consistent even in so far as the direction of changes they elicit in cyclic GMP. As discussed previously, extracellular calcium is a requirement in all brain regions and with all putative transmitters for increases in cyclic GMP to be observed. The conclusion reached by some has been that cyclic GMP seems to be associated more with cellular depolarization and subsequent calcium influx than with any particular neurotransmitter, and that transmitters affect cyclic GMP if and when they elicit depolarizations in some group of neurons (RUBIN and FERRENDELLI 1977, FERRENDELLI 1978).

I. Acetylcholine and Cyclic GMP

Although much of the evidence would indicate that cyclic GMP may not serve as a second messenger for any single transmitter, this is by no means unequivocal. One particular hypothesis is that cyclic GMP is a second messenger for acetylcholine, and in particular in the muscarinic cholinergic system. Acetylcholine increases cyclic GMP levels in cholinergically innervated target organs of the peripheral nervous system such as the heart (GEORGE et al. 1970) and in smooth muscle (LEE et al. 1972). These initial results from peripheral target tissues for ACh lead many investigators to consider the effects of cyclic GMP and muscarinic cholinergics in the nervous system as well (WEIGHT et al. 1974; KEBABIAN et al. 1975a; KUO et al. 1972; LEE et al. 1972; STONE et al. 1975; HOFFER et al. 1977a). However, the hypothesis that cyclic GMP is the second messenger for ACh in the periphery now appears somewhat unlikely. In both the heart and in smooth muscle, the effects of ACh on target cell physiology and on cyclic GMP levels can be dissociated (KATSUKI and MURAD 1977; BROOKER 1977), suggesting that cyclic GMP is not involved. In particular, cyclic GMP appears to be involved in relaxation in smooth muscle, rather than contraction induced by ACh (see MURAD et al. 1979). Thus, the increases in cyclic GMP may occur as a consequence of the physiological response to ACh, rather than to ACh directly.

Nevertheless, this hypothesis has generated considerable interest in an analogous role for cyclic GMP in the nervous system. Oxotremorine was shown in an early study to increase cyclic GMP in cerebellum of mouse (FERRENDELLI et al. 1970) and its effect could be blocked by muscarinic antagonists. In vitro experiments demonstrated similar muscarinic increases in cyclic GMP in a variety of brain regions (cf. DALY 1977a). However, two problems have made this hypothesis somewhat less secure. First, ACh has no effects in vitro in brain slices in the absence of calcium (FERRENDELLI et al. 1973; SCHULTZ et al. 1973; KEBABIAN et al.

1975b), suggesting a lack of direct effect upon the cyclase. Secondly, the effects of oxotremorine in vivo are most likely the result of the activation of cholinergic interneurons which ultimately project to the cerebellum via other brain nuclei, and involving other neurotransmitters. The increases in cerebellar cyclic GMP produced by apomorphine (BIGGIO et al. 1977), are also blocked by cholinergic blockers, suggesting a cholinergic link in this effect. Thus, neither the physiological experiments with ACh and cyclic GMP in the periphery or in the CNS provide much concrete support for the idea that cyclic GMP serves as a second messenger for this transmitter. Until more convincing evidence can be obtained, it would seem that this hypothesis must be seriously questioned.

II. Excitatory Amino Acids and Cyclic GMP

Another possibility is that cyclic GMP serves as a second messenger for some excitatory amino acid (probably glutamate) in the cerebellar cortex (e.g., BIGGIO et al. 1978c). Since the regulation of cyclic GMP levels in this region has been extensively investigated, this provides an opportunity to consider the evidence in favor of this hypothesis in considerable detail.

As mentioned above, the cerebellum has been shown to have endogenous cyclic GMP-dependent kinases and appropriate substrates for phosphorylation, and it also has very high levels of cyclic GMP when compared with other brain regions (at least an order of magnitude higher in mouse cerebellum than in other brain regions; GREENBERG et al. 1978; STEINER et al. 1972). It has been also known for some time that a variety of pharmacologic treatments which influence the electrophysiological activity of the cerebellum can alter the levels of cyclic GMP found in this region. Furthermore, the increases in cyclic GMP evoked in the cerebellum by various treatments are generally larger than those observed in other brain areas, although this may reflect low phosphodiesterase activity rather than a high degree of activation of guanylate cyclase (GREENBERG et al. 1978). Different species also show large differences in the characteristics of cerebellar cyclic GMP systems; almost 60-fold differences can be observed in basal cyclic GMP levels, and similar differences in the magnitude of responses to various test conditions are also observed (KINSCHERF et al. 1976). In sum, the highly variable distribution of cyclic GMP generating systems may suggest an association with particular transmitter systems, rather than being involved with generalized cellular processes common to all neurons. In addition, the apparent concentration of enzymes involved in cyclic GMP systems in cerebellum make this an excellent area to begin an investigation into the role of cyclic GMP.

In vivo, a variety of tremorogenic agents (oxotremorine, harmaline) induce increases in the cyclic GMP levels in cerebellum (FERRENDELLI et al. 1970; OPMEER et al. 1976; MAO et al. 1975a; SPANO et al. 1975); drugs which antagonize these tremors, such as diazepam and pentobarbital, block the increases in cyclic GMP (MAO et al. 1975b; OPMEER et al. 1976). The actions of many of these drugs are clearly indirect, and are not observed in slices of cerebellum maintained in vitro. In particular, excitation or inhibition of a multisynaptic striato-cerebellar pathway seems to be involved in the regulation of cyclic GMP levels in the latter structure. Dopaminergic agents result in elevations of cerebellar cyclic GMP (BURKARD et al.

1976; BIGGIO and GUIDOTTI 1977; GUMULKA et al. 1976), and there is a close correspondence between the affinities of drugs for dopaminergic receptors in the striatum, and their efficacy in regulating cerebellar cyclic GMP (BREESE et al. 1978). Lesions of the caudate nucleus reduce cerebellar cyclic GMP to approximately 25% of control (BIGGIO et al. 1978b), and block the cerebellar cyclic GMP response to the dopminergic agonist, apomorphine (BIGGIO et al. 1977, 1978a). Thus, it would appear that drugs such as apomorphine act indirectly via the caudate to increase cerebellar cyclic GMP levels.

There are at least two pathways into the cerebellum by which these influences on cyclic GMP might be mediated, the mossy fibers and the climbing fibers. The climbing fibers are probably not involved, since lesions of the climbing fibers with 3-acetylpyridine do not block cyclic GMP responses to apomorphine. However, cyclic GMP increases brought about by harmaline, which activates the climbing fibers, *are* blocked by 3-AP lesions (BIGGIO et al. 1977). Thus, it would appear that activation of either excitatory input can increase cerebellar cyclic GMP levels.

On the other hand, drugs which affect GABAergic inhibition can also affect cyclic GMP. Isoniazid, which decreases GABA levels in cerebellum, results in an increase in cyclic GMP. Diazepam, which is thought to potentiate GABA action, can antagonize the effects of isoniazid (BIGGIO et al. 1977).

In sum, the experimental results suggest that cyclic GMP levels in cerebellum are regulated by at least 3 factors; the amount of excitatory input via the mossy fibers, the climbing fibers, and the degree of GABAergic inhibition. Because of the nature of the transmitter systems affected by these drugs, the general conclusions reached in many of these experiments were that transmitters associated with the excitatory pathways (probably glutamate or perhaps aspartate) were involved in the increases in cyclic GMP, and GABA in the decreases (COSTA et al. 1975a, b; MAILMAN et al. 1978). The involvement of glutamate has been supported somewhat by experiments with various glutamate analogs (BRILEY et al. 1979; SHIMIZU and YAMAMURA 1977). The relatively high levels of particulate-bound guanylate cyclase in both hippocampus and cerebellum (GREENBERG et al. 1978), both regions which are thought to possess glutamatergic excitatory pathways, has led to the hypothesis that cyclic GMP acts as a second messenger for glutamate via the activation of specific membrane-bound guanylate cyclases.

While there is little evidence which is contrary to this hypothesis, several aspects of the evidence in favor of this hypothesis make its evaluation rather difficult. In the first place, the actions of glutamate on the central nervous system are exceedingly rapid; on and off times for electrophysiological responses are generally on the order of milliseconds. What, if any, relationship can be drawn between slow biochemical events and fast electrophysiological responses, whose time scale differs by more than 5 orders of magnitude, is unclear. The criterion discussed in the introduction concerning the temporal sequencing of physiological and cyclic nucleotide changes has certainly not been met. Thus, this would hardly seem to be compelling evidence that cyclic GMP mediates these electrophysiological events; it is perhaps just as likely that the cyclic GMP increases are a result of changes in electrophysiological activity.

Another problem is raised by the fact that diazepam can apparently block the increases in cGMP evoked by climbing fiber stimulation (MAO et al. 1975b; but see BIGGIO et al. 1977). If these cyclic GMP increases are mediated directly by excitatory amino acid-coupled guanylate cyclase, it is difficult to see why these increases should be blocked by diazepam, which appears to potentiate GABAergic activity. On the other hand, if cyclic GMP simply reflects generalized neuronal activity, then such an interaction would appear quite probable.

Before leaving this subject, it should also be mentioned that there is also evidence which would seem to indicate that cyclic GMP may *not* serve as a second messenger for glutamate in the cerebellum. To be specific, it has not proven possible to block Ca^{+2}-mediated increases in cerebellar cyclic GMP with glutamate blockers in vitro (OHGA and DALY 1977a, b), even though the same blockers are effective in antagonizing glutamate-induced cyclic GMP increases in vivo (BRILEY et al. 1979). Increases in cerebellar cyclic GMP due to glutamate are not additive with increases in cyclic GMP produced by calcium (OHGA and DALY 1977a), nor does glutamate alone increase cyclic GMP levels to the degree seen with other depolarizing agents such as high potassium (FERRENDELLI et al. 1974). These data suggest that a) calcium influx alone is sufficient to activate guanylate cyclase; b) that depolarizing agents can all increase cyclic GMP via calcium influx directly associated with their depolarizing action; and c) that glutamate blockers are effective in antagonizing only those cyclic GMP increases which involve glutamate. Thus, if cyclic GMP does serve as an intracellular messenger for glutamate, it would appear to do so indirectly by means of changes in intracellular calcium, which are essentially required for activation of guanylate cyclase. The same types of criticisms which have led to a general lack of acceptance for a second messenger role for cyclic GMP in mediating muscarinic cholinergic action (cf. PURVES 1978; KRNJEVIĆ 1978) appear to be equally applicable to the hypothesis of the same role for cyclic GMP in glutamate action. This is not to say that this type of approach has not been extremely productive. The use of cyclic GMP as a biochemical indicant of electrophysiological activity has been essential in uncovering the basic pharmacology of striato-cerebellar pathways. Nevertheless, while it has proved its value as a measure of cellular activity, considerably less has been learned about the actual functional role of cyclic GMP itself.

III. Transmitter Release

The fact that the ionic conditions required to elicit hormone-stimulated increases in cyclic GMP in brain slices correspond quite well to those required for calcium-dependent transmitter release, have led to yet another hypothesis, that cyclic GMP may somehow be involved in the process of transmitter release (FERRENDELLI 1976). In these experiments, the observation was made that depolarization induces increases in cyclic GMP, and that divalent cations which can substitute for Ca^{+2} in the release process (Ba^{2+} and Sr^{2+}) also can produce cyclic GMP changes. Those which cannot substitute for calcium in release processes (Mn^{2+}, Co^{2+} or Mg^{+2}) do not permit and may in fact antagonize Ca^{+2}-dependent accumulations of cyclic GMP.

These experiments all involved depolarization of brain slices; in addition, it has been observed that A-23187, a calcium ionophore, increased cyclic GMP levels in slices of both central and peripheral tissue which have not been depolarized (FER-

RENDELLI et al. 1976; BARTFAI et al. 1978). Thus, depolarization per se does not seem to be an important factor in cyclic GMP increases. The increase in cyclic GMP which results from cellular depolarization under normal conditions would appear to be the result of calcium fluxes secondary to cellular depolarization. The functional role of cyclic GMP increases could be as an intermediary in any process which follows calcium entry into neurons; transmitter release, initiation of synthetic processes, or activation of uptake or pump mechanisms, are all possibilities deserving consideration at this point.

IV. Electrophysiological Effects of Cyclic GMP

As discussed in the previous section, putative transmitters which increase cellular activity generally increase cyclic GMP levels, while those which inhibit cell firing (e.g., GABA) generally do not, although there are some exceptions to this rule (e.g., NE). This has led to the suggestion that cyclic GMP might directly influence electrophysiological activity. This hypothesis receives some support from the work of several groups who have investigated the actions of intracellularly injected cyclic GMP. Although consistent excitatory responses were not observed, intracellular injections of cyclic GMP generally result in increases in membrane conductance (SHINNICK-GALLAGHER et al. 1976; KRNJEVIĆ 1978; KRNJEVIĆ et al. 1976; but see WOODY et al. 1978); intracellular injections of Ca^{+2} can produce somewhat similar effects (KRNJEVIĆ and LISIEWICZ 1972). In addition, intracellular injections of cyclic GMP have been found to "sharpen" spikes by increasing the rate of rise of the depolarizing aspects of the waveform, as well as accentuating the hyperpolarizing phase of the spike. The lack of highly repeatable excitatory effects does not seem to support the idea that cyclic GMP is directly involved in cellular excitation; perhaps a more likely hypothesis is that suggested by KRNJEVIĆ (1978), that cyclic GMP may exert a kind of "restorative" action which would serve to counterbalance changes produced by excessive neuronal activity.

A still different role has been suggested by WOODY (1978). In the pericruciate cortex of the cat, extracellular application of ACh and intracellular injection of cyclic GMP have similar effects upon membrane properties (WOODY et al. 1978). Particular combinations of direct stimulation of neuronal activity coupled with either intracellular injections of cyclic GMP or extracellular iontophoresis of ACh can result in very long-lasting increases in membrane resistance. The hypothesis suggested to account for these results is that cyclic GMP, by an action upon some unspecified cellular process, compiles a hypothetical "record" of the activity of a given cell, which subsequently affects the way that cell responds to subsequent afferent activity. Since cyclic GMP formation is sensitive to calcium influx, and since calcium influx accompanies electrophysiological activity, this could represent a mechanism by which longterm changes in cellular activity could influence other cellular events.

Regardless of whether either of these hypothetical roles for cyclic GMP is correct, it is apparent that there is by no means a uniform action of intracellularly injected cyclic GMP upon any easily measured cellular properties. The biochemical evidence clearly indicates that cyclic GMP and depolarization are closely associated. However, the current experiments would seem to suggest that cyclic GMP does not serve as a second messenger whose function is to depolarize neurons, but rather is formed as a consequence of depolarization, and which may subsequently regulate some more complex aspect of cellular function.

Considering the problems that have developed with intracellular iontophoresis of cyclic GMP, it is not surprising that the effects of extracellular application of cyclic GMP and its analogs have been equally confusing. In the rat cortex, ACh and cyclic GMP have been observed to have parallel actions on corticospinal neurons, exciting 82% of the cells tested (STONE and TAYLOR 1977). Non-pyramidal tract neurons sometimes showed depressant actions to both, and as would be expected, atropine blocked only the responses to ACh. In contrast, responses to cyclic AMP have generally been observed to be in the opposite (i.e., depressant) direction on the same types of cells (STONE et al. 1975). In studies by PHILLIS (1974), cyclic GMP had predominantly excitant actions, with some depressant actions as well; these responses did not appear to correlate well with the effects of ACh in these experiments. Still other experiments have shown depressant actions both in the cortex (PHILLIS et al. 1974) and in the cerebellum (HOFFER et al. 1971b).

In experiments using iontophoretic techniques on isolated in oculo hippocampal transplants, cGMP and acetylcholine have been shown to have excitatory effects on neuronal activity (HOFFER et al. 1977a). Moreover, superfusion of the transplant with phosphodiesterase-resistant cyclic GMP derivatives can elicit clearcut sustained epileptiform activity (FREEDMAN et al. 1979). The possible role of cyclic GMP in initiating and maintaining seizure discharge is presented later in this chapter. In other experiments using the in vitro hippocampal slice preparation, cyclic GMP analogs were found to augment synaptic responses in such a way as to suggest a generalized increase in neuronal excitability (DUNWIDDIE, unpublished results). In addition, nitroprusside, a non-specific activator of the membrane-bound form of guanylate cyclase (MITTAL et al. 1975; NAKAZAWA and SANO 1974) also produced increases in excitability in this preparation (DUNWIDDIE, unpublished results).

In sum, a variety of physiological roles for cyclic GMP have been proposed; as a second messenger, most notably for ACh and glutamate, in neurotransmitter release, and in long- and short-term regulation of cellular excitability, perhaps via an interaction with calcium. The evidence for none of these roles is particularly compelling. While a large variety of agents have been shown to affect cyclic GMP levels, neither the primary events responsible for guanylate cyclase activation nor the subsequent events which occur as a result of the accumulation of this nucleotide are known with any certainty.

D. Cyclic Nucleotides and Disease States

Cyclic nucleotides have been implicated in a number of neuropsychiatric disease states. This portion of the review will focus on two areas where both clinical and basic neurobiological studies have implicated cyclic nucleotides: (1) manic-depressive illness and lithium action; and (2) regulation of neuronal excitability and seizure disorders. More general consideration of these areas can be found in recent reviews (e.g., HAMET and SANDS 1980).

I. Manic-Depressive Illness and Lithium Actions

A major pharmacotherapeutic advance in psychiatric disease has been the use of lithium for treatment of manic-depressive illness. Most recent reviews (DAVIS 1976; GERBINO et al. 1978; SPENCER 1977; COOPER and SIMPSON 1978; KLERMAN 1978, BUNNEY and MURPHY 1976; BUNNEY et al. 1977) continue to emphasize (1) lithium's therapeutic value for patients in the manic phase of manic-depressive psychosis, (2), the existence for a latent period of 7–10 days before the onset of therapeutic effects, (3) reduction of manic symptoms over 7–21 days, and (4) the recurrence of mania within 3–5 days after cessation of lithium (Li). The fact that Li is an active therapeutic agent, which is not metabolized and is easily measured in tissue fluids (COOMBS et al. 1975) provides an experimental treatment paradigm which is extremely useful in both clinical (GERBINO et al. 1978; FRANCIS and TRAILL 1970) and preclinical studies (BUNNEY and MURPHY 1976; SCHOU 1976); patients and animals can be maintained within so-called therapeutic windows (0.7–1.7 mM plasma levels) to determine correlative changes in chemistry and physiology. In clinical studies, longer-term Li treatment appears effective as continuation therapy for recurrent mania (KLERMAN 1978) and for the recurrent depressions of bipolar affective disorder (GERBINO et al. 1978; KLERMAN 1978; BUNNEY and MURPHY 1976). However, Li is regarded as ineffective in the acute treatment of ongoing depression (GERBINO et al. 1978; KLERMAN 1978; BUNNEY and MURPHY 1976; SCHOU 1976). Li has also been found to have therapeutic utility in reducing the alcohol intake by alcoholics diagnosed on rating scales as being depressed, but does not affect the alcohol intake of non-depressed alcoholics (KLINE and COOPER 1975, 1979; REYNOLDS et al. 1979; KLINE et al. 1979). Li may also have some usefulness in antagonizing the psychostimulant phases of opiates or amphetamines, but in man, the latter results are not yet clearcut (VAN KAMMEN and MURPHY 1975; JASINSKI et al. 1977). Although Li was found to have some "anti-euphoric" effects on basal self-perception of moods in drug-free former narcotic abusers, Li did not alter the euphoric responses of these subjects to morphine (JASINSKI et al. 1977). However, in general, Li given in non-toxic doses to normal subjects is reported to produce neither sedation nor psychological impairment (GERBINO et al. 1978; COOPER and SIMPSON 1978; BUNNEY and MURPHY 1976; SCHOU 1976).

There have been a number of observations linking both acute and chronic lithium administration with cyclic nucleotide generating systems.

1. Acute Effects

Earlier observations showed that Li can inhibit adenylate cyclase activation by NE in brain (FORN and VALDECASAS 1971; DOUSA and HECHTER 1970a), by TSH in thyroid (WOLFF et al. 1970), by epinephrine in skeletal muscle (FRAZER et al. 1975), and by vasopressin by distal renal tubules (GEISLER et al. 1972; DOUSA and HECHTER 1970b). It would appear, moreover, that the apparent antagonism by Li of DA-activated adenylate cyclase in vitro (GEISLER and KLYSNER 1977) does not occur when animals are treated first with Li and their brain slices tested in vitro (GEISLER and KLYSNER 1978).

Recently, electrophysiological studies have confirmed these biochemical observations. Both in hippocampus (SEGAL 1974) and in cerebellum (SIGGINS and

SCHULTZ 1979), lithium produces a selective and reversible antagonism of the inhibitory noradrenergic input. Little effect was seen on GABAergic inhibitions.

2. Chronic Effects

It must be realized, however, that the therapeutic effects of Li in mania, or of tricyclic antidepressants in affective psychosis, require treatment periods of 1–2 weeks before therapeutic results occur. In animal experiments, metabolic changes and functional effects were assumed to continue unchanged from the effects of single acute treatments to the effects of chronic treatments. However, as this issue was tested, it became clear that the acute effects do not persist, and are, instead, replaced by changes which may be opposite to those seen after acute treatments (SCHWARTZ et al. 1978). For example, tricyclic antidepressants given in a single acute treatment potentiate the cellular and behavioral effects of norepinephrine by inhibition of the reuptake mechanism (GLOWINSKI and AXELROD 1964). This acute effect has been interpreted within the catecholamine hypothesis of affective disorders (SCHILDKRAUT 1965; SCHILDKRAUT et al. 1977; BUNNEY and POST 1977) to infer that depression was a catecholamine deficiency, and that tricyclics treat depression by bolstering the inadequate amounts of catecholamine seen by the postsynaptic receptor. In animals treated chronically with desmethylimipramine, postsynaptic receptor sensitivity is decreased even though inhibition of presynaptic reuptake remains fully inhibited (VETULANI and SULSER 1975; SCHULTZ 1976; WOLFE et al. 1978; FRAZER et al. 1978).

As far as Li is concerned, W. BUNNEY and colleagues (BUNNEY et al. 1977) have pursued the hypothesis that Li prevents the adaptive responses in receptor-linked adenylate cyclase sensitivity and have searched for receptor selectivity of this hypothetical action. Haloperidol, an antipsychotic drug with some antidopamine actions, leads to supersensitivity of dopamine receptors after chronic treatment; BUNNEY, PERT and their colleagues (GALLAGER et al. 1978; PERT et al. 1978) have observed that if Li is given simultaneously with the haloperidol, this supersensitivity to dopamine is not observed. In these experiments, the Li treatment is stopped 2–3 days before receptor sensitivity is evaluated. Long-term loss of central catecholamine fibers after intraventricular injection of 6-hydroxydopamine results in a supersensitivity of norepinephrine receptors (SPORN et al. 1977; HOFFER et al. 1971a; SEGAL and BLOOM 1974); this effect is also blocked by Li treatments. Tricyclic antidepressants given chronically are reported to produce supersensitivity in cortical α-noradrenergic receptors. Lithium prevents the changes produced by imipramine on α-receptors, but not those produced by imipramine on β-receptors (ROSENBLATT et al. 1978).

Because Li appears to block the regulation of receptor sensitivity following a variety of treatments, these effects could be interpreted to infer a possible pathophysiology in manic-depressive illness. It would appear that the root of the illness may lie in disease-imposed cyclic changes in receptor sensitivity, in which changes in transmitter release alternate against a background of constantly changing but phase-lagged response properties. In this sense, the disease state of affective psychosis could be an enhanced lability of receptor self-regulation, in which case the therapeutic effect of chronic Li might reside in its ability to stabilize the hyperlabile receptor changes (BUNNEY et al. 1977).

Electrophysiological studies by SIGGINS and SCHULTZ (1979) support the marked differential actions of acute and chronic lithium. Long-term LiCl therapy in rat enhances, if anything, noradrenergic input to Purkinje cells, perhaps by an adaptive alteration in β-receptors.

A reasonable body of evidence is thus compatible with the view that acute exposure to Li generally diminishes functional transmission through NE-mediated cyclic nucleotide systems by means of changes in metabolism, decreased release of transmitter and depressed responsivity of postsynaptic receptors associated with depressed ability of NE to activate adenylate cyclase. While this acute anti-NE effect is compatible with a catecholamine hypothesis of mania resulting from excess NE transmission, these acute effects on the metabolism of central NE systems are lost with continuation of treatment for the requisite 7–10 day latent period; by that time, changes in metabolism of other transmitter systems, especially 5-HT (KNAPP and MANDELL 1975) have been reported, as have effects on other enzymes (BERA and CHATTERJEE 1976) and hormone activation of adenylate cyclases in endocrine tissues and muscle (WOLFF et al. 1970; FRAZER et al. 1975; DOUSA and HECHTER 1070b). When viewed from the perspectives of either general psychochemical interactions of Li on receptor regulation (BUNNEY et al. 1977; KAHN 1976) or its possible transmitter-specific effects, Li may be viewed to modify postsynaptic receptor self-regulation, perhaps stabilizing a labile receptor psychopathology as it does stabilize some receptor changes with experimental drug treatments.

II. Regulation of Neuronal Excitability and Seizure Disorders

The role of cyclic nucleotides in seizure disorders had received increasing attention during the past several years. There are three converging lines of evidence suggesting that both cyclic AMP and cyclic GMP are involved in seizures: a) effects of seizures on cyclic nucleotide levels in brain; b) correlation of drug-induced changes in seizures and cyclic nucleotide accumulation; and c) electrophysiological actions of cyclic nucleotides on central neurons.

1. Effects of Seizures on Cyclic Nucleotide Levels in Brain

It is now well established that generalized seizures induced by a number of physical or chemical convulsants elicit elevations of cyclic AMP and cyclic GMP levels in brain (BERTI et al. 1976; FERRENDELLI and KINSCHERF 1977; FOLBERGROVA 1975, 1977; FOLCO et al. 1977; LUST et al. 1976; MAO et al. 1974, 1975a; PALMER et al. 1979; REHNCRONA et al. 1978; SATTIN 1971). Several studies have focused on regional differences in such elevations. Thus, FERRENDELLI and KINSCHERF (1977) showed that pentylenetetrazol elevated cyclic GMP levels in cerebral cortex, hippocampus, thalamus, cerebellum and striatum. Cyclic AMP, on the other hand, was not elevated in striatum, and the increased levels in thalamus and cerebellum returned to normal despite persistence of the seizure.

The temporal relationship between cyclic AMP and GMP changes during seizures has also been investigated. As noted above, both electroshock (LUST et al. 1976, 1978; SATTIN 1971), and chemical convulsants (BERTI et al. 1976; FERRENDELLI and KINSCHERF 1977; MAO et al. 1975a) elevate cyclic nucleotide levels in several brain regions. However, in a number of areas, like striatum and cerebellum, the elevation of cyclic GMP precedes initiation of the seizure whereas increased cyclic AMP follows seizure onset. Support for this differential relationship also comes from dose-response studies (FERRENDELLI 1980). Subconvulsive doses of pentylenetetrazol elicit elevations of cyclic GMP in cerebral cortex, hippocampus, and cerebellum. No changes are seen in cyclic AMP levels, however, unless an overt seizure is elicited.

2. Effects of Drugs Which Modify Seizures

An initial approach to this question utilized anticonvulsant drugs. While agents like phenytoin, phenobarbital, ethosuximide and valproic acid reduce seizure-induced cyclic nucleotide elevations (FERRENDELLI and KINSCHERF 1977; FOLBERGROVA 1975; LUST et al. 1978), this appears to be a direct result of their antiepileptic actions. Hence, little insight could be obtained into the role of cyclic nucleotides in epilepsy using such drugs.

A second approach has been to study drugs which interact with specific neurotransmitter systems. As an example, GROSS and FERRENDELLI (1979) demonstrated that a variety of agents which reduce noradrenergic transmission increased the intensity of pentylenetetrazol-induced seizures. At the same time, pentylenetetrazol-induced elevations of cyclic AMP were reduced whereas elevations of cyclic GMP were unaltered or augmented. These effects were seen using agents which deplete catecholamines (reserpine), agents which destroy catecholamine terminals (6-hydroxydopamine), or drugs which block adrenergic receptors (propranolol). Drugs which block dopamine or 5-HT receptors do not show this effect. On the basis of this data, GROSS and FERRENDELLI (1979) postulated that seizure activity activated adrenergic systems and hence increases cyclic AMP levels as well, and that the consequence of this is a reduction in seizure activity. Cyclic GMP levels appear not to be influenced by adrenergic input during seizures and may thus play a different pathophysiological role.

3. Effects of Cyclic Nucleotide Applications on Neuronal Excitability

Although the electrophysiological actions of cyclic nucleotides remain somewhat controversial (see SIGGINS, this volume), several studies have demonstrated opposite effects of cyclic AMP and cyclic GMP on neuronal excitability in various brain regions. Thus, both in cerebral cortex (STONE et al. 1975) and in hippocampus (HOFFER et al. 1977 b; SEGAL and BLOOM 1974), local application of cyclic GMP excites pyramidal neurons while cyclic AMP depresses them. In hippocampus grafted to the anterior chamber of the eye, superfusion of the 8 bromo- or 8-parachlorophenylthio derivatives of cyclic GMP actually trigger prolonged and clearcut epileptiform activity (FREEDMAN et al. 1979).

The conclusions from these three lines of research have recently been synthesized by FERRENDELLI into a hypothesis concerning the relationship between cyclic nucleotides and epilepsy. Although both cyclic AMP and cyclic GMP levels are elevated during generalized seizures, the time courses and stimuli responsible for the increases appear somewhat different. Cyclic GMP levels are increased by a variety of treatments which trigger not only overt seizures, but also interictal spikes. Stimuli which are subthreshold for convulsant activity are also effective; the magnitude and regional distribution of the cyclic GMP elevation appears related to the intensity of the increases in electrophysiological activity. While the mechanism by which cyclic GMP increases occur is not clear, cellular depolarization and increased intracellular calcium are likely possibilities (FERRENDELLI 1976; FERRENDELLI et al. 1976; TROYER et al. 1978).

Increases in cyclic AMP levels, although also region-specific, appear to require a behaviorally or clinically-evident seizure. The mechanism for the seizure-related cyclic AMP elevation appears to be largely due to transmitter or modulator release into the extracellular space. Biogenic amines, especially norepinephrine and purines, have been particularly implicated (see above). Moreover, pharmacological studies with drugs that alter norepinephrine- or adenosine-induced responses suggest that the elevation in cyclic AMP levels may be inversely related to the intensity of the seizure. Taken together, these data suggest that cyclic GMP may be involved in the transition from interictal spiking to ictus whereas cyclic AMP, perhaps acting as a second messenger at NE or purinergic synapses, may have an antiepileptic or seizure-limiting action.

E. Conclusion

In spite of the effort which has been expended in trying to determine the function of cyclic nucleotides in the nervous system, conclusive evidence for any particular role remains obscure. At the present time, fragmentary knowledge concerning a wide variety of possible roles has been obtained; what remains is to link many individual pieces of information into more comprehensive models of cyclic nucleotide action.

It should be hoped that if this review has not been successful in achieving a coherent synthesis of existing knowledge, at least it may have clarified some of the types of approaches which will be required to significantly advance our understanding of cyclic nucleotide action. First, the complexity of the nervous system is a formidable obstacle to experimental approaches to cyclic nucleotide effects. Because the central nervous system consists of many different types of neurons, with different transmitters and receptors, as well as several different types of glia, presynaptic terminals, vascular elements, etc., cyclic nucleotides are unlikely to have a single "role" even in a very circumscribed brain region. Cyclic AMP (and cyclic GMP) probably have multiple roles, and determining the multiple loci of cyclic nucleotide action is one of the primary challenges to the understanding of their functions in the nervous system. Because of the intrinsic complexity of nervous tissue, the widely-used approach of exogenous application of cyclic nucleotides and their analogs can be a difficult technique to utilize. With many possible sites of cyclic nucleotide action, it becomes difficult to interpret any effects which are observed. The fact that cyclic AMP and some of its derivatives can have potent actions at extracellular sites only complicates matters further. Because of this, experiments in simple systems where the number of sites at which cyclic nucleotides can act are reduced, immunohistochemical localization of cyclic nucleotides to determine where changes are occuring, and using intracellular injection of cyclic nucleotides are all particularly valuable techniques for attacking problems of structural complexity.

The intrinsic complexity of the nervous system is not the only unique difficulty with regard to cyclic nucleotides. The physiological processes of the nervous system also occur at a much faster rate than in many other organ systems. Cyclic nucleotides are implicated in some of the slower processes in the nervous system, but they have also been hypothesized to play essential roles in both the release of neurotransmitters, and in the postsynaptic effects of transmitters as well. If this is the case, then clearly changes in cyclic nucleotide levels would have to occur with extreme rapidity. The experimental evidence that such changes occur is lacking. In the heart, cyclical changes in cyclic AMP levels have been described, with apparently maximal activation of adenylate cyclase occuring within a few hundred milliseconds (BROOKER 1975). Whether the dynamics of cyclic nucleotide formation in the nervous system are similarly rapid is not known. At present, technical difficulties would appear to preclude a high degree of temporal resolution in measuring the formation of cyclic nucleotides in nervous tissue.

In spite of these problems, there appears little question but that cyclic nucleotides play an important role in the function of the nervous system. Presynaptic terminals, postsynaptic cells, and glial cells all possess cyclic nucleotide generating systems responsive to a variety of stimuli. What remains is to develop techniques and strategies which will enable definitive tests to be made of the variety of hypothetical roles for both cyclic AMP and cyclic GMP in the nervous system.

References

Adler-Graschinsky E, Langer SZ (1975) Possible role of a beta-adrenoreceptor in the regulation of noradrenaline release by nerve stimulation through a positive feedback mechanism. Br J Pharmacol 53:43–50

Anagnoste B, Shirron C, Friedman E, Goldstein M (1974) Effect of dibutyryl cyclic adenosine monophosphate on ^{14}C-dopamine biosynthesis in rat brain striatal slices. J Pharmacol Exp Ther 191:370–376

Bandle E, Guidotti A (1978) Studies on the cell location of cyclic 3′,5′-guanosine monophosphate-dependent protein kinase in cerebellum. Brain Res 156:412–416

Bandle E, Guidotti A (1979) Ontogenetic studies of cGMP-dependent protein kinase in rat cerebellum. J Neurochem 32:1343–1347

Bartfai T, Study RE, Greengard P (1978) Muscarinic stimulation and cGMP synthesis in the nervous system. Adv Behav Biol 24:285–295

Beall RJ, Sayers G (1972) Isolated adrenal cells: steroidogenesis and cyclic AMP accumulation in response to ACTH. Arch Biochem Biophys 148:70–76

Bera H, Chatterjee GC (1976) Effect of lithium administration on neural enzymes in rats. Biochem Pharmacol 25:1554–1555

Berti F, Bernareggi V, Folco GC, Fumagalli R, Paoletti R (1976) Prostaglandin E_2 and cyclic nucleotides in rat convulsions and tremors. In: Costa E, Giacobini E, Paoletti R (eds) Advances in psychopharmacology: first and second messengers – new vistas. Raven New York, pp. 367–377

Biggio G, Guidotti A (1977) Regulation of cyclic GMP in cerebellum by a striatal dopaminergic mechanism. Nature 265:240–242

Biggio G, Costa E, Guidotti A (1977) Pharmacologically induced changes in the 3′,5′-cyclic guanosine monophosphate content of rat cerebellar cortex: difference between apomorphine, haloperidol and harmaline. J Pharmacol Exp Ther 200:207–215

Biggio G, Corda MG, Casu M, Gessa GL (1978a) Kainic acid-induced lesion of dopaminergic target cells in the striatum: consequences on the dynamics of cerebellar cGMP. Naunyn Schmiedebergs Arch Pharmacol 304:5–7

Biggio G, Corda MG, Casu M, Gessa GL (1978b) Striato-cerebellar pathway controlling cyclic GMP content in the cerebellum: role of dopamine, GABA and enkephalins. Adv Biochem Psychopharmacol 18:227–244

Biggio G, Corda MG, Casu M, Salis M, Gessa GL (1978c) Disappearance of cerebellar cyclic GMP induced by kainic acid. Brain Res 154:203–208

Blinks JR, Olson CB, Jewell BR, Braveny P (1972) Influence of caffeine and other methylxanthines on mechanical properties of isolated mammalian heart muscle. Circ Res 30:367

Bloom FE (1975) The role of cyclic nucleotides in central synaptic function. Rev Physiol Biochem Pharmacol 74:1–103

Blume AJ (1979) Regulation of mouse neuroblastoma adenylate cyclase by adenosine. In: Baer HP, Drummond GI (eds) Physiological and regulatory functions of adenosine and adenine nucleotides. Raven, New York, pp 249–257

Blume AJ, Foster CJ (1975) Mouse neuroblastoma adenylate cyclase, adenosine and adenosine analogues as potent effectors of adenylate cyclase activity. J Biol Chem 250:5003–5008

Bockaert J (1978) Adenyl-cyclase: a tracer for characterization and location of specific receptors in brain. In: Folco G, Paoletti R (eds) Molecular biology and pharmacology of cyclic nucleotides. Elsevier, Amsterdam Oxford New York

Breckenridge BM, Norman JH (1962) Glycogen phosphorylase in brain. J Neurochem 9:383–392

Breckenridge BM, Burn JH, Matschinsky FM (1967) Theophylline, epinephrine, and neostigmine facilitation of neuromuscular transmission. Proc Natl Acad Sci USA 57:1893–1897

Breese GR, Mailman RB, Ondrusek MG, Harden TK, Mueller RA (1978) Effects of dopaminergic agonists and antagonists on cerebellar guanosine-3′,5′-monophosphate (cGMP). Life Sci 23:533–536

Briley PA, Kouyoumdjian JC, Haidamous M, Gonnard P (1979) Effect of l-glutamate and kainate on rat cerebellar cGMP levels in vivo. Eur J Pharmacol 54:181–184

Brooker G (1975) Implications of cyclic nucleotide oscillations during the myocardial contraction cycle. Adv Cyclic Nucleotide Res 5:435–452

Brooker G (1977) Dissociation of cyclic GMP from the negative inotropic action of carbachol in guinea pig atria. J Cyclic Nucleotide Res 3:407–413

Browning ET, Schwartz JP, Breckenridge BM (1974) Norepinephrine-sensitive properties of C-6 astrocytoma cells. Mol Pharmacol 10:162–174

Bunney WE, Murphy DL (1976) The neurobiology of lithium. Neurosci Res Prog Bull 14:111–207

Bunney WE, Post RM (1977) Catecholamine agonist and receptor hypothesis of affective illness: paradoxical drug effects. In: Usdin E, Hamburg DA, Barchas JD (eds) Neuroregulators and psychiatric disorders. Oxford Press, New York, pp 151–159

Bunney WE, Post RM, Anderson AE, Kopanda RT (1977) A neuronal receptor sensitivity mechanism in affective illness (a review of evidence). Commun Psychopharmacol 1:393–405

Burkard WP (1972) Catecholamine induced increase of cyclic adenosine 3′,5′-monophosphate in rat brain in vivo. J Neurochem 19:2615–2619

Burkard WP, Pieri L, Haefely W (1976) Changes of rat cerebellar guanosine 3′,5′-cyclic phosphate by dopaminergic mechanisms in vivo. Adv Biochem Psychopharmacol 15:315–324

Burnstock G (1972) Purinergic nerves. Pharmacol Rev 24:509–581

Burnstock G (1978) A basis for distinguishing two types of purinergic receptor. In: Bolis L, Straub RW (eds) Cell membrane receptors for drugs and hormones: a multidisciplinary approach. Raven, New York, pp 107–118

Burnstock G (1979) Past and current evidence for the purinergic nerve hypothesis. In: Baer HP, Drummond GI (eds) Physiological and regulatory functions of adenosine and adenine nucleotides. Raven, New York

Bustos G, Roth RH (1979) Does cyclic AMP-dependent phosphorylation account for the activation of tyrosine hydroxylase produced by depolarization of central dopaminergic neurons? Biochem Pharmacol 28:3026–3028

Butcher RW, Sutherland EW (1962) Adenosine 3′,5′-phosphate in biological materials. I. Purification and properties of cyclic 3′,5′-nucleotide phosphodiesterase and use of this enzyme to characterize adenosine 3′,5′-phosphate in human urine. J Biol Chem 237:1244–1250

Casnellie JE, Greengard P (1974) Guanosine 3′,5′-cyclic monophosphate-dependent phosphorylation of endogenous substrate proteins in membranes of mammalian smooth muscle. Proc Natl Acad Sci USA 71:1891–1895

Chapman RA, Miller DJ (1974) The effects of caffeine on the contraction of frog heart. J Physiol (Lond) 242:589–613

Chasin M, Harris DW, Phillips MB, Hess SM (1972) 1-Ethyl-4(isopropylidenehydrazino)-pyrazolo-(3,4b)-pyridine-5-carboxylic acid, ethyl ester, hydrochloride (SQ20009)-A potent new inhibitor of cyclic 3′5′-nucleotide phosphodiesterases. Biochem Pharmacol 21:2443–2450

Chasin M, Mamrak F, Samaniego SG (1974) Preparation and properties of a cell-free, hormonally responsive adenylate cyclase from guinea pig brain. J Neurochem 22:1031–1038

Cheung WY (1980) Calmodulin plays a pivotal role in cellular regulation. Science 207:19–27

Clanachan AS, Johns A, Paton DM (1977) Presynaptic inhibitory actions of adenine nucleotides and adenosine on neurotransmission in the rat vas deferens. Neuroscience 2:597–602

Clark RB, Perkins JP (1971) Regulation of adenosine 3′,5′-cyclic monophosphate concentration in cultured human astrocytoma cells by catecholamines and histamine. Proc Natl Acad Sci USA 68:2757–2760

Clark RB, Gross R, Su Y-F, Perkins JP (1974) Regulation of adenosine 3′,5′-monophosphate content in human astrocytoma cells by adenosine and the adenine nucleotides. J Biol Chem 249:5296–5303

Clark RB, Su Y-F, Ortmann R, Cubeddu L, Johnson GL, Perkins JP (1975) Factors influencing the effect of hormones on the accumulation of cyclic AMP in cultured human astrocytoma cells. Metabolism 24:343–358

Clyman RI, Blacksin AS, Sandler JA, Manganiello VC, Vaughan M (1975) The role of calcium in regulation of cyclic nucleotide content in human umbilical artery. J Biol Chem 250:4718–4721

Cook MA, Hamilton JT, Okwuasaba FK (1978) Coenzyme A is a purine nucleotide modulator of acetylcholine output. Nature 271:768–771

Cook MA, Hamilton JT, Okwuasaba FK (1979) Structure-activity relationship studies of purinergic agonists: some speculations on the source and identity of the purinergic mediator. In: Baer HP, Drummond GI (eds) Physiological and regulatory functions of adenosine and adenine nucleotides. Raven, New York, pp 103–113

Coombs HI, Coombs RRH, Mee UG (1975) Methods of serum lithium estimation. In: Johnson FN (ed) Lithium research and therapy. Academic Press, New York London, pp 165–179

Cooper TB, Simpson GM (1978) Kinetics of lithium and clinical response. In: Lipton MA, DiMascio A, Killam KF (eds) Psychopharmacology – a generation of progress. Raven, New York, pp 928–931

Costa E, Guidotti A, Mao CC (1975a) Evidence for the involvement of GABA in the action of benzodiazepines: studies on rat cerebellum. Adv Biochem Psychopharmacol 14:113–130

Costa E, Guidotti A, Mao CC, Suria A (1975b) New concepts on the mechanism of action of benzodiazepines. Life Sci 17:167–186

Creese I, Burt DR, Snyder SH (1977) Dopamine receptor binding enhancement accompanies lesion-induced behavioral supersensitivity. Science 197:596–598

Cubeddu L, Barnes E, Weiner N (1974) Release of norepinephrine and dopamine-beta-hydroxylase by nerve stimulation. II. Effects of papaverine. J Pharmacol Exp Ther 191:444–457

Cubeddu L, Barnes E, Weiner N (1975) Release of norepinephrine and dopamine-beta-hydroxylase by nerve stimulation. IV. An evaluation of a role for cyclic adenosine monophosphate. J Pharmacol Exp Ther 193:105–127

Daly J (1975) Role of cyclic nucleotides in the nervous system. In: Iversen LL, Iversen SD, Snyder SH (eds) Handbook of psychopharmacology, vol 5, Plenum, New York, pp 47–130

Daly JW (1976) Minireview: the nature of receptors regulating the formation of cyclic AMP in brain tissue. Life Sci 18:1349–1358

Daly JW (1977a) Cyclic nucleotides in the nervous system. Plenum, New York London

Daly JW (1977b) The formation, degradation and function of cyclic nucleotides in the nervous system. Int Rev Neurobiol 20:105–168

Daly JW (1979) Adenosine and cyclic adenosine monophosphate-generating systems in brain tissue. In: Baer HP, Drummond GI (eds) Physiological and regulatory functions of adenosine and adenine nucleotides. Raven, New York, pp 229–241

Davis JM (1976) A review: maintenance therapy in psychiatry: II. Affective disorders. Am J Psychiatry 133:1–13

De Blas AL, Wang VJ, Sorensen R, Mahler H (1979) Protein phosphorylation in synaptic membranes regulated by adenosine 3′,5′-monophosphate. Regional and subcellular distribution of the endogenous substrates. J Neurochem 33:647–659

De Langen DCJ, Mulder AH (1980) On the role of calcium ions in the presynaptic alpha-receptor mediated inhibition of (^{3}H)noradrenaline release from rat brain cortex synaptosomes. Brain Res 185:399–408

Dismukes RK, De Boer AA, Mulder AH (1977) On the mechanism of alpha-receptor mediated modulation of (^{3}H)-noradrenaline release from slices of rat brain neocortex. Naunyn Schmiedebergs Arch Pharmacol 299:115–122

Dousa T, Hechter O (1970a) Lithium and brain adenyl cyclase. Lancet 1:834–835

Dousa T, Hechter O (1970b) Effect of NaCl and LiCl on vasopressin-sensitive adenyl cyclase. Life Sci 9:765–770

Drummond GI, Duncan L, Hertzman E (1966) Effect of epinephrine on phosphorylase b kinase in perfused rat hearts. J Biol Chem 241:5899–5903

Drummond GS, Symchowicz E, Goldstein M, Shenkman L (1978) Activation of rat pheochromocytoma tyrosine hydroxylase by a cyclic AMP-dependent protein-kinase in a cell-free system. J Neural Transm 42:139–144

Dunwiddie TV, Hoffer BJ (1980) Adenine nucleotides and synaptic transmission in the in vitro rat hippocampus. Br J Pharmacol 69:59–68

Ebstein B, Roberge C, Tabachnik J, Goldstein M (1974) The effect of dopamine and of apomorphine on dB-cAMP-induced stimulation of synaptosomal tyrosine hydroxylase. J Pharm Pharmacol 26:975–978

Edelman AM, Raese JD, Lazar MA, Barchas JD (1978) In vitro phosphorylation of a purified preparation of bovine corpus striatal tyrosine hydroxylase. Commun Psychopharmacol 2:461–465

Edstrom JP, Phillis JW (1976) The effects of AMP on the potential of rat cerebral cortical neurons. Can J Physiol Pharmacol 54:787–790

Edwards C, Nahorski SR, Rogers KJ (1974) In vivo changes in cerebral cyclic adenosine 3′,5′-monophosphate induced by biogenic amines: association with phosporylase activation. J Neurochem 22:565–572

Ehrlich YH (1979) Phosphoproteins as specifiers for mediators and modulators in neuronal function. In: Ehrlich YH, Volavka J, Davis LG, Brunngraber EG (eds) Modulators, mediators and specifiers in brain function. Plenum, New York

Ehrlichman J, Rosenfeld R, Rosen OM (1974) Phosphorylation of a cyclic adenosine 3′,5′-monophosphate-dependent protein kinase from bovine cardiac muscle. J Biol Chem 249:5000–5003

Eneroz MA, Saidman BO (1977) Possible feed-back inhibition of noradrenaline release by purine compounds. Naunyn Schmiedebergs Arch Pharmacol 297:39–46

Ferrendelli JA (1976) Cellular depolarization and cyclic nucleotide content in central nervous system. Adv Biochem Psychopharmacol 15:303–313

Ferrendelli JA (1978) Distribution and regulation of cyclic GMP in the central nervous system. Adv Cyclic Nucleotide Res 9:453–465

Ferrendelli JA (1980) Epilepsy and cyclic nucleotides. In: Hamet D, Sands H (eds) Pathophysiological aspects of cyclic nucleotides. Raven, New York

Ferrendelli JA, Kinscherf DA (1977) Cyclic nucleotides in the epileptic brain: effects of pentylenetetrazol on regional cyclic AMP and cyclic GMP levels in vivo. Epilepsia 18:525–531

Ferrendelli JA, Steiner AL, McDougal DB Jr, Kipnis DM (1970) The effect of oxotremorine and atropine on cGMP and cAMP levels in mouse cerebral cortex and cerebellum. Biochem Biophys Res Commun 41:1061–1067

Ferrendelli JA, Kinscherf DA, Kipnis DM (1972) Effects of amphetamine, chlorpromazine and reserpine on cyclic GMP and cyclic AMP levels in mouse cerebellum. Biochem Biophys Res Commun 46:2114–2120

Ferrendelli JA, Kinscherf DA, Chang M-M (1973) Regulation of levels of guanosine cyclic 3′,5′monophosphate in the central nervous system: effects of depolarizing agents. Mol Pharmacol 9:445–454

Ferrendelli JA, Chang MM, Kinscherf DA (1974) Elevation of cyclic GMP levels in central nervous system by excitatory and inhibitory amino acids. J Neurochem 22:535–540

Ferrendelli JA, Kinscherf DA, Chang M-M (1975) Comparison of the effects of biogenic amines on cyclic GMP and cyclic AMP levels in mouse cerebellum in vitro. Brain Res 84:63–77

Ferrendelli JA, Rubin EH, Kinscherf DA (1976) Influence of divalent cations on regulation of cyclic GMP and cyclic AMP levels in brain tissue. J Neurochem 26:741–748

Folbergrova J (1975) Cyclic 3′,5′-adenosine monophosphate in mouse cerebral cortex during homocysteine convulsions and their prevention by sodium phenobarbital. Brain Res 92:165–169

Folbergrova J (1977) Changes of cyclic AMP and phosphorylase a in mouse cerebral cortex during seizures induced by 3-mercaptopropionic acid. Brain Res 135:337–346

Folco GC, Longiave D, Bosisio E (1977) Relations between prostaglandin E_2, $F_{2\alpha}$, and cyclic nucleotide levels in rat brain and induction of convulsions. Prostaglandins 13:893–900

Foote SL, Freedman R, Oliver AP (1975) Effects of putative transmitters on neuronal activity in monkey cortex. Brain Res 86:229–242

Forn J, Greengard P (1978) Depolarizing agents and cyclic nucleotides regulate the phosphorylation of specific neuronal proteins in rat cerebral cortex slices. Proc Natl Acad Sci USA 75:5195–5199

Forn J, Valdecasas FG (1971) Effects of lithium on brain adenyl cyclase activity. Biochem Pharmacol 20:2773–2778

Francis RI, Traill MA (1970) Lithium distribution in the brains of two manic patients. Lancet 2:523–524

Frazer A, Hangaard ES, Mendels J, Hangaard N (1975) Effects of intracellular lithium on epinephrine-induced accumulation of cyclic AMP in skeletal muscle. Biochem Pharmacol 24:2273–2277

Frazer A, Hess ME, Mendels J, Gable B, Kunkel E, Bender A (1978) Influence of acute and chronic treatment with desmethyl imipramine of catecholamine effects in rat. J Pharmacol Exp Ther 207:311–319

Freedman R, Hoffer BJ, Woodward DJ, Puro D (1977) Interaction of norepinephrine with cerebellar activity evoked by mossy and climbing fibers. Exp Neurol 55:269–288

Freedman R, Taylor D, Seiger A, Olson L, Hoffer B (1979) Seizures and related epileptiform activity in hippocampus transplanted to the anterior chamber in the eye. II. Modulation by cholinergic and adrenergic input. Ann Neurol 6:281–293

Gallager DW, Pert A, Bunney WE (1978) Haloperidol-induced presynaptic dopamine supersensitivity is blocked by chronic lithium. Nature 273:309–312

Geisler A, Klysner R (1977) Combined effect of lithium and flupenthixol on striatal adenylate cyclase. Lancet 1:430–431

Geisler A, Klysner R (1978) Influence of lithium on dopamine-stimulated adenylate cyclase activity in rat brain. Life Sci 23:635–636

Geisler A, Wraae O, Oteson OV (1972) Adenylate cyclase activity in kidneys of lithium treated rats. Acta Pharmacol Toxicol (Copenh) 31:203–208

George WJ, Polson JB, O'Toole AG, Goldberg ND (1970) Elevation of guanosine 3′,5′-cyclic phosphate in rat heart after perfusion with acetylcholine. Proc Natl Acad Sci USA 66:398–403

Gerbino L, Oleshansky M, Gershon S (1978) Clinical use and mode of action of lithium. In: Lipton MA, DiMascio A, Killam KF (eds) Psychopharmacology – a generation of progress. Raven, New York, pp 1261–1275

Gilman AG, Nirenberg M (1971) Effect of catecholamines on the adenosine 3′5′-cyclic monophosphate concentrations of clonal satellite cells of neurons. Proc Natl Acad Sci USA 68:2165–2168

Ginsborg BL, Hirst GD (1972) The effect of adenosine on the release of the transmitter from the phrenic nerve of the rat. J Physiol (Lond) 224:629–645

Glowinski J, Axelrod J (1964) Inhibition of uptake of tritiated noradrenaline in intact rat brain by imipramine and structurally related compounds. Nature 204:1318–1319

Goldberg AL, Singer JJ (1969) Evidence for a role for cyclic AMP in neuromuscular transmission. Proc Natl Acad Sci USA 64:134–141

Goldberg ND, Haddox MR (1977) Cyclic GMP metabolism and involvement in biological regulation. Annu Rev Biochem 46:823–896

Goldberg ND, Dietz SB, O'Toole AG (1969) Cyclic guanosine 3′,5′-monophosphate in mammalian tissue and urine. J Biol Chem 244:4458–4466

Goldstein M, Freedman LS, Backstrom T (1970) Inhibition of catecholamine biosynthesis by apomorphine. J Pharm Pharmacol 22:715–717

Goldstein M, Anagnoste B, Shirron C (1973) The effect of trivastal, haloperidol and dibutyryl cyclic AMP on (^{14}C)dopamine synthesis in rat striatum. J Pharm Pharmacol 25:348–351

Gordon AS, Davis CG, Diamond I (1977) Phosphorylation of membrane proteins at a cholinergic synapse. Proc Natl Acad Sci USA 74:263–267

Goridis C, Morgan IG (1973) Guanyl cyclase in rat brain subcellular fractions. FEBS Lett 34:71–73

Goridis C, Massarelli R, Sensenbrenner M, Mandel P (1974) Guanyl cyclase in chick embryo brain cell cultures: evidence of neuronal localization. J Neurochem 23:135–138

Greenberg LH, Troyer E, Ferrendelli JA, Weiss B (1978) Enzymatic regulation of the concentration of cyclic GMP in mouse brain. Neuropharmacology 17:737 –745

Greengard P (1976) Possible role for cyclic nucleotides and phosphorylated membrane proteins in postsynaptic actions of neurotransmitters. Nature 260:101–108

Greengard P (1978a) Phosphorylated proteins as physiological effectors. Science 199:146–152

Greengard P (1978b) Cyclic nucleotides, phosphorylated proteins, and neuronal function. Raven, New York

Greengard P (1979) Cyclic nucleotides, phosphorylated proteins, and the nervous system. Fed Proc 38:2208–2217

Greengard P, Kebabian JW (1974) Role of cyclic AMP in synaptic transmission in the mammalian peripheral nervous system. Fed Proc 33:1059–1067

Greengard P, Kuo JF (1970) On the mechanism of action of cyclic AMP. Adv Biochem Psychopharmacol 3:287–306

Gross RA, Ferrendelli JA (1979) Effects of reserpine, propranolol, and aminophylline on seizure activity and CNS cyclic nucleotides. Ann Neurol 6:296–301

Gumulka SW, Dinnendahl V, Schonhofer PS, Stock K (1976) Dopaminergic stimulants and cyclic nucleotides in mouse brain. Effects of dopaminergic antagonists, cholinolytics, and GABA agonists. Naunyn Schmiedebergs Arch Pharmacol 295:21–26

Hamet P, Sands H (1980) Pathophysiological aspects of cyclic nucleotides. Raven, New York

Harms HH, Wardeh G, Mulder AH (1978) Adenosine modulates depolarization-induced release of ^{3}H-noradrenaline from slices of rat brain neocortex. Eur J Pharmacol 49:305–308

Harris JE, Morgenroth VH, Roth RH, Baldessarini RJ (1974) Regulation of catecholamine biosynthesis in rat brain in vitro by cyclic AMP. Nature 252:156–158

Hartman BK, Zide D, Udenfriend S (1972) Use of dopamine beta-hydroxylase as a marker for the central noradrenergic nervous system in rat brain. Proc Natl Acad Sci USA 69:2722–2726

Hayashi E, Mori M, Yamada S, Kunitomo M (1978) Effects of purine compounds on cholinergic nerves. Specificity of adenosine and related compounds on acetylcholine release in electrically stimulated guinea pig ileum. Eur J Pharmacol 48:297–307

Hedqvist R, Fredholm BB (1976) Effects of adenosine on adrenergic transmission: prejunctional inhibition and postjunctional enhancement. Naunyn Schmiedebergs Arch Pharmacol 293:217–223

Hoeldtke R, Kaufman S (1977) Bovine adrenal tyrosine hydroxylase: purification and properties. J Biol Chem 252:3160–3169

Hoffer BJ, Siggins GR, Bloom FE (1970) Possible cyclic AMP-mediated adrenergic synapses to rat cerebellar Purkinje cells: combined structural, physiological and pharmacological analyses. Adv Biochem Pharmacol 3:349–370

Hoffer BJ, Siggins GR, Woodward DJ, Bloom FE (1971 a) Spontaneous discharge of Purkinje neurons after destruction of catecholamine-containing afferents by 6-hydroxydopamine. Brain Res 30:425–430

Hoffer BJ, Siggins GR, Oliver AP, Bloom FE (1971 b) Cyclic AMP mediation of norepinephrine inhibition in rat cerebellar cortex: a unique class of synaptic responses. Ann NY Acad Sci 185:531–549

Hoffer BJ, Siggins GR, Oliver AP, Bloom FE (1973) Activation of the pathway from locus coeruleus to rat cerebellar Purkinje neurons; pharmacological evidence of noradrenergic central inhibition. J Pharmacol Exp Ther 184:553–569

Hoffer BJ, Seiger A, Freedman R, Olson L, Taylor D (1977 a) Electrophysiology and cytology of hippocampal formation transplants in the anterior chamber of the eye. II. Cholinergic mechanisms. Brain Res 119:107–132

Hoffer BJ, Seiger A, Taylor D, Olson L, Freedman R (1977 b) Seizures and related epileptiform activity in hippocampus transplanted to the anterior chamber of the eye. I. Characterization of seizures, interictal spikes, and synchronous activity. Exp Neurol 54:233–250

Hofmann F, Sold G (1972) A protein kinase activity from rat cerebellum simulated by guanosine 3′,5′-monophosphate. Biochem Biophys Res Commun 49:1100–1107

Horn JP, McAfee DA (1977) Modulation of cyclic nucleotide levels in peripheral nerve without effect on resting or compound action potentials. J Physiol (Lond) 269:753–766

Huang M, Daly JW (1972) Accumulation of cyclic adenosine monophosphate in incubated slices of brain tissue. I. Structure-activity relationships of agonists and antagonists of biogenic amines and of tricyclic tranquilizers and antidepressants. J Med Chem 15:458–462

Huang M, Daly JW (1974) Adenosine elicited accumulation of cyclic AMP in brain slices: potentiation by agents which inhibit uptake of adenosine. Life Sci 14:489–503

Huang M, Shimizu H, Daly J (1971) Regulation of adenosine cyclic 3′,5′-monophosphate formation in cerebral cortical slices: interaction among norepinephrine, histamine and serotonin. Mol Pharmacol 7:155–162

Huang M, Shimizu H, Daly J (1972) Accumulation of cyclic adenosine monophosphate in incubated slices of brain tissue. 2. Effects of depolarizing agents, membrane stabilizers, phosphodiesterase inhibitors, and adenosine analogs. J Med Chem 15:462–466

Huang M, Gruenstein E, Daly JW (1973). Depolarization-evoked accumulation of cyclic AMP in brain slices: inhibition by exogenous adenosine deaminase. Biochim Biophys Acta 329:147–151

Israel M, Lesbats R, Manaranche J, Marsal J, Masteur-Frachon P, Meunier FM (1977) Related changes in amounts of ACh and ATP in resting and active Torpedo nerve electroplaque synapses. J Neurochem 28:1259–1267

Iversen LL, Rogawski MA, Miler RJ (1976) Comparison of the effects of neuroleptic drugs on pre- and postsynaptic dopaminergic mechanisms in the rat striatum. Mol Pharmacol 12:251–262

Jacobs RS, McNiece DM (1977) Motor nerve terminal facilitory action of SQ 20009. J Pharmacol Exp Ther 202:404–410

Jasinski DR, Nutt JG, Haertzen CA, Griffith JD, Bunney WE (1977) Lithium: effects on subjective functioning and morphine-induced euphoria. Science 195:582–584
Jhamandas K, Sawynok J (1976) Methylxantine antagonism of opiate and purine effects on the release of acetylcholine. In: Kosterlitz HW (ed) Opiates and endogenous peptides. Elsevier, Amsterdam Oxford New York, pp 161–168
Joh TH, Park DH, Reis DJ (1978) Direct phosphorylation of brain tyrosine hydroxylase by cyclic AMP-dependent protein kinase: mechanism of enzyme activation. Proc Natl Acad Sci USA 75: 4744–4748
Johnson PN, Inesi G (1969) The effect of methylxanthines and local anaesthetics on fragmented sarcoplasmic reticulum. J Pharmacol Exp Ther 169:308–318
Kahn CR (1976) Membrane receptors for hormones and neurotransmitters. Cell Biol 70:261–286
Kakiuchi S, Rall TW, McIlwain H (1969) The effect of electrical stimulation upon the accumulation of adenosine 3′,5′-monophosphate in isolated cerebral tissue. J Neurochem 16:485–491
Karobath M (1971) Catecholamines and hydroxylation of tyrosine in synaptosomes isolated from rat-brain. Proc Natl Acad Sci USA 68:2370–2373
Katsuki S, Murad F (1977) Regulation of adenosine cyclic 3′,5′-monophosphate and guanosine cyclic 3′,5′-monophosphate levels and contractility of bovine tracheal smooth muscle. Mol Pharmacol 13:330–341
Kebabian JW (1977) Biochemical regulation and physiological significance of cyclic nucleotides in the nervous system. Adv Cyclic Nucleotide Res 8:421–508
Kebabian JW, Calne DB (1979) Multiple receptors for dopamine. Nature 277:93–96
Kebabian JW, Saavedra JM (1976) Dopamine-sensitive adenylate cyclase occurs in a region of substantia nigra containing dopaminergic dendrites. Science 193:683–685
Kebabian JW, Bloom FE, Steiner AL, Greengard P (1975a) Neurotransmitters increase cyclic nucleotides in postganglionic neurons: immunocytochemical demonstration. Science 190:157–159
Kebabian JW, Steiner AL, Greengard P (1975b) Muscarinic cholinergic regulation of cyclic guanosine 3′,5′-monophosphate in autonomic ganglia: possible role in synaptic transmission. J Pharmacol Exp Ther 193:474–488
Kinscherf DA, Chang MM, Rubin EH, Schneider DR, Ferrendelli JA (1976) Comparison of the effects of depolarizing agents and neurotransmitters on regional CNS cyclic GMP levels in various animals. J Neurochem 26:527–530
Klainer LM, Chi Y-M, Friedberg SL, Rall TW, Sutherland EW (1962) The effects of neurohormones on the formation of adenosine 3′,5′-monophosphate by preparations from brain and other tissues. J Biol Chem 237:1239–1243
Klerman GM (1978) Long-term treatment of affective disorders. In: Lipton MA, DiMascio A, Killam KF (eds) Psychopharmacology – a generation of progress. Raven, New York, pp 1303–1311
Kline NS, Cooper TB (1975) Evaluation of lithium therapy in alcoholism. Finn Fed Alcohol Stud 24:143–153
Kline NS, Cooper TB (1979) Lithium therapy in alcoholism. In: Erickson C, Goodwin D (eds) Alcoholism and affective disorders. Plenum, New York London, pp 21–30
Kline NS, Cooper TB, Bennet JA, Calobrisi A, Neidengaard TN, Snyder AF (1979) Lithium in the treatment of chronic alcoholism. In: Cooper TB, Gershon S, Kline NS, Schou M (eds). Lithium: controversies and unresolved issues. Excerpta Med. Amsterdam, pp 117–132
Knapp S, Mandell AJ (1975) Effects of lithium chloride on parameters of biosynthetic capacity for 5-hydroxytryptamine in rat brain. J Pharmacol Exp Ther 193:812–823
Korf J, Sebens JB (1979) Cyclic AMP in the rat cerebral cortex after activation of noradrenaline neurons of the locus coeruleus. J Neurochem 32:463–468
Kostopoulos GK, Phillis JW (1977) Purinergić depression of neurons in different areas of the rat brain. Exp Neurol 55:719–724
Kostopoulos GK, Limacher JJ, Phillis JW (1975) Action of various adenine derivatives on cerebellar Purkinje cells. Brain Res 88:162–165
Krishna G, Forn J, Voight K, Paul M, Gessa GL (1970) Dynamic aspects of neurohormonal control of cyclic 3′,5′-AMP synthesis in brain. Adv Biochem Psychopharmacol 3:155–172

Křivánek J (1977) Brain cyclic adenosine 3′,5′-monophosphate during depolarization of the cerebral cortical cells in vivo. Brain Res 120:493–505

Krnjević K (1974) Chemical nature of synaptic transmission in vertebrates. Physiol Rev 54:418–503

Krnjević K (1978) Acetylcholine and cyclic GMP. Adv Behav Biol 24:261–266

Krnjević K, Lisiewicz A (1972) Injections of calcium ions into spinal motoneurons. J Physiol (Lond) 225:363–390

Krnjević K, Van Meter WG (1976) Cyclic nucleotides in spinal cells. Can J Physiol Pharmacol 54:416–421

Krnjević K, Puil E, Werman R (1976) Is cyclic guanosine monophosphate the internal "second messenger" for cholinergic actions on central neurons? Can J Physiol Pharmacol 54:172–176

Krueger BK, Forn J, Walters JR, Roth RH, Greengard P (1976) Stimulation by dopamine of adenosine 3′,5′-cyclic monophosphate formation in rat caudate nucleus: effect of lesions of nigroneostriatal pathway. Mol Pharmacol 12:639–648

Kuo JF (1974) Guanosine 3′,5′monophosphate-dependent protein kinases in mammalian tissue. Proc Natl Acad Sci USA 71:4037–4041

Kuo JF, Greengard P (1969a) Cyclic nucleotide-dependent protein kinases. IV. Widespread occurrence of adenosine 3′,5′-monophosphate dependent protein kinase in various tissues and phyla of the animal kingdom. Proc Natl Acad Sci USA 64:1349–1355

Kuo JF, Greengard P (1969b) Adenosine 3′,5′-monophosphate-dependent protein kinase from brain. Science 165:63–65

Kuo JF, Greengard P (1970) Cyclic nucleotide-dependent protein kinases. VI. Isolation and partial purification of a protein kinase activated by guanosine 3′,5′-monophosphate. J Biol Chem 245:2493–2498

Kuo JF, Lee TP, Reyes PL, Walton KG, Donnelly TE Jr, Greengard P (1972) Cyclic nucleotide-dependent protein kinases. X. An assay method for the measurement of guanosine 3′,5′-monophosphate in various biological materials and a study of agents regulating its levels in heart and brain. J Biol Chem 247:16–22

Kuroda Y, Kobayashi K (1975) Effects of adenosine and adenine nucleotides on the postsynaptic potential and on the formation of cyclic adenosine 3′,5′-monophosphate from radioactive adenosine triphosphate in guinea pig olfactory cortex slices. Proc Jpn Acad 51:495–500

Kuroda Y, McIlwain H (1974) Uptake and release of (^{14}C)adenine derivatives at beds of mammalian cortical synaptosomes in a superfusion system. J Neurochem 22:691–700

Kuroda Y, Saito M, Kobayashi K (1976) High concentrations of calcium prevent the inhibition of postsynaptic potentials and the accumulation of cyclic AMP induced by adenosine in brain slices. Proc Jpn Acad 52:86–89

Langer SZ (1976) The role of alpha- and beta-presynaptic receptors in the regulation of noradrenaline release elicited by nerve stimulation. Clin Sci Mol Med 51:423s–426s

Langer SZ (1977) Presynaptic receptors and their role in the regulation of transmitter release. Br J Pharmacol 60:481–497

Langer SZ, Enero MA, Adler-Graschinsky E, Dubocovich ML, Celuch SM (1975) Presynaptic regulatory mechanisms for noradrenaline release by nerve stimulation. In: Davies DS, Reid JL (eds) Central action of drugs in the regulation of blood pressure. Pitman Medical, Tunbridge Wells, pp 133–151

Lee TP, Kuo JF, Greengard P (1972) Role of muscarinic cholinergic receptors in regulation of guanosine 3′,5′-cyclic monophosphate content in mammalian brain, heart muscle, and intestinal smooth muscle. Proc Natl Acad Sci USA 69:3287–3291

Lekić D (1977) Presynaptic depression of synaptic response of Renshaw cells by adenosine 5′-monophosphate. Can J Physiol Pharmacol 55:1391–1393

Letendre CH, MacDonnell PC, Guroff G (1977) The biosynthesis of phosphorylated tyrosine hydroxylase by organ cultures of rat adrenal medulla and superior cervical ganglion. Biochem Biophys Res Commun 74:891–897

Levin RM, Weiss B (1976) Mechanism by which psychotropic drugs inhibit cyclic AMP phosphodiesterase of brain. Mol Pharmacol 12:581–589

Lloyd T, Kaufman S (1975) Evidence for the lack of direct phosphorylation of bovine caudate tyrosine hydroxylase following activation by exposure to enzymatic phosphorylating conditions. Biochem Biophys Res Commun 66:907–913

Londos C, Wolff J (1977) Two distinct adenosine sensitive sites on adenylate cyclase. Proc Natl Acad Sci USA 74:5482–5486
Londos C, Wolff J, Cooper DMG (1979) Action of adenosine on adenylate cyclase. In: Baer HP, Drummond GI (eds) Physiological and regulatory functions of adenosine and adenine nucleotides. Raven, New York, pp 271–281
Lovenberg W, Bruckwick EA (1974) Molecular mechanisms in the receptor-mediated regulation of tyrosine hydroxylase. Psychopharmacol Bull 10:26
Lovenberg W, Bruckwick EA, Hanbauer I (1975) ATP, cyclic AMP and magnesium increase the affinity of rat striatal tyrosine hydroxylase for its cofactor. Proc Natl Acad Sci USA 72:2955–2958
Lust WD, Passonneau JV (1976) Cyclic nucleotides in murine brain: effect of hypothermia on adenosine 3′,5′-monophosphate, glycogen phosphorylase, glycogen synthetase and metabolites following maximal electroshock or decapitation. J Neurochem 26:11–16
Lust WD, Goldberg ND, Passonneau JV (1976) Cyclic nucleotides in murine brain: the temporal relationship of changes induces in adenosine 3′,5′-monophosphate and guanosine 3′,5′-monophosphate following maximal electroshock or decapitation. J Neurochem 26:5–10
Lust WD, Kupferberg HJ, Yonekawa WD, Penry JK, Passonneau JV, Wheaton AB (1978) Changes in brain metabolites induced by convulsants or electroshock: effects of anticonvulsant agents. Mol Pharmacol 14:347–356
Mackay AVP, Iversen LL (1972) Increased tyrosine hydroxylase activity of sympathetic ganglia cultured in the presence of dibutyryl cyclic AMP. Brain Res 48:424–426
Mackie C, Richardson MC, Schulster D (1972) Kinetics and dose response characteristics of adenosine 3′,5′-monophosphate production by isolated rat adrenal cells stimulated with adrenocorticotrophic hormone. FEBS Lett 23:345–348
Maeno H, Reyes PL, Ueda T, Rudolph SA, Greengard P (1974) Autophosphorylation of adenosine 3′,5′-monophosphate-dependent protein kinase from bovine brain. Arch Biochem Biophys 164:551–559
Maguire ME, Wiklund RA, Anderson HJ, Gilman AG (1976) Binding of (^{125}I)iodohydroxybenzylpindolol to putative beta-adrenergic receptors of rat glioma cells and other cell clones. J Biol Chem 251:1221–1231
Mah HD, Daly JW (1976) Adenosine-dependent formation of cyclic AMP in brain slices. Pharmacol Res Commun 8:65–79
Mailman RB, Mueller RA, Breese GR (1978) The effect of drugs which alter GABA-ergic function on guanosine-3′5,′-monophosphate content. Life Sci 23:623–627
Malkinson AM (1975) Effect of calcium on cyclic AMP-dependent and cyclic GMP-dependent endogenous protein phosphorylation in mouse brain cytosol. Biochem Biophys Res Commun 67:752–759
Mao CC, Guidotti A, Costa E (1974) The regulation of cyclic guanosine monophosphate in rat cerebellum possible involvement of putative amino acid neurotransmitters. Brain Res 79:510–514
Mao CC, Guidotti A, Costa E (1975a) Evidence for involvement of GABA in the mediation of the cerebellar cGMP decrease and the anticonvulsant action of diazepam. Naunyn Schmiedebergs Arch Pharmacol 289:369–378
Mao CC, Guidotti A, Costa E (1975b) Inhibition by diazepam of the tremor and the increase of cerebellar cGMP content elicited by harmaline. Brain Res 83:516–519
Masserano JM, Weiner N (1979) The rapid activation of adrenal tyrosine hydroxylase by decapitation and its relationship to a cyclic AMP-dependent phosphorylating mechanism. Mol Pharmacol 16:513–528
McAfee DA, Greengard P (1972) Adenosine 3′,5′-monophosphate: electrophysiological evidence for a role in synaptic transmission. Science 178:310–312
McAfee DA, Schorderet M, Greengard P (1971) Adenosine 3′,5′-monophosphate in nervous tissue: increase associated with synaptic transmission. Science 171:1156–1158
McCarthy KD, de Vellis J (1978) Alpha-adrenergic receptor modulation of beta-adrenergic, adenosine, and prostaglandin E_1 increases in adenosine 3′,5′-cyclic monophosphate levels in primary cultures of glia. J Cyclic Nucleotide Res 4:15–26
McGeer EG, Innanen VT, McGeer PL (1976) Evidence on the cellular localization of adenyl cyclase in the neostriatum. Brain Res 118:356–358

McIlwain H (1972) Regulatory significance of the release and action of adenine derivatives in cerebral systems. Biochem Soc Symp 36:69–85
McKenzie SG, Bär HP (1973) On the mechanism of adenyl cyclase inhibition by adenosine. Can J Physiol Pharmacol 51:190–196
Meunier FM, Israel M, Lesbats B (1975) Release of ATP from stimulated nerve electroplaque junctions. Nature 257:407–408
Miech RP, Niedzwicki JG, Smith TR (1979) Effect of theophylline on the binding of cAMP to soluble protein from tracheal smooth muscle. Biochem Pharmacol 28:3687–3688
Minneman KP, Quik M, Emson PC (1978a) Receptor-linked cyclic AMP systems in rat neostriatum: differential localization revealed by kainic acid injection. Brain Res 151:507–521
Minneman KP, Quik M, Emson PC (1978b) Possible glial localization of specific receptor linked cyclic AMP systems in rat striatum: studies with kainic acid. In: Folco G, Paoletti R (eds) Molecular biology and pharmacology of cyclic nucleotides. Elsevier, Amsterdam Oxford New York, pp 207–222
Minneman KP, Hegstrand LR, Molinoff PB (1979a) The pharmacological specificity of beta-1 and beta-2 adrenergic receptors in rat heart and lung in vitro. Mol Pharmacol 16:21–33
Minneman KP, Hegstrand LR, Molinoff PB (1979b) Simultaneous determination of beta-1 and beta-2 adrenergic receptors in tissues containing both receptor subtypes. Mol Pharmacol 16:34
Mittal CK, Kimura H, Murad F (1975) Requirement for a macromolecular factor for sodium azide activation of guanylate cyclase. J Cyclic Nucleotide Res 1:261–269
Miyamoto E, Breckenridge BMcL (1974) A cyclic adenosine monophosphate link in the catecholamine enhancement of transmitter release at the neuromuscular junction. J Gen Physiol 63:609–624
Miyamoto E, Kuo JF, Greengard P (1969) Cyclic nucleotide-dependent protein kinases. I. Purification and properties of adenosine 3′,5′-monophosphate-dependent protein kinase from bovine brain. J Biol Chem 244:6395–6402
Moises HC, Woodward DJ (1980) Potentiation of GABA inhibitory action in cerebellum by locus coeruleus stimulation. Brain Res 182:327–344
Moises HC, Woodward DJ, Hoffer BJ, Freedman R (1979) Interactions of norepinephrine with Purkinje cell responses to putative amino acid neurotransmitters applied by microiontophoresis. Exp Neurol 64:493–515
Morgenroth VH, Boadle-Biber MC, Roth RH (1974) Tyrosine hydroxylase: activation by nerve stimulation. Proc Natl Acad Sci USA 71:4283–4287
Morgenroth VH, Hegstrand L, Roth RH, Greengard P (1975) Evidence for involvement of protein kinase in the activation by adenosine 3′,5′-monophosphate of brain tyrosine 3-monooxygenase. J Biol Chem 250:1946–1948
Mueller AL, Mosimann WF, Weiner N (1979) Effects of adenosine on neurally mediated norepinephrine release from the cat spleen. Eur J Pharmacol 53:329–333
Mulder AH, de Langen CDJ, de Regt V, Hogenboom F (1978) Alpha-receptor mediated modulation of ^{3}H-noradrenaline release from rat brain cortex synaptosomes. Naunyn Schmiedebergs Arch Pharmacol 303:193–196
Murad F, Arnold WP, Mittal CK, Braughler JM (1979) Properties and regulation of guanylate cyclase and some proposed functions for cyclic GMP. Adv Cyclic Nucleotide Res 11:176–204
Murrin LC, Gale K, Kuhar MJ (1979) Autoradiographic localization of neuroleptic and dopamine receptors in the caudate-putamen and substantia nigra: effects of lesions. Eur J Pharmacol 60:229–235
Nahorski SR, Rogers KJ, Edwards C (1975) Cerebral glycogenolysis and stimulation of beta-adrenoceptors and histamine H_2 receptors. Brain Res 92:529–533
Nahorski SR, Howlett DR, Redgrave P (1979) Loss of beta-adrenoceptor binding sites in rat striatum following kainic acid lesions. Eur J Pharmacol 60:249–252
Nakazawa K, Sano M (1974) A new assay method for guanylate cyclase and properties of the cyclase from rat brain. J Biol Chem 249–4207–4211
Nathanson JA (1977) Cyclic nucleotides in nervous system function. Physiol Rev 57:157–256

Nathanson JA (1980) Cerebral microvessels contain a beta-2 adrenergic receptor. Life Sci 26:1793–1799

Nathanson JA, Bloom F (1975) Lead-induced inhibition of brain adenyl cyclase activity. Nature 255:419–420

Newburgh RW, Rosenberg RN (1972) Effect of norepinephrine on glucose metabolism in glioblastoma and neuroblastoma cells in cell culture. Proc Natl Acad Sci USA 69:1677–1680

Ohga Y, Daly JW (1977a) The accumulation of cyclic AMP and cyclic GMP in guinea pig brain slices. Effect of calcium ions, norepinephrine and adenosine. Biochim Biophys Acta 498:46–60

Ohga Y, Daly JW (1977b) Calcium ion-elicited accumulations of cyclic GMP in guinea pig cerebellar slices. Biochim Biophys Acta 498:61–75

Okada Y, Kuroda Y (1975) Inhibitory action of adenosine and adenine nucleotides on the post-synaptic potential of olfactory cortex slices of the guinea pig. Proc Jpn Acad Sci 51:491–494

Okada Y, Saito M (1979) Inhibitory action of adenosine, 5-HT (serotonin), and GABA (gamma-amino butyric acid) on the postsynaptic potential (PSP) of slices from olfactory cortex and superior colliculus in correlation to the level of cyclic AMP. Brain Res 160:368–371

Oliver AP, Segal M (1974) Transmembrane changes in hippocampal neurons: hyperpolarizing actions of norepinephrine, cyclic AMP and locus coeruleus. Proc Soc Neurosci 361

Opler LA, Makman MH (1972) Mediation by cyclic AMP of hormone-stimulated glycogenolysis in cultured rat astrocytoma cells. Biochem Biophys Res Commun 46:1140–1145

Opmeer FA, Gumulka SW, Dinnedahl V, Schonhofer PS (1976) Effects of stimulatory and depressant drugs on cyclic guanosine 3′,5′-monophosphate and adenosine 3′,5′-monophosphate levels in mouse brain. Naunyn Schmiedebergs Arch Pharmacol 292:259–266

Palmer GC, Jones DJ, Medina MA, Stavinoha WB (1979) Anticonvulsant drug actions on in vitro and in vivo levels of cyclic AMP in the mouse brain. Epilepsia 20:95–104

Passoneau JV, Crites SK (1976) Regulation of glycogen metabolism in astrocytoma and neuroblastoma cells in culture. J Biol Chem 251:2015–2022

Paton DM, Bär HP, Clanachan AS, Lanzon PA (1978) Structure-activity relationships for inhibition of neurotransmission in rat vas deferens by adenosine. Neuroscience 3:65–70

Patrick RL, Barchas JD (1974) Regulation of catecholamine synthesis in rat-brain synaptosomes. J Neurochem 23:7–15

Peach MJ (1972) Stimulation of release of adrenal catecholamine by adenosine 3′,5′-cyclic monophosphate and theophylline in the absence of extracellular Ca^{+2}. Proc Natl Acad Sci USA 69:834–836

Penit J, Huot J, Jard S (1976) Neuroblastoma cell adenylate cyclase: direct activation by adenosine and prostaglandins. J Neurochem 26:256–273

Perkins JP (1973) Adenyl cyclase. Adv Cyclic Nucleotide Res 3:1–64

Perkins JP, Moore MM, Kalisker A, Su Y-F (1975) Regulation of cyclic AMP content in normal and malignant brain cells. Adv Cyclic Nucleotide Res 5:641–660

Pert A, Rosenblatt JE, Sivit C, Pert CB, Bunney WE (1978) Long-term treatment with lithium prevents development of dopamine receptor supersensitivity. Science 201:171–173

Phillipson OT, Emson PC, Horn AS, Jessel T (1977) Evidence concerning the anatomical localization of the dopamine stimulated adenylate cyclase in the substantia nigra. Brain Res 136:45–58

Phillis JW (1974) Evidence for cholinergic transmission in the cerebral cortex. Adv Behav Biol 10:57–77

Phillis JW (1977) The role of cyclic nucleotides in the CNS. Can J Neurol Sci 4:151–195

Phillis JW, Edstrom JP (1976) Effect of adenosine analogs on rat cerebral cortical neurons. Life Sci 19:1041–1054

Phillis JW, Kostopoulos GK (1975) Adenosine as a putative transmitter in the cerebral cortex. Studies with potentiators and antagonists. Life Sci 17:1085–1094

Phillis JW, Kostopoulos GK, Limacher JJ (1974) Depression of corticospinal cells by various purines and pyrimidines. Can J Physiol Pharmacol 52:1226–1299

Phillis JW, Kostopoulos GK, Limacher JJ (1975) A potent depressant action of adenine derivatives on cerebral cortical neurons. Eur J Pharmacol 30:125–129

Phillis JW, Edstrom JP, Kostopoulos GK, Kirkpatrick JR (1979a) Effects of adenosine and adenine nucleotides on synaptic transmission in the cerebral cortex. Can J Physiol Pharmacol 57:1289–1312

Phillis JW, Kostopoulos GK, Edstrom JP, Ellis SW (1979b) Role of adenosine and adenine nucleotides in central nervous function. In: Baer HP, Drummond GI (eds) Physiological and regulatory functions of adenosine and adenine nucleotides. Raven, New York, pp 343–359

Poisner AM (1973) Direct stimulant effect of aminophylline on catecholamine release from the adrenal medulla. Biochem Pharmacol 22:469–476

Premont J, Perez M, Bockaert J (1977) Adenosine-sensitive adenylate cyclase in rat striatal homogenates and its relationship to dopamine-sensitive and Ca^{+2}-sensitive adenylate cyclases. Mol Pharmacol 13:662–670

Premont J, Tassin J-P, Blanc G, Bockaert J (1979) Effects of adenosine on adenylate cyclase in broken cell preparations of central nervous system. In: Baer HP, Drummond GL (eds) Physiological and regulatory functions of adenosine and adenine nucleotides. Raven, New York, pp 259–269

Pull I, McIlwain H (1973) Output of (^{14}C)adenine nucleotides and their derivatives from cerebral tissues: tetrodotoxin-resistant and calcium ion-requiring components. Biochem J 136:893–901

Purves RD (1978) The physiology of muscarinic acetylcholine receptors. In: Straub RW, Bolis L (eds) Cell membrane receptors for drugs and hormones: a multidisciplinary approach. Raven, New York, pp 69–79

Quik M, Emson PC, Joyce E 81979) Dissociation between the presynaptic dopamine-sensitive adenylate cyclase and the (^{3}H) spiperone binding sites in rat substantia nigra. Brain Res 167:355–365

Raese J, Patrick RL, Barchas JD (1976) Phospholipid-induced activation of tyrosine hydroxylase from rat brain striatal synaptosomes. Biochem Pharmacol 25:2245–2250

Rall TW (1979) Regulation of cyclic adenosine monophosphate accumulation in brain tissue: interactions of adenosine with other agonists. In: Baer HP, Drummond GI (eds) Physiological and regulatory functions of adenosine and adenine nucleotides. Raven, New York

Rall TW, Sattin A (1970) Factors influencing the accumulation of cyclic AMP in brain tissue. Adv Biochem Psychopharmacol 3:113–133

Rall TW, Sutherland EW (1958) Formation of a cyclic adenine ribonucleotide by tissue particles. J Biol Chem 232:1065–1076

Rall TW, Sutherland EW (1961) The regulatory role of adenosine 3′,5′-phosphate. Cold Spring Harbor Symp Quant Biol 26:347–354

Rasmussen H (1970) Cell communication, calcium ion, and cyclic adenosine monophosphate. Science 170:404–412

Rasmussen H, Jensen P, Lake W, Friedman N, Goodman DBP (1975) Cyclic nucleotides and cellular metabolism. Adv Cyclic Nucleotide Res 5:375–393

Reddington M, Mehl E (1979) Synaptic membrane proteins as substrates for cyclic AMP-stimulated protein phosphorylation in various regions of rat brain. Biochim Biophys Acta 55:230–238

Rehncrona S, Siesjo BK, Westerberg E (1978) Adenosine and cyclic AMP in cerebral cortex of rats in hypoxia, status epilepticus, and hypercapnia. Acta Physiol Scand 104:453–463

Reynolds, CM, Merry J, Coppen A (1979) Prophylactic treatment of alcoholism by lithium carbonate. In: Erickson C, Goodwin D (eds) Alcoholism and affective disorders. Plenum, New York London, pp 31–38

Ribeiro JA (1979) Purinergic modulation of transmitter release. J Theor Briol 80:259–270

Ribeiro JA, Walker J (1973) Action of adenosine triphosphate on endplate potentials recorded from muscle fibers of the rat diaphragm and frog sartorius. Br J Pharmacol 49:725–725

Richards JM, Swislocki NI (1979) Activation of adenylate cyclase by molybdate. J Biol Chem 254:6857–6860

Robison GA, Butcher RW, Sutherland EW (1971) Cyclic AMP. Academic Press, New York London
Rodbard D (1974) Apparent positive cooperative effects in cyclic AMP and corticosterone production by isolated adrenal cells in response to ACTH and analogs. Endocrinology 94:1427
Rodbell M (1980) The role of hormone receptors and GTP-regulatory proteins in membrane transduction. Nature 284:17–22
Rose G, Schubert P (1977) Release and transfer of (^{3}H)adenosine derivatives in the cholinergic septal system. Brain Res 121:353–357
Rosenblatt JE, Pert CB, Tallman JF, Pert A, Bunney WE (1978) Effect of imipramine and lithium on alpha-receptor and beta-receptor binding in rat brain. Brain Res 160:186–191
Roth RH, Morgenroth VH, Salzman PM (1975) Tyrosine hydroxylase: allosteric activation induced by stimulation of central noradrenergic neurons. Naunyn Schmiedebergs Arch Pharmacol 289:327–343
Rubin EH, Ferrendelli JA (1977) Distribution and regulation of cyclic nucleotide levels in cerebellum, in vivo. J Neurochem 29:43–51
Sabol SL, Nirenberg M (1979) Regulation of adenylate cyclase of neuroblastoma-glioma hybrid cells by alpha-adrenergic receptors. 1. Inhibition of adenylate cyclase mediated by alpha receptors. J Biol Chem 254:1913–1920
Salzman PM, Roth RH (1978) Noradrenergic neurons: poststimulation increase in catecholamine biosynthesis. In: Deniker P, Radouco-Thomas C, Villeneuve A (eds) Neuropsychopharmacology. Pergamon Press, Oxford New York, pp 1439–1455
Sattin A (1971) Increase in the content of adenosine 3′,5′-monophosphate in mouse forebrain during seizures and prevention of the increase by methylxanthines. J Neurochem 18:1087–1096
Sattin A, Rall TW (1967) The effect of brain extracts on the accumulation of cyclic 3′,5′-AMP (CA) in slices of guinea pig (GP) cerebral cortex. Fed Proc 26:707
Sattin A, Rall TW (1970) The effect of adenosine and adenine nucleotides on the cyclic adenosine 3′,5′-phosphate content of guinea pig cerebral cortex slices. Mol Pharmacol 6:13–23
Sattin A, Rall TW, Zanella J (1975) Regulation of cyclic adenosine 3′,5′-monophosphate levels in guinea-pig cerebral cortex by interaction of alpha adrenergic and adenosine receptor activity. J Pharmacol Exp Ther 192:22–32
Schildkraut JJ (1965) The catecholamine hypothesis of affective disorders: a review of supporting evidence. Am J Psychiat 122:509–522
Schildkraut JJ, Orsulak PJ, Gudeman JE et al. (1977) Recent studies of role of catecholamines in pathophysiology and classification of depressive disorders. In: Usdin E, Hamburg DA, Barchas JD (eds) Neuroregulators and psychiatric disorders. Oxford Press, New York, pp 122–128
Schlichter DJ, Casnellie JE, Greengard P (1978) An endogenous substrate for cGMP-dependent protein kinase in mammalian cerebellum. Nature 27:61–62
Schmidt MJ, Palmer EC, Dettbarn W-D, Robison GA (1970) Cyclic AMP and adenyl cyclase in the developing rat brain. Dev Psychobiol 3:53–67
Scholfield CN (1978) Depression of evoked potentials in brain slices by adenosine compounds. Br J Pharmacol 63:239–244
Schou M (1976) Pharmacology and toxicology of lithium. Annu Rev Pharmacol 16:231–242
Schubert P, Mitzdorf U (1979) Analysis and quantitative evaluation of the depressive effect of adenosine on evoked potentials in hippocampal slices. Brain Res 172:186–190
Schubert P, Lee K, West M, Deadwyler S, Lynch G (1976) Stimulation dependent release of ^{3}H-adenosine derivatives from central axon terminals to target neurons. Nature 260:541–542
Schubert P, Komp W, Kreutzberg GW (1979) Correlation of 5′-nucleotidase activity and selective trans-neuronal transfer of adenosine in the hippocampus. Brain Res 168:419–424
Schultz G, Hardman JG, Schultz K, Baird CE, Sutherland EW (1973) The importance of calcium ions for the regulation of guanosine 3′,5′-cyclic monophosphate levels. Proc Natl Acad Sci USA 70:3889–3893

Schultz J (1975) Cyclic adenosine 3′,5′-monophosphate in guinea pig cerebral cortical slices: possible regulation of phosphodiesterase activity by cyclic adenosine 3′,5′-monophosphate and calcium ions. J Neurochem 24:495–501

Schultz J (1976) Psychoactive drug effects on a system which generates cyclic AMP in brain. Nature 261:417–418

Schultz J, Daly JW (1973) Cyclic adenosine 3′,5′-monophosphate in guinea pig cerebral cortical slices. I. Formation of cyclic adenosine 3′,5′-monophosphate from endogenous adenosine triphosphate and from radioactive adenosine triphosphate formed during a prior incubation with radioactive adenine. J Biol Chem 248:843–852

Schultz J, Hamprecht B (1973) Adenosine 3′,5′-monophosphate in cultured neuroblastoma cells: effect of adenosine, phosphodiesterase inhibitors and benzodiazepines. Naunyn Schmiedebergs Arch Pharmacol 278: 215–225

Schultz J, Kleefeld G (1979) Cyclic adenosine 3′,5′-monophosphate in rat cerebral cortical slices: effects of methoxamine and clonidine. Pharmacology 18:163–167

Schultz J, Hamprecht B, Daly JW (1972) Accumulation of adenosine 3′,5′-cyclic monophosphate in clonal glial cells: labeling of intracellular adenine nucleotides with radioactive adenine. Proc Natl Acad Sci USA 69:1266–1270

Schwabe U, Daly JW (1977) The role of calcium ions in accumulation of cyclic AMP elicited by alpha- and beta-adrenergic agonists in rat brain slices. J Pharmacol Exp Ther 202:134–143

Schwabe U, Ohga Y, Daly JW (1978) The role of calcium in the regulation of cyclic nucleotide levels in brain slices of rat and guinea pig. Naunyn Schmiedebergs Arch Pharmacol 302:141–151

Schwarcz R, Coyle JT (1977) Neurochemical sequelae of kainate injections in corpus striatum and substantia nigra of the rat. Life Sci 20:431–436

Schwarcz R, Creese I, Coyle JT, Snyder SH (1978) Dopamine receptors localized on cerebral cortical afferents to rat corpus striatum. Nature 271:766–768

Schwartz JC, Costentin J, Martres MP, Protais P, Baudry M (1978) Modulation of receptor mechanisms in CNS: hypersensitivity and hyposensitivity to catecholamines. Neuropharmacology 17:665–685

Segal M (1974) Lithium and monoamine neurotransmitters in rat hippocampus. Nature 250:71–73

Segal M, Bloom FE (1974) The action of norepinephrine in the rat hippocampus. I. Iontophoretic studies. Brain Res 72:79–97

Segal M, Bloom FE (1976) The action of norepinephrine in the rat hippocampus. IV. The effects of locus coeruleus stimulation on evoked hippocampal unit activity. Brain Res 107:513–525

Serck-Hanssen G (1974) Effects of theophylline and propranolol on acetylcholine-induced release of adrenal medullary catecholamines. Biochem Pharmacol 23:2225–2235

Shimizu H (1979) Biochemical characterization of adenosine receptors in brain. In: Baer HP, Drummond GI (eds) Physiological and regulatory functions of adenosine and adenine nucleotides. Raven, New York, pp 243–249

Shimizu H, Yamamura Y (1977) Effects of diaminopropionate, deoxyadenosine, and theophylline on stimulated formation of cyclic AMP and GMP by depolarizing agents in slices of guinea-pig cerebral cortex. J Neurobiol 8:57–65

Shimizu H, Daly JW, Creveling CR (1969) A radioisotopic method for measuring the formation of adenosine 3′,5′-cyclic monophosphate in incubated slices of brain. J Neurochem 16:1609–1619

Shimizu H, Creveling CR, Daly J (1970) Stimulated formation of adenosine 3′,5′-cyclic phosphate in cerebral cortex: synergism between electrical activity and biogenic amines. Proc Natl Acad Sci USA 65:1033–1040

Shinnick-Gallagher P, Williams BJ, Gallagher JP (1976) Biochemical and electrophysiological studies of cyclic nucleotides and their effects in the rat superior cervical ganglion. Neurosci Abstr 2:800

Siggins GR (1977) Electrophysiological effects of cyclic nucleotides on excitable tissues. In: Cramer H, Schultz J (eds) Cyclic nucleotides: mechanisms of action. H. John Wiley and Sons, New York Chichester, pp 317–336

Siggins GR (1979) Neurotransmitters and neuromodulators and their mediation by cyclic nucleotides. In: Ehrlich YH, Volavka J, Davis LG, Brunngraber EG (eds) Modulators, mediators and specifiers in brain function. Plenum, New York London, pp 41–64

Siggins GR, Henriksen SJ (1975) Analogs of cyclic adenosine monophosphate: correlation of inhibition of Purkinje neurons with protein kinase activation. Science 189:559–561

Siggins GR, Schultz JE (1979) Chronic treatment with lithium or desipramine alters discharge frequency and norepinephrine responsiveness of cerebellar Purkinje cells. Proc Natl Acad Sci USA 76:5987–5991

Siggins GR, Hoffer BJ, Bloom FE (1969) Cyclic adenosine monophosphate: possible mediator for norepinephrine effects on cerebellar Purkinje cells. Science 165:1018–1020

Siggins GR, Hoffer BJ, Bloom FE (1971 a) Cyclic adenosine monophosphate and norepinephrine: effect on Purkinje cells in rat cerebellar cortex. Science 174:1258–1259

Siggins GR, Oliver AP, Hoffer BJ, Bloom FE (1971 b) Cyclic adenosine monophosphate and norepinephrine: effects on transmembrane properties of cerebellar Purkinje cell. Science 171:192–194

Siggins GR, Hoffer BJ, Oliver AP, Bloom FE (1971 c) Activation of a central noradrenergic projection to cerebellum. Nature 233:481–483

Siggins GR, Hoffer BJ, Ungerstedt U (1974) Electrophysiological evidence for involvement of cyclic adenosine monophosphate in dopamine responses of caudate neurons. Life Sci 15:779–792

Silinsky EM (1975) On the association between transmitter secretion and the release of adenine nucleotides from mammalian motor nerve terminals. J Physiol (Lond) 247:145–162

Skolnick P, Nimitkitpaisan Y, Stalvey L, Daly JW (1978) Inhibition of brain adenosine deaminase by 2′-deoxyformycin and erythro-9-(2-hydroxy-3-nonyl)-adenine. J Neurochem 30:1579–1582

Smellie FW, Daly JW, Dunwiddie TV, Hoffer BJ (1979 a) The detro- and levorotatory isomers of N-phenyl isopropyladenosine: stereospecific effects on cyclic AMP-formation and evoked synaptic responses in brain slices. Life Sci 25:1739–1748

Smellie FW, Davis CW, Daly JW, Wels JN (1979 b) Alkylxanthines: inhibition of adenosine-elicited accumulation of cyclic AMP in brain slices and of brain phosphodiesterase activity. Life Sci 24:2475–2482

Spano PF, Kumakura K, Govoni S, Trabucchi M (1975) Postnatal development and regulation of cerebellar cyclic guanosine monophosphate system. Pharmacol Res Commun 7:223–237

Spencer HJ (1976) Antagonism of cortical excitation of striatal neurons by glutamic acid diethyl-ester – evidence for glutamic-acid as an excitatory transmitter in rat striatum. Brain Res 102:91–101

Spencer PSJ (1977) Review of the pharmacology of existing antidepressants. Br J Clin Pharmacol 4:57S–68S

Sporn JR, Molinoff PB (1976) Beta-adrenergic receptors in rat brain. J Cyclic Nucleotide Res 2:149–161

Sporn JR, Wolfe BB, Harden TK, Molinoff PB (1977) Supersensitivity in rat cerebral cortex: presynaptic and postsynaptic effects of 6-hydroxydopamine at noradrenergic synapses. Mol Pharmacol 13:1170–1180

Standaert FG, Dretchen KL (1979) Cyclic nucleotides and neuromuscular transmission. Fed Proc 38:2183–2192

Standaert FG, Dretchen KL, Skirboll LR, Morgenroth VH (1976 a) Effects of cyclic nucleotides on mammalian motor nerve terminals. J Pharmacol Exp Ther 199:544–552

Standaert FG, Dretchen KL, Skirboll LR, Morgenroth VH (1976 b) A role of cyclic nucleotides in neuromuscular transmission. J Pharmacol Exp Ther 199:553–564

Steiner AL, Ferrendelli JA, Kipnis DM (1972) Radioimmunoassay for cyclic nucleotides. III. Effects of ischemia, changes during development and regional distribution of adenosine 3′,5′-monophosphate in mouse brain. J Biol Chem 247:1121–1124

Stjärne L (1973) Michaelis-Menten kinetics of secretion of sympathetic neurotransmitter as a function of external calcium: effect of graded alpha-adrenoceptor blockade. Naunyn Schmiedebergs Arch Pharmacol 278:323–327

Stjärne L, Brundin J (1975) Dual adrenoceptor mediated control of noradrenaline secretion from human vasoconstrictor nerves: facilitation by beta-receptors and inhibition by alpha-receptors. Acta Physiol Scand 94:139–141
Stone TW, Taylor DA (1977) Microiontophoretic studies of the effects of cyclic nucleotides on excitability of neurons in the rat cerebral cortex. J Physiol (Lond) 266:523–543
Stone TW, Taylor DA (1978) An electrophysiological demonstration of a synergistic action between norepinephrine and adenosine in the cerebral cortex. Brain Res 147:396–400
Stone TW, Taylor DA, Bloom FE (1975) Cyclic AMP and cyclic GMP may mediate opposite neuronal responses in the rat cerebral cortex. Science 187:845–847
Strömbom U, Forn J, Dolphin AC, Greengard P (1979) Regulation of the state of phosphorylation of specific neuronal proteins in mouse brain by in vivo administration of anaesthetic and convulsant agents. Proc Natl Acad Sci USA 76:4687–4690
Su C (1978) Purinergic inhibition of adrenergic transmission in rabbit blood vessels. J Pharmacol Exp Ther 204:351–361
Sutherland EW, Oye I, Butcher RW (1965) The action of epinephrine and the role of the adenylate cyclase system in hormone action. Recent Prog Horm Res 21:623–642
Sutherland EW, Robison GA, Butcher RW (1968) Some aspects of the biological role of adenosine 3′,5′-monophosphate (cyclic AMP). Circulation 37:279–306
Swartz BE, Woody CD (1979) Correlated effects of acetylcholine and cyclic guanosine monophosphate on membrane properties of mammalian neocortical neurons. J Neurobiol 10:465–488
Szmigielski A, Guidotti A (1979) Action of harmaline and diazepam on the cerebellar content of cyclic GMP and on the activities of two endogenous inhibitors of protein kinase. Neurochem Res 4:189–200
Szmigielski A, Guidotti A, Costa E (1977) Endogenous protein kinase inhibitors: purification, characterization, and distribution in various tissues. J Biol Chem 252:3848–3853
Takai Y, Nishiyama K, Ymamura H, Nishizuka Y (1975) Guanosine 3′,5′-monophosphate-dependent protein kinase from bovine cerebellum. J Biol Chem 250:4690–4695
Takamori M, Ishii M, Mori M (1973) The role of cyclic 3′,5′-adenosine monophosphate in neuromuscular transmission. Arch Neurol 29:420–422
Taneda M, Izumi F, Ika M (1974) Effect of dibutyryl adenosine 3′,5′-monophosphate on catecholamine synthesis in rat brain cortical slices and isolated vasa deferentia. Jpn J Pharmacol 24:934–936
Taylor DA, Stone TW (1978) Neuronal responses to extracellularly applied cyclic AMP: role of the adenosine receptor. Experienta 34:481–482
Taylor DA, Stone TW (1980) The action of adenosine on noradrenergic neuronal inhibition produced by stimulation of locus coeruleus. Brain Res 183:367–376
Troyer EW, Hall IA, Ferrendelli JA (1978) Guanylate cyclase in CNS: enzymatic characteristics of soluble and particulate enzymes from mouse cerebellum and retina. J Neurochem 31:825–833
Tsuzuki J, Newburgh RW (1975) Inhibition of 5′-nucleotidase in rat brain by methylxanthines. J Neurochem 25:895–896
Ueda T, Greengard P (1977) Adenosine 3′,5′-monophosphate-regulated phosphoprotein system of neuronal membranes. J Biol Chem 252:5155–5163
Ueda T, Maeno H, Greengard P (1973) Regulation of endogenous phosphorylation of sepcific proteins in synaptic membrane fractions from rat brain by adenosine 3′,5′-monophosphate. J Biol Chem 248:8295–8305
Ungerstedt U (1971) Stereotaxic mapping of the monoamine pathways in the rat brain. Acta Physiol Scand [Supl] 367:1
Uzunov P, Shein HM, Weiss B (1974) Multiple forms of cyclic 3′,5′-AMP phosphodiesterase of rat cerebrum and cloned astrocytoma and neuroblastoma cells. Neuropharmacology 13:377–392
Van Calker D, Muller M, Hamprecht B (1978) Adenosine inhibits the accumulation of cyclic AMP in cultured brain cells. Nature 276:839–841
Van Kammen DP, Murphy DL (1975) Attenuation of the euphoriant and activating effects of D- and L-amphetamine by lithium carbonate treatments. Psychopharmacologia 44:215–224

Verhaege RH, Vanhoutte PM, Shepherd JT (1977) Inhibition of sympathetic neurotransmission in canine blood vessels by adenosine and adenine nucleotides. Circ Res 40:208–215
Vetulani J, Sulser F (1975) Action of various antidepressant treatments reduces reactivity of noradrenergic cyclic AMP in generating system in limbic forebrain. Nature 257:495–496
Vizi ES, Knoll J (1976) The inhibitory effect of adenosine and related nucleotides on the release of acetylcholine. Neuroscience 1:391–398
Vulliet PR, Langan TA, Weiner N (1980) Tyrosine hydroxylase: a substrate of cyclic AMP-dependent protein kinase. Proc Natl Acad Sci USA 77:92–96
Walsh DA (1978) Role of the cAMP-dependent protein kinase as *the* transducer of cAMP action. Biochem Pharmacol 27:1801–1804
Walsh DA, Ashby CD, Gonzalez C, Calkins D, Fischer EH, Krebs EG (1971) Purification and characterization of a protein inhibitor of adenosine 3′,5′-monophosphate-dependent protein kinases. J Biol Chem 246:1977–1985
Watanabe H, Passonneau JV (1974) The effect of trauma on cerebral glycogen and related metabolites and enzymes. Brain Res 66:147–159
Watanabe H, Passonneau JV (1975) Cyclic adenosine monophosphate in cerebral cortex. Alterations following trauma. Arch Neurol 32:181–184
Waterhouse BD, Woodwar DJ (1980) Interaction of norepinephrine with cerebrocortical activity evoked by stimulation of somatosensory afferent pathways in the rat. Exp Neurol 67:11–34
Waterhouse BD, Moises HC, Woodward DJ (1979) Alpha, beta pharmacological characterization of noradrenergic modulatory actions in rat somatosensory cortex. Neurosci Abstr 5:356
Weber AM, Herz R (1968) The relationship between caffeine contraction of intact muscle and the effect of caffeine on reticulum. J Gen Physiol 52:750–759
Weight FF, Petzold G, Greengard P (1974) Guanosine 3′,5′-monophosphate in sympathetic ganglia: increase associated with synaptic transmission. Science 186:942–944
Weiner N (1975) Factors regulating catecholamine biosynthesis in peripheral and central neurons. In: Brady RO (ed) The basis neurosciences: the nervous system, vol 1. Raven, New York, pp 341–354
Weiner N (1979a) Multiple factors regulating the release of norepinephrine consequent to nerve stimulation. Fed Proc 38:2193–2202
Weiner N (1979b) Tyrosine-3-monooxygenase (tyrosine hydroxylase). In: Youdim MBH (ed) Aromatic amino acid hydroxylases and mental disease. John Wiley and Sons, New York Chichester, pp 141–190
Weiner N, Lee F-L, Barnes E, Dreyer E (1977) Enzymology of tyrosine hydroxylase and the role of cyclic nucleotides in its regulation. In: Usdin E, Weiner N, Youdim MBH (eds) Structure and function of monoamine enzymes. E. Dekker, New York, pp 109–148
Weiner N, Lee F-L, Barnes E, Dreyer E (1978) The activation of tyrosine hydroxylase in noradrenergic neurons during acute nerve stimulation. Life Sci 22:1197–1216
Westfall TC (1977) Local regulation of adrenergic transmission. Physiol Rev 57:659–729
Westfall TC, Kitay D, Wahl G (1976) The effect of cyclic nucleotides on the release of ^{3}H-dopamine from rat striatal slices. J Pharmacol Exp Ther 199:149–157
Wilkening D, Makman MH (1976) Stimulation of glycogenolysis in rat caudate nucleus slices by 1-isopropylnorepinephrine, dibutyryl cAMP and 2-chloroadenosine. J Neurochem 26:923–928
Wilkening D, Makman MH (1977) Activation of glycogen phosphorylase in rat caudate nucleus slices by 1-isopropylnorepinephrine and dibutryl cyclic AMP: J Neurochem 28:1001–1007
Wilkening D, Makman MH (1979) Effects of 1-isopropylnorepinephrine, 3-isobutyl-1-methylxanthine and dibutyryl cyclic AMP on hexose uptake and metabolism by rat striatal slices. J Neurochem 32:1467–1472
Wilson DF (1974) The effects of dibutyryl cyclic AMP, theophylline and aminophylline on neuromuscular transmission in the rat. J Pharmacol Exp Ther 1888:447–452

Wolfe B, Harden TK, Sporn JR, Molinoff PB (1978) Presynaptic modulation of beta-adrenergic receptors in rat cerebral cortex after treatment with antidepressants. J Pharmacol Exp Ther 207:446–457

Wolff J, Berens SC, Jones AB (1970) Inhibition of thryotropin-stimulated adenyl cyclase activity of beef thyroid membranes by low concentration of lithium ion. Biochem Biophys Res Commun 39:77–87

Woodward DJ, Moises HC, Waterhouse BD, Hoffer BJ, Freedman R (1979) Modulatory actions of norepinephrine in the central nervous system. Fed Proc 38:2109–2116

Woody CD (1978) If cyclic GMP is a neuronal second messenger, what is the message? Adv Behav Biol 24:253–260

Woody CD, Swartz BE, Gruen E (1978) Effects of acetylcholine and cyclic GMP on input resistance of cortical neurons in awake cats. Brain Res 158:373–395

Wooten GF, Thoa NB, Kopin IJ, Axelrod J (1973) Enhanced release of dopamine-beta-hydroxylase and norepinephrine from sympathetic nerves by dibutyryl cyclic adenosine monophosphate and theophylline. Mol Pharmacol 9:178–183

Yamauchi T, Fujisawa H (1979) In vitro phosphorylation of bovine adrenal tyrosine hydroxylase by adenosine 3′,5′-monophosphate-dependent protein kinase. J Biol Chem 254:503–507

Zahniser NR, Minneman KP, Molinoff PB (1979) Persistence of beta-adrenergic receptors in rat striatum following kainic acid administration. Brain Res 178:589–595

Zanella J Jr, Rall TW (1973) Evaluation of electrical pulses and elevated levels of potassium ions as stimulants of adenosine 3′,5′-monophosphate (cyclic AMP) accumulation in guinea-pig brain. J Pharmacol Exp Ther 186:241–251

Zivkovic B, Guidotti A, Costa E (1975) The regulation of the kinetic state of striatal tyrosine hydroxylase and the role of postsynaptic dopamine receptors. Brain Res 92:516–521

Zivkovic B, Guidotti A, Costa E (1976) Cyclic AMP and regulation of tyrosine-3-monoxygenase in rat striatum. J Cyclic Nucleotide Res 2:1–10

CHAPTER 26

The Role of Cyclic Nucleotide Metabolism in the Eye

D. B. FARBER

Overview

This chapter summarizes cyclic nucleotide involvement in the eye. While all areas of the eye are discussed, greatest emphasis will be on the retina. The levels of retinal cyclic nucleotides vary according to several factors, including age, type of predominant photoreceptor, conditions of light- or dark-adaptation, states of pathology, etc. The cyclic GMP system is most important in rod visual cells; its principal effector is light, but it responds also to ischemic conditions, free radicals, depolarizing agents, cations and fatty acids. Cyclic AMP metabolism is minimal in rod photoreceptors. In contrast, in cone visual cells, the cyclic AMP system predominates and is responsive to light, with minimal levels of cyclic GMP present.

Cyclic GMP has been proposed to play a role in the visual transduction of rod photoreceptors. Its levels are reduced rapidly by light, and many molecules of cyclic GMP are hydrolyzed for each rhodopsin molecule bleached; this represents a large amplification of the light signal. Cyclic GMP-phosphodiesterase activity is responsible for the light-induced decrease in cyclic GMP. The enzyme is activated by light in the presence of a nucleoside triphosphate, mainly GTP, but photoisomerization of rhodopsin must precede the GTP-dependent step. The function of GTP in this activation is still an unresolved problem. GTP has been suggested to act as an allosteric activator of the phosphodiesterase in a process that involves a light-activated GTPase. This GTPase could hydrolyze the GTP bound to phosphodiesterase and turn off the enzyme. Alternatively, deactivation of phosphodiesterase could occur by transfer of phosphate from GTP (bound to phosphodiesterase) to another protein.

The light-induced changes in cyclic GMP concentration are translated into physiological messages such as specific phosphoproteins. In frog and toad photoreceptors, two proteins of 12,000 and 13,000 molecular weight are the substrates of the cyclic nucleotide-dependent protein kinase. These proteins are dephosphorylated upon illumination of the tissue and are rephosphorylated when illumination ceases. In bovine rods, a protein of 30,000 molecular weight is phosphorylated in a cyclic nucleotide-dependent manner. It has been proposed that the phosphorylated protein could interact with membrane sodium channels to control their conductance, but there is still no evidence to support this hypothesis.

Other studies point to cyclic GMP as an important regulator of rod cell metabolism or function. It has been shown that either perfusion of the retina with cyclic GMP or intracellular injection of cyclic GMP into rod outer segments of isolated retina depolarizes the rod membrane and increases the amplitude of the response. The duration of this depolarization depends upon the amount of cyclic GMP injected and is increased by previous dark adaptation and decreased by previous light adaptation.

A very active cyclic AMP metabolism is found in the inner layers of rod- and cone-dominant retinas. Dopamine, the predominant catecholamine of the retina, is the main stimulator of the adenylate cyclase activity present in the inner layers. The enzyme responds, also, to dopamine agonists and dopamine mimetics, such as ergot alkaloids, and to LSD.

Very little is known about the cyclic nucleotide metabolism of the retinal pigment epithelium. The epithelial cells contain much lower levels of cyclic AMP and cyclic GMP than the rest of the retina.

Abnormalities in cyclic GMP metabolism are associated with the degeneration of rod photoreceptors in some inherited retinal diseases. The *rd* mouse and the Irish setter dog disorders are characterized by elevated levels of cyclic GMP occurring before the onset of visual cell pathological morphology. In both species, a deficiency in the activity of cyclic GMP-phosphodiesterase has been demonstrated; this abnormality is restricted to the photoreceptor cells of the retina. In addition, Ca^{2+} modulation of cyclic GMP metabolism seems to be affected. These disorders have been simulated in vitro by incubating normal retinas with the phosphodiesterase inhibitor IBMX. With this treatment, cyclic nucleotide levels in the eye rudiments of *Xenopus laevis* increase several-fold concomitantly with changes in photoreceptor morphology. In contrast to the diseased retina in the mouse and dog, the dystrophic RCS rat retina shows levels of cyclic GMP which are subnormal prior to the pathological changes in the visual cells. This seems to result from an increased affinity of cyclic GMP-phosphodiesterase for cyclic GMP. Thus, photoreceptors may require specific concentrations of cyclic nucleotides for their normal metabolism or function. Higher or lower levels of cyclic GMP or an altered ratio of cyclic GMP/cyclic AMP may be enough to cause visual cell degeneration.

In addition to the retina, most other ocular tissues also contain cyclic nucleotides. For example, adenylate cyclase activity is suggested to be involved in the regulatory mechanisms of aqueous humor formation in the ciliary body, and cyclic AMP has been shown to participate in the regulation of the aqueous outflow of the eye. Cyclic GMP has no known influence in these processes.

Cyclic AMP inhibits corneal epithelium cell growth, preventing the healing process of the cornea. In contrast, cyclic GMP does not appear to have an effect in the regulation of mitotic activity during wound healing. Cyclic AMP is involved in the activation of the corneal chloride pump; this pump may control the efficient dehydration of the corneal stroma which is indispensable for the maintenance of the transparency of the cornea. Cyclic AMP may also help to reduce ulceration of alkali-burned cornea by causing the suppression of collagenase activity.

The physiological function of cyclic nucleotide metabolism in the lens still remains unknown.

A. Introduction

This chapter summarizes the explorations of cyclic nucleotide involvement in normal or abnormal biochemistry and function of the different components of the eye. In the last decade, our knowledge of this subject has expanded tremendously, and the body of information accumulated has become extensive, especially in the area related to the retina. As a result, the retina may be the best understood constituent of the vertebrate central nervous system.

The review will be divided in four parts; three of them will consider the work on cyclic nucleotides in different kinds of retinas, rod- or cone-dominated, and in retinal degenerations. The fourth part will cover studies on cyclic nucleotides in other tissues of the eye. Throughout this review, it may be helpful for the reader to refer to a source on the anatomy of the eye, such as WALLS (1942).

B. Cyclic Nucleotide Metabolism in the Retina

The sensory retina is the immediate instrument of vision. Its photoreceptor cells receive visual images transmitted through the cornea, lens and vitreous humor and convert them into electrical impulses which are sent to the brain via the optic nerve. However, the retina is much more than an array of photoreceptors. Before the visual signal leaves the eye, it must pass through a neural network made up of different types of nerve cells, where a significant amount of neural processing occurs. The retina can actually be considered part of the brain located within the eye.

In the adult stage, the retina has a layered structure with the photoreceptor cells lying outermost, adjacent to the pigment epithelium. The latter is a cellular lining which separates the retina from the blood capillaries of the choroid. The innermost retinal layer, which is closest to the vitreous, is formed by the ganglion cells. Between these two layers, there is a discrete stratum of neurons formed by bipolar, horizontal and amacrine cells. Glial-like Müller cells extend from the outer nuclear layer (formed by the nuclei of the photoreceptors) to the inner limiting membrane; though their function is not understood, they are in a close cooperative relationship with the nerve cells of the retina, in a manner similar to that which occurs in brain with neurons and glia.

There are two general classes of photoreceptor cells, i.e., rods and cones, each with morphological subclasses (STELL 1972). Rods and cones are sensitive to different levels of illumunation. Rods respond to low intensity light whereas cones require light of high intensity to function. Thus, it is possible to think that, during the evolutionary process, the retinas of different animals acquired the appropriate number of either kind of photoreceptor cell according to the very definite needs for the survival of each species. For example, nocturnal animals (i.e. mice or rats) have retinas with a preponderance of rods, whereas birds, lizards or ground squirrels which are active during daylight evolved to retinas with a majority of cones. Man and most other vertebrates have duplex retinas with a variable mixture of photoreceptors.

In addition to light sensitivity, rods and cones differ by several other morphological, physiological and biochemical criteria. Of interest here is their distinct cyclic nucleotide biochemistry. For the sake of clarity, cyclic GMP and cyclic AMP metabolisms and their function in the rod-dominant and cone-dominant retinas will be reviewed separately. It is, however, important to point out that, exclusive of the photoreceptor cells, cyclic GMP and cyclic AMP metabolism in other retinal cells may be very similar both in rod- and cone-dominated eyes.

I. Cyclic Nucleotides in Rod-Dominant Retinas

1. Cyclic GMP

The photoreceptive part of the rod visual cell, the outer segment, contains an orderly stack of discs formed by bilayered lipid membranes which provide a matrix for protein molecules. The major protein of the outer segment is rhodopsin, the light-catching visual pigment. The discs are encased by but not continuous with the plasmalemma of the cell. The rest of the visual cell is constituted by an inner segment containing mitochondria, a nucleus located in the cell soma, and a synaptic ending joined to the cell soma by a short axon (YOUNG 1969a). When the photoreceptor cell is in the dark, there is a maintained Na^+ flux, referred to as "dark current", which flows out from the cell body and returns across the outer segment membrane (PENN and HAGINS 1969). Upon illumination, light is absorbed by rhodopsin causing a photochemical isomerization of its chromophore 11-cis retinal to the all-trans configuration. This process, known as bleaching of rhodopsin, leads to a reduction in the Na^+ permeability of the plasmalemma which, in vertebrates, is reflected as a hyperpolarization of the photoreceptor cell membrane (WERBLIN 1974). The mechanism which triggers the ionic permeability change remains unknown; photon capture occurs in the disc membrane of the rod outer segment whereas the change in potential takes place across the plasmalemma of the cell. In order to explain this, one must assume that light causes the discs to release a substance which diffuses to the plasma membrane and reduces its conductance for Na^+ (BAYLOR and FUORTES 1970; HAGINS 1972; CONE 1973). This is the basis of the model proposed by HAGINS and YOSHIKAMI (1974), which suggests that Ca^{2+} is the intracellular transmitter of the light signal. Cyclic GMP also may be an intermediate in the visual process, but its role is not clearly established as yet (HUBBELL and BOWNDS 1979).

a) Localization of Cyclic GMP in Rod Photoreceptors

Fully developed, rod-dominant retinas from several species including rat, mouse, rabbit, cow, frog and toad have the highest concentrations of cyclic GMP of any tissue studied (FARBER and LOLLEY 1974, 1977a; GORIDIS et al. 1974, 1977; KRISHNA et al. 1976; FERRENDELLI and COHEN 1976). In fact, the levels of cyclic GMP in retinas dominated by rods are more than tenfold those in cerebellum and about 100 times higher than those in any other regions of the central nervous system (FERRENDELLI 1978). Studies of developing rod-dominant retinas indicate that cyclic GMP is concentrated in the photoreceptors, since its levels rise as the visual cells differentiate and the outer segments grow and mature (FARBER and LOLLEY 1977a). Work with dystrophic retinas of mice (FARBER and LOLLEY 1974, 1977a), rats (LOLLEY and FARBER 1976) and dogs (AGUIRRE et al. 1978), described in Section IV of this chapter, confirm the localization of cyclic GMP in rod photoreceptors. Furthermore, in duplex retinas of human and monkey, cyclic GMP levels are found to vary by area. They are highest in "rod rich" zones (peripheral retina) and lowest in the "cone rich" macula (central retina), also indicating localization in rod photoreceptors (NEWSOME et al. 1980). In addition, quantitative histochemistry of rabbit and monkey retina shows that 90% of the total cyclic GMP is found in the photoreceptor cells, with a great enrichment in rod outer segments. The remaining cyclic GMP (10%) is distributed across the layers of the inner retina (ORR et al. 1976; BERGER et al. 1980). Consistent with these data, isolated rod outer segment preparations from frog and cow retinas have very high levels of cyclic GMP (FLETCHER and CHADER 1976; WOODRUFF et al. 1977).

b) Modulation of Cyclic GMP Concentration by Light

Light lowers the cyclic GMP content of rod-dominant retinas, in vivo and in vitro, and of isolated rod outer segments (GORIDIS et al. 1974, 1977; FLETCHER and CHADER 1976; BRODIE and BOWNDS 1976; FERRENDELLI and COHEN 1976; KRISHNA et al. 1976; FARBER and LOLLEY 1977a; WOODRUFF et al. 1977; COHEN et al. 1978; MITZEL et al. 1978; DE AZEREDO et al. 1978; WOODRUFF and BOWNDS 1979). Microdissection of rabbit retina shows that light affects the cyclic nucleotide content of the whole photoreceptor cells and not only that of the outer segments. Cyclic GMP of the inner retina is unchanged by light (ORR et al. 1976).

If cyclic GMP plays a role in visual transduction (FARBER et al. 1978), the effect of light on the cyclic GMP concentration of the photoreceptor cells must be rapid since rods hyperpolarize within milliseconds of light stimulation. Such an involvement of cyclic GMP in the phototransduction process is evidenced by the studies of WOODRUFF et al. (1977) and WOODRUFF and BOWNDS (1979) on isolated rod outer segments of frog. They found that the decrease in cyclic GMP content of the outer segments caused by illumination has a half-time of approximately 125 milliseconds. With light exposures that bleach less than 100 rhodopsin molecules in each outer segment, at least 10^4 to 10^5 molecules of cyclic GMP are hydrolyzed for each rhodopsin molecule bleached. With continuous illumination, the decrease in cyclic GMP concentration becomes larger as illumination increases, and varies linearly with the logarithm of light intensity at levels that bleach between 5×10^1 and 5×10^4 rhodopsin molecules/outer segment/second. Over this same range of light intensities the ionic permeability of rod outer segments is suppressed, as assayed in vitro by BRODIE and BOWNDS (1976). Therefore, the reduction of cyclic GMP by light in rod outer segments is rapid and it represents a large amplification of the light signal.

An issue that still is unresolved is why experiments in which whole retinas are illuminated give much slower decreases in cyclic GMP content than those using rod outer segments. KILBRIDE and EBREY (1979) and LOLLEY et al. (1979b) showed recently that the decrease of whole retina cyclic GMP levels by light requires several seconds. In experiments of this kind, however, it seems that cyclic GMP levels are maximally influenced by low light intensities, near the physiological working range of the rods. Thus, following a strong flash of light, it takes a full minute before a significant reduction in cyclic GMP levels is observed; whereas a weaker flash causes a fall in cyclic GMP concentration in only 3 s and an almost maximal response after 30 s (GORIDIS et al. 1977); 30–60 s of a continuous bleaching light are required to decrease the cyclic GMP content of incubated mouse retina by 70% (MITZEL et al. 1978).

The time course for the recovery of cyclic GMP content to dark-adapted levels after light exposures varies according to the intensity of the light or the length of the exposure. It is slower the greater the light intensity (WOODRUFF and BOWNDS 1979); for example, after exposure of frog rod outer segments to light bleaching 5×10^5 molecules of rhodopsin per outer segment per second for 2 ms, cyclic GMP recovers in less than 10 s, but after 1 s or 10 s of illumination, 10–20 s are required for recovery of cyclic GMP content. With whole retinas, the time that it takes cyclic GMP to recover to the dark-adapted concentrations is even longer. In frog retinas, it occurs within 30–60 s under continuous, very dim illumination even when the bleaching light remains turned on (KILBRIDE and EBREY 1979). Rat retinas exposed for 2–5 s to light that bleaches about 2% rhodopsin per second, in vivo, recover their cyclic GMP content in approximately 3 min. Longer exposures (30–60 s) cause recovery periods of more than 6 min (LOLLEY et al. 1979a).

c) Other Factors that Affect Cyclic GMP Levels

Several factors that modulate the content of cyclic GMP in rod-dominant retinas or their outer segments have been studied. For example, when dark-adapted retinas of mice are incubated in a medium in which the calcium concentration has been lowered with 3 m*M* EGTA, a 10- to 20-fold increase in the cyclic GMP content is observed, peaking at 2–3 min (COHEN et al. 1978). In contrast, increasing the external calcium levels, even in the presence of the ionophore A 23187, causes no depression of cyclic GMP content. The same kind of results are reported for rod outer segment preparations. WOODRUFF and BOWNDS (1979) have shown that calcium ions at concentrations between 10^{-8} and 10^{-5} *M* lower the level of cyclic GMP; however, increasing the external Ca^{2+} above millimolar concentrations does not influence the cyclic GMP content of isolated rod outer segments. Thus, both cyclic GMP levels and the permeability of the plasma membrane of the rod photoreceptor are functions of Ca^{2+}. Lowering of the Ca^{2+} concentration depolarizes the membrane of the dark-adapted rod (LIPTON et al. 1977a; BROWN et al. 1977) and increases the permeability of the outer segment (BOWNDS and BRODIE 1975). Conversely, the permeability of the rod photoreceptors is suppressed if the Ca^{2+} concentration is raised, mimicking the effect of light.

The effect of phosphodiesterase inhibitors such as papaverine and isobutylmethylxanthine (IBMX) on cyclic GMP levels has also been investigated. Papaverine does not influence cyclic GMP levels in the dark nor reduce the light response in incubated mouse retinas (COHEN et al. 1978). In rod outer segments of frog, addition of papaverine prevents the decay in cyclic GMP levels that usually occurs during the preparation of the samples (BRODIE and BOWNDS 1976); however, papaverine does not influence the amount of illumination required to decrease cyclic GMP levels; in other words, it does not affect the light sensitivity of the cyclic GMP decrease. In contrast, IBMX shows a dose-related inhibition of the light-induced decrease in cyclic GMP content in incubated rat retinas (LOLLEY et al. 1979b), suggesting the involvement of phosphodiesterase in this effect. In addition, COHEN et al. (1978) indicate that the dark and light cyclic GMP levels of mouse retinas are increased when IBMX (1 m*M*) is present in the incubation medium.

Ischemia depresses cyclic GMP levels in dark-adapted retinas of mice in situ, but has no effect in light-adapted retinas (MITZEL et al. 1978). In incubated retinas, anoxia produced by the action of sodium cyanide decreases energy reserves such as ATP and phosphocreatine, regardless of the conditions of illumination, but has little or no effect on the cyclic GMP content. This suggests that cyclic GMP levels are not influenced by changes in the membrane potential of the rod photoreceptor, since potassium cyanide (10 m*M*) abolishes rapidly the "dark current" and photovoltage of rods in incubated rat retina (PENN and HAGINS 1969). Consistent with this observation, agents known to depolarize rods such as high potassium levels or ouabain, when added to the incubation medium of intact mouse retina, do not modify the dark levels of cyclic GMP nor the response to light (COHEN et al. 1978; GORIDIS et al. 1977). Thus, the rod-dominant retina responds differently from other brain regions where depolarizing agents permit the influx of Ca^{2+} and increase cyclic GMP concentration (FERRENDELLI et al. 1976). In addition, neither sodium aspartate, which uncouples the electrical activity of the photoreceptor cells from the inner retinal layers (PENN and HAGINS 1969; SILLMAN et al. 1969), nor taurine, which also depresses the electrical activity of the inner layers (PASANTES-MORALES et al. 1972), has an effect on the dark values or the light-induced decrease of cyclic GMP levels (GORIDIS et al. 1977). These results provide further evidence that the changes in cyclic GMP levels occur specifically in the photoreceptor cells.

d) Synthesis of Cyclic GMP

Guanylate cyclase, the enzyme that catalyzes the synthesis of cyclic GMP from GTP, is found essentially in all tissues studied (GOLDBERG and HADDOX 1977). The highest activity reported thus far is that observed in bovine rod outer segment preparations, which contain approximately 90% of the total retinal guanylate cyclase activity (VIRMAUX et al. 1976). Thus, only minimal levels of cyclic GMP synthesis occur in the inner retinal layers. Quantitative histochemistry of light-adapted rabbit and monkey retinas indicates that guanylate cyclase activity, as well as the concentration of its substrate GTP, are highest in the photoreceptor outer segments (BERGER et al. 1980). Furthermore, FLEISCHMAN and DENISEVICH (1979) have recently shown that the enzyme is localized mainly in the ciliary axonemes, basal bodies and centrioles of bovine rod outer segments. Confirmation of this distribution has been obtained by subjecting retinal homogenates to centrifugation in a continuous sucrose gradient. Under these conditions, guanylate cyclase activity coincides with the peak of rhodopsin content, and it sediments with the rhodopsin-bearing membranes (ZIMMERMAN et al. 1976; VIRMAUX et al. 1976). In addition, developmental studies of mice retina show a close correspondence between differentiation of the photoreceptor cells and growth of their outer segments and the postnatal increases in the activity of guanylate cyclase (FARBER and LOLLEY 1976). There is evidence also which shows that in the inherited retinal degeneration of *rd* mice, guanylate cyclase activity decreases with photoreceptor cell death (FARBER and LOLLEY 1976).

Both soluble and particulate forms of guanylate cyclase have been found in homogenates of several tissues (KIMURA and MURAD 1974). Homogenates of mouse retina contain about three times more particulate than soluble guanylate cyclase (TROYER et al. 1978). However, the enzyme from rod outer segments appears to be entirely membrane-associated. It is not washed off by low or high ionic strength buffers in combination with repeated freezing and thawing (GORIDIS et al. 1976), and it is not solubilized by detergent treatment. In fact, treatment with even a low concentration of Triton X-100 or Ammonyx causes a loss of enzyme activity (KRISHNAN et al. 1978; TROYER et al. 1978; BENSINGER et al. 1974a).

The soluble and particulate guanylate cyclases from mouse retina follow Michaelis-Menten kinetics. The K_m for GTP of the soluble enzyme is 7×10^{-5} *M*, whereas the particulate fraction has two apparent K_m values. One of these is very similar to that of the soluble fraction, 4×10^{-5} *M*, whereas the other is an order of magnitude higher, 2.25×10^{-4} *M* (TROYER et al. 1978). This latter K_m seems to correspond to that of the enzyme from rod outer segments, since the guanylate cyclase of bovine rod outer segments has a K_m for GTP of $2.27–4 \times 10^{-4}$ *M* (BENSINGER et al. 1974a; GORIDIS and WELLER 1976). Rather than suggesting that two K_m values in the outer segments indicate the presence of two separate enzymes, KRISHNAN et al. (1978) consider also the possibility of a single particulate guanylate cyclase exhibiting a negative cooperative interaction with GTP.

Manganese is the preferred cation for retinal guanylate cyclases. Ca^{2+} and Mg^{2+} are only 20–30% as effective as Mn^{2+} with the soluble enzyme (TROYER et al. 1978). With the rod outer segment guanylate cyclase, maximal activity is obtained using a 1:1 ratio between Mn^{2+} and GTP, which indicates that a Mn-GTP complex is the substrate in the reaction rather than GTP alone (KRISHNAN et al. 1978). Ca^{2+} (2–3 m*M*) stimulates the activity of guanylate cyclase in bovine and human rod outer segments, whereas it inhibits at higher concentrations (PANNBACKER 1973a, 1974). Mg^{2+} was the cofactor in these experiments, which allowed the observation of the effect of other cations, since Mg^{2+} supports only 10% of the guanylate cyclase activity determined with Mn^{2+} as cofactor. With Mn^{2+} in the reaction mixture, Ba^{2+}, Ca^{2+}, Mg^{2+} and Co^{2+} inhibit the enzyme when tested in the range of 0.1–0.5 m*M* (KRISHNAN et al. 1978). It remains to be established which cofactor is used by guanylate cyclase of the outer segments in situ. This is an important issue since, in vitro, the presence or absence of Mn^{2+} determines whether Ca^{2+} activates or inhibits the enzyme.

Several agents known to activate guanylate cyclase from brain and other tissues have been tested on the retinal enzyme/s. At 1 m*M* concentrations, ITP is a potent inhibitor of guanylate cyclase from bovine rod outer segment, whereas ATP and UTP inhibit the enzyme by about 30%. Concentrations of 0.1 and 0.01 m*M* ATP appear to stimulate this guanylate cyclase by a mechanism which is unresolved (KRISHNAN et al. 1978). None of the guanylate cyclase fractions from mouse retina is activated or inhibited by sodium azide or hydroxylamine (TROYER et al. 1978). Prostaglandin F_2, carbamylcholine, glutamic acid, insulin and cholera enterotoxin do not affect the activity of the enzyme from frog rod outer segments (BITENSKY et al. 1975, 1978).

The initial reports of guanylate cyclase activity in rod outer segments suggested that the enzyme is inhibited by light (PANNBACKER 1973a; 1974; BENSINGER et al. 1974b; KRISHNA et al. 1976). However, a difficult technical problem has to be overcome in the determination of the light effect on retinal guanylate cyclase. Since the activity of phosphodiesterase in the retina is very high, guanylate cyclase measurements depend upon the ability of phosphodiesterase inhibitors to block the degradation of cyclic GMP during the time of the assay. Inhibitors of phosphodiesterase are not completely effective and, in addition, phosphodiesterase is activated by light in the presence of GTP (see below). Thus, the assay of guanylate cyclase activity reflects degradation as well as synthesis during the time of incubation and it is difficult to distinguish between light-inhibition of guanylate cyclase and light-activation of phosphodiesterase. The inclusion of (^{3}H)-cyclic GMP in the reaction mixture allows correction for the loss of cyclic nucleotide during the assay. Using a variety of conditions for the preparation of rod outer segments, GORIDIS et al. (1975) found no effect of light on guanylate cyclase activity. In some experiments, they first eliminated the phosphodiesterase from outer segments by washing the preparation with hypotonic buffer and then measured guanylate cyclase (GORIDIS et al. 1973). However, the hypotonic conditions could have damaged the rod outer segments with the concomitant loss of light sensitivity. In other experiments, Goridis and Virmaux (1974) prelabeled the nucleotide pool with (^{3}H)-hypoxanthine and measured guanylate cyclase in the presence of the phosphodiesterase inhibitor SQ 20,009. No light effect was observed in any case. Recently, BITENSKY et al. (1978) also reported that, contrary to what they had described before, guanylate cyclase of frog rod outer segments is unchanged by illumination. These authors used 10^{-3} M GTP to irreversibly inhibit phosphodiesterase (see below). Whether light affects guanylate cyclase in situ remains an open question.

e) Degradation of Cyclic GMP

High levels of cyclic nucleotide phosphodiesterase activity are observed in the retina. This activity comprises several classes of phosphodiesterases, as has been shown by developmental studies of animals possessing normal or degenerative retinas (SCHMIDT and LOLLEY 1973; LOLLEY and FARBER 1975; FARBER and LOLLEY 1976). Kinetic analysis of microdissected samples of frozen-dried retinas show two cyclic nucleotide phosphodiesterases in the inner layers and one, or perhaps more, in the photoreceptor cells (LOLLEY and FARBER 1975; PANNBACKER and LOVETT 1977). The enzyme of the rod visual cells, which hydrolyzes cyclic GMP, is the one that has received most of the attention. It has been isolated and purified by different laboratories and characterized in terms of cofactors and light regulation. The phosphodiesterases from the inner layers of the retina have not been studied as yet. They may be very similar to the phosphodiesterases present in the brain; at least, they have comparable K_m values for cyclic AMP and cyclic GMP.

Cyclic GMP phosphodiesterase appears to play a key role in mediating the light regulation of retinal cyclic GMP levels. The enzyme is activated by bleached rhodopsin in the presence of a nucleoside triphosphate (MIKI et al. 1973; GORIDIS and VIRMAUX 1974; CHADER et al. 1974a; MANTHORPE and MCCONNELL 1975) and, in a matter of milliseconds, it reduces the high cyclic GMP content of the dark-adapted photoreceptors. The speed and amplification of the phosphodiesterase reaction (YEE and LIEBMAN 1978) suggest that the light-activated hydrolysis of cyclic GMP could be a stage in visual transduction.

The cyclic nucleotide phosphodiesterase from rod photoreceptors has been localized histochemically in the outer segments; it appears to be on but not between the outer segment lamellae. The adjacent inner segment or the nuclear regions of the rod does not show any phosphodiesterase activity (ROBB 1974a, 1978). PANN-

BACKER and LOVETT (1977) analyzed the cyclic nucleotide phosphodiesterases of the outer layer of the bovine retina using quantitative histochemistry. They found that with either cyclic AMP or cyclic GMP as substrates, the enzyme of the outer segments has the highest specific activity. This has been confirmed by BERGER et al. (1980). Considerable activity is observed also in the outer plexiform layer. However, the phosphodiesterase activity of the outer plexiform layer has different kinetic characteristics than that of the outer segments (PANNBACKER and LOVETT 1977).

Although the rod outer segment phosphodiesterase can hydrolyze cyclic AMP and cyclic GMP in vitro, it displays a marked preference for cyclic GMP. For example, when cyclic nucleotides at a concentration of 10^{-7} M are used as substrates, the hydrolysis of cyclic GMP is 23 times greater than that of cyclic AMP (BITENSKY et al. 1973). Cyclic AMP and cyclic GMP appear to compete for the same active site on the phosphodiesterase molecule, causing inhibition of either substrate when tested in combination (CHADER et al. 1974a). As determined by several laboratories using retinal preparations from different species, K_m values for cyclic GMP are in the 10^{-4} to 10^{-5} M range, whereas the K_m values for cyclic AMP are at least one order of magnitude higher, in the 10^{-3} M range (PANNBACKER et al. 1972; CHADER et al. 1974a; LOLLEY and FARBER 1975; MANTHORPE and MCCONNELL 1975; MIKI et al. 1975; FARBER and LOLLEY 1977a; YEE and LIEBMAN 1978). K_m values are identical for the dark- or light-activated enzyme (YEE and LIEBMAN 1978; MIKI et al. 1975). However, V_{max} values vary with illumination suggesting that light does not change the affinity of phosphodiesterase for cyclic GMP but increases the number of enzyme molecules available for the hydrolysis of cyclic GMP. 2′,3′-GMP monophosphate is not a substrate for the rod phosphodiesterase.

Magnesium or Mn^{2+} is essential for maximal enzyme activity, with Mg^{2+} being the preferred cation. Addition of EDTA to the reaction mixture abolishes phosphodiesterase activity. This effect of EDTA can be reversed by the addition of Mg^{2+} (CHADER et al. 1974b). Unlike cyclic GMP-phosphodiesterase from brain, the rod outer segment phosphodiesterase is not activited by Ca^{2+}, even in the presence of added calmodulin from brain (BITENSKY et al. 1975). In fact, Ca^{2+} inhibits enzyme activity with 90% inhibition observed at 1.0 mM concentration. Addition of EGTA or Mg^{2+} (200 μM) restores phosphodiesterase activity (CHADER et al. 1974b; YEE and LIEBMAN 1978).

The methylxanthines, which usually are very effective inhibitors of phosphodiesterase in most tissues, do not block completely the activity of the enzyme from rod outer segments (PANNBACKER et al. 1972; MIKI et al. 1973; CHADER et al. 1974b, 1974d). However, IBMX, which is more effective than theophylline or caffeine, is the best of all compounds that have been tested including papaverine, SQ 20,009, dipyridamol (Persantine), triiodothyronine and the dibutyryl derivative of cyclic AMP. This, plus the fact that all inhibitors affect similarly cyclic AMP and cyclic GMP hydrolyses, suggests that a single class of phosphodiesterase from rod outer segments is able to degrade in vitro both cyclic nucleotides.

Rhodopsin mediates the effects of light on the rod outer segment phosphodiesterase activity. There is excellent correspondence between the action spectrum for the activation of the disc membrane phosphodiesterase and the absorption spectrum of rhodopsin. Both spectra have a maximum at 500 nm (KEIRNS et al. 1975).

In contrast, all-trans retinal does not mimic the effect of light on phosphodiesterase activity (KEIRNS et al. 1974; GORIDIS et al. 1976).

At low light intensities, bleaching of rhodopsin is proportional to the duration and intensity of the light exposure. KEIRNS et al. (1975) estimated that half-maximal activation of phosphodiesterase from frog rod outer segments is achieved during a light exposure that bleaches 1 in 2,000 rhodopsin molecules (0.05% of the total number of rhodopsin molecules/outer segment). The method used by these authors to assess phosphodiesterase activity quantifies the amount of 5′-GMP or guanosine formed following the quenching of the reaction at a determined period of incubation. KEIRNS et al. (1975) and GORIDIS et al. (1976) also found that it is possible to activate phosphodiesterase by mixing unbleached disc membranes with bleached membranes. In this case, though, the activation of phosphodiesterase is less effective than when direct light bleaches rhodopsin on the membranes, since half-maximal activation occurs with a 1% admixture of bleached membranes (KEIRNS et al. 1975). Regeneration of bleached rhodopsin by addition of 11-cis retinal to illuminated disc membranes blocks the ability of these membranes to activate phosphodiesterase in unilluminated outer segments.

Recently, YEE and LIEBMAN (1978) measured phosphodiesterase activity by monitoring continuously the proton release that accompanies cyclic nucleotide hydrolysis. With this procedure, they determined that half-maximal activation occurs with bleaches of 1 in 80,000 molecules of rhodopsin and they estimated a hydrolytic rate of about 4×10^5 cyclic GMP/second caused when one molecule of rhodopsin is bleached. YEE and LIEBMAN (1978) found also that the ratio between light and dark phosphodiesterase activities is a function of the concentration of the disc membrane suspension. For frog membranes, with a concentration of 16.4 μM rhodopsin, the activity ratio is 66 and, for bovine preparations, with 13.4 μM rhodopsin, it is 230. For each species, however, the light-stimulated phosphodiesterase activity increases linearly with increasing concentrations of rhodopsin, whereas the dark phosphodiesterase activity remains low.

Activation of phosphodiesterase by light requires the presence of a nucleoside triphosphate (CHADER et al. 1974c; BITENSKY et al. 1975; MANTHORPE and MCCONNELL 1975). In general, the purine nucleotides support the light activation of phophodiesterase better than the pyrimidine triphosphates. GTP is the most effective, and it causes maximal activation at very low concentrations, in the 10^{-7} to 10^{-8} M range (WHEELER and BITENSKY 1977; YEE and LIEBMAN 1978). ITP is less effective by threefold than GTP; XTP and ATP required 100-fold higher concentrations. GDP is also effective, although it is not clear if the activation is produced by GDP itself or by GTP present as a contaminant or produced by enzymatic conversion of GDP. The methylene and imido analogs of ATP do not support phosphodiesterase activation by light, but GMP-PNP can substitute for GTP, suggesting that GTP is an allosteric effector rather than an energy or phosphate donor (WHEELER and BITENSKY 1977; YEE and LIEBMAN 1978). Other triphosphates or high energy phosphates such as thiamine triphosphate, tripolyphosphate, phosphoenol pyruvate or creatine phosphate have no effect (BITENSKY et al. 1975).

The maximal rate of phosphodiesterase activity is not achieved immediately. The enzyme activity increases gradually from the dark level with a lag time that depends upon the species of nucleoside triphosphate used in the reaction, its concentration, and the amount of bleach caused by light. For example, at 200 μ*M* GTP, lag time is $\leqq 100$ ms with light intensities that produce a 0.4–4.0% bleach. Increasing either the concentration of the nucleoside triphosphate or the bleach shortens the lag time (YEE and LIEBMAN 1978). In these studies, it is observed that once the lag is over, the hydrolysis of cyclic nucleotide increases linearly with time. Thus, enzyme activation appears to follow zero-order kinetics. In addition, a spontaneous deactivation of light-GTP-activated phosphodiesterase occurs following first-order kinetics, which is attributed to a light-activated reaction that consumes GTP. This is supported by the fact that activation with the non-hydrolyzable analogue of GTP, GMP-PNP, does not exhibit the phosphodiesterase activity decay (WHEELER and BITENSKY 1977).

YEE and LIEBMAN (1978) calculated from a specific activity of phosphodiesterase of 4×10^5 cyclic GMP/second/molecule of bleached rhodopsin and a turnover number of 800/s (MIKI et al. 1973) that 500 phosphodiesterase molecules are activated by bleaching one molecule of rhodopsin. This multiplier mechanism could provide extraordinary gain to the system. Furthermore, the activity of phosphodiesterase is compatible with the high rate of cyclic GMP hydrolysis observed in outer segments following illumination (WOODRUFF and BOWNDS 1979).

Free sulfhydryl groups are implicated in the activation by light and nucleoside triphosphate of phosphodiesterase. Activation can be blocked by organic mercurials; this effect can be reversed by the addition of dithiothrietol or other sulfhydryl donors (CHADER et al. 1974d, BITENSKY et al. 1975). Also, aging of the disc membranes prevents activation by light-nucleotide triphosphate; this is similarly reversed by dithiothreitol. This suggests that the labile sulfhydryl group must be in a reduced form for activation to occur.

Other agents such as non-ionic detergents can activate the phosphodiesterase of rod outer segments without the need of light. Triton X-100 (0.01%) increases by twofold the hydrolysis of cyclic GMP, but higher concentrations inhibit phosphodiesterase activity (CHADER et al. 1974b). Lubrol also increases cyclic nucleotide hydrolysis (PANNBACKER et al. 1972). Homogenization of dark-adapted rod outer segments with a glass-on-glass homogenizer renders phosphodiesterase fully activated. This activation is shown to be caused by silicate released from the homogenizer. Another polyanion, heparin, also fully activates phosphodiesterase in the absence of light and nucleoside triphosphate. In contrast, polyglutamine and anions such as chloride, sulfate, and phosphate do not increase phosphodiesterase activity (BITENSKY et al. 1975). Several polycations, including protamine, histone, polylysine and polyarginine, also activate phosphodiesterase (BITENSKY et al. 1975).

Phosphodiesterase is firmly bound to the disc membranes, but can be eluted from the membranes by hypoosmotic shock. The omission of Mg^{2+} from the buffer or the sequestering of Mg^{2+} by EDTA facilitates the extraction (MIKI et al. 1975; COQUIL et al. 1975). Magnesium appears to promote binding of the enzyme to the disc membranes (BITENSKY et al. 1975). MANTHORPE and MCCONNELL (1975) released the enzyme by homogenization of the rod outer segments in isotonic sucrose, and BIGNETTI et al. (1978) used mannitol. This eluted phosphodiesterase has reduced activity, but can be activated by polycations. Protamine appears to aggregate the soluble phosphodiesterase at the same time that it activates the enzyme, since more than 95% of protamine-stimulated activity is removed from solution by centrifugation at 10,000 × g for 15 min. Protamine increases the V_{max} without changing the K_m for cyclic GMP (MIKI et al. 1975). In contrast, light and nucleoside triphosphates do not increase the solubilized phosphodiesterase activity (MANTHORPE and MCCONNELL 1975), and neither do polyanions or N-ethylmaleimide (BITENSKY et al. 1975). SITARAMAYYA et al (1977a) reported that whereas phosphodiesterase has to be in the rod outer segment membranes to be activated by light, bleached rhodopsin in the presence of ATP can activate the soluble enzyme once it has been extracted from the discs. Both the extracted phosphodiesterase and the enzyme in the discs can be activated also by potassium fluoride (SITARAMAYYA et al. 1977b). More than 50% of the released phosphodiesterase activity can be restored to the disc membranes when incubated with $MgCl_2$ (2 m*M*) and KCl (100 m*M*). However, some controlling elements may be lost during the off-on process, because when back on the membranes, the enzyme can be only partially reactivated by light and nucleoside triphosphate, i.e., sensitivity to light is reduced (BITENSKY et al. 1975).

Cyclic GMP-phosphodiesterase from frog rod outer segments has been purified by binding the eluted enzyme to agarose-polyhistidine (MIKI et al. 1975) after subjecting it to a continuous sucrose gradient (5–20% w/v). Rod outer segment phosphodiesterase does not bind to carboxymethyl-cellulose; it binds but does not elute from DEAE-cellulose with buffers of pH from 4.5–10. Phosphodiesterase is eluted from the agarose-polyhistidine column with imidazole buffer (100 m*M*). The overall purification of the enzyme is 185-fold if the phosphodiesterase eluted from the rod outer segments is considered as the starting material. The enzyme accounts for approximately 0.5% of the disc membrane protein; it has an isoelectric point of 5.7 and a sedimentation coefficient of 12.4 S which corresponds to a molecular weight of about 240,000. SDS-gel electrophoresis separates the purified enzyme into two subunits of 120,000 and 110,000 molecular weight. The K_m value of this phosphodiesterase for cyclic GMP is 70 μ*M*, lower than that of the enzyme bound to the disc membranes. The solubilized enzyme has also a lower pH optimum (7.5) than the disc-bound phosphodiesterase (8.0), and one-fourth of its total amino acid residues is contributed by aspartic and glutamic acids or their amides.

Partial proteolysis activates the purified phosphodiesterase to a greater extent than protamine. The trypsin-treated enzyme has a sedimentation coefficient of 7.8 S, which corresponds to an approximate molecular weight of 170,000. Only the 110,000-dalton subunit is affected by trypsin, and it is replaced by smaller fragments. MIKI et al. (1975) calculate a catalytic constant of 48,000 molecules of cyclic GMP hydrolyzed/min/mol of enzyme, based on a specific activity of 185 μmol of cyclic GMP hydrolyzed/min/mg of protein obtained after purification (using 2 m*M* cyclic GMP as substrate) and a molecular weight of 240,000.

Mammalian rod outer segments possess a cyclic GMP phosphodiesterase with some characteristics apparently different from those of the phosphodiesterase from frog rod outer segments. The enzyme from bovine photoreceptors has been partially purified using, sequentially, DEAE-cellulose and G-100 Sephadex chromatography (COQUIL et al. 1975). The resulting phosphodiesterase has a specific activity of 1.1–7.0 μmol cyclic GMP hydrolyzed/min/mg protein at 10 μ*M* substrate measured without the addition of activators. Freezing and thawing causes loss of enzyme activity; the same kind of observation has been made for crude rod outer segment phosphodiesterase (CHADER et al. 1974b; MANTHORPE and MCCONNELL 1975).

Polyacrylamide gel electrophoresis of the partially purified phosphodiesterase separates one major and three minor proteins (COQUIL et al. 1975). All of the activity is associated with the major band. SDS-gel electrophoresis of the enzyme eluted from the native gel shows a molecular weight of 105,000, which is approximately the same as that obtained by gel filtration on the G-100 Sephadex column. In contrast to the phosphodiesterase from frog rod outer segments, the bovine enzyme purified by COQUIL et al. (1975) does not give a doublet on SDS-gel electrophoresis. In addition, complex kinetics for cyclic GMP hydrolysis are observed with the purified enzyme. The plot of velocity vs. substrate concentration is hyperbolic at concentrations lower than 3 μM and sigmoidal at higher concentrations. These investigators could not estimate a K_m value because of the complex shape of the curve. They speculated that the anomalous kinetics could arise from phosphodiesterase showing negative cooperativity at low and positive cooperativity at higher concentrations. This means that a build-up of cyclic GMP levels would be favored by the negatively cooperative kinetics, whereas higher concentrations of cyclic GMP would prevent a further rise. Upon storage of the purified enzyme at 4 °C, the complex kinetics change, approaching Michaelis-Menten behavior, and the phosphodiesterase activity increases. These characteristics are not described for the phosphodiesterase from frog rod outer segments. However, MIKI et al. (1975) may not have used concentrations low enough to reveral the unusual kinetics. With cyclic AMP as substrate, the purified enzyme displays normal kinetics, with an apparent K_m of 0.1 mM.

Recently, similar purification of bovine phosphodiesterase by DEAE-cellulose and G-100 or G-200 Sephadex chromatography has been reported (BAEHR et al. 1979; HURLEY and EBREY 1979). Some of the characteristics of the enzyme isolated by BAEHR et al. (1979) differ from those reported by COQUIL et al. (1975). For example, the molecular weight of phosphodiesterase assessed by sucrose gradient centrifugation and analytical ultracentrifugation is 170,000, similar to the molecular weight of the frog phosphodiesterase after trypsin treatment (MIKI et al. 1975). In addition, two subunits (doublet, 88,000 and 84,000), and a third polypeptide (13,000 daltons) could be separated by SDS-gel electrophoresis. These authors also determined an isoelectric pH of 5.0–5.5 for the bovine phosphodiesterase. HURLEY and EBREY (1979) also found the doublet at 84,000 and 88,000 daltons on SDS gel electrophoresis, but their phosphodiesterase elutes from a Sephadex G-200 column with an apparent molecular weight of 340,000. Probably two phosphodiesterase molecules aggregate to form a dimer, since the molecular weight is exactly double that reported by BAEHR et al. (1979).

There is an obligatory sequence in the activation of phosphodiesterase: photoisomerization of rhodopsin must precede the GTP-dependent step (WHEELER and BITENSKY 1977). The function of GTP in this activation is still an unresolved problem, but several studies on this subject have provided valuable information. For example, it has been shown that the nucleoside triphosphate does not participate in the activation of phosphodiesterase by phosphorylating bleached rhodopsin (SITARAMAYYA et al. 1977a). In addition, CHADER et al. (1976) have shown that no radioactivity is associated with phosphodiesterase following light-stimulated incubation with (α^{32}P)-GTP or (α^{32}P)-ATP, and MIKI et al. (1973) indicated that exogenous kinases do not mimic the effects of illumination when added to the unilluminated rod outer segments nor stimulate phosphodiesterase in lighted photoreceptor material. Furthermore, SITARAMAYYA et al. (1977a) have reported that phosphorylated opsin does not activate solubilized phosphodiesterase and that phosphodiesterase is not adenylated by ATP. GTP may be involved in the production of an activator molecule, which could cause full expression of the hydrolytic activity, or GTP could be related to a mechanism of "disinhibition" of phosphodiesterase by causing the release of an inhibitory molecule attached to the enzyme.

Several laboratories have reported the finding of either an activator or an inhibitor of rod outer segment phosphodiesterase. GORIDIS et al. (1976) have observed that an endogenous soluble factor is lost during the isolation of rod outer segments. This soluble factor seems to be required for full expression of the light effect. Illumination appears to produce an activator which is resistant to digestion by trypsin, subtilisin, chymotrypsin or phospholipase C and to dialysis against EGTA (BITENSKY et al. 1975). Heating at 90 °C for 10 min and treatment with 0.5% Triton X-100 or 1.0% digitonin destroy the activator. The macromolecular activator remains associated with the disc membranes when these are sedimented to their equilibrium position in a sucrose density gradient; thus, it seems that the activator may be closely associated with bleached rhodopsin. In the presence of nucleoside triphosphate (0.75 m*M*), this activator causes a greater than fivefold increase in the V_{max} of the rod outer segment phosphodiesterase without changing the K_m. In contrast, the activator does not have any effect on the phosphodiesterase of other tissues such as rat liver, myocardium or brain.

Calmodulin, the calcium-dependent activator of phosphodiesterase, has been found in all subcellular fractions of bovine retina and outer segments (LIU and SCHWARTZ 1978). However, the phosphodiesterase activity measured in rod outer segments is calcium independent, since EGTA causes minimal or no depression of enzyme activity. Thus, the calmodulin of photoreceptors may have functions other than activating phosphodiesterase.

DUMLER and ETINGOF (1976) found that when retina or rod outer segments of oxen are treated in conditions identical to those used to extract calmodulin from brain (CHEUNG 1970), a protein inhibitor of phosphodiesterase is obtained instead of an activator. In the process of purification of this protein by gel filtration and anion exchange chromatography, an activator factor elutes in some fractions separated from the inhibitor. This activator has a molecular weight (15,000) similar to that of calmodulin and seems to be a necessary subunit of the whole inhibitory complex. In fact, addition of the activator to the purified inhibitor increases its inhibitory action on phosphodiesterase.

The inhibitory complex is trypsin-sensitive, and it is not tissue specific; that is, it inhibits phosphodiesterase from rod outer segments as well as other phosphodiesterases. This inhibitor has a molecular weight of 38,000 and it decreases the V_{max} but has no effect on the K_m of phosphodiesterase for cyclic AMP. The phosphodiesterase activity measured using cyclic AMP as substrate is more susceptible to inhibition than that determined with cyclic GMP as substrate. Furthermore, the soluble form of phosphodiesterase from rod outer segments is more sensitive to the inhibitor than the membrane bound enzyme. BERMAN and USOVA (1978) reported that this protein inhibitor of phosphodiesterase is localized in bovine rod outer segments, and it is not observed in the other retinal layers. Recently, HURLEY and EBREY (1979) studied a phosphodiesterase inhibitor from bovine retina which has properties similar to those of the compound described by DUMLER and ETINGOF (1976).

There are several characteristics of the phosphodiesterase from rod outer segments that seem to indicate the possibility for the enzyme to exist as a complex of a phosphodiesterase catalytic subunit and a regulatory subunit with inhibitory properties. For example, as mentioned above, purified phosphodiesterase is usually found as a doublet on SDS-polyacrylamide gels, and it is activated by protamine, which could act by dissociating the inhibitory subunit from the enzyme. In addition, anomalous concentration dependence of phosphodiesterase has been observed by YEE and LIEBMAN (1978), SITARAMAYYA et al. (1977b) and LOLLEY and FARBER (1978). At high concentrations of the enzyme, its specific activity becomes lower. Furthermore, BAEHR et al. (1979) found another protein of rod outer segments which inhibits phosphodiesterase activity. This compound is membrane-bound and is extracted with phosphodiesterase under hypotonic conditions in approximately equal molar amounts. It has two subunits of 39,000 and 37,000 molecular weight and, by gel filtration, the native protein elutes with an approximate molecular weight of 80,000. When this protein is added to purified phosphodiesterase from bovine rod outer segments in a 1:1 molar ratio, it inhibits 50% of the enzyme activity.

Another possible participation of GTP in the mechanism of activation of phosphodiesterase has been suggested by studies in several laboratories. GTP could function as an allosteric activator of the photoreceptor phosphodiesterase in a process that involves a light-activated GTPase (WHEELER et al. 1977). This GTPase shows remarkable sensitivity to light. Also, the action spectrum of GTPase corresponds perfectly to the absorption spectrum of rhodopsin. Half-maximal activation is observed when only 1 in 2,000–2,500 rhodopsin molecules is photoisomerized (BITENSKY et al. 1978; CARETTA et al. 1979). The enzyme can also be activated by mixing the unilluminated membranes with 1.0% of fully bleached discs, similar to that described for phosphodiesterase. BITENSKY et al. (1978) estimated that a single bleached rhodopsin molecule could activate both a GTPase and a phosphodiesterase molecule. The range of GTP concentrations over which light activation is observed is from 0.01–5.0 μM. The apparent K_m of the enzyme for GTP is 0.5 μM, with a V_{max} of about 500 pmoles of GTP hydrolyzed/min/mg protein. It is interesting to mention that the photoreceptor rod outer segments also have light insensitive GTPase activity. The requirements of GTP for this enzyme are much higher though than those for the light-activated GTPase; it has a K_m of 90 μM GTP and a V_{max} of 12 nmoles of GTP hydrolyzed/min/mg protein (WHEELER et al. 1977). The ionic requirements of the light-activated GTPase are not specific. The hydrolysis of GTP occurs in the presence or absence of magnesium and with or without calcium in the medium (BIGNETTI et al. 1978). WHEELER and BITENSKY (1977) have reported that the activation of phosphodiesterase by GTP shows a time-dependent decay which correlates with the light-activated GTPase activity. At a concentration of 0.2 μM, GMP-PNP completely inhibits the light-activated

GTPase and fully activates the rod outer segment phosphodiesterase. Under these conditions, the phosphodiesterase decay is not observed, since the levels of GTP remain high. These observations together with the analogous kinetic data of phosphodiesterase and light-activated GTPase led WHEELER and BITENSKY (1977) to conclude that the allosteric site at which GTP activates phosphodiesterase may correspond to the catalytic site of the light-activated GTPase.

The light-activated GTPase, together with cyclic GMP-phosphodiesterase can be quantitatively removed from the unilluminated rod outer segment disc membranes by washing with 1.0 mM EDTA (WHEELER et al. 1977) or with a low-salt mannitol (220 mM) solution (BIGNETTI et al. 1978). Both enzyme activities can be restored to the depleted disc membranes by addition of Mg^{2+} (5 mM) and the supernatant obtained by centrifugation of the washed rods, in the presence of light. The supernatant of the washed rods alone does not show GTPase activity, suggesting that the GTPase needs the integrity of the membrane to express itself, or that a soluble factor is released from the disc membranes when they are suspended in a low salt solution, leaving the membrane-bound GTPase inactive. However, a protein of 32,000 molecular weight in SDS-polyacrylamide gel electrophoresis, which is heat-labile and does not have phosphodiesterase activity, is associated with the GTPase activity of the supernatant as determined by gel filtration of the supernatant (WHEELER et al. 1977).

Other laboratories have reported similar and additional characteristics of the light-activated GTPase (ROBINSON and HAGINS 1977; KÜHN 1978, 1980a; GODCHAUX and ZIMMERMAN 1979). For example, GTPase is extracted from dark-kept rod outer segments with aqueous buffer either at low or very high ionic strength (5 mM Tris buffer or 1.0 M NH_4Cl) but not at moderate ionic strength. This suggests that the enzyme is a peripherally bound membrane protein, which needs extremes of ionic strength to be solubilized. Upon illumination, GTPase activity disappears from the supernatant and is again found on the rod outer segments membranes. This light-induced binding of GTPase is completely inhibited if GTP (0.1–1.0 mM) is present during illumination, and is quickly reversed if GTP is added in the dark after illumination (KÜHN 1980a). Taking advantage of these properties, it was possible to purify the enzyme in a relatively simple way. SDS-polyacrylamide gel electrophoresis showed three polypeptide subunits of the GTPase with molecular weights of 37,000, 35,000 and 5,000 (KÜHN 1980b). It is unclear whether the one versus three GTPase subunits reported by BITENSKY et al. (1978) and KÜHN (1980b), respectively, indicate species differences (frog vs. cow) or differences in the resolution of the SDS-gel electrophoresis experiments.

The concentrations of GTP found in illuminated rod outer segments are sufficient to support the full activation of phosphodiesterase. DE AZEREDO et al. (1978) have estimated that in vivo the GTP concentrations are 400 μM in dark-adapted rod outer segments, and 170 μM after 2 min of exposure to light. BIERNBAUM and BOWNDS (1979) have found that, in isolated rod outer segments, the light-induced decrease in GTP can be as large as 70%, it has a half-time of 7 s, and it is a linear function of the logarithm of continuous light intensity at levels which bleach between 5×10^2 and 5×10^6 rhodopsin molecules/outer segment/second. ROBINSON and HAGINS (1979) have obtained similar results. In addition, GTP concentration in dark-adapted rod outer segments can fall to the same level as that caused by light when the external Ca^{2+} is reduced to 10^{-8} *M*; restoration of millimolar levels of Ca^{2+} causes net synthesis of GTP (BIERNBAUM and BOWNDS 1979).

The loss of GTP in the deactivation step of phosphodiesterase is harder to explain. It has been proposed that bleached rhodopsin activates light-dependent GTPase which in turn hydrolyzes the GTP bound to phosphodiesterase and turns the enzyme off (BITENSKY et al. 1978). However, the activation of GTPase occurs only at GTP levels of 5 μ*M* or less, a value far below the concentration of GTP in vivo (DE AZEREDO et al., 1978). The only way of possibly interpreting the GTPase action would be to assume that GTP is compartmentalized in such a fashion that 98% of it is unavailable to the enzyme. Alternatively, phosphoryl transfer from the nucleoside triphosphate bound to phosphodiesterase (to bleached rhodopsin?) might be associated with deactivation. LIEBMAN and PUGH (1979) have described an ATP-mediated phosphodiesterase shut-off mechanism. When both ATP (0.5 m*M*) and GTP (0.25 m*M*) are present in the reaction medium, with cyclic GMP (1 m*M*) as substrate, individual flashes which bleach 10^{-4} molecules of rhodopsin cause only an approximate 100 μ*M* cyclic GMP turnover. If 0.25 m*M* GTP alone is present in the reaction, the same 10^{-4} bleach causes hydrolysis of all the cyclic GMP. The non-hydrolyzable GTP analogs that support activation cannot support turn-off. Furthermore, BIERNBAUM and BOWNDS (1979) found that only a small fraction (less than 5%) of the GTP degraded upon illumination is used to phosphorylate bleached rhodopsin. The phosphate group used for this purpose could be that provided by the shut-off mechanism of phosphodiesterase. Thus, both allosteric and phosphate transfer regulation appear to be involved in phosphodiesterase control.

f) Modulation of Protein Phosphorylation by Cyclic GMP

Cyclic nucleotides are known to express their actions through the activation of protein kinases which phosphorylate proteins selectively (GREENGARD 1976). These phosphoproteins, in turn, may be specifically involved in the regulation of functions that are fundamental to the cell, e.g. in neurons they have been implicated in the control of membrane permeability to certain ions (NATHANSON 1977).

Rod outer segments possess the necessary biochemical components for translating light-induced changes in cyclic GMP concentration into a physiologically significant message, i.e. a rod outer segment-specific phosphoprotein (LOLLEY et al. 1977a). In addition to the cyclic nucleotide-dependent phosphorylating system, rod outer segments have also a cyclic nucleotide-independent protein kinase which phosphorylates rhodopsin in a reaction that is strongly stimulated by light (BOWNDS et al. 1972; FRANK et al. 1973; KÜHN and DREYER 1972; KÜHN et al. 1973; WELLER et al. 1975, 1976; CHADER et al. 1976). The cyclic nucleotide independent phosphorylation of rhodopsin will not be considered in this chapter. For a review of the subject, see FARBER and LOLLEY (1979).

The first report indicating the presence of a cyclic nucleotide-dependent phosphorylation reaction in rod outer segment preparations is that of PANNBACKER (1973b). However, most of the work done on protein kinases of rod outer segments failed to corroborate any involvement of cyclic nucleotides in the incorporation of phosphate molecules into protein. The reason for this lack of effect of cyclic nucleotides on the protein kinases studied is simple. Cyclic nucleotides stimulate a protein kinase of the rod outer segments only when it is in soluble form, but do not activate the enzyme when it is associated with the disc membranes (LOLLEY et al. 1977a).

When isolated bovine rod outer segments are extracted with Tris buffer, pH 7.6, protein kinase activity is partitioned, after centrifugation at $100{,}000 \times g$, into a soluble and a membrane-bound form, and the membrane kinase can be solubilized by the detergent Lubrol PX. The soluble and membrane-solubilized activities are both unaffected by light and stimulated by cyclic nucleotides, and they phosphorylate exogenous histones used as substrates (LOLLEY et al. 1977a). Half-maximal stimulation is observed at 1×10^{-7} M cyclic AMP and $4\text{–}5 \times 10^{-6}$ M cyclic GMP (FARBER et al. 1979a). The Lubrol PX-solubilized kinase is activated 5–6 times by cyclic AMP and 4–5 times by cyclic GMP. This degree of activation is higher than that observed with the soluble, Tris-extracted enzyme, suggesting that detergents extract predominantly the holoenzyme from the rod outer segment membranes. The soluble enzyme may be already dissociated in situ, since cyclic GMP levels are high in dark-adapted rod outer segments.

DEAE-cellulose chromatography of the Tris-extract of rod outer segment resolves three peaks which show kinase activity; two of them correspond to the Type I and Type II cyclic AMP-dependent protein kinases described in most tissues (CORBIN et al. 1975). The third is a cyclic nucleotide-independent peak that elutes with the flow-through volume and is probably free catalytic subunit of the cyclic nucleotide-dependent enzyme. These data, together with the observations that the soluble enzyme is responsive to lower concentrations of cyclic AMP than cyclic GMP, in vitro, and that the apparent level of activation is greater with cyclic AMP, suggest that the soluble protein kinase of rod outer segments has the characteristics of a cyclic AMP-dependent enzyme (FARBER et al. 1979a). However, it is probable that in rod-dominant retinas, this protein kinase is modulated by the light-induced changes in cyclic GMP concentrations. For example, frog rod outer segments exhibit about a tenfold higher capacity for binding cyclic GMP (25 pmol/mg protein) than cyclic AMP, and the dissociation constant is ten times smaller for cyclic GMP (2×10^{-7} M) than for cyclic AMP (BITENSKY et al. 1975). What is not clear is why the presumed regulatory subunit of cyclic nucleotide-dependent protein kinase shows a preference for cyclic GMP whereas the protein kinase activity is more sensitive to activation by cyclic AMP.

The soluble fraction of rod outer segments contains also phosphoprotein phosphatase activity, indispensable for the turnover of phosphorylated proteins in vivo (FARBER et al. 1979a).

When the soluble, Tris-extracted kinase is incubated with rod outer segment membranes that had been depleted of kinase activity but enriched in purified rhodopsin (WELLER et al. 1975), an apparent reassociation of the enzyme with the membranes occurs (FARBER et al. 1979a). Once on the membrane, the kinase phosphorylates bleached rhodopsin independent of cyclic nucleotides. Thus, it seems that soluble and membrane-associated protein kinases are interchangeable. What it is that controls their being "on" or "off" the membrane still remains an open question.

The physiological action of cyclic GMP could be expressed through the mediation of the soluble, cyclic nucleotide-dependent protein kinase and specific phosphoproteins. From the several proteins of the soluble fraction of rod outer segments that are phosphorylated by the kinase, only one protein is phosphorylated in a cyclic nucleotide-dependent manner (LOLLEY et al. 1977a; FARBER et al. 1979a). This soluble protein, molecular weight 30,000 on SDS gels, is present in the Tris-extracts of rod outer segments of bovine, mouse and rat. PANNBACKER (1974) also observes a similar protein in human rod outer segments, with an estimated molecular weight of 25,000. In rod outer segments of frog (POLANS et al. 1979) and toad (FARBER and LOLLEY, unpublished observations), the 30,000-dalton protein is not detected but, instead, two proteins of molecular weight 12,000 and 13,000 are phosphorylated in a cyclic nucleotide-dependent manner. These proteins are also observed in intact retinas of the frog. They are dephosphorylated when the retinas are illuminated (POLANS et al 1979) and are rephosphorylated when illumination ceases. The light-induced dephosphorylation increases with higher intensities of illumination, and it is maximal with light which bleaches 5.0×10^5 rhodopsin molecules/outer segment/second. Half-maximal dephosphorylation occurs with the bleaching of 5.0×10^3 rhodopsin molecules/outer segment/second. This same level of illumination causes half-maximal decrease of cyclic GMP content and of permeability in isolated outer segments (WOODRUFF et al. 1977; BRODIE and BOWNDS 1976). However, the dephosphorylation process is not observed in the isolated outer segments.

Drugs that influence the concentration of cyclic GMP also alter the levels of phosphorylation of the 12,000 and 13,000 molecular weight proteins of frog retina (POLANS et al. 1979). For example, lowering Ca^{2+} with EGTA increases the phosphorylation threefold; IBMX, sixfold; IBMX plus dibutyryl-cyclic GMP, eightfold. Addition of Ca^{2+} elicits a 50% decrease in the incorporation of phosphate.

On the basis of all the data that is available, a model has been proposed by FARBER et al. (1978) which suggests that the phosphorylation of specific proteins in the rod outer segment cytosol or membrane compartments could regulate separately the amplitude of the visual response and the sensitivity of the visual pigment to light.

The key point of the cytoplasmic events, in bovine rod outer segments, is how much of the 30,000-dalton protein is phosphorylated or unphosphorylated. It is proposed that the phosphorylated protein interacts with the rod outer segment plasmalemma alone or in conjunction with Ca^{2+}, facilitating in this way the free movement of ions across the open channels of the membrane and providing a mechanism for the sustained state of depolarization that characterized dark-adapted rod outer segments. When light bleaches rhodopsin, the levels of cyclic GMP are rapidly reduced as a consequence of the activation of cyclic GMP-phosphodiesterase. This fall in cyclic GMP concentration reduces the activity of the soluble protein kinase and slows the rate of phosphorylation of the 30,000-dalton protein. This, together with the continued activity of the phosphoprotein phosphatase, will decrease the concentration of the 30,000-dalton phosphoprotein. The net result will be a reverse of the dark state, e.g. closure of the ion channels and hyperpolarization of the visual cell.

The model shows also that bleached rhodopsin is phosphorylated by the membrane-associated protein kinase, which is interchangeable with the soluble protein kinase. The time-course of the phosphorylation-dephosphorylation reactions suggests that these events may be related to the mechanisms of dark/light adaptation.

The phosphorylation of rhodopsin could be a means for reducing the sensitivity of the visual pigment to light.

Thus, specific phosphoproteins of rod photoreceptor cell outer segments may modulate, and perhaps regulate, the physiological response of visual cells.

g) Other Physiological Effects of Cyclic GMP

Cyclic GMP has been linked to changes in the permeability of the photoreceptor cells that are initiated by light. BRODIE and BOWNDS (1976) measured changes in the swelling of isolated rod outer segments as a function of light and in the presence of phosphodiesterase inhibitors. They reported that the addition of papaverine to the rod outer segment suspension raises intracellular cyclic GMP levels and increases the magnitude of the dark permeability, but does not have a large influence on the amount of illumination required for suppression of this permeability. They concluded that cyclic nucleotides modulate the amplitude of the in vitro response to light rather than affecting the sensitivity control mechanism. CARETTA et al. (1979) also tested the effect of cyclic GMP on membrane permeability. They perfused broken rod outer segments with a solution containing $^{22}Na^{+}$, $^{42}K^{+}$ or $^{36}Cl^{-}$. Addition of cyclic GMP to the perfusing medium increases the Na^{+} and K^{+} effluxes, but not the efflux of Cl^{-}. Cyclic AMP is able to increase the Na^{+} efflux to some extent, even though less than cyclic GMP, but guanosine, GMP and GTP are ineffective. The effect of cyclic GMP on the membrane permeability is independent of the ionic strength of the perfusing medium, and of the presence or absence of Ca^{2+}.

The first report on the effects of cyclic nucleotides on the electrical activity of photoreceptors is that by HOOD and EBREY (1974). These authors applied cyclic AMP, dibutyryl-cyclic AMP and cyclic GMP to a frog retina while recording the receptor potential extracellularly and found no effects of any of the cyclic nucleotides on the receptor potential. However, using phosphodiesterase inhibitors, they showed decreased receptor potential amplitudes (EBREY and HOOD 1973). In contrast, GOVARDOVSKII and BERMAN (1977) found that in dark-adapted frogs, cyclic GMP or cyclic AMP affect the electrical response, increasing the amplitude of the late receptor potential without a sharp change in its time-course. Papaverine or theophylline present in the solutions containing the cyclic nucleotides causes even stronger effects, whereas GMP does not produce any change.

When the retina is superfused continually with cyclic GMP, dibutyryl-cyclic GMP, IBMX or the prostaglandin $PGF_{2\alpha}$, the effects obtained in the rods closely match those observed when extracellular calcium levels are lowered (LIPTON et al. 1977a, b). For example, short exposure of the retina (6 min) to these drugs causes depolarization of the membrane potential, increases in response amplitudes and some changes in waveform, but no changes in receptor sensitivity are observed in either the dark- or the partially light-adapted retina. However, these drugs, like lowered extracellular Ca^{2+}, affect the time required for both membrane potential and sensitivity to recovery during dark adaptation. With prolonged exposure of a dark-adapted retina to IBMX and cyclic GMP, just like after long-term exposure to low Ca^{2}, the rods show diminished response amplitude and sensitivity, mimicking light adaptation. Application of high Ca^{2+} to the retina blocks the effect of applied dibutyryl-cyclic GMP. Thus, increased cyclic GMP and lowered Ca^{2+} produce similar alterations in the electrical activity of rods.

Recently, cyclic GMP has been injected intracellularly through the recording pipette into rod outer segments of the isolated retina of the toad, *Bufo marinus* (NICOL and MILLER 1978; MILLER and NICOL 1979; WALOGA and BROWN 1979). Excess cyclic GMP in dark-adapted preparations increases both the latency and amplitude of the response and depolarizes the rod membrane to a potential close to the equilibrium potential for sodium. MILLER and NICOL (1979) show that the length of time for which the potential is decreased is directly proportional to the amount of injected cyclic GMP and is increased by previous dark adaptation and decreased by previous light adaptation. Depolarization is abolished if the injection of cyclic GMP is preceded by a strong light flash. The increased length of latency and amplitude of the response are observed only when the light is delivered during the time when the membrane is depolarized. No increase in latency or amplitude is observed after the membrane has repolarized. The intracellular injection of cyclic AMP or 5′-GMP does not mimic the effects of injection of cyclic GMP. Thus, it seems that cyclic GMP must be hydrolyzed by light-activated phosphodiesterase to produce the normal hyperpolarizing response to illumination.

WALOGA and BROWN (1979) indicate that even when there are similarities in the effects of lowering extracellular Ca^{2+} concentration and increasing intracellular levels of cyclic GMP, there are also differences which show that these factors do not produce the same changes in the physiology of rods. For example, they cause different effects on the kinetics of receptor potentials. The falling phase of the receptor potential is slightly accelerated in low Ca^{2+} whereas it is greatly slowed both with IBMX in the media and by cyclic GMP injection.

h) Other Components of the Cyclic GMP System

5′-Nucleotidase, the enzyme that catalyzes the conversion of 5′-GMP to guanosine, also seems to be concentrated in the photoreceptor cells. Developmental studies indicate that the 5′-nucleotidase activity increases steadily from birth in normal mouse retina but, in the *rd* retinas, it decreases sharply, as the photoreceptor population is depleted (FARBER and LOLLEY 1976).

Guanylate kinase, the enzyme that converts 5′-GMP to GDP, has a different distribution in the retina. Its activity is very low in the outer segments and very high in the rest of the photoreceptor cell. Guanylate kinase is almost absent from the inner retinal layers (BERGER et al. 1980).

Nucleoside diphosphokinase catalyzes the phosphorylation of GDP to GTP. Similar to guanylate kinase, the activity of nucleoside diphosphokinase is very low in the outer segments and higher in the inner segments and outer plexiform layer (BERGER et al. 1980).

Inorganic pyrophosphatase degrades the inorganic pyrophosphate, product of the guanylate cyclase reaction, to inorganic phosphate. This enzyme has very high activity in all photoreceptor cell layers, except the outer segments (LOWRY 1964).

2. Cyclic AMP

a) Distribution and Factors that Affect its Levels

The cyclic AMP content of rod-dominant retinas is considerably lower than that of cyclic GMP and is uniformly distributed throughout the layers of the retina with the exception of the rod outer segments, which contain the lowest cyclic AMP concentration (ORR et al. 1976). Light does not affect the levels of cyclic AMP of the outer segments (FLETCHER and CHADER 1976; KRISHNA et al. 1976; ORR et al. 1976), but reduces the cyclic AMP content of the outer nuclear layer and mainly of the outer plexiform layer, as has been shown by quantitative histochemistry studies of rabbit retina (ORR et al. 1976). Probably, the 40% reduction by light of cyclic AMP levels observed in intact mouse retina occurs in the same retinal layer (DE VRIES et al. 1978). Since it is thought that photoreceptor terminals are more active in the dark, releasing larger amounts of depolarizing transmitter (BYZOV and TRIFONOV 1968; DOWLING and RIPPS 1973; CERVETTO and PICCOLINO 1974), the presence of higher dark-cyclic AMP levels in the layer that contains the photoreceptor terminals and post-synaptic elements could be related to the increased amount of photoreceptor synaptic transmission in the dark (ORR et al. 1976). However, it has not been established as yet whether the dark accumulation of cyclic AMP in the outer plexiform layer occurs in visual cell terminals and/or in horizontal or bipolar cell processes.

Several putative neurotransmitters are present in the inner retina including acetylcholine (NEAL 1976; MASLAND and LIVINGSTONE 1976; BAUGHMAN and BADER 1977; MASSEY and NEAL 1979), glycine and γ-aminobutyric acid (VOADEN 1976; EHINGER 1976), serotonin (SUZUKI et al. 1978) and dopamine (EHINGER 1978). All of these compounds are concentrated in amacrine cells; dopamine is the only endogenous neurotransmitter that appears to modulate the retinal level of cyclic AMP (KRAMER 1976).

The dopaminergic system in the retina may be very sensitive to light of low intensity. DE VRIES et al. (1978) reported that cyclic AMP levels are lower in retinas isolated under dim red light than in those isolated under infrared illumination; a decrease in cyclic GMP content under such conditions is not observed. The authors suggest that levels of illumination that are too low to generate measurable photoreceptor responses may cause many very small responses in cells of the inner retina, and their summation could be reflected in alterations of cyclic AMP concentration before changes in cyclic GMP could be measured. However, WOODRUFF et al. (1977) observe lower levels of cyclic GMP in isolated rod outer segments of frog when the dissections are carried out under dim red light instead of under infrared illumination.

As in other neural tissue, anoxia or ischemia elevates cyclic AMP levels in rabbit (ORR et al. 1976) and mouse retina (MITZEL et al. 1978). These cyclic AMP changes occur predominantly in the inner layers of the retina. They are more pronounced in dark-adapted tissue, probably as a consequence of increased release of neurotransmitter which may increase the metabolic rate of some cells of the inner retina. The need for glycogenolysis in these cells would be increased if the blood supply is shut off by the ischemic condition. After five minutes of ischemia, the distribution of cyclic AMP in the dark-adapted rabbit retinas closely parallels the distribution of glycogen (MATSCHINSKY 1970). The increased cyclic AMP levels suggest phosphorylase b activation and provide a mechanism for the more rapid breakdown of glycogen (ORR et al. 1976).

Alteration of calcium levels has been reported not to affect the concentration of retinal cyclic AMP (COHEN et al. 1978). BROWN and MAKMAN (1972) reported that depolarizing agents such as ouabain and high potassium cause a twofold elevation in the cyclic AMP content of intact bovine retina.

b) Cyclic AMP Synthesis

Adenylate cyclase, the enzyme that synthesizes cyclic AMP from ATP, has been localized in the inner layers of the retina through use of developmental studies (FARBER and LOLLEY 1977b) and by work with dystrophic retinas which are devoid of photoreceptor cells (LOLLEY et al. 1974; MAKMAN et al. 1975a). In addition, the treatment of neonatal rats with glutamate, which selectively destroys the inner retina while leaving the photoreceptor cells intact, decreases adenylate cyclase activity (MAKMAN et al. 1975a). Consistent with these data, the P_1 and P_2 subcellular fractions of rabbit retina show adenylate cyclase activity (CLEMENT-CORMIER and REDBURN 1978). The highest specific activity is found in the P_2 fraction, which is enriched in synaptosomes from amacrine cells, and, to a lesser extent, from bipolar and horizontal cells. The P_1 fraction contains synaptosomes from photoreceptor cells. This P_1 adenylate cyclase activity may correspond to that which in the early seventies was reported by BITENSKY et al. (1971) and by HENDRIKS et al. (1973) to be inhibited by light. The light effect on adenylate cyclase activity remained controversial for quite a while. MANTHORPE and MCCONNELL (1974) separated various fractions derived from retinal homogenates and found that as unbleached rhodopsin concentration rises during fractionation, adenylate cyclase activity declines, whereas the fractions that have high adenylate cyclase activity are poor in rhodopsin content. They also showed that most of the adenylate cyclase activity is confined to membranes and that it is not affected by bleaching. The studies of MIKI et al. (1973) confirmed that, in fact, the loss of radioactive cyclic AMP from suspensions of rod outer segments is far greater when membranes have been illuminated, indicating the presence of a light-activated phosphodiesterase instead of a light-inhibited adenylate cyclase.

Retinal adenylate cyclase is stimulated by dopamine but it is not affected by serotonin, histamine or GABA (BROWN and MAKMAN 1972, 1973; BUCHER and SCHORDERET 1975). Epinephrine and norepinephrine are about one-tenth as potent as dopamine in the activation of the enzyme from calf and rat (BROWN and MAKMAN 1972). Only the adenylate cyclase from the P_2 subcellular fraction is sensitive to dopamine (CLEMENT-CORMIER and REDBURN 1978).

Dopamine-stimulated adenylate cyclase has been found in retina of many species, including primates (MISHRA et al. 1974), fishes (WATLING et al. 1980), avian (SCHWARCZ and COYLE 1976) and invertebrates such as octopus (MAKMAN et al. 1975a). In mice and rats, its activity increases markedly during the early postnatal period, as retinal maturation occurs (LOLLEY et al. 1974; BROWN et al. 1973). In rhesus monkeys, which are born with a well-developed and functional retina, the dopamine-stimulated adenylate cyclase activity 30 h after birth is more than one-half that attained by adulthood (MAKMAN et al. 1975a). In chick embryonic retina, a sharp threefold increase in cyclic AMP levels is observed between the 16th and 18th embryonic day and remains constant thereafter. However, a dopamine-dependent increase in cyclic AMP of the chick retina is already present in 7-day-old embryos (DE MELLO 1978).

The dopamine-sensitive adenylate cyclase from the inner retinal layers responds to changes in the conditions of illumination (WATLING et al. 1980). It has been shown that in carp retina, the interplexiform cells are optimally stimulated by bright, flashing, red light (HEDDEN and DOWLING 1978), whereas continuous red light of the same intensity activates preferentially the photoreceptor cells. WATLING et al. (1980) found that cyclic AMP levels increase in pieces of retina exposed to flashing light as compared to their equivalent pieces left in darkness. In contrast, pieces of retina exposed to continuous red light showed a decline in cyclic AMP content.Thus, the cyclic AMP increase induced by flickering light reflects changes mediated by the dopamine-containing neurons, whereas the cyclic AMP decrease occurs in the photoreceptors, was confirmed by incubation of pieces of retina under analogous conditions of illumination, but in the presence of haloperidol. Since the effect of haloperidol is to block dopamine action, the decline in cyclic AMP levels observed in haloperidol-treated pieces with either light condition indicates that the increase in cyclic AMP level following stimulation with flashes results from activation of the dopamine-containing neurons. WATLING et al. (1980) concluded that perhaps the appropriate comparison to make is not between dark- and light-exposed retinas but between retinas exposed to flickering and continuous illumination. If this is done, the increase in retinal cyclic AMP obtained is close to 50%.

Depolarizing agents such as ouabain (0.01 m*M*) and potassium (10–83 m*M*) can stimulate the synthesis of cyclic AMP in intact incubated retinas as well as in homogenates (WASSENAAR and KORF 1976; BROWN and MAKMAN 1972). In brain slices, depolarizing agents cause a larger increase in cyclic AMP levels than in retina. These increases are believed to be mediated by the release of adenosine and are blocked by the methylxanthines (SHIMIZU et al. 1970). Since adenosine does not stimulate adenylate cyclase in retina, the mechanism of activation proposed for brain may not be functional in retina. Furthermore, BROWN and MAKMAN (1972) showed that the effects of dopamine and of the depolarizing agents in intact retina appear to be additive. This indicates that dopamine and depolarizing agents cause an increase in cyclic AMP synthesis by different mechanisms. However, WATLING et al. (1979) reported that K^+ and veratridine appear to increase cyclic AMP levels in the retina via dopamine. These agents probably depolarize the dopamine-containing cells causing a release of dopamine from presynaptic terminals. Co^{2+}, which inhibits the release of substances from presynaptic terminals, and haloperidol, which inhibits dopamine action, both effectively block the K^+-mediated increase of cyclic AMP. On the other hand, tetrodotoxin entirely abolishes the retinal response to veratridine, as it does in other tissues, and most likely exerts its effect by depolarizing the dopamine-containing neurons. It seems possible that the effect of ouabain is due to inhibition of sodium potassium ATPase activity, which would preserve ATP for the use in the adenylate cyclase reaction (BROWN and MAKMAN 1972).

c) Influence of Dopamine Agonists on Adenylate Cyclase Activity

The retinal dopamine-sensitive adenylate cyclase has pharmacological properties that clearly distinguish it from either of the α- or β-adrenoceptor classes found in the CNS. For example, the dopamine system is not activated by the potent β-adrenergic stimulant isoproterenol nor is it blocked by the β-adrenoceptor antagonist propanolol (BROWN and MAKMAN 1972; BUCHER and SCHORDERET 1974).

There is a high degree of specificity for agonists at retinal dopamine receptors. Among simple β-phenethyl-amine analogs of dopamine, only the N-methyl derivative epinine is equipotent with the parent compound (SCHORDERET 1978a). Half-maximal stimulation of retinal adenylate cyclase is achieved with dopamine at a concentration of 1 μM (BUCHER and SCHORDERET 1975). The α-methyl analog of dopamine is also considerably less potent than dopamine. Compounds that lack the catechol hydroxyl groups of dopamine or substances in which the side chain contains one or three carbon atoms, instead of the usual two, are without activity (IVERSEN 1975). Epinephrine and norepinephrine are as potent as dopamine at 10^{-4} M, whereas no agonist activity is detected at 10^{-6} M. WATLING et al. (1979) have evidence which suggests that both compounds stimulate adenylate cyclase activity by interacting with dopamine receptors, rather than with α- or β-adrenoceptors. For example, isoproterenol and phenylephrine, which are specific β- and α-adrenoceptor agents, respectively, cause no increase in the adenylate cyclase activity of carp homogenates. In addition, dopamine and norepinephrine added together at concentrations sufficient for each to maximally activate adenylate cyclase do not increase activity in the homogenate. Furthermore, the response to norepinephrine is blocked by low doses of dopamine antagonists.

A variety of compounds in which the side chain of dopamine is held in a rigid conformation in a second ring have been tested as potential agonists. Among these, the alkaloid apomorphine has been shown to be an even better stimulator than dopamine on the adenylate cyclase activity of intact retinas of the rabbit, whereas it caused a smaller effect in homogenates and a comparable effect to that of dopamine in calf retina (BUCHER and SCHORDERET 1974; BROWN and MAKMAN 1973). Among tetrahydroisoquinolines, there are rigid analogs in which the side chain of dopamine is locked in a folded rather than an extended conformation; these compounds are only weakly effective as dopamine agonists (IVERSEN 1975). In contrast, 2-amino-6,7-dihydroxy-1,2,3,4-tetrahydronaphthalene, which represents the fully extended conformation of the dopamine side chain with the amino group trans to the phenyl ring, is equipotent with dopamine as an agonist in rabbit retina (SCHORDERET et al. 1978). In addition to the trans β-rotamer conformation, dopamine can also exist in a trans α-rotamer conformation. This 5,6-dihydroxy-substituted aminotetralin is not optimal for dopamine-like activity. However, its dopamine-mimetic activity can be improved by dialkylation of the nitrogen or practically abolished by cyclization of substituents on the nitrogen (SCHORDERET et al. 1978). It is interesting that the effectiveness of its monohydroxyl analog is stereospecific. The dextro enantiomer is inactive, whereas the levo enantiomer, even at a concentration of 5×10^{-6} M, induces a significant accumulation of cyclic AMP. Stereochemical dependency of drugs interacting with retinal dopamine receptors has been also shown for antagonists (SCHORDERET et al. 1978).

The dopamine precursor L-dopa at 10^{-4} M also is a potent inducer of cyclic AMP accumulation in intact rabbit retina (SCHORDERET 1977b). Presumably, L-dopa is converted by aromatic amino acid decarboxylase to dopamine, which in turn stimulates dopamine-sensitive adenylate cyclase (MAKMAN et al. 1975b). Another dopamine agonist is S 584, a catechol metabolite of the antiparkinsonian drug piribedil (MAKMAN et al. 1975b; SCHORDERET 1975). Piribedil has dopamine agonist activity in vivo (CORRODI et al. 1971) but has no effect on slices or homogenates of retina. The maximal response to S 584, measured at 1 μM, is equivalent to that of 10 μM dopamine in calf retina.

Several ergot alkaloid derivatives have been found to have dopamine-mimetic activity in intact rabbit retina (SCHORDERET 1976; 1978a, b). Agroclavine, ergometrine, 2-bromo-α-ergocryptine, lisuride and α- or β-DH-ergocryptine produce effects similar to those of dopamine: half-maximal stimulation at 10^{-4} M and inhibition of cyclic AMP accumulation by antipsychotic drugs. Other alkaloids like mescaline and drugs such as amantadine and (+) or (±) amphetamines, at a concentration at 10^{-6} M, do not activate retinal adenylate cyclase (SCHORDERET 1978a).

d-LSD (lysergic acid diethylamide) exerts a significant stimulatory effect, about twofold, on the activity of the retinal adenylate cyclase of several species including rat, rabbit, cat and calf (SPANO et al. 1976). This LSD stimulation is totally abolished by neuroleptics. d-LSD inhibits the activation by dopamine of adenylate cyclase in vitro and in vivo, and this effect is dose-dependent (SCHORDERET and MAGISTRETTI 1980). This indicates a common site of action for dopamine and d-LSD on the dopamine-sensitive adenylate cyclase and suggests a central interaction of d-LSD with dopamine.

d) Influence of Dopamine Antagonists on Adenylate Cyclase Activity

The retinal dopamine-sensitive adenylate cyclase is extremely responsive to inhibition by antipsychotic drugs. These drugs selectively antagonize a number of behavioral and physiological actions of dopamine in the central nervous system and are believed to exert these effects through specific postsynaptic blockade of the dopamine receptors (BROWN and MAKMAN 1973). Their action is selective for the dopamine receptor in the adenylate cyclase system with essentially no effect on basal or sodium fluoride-stimulated activity. The potency of these drugs as inhibitors of dopamine-sensitive adenylate cyclase can be expressed as inhibition constants for drug interaction with the dopamine receptor sites. The most potent are the phenothiazine derivative fluphenazine and the thioxanthene derivatives α-piflutixol and α-flupenthixol (K_i's of $3–7 \times 10^{-9}$ M). (+) Butaclamol, chlorpromazine, thioridazine and haloperidol have K_i's of $2–9 \times 10^{-8}$ M. Among other effective antagonists of the retinal dopamine-sensitive adenylate cyclase are drugs like spiroperidol, pimozide, clozapine, pipamperone and spiperone (BROWN and MAKMAN 1973; SCHORDERET 1977b; WATLING et al. 1980).

The stereochemical conformation of neuroleptics is of decisive importance for an interaction with dopamine receptors leading to biological activity. For example, the cis isomers of the thioxanthenes are more potent than the trans isomers in various animal tests for antipsychotic activity. Similarly, in intact rabbit retina, the cis isomers of thioxanthenes such as flupenthixol, clopenthixol and chlorprothixene are very good inhibitors of cyclic AMP formation induced by dopamine, in contrast to the lack of blocking effects of trans isomers (SCHORDERET et al. 1978a, b). In another case of stereospecificity, (+) butaclamol completely inhibits the dopamine action, whereas the (−) enantiomer of the drug is inactive (SCHORDERET 1977b).

WASSENAAR and ROELSE (1980) have indicated recently that fluphenazine and haloperidol, which block completely the response to dopamine of adenylate cyclase, cause instead an enhancement of cyclic AMP formation by norepinephrine with an inhibition of phosphodiesterase activity. These authors suggest the existence in rat retina of a neuroleptic-sensitive phosphodiesterase, belonging to a norepinephrine-cyclic AMP system. This enzyme would be in a special compartment in the retina to which dopamine or cyclic AMP synthesized in a dopamine-stimulated manner would have no access.

Lithium has been found to be an effective antagonist of retinal dopamine-sensitive adenylate cyclase. This anti-manic drug, with possible mechanism of action related to dopaminergic systems (SMITH 1976), at a concentration of 50 m*M*, can completely inhibit the dopamine-, apomorphine-, epinine-, ergometrine- and lisuride-elicited production of cyclic AMP in intact retina of the rabbit (SCHORDERET 1977a, b). The lowest effective dose of lithium is 2 m*M* (SCHORDERET 1977a). Therapeutic concentrations of lithium in human plasma can easily reach 2 m*M* during the treatment of acute mania with lithium salts (FORN and VALDECASAS 1971).

α- or β-Adrenergic antagonists such as phentolamine or propanolol, at concentrations which are maximally effective in blocking adenylate cyclase of brain (PERKINS and MOORE 1973), do not inhibit the cyclic AMP accumulation induced by dopamine in retina (SCHORDERET 1977b). Phentolamine is effective only at concentrations 50–100 times those necessary for blockade with the neuroleptic agents and propanolol fails to produce greater than 50% inhibition even at concentrations 25 times those of dopamine (BROWN and MAKMAN 1973).

Two types of dopamine receptors have been described in many areas of the central nervous system (COOLS and VAN ROSSUM 1976; IVERSEN 1975): the D_1 receptor type is linked to adenylate cyclase whereas the D_2 is not (KEBABIAN and CALNE 1979). Binding studies with ^{3}H-domperidone, which is a very weak antagonist of the dopamine-sensitive adenylate cyclase (LADURON and LEYSEN 1979) and appears to bind only to D_2 receptors, suggest that all dopamine receptors in the retina are linked to adenylate cyclase, that is, are of the D_1 type (WATLING et al. 1979). A similar conclusion had been reported by MAGISTRETTI and SCHORDERET (1978) from their studies of the effect of the neuroleptic sulpiride upon dopamine-sensitive adenylate cyclase of intact rabbit retina.

e) Effects of Light Deprivation, Aging and Degenerative Diseases on Cyclic AMP Metabolism

Light deprivation increases by approximately 100% the formation of cyclic AMP stimulated by dopamine and LSD in retinal homogenates from rats kept in the dark for 65 h, compared to those from rats under a light cycle of 12 h/day (TRABUCCHI et al. 1976). Similarly, retinal cyclic AMP synthesis increases when dopamine is depleted from the nerve terminals of rats injected with reserpine, as compared to the cyclic AMP levels in control animals. Since dopamine in the retina appears to be released mainly as a consequence of light stimulation, TRABUCCHI et al. (1976) speculate that light deprivation is a sort of functional denervation. Thus, the enhancement of dopamine-stimulated adenylate cyclase activity, after maintaining the rats in the dark, as well as that observed after the chemical lesion of dopamine terminals induced by reserpine, may indicate that the postsynaptic dopamine receptors have developed supersensitivity.

On the same line of thought, SPANO et al. (1977) showed that dopamine-stimulated formation of cyclic AMP in homogenates of rat retina is greater at 9 postnatal days than at 21 days of age. The authors suggested that at 9 days of age, since the rats have not opened their eyes, the dopaminergic neurons are releasing only a small amount of transmitter, and dopamine receptors are in a state of functional supersensitivity. As soon as light enters the eyes, the dopamine receptor sensitivity adjusts to a new steady state. This is supported by the fact that the turnover rate of dopamine in retina is low at 9–10 days but increases drastically when the animals open their eyes (DA PRADA 1977). In addition, it has been shown that the activation of dopamine-sensitive adenylate cyclase in retinal homogenates of senescent rats is higher than that observed with mature rats (GOVONI et al. 1977). This may reflect a reduced function with aging of retinal dopaminergic neurons to which the receptor and the adenylate cyclase system react with a supersensitive response.

Studies of photoreceptor degeneration in mouse and rat retinas (FARBER and LOLLEY 1977b) suggest that the synaptic relationship between photoreceptor cells and the neurons of the inner retina can modify the metabolism of cyclic AMP in the inner layers of the mature retina. The different responses of pre- and post-differentiated neurons of the inner retina to deafferentiation have a critical period of development in which contact with photoreceptor cells can modulate the long-term metabolism of cyclic AMP. For example, the photoreceptor cells of the RCS rat retina (see section IV.4) are mature before they degenerate and, in this retina, the content of cyclic AMP and the activity of adenylate cyclase are unchanged from that of the control at all times during development, even when all the photoreceptor cells have degenerated. In contrast, in the *rd* mouse retina, the photoreceptor cell degeneration occurs during the period of inner neuron maturation and synapse formation (BLANKS et al. 1974). In this retina, the content of cyclic AMP and the activity of adenylate cyclase increase above that of the control during development, and both parameters remain elevated in the adult retina after photoreceptor cells have degenerated.

f) Physiological Effects of Cyclic AMP

Cyclic AMP has been implicated in the modulation of several metabolic processes in the retina. For example, cyclic AMP seems to activate phosphorylase b kinase and to inactivate glycogen synthetase I, thereby increasing retinal glycogenolysis and glycolysis (ORR et al. 1976). Cyclic AMP has been shown also to increase dopamine formation through activation of the biosynthetic enzyme, tyrosine hydroxylase: incubation of intact chick retina with 1 m*M* dibutyryl-cyclic AMP causes a 41% stimulation of tyrosine hydroxylase activity (TUNNICLIFF 1977). In addition, cyclic AMP induces glutamine synthetase activity in embryonic chick retina (CHADER 1971).

BROWN and MAKMAN (1972) reported the presence of protein kinase from bovine retina that is stimulated more than 20-fold by the addition of 1 μ*M* cyclic AMP. Similar concentrations of the cyclic nucleotide also stimulate by several fold the cyclic AMP-dependent protein kinase from bovine rod outer segments (FARBER et al. 1979a). Recently, some other retinal proteins have been shown to be phosphorylated in a cyclic nucleotide-dependent manner. HESKETH et al. (1978) reported that the phosphorylation of three proteins from a crude retinal actomyosin fraction, with molecular weights of 22,000, 33,000 and 200,000, is markedly increased by the addition of 10 μM cyclic AMP. The 200,000 molecular weight protein has been identified as the heavy chain of the retinal myosin molecule.

Cyclic AMP has been reported to enhance a release of sodium ions from isolated bovine rod outer segments maintained at 20 °C, whereas potassium ions are not affected (DUMLER and ETINGOF 1973). This enhanced release of sodium ions is more pronounced in light- than in dark-adapted rod outer segments and is not changed by addition of 10 mM theophylline to the incubation mixture. However, reducing the temperature of the medium to 2 °C causes a three to fourfold decrease in the stimulatory effect of cyclic AMP on the sodium ion release.

The work of WIGLUSZ (1973, 1975a, b) has pointed out some correlations between the amplitude of the action potentials of rabbit and frog retinas and active sodium transport across cell membranes. Cyclic AMP and drugs which increase the concentration of cyclic AMP in the retina raise the amplitude of the b wave of the electroretinogram (ERG) and stimulate active sodium transport. Similar effects are obtained after retrobulbar injection of dibutyryl-cyclic AMP. On the other hand, imidazole, which stimulates phosphodiesterase and thereby the reduction of cyclic AMP levels, decreases both the amplitude of the action potentials and the active sodium transport. Ouabain also inhibits both the bioelectrical responses to light as well as the active sodium transport, indicating that the action of cyclic AMP is effective only in the presence of full activity of Na^+-K^+-ATPase.

II. Cyclic Nucleotides in Cone-Dominant Retinas

1. Cyclic AMP and Cyclic GMP Content

In contrast to rods, cone visual cells have received relatively little attention despite the fact that they play a major role in human vision. It is only in the last couple of years that studies on the cyclic nucleotide metabolism of retinas dominated by cones have been started. FARBER and LOLLEY (1978) reported that the cone-dominant retina of the ground squirrel has considerably higher levels of cyclic AMP than of cyclic GMP (91.0 ± 5.0 vs. 11.1 ± 0.8 pmol/mg protein). The cyclic AMP/cyclic GMP ratio (8.2) is 35–40 times higher than that of rod-dominant retinas, which is less than 1.0. Additionally, the Western fence lizard, another vertebrate with a cone-dominant retina, also has higher levels of cyclic AMP than of cyclic GMP, with a cyclic AMP/cyclic GMP ratio of 2.2 (FARBER et al. 1980).

2. Modulation of Cyclic AMP Levels by Light

Light appears to affect cyclic AMP metabolism in cone-dominant retinas. For example, the content of cyclic AMP in dark-adapted ground squirrel retina is reduced approximately 55% by exposure to light, whereas cyclic GMP levels are unaffected (FARBER et al. 1981). Similar results are observed with the Western fence lizard. All of the cyclic nucleotide levels given in these reports correspond to measurements made on freshly dissected retinas. In the isolation of the ground squirrel retina, there is always the possibility of losing many of the outer segments, since the cone cells break very easily at the base of the outer segments, and these adhere firmly to the pigment epithelium cells. This has been confirmed by electron microscopy. When cyclic nucleotide levels are measured in retinal pigment epithelium of dark-adapted ground squirrels, a considerable concentration of cyclic AMP is found, probably contributed by the outer segments. This cyclic AMP (24.3 pmol/mg protein) is reduced by 35% after exposure to light. In contrast, the levels of cyclic GMP in the pigment epithelium are minimal and do not change during illumination (FARBER et al. 1981).

In order to increase the speed of dissection and reduce the trauma imposed on the retina, the cyclic nucleotide content from the intact eyes of dark- and light-adapted ground squirrels has been measured (FARBER et al. 1980). It is calculated that 65% of the cyclic AMP and 80–90% of the cyclic GMP of the eye is localized in the retina. Similar to what is observed with the dissected retina, light reduces by 50% the cyclic AMP content of the dark-adapted ground squirrel eye, whereas the levels of cyclic GMP are not significantly affected.

3. Effect of Freezing

Freezing of the ground squirrel retina or whole eye modifies the content of cyclic AMP by a process which is unknown. It reduces the levels of cyclic AMP in the dark- or light-adapted tissues by about 60%, whereas the levels of cyclic GMP are minimally affected (FARBER et al. 1979 b). This is surprising because, in brain tissue, freezing is used to prevent an anoxia-induced increase of cyclic AMP (STEINER et al. 1972). Furthermore, light reduces cyclic AMP levels in fresh as well as frozen dark-adapted retinas of the ground squirrel (FARBER et al. 1981). For example, microdissected retinal samples which had been frozen in the dark and freeze-dried in the light contain less than 20% of the cyclic AMP present in dark-adapted retinas. These observations explain why DE VRIES et al. (1979), based on their studies of microdissected retinal layers, indicated that cyclic GMP is the predominant cyclic nucleotide of cone photoreceptors. Moreover, these authors do not observe a difference between the cyclic nucleotide content of eyes frozen in the dark, before freeze-drying in the light, and those exposed to light from the onset of enucleation, because all their microdissected samples are "light-adapted" layers of ground squirrel retina. Also from studies on microdissected retinas, it has been reported that guanylate cyclase activity is highest in the outer segments, whereas adenylate cyclase activity is associated with the inner portions of the ground squirrel retina (FERRENDELLI et al. 1980); both cyclic GMP- and cyclic AMP-phosphodiesterase activities are higher in the outer segments than in any other layer of the retina.

4. Effect of Hibernation

Partial or total loss of cone outer segments is found naturally in the hibernating ground squirrel. Upon entering hibernation, cone outer segments become shorter (RÉME and YOUNG 1977) or eventually disappear (KUWABARA 1975), and the diameter of the discs decreases. The mitochondria of the ellipsoid region are reduced in number and length, and the number of synaptic vesicles and synaptic ribbons is decreased. The synaptic ribbons tend to be displayed from their normal position along the presynaptic membrane and are found in "ribbon fields", which are aggregates of short, randomly arranged segments of synaptic ribbons and synaptic vesicles. Changes in synaptic ribbon morphology are specific to visual cells because synaptic ribbons of the bipolar terminals are unchanged during hibernation (FARBER et al. 1979c). After arousal, cones recover and restore their morphology within a few days.

During the first days of hibernation, cyclic AMP levels of the ground squirrel retina rise to values above those found in dark-adapted, non-hibernating animals (FARBER et al. 1980). Then, as the photoreceptor cell undergoes the morphological changes associated with hibernation, cyclic AMP levels fall to about 45% of the dark-adapted value. Following one and up to three months in hibernation, retinal cyclic AMP content is stabilized at a value (42.3 ± 1.4 pmol/mg protein) which is similar to that of non-hibernating animals in the light. In contrast, cyclic GMP levels do not change during hibernation.

Within 3 days after arousal, cyclic AMP levels return to pre-hibernation values, coinciding with the re-forming of cone photoreceptors. Thus, hibernation alters both the morphology and the metabolism of cyclic AMP in cone photoreceptors, indicating that at least 50% of the cyclic AMP content of dark-adapted, non-hibernating retinas may be localized in the cone photoreceptor layer.

5. Effect of Iodoacetic Acid-Induced Degeneration of Cone Visual Cells

Intravenous injections of sodium iodoacetate produce a characteristic visual cell degeneration in several species of animals (SCHUBERT and BORNSCHEIN 1951; NÖELL 1952a). All other cells of the retina remain undamaged morphologically, unless high doses of this poison are used. Iodoacetate has been successfully employed to destroy the photoreceptors of the ground squirrel retina (FARBER et al. 1981).

Eleven days after a single intracardiac injection of iodoacetate, intact cone cells are replaced by a layer of macrophages containing large, irregular, dense material. These masses are identified by electron microscopy as the partially degraded residue of photoreceptors. In sparse patches of the retina, cones, debris and macrophages are absent altogether, so that the pigment epithelium lies directly on the inner nuclear layer. The inner layers of the ground squirrel retina remain apparently unchanged.

The level of cyclic AMP in the dark-adapted retina of the iodoacetate-treated ground squirrel is reduced by approximately 46% (from 91.0 ± 5.0 to 49.2 ± 0.2 pmol/mg protein), and that of cyclic GMP by 94% (from 11.1 ± 0.7 to less than 1.0 pmol/mg protein). Thus, both cyclic nucleotides are located in cone visual cells, with most of cyclic GMP present in the photoreceptors. The absolute loss of cyclic AMP after iodoacetic acid treatment is about four times greater than that of cyclic GMP. Therefore, a reasonable estimate is that cone photoreceptors contain four times more cyclic AMP than cyclic GMP (FARBER et al. 1981).

III. Cyclic Nucleotides in Retinal Pigment Epithelium

The pigment epithelium is essential for the survival of the photoreceptor cells and for the maintenance of retinal responsiveness to light. It is involved in the mechanism of renewal of the photoreceptors (YOUNG and BOK 1969), and it regulates the flow of molecules and ions between the choroidal blood and the retina (NÖELL 1952b, 1963; LASANSKY and DEFISCH 1966; STEINBERG and MILLER 1973; MILLER and STEINBERG 1976, 1977a, b).

Cyclic GMP levels in monkey and human pigment epithelium vary by area (NEWSOME et al. 1980) following an inverse pattern to that observed for cyclic GMP in the retina. Higher concentrations of cyclic GMP are found in the macula than in the more peripheral regions. In contrast, cyclic AMP is uniformly distributed in all areas of the pigment epithelium.

The dibutyryl derivative of cyclic AMP (0.1 m*M*), in the presence of the phosphodiesterase inhibitor, IBMX, seems to increase the pigmentation of retinal pigment epithelial cells in culture (REDFERN et al. 1976). After 13 days in culture, melanin synthesis is increased by 40%. Furthermore, cells appear more differentiated, with increased numbers of mature pigment granules and other organelles. The cyclic nucleotide seems to favor also the elongation of microvilli. Similar data is reported by TAKEUCHI and KAJISHIMA (1976), who focused their studies mainly on the depigmentation of the pigment epithelium cells. When pigment epithelial cells of chick embryo are cultured in monolayers, the pigment granules degrade forming organelles called dense bodies and melanosome complexes. Dibutyryl-cyclic AMP as well as theophylline prevent the transformation of pigment granules and enhance their synthesis. These observations differ from those reported by NEWSOME et al. (1974) regarding the effect of dibutyryl-cyclic AMP on the cultured pigment epithelial cells. These authors found that the cyclic AMP derivatives retarded the rate of increase in cell number, decreased the final number of cells per culture and considerably reduced visible pigmentation of normal pigment epithelium cells. However, in this case, NEWSOME et al. (1974) had not included IBMX in their incubation medium and, thus, phosphodiesterase activity could have reduced the specific pools of cyclic AMP that are involved in the processes in question. Cyclic GMP and its dibutyryl derivative have little effect on visible pigmentation of pigment epithelium cells in culture; that is, they are ineffective both in the prevention of transformation and in the synthesis of pigment granules (REDFERN et al. 1976; TAKEUCHI and KAJISHIMA 1976).

Cyclic nucleotides do not have an effect on the release of enzymes from lysosomes of the retinal pigment epithelium (HAYASAKA et al. 1977); but cyclic AMP seems to enhance phagocytosis in pigment epithelium explants, in culture. After 22 h in the continuous presence of cyclic AMP and latex beads, more pigment epithelial cells contain large numbers of latex spheres than pigment epithelial cells cultured without the cyclic nucleotide (FEENEY and MIXON 1976).

IV. Abnormalities in Cyclic Nucleotide Metabolism and Retinal Degenerations

Retinal degenerations that cause blindness occur in several species of animals including man. The etiology of these diseases is not completely understood, but abnormalities in cyclic nucleotide metabolism have been shown to be involved in the process of degeneration that affects preferentially the rod visual cells of the *rd* mouse, the Irish Setter dog, and several strains of rat retinas.

1. *rd* (Retinal Degeneration) Mouse

The occurrence of an inherited disorder of retinal development in mice was first reported by BRÜCKNER in 1951. The *rd* mutation is carried as an autosomal recessive characteristic (SIDMAN and GREEN 1965; LAVAIL and SIDMAN 1974), and it affects specifically the visual cells of the retina. The photoreceptor cells appear to form normally during the prenatal and early postnatal period and to achieve some degree of differentiation, as indicated by the development of rudimentary rod outer segments and a synaptic ribbon complex (LAVAIL and SIDMAN 1974; BLANKS et al. 1974). They are responsive to high intensity illumination, and they exhibit an attenuated ERG (NÖELL 1965). The pigment epithelium is morphologically and functionally normal in this disorder (LAVAIL and SIDMAN 1974). The first sign of ultrastructural pathology in the *rd* photoreceptors has been observed on the 8th postnatal day as a swelling of mitochondria of the inner segments (SONOHARA and SHIOSE 1968). Cellular death is apparent by the 10th day and, by the 20th, virtually all of the rod visual cells have degenerated (NÖELL 1965). The rate of the degenerative process is not accelerated by the level of illumination in which the mice are reared. Loss of photoreceptor cells is reflected in the loss of protein from the retina (FARBER and LOLLEY 1973). The few cells that remain after 20 days of age appear to be cones (CARTER-DAWSON et al. 1978). It has been proposed that the *rd* defect results from a failure of photoreceptor cells to fully differentiate (TANSLEY 1951; SORSBY et al. 1954).

An abnormality in cyclic GMP metabolism occurs about two days before the *rd* photoreceptor cells begin to degenerate (FARBER and LOLLEY 1974). The photoreceptor cells are able to synthesize cyclic GMP via the guanylate cyclase reaction from the onset of differentiation but they are always deficient in the capacity to hydrolyze cyclic GMP via the cyclic GMP-phosphodiesterase reaction (FARBER and LOLLEY 1976). As a consequence, the levels of cyclic GMP become greatly elevated in the *rd* retina, especially when compared to the levels of cyclic GMP present in retina of control mice (FARBER and LOLLEY 1974). Cyclic GMP levels start to accumulate by the 6th postnatal day and peak at day 14. Kinetic studies have shown that the *rd* retina possesses a cyclic GMP-phosphodiesterase, the activity of which, when assayed in retinal homogenates of freshly dissected tissue, cannot be demonstrated at any age. But, if the *rd* retina is freeze-dried, this phosphodiesterase is stabilized and shows a K_m similar to that of photoreceptor cells of control retina; however, its apparent V_{max} is quite below normal (FARBER and LOLLEY 1977a). This enzyme has been localized by histochemical techniques within the *rd* outer segments (ROBB 1974b). In vivo, the cyclic GMP-phosphodiesterase of *rd* rod visual cells is responsive to light. This is indicated by a reduction in cyclic GMP content during light adaptation; the response to light is present in the *rd* retina only during the postnatal period when the visual cells have morphologically intact outer segments (FARBER and LOLLEY 1977a). The amount of cyclic GMP in the *rd* retina that is hydrolyzed by phosphodiesterase after light activation corresponds to a small fraction; the major portion of the retinal cyclic GMP is not affected by light. The high levels of cyclic GMP in the *rd* retina do not decrease immediately following the degeneration of the outer segments. This suggests that the light-insensitive cyclic GMP is present in the inner segments, in the soma or in the synaptic terminals of the visual cells.

The abnormality in cyclic GMP hydrolysis is restricted to visual cells of the *rd* retina. Several body tissues of the *rd* mouse such as blood components, muscle, brain and skin have been evaluated for phosphodiesterase activity, and all of them appear normal (LOLLEY and FARBER 1980).

Recent findings have indicated that the levels of cyclic GMP in normal visual cells of mice are modulated by calcium (COHEN et al. 1978). For example, when dark-adapted retinas are incubated in calcium-free medium plus EGTA, cyclic GMP levels increase ten- to twenty-fold. This increase in cyclic GMP content is reversible. If retinas are placed back in media containing normal calcium, cyclic GMP content falls to the dark-adapted levels.

The retinas of *rd* mice contain a subnormal concentration of calcium in the period of postnatal development during which the photoreceptors differentiate and degenerate (FARBER and LOLLEY 1976). The developing *rd* retinas respond to EGTA treatment in vitro by accumulating cyclic GMP only after rod visual cells have differentiated and before they degenerate, but the increase in the cyclic nucleotide level is much less than that observed in normal retinas of developing mice (LOLLEY et al. 1980). The total accumulation of cyclic GMP (mutation plus EGTA-stimulated accumulation) in *rd* retinas is similar to that observed in normal retinas treated with EGTA. Moreover, if 13-day-old *rd* retinas are incubated in media containing 5.0 m*M* Ca^{2+}, cyclic GMP levels decrease by about 43%. Thus, it seems that the *rd* mutation and EGTA treatment probably act by the same mechanism. In addition to the cyclic GMP-phosphodiesterase deficiency and the low levels of calcium, the *rd* photoreceptors may have a reduced ability to utilize the available calcium.

All of the observations above imply that an accumulation of cyclic GMP in rod visual cells is an early and perhaps causative factor in the inherited disease of *rd* mice. But how cyclic GMP is involved in the degenerative process is still unresolved. If cyclic GMP is associated with the visual transducer mechanism regulating ion permeability of the photoreceptor (FARBER et al. 1978), an accumulation of cyclic GMP might increase the free passage of ions into the cell, leading to osmotic imbalance and eventual death. Alternatively, cyclic GMP may regulate other processes of the photoreceptors such as disc membrane assembly or protein translocation. Accumulation of cyclic GMP in the visual cells of the *rd* retina could then disrupt those processes and lead to degenerative conditions.

Studies of mice heterozygous for the *rd* gene have shown that they also have an abnormality in retinal cyclic GMP metabolism (FERRENDELLI and COHEN 1976). Light- or dark-adapted retinas of heterozygotes have 40% less cyclic GMP than those of control animals, even when the number of photoreceptor cells is the same in both experimental groups.

2. Irish Setter Dog

Irish Setters carry an autosomal recessive mutation (PARRY 1953) that causes retinal degeneration (rod-cone dysplasia) in homozygous animals (AGUIRRE and RUBIN 1975). The early onset of the disease leads to night blindness within 6–8 weeks and subsequent complete blindness. Neither the rods nor the cones of the Irish Setter retina shows a normal electrophysiological response, not even during the first postnatal weeks, indicating that the photoreceptors never reach functional maturity. Nor do they achieve the final length that is characteristic of the photoreceptors of the normal retina, Thus, the disease in the Setters is best classified as a "dysplasia" (abnormal development) rather than a degeneration (AGUIRRE and RUBIN 1975).

Following their initial differentiation, the visual cells of the affected retina form only small and disorganized rod outer segments. The morphological abnormalities are already apparent in the second postnatal week. By two months of age, the retinas have lost the majority of the rod outer segments as well as many of the rod visual cells. By 18–20 weeks, all rod photoreceptors have degenerated leaving the retina with only a small number of cones in the photoreceptor layer. The inner retinal layers remain unchanged. Thus, in the Irish Setter disease, the early onset of rod degeneration and the maintenance of cone integrity is similar to the pattern of visual cell degeneration observed in retinas of *rd* mice.

An abnormality in cyclic GMP metabolism has been demonstrated in the Irish Setter dog disorder (AGUIRRE et al. 1978). As in *rd* mice, the levels of cyclic GMP in the affected retinas are higher than in control retinas even by 9–12 days, a time when photoreceptor outer segments are in their earliest stages of formation (CHADER et al. 1980). By 8–18 weeks, cyclic GMP levels are ten-fold higher than in control retinas (AGUIRRE et al. 1978). Cyclic AMP levels remain normal in affected retinas throughout development. Similar to *rd* mice, the Irish Setter dog retinas are deficient in the cyclic GMP-phosphodiesterase activity characteristic of rod visual cells. This deficiency is specific for the photoreceptors and does not alter the concentration of cyclic GMP of liver, brain or the pigment epithelium.choroid unit. By the 9th postnatal day, cyclic GMP-phosphodiesterase activity is already lower in dystrophic than in control dog retina. In addition, the endogenous calcium-dependent protein activator for cyclic GMP-phosphodiesterase, calmodulin, measured using activator-deficient brain phosphodiesterase, is lower in affected than in control retinas at all ages (LIU et al. 1979). Exogenous brain activator increases whereas EGTA decreases the cyclic GMP-phosphodiesterase activity both in control and affected retinas of 9-day-old dogs. This indicates that the phosphodiesterase that is present in the retina at this stage of development is calmodulin-dependent. By 5–7 weeks, however, neither brain activator nor EGTA have any effect on phosphodiesterase activity in the control retina although the effects are yet evident in the affected retinas. LIU et al. (1979) suggest that there is a switch in phosphodiesterase type (calmodulin-dependent to -independent) in the control retinas, whereas the affected retinas remain activator-dependent. This, and the lowered level of calmodulin in the affected Irish Setter retinas, can lead to greatly increased levels of cyclic GMP and photoreceptor cell degeneration.

3. Drug-Induced Photoreceptor Cell Degeneration in Normal Eyes

A retinal degeneration that resembles all of the morphological changes caused by the recessive mutation occurring in *rd* mice and Irish Setter dogs has been induced by the use of phosphodiesterase inhibitors in the eye rudiments of *Xenopus laevis* embryos (LOLLEY et al. 1977b). These eye rudiments differentiate and grow in hanging-drop cultures using a simple salt solution, since the intracellular food reserves that are distributed among all cells of the amphibian embryo are sufficient to sustain development in vitro for several days (HOLLYFIELD et al. 1975). Photoreceptors of the retinal neuroepithelium from stage 31 embryos are undifferentiated when placed in culture but, during three days in vitro, rods and cones develop morphologically and form outer segment membranes as well as synaptic contacts with second-order neurons in the outer plexiform layer. The normal eye rudiments can undergo the same process in cultures containing low concentrations ($<10^{-5}$ M) of phosphodiesterase inhibitors such as IBMX or Squibb 65,422 (LOLLEY et al. 1977b). However, with concentrations of inhibitor between 10^{-5} to 10^{-3} M in the cultures, rod visual cells become degenerative selectively as the levels of cyclic GMP increase within the rudiment; higher concentrations of the drugs result in cell death throughout the retina. For example, in the presence of 9×10^{-4} M IBMX, cyclic GMP content in the eye rudiments increases about 80% above that of the control after one day in culture, and it becomes greater throughout day 2. During this period of time, the developing photoreceptors elaborate disorganized outer segment membranes and many of the cells undergo a change in shape, becoming spherical, and are extruded from the retinal surface. By day 3, the concentration of cyclic GMP in the eye rudiments drops considerably and is very high in the incubation medium, suggesting the release of cyclic GMP from the photoreceptors upon degeneration. At this time, most of the extruded visual cells are necrotic and only a few photoreceptors remain in the outer retina (LOLLEY et al. 1977b). All of these observations indicate that an abnormality in cyclic GMP hydrolysis can cause degeneration of rod visual cells in normal retina.

With the use of phosphodiesterase inhibitors in the culture, FARBER et al. (1979d) have shown that the levels of cyclic AMP also increase during the 3 days of incubation of *Xenopus laevis* eye rudiments. The increase in cyclic AMP content is about one-half of that observed in cyclic GMP content. These authors assessed the effect of high levels of each cyclic nucleotide on photoreceptor viability by growing the eye rudiments in medium containing the dibutyryl or 8-bromo derivatives of cyclic AMP and cyclic GMP. After 3 days in vitro, retinal morphology was affected differently by each compound. Below 1 mM concentration, 8-bromo-cyclic AMP was non-toxic but, above 1 mM, it produces widespread cell death throughout all retinal layers. 8-Bromo-cyclic GMP at 2 mM concentration prevents the elaboration of photoreceptor outer segments, in the absence of cell death. Dibutyryl-cyclic AMP (8–16 mM) causes widespread destruction of cells throughout the retina with some localized photoreceptor cell death evident at lower concentrations (4 mM). Dibutyryl-cyclic GMP blocks retinal differentiation when applied to stage 31 eye rudiments but destroys specifically the photoreceptor layer when applied to stage 37 retinas, just as occurred when the phosphodiesterase inhibitors were used. Non-toxic levels of dibutyryl-cyclic GMP and IBMX, when added together in the incubation medium, act synergistically to cause selective photoreceptor cell death. Thus, elevated levels of cyclic AMP or cyclic GMP both are toxic to neurons of the retina, but only elevated levels of cyclic GMP cause the specific destruction of photoreceptor cells.

4. Retinal Degeneration in Several Strains of Rats

The inherited diseases affecting the retina of rats from strains such as the Royal College of Surgeons (RCS), the Hunter and the Campbell arise probably from an inborn error of metabolism completely different from that occurring in *rd* mice and Irish Setter dogs. In the rat disorder, the defective gene appears to interrupt the process of photoreceptor renewal by altering the ability of the pigment epithelium to phagocytize the sheddings of the photoreceptor cell outer segments (BOK and HALL 1971; HERRON et al. 1969; LAVAIL et al., 1972).

In normal retina, membrane components of the outer segment discs are synthesized in the inner segment, transported to the outer segment and assembled at their base into the discs (YOUNG 1969 b). The discs are then displaced proximally by the addition of new discs and, after a period of time which varies with the species (for rats it takes about nine days), the discs reach the tip of the outer segment and then are shed. For rod photoreceptors, this occurs every day at dawn (LAVAIL 1976). The sheddings are then engulfed and phagocytized by the pigment epithelium (YOUNG and BOK 1969). This constitutes the normal mechanism of rod outer segment renewal (YOUNG 1967, 1969 b; YOUNG and BOK 1969). Cyclic nucleotides may be involved in this process, since it has been reported by FEENEY and MIXON (1976) that they can alter the morphology and perhaps the function of bovine and human pigment epithelium cells.

In the dystrophic RCS rat retina, synthesis, assemblage and displacement of rod outer segment discs are apparently normal during the early phases of the disease (BOK and HALL 1971; HERRON et al. 1971). The failure of the pigment epithelium to remove and phagocytize the outer segment membranes results in a build-up of debris in the space between the tip of the rod outer segment and the pigment epithelium. This debris constitutes the morphological characteristic of the RCS disorder (DOWLING and SIDMAN 1962; BOK and HALL 1971).

The abnormality in the function of the pigment epithelium was suggested by MULLEN and LAVAIL (1976), from their studies of chimeric rats of normal and RCS parentage. In addition, it has been shown in vivo (GOLDMAN and O'BRIEN 1978) and in vitro (EDWARDS and SZAMIER 1977; HALL 1978) that the pigment epithelial cells of the dystrophic retina have a reduced ability to ingest the rod outer segment material. The question that comes up immediately is why do the photoreceptor cells of the dystrophic rat retinas degenerate if the genetic abnormality resides in the pigment epithelium. At present, there is no definitive answer, but it has been suggested that cyclic GMP metabolism may be disrupted by the accumulation of debris (LOLLEY and FARBER 1975).

The activities of both guanylate cyclase and cyclic GMP-phosphodiesterase are normal in the RCS retinas until 12–14 postnatal days, as debris has not yet appeared (LOLLEY and FARBER 1976). But, thereafter, the synthesis of cyclic GMP is reduced and its hydrolysis is altered; at least in vitro, the cyclic GMP-phosphodiesterase of the RCS retina appears to increase its affinity for cyclic GMP. A heat-denaturable, non-dialyzable protein in the debris seems to cause the kinetic modification of the photoreceptor phosphodiesterase (LOLLEY and FARBER 1975, 1976). In vivo, the levels of cyclic GMP in retinas of RCS rats are decreased by light but, after debris starts to accumulate, the cyclic GMP content of the dark- or light-adapted dystrophic retinas is always below that of the comparable control (FARBER and LOLLEY 1977 a). The light-accelerated visual cell degeneration which occurs in the RCS disease (LAVAIL and BATTELLE 1975) might be related to the subnormal levels of cyclic GMP found in the light-adapted RCS retinas. The reduced level of cyclic GMP is the only biochemical defect that has been described so far which occurs prior to pathological changes in the visual cells.

Phosphodiesterase activity in the albino, dystrophic Campbell strain (BOURNE et al. 1938) and in the pigmented Hunter dystrophic rat retinas has been studied by DEWAR et al. (1975a, b) using cyclic AMP as substrate. The affected albino retina appears to be deficient in the activity of the photoreceptor phosphodiesterase before the first signs of histological degeneration are observed. In contrast, the pigmented, dystrophic Hunter retina shows a reduction in phosphodiesterase activity secondary to the degeneration of the photoreceptor cells. In ox retina, a thermostable protein component of the pH 5.9 fraction inhibits the cyclic GMP-phosphodiesterase (DUMLER and ETINGOF 1976). A similar factor/effect is found in normal rat retina, but the thermostable protein from Campbell rat retina activates, rather than inhibits, phosphodiesterase activity, and the component from Hunter rat retina has no effect on the enzyme (ETINGOF and OSTAPENKO 1978; USOVA et al. 1978). Studies of rhodopsin content, ERG changes after debris accumulation (GOVARDOVSKII et al. 1977; ETINGOF 1978), and the possible involvement of lysosomal enzymes (DEWAR et al. 1977) in the etiology of these diseases of the rat retina have not as yet clarified the cause of photoreceptor cell degeneration.

C. Cyclic Nucleotide Metabolism in Ocular Tissues Other Than Retina

Cyclic AMP is present in the ocular tissues of many species and is certainly involved in at least the aqueous outflow regulation of the eye (NEUFELD and SEARS 1974; BONOMI and APPIANI 1975). In contrast, very little is known about cyclic GMP levels or function outside of the retina. The next sections will attempt to provide a summarized review of the available literature.

I. Ciliary Body-Iris-Aqueous Humor

The aqueous humor occupies the space between the vitreous and the cornea in the anterior segment of the eye. The anterior segment is incompletely divided into two unequal parts by the iris, to form the anterior and posterior chambers. Behind the iris, the lens occupies the greater part of the anterior segment and, therefore, the volume of aqueous humor in the posterior chamber is less than in the anterior chamber. The two chambers are connected by the opening of the iris, the pupil, and the aqueous humor which is produced in the posterior chamber flows through the pupil into the anterior chamber. The pupil can be reduced or expanded through the contraction or relaxation of the constrictor and dilator muscles, respectively. The ciliary epithelium covering the ciliary process is continuous with the epithelium of the posterior surface of the iris. The ciliary muscle together with the stroma and epithelium form the ciliary body from which the lens is suspended.

It is generally accepted that the site of aqueous humor formation is in the ciliary process and that the non-pigmented epithelium of the ciliary process is involved in its secretion (SEARS 1975). Ciliary process tissue contains both adenylate cyclase (WAITZMAN and WOODS 1971) and cyclic AMP-phosphodiesterase (SHANTA et al. 1966). The adenylate cyclase of ciliary body has been localized cytochemically

(TSUKAHARA and MAEZAWA 1978). Its activity is distributed almost exclusively on the plasma membrane of non-pigmented epithelial cells and capillary endothelial cells located in the stroma of the ciliary process. No reaction product has been found on the plasma membrane of pigmented epithelial cells nor in the epithelial cells of the iridial portion of the ciliary process. This suggests that adenylate cyclase activity on the plasma membrane of the non-pigmented epithelial cells could be involved in the regulatory mechanisms of aqueous humor formation (see also NATHANSON 1980).

Adenylate cyclase activity from rabbit ciliary process is activated by KCl, NaF, catecholamines and prostaglandin E_1 (WAITZMAN and WOODS 1971). The effect of epinephrine is blocked by propanolol, a β-adrenergic antagonist, but phenoxybenzamine, the α-antagonist, is ineffective. LAHAV et al. (1978) showed that a fluorescent analogue of propanolol, systemically delivered, was localized in the ciliary process of the rat. In addition, β-adrenergic receptors have been identified in preparations of rabbit iris-ciliary body (NEUFELD and PAGE 1977; NATHANSON 1980), and BROMBERG et al. (1980) characterized β-adrenergic receptors in a membrane fraction from isolated ciliary processes of rabbit eyes. In this study, adenylate cyclase activity was recovered from a discontinuous sucrose density gradient in the same fraction as the binding sites for ^{125}I-hydroxybenzylpindolol (a β-adrenergic antagonist). Prostaglandin E_1 activation seems to be additive with β-adrenergic activation and to oppose α-adrenergic antagonism in a competitive manner (WAITZMAN and WOODS 1971).

Cyclic AMP is present in the ciliary body as well as in iris and aqueous humor (NEUFELD and SEARS 1974). DUTTON et al. (1979) reported an active uptake and rapid metabolism of cyclic AMP in isolated rabbit ciliary body-iris preparation.

Guanylate cyclase activity from iris is inhibited in vitro by concentrations of secretin that activate the enzyme from several different tissues (THOMPSON et al. 1974). However, lower concentrations of the hormone do not cause any effect on the activity of the enzyme. THOMPSON et al. (1974) suggest that guanylate cyclase from rat iris may have different receptor characteristics from that of other tissues, probably related to the dense automatic innervation of the iris.

Traumatic stimuli such as topical application of prostaglandins E_2 or E_1, infrared irradiation of the iris, subcutaneous injection of α-melanocyte-stimulating hormone (α-MSH), paracentesis or intravitreal injection of Shigella or *E. coli* endotoxins cause a disruption of the blood-aqueous barrier in the eye. Imidazole, an activator of cyclic AMP-phosphodiesterase, antagonizes the damage of the barrier (ZINK et al. 1975; BENGTSSON 1976; KASS et al. 1977). However, in rabbit, systemically administered imidazole has no effect on the aqueous humor concentration of cyclic AMP or cyclic GMP (KASS et al. 1977); neither does imidazole, at a concentration of 10^{-3} *M*, in vitro, activate the rabbit ciliary body-iris phosphodiesterase. High levels of prostaglandins have been shown in aqueous humor of human and laboratory animals in different forms of ocular inflammation. BENGTSSON (1977) suggested that imidazole probably acts by promoting the prostaglandin uptake in the iris and ciliary body. The protein leakage caused by PGE_2 and α-MSH is potentiated by pretreatment with intravenous theophylline (BENGTSSON 1977). In fact, theophylline itself can cause a barrier damage. This effect is not inhibited by pretreatment with indomethacin, which indicates that it is the increased intraocular concentration of cyclic AMP, without any increase in the intraocular prostaglandin synthesis, that elicits the barrier disruption. BENGTSSON (1977) suggested that cyclic AMP might be the common effector of the barrier breakdown caused by prostaglandin and by non-prostaglandin agents.

Tetanus toxin blocks the cholinergic nerve terminals of the sphincter pupillary muscles producing pupillary paralysis. Pharmacological agents injected intraocularly into the anterior chamber can modify the degree of paralysis. For example, both theophylline and glycine can temporarily reverse tetanus toxin-induced paralysis of rabbit sphincter pupillary muscles and also shorten the recovery period. It has been shown that the adrenergic system is not involved in these reactions of the rabbit iris and that the cholinergic system is the site of toxin action (FEDINEC and KING 1969; FEDINEC 1975; FEDINEC et al. 1976; AMBACHE et al. 1948a, b). Cyclic nucleotides have no marked effect on the pupillary muscles of normal rabbit eyes. However, when the muscles are denervated by tetanus toxin, they become very responsive to cyclic GMP. Injections of either cyclic GMP or dibutyryl-cyclic GMP can temporarily reverse the paralysis of sphincter pupillary muscles (KING et al. 1978).

Cyclic AMP has been shown to alter the configuration of cultured iris epithelial cells. The lamellar iris epithelial cells take a stellate configuration when cyclic AMP, dibutyryl-cyclic AMP, monobutyryl-cyclic AMP or theophylline is added to the culture medium. Thus, the stellate effect seems to be an expression of the increase in intracellular level of cyclic AMP (ORTIZ et al. 1973). To test this hypothesis, YAMADA (1977) microinjected cyclic AMP into iris epithelial cells kept in culture. The injecion of 0.005–0.5 pmol per cell of cyclic AMP in medium containing 1 m*M* theophylline caused a reduction in the area of cell-substrate contact: the lammelar cytoplasm retracted toward the nucleus and the stellate configuration appeared. With higher levels of cyclic AMP injected, further retraction was obtained and the cell became a compact sphere. In the absence of theophylline in the medium, the reduction of the area of cell-substrate contact was less. Injection of theophylline did not alter the cell configuration. Thus, the major effect of cyclic AMP is to shift the cell surface from the expanded to contracted condition.

Dibutyryl-cyclic GMP in the culture medium does not change the lamellar configuration of the iris epithelial cells. However, it seems that when the iris epithelial cells are in the contracted state, addition to the culture medium of dibutyryl-cyclic GMP makes the cells expand. This suggests that cyclic AMP and cyclic GMP may control cell configuration in an antagonistic way. Furthermore, YAMADA (1977) refers to an unpublished experiment of Ortiz, who observed that the stellate effect of dibutyryl-cyclic AMP on lamellar iris epithelial cells is suppressed by the addition of dibutyryl-cyclic GMP.

II. The Aqueous Outflow System

The significant resistance to aqueous outflow is localized in the small channels which communicate through the wall of the eye at the "chamber angle". These channels form two communicating networks, an inner trabecular meshwork of small channels and an outer intrascleral plexus of larger channels, which are separated in man and primates by the canal of Schlemm. This canal of Schlemm is like a sink for the aqueous humor percolating through the meshwork (LANGHAM 1963). Other animals do not have a canal of Schlemm and the aqueous humor flowing through the trabecular meshwork is collected directly into the veins of the intrascleral plexus. These can be filled with blood, with aqueous humor or with a mixture of blood and aqueous humor. In all species, the mixed blood and aqueous humor leaves the intrascleral plexus and drains to the heart through the episcleral, anterior ciliary and ophthalmic veins (ASHTON 1951, 1952; RUSKELL 1961).

The in vivo outflow resistance could be considered as having two components: a mechanical one derived from the small caliber of the flow channels and a vascular component that arises from the flow of both blood and aqueous humor through the intrascleral plexus; the channel space for aqueous humor depends then on the amount of blood that is filling the plexus (HART 1972).

In the living eye, outflow resistance and aqueous humor formation change with increasing intraocular pressure (LANGHAM 1959; BILL and BÁRÁNY 1966). Thus, glaucomatous eyes have in general a very high outflow resistance, contributed mainly by the veins of the intrascleral plexus (LANGHAM 1977).

Both α- and β-adrenergic receptors are present in the outflow system, and their stimulation may induce specific responses in the intraocular pressure and outflow resistance. For example, a single topical application of salbutamol (a synthetic β_2-adrenergic agonist) or of isoproterenol (which shows in the eye β_1-, β_2-, and α-agonist activities) decreases intraocular pressure and decreases both the rate of formation of aqueous humor and the outflow resistance (LANGHAM and DIGGS 1974). Epinephrine, the most common catecholamine in the treatment of glaucoma, is also a mixed agonist which decreases the rate of aqueous humor outflow resistance and formation. Its effect on the outflow resistance is determined by α-agonist activity only (LANGHAM 1977).

Adrenergic agonists increase the cyclic AMP concentration in the aqueous humor of the treated eye. NEUFELD et al. (1972) showed that epinephrine is more potent than norepinephrine and isoproterenol both for reducing intraocular pressure and increasing cyclic AMP levels. Intravenous injection of the α-antagonist, phenoxybenzamine (30 mg/kg) partially inhibits the response to topical epinephrine or norepinephrine, whereas the β-antagonist propanolol is ineffective. Topically applied phosphodiesterase inhibitors such as aminophylline or theophylline, and dibutyryl-cyclic AMP are also ineffective. In contrast, intravenous injection of bupranolol, another β-adrenergic blocking agent, inhibits the increase of cyclic AMP levels in the aqueous humor due to topical application of isoproterenol (TAMURA et al. 1978). Intracameral injection of high concentrations of cyclic AMP ($4 \times 10^{-4}\,M$) causes a marked decrease in intraocular pressure and also increases the outflow facility (NEUFELD et al. 1975; NEUFELD and SEARS 1975). Neufeld and collaborators interpreted these observations to indicate that cyclic AMP mediates the action of catecholamines on aqueous humor dynamics. These authors showed, further (NEUFELD et al. 1973), another correlation between cyclic AMP levels and intraocular pressure. They altered the intraocular pressure response of the eye to epinephrine in two ways: (1) decreased responsiveness to the drug by repeated, daily topical administration of epinephrine, which results also in a smaller increase in cyclic AMP in the aqueous humor, when compared to the response of an untreated eye, and (2) increased responsiveness to epinephrine by unilateral superior cervical ganglionectomy, which causes a denervation supersensitivity to adrenergic agonists. In fact, topical application or intravitreal injections of epinephrine produce a greater decrease in intraocular pressure and a greater increase in cyclic AMP in the aqueous humor of the denervated eye than in that of the control. In a similar study using bilaterally superior cervical sympathetic ganglionectomized rabbits, WAITZMAN (1978) also showed an increase in cyclic AMP levels in aqueous humor when compared to those of sham-operated controls. Furthermore, it has been observed that sympathetic denervation by destruction of the nerve terminals with 6-hydroxydopamine or treatment with a β-adrenergic antagonist cause, in the ciliary body-iris preparations, an increase in the density of β-adrenergic receptors; that is, a denervation supersensitivity response similar in magnitude to that obtained by treatment with an adrenergic agonist in a denervated eye (NEUFELD et al. 1978).

RADIUS and LANGHAM (1973) confirmed that in rabbits, phenoxybenzamine (10 mg/kg) blocks the physiological response to norepinephrine applied after the injection of antagonist. However, they observed high levels of cyclic AMP both in the untreated and norepinephrine-treated eyes compared to rabbits not given phenoxybenzamine, which indicates that phenoxybenzamine itself causes a significant accumulation of cyclic AMP in the aqueous humor. Thus, these results do not support the suggestion of NEUFELD et al. (1973) that cyclic AMP accumulation in the aqueous humor directly mediates the hypotensive response. Nevertheless, another series of studies have shown that analogues of cyclic AMP such as dibutyryl- and 8-methylthio-cyclic AMP, injected into the anterior chamber of the eye of the vervet monkey, cause a two-fold increase in outflow facility (NEUFELD 1978). This increase does not occur, however, if the treatment with the cyclic AMP derivative is preceded by intracamerally or topically administered epinephrine. This suggests that once epinephrine has stimulated the β-mechanism, cyclic AMP is no longer effective, and indicates again that the primary action of catecholamines on outflow facility is mediated by cyclic AMP.

Results are not so clear when the cyclic AMP derivatives are applied to enucleated eyes. This was done in order to establish if an intact vascular supply or formation of aqueous humor is necessary for the decrease in outflow resistance that is observed following intracameral administration of the cyclic AMP derivative (NEUFELD 1978). Contrary to what is observed in vivo, perfusion of the anterior chamber of the enucleated eye with 8-methylthio-cyclic AMP causes a decrease in outflow facility. This may be due to relaxation of the ciliary muscle, since BILL (1970) suggested that β-adrenergic stimulation leads to relaxation of the ciliary muscle with consequent decrease in outflow facility. Possibly, if the ciliary muscle is relaxed by intracameral injection of 8-methylthio-cyclic AMP in vivo, then the observed increase in outflow facility in vivo is much greater than what is measured. This topic is still unclear.

In addition to disrupting the blood-aqueous barrier, prostaglandins (mainly the PGEs), administered topically, systemically or intracamerally, increase the intraocular pressure in rabbit, cat and monkey (WAITZMAN and KING 1967; BEITCH and EAKINS 1969; EAKINS 1970; KELLY and STARR 1971; KASS et al. 1972; CASEY 1974). The mechanism of the intraocular pressure response appears to be increased aqueous humor formation. The levels of cyclic AMP in aqueous humor of PGE_2-treated eyes are significantly higher than in the contralateral eyes treated with diluent (PODOS 1976). Thus, epinephrine and PGE_2, both of which induce elevations of aqueous humor cyclic AMP, cause opposite results on the intraocular pressure: epinephrine induces a fall and PGE_2 induces a rise.

The constrictor pupillae and ciliary muscles are innervated by cholinergic nerves. The concept that cholinergic compounds decrease the mechanical components of the outflow resistance was supported by studies on the ocular response to pilocarpine, the drug most widely used in the treatment of glaucoma (BÁRÁNY 1966). To test whether cyclic GMP, which has been implicated as a mediator of cholinergic stimulation, has an influence on outflow facility, NEUFELD (1978) administered 8-bromo-cyclic GMP to the eyes of vervet monkeys intracamerally. He observed no effect of the cyclic GMP derivative on outflow facility in eyes which subsequently responded to pilocarpine treatment. Furthermore, atropine, pilocarpine and eserine fail to produce any variation in the normally high cyclic GMP content of the rabbit aqueous humor (BONOMI et al. 1977). KASS et al. (1977) reported a similar cyclic GMP concentration (about 13 pmol/ml).

Guanylate cyclase activity is increased in vitro by sodium azide or sodium nitroprusside (KIMURA et al. 1975; KATSUKI et al. 1977). These compounds, applied topically to rabbit eyes, increase the intraocular pressure in a dose-dependent manner and elevate the levels of cyclic GMP in the aqueous humor (KRUPIN et al. 1977). The outflow facility remains unchanged, suggesting that an increase in aqueous humor production is the cause for the elevation of intraocular pressure. Topical application of atropine or systemic β-adrenergic blockade with epinephrine does not modify the increase in intraocular pressure following sodium azide or sodium nitroprusside treatment. The α-adrenergic agent, phenoxybenzamine, also does not prevent the increase in aqueous humor cyclic GMP content but it does block the elevation of intraocular pressure.

III. Lens

Only a few studies have been reported on cyclic nucleotide metabolism in lens, and its physiological function in this tissue still remains unknown.

The content of cyclic nucleotides in lens is very low. BONOMI et al. (1977) report a cyclic GMP level of 0.042 pmol/mg protein in rabbit. However, cyclic AMP-dependent protein kinase activity has been demonstrated in extracts of epithelial cells and cortical fibers of bovine lens (TAKÁTS et al. 1978). The catalytic properties of the enzymes from these two cell types are very similar. They have identical substrate specificity (highest incorporation of phosphate is obtained with f_{2b} and f_1 histone fractions), similar affinity for ATP, similar pH optima and similar concentration of cyclic AMP required for half-maximal activation ($5–9 \times 10^{-8}$ *M*). The magnitude of activation, however, is very different. The cyclic AMP-stimulated increase in activity of the epithelial protein kinase is five-to ten-fold, whereas the cortical enzyme shows a 20- to 25-fold activation by cyclic AMP. It seems that the reason for the low basal activity of the cortical protein kinase is that it is present mainly as the holoenzyme. In fact, the cortical extract of lens contains three times more cyclic AMP-binding protein per unit of enzyme activity than the epithelial extract.

The hydrolysis of cyclic AMP is much faster than that of cyclic GMP in the bovine lens (LIU and SCHWARTZ 1978). When the homogenate of lens is separated into a particulate and a $105,000 \times g$ supernatant fraction, most of the cyclic AMP- and cyclic GMP-phosphodiesterase activities are found in the supernatant fraction. Kinetic analysis reveals two apparent K_m values for each cyclic AMP- and cyclic GMP-phosphodiesterase in the 10^{-6} and 10^{-5} M range. The calcium-dependent protein activator of phosphodiesterase is also present in the bovine lens.

IV. Cornea

The outer coat of the wall of the eyeball, which gives the organ its form and protects its inner delicate structures, consists of a large, opaque, posterior portion – the sclera – and a smaller anterior, transparent segment – the cornea.

The epithelium of the cornea is extremely sensitive and contains numerous free nerve endings. It has a remarkable capacity for regeneration. Healing occurs rapidly, by flattening and by a gliding movement of the adjacent epithelial cells. Mitotic activity may be found at considerable distances from a wound.

Systemic administration of epinephrine in high doses in rats inhibits the cell movement that follows injury, preventing the healing process (FRIEDENWALD and BUSCHKE 1944a). In addition, superior cervical ganglionectomy, as well as excitement and pain stimuli, decrease the mitotic activity in the corneal epithelium of rats (FRIEDENWALD and BUSCHKE 1944b) and of rabbits (MISHIMA 1957). Cyclic AMP seems to be involved in these processes. NEUFELD and SEARS (1974) showed that epinephrine and norepinephrine, in vitro, increase about twofold the levels of cyclic AMP in incubated corneas of rabbits, monkeys and humans and that this effect is blocked specifically by the β-adrenergic antagonist propanolol. In addition, CAVANAGH (1975) reported that cyclic AMP inhibits corneal epithelium cell growth, in culture. Furthermore, BUTTERFIELD and NEUFELD (1977) found that twenty hours after superior cervical ganglionectomy, norepinephrine, which is released from the degenerating adrenergic nerve terminals, causes the levels of cyclic AMP to increase in the corneal epithelium of rabbit. This effect parallels a decrease in mitotic activity in the corneal epithelium cells. Intravenous propanolol administered after surgery blocks both the increase in cyclic AMP levels and the decrease in mitotic activity.

The density of β-adrenergic receptors on membranes from homogenized corneas has been determined by measuring the specific binding of ^{3}H-dihydroalprenolol (NEUFELD et al. 1978). Sympathetic denervation of the eye, either by superior cervical ganglionectomy or by subconjunctival treatment with 6-hydroxydopamine, does not alter the density of β-adrenergic receptors in the cornea. In contrast, the in vivo treatment with epinephrine causes a marked decrease (40%) in the corneal β-adrenergic receptors which is associated with a decreased capacity to synthesize cyclic AMP. Similar topical treatment with timolol, the potent β-adrenergic antagonist, results in an increase in receptor density. However, the increased number of receptors in the membrane apparently does not alter the coupling between β-adrenergic receptors and adenylate cyclase, possibly because the amount of adenylate cyclase is limiting. Thus, the tissue does not make more cyclic AMP even when it has more receptors available (NEUFELD et al. 1978).

Cyclic GMP does not appear to have an effect in the regulation of mitotic activity during wound healing. This is compatible with the very low levels of cyclic GMP in the cornea (BUTTERFIELD and NEUFELD 1977).

The mitotic activity of corneal epithelial cells is also modulated by epidermal growth factor. This is a polypeptide which stimulates both proliferation and differentiation of epithelial tissues. FRATI et al. (1972) and SAVAGE and COHEN (1973) have shown that the epidermal growth factor, when applied to wounded corneas of rabbit, causes re-epithelialization by inducing hyperplasia of epithelial cell layers. The mechanism by which epidermal growth factor modulates cell proliferation is unknown, but it seems to be associated with changes in the levels of cyclic nucleotides. The cyclic AMP content of isolated corneal epithelium, when incubated in vitro with the factor (10^{-6} *M*), increases rapidly but transiently, whereas the cyclic GMP levels are slightly depressed first but elevated in the following minutes (FRATI et al. 1977).

The transparency of the cornea is a function of its hydration (MAURICE 1969), and corneal hydration seems to be regulated by electrolyte transport across the cellular layers of this tissue. Active chloride and sodium transport systems have been reported in frog, rabbit, monkey and human corneas (ZADUNAISKY and LANDE 1971; DICKSTEIN and MAURICE 1972; KLYCE et al. 1973; DONN et al. 1959; FISCHER et al. 1978).

Cyclic AMP is involved in the regulation of the corneal chloride pump. CHALFIE et al. (1972) showed that epinephrine stimulates transport in the frog corneal epithelium. KLYCE et al. (1973) demonstrated that the addition of epinephrine or phosphodiesterase inhibitors (both of which increase cyclic AMP levels) or of dibutyryl-cyclic AMP to the solution that bathes the epithelial side of the isolated rabbit cornea increases the net transport of chloride ions from the endothelial to the epithelial side. Cyclic AMP appears to change the permeability of the epithelial cells with a secondary increase in pump activity. Both in frog and rabbit, the chloride pump activated by cyclic AMP is located in the corneal epithelium and transports chloride ions toward the tear side (ZADUNAISKY 1966; ZADUNAISKY and LANDE 1971; KLYCE et al. 1973). This could be a mechanism for efficient dehydration of the corneal stroma. In the human cornea, cyclic AMP increases the unidirectional efflux of both sodium and chloride from aqueous humor to the tear side. This can be achieved without the use of dibutyryl-cyclic AMP (which is needed with the rabbit cornea) and probably reflects a higher permeability of human than rabbit corneal cells to cyclic AMP (FISCHER et al. 1978).

Low concentrations of ascorbic acid (10^{-5} *M*) stimulate the active transport of chloride of the toad corneal epithelium (SCOTT and FRIEDENTHAL 1973). It has been shown by GILMOUR-BUCK and ZADUNAISKY (1975) that the effect of ascorbic acid is not demonstrable if the isolated corneas are previously stimulated with theophylline. Similarly, theophylline has no action on the chloride flux after stimulation of the corneas with ascorbic acid, suggesting an inhibitory effect of ascorbic acid on the corneal cyclic AMP-phosphodiesterase. In fact, this inhibition of phosphodiesterase activity by ascorbic acid has been shown in soluble and in particulate fractions of corneal epithelium from frog, toad and rabbit (GILMOUR-BUCK and ZADUNAISKY 1975).

Corneal ulceration or regeneration depends upon the balance of collagen production by stromal fibroblasts and the collagenolysis which is induced primarily by the corneal epithelium (BROWN and WELLER 1970; ITOI et al. 1969; DOHLMAN 1971). When dibutyryl-cyclic AMP or theophylline is added to cultures of alkali-burned cornea, there is a partial inhibition of collagenase activity and of the degradation of collagen (BERMAN et al. 1976). 5′-AMP is also very effective in producing the same effects. The mechanism by which these drugs regulate collagenase activity is still unknown, but the observations above suggest that endogenous cyclic AMP may affect the synthesis or the secretion of collagenase in the cornea, in vivo. Inhibition of phosphodiesterase activity by theophylline or by the competitive inhibitor 5′-AMP would then increase cyclic AMP levels causing the suppression of collagenase activity (BERMAN et al. 1976). In agreement with these observations, CRABB (1977) showed that dibutyryl-cyclic AMP applied subconjunctivally produces a significant reduction of ulceration in the alkali-burned rabbit cornea, with an acceleration of corneal neovascularization in the first two weeks postburn.

D. Concluding Remarks

This review of the vast literature on cyclic nucleotides in the eye is intended only to provide a summarized account of the information currently available. The rate of growth of knowledge about each individual component of the eye, be it tissue or differentiated cellular type, makes any other kind of approach impossible.

In the last decade, cyclic nucleotides have been shown to be involved in one way or another in the metabolism, normal function, and disease states of most of the tissues of the eye. Learning more about how cyclic nucleotides modulate all of these conditions is a challenge, therefore, for the cell biologist, the biochemist, the pharmacologist, the physiologist and the clinician. Perhaps, in the next decade, the collaborative efforts of all of these individuals will provide the means to understand the mechanisms which operate in the normal and diseased eye.

Acknowledgements. My appreciation to Drs. BRUCE L. BASTIAN, RICHARD N. LOLLEY and MICHAEL L. WOODRUFF for their constructive criticism of the manuscript. Special thanks to LOUISE V. EATON, TUNDE CSISZAR, INGA ANDERSON and PATRICIA SHAMBLIN for their help in manuscript preparation. I want also to acknowledge the dedicated assistance of my Research Associate, DENNIS SOUZA and the support from the National Eye Institute (Grant EY2651 and RCDA K04EY144).

References

Aguirre GD, Rubin LF (1975) Pathology of hemeralopia in the Alaskan malamute dog. J Am Vet Med Assoc 166:257–259

Aguirre G, Farber D, Lolley R, Fletcher RT, Chader GJ (1978) Rod-Cone dysplasia in Irish setters: a defect in cyclic GMP metabolism in visual cells. Science 201:1133–1134

Ambache N, Morgan RS, Wright GP (1948 a) The action of tetanus toxin on the rabbit's iris. J Physiol (Lond) 107:45–53

Ambache N, Morgan RS, Wright GP (1948 b) The action of tetanus toxin on the acetylcholine and cholinesterase contents of the rabbit's iris. Br J Exp Pathol 29:408–418

Ashton N (1951) Anatomical study of Schlemm's canal and aqueous veins by means of neoprene casts. I. Aqueous veins. Br J Ophthalmol 35:291–303

Ashton N (1952) Anatomical study of Schlemm's canal and aqueous veins by means of neoprene casts. II. Aqueous veins. Br J Ophthalmol 36:265–267

Baehr W, Devlin MJ, Applebury M (1979) Isolation and characterization of cGMP phosphodiesterase from bovine rod outer segments. J Biol Chem 254:11669–11677

Bárány EH (1966) The mode of action of miotics on outflow resistance. Trans Ophthalmol Soc UK 86:539–578

Baughman R, Bader C (1977) Biochemical characterization and cellular localization of the cholinergic system in the chicken retina. Brain Res 138:469–485
Baylor DA, Fuortes MGF (1970) Electrical responses of single cones in the retina of the turtle. J Physiol (Lond) 207:77–92
Beitch BR, Eakins KE (1969) The effects of prostaglandins on the intraocular pressure of the rabbit. Br J Pharmacol 37:158–167
Bengtsson E (1976) The effect of imidazole on the disruption of the blood-aqueous barrier in the rabbit eye. Invest Ophthalmol Vis Sci 15:315–320
Bengtsson E (1977) The effect of theophylline on the breakdown of the blood-aqueous barrier in the rabbit eye. Invest Ophthalmol Vis Sci 16:636–640
Bensinger RE, Fletcher RT, Chader GJ (1974a) "Piggyback" chromatography: assay for guanylate cyclase in retina and other neural tissue. J Neurochem 22:1131–1134
Bensinger RE, Fletcher RT, Chader GJ (1974b) Guanylate cyclase: inhibition by light in retinal photoreceptors. Science 183:86–87
Berger SJ, De Vries GW, Carter JG, Schulz DW, Passoneau PW, Lowry OH, Ferrendelli JA (1980) The distribution of the components of the cyclic GMP cycle in retina. J Biol Chem 255:3128–3133
Berman AL, Usova AA (1978) Protein inhibitor of the retinal cyclic nucleotide phosphodiesterase: its localization in the outer segment of a photoreceptor (in Russian). Biokheimiia 43:486–490
Berman MB, Cavanagh HD, Gage J (1976) Regulation of collagenase activity in the ulcerating cornea by cyclic AMP. Exp Eye Res 22:209–218
Biernbaum MS, Bownds MD (1979) Influence of light and calcium on guanosine 5′-triphosphate in isolated frog rod outer segments. J Gen Physiol 74:649–669
Bignetti E, Cavaggioni A, Sorbi RT (1978) Light-activated hydrolysis of GTP and cyclic GMP in the rod outer segments. J Physiol (Lond) 279:55–69
Bill A (1970) Effects of norepinephrine, isoproterenol and sympathetic stimulation on aqueous humor dynamics in vervet monkeys. Exp Eye Res 10:31–46
Bill A, Bárány EH (1966) Gross facility, facility of conventional routes, and pseudofacility of aqueous humor outflow in the Cynomolgus monkey. Arch Ophthalmol 75:665–673
Bitensky MW, Gorman RE, Miller WH (1971) Adenyl cyclase as a link between photon capture and changes in membrane permeability of frog photoreceptors. Proc Natl Acad Sci USA 68:561–562
Bitensky MW, Miki N, Marcus FR, Keirns JJ (1973) The role of cyclic nucleotides in visual excitation. Life Sci 13:1451–1472
Bitensky MW, Miki N, Keirns JJ et al. (1975) Activation of photoreceptor disk membrane phosphodiesterase by light and ATP. Adv Cyclic Nucleotide Res 5:213–240
Bitensky MW, Wheeler GL, Aloni B, Vetury S, Matuo Y (1978) Light- and GTP-activated photoreceptor phosphodiesterase: regulation by a light-activated GTPase and identification of rhodopsin as the phosphodiesterase binding site. Adv Cyclic Nucleotide Res 9:553–572
Blanks JC, Adinolfi AM, Lolley RN (1974) Photoreceptor degeneration and synaptogenesis in retinal-degenerative (rd) mice. J Comp Neurol 156:95–106
Bok D, Hall MD (1971) The role of the pigment epithelium in the etiology of inherited retinal dystrophy in the rat. J Cell Biol 49:664–682
Bonomi L, Appiani S (1975) Comportamento dell AMP cyclico nei tessuti e fluidi oculari sotto vari stimoli farmacologici. Atti 54° Congr Soc Ital Oftalmol, pp 196–200
Bonomi L, Fregona I, Tomazzoli L (1977) Cyclic guanosine monophosphate (GMP) levels in ocular tissues. Albrecht Von Graefes Arch Klin Exp Ophthalmol 205:23–27
Bourne MC, Campbell DA, Tansley K (1938) Hereditary degeneration of the rat retina. Br J Ophthalmol 22:613–623
Bownds D, Brodie AE (1975) Light-sensitive swelling of isolated frog rod outer segments as an in vitro assay for visual transduction and dark adaptation. J Gen Physiol 66:407–425
Bownds D, Dawes L, Miller J, Stahlman M (1972) Phosphorylation of frog photoreceptor membranes induced by light. Nature New Biol 237:125–127
Brodie AE, Bownds D (1976) Biochemical correlates of adaptation processes in isolated frog photoreceptor membranes. J Gen Physiol 63:1–11

Bromberg BB, Gregory DS, Sears ML (1980) Beta-adrenergic receptors in ciliary processes of the rabbit. Invest Ophthalmol Vis Sci 19:203–207

Brown JE, Coles JA, Pinto LH (1977) Effects of injections of calcium and EGTA into the outer segments of retinal rods of *Bufo marinus*. J Physiol (Lond) 269:707–722

Brown JH, Makman MH (1972) Stimulation by dopamine of adenylate cyclase in retinal homogenates and of adenosine-3′:5′-cyclic monophosphate formation in intact retina. Proc Natl Acad Sci USA 69:539–543

Brown JH, Makman MH (1973) Influence of neuroleptic drugs and apomorphine on dopamine-sensitive adenylate cyclase of retina. J Neurochem 21:477–479

Brown JH, Makman MH, Opler LA (1973) Development and localization of dopamine-sensitive adenylate cyclase of mammalian retina. Fed Proc 32:679

Brown SI, Weller CA (1970) Pathogenesis and treatment of collagenase induced diseases of the cornea. Trans Am Acad Ophthalmol Otolaryngol 74:375–383

Brückner R (1951) Spaltlampenmikroskopie und Ophthalmoskopie am Auge von Ratte und Maus. Doc Ophthalmol 5–6:452–554

Bucher MB, Schorderet M (1974) Apomorphine-induced accumulation of cyclic AMP in isolated retinas of the rabbit. Biochem Pharmacol 23:3079–3082

Bucher MB, Schorderet M (1975) Dopamine- and apomorphine-sensitive adenylate cyclase in homogenates of rabbit retina. Naunyn Schmiedebergs Arch Pharmacol 288:103–107

Butterfield LC, Neufeld AH (1977) Cyclic nucleotides and mitosis in the rabbit cornea following superior cervical ganglionectomy. Exp Eye Res 25:427–433

Byzov AL, Trifonov YA (1968) The response to electric stimulation of horizontal cells in the carp retina. Vision Res 8:817–822

Caretta A, Cavaggioni A, Sorbi RT (1979) Cyclic GMP and the permeability of the disks of the frog photoreceptors. J Physiol (Lond) 295:171–178

Carter-Dawson LD, LaVail MM, Sidman RL (1978) Differential effect of the *rd* mutation on rods and cones in the mouse retina. Invest Ophthalmol Vis Sci 7:489–498

Casey WJ (1974) Prostaglandin E_2 and aqueous humor dynamics in the rhesus monkey eye. Prostaglandins 8:327–337

Cavanagh HD (1975) Herpetic ocular disease: therapy of persistent epithelial defects. Int Ophthalmol Clin 15:67–88

Cervetto L, Piccolino M (1974) Synaptic transmission between photoreceptors and horizontal cells in the turtle retina. Science 183:417–419

Chader GJ (1971) Hormonal effects on the neural retina: induction of glutamine synthetase by cyclic-3′,5′-AMP. Biochem Biophys Res Commun 43:1102–1105

Chader G, Johnson M, Fletcher R, Besinger R (1974a) Cyclic nucleotide phosphodiesterase of the bovine retina: activity, subcellular distribution and kinetic parameters. J Neurochem 22:93–99

Chader G, Fletcher R, Johnson M, Bensinger R (1974b) Rod outer segment phosphodiesterase: factors affecting the hydrolysis of cyclic-AMP and cyclic-GMP. Exp Eye Res 18:509–515

Chader GJ, Herz LR, Fletcher RT (1974c) Light activation of phosphodiesterase activity in retinal rod outer segments. Biochim Biophys Acta 347–491–493

Chader GJ, Herz L, Fletcher RT (1974d) Cyclic nucleotide hydrolysis: some possible natural regulators in retina and rod outer segments. J Neurochem 23:873–874

Chader GJ, Fletcher RT, O'Brien PJ, Krishna G (1976) Differential phosphorylation by GTP and ATP in isolated rod outer segments of the retina. Biochemistry 15:1615–1620

Chader G, Liu Y, O'Brien P, Fletcher R, Krishna G, Aguirre G, Farber D, Lolley R (1980) Cyclic GMP phosphodiesterase activator: involvement in a hereditary retinal degeneration. In: Bazán NG, Lolley RN (eds) Neurochemistry of the retina. Pergamon, Oxford New York Paris Toronto Frankfurt Sydney, pp 441–458

Chalfie M, Neufeld AH, Zadunaisky JA (1972) Action of epinephrine and other cyclic AMP-mediated agents on the chloride transport of the frog cornea. Invest Ophthalmol 11:644–650

Cheung WY (1970) Cyclic 3′,5′-nucleotide phosphodiesterase. Evidence for and properties of a protein activator. J Biol Chem 246:2859–2869

Clement-Cormier YC, Redburn DA (1978) Dopamine-sensitive adenylate cyclase in retina – subcellular distribution. Biochem Pharmacol 27:2281–2282

Cohen AI, Hall IA, Ferrendelli JA (1978) Calcium and cyclic nucleotide regulation in incubated mouse retinas. J Gen Physiol 71:595–612
Cone RA (1973) The internal transmitter model for visual excitation: some quantitative implications. In: Langer H (ed) Biochemistry and physiology of visual pigments. Springer, Berlin Heidelberg New York, pp 275–282
Cools AR, van Rossum JM (1976) Excitation and inhibition mediating dopamine receptors. Psychopharmacology (Berlin) 45:243–254
Coquil JF, Virmaux N, Mandel P, Goridis C (1975) Cyclic nucleotide phosphodiesterase of retinal photoreceptors. Partial purification and some properties of the enzyme. Biochim Biophys Acta 403:425–437
Corbin JD, Keely S, Park CR (1975) Distribution and dissociation of cyclic adenosine 3′:5′-monophosphate-dependent protein kinases in adipose, cardiac and other tissues. J Biol Chem 250:218–225
Corrodi H, Fuxe K, Ungerstedt U (1971) Evidence for a new type of dopamine receptor stimulating agent. J Pharm Pharmacol 23:989–991
Crabb CV (1977) Endocrine influences on ulceration and regeneration in the alkali-burned cornea. Arch Ophthalmol 95:1866–1870
Da Prada M (1977) Dopamine content and synthesis in retina and N. accumbens septi: pharmacological and light-induced modifications. Adv Biochem Psychopharmacol 16:311–319
De Azeredo FA, Lust WD, Passonneau JV (1978) Guanine nucleotide concentrations in vivo in outer segments of dark and light adapted frog retina. Biochem Biophys Res Commun 85:293–300
De Mello FG (1978) The ontogeny of dopamine-dependent increase of adenosine 3′,5′-cyclic monophosphate in the chick retina. J Neurochem 31:1049–1053
De Vries GW, Cohen AI, Hall IA, Ferrendelli JA (1978) Cyclic nucleotide levels in normal and biologically fractionated mouse retina: effects of light and dark adaptation. J Neurochem 31:1345–1351
De Vries GW, Cohen AI, Lowry OH, Ferrendelli JA (1979) Cyclic nucleotides in the cone-dominant ground squirrel retina. Exp Eye Res 29:315–321
Dewar AJ, Barron G, Richmond J (1975a) Adenosine 3′:5′-cyclic monophosphate phosphodiesterase activity in the dystrophic rat retina. Biochem Soc Trans 3:265–268
Dewar AJ, Barron G, Richmond J (1975b) Retinal cyclic-AMP phosphodiesterase activity in two strains of dystrophic rat. Exp Eye Res 21:299–306
Dewar AJ, Barron G, Reading HW (1977) The effect of anti-inflammatory drugs on retinal dystrophy in the rat. Toxicol Appl Pharmacol 42:65–74
Dickstein S, Maurice DM (1972) The metabolic basis of the fluid pump in the cornea. J Physiol (Lond) 221:29–41
Dohlman CH (1971) The function of the corneal epithelium in health and disease. Invest Ophthalmol 10:383–407
Donn H, Maurice DM, Mills NL (1959) Studies on the living cornea in vitro. II. The active transport of sodium across the epithelium. Arch Ophthalmol 62:748–757
Dowling JE, Ripps H (1973) Effect of magnesium on horizontal cell activity in the skate retina. Nature 242:101–103
Dowling JE, Sidman RL (1962) Inherited retinal dystrophy in the rat. J Cell Biol 14:73–109
Dumler IL, Etingof RN (1973) The effect of cyclic 3′,5′-adenosine monophosphoric acid on release of Na and K from the external segments of retinal rods (in Russian). Biokhimiia 38:408–411
Dumler IL, Etingof RN (1976) Protein inhibitor of cyclic adenosine 3′:5′-monophosphate phosphodiesterase in retina. Biochim Biophys Acta 429:474–478
Dutton JJ, Krupin T, Becker B (1979) Uptake and metabolism of cyclic-AMP in isolated rabbit ciliary body-iris preparations. ARVO Abstracts, Supplement to Invest Ophthalmol Vis Sci, p 21
Eakins KE (1970) Increased intraocular pressure produced by prostaglandins E_1 and E_2 in the cat eye. Exp Eye Res 10:87
Ebrey TG, Hood DC (1973) The effects of cyclic nucleotide phosphodiesterase inhibitors on the frog rod receptor potential. In: Langer H (ed) Biochemistry and physiology of visual pigments. Springer, Berlin Heidelberg New York, pp 341–350

Edwards RB, Szamier RB (1977) Defective phagocytosis of isolated rod outer segments by RCS rat retinal pigment epithelium in culture. Science 197:1001–1003

Ehinger B (1976) Biogenic monoamines as transmitters in the retina. In: Bonting SL (ed) Transmitters in the visual process. Pergamon, Oxford New York Toronto Sydney Paris Frankfurt, pp 145–163

Ehinger B (1978) Biogenic monoamines and amino acids as retinal neurotransmitters. In: Cool SJ, Smith EL III (eds), Frontiers in visual science. Springer, Berlin Heidelberg New York, pp 42–53

Etingof RN (1978) Enzymes of the outer segments of the retinal rods: the problem of localization and coupling with rhodopsin (in Russian). Tsitologiia 20:5–17

Etingof RN, Ostapenko IA (1978) Changes in the proteins of the outer segments of retinal rods in rats with tapeto-retinal dystrophies (in Russian). Vestn Akad Med Nauk SSSR 10:3–8

Farber DB, Lolley RN (1973) Proteins in the degenerative retina of C_3H mice: deficiency of a cyclic-nucleotide phosphodiesterase and opsin. J Neurochem 21:817–828

Farber DB, Lolley RN (1974) Cyclic guanosine monophosphate: Elevation in degenerating photoreceptor cells of the C_3H mouse retina. Science 186:449–451

Farber DB, Lolley RN (1976) Enzymic basis for cyclic GMP accumulation in degenerative photoreceptor cells of mouse retina. J Cyclic Nucleotide Res 2:139–148

Farber DB, Lolley RN (1977a) Light-induced reduction in cyclic GMP of retinal photoreceptor cells in vivo: abnormalities in the degenerative diseases of RCS rats and *rd* mice. J Neurochem 28:1089–1095

Farber DB, Lolley RN (1977b) Influence of visual cell maturation or degeneration on cyclic AMP content of retinal neurons. J Neurochem 29:167–170

Farber DB, Lolley RN (1978) Cyclic-AMP and cyclic-GMP content of cone-dominant retinas of ground squirrel. ARVO Abstracts, Supplement to Invest Ophthalmol Vis Sci, p 255

Farber DB, Lolley RN (1979) Phosphoproteins as proposed modulators of visual function. Adv Exp Med Biol 116:103–115

Farber DB, Brown BM, Lolley RN (1978) Cyclic GMP: proposed role in visual cell function. Vision Res 18:497–499

Farber DB, Brown BM, Lolley RN (1979a) Cyclic nucleotide dependent protein kinase and the phosphorylation of endogenous protein of retinal rod outer segments. Biochemistry 18:370–378

Farber DB, Souza D, Lolley RN (1979b) Cyclic nucleotides in the cone-dominant retina of ground squirrel. Trans Am Soc Neurochem 10:105

Farber DB, Chase D, Souza D, Lolley RN (1979c) Cyclic nucleotides in the cone-dominant retina of hibernating ground squirrel. Society for Neuroscience, Abstracts 9th Annual Meeting, p 402

Farber DB, Lolley RN, Rayborn ME, Hollyfield JG (1979d) Cyclic nucleotide modulation of visual cell morphology. ARVO Abstracts, Supplement to Invest Ophthalmol Vis Sci, p 260

Farber D, Chase DG, Lolley RN (1980) Cyclic nucleotides in rod- and cone-dominant retinas. In: Bazán NG, Lolley RN (eds) Neurochemistry of the retina. Pergamon, Oxford New York Paris Toronto Frankfurt Sydney, pp 327–336

Farber DB, Souza DW, Chase DG, Lolley RN (1981) Cyclic nucleotides of cone-dominant retinas: reduction of cyclic AMP levels by light and by cone degeneration. Invest Ophthalmol Vis Sci 20:24–31

Fedinec AA (1975) Tetanospasmin spreading, metabolism and possibilities of neutralization. In: Proceedings of the Fourth International Conference on Tetanus, vol 1. Fondation Merieux, Lyon, p 123

Fedinec AA, King LE Jr (1969) Glycine's reversal of tetanus toxin induced mydriasis in rabbit eyes. Physiologist 12:331–333

Fedinec AA, King LE Jr, Latham WC (1976) Glycine, theophylline and antitoxin effects on rabbit sphincter pupillae muscle paralyzed by tetanus toxin. In: Ohsaka A, Hayashi K, Sawai Y (eds) Animal, plant and microbiology toxins, vol 2. Plenum, New York, p 351

Feeney L, Mixon RN (1976) An in vitro model of phagocytosis in bovine and human retinal pigment epithelium. Exp Eye Res 22:533–548

Ferrendelli JA (1978) Distribution and regulation of cyclic GMP in the central nervous system. Adv Cyclic Nucleotide Res 9:453–464
Ferrendelli JA, Cohen AI (1976) The effects of light and dark adaptation on the levels of cyclic nucleotides in retinas of mice heterozygous for a gene for photoreceptor dystrophy. Biochem Biophys Res Commun 74:421–427
Ferrendelli JA, Rubin EH, Kinscherf DA (1976) Influence of divalent cations on the regulation of cyclic GMP and cyclic AMP levels in brain tissue. J Neurochem 26:741–748
Ferrendelli JA, DeVries GW, Cohen AI, Lowry OH (1980) Localization and roles of cyclic nucleotide systems in retina. In: Bazán NG, Lolley RN (eds) Neurochemistry of the retina. Pergamon, Oxford New York Paris Toronto Frankfurt Sydney, pp 311–326
Fischer FH, Schmitz L, Hoff W, Schartl S, Liegl O, Wiederholt M (1978) Sodium and chloride transport in the isolated human cornea. Pfluegers Arch 373:179–188
Fleischman D, Denisevich M (1979) Guanylate cyclase of isolated bovine retinal rod axonemes. Biochemistry 18:5060–5066
Fletcher RT, Chader GJ (1976) Cyclic GMP: control of concentration by light in retinal photoreceptors. Biochem Biophys Res Commun 70:1297–1302
Forn J, Valdecasas FG (1971) Effects of lithium on brain adenyl cyclase activity. Biochem Pharmacol 20:2773–2779
Frank RN, Cavanagh HD, Kenyon KR (1973) Light stimulated phosphorylation of bovine visual pigments by ATP. J Biol Chem 218:596–609
Frati L, Daniele S, Delogu A, Covelli I (1972) Selective binding of the epidermal growth factor and its specific effects on the epithelial cells of the cornea. Exp Eye Res 14:135
Frati L, D'Armiento M, Gulletta E, Verna R, Covelli I (1977) The control of epidermis proliferation by epidermal growth factor (EGF). Relationship with cyclic nucleotides systems. Pharmacol Res Commun 9:815–822
Friedenwald JS, Buschke W (1944a) Influence of some experimental values on epithelial movements in healing of corneal wounds. J Comp Cell Physiol 23:95–107
Friedenwald JS, Buschke W (1944b) The effects of excitement, of epinephrine and of sympathectomy on the mitotic activity of the corneal epithelium in rats. Am J Physiol 141:689–694
Gilmour-Buck M, Zadunaisky JA (1975) Stimulation of ion transport by ascorbic acid through inhibition of 3′:5′-cyclic-AMP phosphodiesterase in the corneal epithelium and other tissues. Biochim Biophys Acta 389:251–260
Godchaux W III, Zimmerman WF (1979) Membrane-dependent guanine nucleotide binding and GTPase activities of a soluble protein from bovine rod outer segments. ARVO Abstracts, Supplement to Invest Ophthalmol Vis Sci, p 269
Goldberg ND, Haddox MK (1977) Cyclic GMP metabolism and involvement in biological regulation. Annu Rev Biochem 46:823–896
Goldman AI, O'Brien PJ (1978) Phagocytosis in the retinal pigment epithelium of the RCS rat. Science 201:1023–1025
Goridis C, Virmaux N (1974) Light-regulated guanosine 3′,5′-monophosphate phosphodiesterase of bovine retina. Nature 248:57–58
Goridis C, Weller M (1976) A role for cyclic nucleotides and protein kinase in vertebrate photoreception. Adv Biochem Psychopharmacol 15:391–412
Goridis C, Virmaux N, Urban PF, Mandel P (1973) Guanyl cyclase in a mammalian photoreceptor. FEBS Lett 30:163–166
Goridis C, Virmaux N, Cailla HL, DeLaage MA (1974) Rapid, light-induced changes of retinal cyclic GMP levels. FEBS Lett 49:167–169
Goridis C, Virmaux N, Weller M, Coquil JF, Mandel P (1975) Guanylate cyclase and cyclic GMP phosphodiesterase in vertebrate photoreceptor organelles. In: Boissier JR, Hippius H, Pichot P (eds) Proceedings of the IXth Congress of the Collegium Internationale Neuropsychopharmacologicum, Paris 1974. Excerpta Medica, Amsterdam London New York, pp 920–931
Goridis C, Virmaux N, Weller M, Urban PF (1976) Role of cyclic nucleotides in photoreceptor function. In: Bonting SL (ed) Transmitters in the visual process. Pergamon, Oxford New York Toronto Sydney Paris Frankfurt, pp 27–58
Goridis C, Urban PF, Mandel P (1977) The effect of flash illumination on the endogenous cyclic GMP content in isolated frog retinae. Exp Eye Res 24:171–177

Govardovskii I, Berman AL (1977) Mechanism of vertebrate photoreceptor excitation: possible role of cyclic nucleotides. (in Russian). Dokl Akad Nauk SSSR 237:739–742
Govardovskii VI, Ostapenko IA, Shabanova ME, Fuks BB, Etingof RN (1977) Changes in the electroretinogram and in the content of rhodopsin of Hunter rats during the development of retinal degeneration (in Russian). Neirofiziologiia 9:527–531
Govoni S, Loddo P, Spano PF, Trabucchi M (1977) Dopamine receptor sensitivity in brain and retina of rats during aging. Brain Res 138:565–570
Greengard P (1976) Possible role for cyclic nucleotides and phosphorylated membrane proteins in postsynaptic actions of neurotransmitters. Nature 260:101–108
Hagins WA (1972) The visual process: excitatory mechanisms in the primary photoreceptor cells. Annu Rev Biophys Bioeng 1:131–158
Hagins WA, Yoshikami S (1974) A role for calcium in excitation of retinal rods and cones. Exp Eye Res 18:299–305
Hall MO (1978) Phagocytosis of light- and dark-adapted rod outer segments by cultured pigment epithelium. Science 202:526–528
Hart R (1972) Theory of neural mediation of intraocular dynamics. Bull Math Biophys 34:113–140
Hayasaka S, Hara S, Mizuno K (1977) In vitro effect of prostaglandins and cyclic nucleotides on differential release of enzyme from lysosomes of the bovine retinal pigment epithelium. Exp Eye Res 24:633–639
Hedden WL, Dowling JE (1978) The interplexiform cell system. II. Effects of dopamine on goldfish retinal neurons. Proc R Soc Lond [Biol] 201:27–55
Hendriks T, De Pont JJ, Daemen FJ, Bonting SL (1973) Biochemical aspects of the visual process. XXIV. Adenylate cyclase and rod photoreceptor membranes: a critical appraisal. Biochim Biophys Acta 330:156–166
Herron WL Jr, Riegel BW, Meyers OE, Rubin ML (1969) Retinal dystrophy in the rat: a pigment epithelial disease. Invest Ophthalmol 8:595–604
Herron WL Jr, Riegel BW, Rubin ML (1971) Outer segment production and removal in the degenerating retina of the dystrophic rat. Invest Ophthalmol 10:54–63
Hesketh JE, Virmaux N, Mandel P (1978) Evidence for a cyclic nucleotide-dependent phosphorylation of retinal myosin. FEBS Lett 94:357–360
Hollyfield JG, Mottow LS, Ward A (1975) Autoradiographic study of [^{3}H] glucosamine incorporation by the developing retina of the clawed toad, Xenopus laevis. Exp Eye Res 20:383–391
Hood DC, Ebrey TG (1974) On the possible role of cyclic AMP in receptor dark adaptation. Vision Res 14:437–439
Hubbell WL, Bownds MD (1979) Visual transduction in vertebrate photoreceptors. Annu Rev Neurosci 2:17–34
Hurley JB, Ebrey TG (1979) Regulation of rod outer segment phosphodiesterase. Biophys J 25:314a
Itoi M, Gnadinger MC, Slansky HH et al. (1969) Collagenase in the cornea. Exp Eye Res 8:369–373
Iversen LL (1975) Dopamine Receptors in the brain. Science 188:1084–1089
Kass MA, Podos SM, Moses RA, Becker B (1972) Prostaglandin E_1 and aqueous humor dynamics. Invest Ophthalmol 11:1022–1027
Kass MA, Palmberg P, Becker B (1977) The ocular anti-inflammatory action of imidazole. Invest Ophthalmol Vis Sci 16:66–69
Katsuki S, Arnold W, Mittal C, Murad F (1977) Stimulation of guanylate cyclase by sodium nitroprusside, nitroglycerin and nitric oxide in various tissue preparations and comparison to the effects of sodium azide and hydroxylamine. J Cyclic Nucleotide Res 3:23–35
Kebabian JW, Calne DB (1979) Multiple receptors for dopamine. Nature 277:93–96
Keirns JJ, Wheeler MA, Bitensky MW (1974) Isolation of cyclic AMP and cyclic GMP by thin-layer chromatography. Application to assay of adenylate cyclase, guanylate cyclase, and cyclic nucleotide phosphodiesterase. Anal Biochem 61:336–348
Keirns JJ, Miki N, Bitensky MW, Keirns M (1975) A link between rhodopsin and disc membrane cyclic nucleotide phosphodiesterase. Action spectrum and sensitivity to illumination. Biochemistry 14:2760–2766

Kelly RG, Starr MS (1971) Effects of prostaglandins and a prostaglandin antagonist on intraocular pressure and protein in the monkey eye. Can J Ophthalmol 6:205–211
Kilbride P, Ebrey TG (1979) Light initiated changes of cyclic GMP levels in the frog retina measured with quick freezing techniques. J Gen Physiol 74:415–426
Kimura H, Murad F (1974) Evidence for two different forms of guanylate cyclase in rat heart. J Biol Chem 249:6910–6916
Kimura H, Mittal CK, Murad F (1975) Increases in cyclic GMP levels in brain and liver with sodium azide, an activator of guanylate cyclase. Nature 257:700–702
King LE Jr, Fedinec AA, Latham WC (1978) Effects of cyclic nucleotides on tetanus toxin paralyzed rabbit sphincter pupillae muscles. Toxicon 16:625–631
Klyce SD, Neufeld AH, Zadunaisky JA (1973) The activation of chloride transport by epinephrine and Db-cyclic AMP in the cornea of the rabbit. Invest Ophthalmol 12:127–139
Kramer SG (1976) Dopamine in retinal neurotransmission. In: Bonting SL (ed) Transmitters in the visual process. Pergamon, Oxford New York Toronto Sydney Paris Frankfurt, pp 165–198
Krishna G, Krishnan N, Fletcher RT, Chader G (1976) Effects of light on cyclic GMP metabolism in retinal photoreceptors. J Neurochem 27:717–722
Krishnan N, Fletcher RT, Chader GJ, Krishna G (1978) Characterization of guanylate cyclase of rod outer segments of the bovine retina. Biochim Biophys Acta 523:506–515
Krupin T, Weiss A, Becker B, Holmberg N, Fritz C (1977) Increased intraocular pressure following topical azide or nitroprusside. Invest Ophthalmol Vis Sci 16:1002–1007
Kühn H (1978) Light-regulated binding of rhodopsin kinase and other proteins to cattle photoreceptor membranes. Biochemistry 17:4389–4395
Kühn H (1980a) Light-induced reversible binding of proteins to bovine photoreceptor membranes. Influence of nucleotides. In: Bazán N, Lolley RN (eds) Neurochemistry of the retina. Pergamon, Oxford New York Paris Toronto Frankfurt Sydney, pp 269–286
Kühn H (1980b) Light- and GTP-regulated interaction of GTPase and other proteins with bovine photoreceptor membranes. Nature 283:587–589
Kühn H, Dreyer WJ (1972) Light-dependent phosphorylation of rhodopsin by ATP. FEBS Lett 20:1–6
Kühn H, Cook JH, Dreyer WJ (1973) Phosphorylation of rhodopsin in bovine photoreceptor membranes: a dark reaction after illumination. Biochemistry 12:2495–2502
Kuwabara T (1975) Cytologic changes of the retina and pigment epithelium during hibernation. Invest Ophthalmol 14:457–467
Laduron PM, Leysen JE (1979) Domperidone, a specific in vitro dopamine antagonist devoid of in vivo central dopaminergic activity. Biochem Pharmacol 28:2161–2165
Lahav M, Melamed E, Dafna Z, Atlas D (1978) Localization of beta receptors in the anterior segment of the rat eye by a fluorescent analogue of propranolol. Invest Ophthalmol Vis Sci 17:645–651
Langham ME (1959) Influence of the intraocular pressure on the formation of the aqueous humor and the outflow resistance in the living eye. Br J Ophthalmol 43:705–732
Langham ME (1963) A new procedure for the analysis of intraocular dynamics in human subjects. Exp Eye Res 2:314–324
Langham ME (1977) The aqueous outflow system and its response to autonomic receptor agonists. Exp Eye Res [Suppl] 311–322
Langham ME, Diggs E (1974) Beta-adrenergic responses in the eyes of rabbits, primates and man. Exp Eye Res 19:281–295
Lasansky A, DeFisch FW (1966) Potential, current and ionic fluxes across the isolated retinal pigment epithelium and choroid. J Gen Physiol 49:913–924
LaVail MM (1976) Rod outer segment disk shedding in rat retina: relationship to cyclic lighting. Science 194:1071–1074
LaVail MM, Battelle BA (1975) Influence of eye pigmentation and light deprivation on inherited retinal dystrophy in the rat. Exp Eye Res 21:167–192
LaVail MM, Sidman RL (1974) Retinal degeneration in the mouse. Arch Ophthalmol 91:394–400
LaVail MM, Sidman RL, O'Neil D (1972) Photoreceptor-pigment epithelial cell relationships in rats with inherited retinal degeneration: ratio-autographic and electron microscope evidence for a dual source of extra lamellar material. J Cell Biol 53:185–209

Liebman PA, Pugh EN Jr (1979) The control of phosphodiesterase in rod disk membranes – kinetics, possible mechanisms and significance for vision. Vision Res 19:375–380

Lipton SA, Ostroy SE, Dowling JE (1977a) Electrical and adaptive properties of rod photoreceptors in *Bufo marinus*. I. Effects of altered extracellular Ca^{2+} levels. J Gen Physiol 70:747–770

Lipton SA, Rasmussen H, Dowling JE (1977b) Electrical and adaptive properties of rod photoreceptors in *Bufo marinus*. II. Effects of cyclic nucleotides and prostaglandins. J Gen Physiol 70:771–791

Liu YP, Schwartz HS (1978) Protein activator of cyclic AMP phosphodiesterase and cyclic nucleotide phosphodiesterase in bovine retina and bovine lens. Activity, subcellular distribution and kinetic parameters. Biochim Biophys Acta 526:186–193

Liu YP, Krishna G, Aguirre G, Ghader GJ (1979) Involvement of cyclic GMP phosphodiesterase activator in an hereditary retinal degeneration. Nature 280:62–64

Lolley RN, Farber DB (1975) Cyclic nucleotide phosphodiesterase in dystrophic rat retinas: Guanosine 3′,5′-cyclic monophosphate anomalies during photoreceptor cell degeneration. Exp Eye Res 20:585–597

Lolley RN, Farber DB (1976) A proposed link between debris accumulation, guanosine 3′,5′-cyclic monophosphate changes and photoreceptor cell degeneration in retina of RCS rats. Exp Eye Res 22:477–486

Lolley RN, Farber DB (1978) An endogenous cyclic nucleotide phosphodiesterase inhibitor of bovine rod outer segment. ARVO Abstracts, p 255

Lolley RN, Farber DB (1980) Cyclic GMP metabolic defects in inherited disorders of *rd* mice and RCS rats. In: Bazán NG, Lolley RN (eds) Neurochemistry of the retina. Pergamon, Oxford New York Paris Toronto Frankfurt Sydney, pp 427–441

Lolley RN, Schmidt SY, Farber DB (1974) Alterations in cyclic AMP metabolism associated with photoreceptor cell degeneration in the C_3H mouse. J Neurochem 22:701–707

Lolley RN, Brown BM, Farber DB (1977a) Protein phosphorylation in rod outer segments from bovine retina: cyclic nucleotide-activated protein kinase and its endogenous substrate. Biochem Biophys Res Commun 78:572–578

Lolley RN, Farber DB, Rayborn ME, Hollyfield JG (1977b) Cyclic GMP accumulation causes degeneration of photoreceptor cells: Simulation of an inherited disease. Science 196:664–666

Lolley RN, Racz E, Farber DB (1979a) Recovery of retinal cyclic GMP content after light or drug treatment. ARVO Abstracts, Supplement to Invest Ophthalmol Vis Sci, p 21

Lolley RN, Racz E, Farber DB (1979b) Modulation of retinal cyclic GMP levels by light. Trans Am Soc Neurochem 10:87

Lolley RN, Rayborn ME, Hollyfield JG, Farber DB (1980) Cyclic GMP and visual cell degeneration in the inherited disorder of *rd* mice: a progress report. Vision Res 20:1157–1161

Lowry OH (1964) Biochemical studies on layered structures. In: Cohen MM, Snider RS (eds) Morphological and biochemical correlates of neural activity. Harper & Row, New York, pp 178–191

Magistretti P, Schorderet M (1978) Differential effects of benzamides and thioxanthenes on dopamine-elicited accumulation of cyclic AMP in isolated rabbit retina. Naunyn Schmiedebergs Arch Pharmacol 303:189–191

Makman MH, Brown JH, Mishra RK (1975a) Cyclic AMP in retina and caudate nucleus: influence of dopamine and other agents. Adv Cyclic Nucleotide Res 5:661–679

Makman MH, Mishra RK, Brown JH (1975b) Drug interactions with dopamine-stimulated adenylate cyclases of caudate nucleus and retina: direct agonist effect of a piribedil metabolite. Adv Neurol 9:213–222

Manthorpe M, McConnell DG (1974) Adenylate cyclase in vertebrate retina. Relationship to specific fractions and to rhodopsin. J Biol Chem 249:4608–4613

Manthorpe M, McConnell DG (1975) Cyclic nucleotide phosphodiesterases associated with bovine retinal outer-segment fragments. Biochim Biophys Acta 403:438–445

Masland RH, Livingstone CJ (1976) Effect of stimulation with light on synthesis and release of acetylcholine by an isolated mammalian retina. Neurophysiology 39:1210–1219

Massey SC, Neal MJ (1979) The light evoked release of acetylcholine from the rabbit retina in vivo and its inhibition by gamma-aminobutyric acid. J Neurochem 132:1327–1329

Matschinsky FM (1970) Energy metabolism of the microscopic structures of the cochlea, the retina and the cerebellum. Adv Biochem Psychopharmacol 2:217–243

Maurice DM (1969) The cornea and sclera. In: Davson H (ed) The eye, vol 1. Academic Press, New York London, pp 489–600

Miki N, Keirns JJ, Marcus FR, Freeman J, Bitensky MW (1973) Regulation of cyclic nucleotide concentrations in photoreceptors: an ATP-dependent stimulation of cyclic nucleotide phosphodiesterase by light. Proc Natl Acad Sci USA 70:3820–3824

Miki N, Baraban JM, Keirns JJ, Boyce JJ, Bitensky MW (1975) Purification and properties of the light-activated cyclic nucleotide phosphodiesterase of rod outer segments. J Biol Chem 250:6320–6327

Miller SS, Steinberg RH (1976) Transport of taurine, L-methionine and 3-O-methyl-D glucose across frog retinal pigment epithelium. Exp Eye Res 23:177–189

Miller SS, Steinberg RH (1977a) Active transport of ions across frog retinal pigment epithelium. Exp Eye Res 25:235–248

Miller SS, Steinberg RH (1977b) Passive ionic properties of frog pigment epithelium. J Membr Biol 36:337–372

Miller WH, Nicol GD (1979) Evidence that cyclic GMP regulates membrane potential in rod photoreceptors. Nature 280:64–66

Mishima S (1957) The effects of the denervation and the stimulation of the sympathetic and the trigeminal nerve on the mitotic rate of the corneal epithelium in the rabbit. Jpn J Ophthalmol 1:65–74

Mishra RK, Katzman R, Makman MH (1974) Dopamine-stimulated adenylate cyclase of corpus striatum and retina: activity in the cebus monkey and other species. Fed Proc 33:494

Mitzel DL, Hall IA, DeVries GW, Cohen AI, Ferrendelli JA (1978) Comparison of cyclic nucleotide and energy metabolism of intact mouse retina in situ and in vitro. Exp Eye Res 27:27–37

Mullen RJ, LaVail MM (1976) Inherited retinal dystrophy: a primary defect in pigment epithelium determined with experimental rat chimeras. Science 192:799–801

Nathanson JA (1977) Cyclic nucleotides and nervous system function. Physiol Rev 57:157–256

Nathanson JA (1980) Adrenergic regulation of intraocular pressure: identification of beta$_2$-adrenergic-stimulated adenylate cyclase in ciliary process epithelium. Proc Natl Acad Sci USA 77:7420–7424

Neal MJ (1976) Acetylcholine as a retinal transmitter substance. In: Bonting SL (ed) Transmitters in the visual process. Pergamon, Oxford New York Toronto Sydney Paris Frankfurt, pp 127–143

Neufeld AH (1978) Influences of cyclic nucleotides on outflow facility in the Vervet monkey. Exp Eye Res 27:387–397

Neufeld AH, Page ED (1977) In vitro determination of the ability of drugs to bind to adrenergic receptors. Invest Ophthalmol Vis Sci 16:1118–1124

Neufeld AH, Sears ML (1974) Cyclic AMP in ocular tissues of the rabbit, monkey and human. Invest Ophthalmol 13:475–477

Neufeld AH, Sears ML (1975) Adenosine 3′,5′-monophosphate increases the outflow facility of the primate eye. Invest Ophthalmol 14:688–689

Neufeld AH, Jampol LM, Sears ML (1972) Cyclic AMP in the aqueous humor: the effects of adrenergic agents. Exp Eye Res 14:242–250

Neufeld AH, Chavis RM, Sears ML (1973) Cyclic AMP in the aqueous humor: the effects of repeated topical epinephrine administration and sympathetic denervation. Exp Eye Res 16:265–272

Neufeld AH, Dueker DK, Vegge T, Sears ML (1975) Adenosine 3′,5′-monophosphate increases the outflow of aqueous humor from the rabbit eye. Invest Ophthalmol 14:40–42

Neufeld AH, Zawistowski KA, Page ED, Bromberg BB (1978) Influences on the intensity of beta-adrenergic receptors in the cornea and iris – ciliary body of the rabbit. Invest Ophthalmol Vis Sci 17:1069–1075

Newsome DA, Fletcher RT, Robison WG Jr, Kenyon KR, Chader GJ (1974) Effects of cyclic AMP and Sephadex fractions of chick embryo extract on cloned retinal pigmented epithelium in tissue culture. J Cell Biol 61:369–382

Newsome DA, Fletcher RT, Chader GJ (1980) Cyclic nucleotides vary by area in the human retina and pigmented epithelium of the human and monkey. Invest Ophthalmol Vis Sci 19:864–869
Nicol GD, Miller WH (1978) Cyclic GMP injected into retinal rod outer segments increases latency and amplitude of response to illumination. Proc Natl Acad Sci USA 75:5217–5220
Nöell WK (1952a) The impairment of visual cell structure by iodoacetate. J Cell Comp Physiol 40:25–55
Nöell WK (1952b) Azide sensitive potential differences across the eye bulb. Am J Physiol 170:217–238
Nöell WK (1963) Cellular physiology of the retina. J Opt Soc Am 53:36–48
Nöell WK (1965) Aspects of experimental and hereditary retinal degeneration. In: Graymore CN (ed) Biochemistry of the retina. Academic Press, New York London, pp 51–72
Orr HT, Lowry OH, Cohen AI, Ferrendelli JA (1976) Distribution of 3′:5′-cyclic AMP and 3′:5′-cyclic GMP in rabbit retina in vivo: selective effects of dark and light adaptation and ischemia. Proc Natl Acad Sci USA 73:4442–4445
Ortiz JR, Yamada J, Hsie AW (1973) Induction of the stellate configuration in cultured iris epithelial cells by adenosine and compounds related to adenosine 3′:5′-cyclic monophosphate. Proc Natl Acad Sci USA 70:2286–2290
Pannbacker RG (1973a) Control of guanylate cyclase activity in the rod outer segment. Science 182:1138–1140
Pannbacker RG (1973b) Protein kinases and protein phosphorylation in the rod outer segment. In: Kahn RH, Lands WE (eds) Prostaglandins and cyclic AMP. Academic Press, New York London, pp 251–252
Pannbacker RG (1974) Cyclic nucleotide metabolism in human photoreceptors. Invest Ophthalmol 13:535–538
Pannbacker RG, Lovett K (1977) Localization of cyclic nucleotide phosphodiesterase activity within the bovine photoreceptor cell. Invest Ophthalmol Vis Sci 16:166–168
Pannbacker RG, Fleischman DE, Reed DW (1972) Cyclic nucleotide phosphodiesterase: high activity in a mammalian photoreceptor. Science 175:757–758
Parry H (1953) Degenerations of dog retina, generalized progressive atrophy of hereditary origin. Br J Ophthalmol 37:487–502
Pasantes-Morales H, Klethi J, Urban PF, Mandel P (1972) The physiological role of taurine in retina uptake and effect on electroretinogram (ERG). Physiol Chem Phys 4:339–348
Penn RD, Hagins WA (1969) Signal transmission along retinal rods and the origin of the electroretinographic a-wave. Nature 223:201–205
Perkins JP, Moore MM (1973) Characterization of the adrenergic receptors mediating a rise of cyclic 3′-5′-adenosine monophosphate in rat cerebral cortex. J Pharmacol Exp Ther 185:371–378
Podos SM (1976) Prostaglandins, nonsteroidal anti-inflammatory agents and eye disease. Trans Am Ophthalmol Soc 74:637–660
Polans AS, Hermolin J, Bownds MD (1979) Light-induced dephosphorylation of two proteins in frog rod outer segments. Influence of cyclic nucleotides and calcium. J Gen Physiol 74:595–613
Radius R, Langham ME (1973) Cyclic-AMP and the ocular responses to norepinephrine. Exp Eye Res 17:219–229
Redfern N, Israel P, Bergsma D, Robison WG Jr, Whikehart D, Chader G (1976) Neural retinal and pigment epithelial cells in culture: patterns of differentiation and effects of prostaglandins and cyclic AMP on pigmentation. Exp Eye Res 22:559–568
Remé C, Young RW (1977) The effect of hibernation on cone visual cells in the ground squirrel. Invest Ophthalmol Vis Sci 16:815–840
Robb RM (1974a) Histochemical evidence of cyclic nucleotide phosphodiesterase in photoreceptor outer segments. Invest Ophthalmol 13:740–747
Robb RM (1974b) Electron microscopic histochemical studies of cyclic 3′,5′-nucleotide phosphodiesterase in the developing retina of normal mice and mice with hereditary retinal degeneration. Trans Am Ophthalmol Soc 72:650–669
Robb RM (1978) Histochemical demonstration of cyclic guanosine 3′,5′-monophosphate phosphodiesterase activity in retinal photoreceptor outer segments. Invest Ophthalmol Vis Sci 17:476–480

Robinson WE, Hagins WA (1977) A light-activated GTPase in retinal rod outer segments. Biophys J 17:196a
Robinson WE, Hagins WA (1979) GTP hydrolysis: a possible source of free energy for the transmitter cycle in visual excitation. Biophys J 25:318a
Ruskell GL (1961) Aqueous drainage paths in the rabbit. A neoprene latex cast study. Arch Ophthalmol 66:861–870
Savage CR Jr, Cohen S (1973) Proliferations of corneal epithelium induced by epidermal growth factor. Exp Eye Res 15:361–366
Schmidt SY, Lolley RN (1973) Cyclic-nucleotide phosphodiesterase: an early defect in inherited retinal degeneration of C_3H mice. J Cell Biol 57:117–123
Schorderet M (1975) The effects of dopamine, piribedil (ET-495) and its metabolite S-584 on retinal adenylate cyclase. Experientia 31:1325–1327
Schorderet M (1976) Direct evidence for the stimulation of rabbit retina dopamine receptors by ergot alkaloids. Neurosci Lett 2:87–91
Schorderet M (1977a) Lithium inhibition of cyclic AMP accumulation induced by dopamine in isolated retinae of the rabbit. Biochem Pharmacol 26:167–170
Schorderet M (1977b) Pharmacological characterization of the dopamine-mediated accumulation of cyclic AMP in intact retina of rabbit. Life Sci 20:1741–1747
Schorderet M (1978a) The interrelationship between dopamine receptors and cyclic AMP metabolism in rabbit retina and its importance for the mechanism of action of centrally active drugs. In: Folco G, Paoletti R (eds) Molecular biology and pharmacology of cyclic nucleotides. Elsevier/North-Holland, Amsterdam Oxford New York, pp 259–263
Schorderet M (1978b) Dopamine-mimetic activity of ergot derivatives, as measured by the production of cyclic AMP in isolated retinae of the rabbit. Gerontology 24:86–93
Schorderet M, Magistretti PJ (1980) The isolated retina of mammals: a useful preparation for enzymatic-(adenylyl cyclase) and/or binding studies of dopamine receptors. In: Bazán NG, Lolley RN (eds) Neurochemistry of the retina. Pergamon, Oxford New York Paris Toronto Frankfurt Sydney, pp 337–354
Schorderet M, McDermod J, Magistretti P (1978) Dopamine receptors and cyclic AMP in rabbit retina: a pharmacological and stereochemical analysis using semi-rigid analogs of dopamine (aminotetralins) and thioxanthene isomers. J Physiol (Paris) 74:509–513
Schubert G, Bornschein H (1951) Specific damage to retinal elements by iodine acetate. Experientia 7:461–462
Schwarcz R, Coyle JT (1976) Adenylate cyclase activity in chick retina. Gen Pharmacol 7:349–354
Scott WN, Friedenthal DF (1973) A proposed role of ascorbate in the transport of amino acids and ions in the cornea. Exp Eye Res 15:683–689
Sears ML (1975) The aqueous. In: Moses RA (ed) Adler's physiology of the eye. Mosby, St. Louis, pp 232–252
Shanta TR, Woods WD, Waitzman MB, Bourne GM (1966) Histochemical method for localization of cyclic 3′,5′-nucleotide phosphodiesterase. Histochemie 7:177–190
Shimizu H, Creveling CR, Daly J (1970) Stimulated formation of adenosine 3′,5′-cyclic phosphate in cerebral cortex: synergism between electrical activity and biogenic amines. Proc Natl Acad Sci USA 65:1033–1040
Sidman RL, Green MC (1965) Retinal degeneration in the mouse; location of the *rd* locus in linkage group XVII. J Hered 56:23–29
Sillman AJ, Ito H, Tomita T (1969) Studies on the mass receptor potential of isolated frog retina. I. General properties. Vision Res 9:1435–1448
Sitaramayya A, Virmaux N, Mandel P (1977a) On a soluble system for studying light activation of rod outer segment cyclic GMP phosphodiesterase. Neurochem Res 2:1–10
Sitaramayya A, Virmaux N, Mandel P (1977b) On the mechanism of light activation of retinal rod outer segments cyclic GMP phosphodiesterase (light activation-influence of bleached rhodopsin and KF-deinhibition). Exp Eye Res 25:163–169
Smith DF (1976) Antagonistic effect of lithium chloride on l-dopa-induced locomotor activity in rats. Pharmacol Res Commun 8:575–579
Sonohara O, Shiose Y (1968) Electron microscopic study of the visual cell of inherited retinal dystrophic mice. Folia Ophthalmol Jpn 19:77–86
Sorsby A, Koller PC, Attfield M (1954) Retinal dystrophy in the mouse: histological and genetic aspects. J Exp Zool 125:171–197

Spano PF, Kumakura K, Trabucchi M (1976) Dopamine-sensitive adenylate cyclase in the retina: a point of action for D-LSD. Adv Biochem Psychopharmacol 15:357–365

Spano PF, Govoni S, Hofmann M, Kumakura K, Trabucchi M (1977) Physiological and pharmacological influences on dopaminergic receptors in the retina. Adv Biochem Psychopharmacol 16:307–310

Steinberg RH, Miller SS (1973) Aspects of electrolyte transport in frog pigment epithelium. Exp Eye Res 16:365–372

Steiner AL, Ferrendelli JA, Kipnis DM (1972) Radioimmunoassay for cyclic nucleotides. J Biol Chem 247:1121–1124

Stell WK (1972) The morphological organization of the vertebrate retina. In: Fuortes MFG (ed) Handbook of sensory physiology, vol 7/2. Springer, Berlin Heidelberg New York, pp 111–213

Suzuki O, Noguchi E, Yagi K (1978) Uptake of 5-hydroxytryptamine by chick retina. J Neurochem 30:295–296

Takáts A, Antoni F, Faragó A, Kertész P (1978) Some properties of the cyclic AMP dependent protein kinase of epithelial cells and cortical fibers of bovine eye lens. Exp Eye Res 26:389–397

Takeuchi YK, Kajishima T (1976) Inhibitory effects of dibutyryl cyclic AMP and theophylline on the melanosome transformation in the embryonic chick pigmented retina cultured in vitro. Dev Biol 53:178–189

Tamura T, Osada E, Ueno K (1978) Effect of bupranolol hydrochloride (KL 255) on cyclic AMP level of aqueous humor, iris and ciliary body of albino rabbit. Nippon Ganka Gakkai Zasshi 82:517–521

Tansley K (1951) Hereditary degeneration of the mouse retina. Br J Ophthalmol 35:573–582

Thompson WJ, Johnson DG, Lavis VR, Williams RH (1974) Effects of secretin on guanyl cyclase of various tissues. Endocrinology 94:276–278

Trabucchi M, Govoni S, Tonon GC, Spano PF (1976) Dopamine receptor supersensitivity in rat retina after light deprivation. In: Usdin E (ed) Catecholamines and stress. Pergamon, Oxford New York Toronto Sydney Paris Frankfurt, pp 225–234

Troyer EW, Hall IA, Ferrendelli JA (1978) Guanylate cyclases in CNS: enzymatic characteristics of soluble and particulate enzymes from mouse cerebellum and retina. J Neurochem 31:825–833

Tsukahara S, Maezawa N (1978) Cytochemical localization of adenyl cyclase in the rabbit ciliary body. Exp Eye Res 26:99–106

Tunnicliff G (1977) Increase in the tyrosine hydroxylase activity of the chick retina by an apparent phosphorylation. Union Med Can 106:472–474

Usova AA, Ostapenko IA, Etingof RN (1978) Protein inhibitor of cyclic nucleotide phosphodiesterase in the retina in hereditary degeneration (in Russian). Vopr Med Khim 2:227–232

Virmaux N, Nullans G, Goridis C (1976) Guanylate cyclase in vertebrate retina: evidence for specific association with rod outer segments. J Neurochem 26:233–235

Voaden M (1976) Gamma aminobutyric acid and glycine as retinal neurotransmitters. In: Bonting SL (ed) Transmitters in the visual process. Pergamon, Oxford New York Toronto Sydney Paris Frankfurt, pp 107–126

Waitzman MB (1978) Effects of cervical sympathetic ganglionectomy on cyclic AMP and prostaglandins in brain and eye tissues and fluids. Prostaglandins Med 1:139–150

Waitzman MB, King CD (1967) Prostaglandin influences on intraocular pressure and pupil size. Am J Physiol 212:329–334

Waitzman MB, Woods WD (1971) Some characteristics of an adenyl cyclase preparation from rabbit ciliary process tissue. Exp Eye Res 12:99–111

Walls GL (1942) The vertebrate eye and its adaptive radiation. Cranbrook Inst Sci, Bull 19. Cranbrook Press, Bloomfield Hills, Michigan

Waloga G, Brown JE (1979) Effects of cyclic nucleotides and calcium ions on *Bufo* rods. Supplement to Invest Ophthalmol Vis Sci 18:5

Wassenaar JS, Korf J (1976) Characterization of catecholamine receptors in rat retina. In: Bonting SL (ed) Transmitters in the visual process. Pergamon, Oxford New York Toronto Sydney Paris Frankfurt, pp 199–218

Wassenaar JS, Roelse H (1980) The action of psychotropic drugs on adenylate cyclases and phosphodiesterases in the rat retina. In: Bazán NG, Lolley RN (eds) Neurochemistry of the retina. Pergamon, Oxford New York Paris Toronto Frankfurt Sydney, pp 367–380
Watling KJ, Dowling JE, Iversen LL (1979) Dopamine receptors in the retina may all be linked to adenylate cyclase. Nature 281:578–580
Watling KJ, Dowling JE, Iversen LL (1980) Dopaminergic mechanisms in the carp retina: effects of dopamine, K^+ and light on cyclic AMP synthesis. In: Bazán NG, Lolley RN (eds) Neurochemistry of the retina. Pergamon, Oxford New York Paris Toronto Frankfurt Sydney, pp 519–537
Weller M, Virmaux N, Mandel P (1975) Light-stimulated phosphorylation of rhodopsin in the retina: the presence of a protein kinase that is specific for photobleached rhodopsin. Proc Natl Acad Sci USA 72:381–385
Weller M, Virmaux N, Mandel P (1976) The relative specificity of opsin kinase towards ATP and GTP and the lack of effect of cyclic nucleotides on the activity of the enzyme. Exp Eye Res 23:65–67
Werblin FS (1974) Organization of the vertebrate retina: receptive fields and sensitivity control. In: Davson H, Graham LT Jr (eds) The eye, vol 6. Academic Press, New York London, pp 257–281
Wheeler GL, Bitensky MW (1977) A light-activated GTPase in vertebrate photoreceptors: regulation of light-activated cyclic GMP phosphodiesterase. Proc Natl Acad Sci USA 74:4238–4242
Wheeler GL, Matuo Y, Bitensky MW (1977) Light-activated GTPase in vertebrate photoreceptors. Nature 269:822–824
Wiglusz Z (1973) Investigations on the role of cyclic 3′,5′-AMP and active sodium transport in generation of action potential in vivo (in Polish). Acta Biol Med Soc Sci Gedan 17:7–63
Wiglusz Z (1975a) The influence of pharmacological agents acting by lowering the membrane potential difference on the amplitude of b wave in ERG of frog isolated eye (in Polish). Klin Oczna 45:1297–1304
Wiglusz Z (1975b) Investigations of the role of cyclic AMP in generation of action potential of frog isolated retina. (in Polish). Klin Oczna 45:765–771
Woodruff ML, Bownds MD (1979) Amplitude, kinetics, and reversibility of a light-induced decrease in guanosine 3′,5′-cyclic monophosphate in frog photoreceptor membranes. J Gen Physiol 73:629–653
Woodruff ML, Bownds D, Green SH, Morrisey JL, Shedlovsky A (1977) Guanosine 3′,5′-cyclic monophosphate and the in vitro physiology of frog photoreceptor membranes. J Gen Physiol 69:667–679
Yamada T (1977) Control mechanisms in cell-type conversion in newt lens regeneration. Monogr Dev Biol 13:1–126
Yee R, Liebman PA (1978) Light-activated phosphodiesterase of the rod outer segment. Kinetics and parameters of activation and deactivation. J Biol Chem 253:8902–8909
Young RW (1967) The renewal of photoreceptor cell outer segments. J Cell Biol 33:61–72
Young RW (1969a) The organization of vertebrate photoreceptor cells. In: Straatsma BR, Hall MO, Allen RA, Crescitelli F (eds) The retina: morphology, function and clinical characteristics. University of California Press, Los Angeles, pp 177–210
Young RW (1969b) A difference between rods and cones in the renewal of outer segment protein. Invest Ophthalmol 8:222–231
Young RW, Bok D (1969) Participation of the retinal pigment epithelium in the rod outer segment renewal process. J Cell Biol 42:392–403
Zadunaisky JA (1966) Active transport of chloride in frog cornea. Am J Physiol 211:506–512
Zadunaisky JA, Lande MA (1971) Active chloride transport and control of corneal transparency. Am J Physiol 221:1837–1844
Zimmerman WF, Daemen FJ, Bonting SL (1976) Distribution of enzyme activities in subcellular fractions of bovine retina. J Biol Chem 251:4700–4705
Zink HA, Podos SM, Becker B (1975) Modification by imidazoles of ocular inflammatory and pressure responses. Invest Ophthalmol 14:280–285

CHAPTER 27

The Role of Cyclic Nucleotides in the Control of Anterior Pituitary Gland Activity

F. LABRIE, P. BORGEAT, J. DROUIN, L. LAGACE, V. GIGUERE, V. RAYMOND, M. GODBOUT, J. MASSICOTTE, L. FERLAND, N. BARDEN, M. BEAULIEU, J. COTE, J. LEPINE, H. MEUNIER, and R. VEILLEUX

Overview

The anterior pituitary gland secretes six known polypeptide hormones: ACTH (adrenocorticotropin), GH (growth hormone), PRL (prolactin), TSH (thyrotropin), LH (luteinizing hormone), and FSH (follicle-stimulating hormone). The rate of secretion of these individual polypeptides is specifically controlled by neurohormones released from the hypothalamus and transported to their adenohypophyseal site of action by a short portal blood system (SCHALLY et al. 1968). The secretion of LH, FSH, and ACTH is known to be under only positive hypothalamic control, whereas that of GH, TSH, and PRL results from the balance of action of inhibitory and stimulatory neurohormones (Fig. 1). The overall influence of the hypothalamus on GH and TSH secretion is stimulatory, whereas it is inhibitory on PRL secretion.

Only recently has the concept of neurohormonal control of adenohypophyseal function been translated into biochemical and chemical terms. This new era of neuroendocrinology started with the elucidation of the structure of porcine and ovine TRH (TSH-releasing hormone), the neurohormone controlling the activity of the TSH-secreting cells, as (pyro)Glu-His-Pro-NH_2 (BOLER et al. 1969; BURGUS et al. 1969). This achievement was soon followed by the isolation of LHRH, the neurohormone which stimulates the release of both LH and FSH. LHRH is a decapeptide having the structure: (pyro)Glu-His-Trp-Ser-Tyr-Gly-Leu-Arg-Pro-Gly-NH_2 (MATSUO et al. 1971; BURGUS et al. 1971). The tetradecapeptide H-Ala-Gly-Cys-Lys-Asn-Phe-Phe-Trp-Lys-Thr-Phe-Thr-Ser-Cys-OH has been isolated from ovine and porcine hypothalami (BRAZEAU et al. 1973; SCHALLY et al. 1975) on the basis of its ability to inhibit GH release; this peptide has been named somatostatin. More recently, peptide with potent ACTH-releasing activity (CRF) has been isolated from ovine hypothalami (VALE et al. 1981).

The relative ease of synthesis of these peptides and their analogues opened new possibilities for studies of their mechanism of action and has led to a rapid expansion of our knowledge of the physiology of the hypothalamo-pituitary complex. These studies were much facilitated by another important recent development, the pituitary cell culture system (VALE et al. 1972; LABRIE et al. 1973a). In fact, adenohypophyseal cells in primary culture have been extremely useful, not only for assessment of the biological activity of analogs of TRH, LHRH and somatostatin (LABRIE et al. 1973a, 1976a; BÉLANGER et al. 1974; CARON et al. 1978)

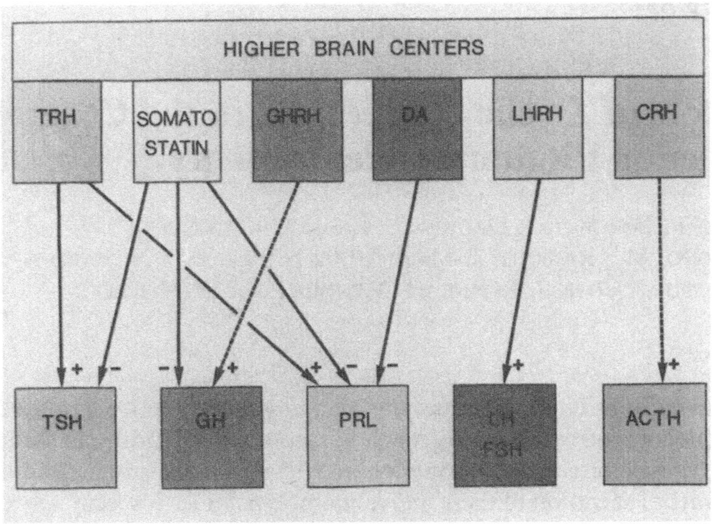

Fig. 1. Schematic representation of the hypothalamo-adenohypohyseal complex. *TSH*, thyrotropin; *LH*, luteinizing hormone; *ACTH*, adrenocorticotropin; *FSH*, follicle-stimulating hormone; GH, growth hormone; *PRL*, prolactin; *TRH*, thyrotropin-releasing hormone; *GH-RH*, growth hormone-releasing hormone. *CRH*, corticotropin-releasing hormone; *DA*, dopamine; *LHRH*, luteinizing hormone-releasing hormone and somatostatin, GH-release inhibiting hormone

but also for determination of the characteristics of interaction between hypothalamic and peripheral hormones at the adenohypophyseal level (DROUIN and LABRIE 1976a, b; DROUIN et al. 1976a, b, c, 1978; CARON et al. 1978). Although peripheral hormones were known to play a major role in the control of adenohypophyseal activity in man and experimental animals, in vivo approaches could not dissociate between hypothalamic and pituitary sites of action.

This presentation will summarize the available evidence about cyclic AMP accumulation in the anterior pituitary gland in response to the synthetic hypothalamic hormones, TRH, LHRH, CRF and somatostatin, as well as a catecholamine, dopamine, and a purified "inhibin" preparation. This review will summarize the evidence available for a role of prostaglandins (PGs) in the control of GH and TSH secretion at the pituitary level. Since the characteristics of binding of TRH and the properties of cyclic AMP-dependent adenohypophyseal protein kinase and some of its substrates have been described in relatively recent reviews (LABRIE et al. 1975a, b), these aspects will not be included in the present discussion. Recent knowledge gained on the characteristics of the pituitary LHRH receptor will however be presented.

Knowing that LHRH stimulates the secretion of both LH and FSH (BORGEAT et al. 1972), the divergence frequently observed in vivo between the rate of secretion of the two gonadotropins can be best explained by differential effects of gonadal steroids at the pituitary level on the secretion of these two hormones. Thus, emphasis will be given to the specific effects of androgens, estrogens and progesterone on basal and LHRH-induced secretion of LH and FSH in anterior pituitary cells in culture. Data describing the effects of "inhibin" of testicular and ovarian origin at the pituitary level on gonadotropin secretion will also be presented.

Since estrogens are potent stimulators of prolactin secretion, the interaction of estrogens with dopaminergic action will then be studied at the pituitary level both in vitro and in vivo. Estrogens were found to act directly at the pituitary level and, more surprisingly, to have potent antidopaminergic activity on prolactin secretion. Finally, data will be presented on the α-adrenergic control of secretion of β-LPH and β-endorphin-like peptides in rat anterior pituitary gland.

A. Role of Cyclic AMP in the Action of LHRH, TRH, CRF Somatostatin, Dopamine and "Inhibin" in the Adenohypophysis

I. Indirect Evidence for a Role of Cyclic AMP in Adenohypophyseal Function

The first indirect evidence for a role of cyclic AMP as mediator of the action of the hypothalamic regulatory hormones in the anterior pituitary gland was the observations that either cyclic AMP derivatives or theophylline, an inhibitor of cyclic nucleotide phosphodiesterase, stimulates the release of all six main anterior pituitary hormones. SCHOFIELD (1967) first reported the stimulatory effect of theophylline on GH release from bovine pituitary gland. This effect was soon confirmed in rat anterior pituitary gland by WILBER et al. (1968). Theophylline also stimulates the in vitro release of TSH (WILBER et al. 1968; LABRIE et al. 1975b, 1976b) and PRL (LEMAY and LABRIE 1972).

Cyclic AMP derivatives substituted at either the N-6 or the C-8 positions stimulate release, in vitro, of GH (CEHOVIC et al. 1970; LABRIE et al. 1971a; LEMAY and LABRIE 1972), TSH (CEHOVIC 1969; WILBER et al. 1969; WILBER and SEIBEL 1973), ACTH (FLEISCHER et al. 1969), LH (RATNER 1970; LABRIE et al. 1973a), and PRL (LEMAY and LABRIE 1972; WAKABAYASHI et al. 1973). Data obtained with methylxanthines and cyclic AMP derivatives suggest that cyclic AMP has a stimulatory role in the control of the secretion of all six main anterior pituitary hormones. Stimulation or inhibition of adenylate cyclase activity in specific pituitary cell types by the corresponding stimulatory and inhibitory hypothalamic regulatory hormones could thus provide a mechanism of control of adenohypophyseal hormone secretion.

II. Stimulatory Effect of LHRH on Cyclic AMP Accumulation

The observation that theophylline and cyclic AMP derivatives (RATNER 1970; LABRIE et al. 1973a; DROUIN et al. 1978; GOODYER et al. 1977; ADAMS et al. 1979) have a stimulatory effect on LH release and the potentiation by theophylline of the effect of a crude preparation of FSH-releasing hormone on FSH release (JUTISZ and PALOMA DE LA LLOSA 1970) suggested that cyclic AMP plays a role in the control of gonadotropin secretion. Definitive proof that the adenylate cyclase system is a mediator of the action of LHRH was obtained, however, by determination of the effect of the neurohormone on either adenohypophyseal adenylate cyclase activity or cyclic AMP concentration.

LHRH stimulates cyclic AMP accumulation in rat anterior pituitary gland in vitro (BORGEAT et al. 1972, 1974a; KANEKO et al. 1973; MAKINO 1973; NAOR et al. 1975a). The concentration of LHRH required for half-maximal stimulation of cyclic AMP accumulation is 0.1 to 1.0 ng/ml or 1×10^{-10} to 1×10^{-9} M LHRH (BORGEAT et al. 1972). In ovine adenohypophyseal cells (incubated in the presence of dopamine to minimize the contribution of mammotrophs to basal cyclic AMP levels) LHRH increases cyclic AMP release into the incubation medium (ADAMS et al. 1979). The enhanced release of either LH or cyclic AMP in response to LHRH were potentiated by the cyclic nucleotide phosphodiesterase inhibitor IBMX, 3-isobutyl-1-methyl-xanthine.

In rat hemipituitaries, changes in the rate of gonadotropin release parallel cyclic AMP content as a function of either duration of incubation or concentration of gonadotropin-releasing peptides (BORGEAT et al. 1972; MENON et al. 1977). In a more precise system, ovine adenohypophyseal cells in culture, a similar close correlation has been observed between changes of cyclic AMP and LH release into the incubation medium (ADAMS et al. 1979).

When LHRH analogues having biological activity between 0.001% and 1000% the activity of LHRH itself were used, the same close parallelism between stimulation of cyclic AMP accumulation and both LH and FSH release was found under all experimental conditions (BORGEAT et al. 1974a). A similar effect of LHRH was observed in the presence or absence of theophylline or IBMX (BORGEAT et al. 1972; ADAMS et al. 1979), thereby suggesting that LHRH exerts its action by activating adenylate cyclase and not by inhibiting cyclic nucleotide phosphodiesterase.

The possibility of developing a contraceptive method based on inhibitory LHRH analogues has led to the synthesis of many such substances, some of which are potent inhibitors of LHRH action both in vivo (FERLAND et al. 1975a) and in vitro (LABRIE et al. 1976c). The availability of LHRH antagonists offered the possibility of investigating the correlation between their inhibitory effect on LHRH-induced cyclic AMP accumulation and LH and FSH release.

As an example, Fig. 2 shows the inhibitory effect of increasing concentrations of [D-Phe^2, D-Leu^6]LHRH on cyclic AMP accumulation and LH and FSH release in rat anterior pituitary gland in vitro. The close correlation between inhibition of LHRH-induced cyclic AMP accumulation and LH and FSH release adds strong support to the concept of an obligatory role of the adenylate cyclase system as mediator of LHRH action in the anterior pituitary gland.

As direct evidence for a stimulatory effect of LHRH on pituitary adenylate cyclase activity, the neurohormone has been found to stimulate cyclic AMP formation in rat anterior pituitary homogenate (DEERY and HOWELL 1973; SPONA 1975) and membrane fractions (MAKINO 1973). A stimulatory effect of LHRH on adenylate cyclase activity has also been reported in homogenate from the ventral lobe of the pituitary of the dogfish (DEERY and JONES 1975) and fresh rat pituitary while the stimulatory effect was lost when the adenylate cyclase assay was delayed (BAUMANN and KUHL 1980).

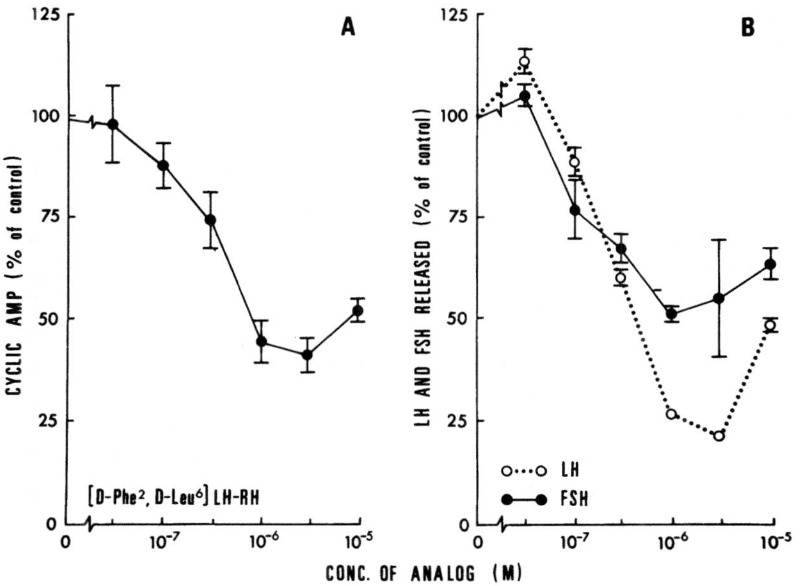

Fig. 2A and B. Effect of increasing concentrations of [D-Phe^2, D-Leu^6]LH-RH on 3×10^{-9} *M* LH-RH-induced cyclic AMP accumulation **A** and LH and FSH **B** release in rat hemipituitaries in vitro. (BEAULIEU et al. 1975)

Some groups have not detected changes of pituitary cyclic AMP levels accompanying LHRH-induced LH release (NAOR et al. 1975b, 1978; RATNER et al. 1974; CONN et al. 1979; RIGLER et al. 1978). No stimulatory effect of LHRH could be detected in ovine (THEOLEYRE et al. 1976), bovine, or rat (CLAYTON et al. 1978) pituitary membranes. Moreover, cholera toxin and prostaglandins increase pituitary cyclic AMP levels without affecting LH release (SUNDBERG et al. 1976; CONN et al. 1979).

Since gonadotrophs represent about 5% of the total cell population in the anterior pituitary gland, it is not surprising that addition of LHRH leads to only a 100 to 300% stimulation (over control) of anterior pituitary cyclic AMP concentration (BORGEAT et al. 1972, 1974a; LABRIE et al. 1973a; NAOR et al. 1975a, b). In order to induce this significant increase of total cyclic AMP accumulation, LHRH must stimulate specific cyclic AMP formation at least twenty- to sixty-fold in gonadotrophs. Moreover, DROUIN et al. (1976a) found that estrogens increase the sensitivity of gonadotrophs to LHRH by a direct action upon the pituitary gland, while androgens have the opposite effect. Such a gonadal hormone-induced change of pituitary responsiveness to LHRH may explain why pituitaries obtained from male rats show a consistent increase of pituitary cyclic AMP levels under the influence of LHRH (BORGEAT et al. 1972, 1974a; LABRIE et al. 1973a, 1975a, b; NAOR et al. 1975a, b), while no significant effect could be observed using female rat pituitaries (NAOR et al. 1979; P. BORGEAT, M. BEAULIEU, and F. LABRIE, unpublished work). Conceivably, the higher sensitivity to LHRH in female animals requires lower (undetectable) changes of the intracellular cyclic AMP concentration; conversely, the lower sensitivity to LHRH in male pituitary glands might require higher (detectable) changes of cyclic AMP content.

Suggestions against an obligatory role of cyclic AMP as mediator of LHRH action derive mainly from the findings that nonspecific agents leading to changes of total pituitary cyclic AMP accumulation (such as theophylline, prostaglandins, inhibitors of prostaglandin synthesis, and cholera toxin) do not always lead to parallel changes of LH release (NAOR et al. 1975a; SUNDBERG et al. 1976; CONN et al. 1979). Since prostaglandins are not involved in LHRH action at the level of the anterior pituitary gland (DROUIN and LABRIE 1976b; DROUIN et al. 1976c; LABRIE et al. 1976b; BARDEN et al. 1976), and, as mentioned earlier, gonadotrophs represent only 5% of the total cell population in the anterior pituitary gland, the changes of cyclic AMP levels observed with the above-mentioned compounds may take place in cell types other than gonadotrophs. In fact, somatotrophs represent approximately 50% of the total adenohypophyseal cell population and are highly sensitive to all the substances tested in the above-mentioned studies (DROUIN and LABRIE 1976b; LABRIE et al. 1975a, b, 1976a, b; BARDEN et al. 1976). All these negative attempts to correlate changes of cyclic AMP levels with alterations of LH release can be explained by the lack of specificity of the substances used and the failure to take into account the heterogeneity of the pituitary cell population. In fact, all above-mentioned non-specific compounds act on somatotrophs; this extragonadotropic action could explain all the reported changes of cyclic AMP levels which were not accompanied by specific effects on LH secretion (NAOR et al. 1975a, b; SUNDBERG et al. 1976; CONN et al. 1979).

Prolactin-secreting cells represent a high proportion of pituitary cells (30–75%) and are likely to be responsible for a major proportion of the pool of total pituitary cyclic AMP, thus masking the specific stimulatory effect of LHRH action on only a small population of cells. This is well supported by the elegant study of ADAMS et al. (1979) who have found, using ovine anterior pituitary cells in culture, that incubation with a specific inhibitor of prolactin secretion, dopamine, was required to permit demonstration of the stimulatory effect of LHRH on cyclic AMP release.

Although cyclic GMP derivatives do not stimulate adenohypophyseal hormone release, cyclic GMP has also been suggested as a possible intracellular nucleotide responsible for modulating LH and FSH release (NAKANO et al. 1978; NAOR et al. 1978; RIGLER et al. 1978). For example, in pentobarbital-anesthetized proestrus or estrogen-primed ovariectomized rats, increased pituitary cyclic GMP levels were also found after LHRH administration (KAWAKAMI and KIMURA 1980). The absence of elevated cyclic AMP levels in these animals under the influence of LHRH is in agreement with our findings and the findings of other groups demonstrating that LHRH induces stimulatory effects on pituitary cyclic AMP levels in male or castrated female rats but not in intact female animals. As discussed earlier, the increased LH and FSH responsiveness to LHRH under the influence of estrogens can probably explain the need for smaller changes of cyclic AMP levels to induce gonadotropin secretion in female animals.

LHRH acting upon similar, or perhaps identical, receptors may either enhance or inhibit adenylate cyclase in different tissues. Thus, LHRH binding to the pituitary LHRH receptors leads to stimulation of cyclic AMP formation (BORGEAT et al. 1972); however binding of LHRH to its ovarian receptor inhibits cyclic AMP accumulation (MASSICOTTE et al. 1980). LHRH may thus represent the first example of a peptide hormone binding to similar or identical receptors in two tissues (anterior pituitary and ovary) with opposite effects on adenylate cyclase activity.

The finding of an inhibitory effect of LHRH on LH-induced cyclic AMP accumulation in porcine granulosa cells lends support to the previously proposed LHRH-receptor adenylate cyclase system in the anterior pituitary gland (BORGEAT et al. 1972).

III. Stimulatory Effect of TRH on Cyclic AMP Accumulation

Many groups have reported a TRH-induced increase in pituitary cyclic AMP levels accompanying the TRH-induced TSH release. Thus, after 30 min of incubation with TRH, rat hemipituitaries demonstrate a 30% increase of their cyclic AMP content and an increased TSH release (LABRIE et al. 1975a, b). The maximal effect, 50% increase above control, was found after 2 h of incubation. Similarly, BOWERS (1971) reported a stimulatory effect of TRH on cyclic AMP levels in intact rat pituitaries; ROSE and CONKLIN (1978) have found a maximal increase (50%) of cyclic AMP levels 10–20 min after addition of TRH to pituitary fragments. Moreover, a close correlation could be observed between cyclic AMP accumulation and TSH release as a function of TRH concentration. In enriched thyrotrophs, BARNES et al. (1978) found a small (11 and 21%) increase in cyclic AMP in two out of three experiments; NAOR et al. (1979) found a 70% increase 30 min after addition of TRH in one of two populations of enriched thyrotrophs. Since our experiments (LABRIE et al. 1975a, b) were performed in the presence of 5 m*M* theophylline, it is likely that the observed changes of cyclic AMP concentrations are secondary to parallel modifications of adenylate cyclase activity rather than to inhibition of cyclic nucleotide phosphodiesterase.

Other groups have been unable to find a correlation between TRH-induced changes of cyclic AMP levels and TRH release in normal pituitary tissue (TAL et al. 1974; TAL and FRIEDMAN 1978; SUNDBERG et al. 1976) or in normal pituitary or tumor (ETO and FLEISCHER 1976; GERSHENGORN et al. 1980) cells.

With the knowledge gained in other systems, and the known heterogeneity of the anterior pituitary gland, it is not surprising that changes of pituitary hormone release are not always accompanied by measurable parallel changes of total pituitary cyclic AMP content. Such a dissociation occurs in the corpus luteum where changes of steroid secretion occur at low concentrations of gonadotropin which do not cause detectable changes of cyclic AMP levels (DUFAU et al. 1978). Such findings indicate a compartimentalization of cyclic AMP into pools of different biological importance and that the elevation of cyclic AMP levels in a small cellular compartment not reflected by measurements of total cellular cyclic AMP, is sufficient for hormone-induced cellular activation. The presence of pituitary cyclic AMP pools, analogous to those in the corpus luteum, is also suggested by the finding that increased TSH and ACTH release induced by TRH and lysine-vasopressin, respectively, can occur at low concentrations, in the absence of detectable changes of cyclic AMP levels while higher concentrations lead to an increase of both hormone release and cyclic AMP levels (ROSE and CONKLIN 1978).

IV. Stimulatory Effect of CRF on Cyclic AMP Accumulation

Recent isolation and elucidation of the structure of a peptidic CRF (corticotropin-releasing factor) having potent ACTH-releasing activity in vivo and in vitro in the rat (VALE et al. 1981) opens new possibilities for studies of the control of

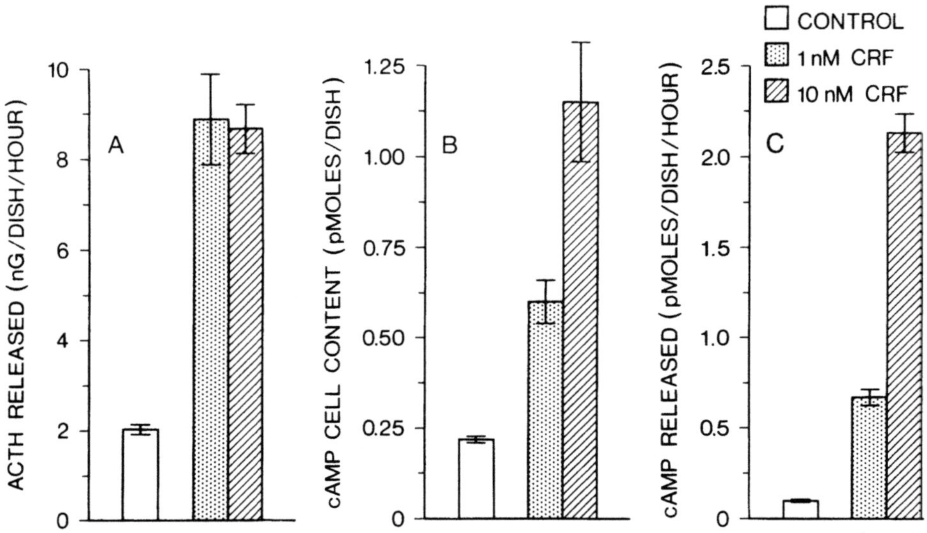

Fig. 3. Effect of synthetic ovine CRF on ACTH release and cyclic AMP content and release in an enriched population of rat corticotrophs. ACTH and cyclic AMP were measured by specific radioimmunoassays after a 1-h incubation in the absence or presence of 1 or 10 n*M* CRF

adrenocortical activity and for a better understanding of the mechanisms controlling the pituitary response to stress. The first suggestive evidence for a role of cyclic AMP as intracellular mediator of pituitary ACTH secretion originated from the observation that theophylline, an inhibitor of cyclic nucleotide phosphodiesterase, stimulated ACTH release in intact pituitary glands (FLEISCHER et al. 1969). In addition, cyclic AMP derivatives are powerful stimuli of ACTH secretion in intact pituitaries (FLEISCHER et al. 1969) and in pituitary cells in culture (RAYMOND et al. 1979). Although the observation of a stimulatory effect of theophylline and cyclic AMP derivatives on ACTH release was suggestive of a role of the cyclic nucleotide in the control of ACTH secretion, definitive proof of the role of the adenylate cyclase system had to be obtained by measurements of changes of cyclic AMP levels or adenylate cyclase activity. The present data are the first demonstration of the potent stimulatory effect of CRF on cyclic AMP accumulation in a purified fraction of rat corticotrophs.

After a 1-h incubation with an enriched population of rat corticotrophs, 1 n*M* CRF stimulates ACTH release by approximately 3.5-fold while cyclic AMP content and release are increased 2- and 7-fold above control, respectively (Fig. 3). A 10-fold higher concentration of CRF (10 n*M*) leads to no further stimulation of ACTH release while cyclic AMP content and release are further increased to 5- and 20-fold above control, respectively.

The present data clearly show that synthetic ovine CRF leads to a rapid and marked stimulation of cyclic AMP accumulation in an enriched population of rat corticotrophs. The 100% stimulation of cyclic AMP cellular content measured as early as 60 s after addition of the peptide strongly suggests that the changes of cyclic AMP accumulation coincide with or precede ACTH release induced by CRF.

V. Inhibitory Effect of Somatostatin on Cyclic AMP Accumulation

Since we had found that a purified fraction of GH-RH led to a marked stimulation of pituitary cyclic AMP accumulation and GH release (BORGEAT et al. 1973), it was of interest to study the effect of somatostatin on pituitary cyclic AMP accumulation. Somatostatin inhibits cyclic AMP accumulation in anterior pituitary gland in vitro (KANEKO et al. 1973; BORGEAT et al. 1974b), and reduces the release of both GH and TSH (BORGEAT et al. 1974b). The effect of somatostatin on cyclic AMP accumulation in rat hemipituitaries is well illustrated by a maximal inhibition (to approximately 35% of the control level) 10 min after adding the peptide (BORGEAT et al. 1974).

Since growth hormone (GH)- and TSH-secreting cells account for 50–70% of the total adenohypophyseal cell population in adult male rats, the 50% inhibition of cyclic AMP accumulation in total pituitary tissue suggests an almost complete inhibition of cyclic AMP accumulation in the GH- and TSH-secreting cells. The inhibitory effect of somatostatin is observed under both basal and prostaglandin E_2 (PGE_2)- or theophylline-induced conditions, thus suggesting an inhibitory action of somatostatin on adenylate cyclase. Using a similar in vitro system, LIPPMAN et al. (1976) have shown that somatostatin and its agonistic analogues exert parallel inhibitory effects on prostaglandin E_2-induced pituitary cyclic AMP accumulation and growth hormone release.

The correlation between inhibition of cyclic AMP levels and GH release is well illustrated by an experiment performed in pituitary cells in primary culture (Fig. 4). The approximate ten-fold increase of cyclic AMP levels induced by 10^{-5} *M* PGE_2 is inhibited 60% by somatostatin at an ED_{50} value of 0.3 n*M*. Under the same experimental conditions, GH release is 90–95% inhibited at maximal concentrations of somatostatin. The inhibitory effect of somatostatin on cyclic AMP levels and GH release is observed at the same ED_{50} value (0.3 n*M*). The absence of a significant effect of somatostatin on basal cyclic AMP levels in cells in culture although it causes an approximate 50% inhibition of basal GH release can possibly be explained by the presence of fibroblasts in the culture. Besides its own interest, this system could be advantageous as a model for studies of the mechanisms of action of substances (PGE, GHRH and somatostatin) having opposite effects on cyclic AMP accumulation in the same cell type.

The data presented so far clearly show that three stimulatory hypothalamic hormones, TRH, CRF, and LHRH, lead to parallel stimulation of cyclic AMP accumulation and specific hormone release, while one inhibitory peptide, somatostatin, leads to parallel inhibition of cyclic AMP accumulation and GH and TSH release. Such findings strongly suggest that changes of adenylate cyclase activity are involved in the mechanism of action of these four peptides in the anterior pituitary gland.

VI. Inhibitory Effect of Dopamine on Cyclic AMP Accumulation

Much evidence obtained in the rat indicates that dopamine (DA) secreted by the tuberoinfundibular system is the main factor involved in the control of prolactin secretion (MACLEOD and LEHMEYER 1974; LABRIE et al. 1978a; SHAAR and CLEMENS

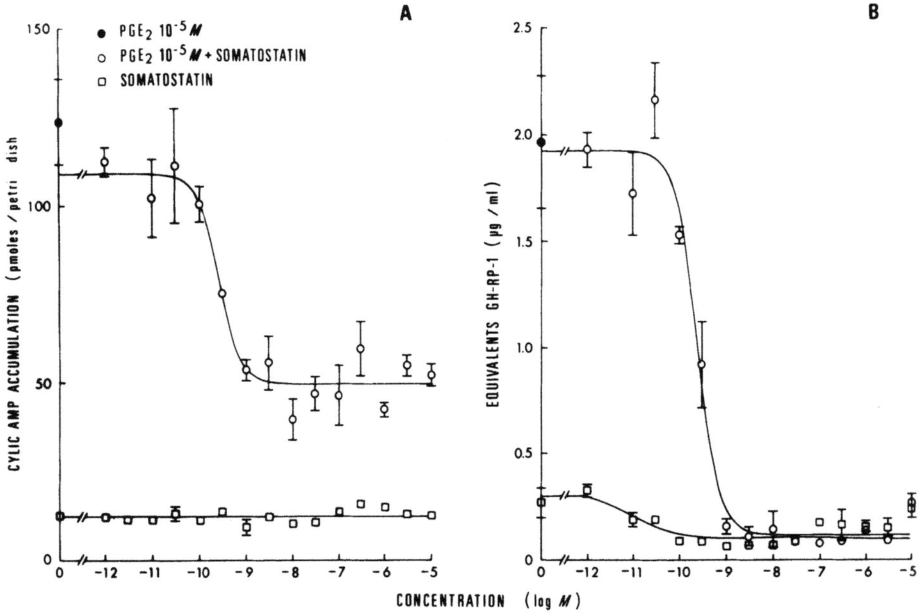

Fig. 4A and B. Effect of increasing concentrations of somatostatin alone or in the presence of 10^{-5} M PGE_2 on cyclic AMP accumulation **A** and GH release **B** in rat anterior pituitary cells in primary culture. Cells were incubated for 30 min in the presence of the indicated substances as described (LABRIE et al. 1973 a) and cyclic AMP measured by RIA

1974; TAKAHARA et al. 1974). DA, released from nerve endings in the median eminence, is transported to the pituitary prolactin-secreting cells by the hypothalamo-adenohypophyseal portal blood system. In support of such a physiological role of DA at the pituitary level on prolactin secretion, DA has recently been detected in portal blood (BEN-JONATHAN et al. 1977) and a typical dopaminergic receptor has been characterized in anterior pituitary gland (CARON et al. 1978; CALABRO and MACLEOD 1978).

The first suggestive evidence for a role of cyclic AMP in the control of prolactin secretion originated from the observations that a cyclic AMP derivative (LEMAY and LABRIE 1972) or theophylline, an inhibitor of cyclic nucleotide phosphodiesterase (Lemay and LABRIE 1972; WAKABAYASHI et al. 1973), stimulated prolactin release. These data obtained with theophylline and cyclic AMP derivatives already suggested that the cyclic nucleotide has a stimulatory role in the control of prolactin secretion.

More convincing evidence supporting a role of cyclic AMP in the action of dopamine on prolactin secretion had to be obtained, however, by measurement of adenohypophyseal adenylate cyclase activity or cyclic AMP concentration under the influence of the catecholamine. As illustrated in Fig. 5, addition of 100 nM dopamine to male rat hemipituitaries led to a rapid inhibition of cyclic AMP accumulation, a maximal effect (30% inhibition) being already obtained 5 min after addition of the catecholamine. Thus, while dopamine is well known to stimulate adenylate cyclase activity in the striatum (KEBABIAN 1973; KEBABIAN et al. 1977), its

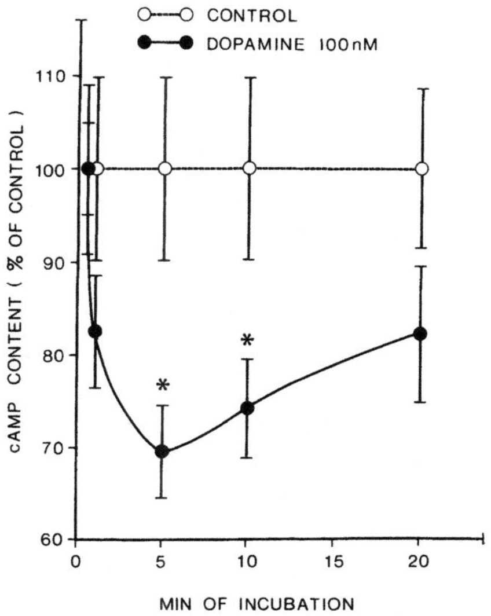

Fig. 5. Effect of dopamine (100 n*M*) on cyclic AMP accumulation in male rat anterior pituitaries. The experiment was performed as described. (BORGEAT et al. 1972)

effect at the adenohypophyseal level in intact cells is inhibitory. Dopamine has also been found to exert parallel inhibitory effects on cyclic AMP and prolactin release in ovine adenohypophyseal cells in culture (ADAMS et al. 1979), a significant inhibitory effect being observed at 0.5 μ*M* dopamine.

Since cyclic AMP derivatives and inhibitors of cyclic nucleotide phosphodiesterase stimulate prolactin release (Lemay and LABRIE 1972; LABRIE et al. 1973a; PELLETIER et al. 1972), and dopamine is a potent inhibitor of prolactin release (LABRIE et al. 1978a), it is not surprising that the catecholamine does not stimulate the adenylate cyclase system. On the contrary, the present data and those of DE CAMILLI et al. (1979) indicate that the pituitary DA receptor is negatively coupled to adenylate cyclase. Although it is quite possible that some brain DA receptors do not act through the adenylate cyclase system and could be called D-2 receptors (KEBABIAN and CALNE 1979), this terminology does not apply to pituitary receptors. In order to avoid possible confusion with vitamin D receptors, we suggest the terminology DA_+, DA_- and DA_0 to correspond to DA receptors positively, negatively or uncoupled to adenylate cyclase. The pituitary DA receptor is thus a typical DA_--receptor. This proposed classification of dopamine receptors is based exclusively on their association with the adenylate cyclase system as second messenger. SEEMAN and collaborators have proposed that dopamine receptors be called D_1, D_2, and D_3 on the basis of their binding properties (TITELER et al. 1980).

VII. Inhibitory Effect of "Inhibin" on Cyclic AMP Accumulation

In addition to LHRH and sex steroids, an inhibitory substance of ovarian and testicular origin called "inhibin" could be involved in the control of LH and FSH secretion (FRANCHIMONT 1972; BAKER et al. 1976; LABRIE et al. 1978b; FRANCHIMONT et al. 1979; LAGACÉ et al. 1979a, b). The action of "inhibin" on spontaneous gonadotropin secretion is specific for FSH, no effect being exerted on basal LH release in rat anterior pituitary cells in culture. However, when the LH and FSH responses to LHRH are measured, a marked inhibitory effect is observed on the secretion of both gonadotropins. Moreover, "inhibin" interacts with sex steroids by reversing all their stimulatory effects and by potentiating all their inhibitory effects at the anterior pituitary level (LAGACÉ et al. 1979b; J. MASSICOTTE, L. LAGACÉ, V. GIGUÈRE, M. GODBOUT and F. LABRIE, unpublished work).

Since LHRH stimulates cyclic AMP accumulation in rat anterior pituitary gland in vitro (BORGEAT et al. 1972, 1974a; MAKINO 1973; KANEKO 1973; NAOR et al. 1975a), "inhibin" may exert an inhibitory effect on LHRH-induced cyclic AMP accumulation. In order to avoid the delay of "inhibin" action under in vitro conditions, the cyclic AMP response to LHRH was measured in vitro in pituitaries obtained from male rats at different time intervals after injection of "inhibin".

Single injection of a purified fraction of "inhibin" by the intravenous route led to a progressive and long-lasting inhibition of basal plasma FSH levels in both immature and mature male rats. In both groups, a maximal (30–40%) inhibition ($p<0.01$) of plasma FSH levels was observed at 6 and 12 h after injection of "inhibin" with a return toward control values at 18 h. No effect of "inhibin" was detected on plasma LH levels (GODBOUT and LABRIE 1982).

The stimulation of cyclic AMP levels induced in anterior pituitary tissue after 4 h of incubation with 10 n*M* LHRH was reduced 30–35% ($p<0.01$) in pituitaries obtained from either immature or mature male rats injected 6 or 12 h previously with "inhibin". Cyclic AMP levels in control basal and LHRH-treated hemipituitaries were 7.24 ± 0.90 and 18.2 ± 1.0 pmoles/mg protein, respectively, in immature animals. The control basal and LHRH-induced cyclic AMP levels in mature animals were 10.70 ± 0.40 and 17.60 ± 1.33 pmoles/mg protein, respectively.

The cyclic AMP accumulation induced by LHRH is decreased in hemipituitaries obtained from animals treated previously with a purified fraction of porcine follicular fluid "inhibin". The time-course of the effect of "inhibin" on plasma FSH levels and on the in vitro cyclic AMP response to LHRH is parallel, thus suggesting that the action of "inhibin" on gonadotropin secretion is mediated by a decrease of cyclic AMP accumulation in gonadotrophs, both in immature and adult male rats.

Based on the present findings, it is tempting to suggest that the rate of LH and FSH secretion is under two opposite influences acting through adenylate cyclase: stimulation by LHRH and inhibition by "inhibin". Assuming that "inhibin" reaches the pituitary by the general circulation and acts as an inhibitory hormone, it could possibly be added to the rapidly elongating list of peptides and neurotransmitters which are negatively coupled to adenylate cyclase such as somatostatin (BORGEAT et al. 1974b), norepinephrine (JAKOBS 1979) and dopamine (Fig. 5).

The data presented so far show that three stimulatory hypothalamic hormones, TRH, CRF, and LHRH, lead to parallel stimulation of cAMP accumulation and specific hormone release while somatostatin, "inhibin" and dopamine lead to parallel inhibition of cAMP accumulation and specific hormone release. Such findings suggest strongly that changes of adenylate cyclase activity are involved in the mechanism of action of these six substances in the anterior pituitary gland.

B. Role of Prostaglandins in the Adenohypophysis

I. Prostaglandins and Adenohypophyseal Cyclic AMP

Prostaglandins (PGs) are biologically active substances widely distributed in the body, including the hypothalamus and anterior pituitary gland (ORCZYK and BEHRMAN 1972; OJEDA et al. 1978). PGs may control hypothalamic hormone secretion and act as potential mediators of the action of the neurohormones in the anterior pituitary gland. Using combined in vivo and in vitro approaches, this review will summarize the evidence available for a role of PGs at the pituitary level in the control of GH and TSH secretion and for their effect on LHRH, TRH and CRH secretion.

Prostaglandins (PGs) are well known to stimulate cAMP accumulation in anterior pituitary tissue (ZOR et al. 1969, 1970; MACLEOD and LEHMEYER 1970; MAKINO 1973; LABRIE et al. 1973b; RATNER et al. 1974; BORGEAT et al. 1975b). At concentrations from 10^{-7} to 10^{-4} M, the various PGs exhibit markedly different potencies to induce cAMP accumulation in rat adenohypophysis after 120 min of incubation. The order of potency is: $PGE \simeq E_2 > A_1 \simeq A_2 > F_{1\alpha} \simeq F_{1\beta}$ (BORGEAT et al. 1975b). As mentioned earlier, the stimulatory effect of PGE_2 on adenohypophyseal cyclic AMP accumulation is also observed in anterior pituitary cells in culture (Fig. 4). Somatostatin can also inhibit the PGE-induced stimulation of adenylate cyclase activity in rat anterior pituitary gland homogenate, an half-maximal inhibition being observed at 15 nM somatostatin.

II. Fatty Acids and Changes of Adenohypophyseal Cyclic AMP Accumulation in vitro

In agreement with the specificity of PGE_1 and PGE_2 to stimulate adenohypophyseal rat hemipituitaries and pituitary cells in culture (BORGEAT et al. 1975b; LABRIE et al. 1976b), of all the fatty acids tested on pituitary cyclic AMP levels, only arachidonic and cis-8,11,14-eicosatrienoic acids showed a stimulatory effect (BERGERON and BARDEN 1975). At concentrations of 10^{-4} M, either arachidonic or 8,11,14-eicosatrienoic acids increased cyclic AMP levels within the first min of incubation. After 10–15 min of incubation, the concentration of cyclic AMP was almost 5 times the control value in the case of arachidonic acid and approximately 4 times the control level with cis-8,11,14-eicosatrienoic acid. If incubations were continued, cyclic AMP levels began to fall and reached control values after 60–90 min. At a concentration of 10^{-4} M, and under the same incubation conditions, *cis*-11,14,17-eicosatrienoic acid was without effect on cyclic AMP levels. Thus, both arachidonic acid and cis-8,11,14-eicosatrienoic acid can stimulate anterior pituitary gland cyclic AMP accumulation. The presence of theophylline potentiates the effect of these immediate precursors of PGE_1 and PGE_2 on cyclic AMP levels. However, theophylline has no effect on the time-course of stimulation (data not shown). Thus, arachidonic acid appears to exert its effect on cyclic AMP formation rather than by inhibition of cyclic nucleotide phosphodiesterase activity.

The PGs of the E type stimulate cyclic AMP accumulation in the anterior pituitary gland. This stimulation is maximal after 10–30 min of incubation and thereafter decreases; furthermore, the effects of the PGs are unchanged by theophylline

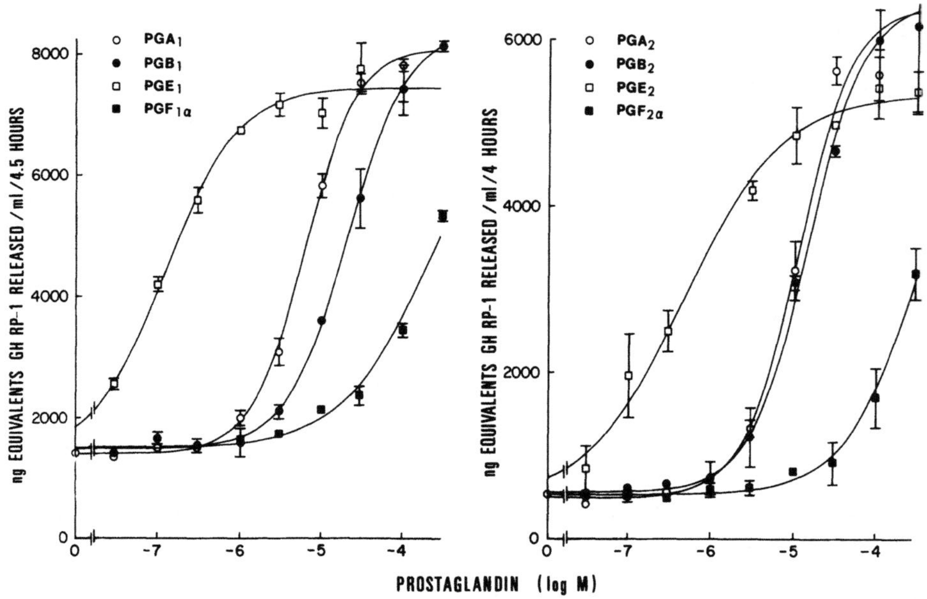

Fig. 6. Effect of increasing concentrations of prostaglandins E_1, A_1, B_1, $F_{1\alpha}$, E_2, A_2, B_2, and $F_{2\alpha}$ on growth hormone (GH) release in anterior pituitary cells in culture. After 3 days in culture, the cells were incubated for 4 h with the indicated prostaglandin concentrations. (DROUIN et al. 1976b)

and show no requirement for Ca^{2+} (BORGEAT et al. 1975b). The similarity between these findings and the stimulation of cyclic AMP accumulation induced by arachidonic or cis-8,11,14-eicosatrienoic acids strongly suggests that these fatty acids may exert their action via prostaglandin formation. This possibility is supported by the effects of prostaglandin synthetase inhibitors; both aspirin and indomethacin significantly inhibited the stimulatory effect of arachidonic acid on cyclic AMP accumulation (BERGERON and BARDEN 1975). This suggests that the active fatty acids do not directly stimulate a PG receptor; rather, their conversion to the corresponding PGs is essential for their activity. In agreement with evidence for fatty acid availability being the rate-limiting factor of prostaglandin formation (KUNZE 1970; PACE-ASCIAK and WOLFE 1970), the effects of arachidonic and cis-8,11,14-eicosatrienoic acids on cyclic AMP levels have been noted within 30 s of incubation, this time course of stimulation being similar to that seen in the presence of PGE_1 or PGE_2 (PACE-ASCIAK and WOLFE 1970).

III. Prostaglandins and Adenohypophyseal Hormone Release

1. PGs and Growth Hormone Release

In vitro studies using ox pituitary slices (SCHOFIELD 1970; COOPER et al. 1972) and rat hemipituitaries (MACLEOD and LEHMEYER 1970; HERTELENDY 1971; HERTELENDY et al. 1971, 1972; KATO et al. 1973; BÉLANGER et al. 1974; RATNER et al. 1974; BORGEAT et al. 1975b; BETTERIDGE and WALLIS 1977, 1978, 1979) show that PGs of the E series stimulate GH release. As shown in Fig. 6, the order of potency of various PGs in stimulating GH release from rat anterior pituitary cells in culture closely parallels the potency previously observed on cAMP accumulation (BORGEAT et al. 1975b). In fact, half-maximal stimulation of GH release by PGE_1 and PGE_2 is observed at 5×10^{-7} *M*, 8 to 10×10^{-6} *M* for PGA_1 and PGA_2, and approximately 3×10^{-4} *M* for $PGF_{1\alpha}$ and $PGF_{2\alpha}$. This in vitro stimulatory effect of PGE_1 and PGE_2 on GH release was confirmed in vivo (LABRIE et al. 1976b). Either PGE_1 or PGE_2, injected into the right superior vena cava in conscious rats, led to a rapid elevation of plasma GH levels; the effect of PGE_2 was approximately twice that of PGE At doses up to 250 µg, PGA_1 and PGA_2 have no effect on plasma GH levels (data not shown). These data, obtained in unanesthetized animals, agree with the stimulatory effect of PGE_1 on plasma GH levels found in rats anesthetized with pentobarbital (HERTELENDY et al. 1972) or urethane (KATO et al. 1973).

A partially purified fraction of GH-releasing hormone (GHRH) causes a rapid and concomitant stimulation of cAMP accumulation and GH release in rat anterior pituitary tissue (BORGEAT et al. 1973); comparable data have been obtained using a crude hypothalamic extract (STEINER et al. 1970). This close parallelism between PG-induced changes of cAMP levels and GH release and purified GHRH may well indicate a role of PGs and cAMP in the control of GH secretion. However, definite proof of the role of PGs in the control of the activity of the somatotrophs will be only obtained by direct measurement of the synthesis or mobilization of PGs under the influence of the corresponding neurohormones.

2. PGs and Gonadotropin Release

PGs of the E type stimulate LH release after in vivo administration. In fact, PGEs increase plasma LH levels in pentobarbital-blocked, proestrous rats (TSAFRIRI et al. 1973) as well as in steroid-primed ovariectomized animals (HARMS et al. 1974; SATO et al. 1975) and in intact male animals (RATNER et al. 1974). These data do not, however, differentiate between an effect of PGs at the hypothalamic level on LHRH release and a direct pituitary site of action on LH secretion.

Since the reports concerning the in vitro effects of PGs on LH release were conflicting (RATNER et al. 1974; ZOR et al. 1970; MAKINO 1973; SATO et al. 1975; BORGEAT et al. 1975b), it was of interest to study, in more detail, the effect of PGs on basal and LHRH-induced LH release in vitro using adenohypophaseal cells in culture and to examine the in vivo site of action of PGs using a LHRH antiserum. In the event of an hypothalamic site of action of PGs, administration of the antiserum should neutralize LHRH release by PGs and thus prevent the PG-induced increase of plasma LH levels.

In anterior pituitary cells in primary culture, the presence of 10^{-6} *M* PGE_1 had no influence on the ability of LHRH to stimulate LH release. In both control and PGE_1-treated cells, a 45-fold stimulation of LH release was found at 1×10^{-8} *M* LHRH, a half-maximal response being measured at 3×10^{-10} *M*. Moreover, PGE_2 (10^{-6} *M*) did not alter the time-course of basal or LHRH-induced LH release in cells in culture up to 10 h of incubatioh (DROUIN et al. 1976b).

Since PGEs do not stimulate LH release and do not change the responsiveness to LHRH in cultured cells, it became of great interest to study the site of action of PGs injected in vivo. The availability of a specific LHRH antiserum offered the ideal means of assessing the role of LHRH in the previously observed PG-induced

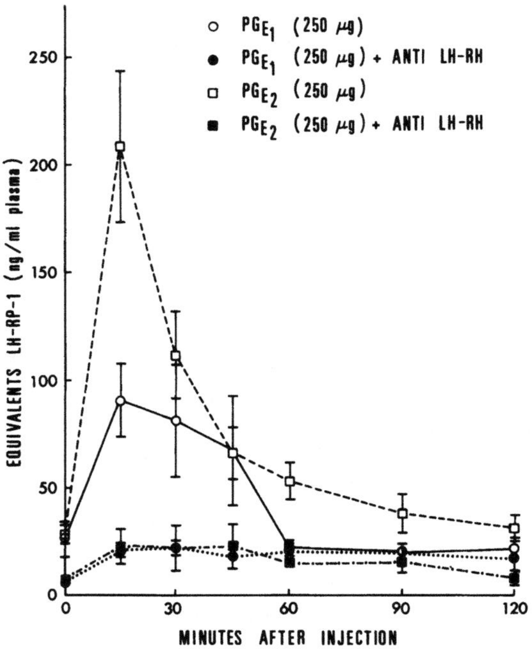

Fig. 7. Effect of 1 ml of anti-LHRH serum on PGE_2-induced LH release in anesthetized female rats on the afternoon of proestrus. The antiserum was injected 1 h before PGE_2 through a cannula inserted into the right superior vena cava. Plasma LH concentrations are plotted as mean ±SEM of 6–8 rats. (DROUIN and LABRIE 1976b)

LH release and to discriminate between a hypothalamic or pituitary site of action of PGEs on LH release. Under appropriate conditions, the presence of excess circulating LHRH antiserum should neutralize any PG-induced LHRH secretion. As can be seen in Fig. 7, not only was the basal plasma LH concentration reduced by approximately 75% 1 h after injection of the antiserum, but the treatment almost completely obliterated the plasma LH rise observed after injection of PGE_1 or PGE_2.

The absence of a direct effect of PGEs at the pituitary level on LH release is confirmed by the in vivo experiments using LHRH antiserum. In fact, the almost complete inhibition of the PGE_1- or PGE_2-induced rise of plasma LH in animals treated 1 h previously with sheep anti-LHRH serum leaves little doubt that the increased plasma LH levels observed in vivo after PGE administration are secondary to a stimulatory action of PGs on LHRH release at the hypothalamic level. Similar findings have been obtained when plasma LH was measured 15 min after injection of PGE_2 (CHOBSIENG et al 1975).

3. PGs and TSH and PRL Release

The effect of PGs on TSH release (SUNDBERG et al. 1976; BROWN and HEDGE 1974; TAL et al. 1974) and PRL release (SUNDBERG et al. 1976; LABRIE et al. 1973b; OJEDA et al. 1974; HARMS et al. 1973) were conflicting. The effect of the eight primary PGs

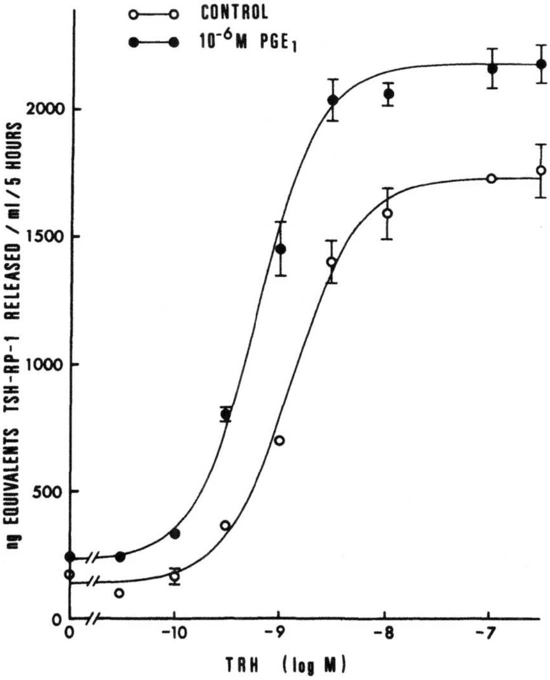

Fig. 8. TSH dose-response curve to TRH in the presence (●) or the absence (○) of 10^{-6} *M* PGE_1. The experiment was performed as described. (DROUIN et al. 1976b)

was then studied on the release of these two hormones in anterior pituitary cells in primary culture. At concentrations as high as 3×10^{-4} *M*, PGE_1 had no effect on basal PRL release; TSH release was slightly but reproducibly stimulated (170% of control) at concentrations above 10^{-6} *M* (DROUIN and LABRIE 1976b).

Further investigations of the effect of the PGEs on TSH release were based on in vivo results (BROWN and HEDGE 1974), demonstrating a potentiation of TRH-induced TSH release after intrapituitary injection of PGs. We examined the effect of PGE_1 on the TSH response to TRH in pituitary cells in culture. As illustrated in Fig. 8, PGE_1 (10^{-6} *M*) increased the responsiveness of the thyrotrophs to TRH by increasing both the basal and the TRH-stimulated release of TSH as well as by decreasing the TRH ED_{50} value from 1.3×10^{-9} *M* to 6.2×10^{-10} *M*.

The present data show that PGs can have two effects on hormone release by anterior pituitary cells in culture: a direct stimulatory effect on GH and TSH release and a potentiation of the stimulatory effect of TRH on TSH release. The effect of PGs appears to be specific for somatotrophs and thyrotrophs, no effect being detected on LH, FSH or PRL release.

4. PGS and ACTH Release

In rats pretreated with a small dose of dexamethasone (25 μg/100 g body weight) and anesthetized with pentobarbital, the injection into the median eminence of

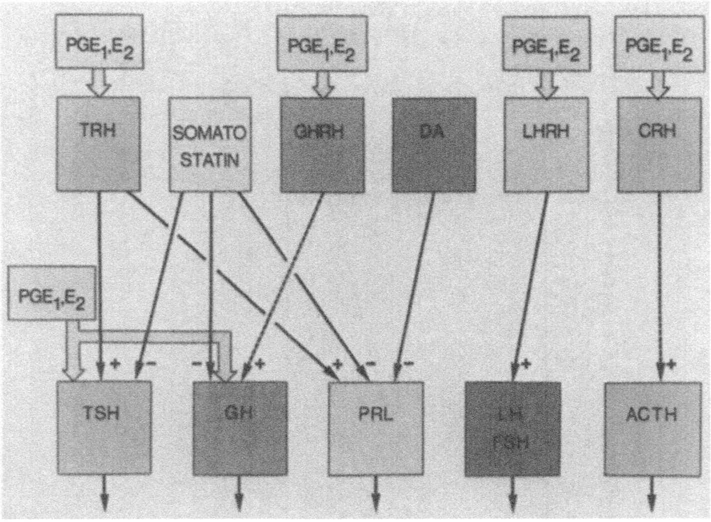

Fig. 9. Schematic representation of the stimulatory effect of PGE_1 and PGE_2 on hypothalamic and adenohypophyseal hormone secretion

small doses of PGE_1, $PGF_{1\alpha}$ or $PGF_{2\alpha}$ increased ACTH secretion as estimated by changes of plasma corticosterone levels (HEDGE 1972). Intravenous injections and injections into the lateral hypothalamus or pituitary had no effect. In animals treated with pentobarbital only, ACTH secretion is very sensitive to the injection of PGE_1, a maximal response of plasma corticosterone being obtained at a dose of 1 µg; $PGF_{2\alpha}$ is much less potent by this route. These data confirm those of PENG et al. (1970) who found that under similar conditions, PGE_1 produced maximal adrenal ascorbic acid depletion at a dose of 2 µg intravenously. PGA_1 or $PGF_{2\alpha}$ were not effective at even higher doses (5 µg/rat). DE WIED et al. (1969) also found that in rats pretreated with pentobarbital and chlorpromazine, a dose of 10 µg PGE_1 or PGE_2 (but not $PGF_{1\alpha}$ or $PGF_{2\alpha}$) stimulated plasma corticosterone levels. The possibility of a direct stimulatory effect of PGs at the adrenal level was ruled out since the response was abolished by hypophysectomy.

Since morphine, a drug believed to act mainly at the level of the CNS, inhibited the stimulatory response of ACTH secretion to PGs injected into the median eminence or intravenously (BROWN and HEDGE 1974; PENG et al. 1970; DE WIED et al. 1969), it is quite likely that PGs act at the hypothalamic level to stimulate the release of corticotropin-releasing hormone (CRH), which secondarily increases ACTH secretion. Moreover, DE WIED et al. (1969) found that PGE_1 had a stimulatory effect on ACTH secretion in several systems commonly used for CRH assays, but that the response was abolished in rats with median eminence lesions. Furthermore, the same authors found that the addition of PGs had no effect on rat pituitaries incubated in vitro. The lower activity of $PGF_{1\alpha}$ and $PGF_{2\alpha}$ relative to PGE_1 when injected intravenously was attributed to a more rapid inactivation of PGs of the F than E types by plasma (OJEDA et al. 1974). Thus, PGs appear to stimulate ACTH secretion in vivo by an action at the hypothalamic level leading to release of CRH(s) (Fig. 9).

C. Role of Ca^{2+} in the Adenohypophysis

Extracellular Ca^{2+} is required for the stimulated release of all pituitary hormones examined, including LH and FSH (SAMLI and GESCHWIND 1968; WAKABAYASHI et al. 1969; ADAMS and NETT 1979; JUTISZ and PALOMA DE LA LLOSA 1970; BORGEAT et al. 1975a), prolactin (PARSONS 1969), somatotrophs (GAUTVIK and TASHJIAN 1973; MILLIGAN et al. 1972), ACTH (KRAICER et al. 1969; ZIMMERMAN and GLEISCHER et al. 1970; MORIARTY 1977) and TSH (VALE et al. 1967; VALE and GUILLEMIN 1967). The ionophore A 23187 which increases membrane permeability to Ca^{2+} (SCARPA et al. 1972) increases growth hormone release in rat anterior pituitary tissue (BICKNELL and SCHOFIELD 1976). Ca^{2+} is also required for GH release induced by cyclic nucleotide phosphodiesterase inhibitors (STEINER et al. 1970; MIRA-MOSER et al. 1976; SPENCE et al. 1980) and PGs (HERTELENDY 1971; COOPER et al. 1972; HERTELENDY et al. 1978). Since the increase of pituitary cyclic AMP levels induced by PGs and phosphodiesterase inhibitors in total pituitary tissue (STEINER et al. 1970; COOPER et al. 1972) and purified somatotrophs (SPENCE et al. 1980) is increased in low Ca^{2+} medium, it appears that at least in somatotrophs, the Ca^{2+}-dependent step is needed for the expression of cyclic AMP while the cation is not required for PG-induced activation of adenylate cyclase (BORGEAT et al. 1975b).

Since Ca^{2+} was required for the hypothalamic extract-induced release of LH (SAMLI and GESCHWIND 1968; WAKABAYASHI et al. 1969), and FSH (WAKABAYASHI et al. 1969; JUTISZ and PALOMA DE LA LLOSA 1970), it was felt important to study a possible requirement of Ca^{2+} at a step preceding activation of adenylate cyclase by LHRH (BORGEAT et al. 1975a). Such an early site of action in the LH and FSH secretory cells would then be added to the already suspected late site of Ca^{2+} requirement observed during high K^+-induced release of LH and FSH (SAMLI and GESCHWIND 1968; WAKABAYASHI et al. 1969; JUTISZ and PALOMA DE LA LLOSA 1970). Ca^{2+} is required for activation by ACTH of adenylate cyclase activity in adrenal cell membrane particles (LEFKOWITZ et al. 1970). The observed Ca^{2+} requirement for LHRH-induced cyclic AMP accumulation (BORGEAT et al. 1975a) could be on the LHRH receptor, on the adenylate cyclase, on cyclic nucleotide phosphodiesterase, at some intermediate step between binding of LHRH and activation of adenylate cyclase, or at a combination of these sites. Since the binding of LHRH is not increased by Ca^{2+}, and 1 mM EDTA does not affect fluoride-stimulated adenohypophyseal adenylate cyclase activity, it appears more likely that Ca^{2+} is required at some step(s) between binding of LHRH and activation of adenylate cyclase, although an action at other sites remains possible.

In view of the ubiquity of Ca^{2+}-dependent regulatory proteins in mammalian tissues (WOLFE and BROSTROM 1979; CHEUNG et al. 1978) and the finding of protein kinases activated by calmodulin and Ca^{2+} (WOLFE and BROSTROM 1979; WAISMAN et al. 1978), it is quite possible that both cyclic AMP and Ca^{2+} have additive effects on the phosphorylation of specific proteins (Fig. 10).

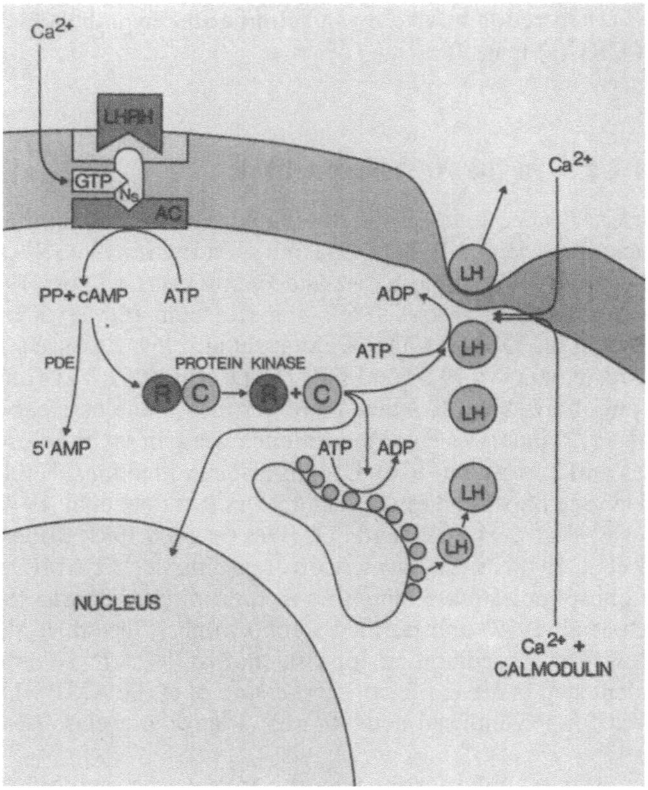

Fig. 10. Schematic representation of a proposed mode of action of hypothalamic regulatory hormones in the adenohypophyseal cell. First, binding of the neurohormone to a receptor located on the plasma membrane stimulates (LHRH, CRF or TRH) or inhibits (somatostatin, "inhibin" or dopamine), adenylate cyclase activity. Changes in intracellular cyclic AMP levels then modulate cyclic AMP-dependent protein kinase activity and lead to changes of the levels of phosphorylation of different intracellular protein substrates. Increased (under the influence of TRH, CRF or LHRH) or decreased (under the influence of somatostatin, inhibin or dopamine) cyclic AMP levels could then lead to changes in the activity of the various specialized processes of the corresponding adenohypophyseal cells. Much evidence suggests that Ca^{2+} is also involved at the receptor-adenylate cyclase step and/or in the release process

D. Adenohypophyseal Cyclic AMP-Dependent Protein Kinase and Its Substrates

The finding of a cyclic AMP-dependent protein kinase that catalyzes the phosphorylation of phosphorylase kinase (DE LANGE et al. 1968) and glycogen synthetase (SCHLENDER et al. 1969), with respective stimulation and inhibition of enzymatic activity, led to the explanation of how cyclic AMP acts on glycogen metabolism at the chemical level (see EXTON, this volume). Convincing evidence supports the hypothesis that in many systems, cyclic AMP-dependent protein kinase mediates

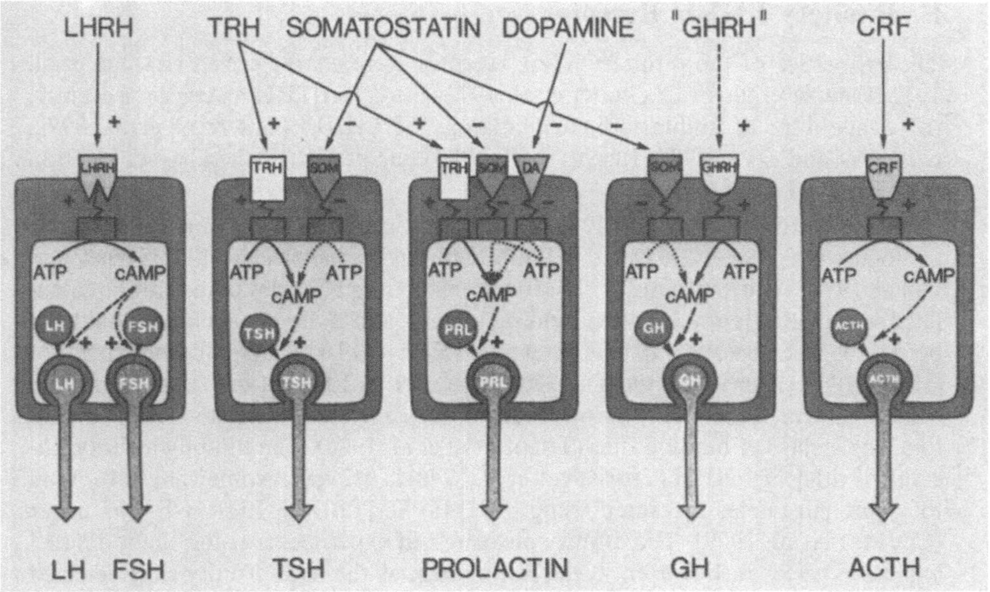

Fig. 11. Schematic representation of the interaction between stimulatory and inhibitory hypothalamic hormones in the control of anterior pituitary gland activity. Ca^{2+} is also known to play a major role in the coupling of hormone receptors with adenylate cyclase and/or release mechanisms in all pituitary cell types. The major role of peripheral hormones (sex steroids, thyroid hormones, and "inhibin") is not indicated

the intracellular effects of the cyclic nucleotide. In fact, besides the well-known effect of cyclic AMP-dependent phosphorylation of phosphorylase kinase and glycogen synthetase, there is evidence that cyclic AMP stimulates the phosphorylation of other physiologically important protein substrates.

Properties of adenohypophyseal protein kinase, including interaction of the catalytic and receptor subunits with various nucleotides including cyclic AMP and GTP, have been described in detail (LABRIE et al. 1971 a, b; LEMAIRE et al. 1971, 1974). Moreover, cyclic AMP-dependent phosphorylation of proteins from the ribosomes (BARDEN and LABRIE 1973), secretory granules (LABRIE et al. 1971 b), plasma membranes (LEMAY et al. 1974), and nuclei (JOLICOEUR and LABRIE 1964) have been described (Fig. 11). Since this information has been presented in previous reviews (LABRIE et al. 1975 a, b), it will not be discussed in this presentation. It should be mentioned that SHETERLINE and SCHOFIELD (1975) have reported the presence of cyclic AMP-dependent protein kinase associated with microtubules in bovine adenohypophysis. Moreover, BRATTIN and PORTANOVA (1981) have found that dbcAMP stimulates ^{32}P incorporation into three major proteins separated by two-dimensional gel electrophoresis in rat adenohypophysis. The time-course and dose-dependency of the effect of dbcAMP on protein phosphorylation was similar to that on hormone secretion, thus suggesting that increased phosphorylation is involved in the secretory processes.

E. Pituitary LHRH Receptor

The properties of the pituitary TRH receptor were characterized (LABRIE et al. 1972; POIRIER et al. 1972; GRANT et al. 1972) using [^{3}H]TRH as tracer. Recently, the availability of stable iodinated analogs of LHRH (CLAYTON et al. 1979; CLAYTON and CATT 1980; REEVES et al. 1980) has permitted the characterization of the LHRH receptor.

In early studies using [^{125}I]LHRH as tracer, active agonistic and antagonistic analogues of LHRH were found to inhibit binding (PEDROSA et al. 1977; HEBER and ODELL 1978; WAGNER et al. 1979). However, binding affinities could not be calculated and a correlation between binding affinity and biological activity could not be established because of the presence of two classes of binding sites for [^{125}I]LHRH (HEBER and ODELL 1978; SPONA 1973, 1975; MARSHALL et al. 1976; MARSHALL and ODELL 1975). Low levels of [^{3}H]LHRH (GRANT et al. 1973) bound to a single class of binding sites (THEOLEYRE et al. 1976). The binding affinity calculated with [^{3}H]LHRH (THEOLEYRE et al. 1976) is, however, somewhat lower than the same parameter measured using [^{125}I] [D-Ser(TBU)^6], LHRH-EA as tracer (CLAYTON et al. 1979). The affinity measured in experiments using the iodinated analog as tracer is, however, in the same range as the high affinity sites detected with [^{125}I]LHRH (MARSHALL et al. 1976; HEBER and ODELL 1978; CLAYTON et al. 1978).

In order to gain a better understanding of the action of LHRH agonists on the anterior pituitary, a large series of LHRH agonists and antagonists were used to compare the specificity of the LHRH receptor in the rat anterior pituitary gland and ovary. The LHRH agonist, [D-Ser(TBU)^6]LHRH-EA, was used as the iodinated tracer. [^{125}I] [D-Ser(TBU)^6]LHRH-EA binds to a single class of high affinity sites in both anterior pituitary and ovarian homogenates with an apparent dissociation constant of 0.2 n*M* in either tissue (REEVES et al. 1980). No specific binding was obtained in other control tissues tested. The homologous unlabeled peptide binds to the site with an apparent K_D value of 0.1 and 0.17 n*M* in the pituitary gland and the ovary, respectively. These data indicate that unlabeled and [^{125}I] [D-Ser(TBU)^6]LHRH-EA bind with similar affinities in both tissues and help to validate the use of the radioiodinated analog for binding studies of the LHRH receptor. The binding capacity was 30 and 10 fmol/mg fresh tissue for the pituitary gland and ovary, respectively.

As illustrated in Fig. 12, [D-Ser(TBU)^6]-LHRH-EA and LHRH displace [^{125}I]-[D-Ser(TBU)^6]LHRH-EA with ED_{50} values of 0.32 and 48 n*M*, respectively, in rat anterior pituitary homogenates, while LHRH-EA had an intermediate value of 7.9 n*M*. The superagonist, [D-Leu^6]LHRH-EA, has a high affinity; the weak LHRH agonists [Glu^1]LHRH and [D-Leu^2]LHRH displace the labeled tracer at high concentrations. The affinity of all the LHRH agonists for the LHRH receptor in both pituitary and ovarian tissue correlates well with their ability to stimulate LH release in rat anterior pituitary cells in primary culture (REEVES et al. 1980).

The LHRH antagonists [Des-His^2, D-Phe^6]LHRH and [D-pGlu^1, D-Phe^2, D-Trp^3, D-Phe^6]LHRH displaced the iodinated ligand from both adenohypophyseal and ovarian homogenates at concentrations lower than LHRH itself, while [D-Phe^2, D-Phe^3, D-Phe^6]LHRH, [D-His^2, D-Leu^6]LHRH and [Des-His^2, D-

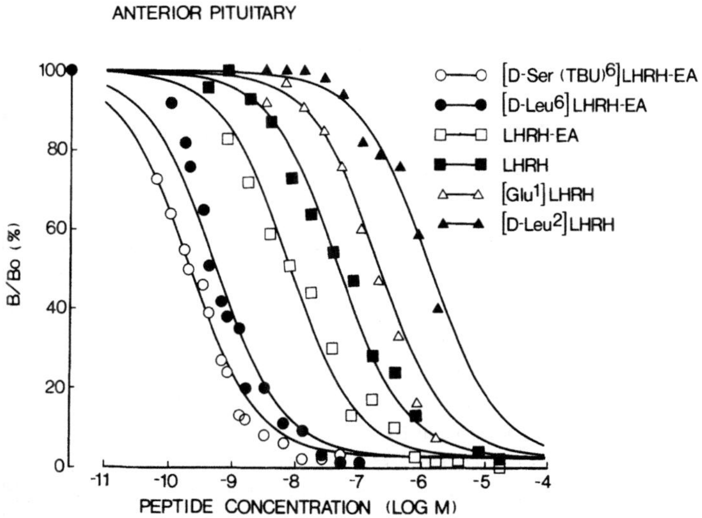

Fig. 12. Displacement of [^{125}I] [D-Ser(TBU)^6]LHRH-EA binding from rat anterior pituitary homogenate by a representative group of LHRH agonists. (REEVES et al. 1980)

Ala^6]LHRH were almost equipotent and [D-Phe^2, D-Phe^6, D-Trp^8]LHRH, [D-Phe^2, D-Phe^3, D-Phe^6, D-Leu^7]LHRH and [Des-His^2]LHRH were less potent than the natural hormone. As noticed previously for the LHRH agonists, the biological activity of all the antagonists tested corresponded well with their binding activity. The biologically inactive peptides, [D-Glu^1, desHis^2]LHRH-EA, [DesHis^2, Leu^3]LHRH-EA, H-Glu-His-OH, H-Glu-His-Trp-Ser-TyrOH, H-Glu-His-Trp-Ser-Trp-Gly-OH, H-Glu-His-Trp-Ser-Tyr-Gly-Leu-Arg-OH, [His^3]LHRH, oxytocin and somatostatin were also inactive in the receptor assay up to 10 μ*M*. The present data clearly demonstrate a close relationship between the binding activity of a large series of LHRH agonists and antagonists in the anterior pituitary gland and their biological activity as modulators of LH release from pituitary cells in culture. This information supports and extends recent findings (CLAYTON et al. 1979) obtained in these two tissues and clearly indicates that the specificity of the LHRH receptor is similar in the anterior pituitary and ovary.

The close correlation observed between the relative potency of the binding of the LHRH agonists to the LHRH receptor and their LH-releasing potency in pituitary cell cultures suggests that the affinity of the various peptides for the pituitary receptor rather than their resistance to enzymatic degradation can account for the increase of biological activity.

Although the order of potency of the various antagonists was similar in both the receptor- and bioassays, these peptides showed a 100- to 300-fold higher affinity in the receptor- than in the bioassay. This finding is analogous to the binding specificity of the dopaminergic agonist [^{3}H]-dihydroergocryptine in bovine anterior pituitary membranes (CARON et al. 1978). In that system, although dopaminergic drugs compete for [^{3}H]dihydroergocryptine binding according to the order of their known agonistic and antagonistic potencies, antagonists are relatively more potent than agonists. This finding of a relatively greater potency of LHRH antagonists than agonists to displace [^{125}I] [D-Ser-(TBU)^6]LHRH-EA may well indicate the presence of multiple LHRH binding sites.

F. Interactions Between LHRH, Sex Steroids and "Inhibin" in the Control of LH and FSH Secretion

Although the influence of the hypothalamus on the secretion of both gonadotropins is probably exerted exclusively through LHRH, it is well recognized that gonadal steroids can have a marked influence on LH and FSH secretion. The recent observation that LHRH can potentiate the LH response to subsequent injection of the neurohormone (AIYER et al. 1973; CASTRO-VASQUEZ and MCCANN 1975; FERLAND et al. 1976) illustrates the difficulty in discriminating between hypothalamic and pituitary sites of steroid action under in vivo conditions. In fact, a stimulatory effect of gonadal steroids on LHRH secretion should lead to an increased LH responsiveness to the neurohormone (in the absence of any direct effect of the steroid at the pituitary level) while the opposite situation should follow the inhibitory effect of a steroid on LHRH secretion.

As shown in Fig. 13, preincubation of male rat anterior pituitary cells for 40 h in medium containing 1×10^{-8} *M* 17β-estradiol (E_2) increased the LH responsiveness to LHRH. The LHRH concentration required to produce a half-maximal stimulation (ED_{50}) of LH release is decreased by E_2 pretreatment from 2.30 ± 0.03 to 1.20 ± 0.01 n*M* ($p < 0.01$). Preincubation with E_2 increased the basal LH release from 120 ± 8 ng LH-RP-1 per ml per 4 h to 205 ± 10 ng per ml per 4 h ($p < 0.01$). Moreover, in this and similar experiments performed with adenohypophyseal cells obtained from male and female animals (DROUIN et al. 1976a), the maximal LH response to LHRH is slightly, but not significantly increased. E_2 pretreatment increased both the basal FSH release and the maximal response of the hormone to LHRH (Fig. 13B). Similar effects have been previously obtained in anterior pituitary cells obtained from female rats (DROUIN et al. 1976a).

This stimulatory effect of E_2 at the adenohypophyseal level may well be, at least partly, responsible for the increased LH and FSH sensitivity to LHRH observed at proestrus in the rat (FERLAND et al. 1975b; GORDON and REICHLIN 1974) and during the preovulatory period in the human (NILLIUS and WIDE 1971; YEN et al. 1972).

As illustrated in Fig. 14, pretreatment of cultured anterior pituitary cells with 10^{-8} *M* testosterone led to a marked inhibition of the LH responsiveness to LHRH. The LHRH ED_{50} was increased from 1 to 3 n*M* in the presence of the androgen ($p < 0.01$). Testosterone did not affect basal LH release but slightly decreased the maximal response to the neurohormone. In contrast with the LH data, testosterone did not significantly affect the LHRH ED_{50} (1 n*M*) for FSH release. Both the spontaneous and maximal release of FSH were, however, slightly (30–40%) but consistently increased after androgen pretreatment ($p < 0.01$).

These data clearly show that androgens have not only specific but also opposite effects at the pituitary level on LH and FSH secretion. In fact, pretreatment of pituitary cells with androgens can markedly inhibit the LH response to LHRH while the effect on FSH secretion is stimulatory. Qualitatively similar results have been

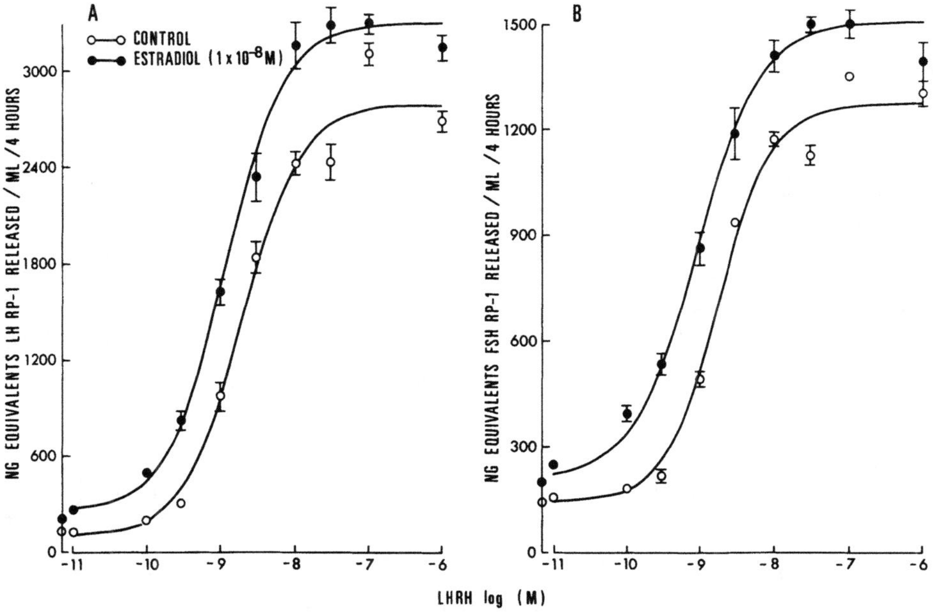

Fig. 13A and B. Effect of increasing concentrations of LHRH on LH **A** and FSH **B** release by anterior pituitary cells in primary culture preincubated for 40 h in the presence of 1×10^{-8} *M* 17*β*-estradiol (●) or control medium (○). Anterior pituitary cells were obtained from adult male rats. The response to LHRH was performed during a 4 h-period after preincubation in the presence or absence of the estrogen. The results are presented as means ±S.E.M. of data obtained from triplicate dishes

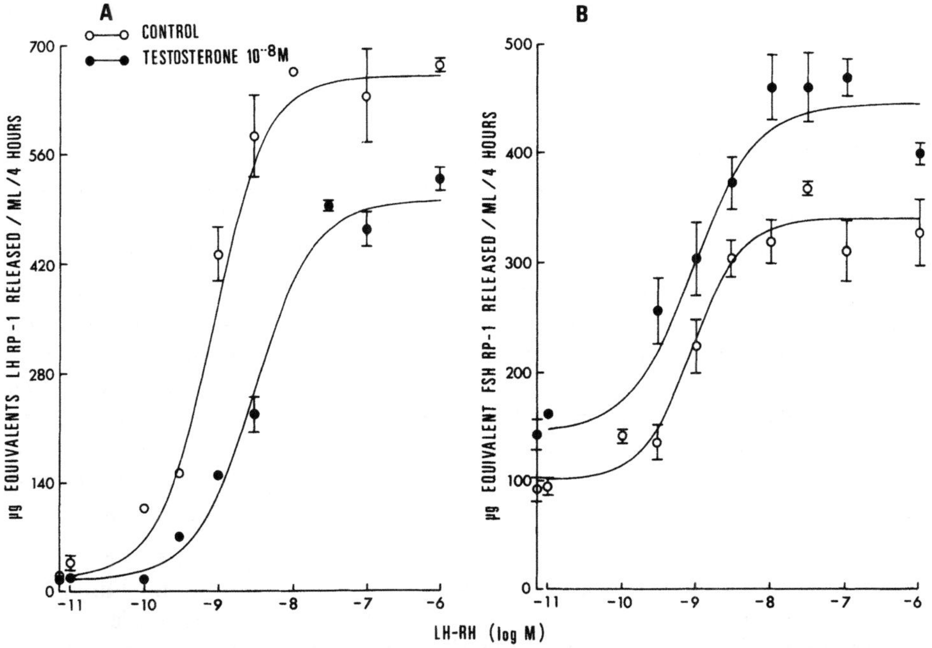

Fig. 14A and B. Effect of increasing concentrations of LHRH on LH **A** and FSH **B** release by anterior pituitary cells in primary culture preincubated for about 40 h in the presence (●) or absence (○) of 1×10^{-8} *M* testosterone. Results are expressed as means ±S.E.M. of triplicate determinations

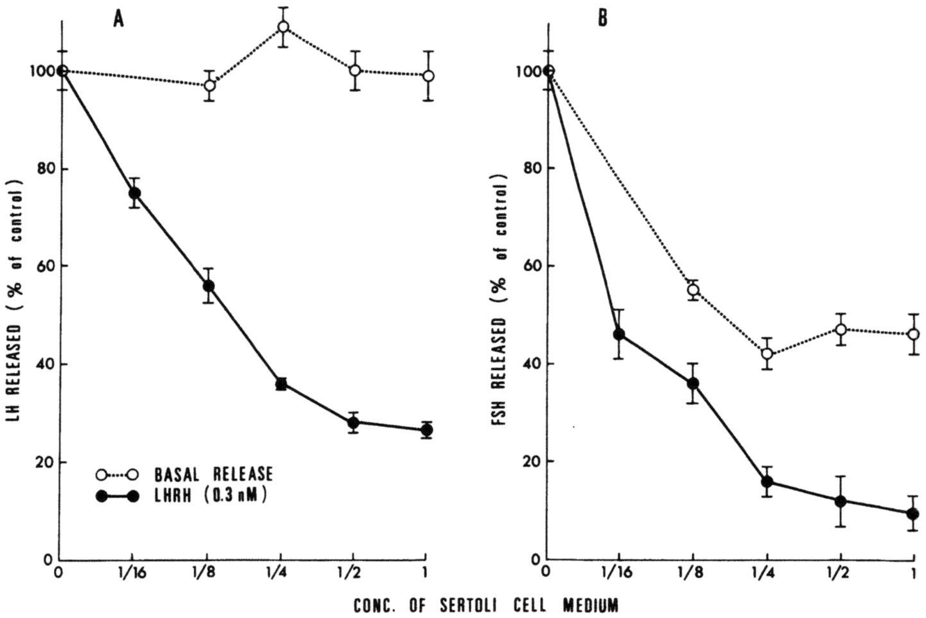

Fig. 15A and B. Effect of increasing concentrations of Sertoli cell culture medium (days 5–8 in culture, 35-day old animals, 1.5 mg protein/7.5 ml culture medium) on basal (○--○) and 0.3 n*M* LHRH-induced (●--●) LH **A** and FSH **B** release. The response to LHRH was performed during a 4 h-period after a 72 h preincubation in the presence of the indicated concentrations of Sertoli cell culture medium. The results are presented as % of control (mean ± SEM of triplicate determinations). Hormone release in control cells under basal and LHRH-induced conditions was: 25 ± 2 and 710 ± 21 (LH) and 20 ± 2 and 110 ± 5 (FSH) ng/ml, respectively

obtained when anterior pituitary cells obtained from male or female rats were used. These findings can offer an explanation for the observations in rat (SWERDLOFF et al. 1970) and man (SWERDLOFF and ODELL 1968) of a greater sensitivity of LH than FSH release to the inhibitory action of androgen administration in vivo.

The data summarized above show differential and specific effects of sex steroids on LH and FSH secretion: while estrogens stimulate both basal and LH-induced secretion of both LH and FSH, androgens and progesterone (in the presence of estrogens) inhibit LH secretion but stimulate FSH secretion. Thus, the action of the three classes of sex steroids on FSH secretion at the adenohypophyseal level appears to be exclusively stimulatory. These data provide some support to the concept, first proposed by MCCULLAGH (1932), of an inhibitory substance of testicular origin which could be involved in the specific inhibition of FSH secretion.

As illustrated in Fig. 15, incubation of female rat anterior pituitary cells for 72 h in the presence of increasing concentrations of Sertoli cell culture medium (days 5–8 in culture) led to a maximal 45% inhibition of spontaneous FSH release while basal LH release was not affected. The LHRH-induced release of both gonadotropins was inhibited by Sertoli cell culture medium. Porcine follicular fluid exerts

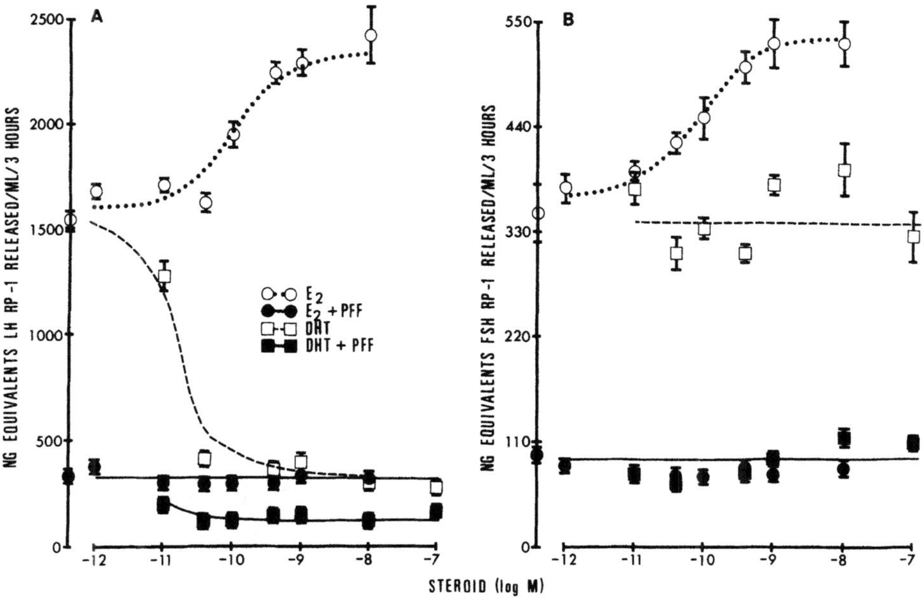

Fig. 16A and B. Effect of increasing concentrations of estradiol (E_2) (○--○) (●--●) and DHT (□--□) (■--■) in the presence (filled symbols) or absence (open symbols) of porcine follicular fluid on the LH **A** and FSH **B** responses to 0.1 n*M* LHRH. LHRH was present during a 3 h-incubation period after a 40 h-preincubation with the indicated steroids or porcine follicular fluid

similar effects on both basal and LHRH-induced gonadotropin secretion (LAGACÉ et al. 1979b).

The interaction between estrogens, dihydrotestosterone (DHT) and a constituent of porcine follicular fluid is illustrated in Fig. 16. A 48-h incubation with 17β-estradiol (10 n*M*) led to a stimulation of the LH and FSH responses to LHRH while a similar preincubation with DHT (10 n*M*) led to a marked inhibition of the LH response to LHRH. Preincubation with porcine follicular fluid led to a marked inhibition of the LHRH-induced release of both LH and FSH in the absence of steroids and completely abolished the stimulatory effect of estradiol on the secretion of the two gonadotropins. Moreover, addition of both porcine follicular fluid and DHT led to a greater inhibition of LHRH-induced LH release than that observed in the presence of porcine follicular fluid or DHT alone.

Estradiol, androgens, progesterone and substances of rat Sertoli cell culture medium and porcine follicular fluid selectively alter LH and FSH secretion by a direct action at the anterior pituitary level (Fig. 17). These findings suggest that testicular and ovarian "inhibin" could interact with sex steroids and LHRH in the differential control of LH and FSH secretion and explain the changes of ratio of LH and FSH secretion frequently observed in man (GRUMBACH et al. 1974; FRANCHIMONT et al. 1975) and experimental animals (FERLAND et al. 1976).

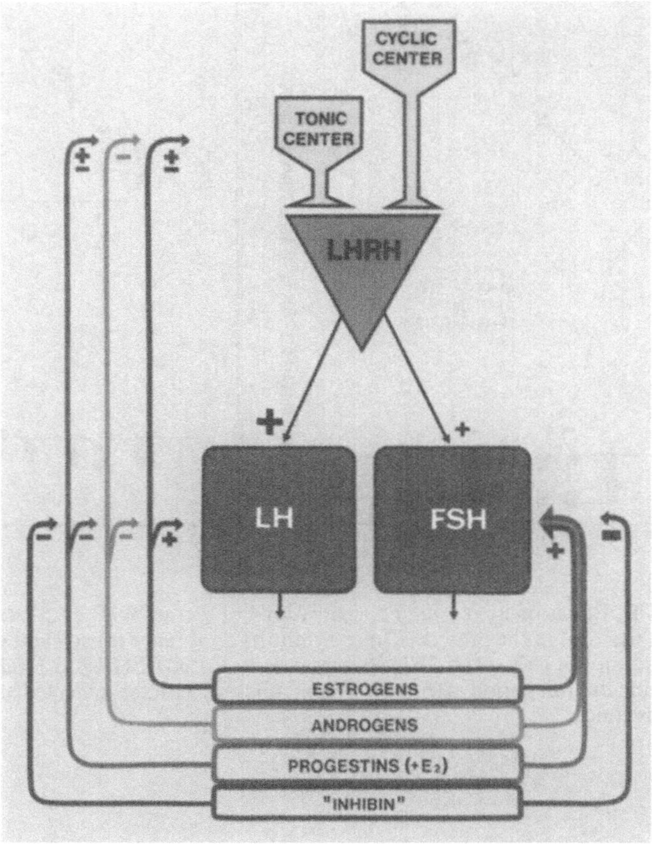

Fig. 17. Schematic representation of the interactions between LHRH, estrogens, androgens, progestins and "inhibin" in the control of LH and FSH secretion in the rat

G. Interactions Between Sex Steroids and Dopamine in the Control of Prolactin Secretion

In vivo treatment with estrogens is well known to lead to a stimulation of prolactin secretion in both man (FRANTZ et al. 1972) and rat (CHEN and MEITES 1970). At least in part, estrogens were acting at the pituitary level to enhance prolactin secretion. Recently, we have found that 17β-estradiol not only stimulates basal and TRH-induced prolactin secretion in rat anterior pituitary cells in primary culture but, somewhat surprisingly, reverses almost completely the inhibitory effect of DA agonists on prolactin release (RAYMOND et al. 1978). The present paper extends these previous findings and investigates in more detail the antidopaminergic action of estrogens and their interaction with progestins and androgens on the pituitary DA receptor controlling prolactin secretion.

The antidopaminergic action of estrogens, first observed at the anterior pituitary level (RAYMOND et al. 1978; LABRIE et al. 1978a), also occurs in the central

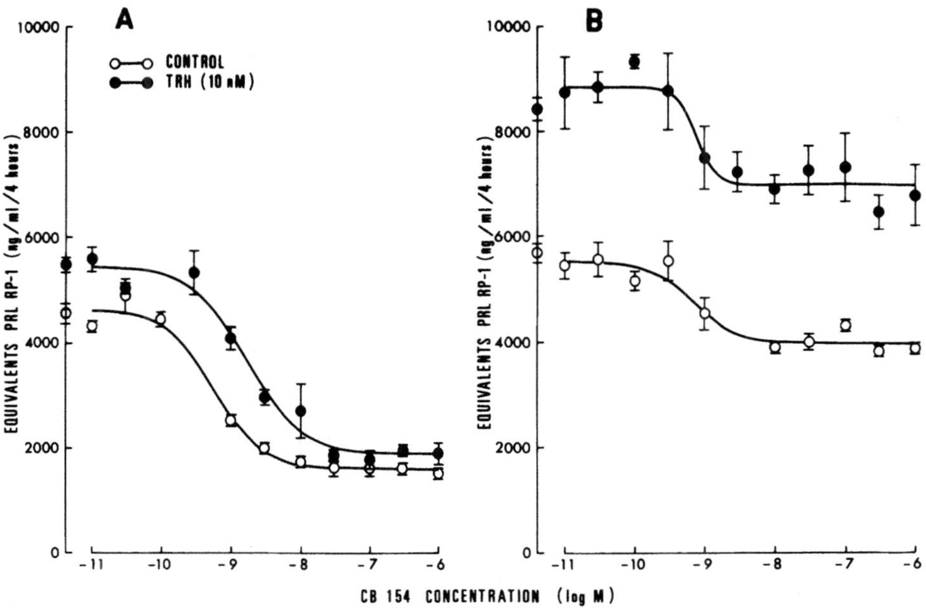

Fig. 18A and B. Effect of 17β-estradiol on the prolactin response to increasing concentrations of the DA agonist CB-154 in rat adenohypophyseal cells in culture. The cells were preincubated for 5 days in the presence **B** or absence **A** of 1 nM 17β-estradiol before a 4 h-incubation in the presence or absence of 10 nM TRH and the indicated concentrations of CB-154

nervous system. Thus, estrogen treatment decreases the circling behavior induced by apomorphine administration in rats having an unilateral lesion of the entopedoncular nucleus (Bédard et al. 1978) and inhibits the apomorphine-induced accumulation of acetylcholine in rat striatum (Euvrard et al. 1979). Moreover, clinical studies have recently shown that estrogens have a beneficial effect on L-dopa- and neuroleptic-induced dyskinesias (Bédard et al. 1977). Thus, the pituitary cell culture system may be a model for other less accessible brain dopaminergic systems.

A detailed analysis of the inhibitory effect of estrogens on the activity of the DA receptor is presented in Fig. 18. The dopaminergic ergot, CB-154, inhibited prolactin release by as much as 70% with an ED_{50} value of approximately 3 nM in both the presence and absence of 10 nM TRH in control cells. However, preincubation for 5 days with 17β-estradiol led to a small stimulation (approximately 20%) of spontaneous prolactin release while the maximal response to TRH was increased by 70%. The most dramatic effect of estrogen treatment was observed in the presence of CB-154: the 70% inhibition of prolactin release induced by the DA agonist in control cells was reduced to 20% in 17β-estradiol-treated cells.

Since progestins and androgens are well known to exert antiestrogenic activity at the uterine level, we next studied the possibility of a similar effect on prolactin secretion in rat anterior pituitary cells in culture. As illustrated in Fig. 19, while preincubation for 10 days with 10 nM progesterone alone had no effect on prolactin release, the stimulatory effect of 17β-estradiol was 40–50% reversed by the

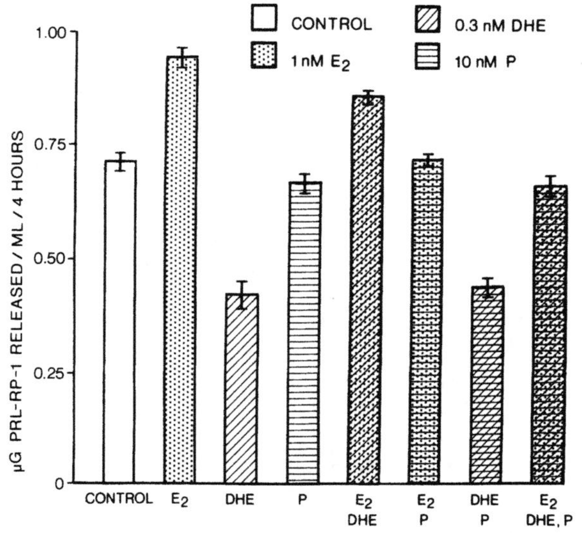

Fig. 19. Effect of preincubation for 10 days with 17β-estradiol (E_2, 1 n*M*) or progesterone (P, 10 n*M*) alone or in combination on spontaneous prolactin release in the presence or absence of dihydroergocornine (DHE, 0.3 n*M*). Prolactin release was measured during a 4 h-incubation

progestin in both the presence and absence of the dopamine agonist dihydroergocornine. We could also find that 5α-dihydrotestosterone exerted antiestrogenic effects almost superimposable to those observed with progesterone (data not shown).

Following our in vitro data showing a potent antidopaminergic effect of estrogens on prolactin secretion, it then became of interest to investigate if such a potent activity of estrogens occurs under in vivo conditions. The present study was facilitated by our recent findings that the endogenous inhibitory dopaminergic influence on prolactin secretion can be eliminated by administration of opiates, thus making possible study of the effect of exogenous dopaminergic agents without interference by endogenous dopamine.

The subcutaneous administration of 100 μg or 400 μg of dopamine completely prevented the increase of plasma prolactin levels following morphine injection in rats ovariectomized two weeks previously (FERLAND et al. 1979). Treatment with estradiol benzoate (20 μg/day) for seven days led to a stimulation of basal plasma prolactin levels from 14 ± 1 to 56 ± 8 ng/ml and to a marked increase of the maximal plasma prolactin response to morphine from 215 ± 60 to 2175 ± 390 ng/ml plasma. The most interesting finding was however that the 100 μg and 400 μg doses of dopamine which could maintain plasma prolactin levels at undetectable levels after morphine injection in control rats led only to 40 and 85% inhibition of prolactin levels, respectively, in animals treated with estrogens.

These studies clearly demonstrate that estrogens have potent antidopaminergic activity on prolactin secretion, not only in anterior pituitary cells in culture but also in vivo, the effect being qualitatively similar in both female and male animals. As reflected by an increase of the ED_{50} value of dopamine agonists, the in vitro effect of estrogens was due to a decreased sensitivity of prolactin release to dopamine action at the anterior pituitary level. Such findings indicate that higher concentrations of dopamine in the hypothalamo-hypophyseal portal blood system are likely to be required to inhibit prolactin secretion under conditions of high estrogenic influence. The almost complete reversal of the inhibitory effect of low doses of dopamine by estrogen treatment clearly indicates an important interaction between sex steroids and dopamine agonists at the adenohypophyseal level.

H. Alpha-Adrenergic Control of ACTH and Beta-Endorphin Secretion

Most of the substances known to modulate ACTH secretion at the pituitary level (YATES and MARAN 1974; VALE and RIVIER 1977; SCHALLY et al. 1978) have recently been found to exert a parallel effect on the release of both ACTH and β-endorphin (β-LPH_{61-91}) immunoreactive material in rat anterior pituitary cells in culture (RAYMOND et al. 1979). These findings are well supported by the earlier demonstration of a common precursor for ACTH and β-LPH and other related peptides by MAINS et al. (1977) and ROBERTS and HERBERT (1977) and by the finding that ACTH, β-melanotropin (β-MSH, β-LPH_{41-58}) and β-LPH are contained not only in the same cells of the pituitary (MORIARTY 1973; DUBOIS et al. 1973; PHIFER et al. 1974) but also in the same secretory granules (PELLETIER et al. 1977).

At high concentrations, the catecholamine norepinephrine has been shown to stimulate the release of ACTH and β-endorphin immunoreactive material, this effect being reversed by the α-adrenergic antagonist, phentolamine (VALE et al. 1978; VALE and RIVIER 1977). Following our preliminary findings of up to a 10-fold stimulation of ACTH release by norepinephrine and epinephrine and the possible physiological importance of this α-adrenergic mechanism in the control of ACTH secretion, we have studied in more detail the characteristics of the stimulatory effect of α-adrenergic agents on ACTH, β-endorphin + β-LPH and α-MSH secretion in rat anterior pituitary cells in culture (GIGUERE et al. 1981).

As illustrated in Fig. 20A, maximal concentrations of (−)epinephrine and (−)norepinephrine lead to a 8- to 10-fold stimulation of ACTH release at ED_{50} values of 20 and 50 n*M*, respectively while dopamine is not active below 1 μ*M*. The α-adrenergic agonist, phenylephrine, stimulates ACTH release at an ED_{50} value of 200 n*M* while the β-adrenergic agonist isoproterenol is not active below 1 μ*M* (Fig. 20B). In various experiments, the following order of potency of a series of catecholaminergic agents was found: (−)epinephrine (20 n*M*) > (−)norepinephrine (50 n*M*) > phenylephrine (200 n*M*) > isoproterenol (6,000 n*M*) while dopamine had only a slight stimulatory effect at 10 μ*M*. A similar potency of all these agents was found on ACTH, β-endorphin + β-LPH and α-MSH secretion.

Specificity of the α-adrenergic stimulation of ACTH release was next studied with a series of catecholamine antagonists. The highly α_1-selective antagonist, prazosin (HOFFMAN et al. 1979) which is 10,000-fold more potent on α_1- than α_2-receptors, inhibits both (−)epinephrine and phenylephrine-induced ACTH release at low ED_{50} values of 0.06 and 0.2 n*M*, respectively. The α_2-antagonist yohimbine exerts a similar effect at much higher concentrations [ED_{50} values = approximately 100 n*M* for phenylephrine (100 n*M*) and 250 n*M* for (−)epinephrine (100 n*M*)].

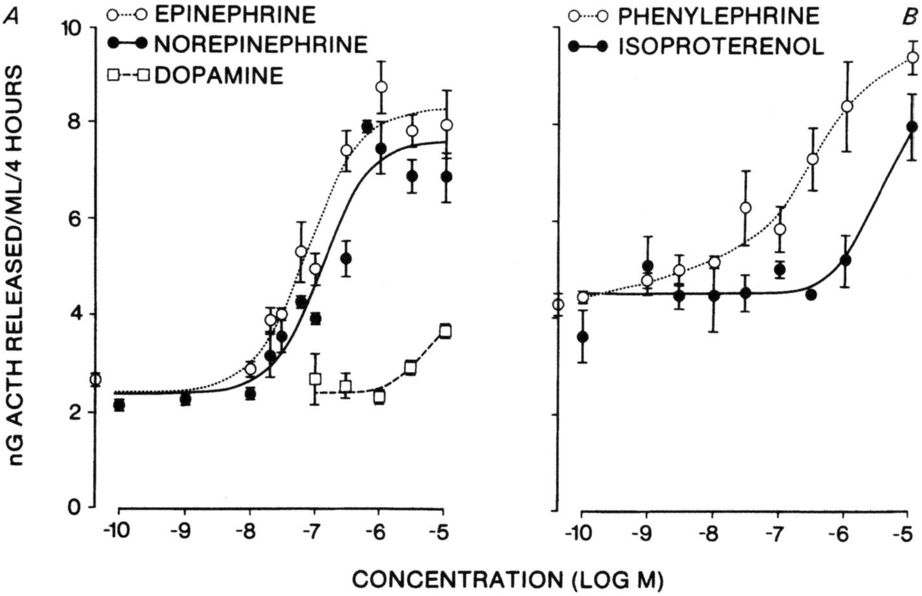

Fig. 20A and B. Effects of increasing concentrations of (−) epinephrine, (−)norepinephrine and dopamine **A** as well as phenylephrine and isoproterenol **B** on ACTH release in rat anterior pituitary cells in culture. Five days after plating, cells were incubated for 4 h in the presence of the indicated concentrations of catecholamines

When the concentrations and potencies of phenylephrine and epinephrine are taken into account, the K_D values of prazosin and yohimbine are 0.1 and 100 n*M*, respectively. WB-4101, an α-antagonist, is also a potent inhibitor of (−)epinephrine-induced ACTH release at a K_D value of 1 n*M*.

The above-mentioned study clearly demonstrates that α-adrenergic agents exert a potent and coordinate stimulatory effect on the secretion of ACTH, β-endorphin and α-MSH by a direct action at the anterior pituitary level. The stereospecificity and the order of potency of the catecholaminergic agonists in stimulating ACTH, α-MSH, and β-endorphin + β-LPH secretion and the specificity of the interaction of antagonists with this process are consistent with the characteristics of an α-adrenergic mechanism. In agreement with other tissues where an α-adrenergic receptor has been studied in correlation with a physiological response (STRITTMATTER et al. 1977a, b; WILLIAMS et al. 1978), the stereospecificity is illustrated by the greater potency of the (−) isomers of epinephrine and norepinephrine and by the following order of potency: epinephrine > norepinephrine > phenylephrine > isoproterenol.

The present data show that the concentration at which epinephrine and norepinephrine stimulate the release of ACTH and other related peptides directly at the pituitary level as measured by ED_{50} values is in the same order of potency as the ID_{50} value of dopamine (35 n*M*) for inhibition of prolactin release measured under similar conditions in anterior pituitary cells in culture (CARON et al. 1978) or ever lower than the ED_{50} values of the natural catecholamines for the stimulation of α- and β-adrenergic mechanisms in smooth muscle contraction (LEFKOWITZ and

WILLIAMS 1976; WILLIAMS et al. 1978) or for catecholamine-stimulated K^+ efflux (STRITTMATTER et al. 1977a) and adenylate cyclase activation (LEVITZKI et al. 1974; MUKHERJEE et al. 1975; BROWN et al. 1976).

These data are also in agreement with those of VALE et al. (1978) who have described parallel changes of ACTH and β-endorphin release in the same cell culture system under the influence of various secretory modulators. They add moreover that a typically α-adrenergic mechanism is stimulating the secretory process in pituitary corticotrophs at concentrations of physiological significance. In analogy with dopamine controlling prolactin secretion (MACLEOD and LEHMEYER 1974; LABRIE et al. 1978a), it is tempting to suggest that norepinephrine or epinephrine of central and/or peripheral origin is (are) involved in the regulation of ACTH secretion. It would be surprising to find that such a functional and highly specific α-adrenergic receptor is not involved in the physiological control of secretion of ACTH and its related peptides.

References

Adams TE, Nett TM (1979) Interaction of GnRH with anterior pituitary. III. Role of divalent cations, microtubules and microfilaments in the GnRH activated gonadotroph. Biol Reprod 21:1073–1086

Adams TE, Wagner TOF, Sawyer HR, Nett TM (1979) GnRH interaction with anterior pituitary. II. Cyclic AMP as an intracellular mediator in the GnRH activated gonadotroph. Biol Reprod 21:735–747

Aiyer BS, Chiappa SA, Fink G, Greig FJ (1973) A priming effect of luteinizing hormone releasing factor on the anterior pituitary gland in the female rat. J Physiol (Lond) 234:81P–82P

Baker HWG, Bremner WJ, Burger HG et al. (1976) Recent Prog Horm Res 32:429–476

Barden N, Labrie F (1973) Cyclic adenosine 3′,5′-monophosphate-dependent phosphorylation of ribosomal proteins from bovine anterior pituitary gland. Biochemistry 12:3096–3102

Barden N, Bergeron L, Betteridge A (1976) Effects of prostaglandin synthetase inhibitors and prostaglandin precursors on anterior pituitary cyclic AMP and hormone secretion. In: Samuelson B and Paoletti R (eds) Advances in Prostaglandin Thromboxane Res. Raven Press NY, p 341

Barnes GD, Brown BL, Gard TG, Atkinson D, Ekins RP (1978) Effect of TRH and dopamine on cyclic AMP levels in enriched mammotroph and thyrotroph cells. Mol Cell Endocrinol 12:273–275

Baumann R, Kuhl H (1980) Effect of LHRH and of a highly potent LHRH analog upon pituitary adenyl cyclase activity. Horm Metab Res 12:128–130

Beaulieu M, Labrie F, Coy DH, Coy EJ, Schally AV (1975) Parallel inhibition of LHRH-induced cyclic AMP accumulation and LH and FSH release by LHRH antagonists in vitro. J Cyclic Nucleotide Res 1:243–250

Bédard P, Langelier P, Villeneuve A (1977) Estrogens and the extra-pyramidal system. Lancet 1:1367

Bédard P, Dankova J, Boucher R, Langelier P (1978) Effect of estrogens on apomorphine-induced circling behavior in the rat. Can J Physiol Pharmacol 56:538–541

Bélanger A, Labrie F, Borgeat P et al. (1974) Inhibition of growth hormone and thyrotropin release by growth hormone-release inhibiting hormone. J Mol Cell Endocrinol 1:329–339

Ben-Jonathan N, Oliver C, Weiner HJ, Mical RS, Porter JC (1977) Dopamine in hypophyseal portal plasma of the rat during the estrous cycle and throughout pregnancy. Endocrinology 100:452–458

Bergeron L, Barden N (1975) Stimulation of cyclic AMP accumulation by arachidonic and 8,11,14-eicosatrienoic acids in rat anterior pituitary gland. Mol Cell Endocrinol 2:253–260

Betteridge A, Wallis M (1977) Role of prostaglandins and adenosine 3′,5′-cyclic monophosphate in the control by insulin of growth hormone synthesis in vitro. Biochem Soc Trans 5:224–226
Betteridge A, Wallis M (1978) Stimulation of anterior pituitary prostaglandin E content and somatotropin (growth hormone) synthesis by phospholipase A. Biochem J 176:319–323
Betteridge A, Wallis M (1979) Involvement of prostaglandins in the inhibition of growth hormone production in cultured pituitary cells by insulin. J Endocrinol 80:239–248
Bicknell RJ, Schofield JG (1976) Mechanism of action of somatostatin: inhibition of ionophore A 23187-induced release of growth hormone from dispersed bovine pituitary cells. FEBS Lett 68:23–26
Boler J, Enzman F, Folkers K, Bowers CY, Schally AV (1969) The identity of chemical and hormonal properties of the thyrotropin-releasing hormone and pyroglutamyl-histidyl-proline amide. Biochem Biophys Res Commun 37:705–710
Borgeat P, Chavancy G, Dupont A, Labrie F, Arimura A, Schally AV (1972) Stimulation of adenosine 3′,5′-cyclic monophosphate accumulation in anterior pituitary gland in vitro by synthetic luteinizing hormone-releasing hormone/follicle-stimulating hormone (LHRH/FSH-RH). Proc Natl Acad Sci USA 69:2677–2681
Borgeat P, Labrie F, Poirier G, Chavancy G, Schally AV (1973) Stimulation of adenosine 3′,5′-cyclic monophosphate accumulation in anterior pituitary gland by purified growth hormone-releasing hormone. Trans Assoc Am Physicians 86:284–299
Borgeat P, Labrie F, Côté J et al. (1974a) Parallel stimulation of cyclic AMP accumulation and LH and FSH release by analogs of LHRH in vitro. J Mol Cell Endocrinol 1:7–20
Borgeat P, Labrie F, Drouin J et al. (1974b) Inhibition of adenosine 3′,5′-monophosphate accumulation in anterior pituitary gland in vitro by growth hormone release-inhibiting hormone. Biochem Biophys Res Commun 56:1052–1059
Borgeat P, Garneau P, Labrie F (1975a) Calcium requirement for stimulation of cyclic AMP accumulation in anterior pituitary by LHRH. Mol Cell Endocrinol 2:117–124
Borgeat P, Labrie F, Garneau P (1975b) Characteristics of action of prostaglandins on cyclic AMP accumulation in rat anterior pituitary gland. Can J Biochem 53:455–460
Bowers CY (1971) The role of cyclic AMP in the release of anterior pituitary hormones. Ann NY Acad Sci 185:263–290
Brattin WJ Jr, Portanova R (1981) Dibutyryl cyclic AMP-induced phosphorylation of specific proteins in adenohypophysial cells. Mol Cell Endocrinol 23:77–90
Brazeau P, Vale W, Burgus R, Ling N, Butcher M, Rivier J, Guillemin R (1973) Hypothalamic polypeptide that inhibits the secretion of immunoreactive growth hormone. Science 179:77–79
Brown MR, Hedge GA (1974) In vivo effects of prostaglandins on TRH-induced TSH secretion. Endocrinology 95:1392–1397
Brown GM, Seeman P, Lee T (1976) Dopamine neuroleptics receptors in basal hypothalamus and pituitary. Endocrinology 99:1407–1410
Burgus R, Dunn TF, Desiderio D, Guillemin R (1969) Structure moléculaire du facteur hypothalamique TRF d'origine ovine: mise en évidence par spectrométrie de masse de la séquence PCP-His-Pro, NH_2. CR Acad Sci [D] (Paris) 269:1870–1873
Burgus R, Butcher M, Ling N et al. (1971) Structure moléculaire du facteur hypothalamique (LRF) d'origine ovine contrôlant la sécrétion de l'hormone gonadotrope hypophysaire. CR Acad Sci [D] (Paris) 273:1611–1613
Calabro MA, MacLeod RM (1978) Binding of dopamine to bovine anterior pituitary gland membranes. Neuroendocrinology 25:32–46
Caron MG, Beaulieu M, Raymond V, Gagné B, Drouin J, Lefkowitz RJ, Labrie F (1978) Dopaminergic receptors in the anterior pituitary gland. Correlation of [^{3}H]dihydroergocryptine binding with the dopaminergic control of prolactin release. J Biol Chem 254:2244–2253
Castro-Vasquez A, McCann SM (1975) Cyclic variations in the increased responsiveness of the pituitary to luteinizing hormone releasing hormone (LHRH) indicated by LHRH. Endocrinology 97:13–19
Cehovic G (1969) Role de l'adénosine 3′,5′-monophosphate cyclique dans la libération de TSH hypophysaire. CR Acad Sci [D] (Paris) 268:2929–2931

Cehovic G, Lewis UJ, Vander Laan WP (1970) Etude de l'action adénosine 3',5'-monophosphate cyclique sue la libération de l'hormone de croissance et de la prolactine in vitro. CR Acad Sci [D] (Paris) 270:3119–3122

Chen L, Meites J (1970) Effects of estrogen and progesterone on serum and pituitary prolactin levels in ovariectomized rats. J Endocrinol 86:503–505

Cheung WY, Lynch TJ, Wallace RW (1978) An endogenous Ca^{2+}-dependent activator protein of brain adenylate cyclase and cyclic nucleotide phosphodiesterase. Adv Cyclic Nucleotide Res 9:233–251

Chobsieng P, Naor Z, Koch Y, Zor U, Lindner HR (1975) Stimulatory effect of prostaglandin E_2 on LH release in the rat: evidence for hypothalamic site of action. Neuroendocrinology 17:12–17

Clayton RN, Catt KJ (1980) Receptor binding affinity of gonadotropin-releasing hormone analogs: analysis by radioligand-receptor assay. Endocrinology 106:1154–1159

Clayton RN, Shakespear RA, Marshall JC (1978) LHRH binding to purified pituitary plasma membranes: absence of adenylate cyclase activation. Mol Cell Endocrinol 11:63–78

Clayton EN, Shakespear RA, Duncan JA, Marshall JC (1979) Radioiodinated nondegradable gonadotropin-releasing hormone analogs: new probes for the investigation of pituitary gonadotropin-releasing hormone receptors. Endocrinology 105:1369–1381

Conn PM, Morrell DV, Dufau ML, Catt KJ (1979) Gonadotropin-releasing action in cultured pituicytes: independence of luteinizing hormone release and adenosine 3',5'-monophosphate production. Endocrinology 104:448–453

Cooper RH, McPherson M, Schofield JG (1972) The effect of prostaglandins on pituitary content of adenosine 3',5'-cyclic monophosphate and the release of growth hormone. Biochem J 127:143–154

De Camilli P, Macconi D, Spada A (1979) Dopamine inhibits adenylate cyclase in human prolactin-secreting pituitary adenomas. Nature 278:252–254

De Lange RJ, Kamp RG, Riley WD, Cooper WD, Krebs RG (1968) Activation of skeletal muscle phosphorylase kinase by adenosine 3',5'-monophosphate. J Biol Chem 243:2200–2208

Deery DJ, Howell SL (1973) Rat anterior pituitary adenyl cyclase activity. GTP requirement of prostaglandin E_1 and E_2 and synthetic luteinizing hormone-releasing hormone activation. Biochim Biophys Acta 329:17–22

Deery DJ, Jones AC (1975) Effects of hypothalamic extracts, neurotransmitters and synthetic hypothalamic releasing hormones on adenylyl cyclase activity in the lobes of the pituitary of the dogfish (Scylrorhinus canicula L.). J Endocrinol 64:49–57

De Wied D, Witter A, Versteeg DHG, Mulder AH (1969) Release of ACTH by substances of central nervous system origin. Endocrinology 85:561–569

Drouin J, Labrie F (1976a) Selective effect of androgens on LH and FSH release in anterior pituitary cells in culture. Endocrinology 98:1528–1524

Drouin J, Labrie F (1976b) Specificity of the stimulatory effect of prostaglandins on hormone release in anterior pituitary cells in culture. Prostaglandins 11:355–366

Drouin J, Lagacé L, Labrie F (1976a) Estradiol-induced increase of the LH responsiveness to LHRH in anterior pituitary cells in culture. Endocrinology 99:1477–1481

Drouin J, De Léan A, Rainville R, Lachance R, Labrie F (1976b) Characteristics of the interaction between TRH and somatostatin for thyrotropin and prolactin release. Endocrinology 98:514–521

Drouin J, Ferland L, Bernard J, Labrie F (1976c) Site of the in vivo stimulatory effect of prostaglandins on LH release. Prostaglandins 11:367–376

Drouin J, Lavoie M, Labrie F (1978) Effect of gonadal steroids on the LH and FSH response to 8-Br cyclic AMP in anterior pituitary cells in culture. Endocrinology 102:358–361

Dubois P, Varques-Regairas H, Dubois MP (1973) Human foetal anterior pituitary immunofluorescent evidence for corticotropin and melanotropin activities. Z Zellforsch Mikrosk Anat 145:131–143

Dufau ML, Horner KA, Yayashi K, Tsuruhara T, Conn PM, Catt KJ (1978) Actions of choleragen and gonatropin in isolated Leydig cells. Functional compartimentalization of the hormone-activated cyclic AMP response. J Biol Chem 253:3721–3729

Eto S, Fleischer N (1976) Regulation of thyrotropin (TSH) release and production in monolayer cultures of transplantable TSH-producing mouse tumors. Endocrinology 98:114–122

Euvrard C, Labrie F, Boissier JR (1979) Antagonism between estrogens and dopamine in the rat striatum. In: Usdin E (ed) Catecholamines: basic and clinical frontiers. Pergamon, Oxford New York, p 1263

Ferland L, Labrie F, Coy DH, Coy EJ, Schally AV (1975a) Inhibitory activity of four analogs of luteinizing hormone-releasing hormone in vivo. Fertil Steril 26:889–893

Ferland L, Borgeat P, Labrie F, Bernard J, De Léan A, Raynaud JP (1975b) Changes in pituitary sensitivity to LHRH during the estrous cycle. Mol Cell Endocrinol 2:107–115

Ferland L, Drouin J, Labrie F (1976) Role of sex steroids on LH and FSH secretion in the rat. In: Labrie F, Meites J, Pelletier G (eds) Hypothalamus and endocrine functions. Plenum, Oxford New York, p 191

Ferland L, Labrie F, Euvrard C, Raynaud JP (1979) Antidopaminergic activity of estrogens on prolactin release at the pituitary level in vivo. Mol Cell Endocrinol 14:199–204

Fleischer H, Donald RA, Butcher RW (1969) Involvement of adenosine 3′,5′-monophosphate in release of ACTH. Am J Physiol 5:1287–1291

Franchimont P (1972) Human gonadotropin secretion. J R Coll Physicians Lond 6:283–295

Franchimont P, Chari S, Demoulin A (1975) Hypothalamus-pituitary-testis interaction. J Reprod Fertil 44:335–350

Franchimont P, Verstraelen-Proyard J, Hazee-Hagelstein MT, Renard CH, Demoulin A, Bourguignon JP, Hustin J (1979) Inhibin. From concept to reality. Vitam 37:243–302

Frantz AG, Kleinberg DL, Noel GL (1972) Studies on prolactin in man, Recent Prog Horm Res 28:527–590

Gautvick KM, Tashjian AH Jr (1973) Effects of cations and colchicine on the release of prolactin and growth hormone by functional pituitary cells in culture. Endocrinology 93:793–799

Gershengorn MC, Rebecchi MJ, Geras E, Arevalo CO (1980) Thyrotropin-releasing hormone (TRH) action in mouse thyrotropic tumor cells in culture: evidence against a role for adenosine 3′,5′-monophosphate as a mediator of TRH-stimulated thyrotropin release. Endocrinology 107:665–670

Giguere V, Cote J, Labrie F (1981) Characteristics of the α-adrenergic stimulation of adrenocorticotropin secretion in rat anterior pituitary cells. Endocrinology 109:757–762

Godbout M, Labrie F (1982) Inhibitory effects of porcine follicular fluid "inhibin" on pituitary cyclic AMP levels. Mol Cell Endocrinol, in press

Goodyer CG, St George Hall C, Guyda H, Robert F, Giroud CJP (1977) Human fetal pituitary in culture: hormone secretion and response to somatostatin, luteinizing hormone releasing factor, thyrotropin-releasing factor and dibutyryl cyclic AMP. J Clin Endocrinol Metab 45:73–85

Gordon JH, Reichlin S (1974) Changes in pituitary responsiveness to luteinizing hormone-releasing factor during the estrous cycle. Endocrinology 94:974–978

Grant G, Vale W, Guillemin R (1972) Interaction of thyrotropin releasing factors with membrane receptors of pituitary cells. Biochem Biophys Res Commun 46:28–30

Grant G, Vale W, Rivier J (1973) Pituitary binding sites for [^{3}H]labelled luteinizing hormone-releasing factor (LRF). Biochem Biophys Res Commun 50:771–778

Grumbach M, Roth JC, Kaplan SL, Kelch P (1974) Hypothalamic-pituitary regulation of puberty: evidence and concepts derived from clinical research, In: Grumbach G, Grave G, Mayer FE (eds) The Control of the onset of puberty. John Wiley and Sons, New York Chichester, p 115

Harms PG, Ojeda SR, McCann SM (1973) Prostaglandin involvement in hypothalamic control of gonadotropin and prolactin release. Science 181:760–761

Harms PG, Ojeda SR, McCann SM (1974) Prostaglandin-induced release of pituitary gonadotropins: central nervous system and pituitary sites of action. Endocrinology 94:1459–1464

Heber D, Odell WD (1978) Pituitary receptor binding activity of active, inactive, superactive and inhibitory analogs of gonadotropin-releasing hormone. Biochem Biophys Res Commun 82:67–73

Hedge GA (1972) The effects of prostaglandins on ACTH secretion. Endocrinology 91:925–933
Hertelendy F (1971) Studies on growth hormone secretion. II. Stimulation by prostaglandins in vitro. Acta Endocrinol (Copenh) 68:355–362
Hertelendy P, Peake GT, Todd H (1971) Studies on growth hormone secretion: inhibition of prostaglandin, theophylline and cyclic AMP stimulated growth hormone release by valinomycin in vitro. Biochem Biophys Res Commun 44:253–260
Hertelendy F, Todd H, Ehrhart K, Blute R (1972) Studies on growth hormone secretion. IV. In vivo effects of prostaglandin E_1. Prostaglandins 2:79–91
Hertelendy F, Todd H, Marconis RJ Jr (1978) Studies on growth hormone secretion. IX. Prostaglandins do not act like ionophores. Prostaglandins 15:575–581
Hoffman BB, De Léan A, Wood CL, Schocken DO, Lefkowitz RJ (1979) Alpha-adrenergic receptor subtypes: quantitative assessment by ligand binding. Life Sci 24:1739–1746
Jakobs KH (1979) Inhibition of adenylate cyclase by hormones and neurotransmitters. Mol Cell Endocrinol 16:147–156
Jolicoeur P, Labrie F (1974) Phosphorylation of nuclear proteins from bovine anterior pituitary gland induced by adenosine 3′,5′-monophosphate. Eur J Biochem 48:1–9
Jutisz M, Paloma de la Llosa M (1970) Requirement of Ca^{++} and Mg^{++} ions for the in vitro release of follicle-stimulating hormone from rat pituitary gland and its subsequent biosynthesis. Endocrinology 86:761–768
Kaneko T, Saito S, Oka H, Oda T, Yanaihara N (1973) Effects of synthetic LHRH and its analogs on rat anterior pituitary cyclic AMP and LH and FSH release. Metabolism 22:77–78
Kato Y, Dupré J, Beck JC (1973) Plasma growth hormone in the anesthetized rat: effects of dibutyryl cyclic AMP, prostaglandin E, adrenergic agents, vasopressin, chlorpromazine, amphetamine and L-Dopa. Endocrinology 93:135–146
Kawakami M, Kimura F (1980) Stimulation of guanosine 3′,5′-monophosphate accumulation in anterior pituitary glands in vivo by synthetic luteinizing hormone-releasing hormone. Endocrinology 106:626–630
Kebabian JW (1973) Biochemical regulation and physiological significance of cyclic nucleotides in the nervous system, Cyclic Nucleotide Res 8:421
Kebabian JW, Calne DB (1979) Multiple receptors for dopamine. Nature 277:93–96
Kebabian JW, Petzold GL, Greengard P (1977) Dopamine sensitive adenylate cyclase in caudate nucleus of rat brain and its similarity to the dopamine receptor. Proc Natl Acad Sci USA 69:2145–2149
Kraicer J, Milligan JV, Gosbee JL, Conrad RG, Branson CM (1969) In vitro release of ACTH: effects of potassium, calcium and corticosterone. Endocrinology 85:1144–1153
Kunze H (1970) Formation of [I-14C]prostaglandin E_2 and two prostaglandins metabolites from [I-14C] arachidonic acid during vascular perfusion of the frog intestine. Biochim Biophys Acta 202:180–183
Labrie F, Béraud G, Gauthier M, Lemay A (1971 a) Actinomycin-insensitive stimulation of protein synthesis in rat anterior pituitary in vitro by dibutyryl adenosine 3′,5′-monophosphate. J Biol Chem 246:1902–1908
Labrie F, Lemaire S, Courte C (1971 b) Adenosine 3′,5′-monophosphate-dependent protein kinase from bovine anterior pituitary gland. I. Properties. J Biol Chem 246:7293–7302
Labrie F, Barden N, Poirier G, De Léan A (1972) Characteristics of binding of [^{3}H]thyrotropin-releasing hormone to plasma membranes of bovine anterior pituitary gland. Proc Natl Acad Sci USA 69:283–287
Labrie F, Pelletier G, Lemay A et al. (1973 a) Control of protein synthesis in anterior pituitary gland. Karolinska Symp Res Methods Reprod Endocrinol: 301
Labrie F, Gauthier M, Pelletier G, Borgeat P, Lemay A, Gouge JJ (1973 b) Role of microtubules in basal and stimulated release of growth hormone and prolactin in rat adenohypophysis in vitro. Endocrinology 93:903–914
Labrie F, Pelletier G, Borgeat P, Drouin J, Savary M, Côté J, Ferland L (1975 a) Aspects of the mechanism of action of hypothalamic hormone (LHRH), In: Thomas JA, Singhal RL (eds) Gonadotropins and gonadal functions, vol 1. University Park Press, Baltimore, p 77

Labrie F, Borgeat P, Lemay A et al. (1975b) Role of cyclic AMP in the action of hypothalamic regulatory hormones. Adv Cyclic Nucleotide Res 5:787

Labrie F, De Léan A, Drouin J et al. (1976a) New aspects of the mechanism of action of hypothalamic regulatory hormones. In: Labrie F, Meites J, Pelletier G (eds) Hypothalamus and endocrine functions. Raven, New York, p 147

Labrie F, Pelletier G, Borgeat P, Drouin J, Ferland L, Bélanger A (1976b) Mode of action of hypothalamic regulatory hormones. Neuroendocrinol 4:63

Labrie F, Savary M, Coy DH, Coy EJ, Schally AV (1976c) Inhibition of LH release by analogs of LH-releasing hormone (LHRH) in vitro. Endocrinology 98:289–294

Labrie F, Beaulieu M, Caron MG, Raymond V (1978a) The adenohypophyseal dopamine receptor: specificity and modulation of its activity by estradiol. In: Robyn C, Harter M (eds) Progress in prolactin physiology and pathology. Elsevier North-Holland Biomedical, Amsterdam Oxford New York, p 121

Labrie F, Lagacé L, Ferland et al. (1978b) Interactions between LHRH, sex steroids and "inhibin" in the control of LH and FSH secretion. Int J Andrology [Suppl] 2:81

Lagacé L, Labrie F, Lorenzen J, Schwartz NB, Channing CP (1979a) Selective inhibitory effect of porcine follicular fluid on FSH secretion in anterior pituitary cells in culture. Clin Endocrinol 10:401–406

Lagacé L, Massicotte J, Drouin J, Giguère V, Dupont A, Labrie F (1979b) Interactions between LHRH, sex steroids and "inhibin" at the pituitary level in the control of LH and FSH secretion in the rat. In: Talwar GP (ed) Recent advances in reproduction and regulation of fertility. Elsevier North-Holland Biochemical, Amsterdam Oxford New York, p 73

Lefkowitz RJ, Williams LT (1976) Alpha-adrenergic receptor identification by [^{3}H]dihydroergocryptine. Science 192:791–793

Lefkowitz RJ, Roth J, Pastan I (1970) Effects of calcium on ACTH stimulation of the adrenal separation of hormone binding from adenyl cyclase activation. Nature 228:864–866

Lemaire S, Pelletier G, Labrie F (1971) Adenosine 3′,5′-monophosphate-dependent protein kinase from bovine anterior pituitary gland. II. Subcellular distribution. J Biol Chem 246:7303–7310

Lemaire S, Labrie F, Gauthier M (1974) Adenosine 3′,5′-monophosphate-dependent protein kinase from bovine anterior pituitary gland. III. Structural specificity of the ATP site of the catalytic subunit. Can J Biochem 52:137–141

Lemay A, Labrie F (1972) Calcium-dependent stimulation of prolactin release in rat anterior pituitary in vitro by N^6-monobutyryl adenosine 3′,5′-monophosphate. FEBS Lett 20:7–10

Lemay A, Deschenes M, Lemaire S, Poirier G, Poulin L, Labrie F (1974) Phosphorylation of adenohypophyseal plasma membranes and properties of associated protein kinase. J Biol Chem 248:323–328

Levitzki A, Atlas D, Steer ML (1974) The binding characteristics and number of β-adrenergic receptors on the turkey erythrocyte. Proc Natl Acad Sci USA 71:2773–2776

Lippmann W, Sestanj K, Nelson VR, Immer HV (1976) Antagonism of prostaglandin-induced cyclic AMP accumulation in the rat anterior pituitary in vitro by somatostatin analogues. Experientia 32:1034–1036

MacLeod RM, Lehmeyer JE (1970) Release of pituitary growth hormone by prostaglandins and dibutyryl adenosine cyclic 3′,5′-monophosphate in the absence of protein synthesis. Proc Natl Acad Sci USA 67:1172–1179

MacLeod RM, Leymeyer JE (1974) Restoration of prolactin synthesis and release by the administration of monoaminergic blocking agents to pituitary tumor-bearing rats. Cancer Res 34:345–350

Mains RE, Eipper BA, Ling N (1977) Common precursor to corticotropins and endorphins. Proc Natl Acad Sci USA 74:3014–3018

Makino T (1973) Study of the intracellular mechanism of LH release in the anterior pituitary. Am J Obstet Gynecol 115:606–614

Marshall JC, Odell WD (1975) Preparation of biologically active ^{125}I-LHRH suitable for membrane binding studies. Proc Soc Exp Biol Med 149:351–355

Marshall JC, Shakespear RA, Odell WD (1976) LHRH-pituitary membrane binding: the presence of specific binding sites in other tissues. Clin Endocrinol 5:671–677

Massicotte J, Veilleux R, Lavoie M, Labrie F (1980) An LHRH agonist inhibits FSH-induced cyclic AMP accumulation and steroidogenesis in porcine granulosa cells in culture. Biochem Biophys Res Commun 94:1362–1366

Matsuo H, Baba Y, Nair RMG, Arimura A, Schally AV (1971) Structure of the porcine LH- and FSH-releasing hormone. I. The proposed amino acid sequence. Biochem Biophys Res Commun. 43:1334–1339

McCullagh DR (1932) Dual endocrine activity of the testis. Science 76:19–20

Menon KMJ, Guanaja KP, Azhar S (1977) GnRH action in rat anterior pituitary gland: regulation of protein glycoprotein and LH synthesis. Acta Endocrinol (Copenh) 86:473–481

Milligan JV, Kraicer J, Fawcett CP, Illner P (1972) Purified growth hormone releasing factor increases 45Ca uptake into pituitary cells. Can J Physiol Pharmacol 50:613–619

Mira-Moser F, Schofield JG, Orci L (1976) Modification in the release of rat growth hormone in vitro and the morphology of rat anterior pituitaries incubated in various ionophores. Eur J Clin Invest 6:103–111

Moriarty G (1973) Adenohypophysis: ultrastructural cytochemistry. A review. J Histochem 21:855–894

Moriarty CM (1977) Involvement of intracellular calcium in hormone secretion from rat pituitary cells. Mol Cell Endocrinol 6:349–361

Mukherjee C, Caron MG, Coverstone M, Lefkowitz RJ (1975) Identification of adenylate cyclase-coupled beta-adrenergic receptors in frog erythrocytes with (minus)-[^{3}H]alprenolol. J Biol Chem 250:5849–4876

Nakano H, Fawcett CP, Kimura F, McCann SM (1978) Evidence for the involvement of guanosine 3′,5′-cyclic monophosphate in the regulation of gonadotropin release. Endocrinology 103:1527–1533

Naor Z, Koch Y, Chobsieng P, Zor U (1975a) Pituitary cyclic AMP production and mechanism of luteinizing hormone release. FEBS Lett 58:318–321

Naor F, Koch Y, Bauminger S, Zor U (1975b) Action of luteinizing hormone and synthesis of prostaglandins in the pituitary gland. Prostaglandins in the pituitary gland. Prostaglandins 9:211–219

Naor Z, Snyder G, Fawcett CP, McCann SM (1978) A possible role for cyclic GMP in mediating the effect of luteinizing hormone releasing hormone on gonadotropin release in dispersed pituitary cells of the female rat. J Cyclic Nucleotide Res 4:475–486

Naor Z, Fawcett CP, McCann SM (1979) Differential effects of castration and testosterone replacement on basal and LHRH-stimulated cAMP and cGMP accumulation and on gonadotropin release from the pituitary of the male rat. Mol Cell Endocrinol 14:191–198

Nillius SJ, Wide L (1971) Induction of a midcycle-like peak of luteinizing hormone in young women by exogenous estradiol-17β. J Obstet Gynaecol Br Commonw 78:822–827

Ojeda SR, Harms PG, McCann SM (1974) Central effect of prostaglandin E_1 (PGE_1) on prolactin release. Endocrinology 95:613–618

Ojeda SR, Naor Z, McCann S (1978) Prostaglandin E levels in hypothalamus, median eminence and anterior pituitary of rats of both sexes. Brain Res 149:274–277

Orczyk GP, Behrman HR (1972) Ovulation blockade by aspirin or indomethacin. In vivo evidence for a role of prostaglandin in gonadotropin secretion. Prostaglandins 1:3–20

Pace-Asciak C, Wolfe LS (1970) Biosynthesis of prostaglandins E_2 and $F_{2\alpha}$ from tritium-labelled arachidonic acid by rat stomach homogenates. Biochim Biophys Acta 218:539–542

Parsons JA (1969) Calcium ion requirement for prolactin secretion by rat adenohypophyses in vitro. Am J Physiol 217:1599–1603

Pedroza E, Vilchez-Martinez JA, Fishback J, Arimura A, Schally AV (1977) Binding capacity of luteinizing hormone-releasing hormone and its analogues for pituitary receptor sites. Biochem Biophys Res Commun 79:234–238

Pelletier G, Lemay A, Béraud G, Labrie F (1972) Ultrastructural changes accompanying the stimulatory effect of N^6-monobutyryl adenosine 3′,5′-monophosphate on the release of growth hormone, prolactin, and adrenocorticotropic hormone in rat anterior pituitary gland in vitro. Endocrinology 91:1355–1371

Pelletier G, Leclerc R, Labrie F, Côté J, Chretien M, Lis M (1977) Immunohistochemical localization of β-lipotropic hormone in the pituitary gland. Endocrinology 100:770–776

Peng TS, Six KM, Munson PK (1970) Effects of prostaglandin E_1 on the hypothalamo-hypophyseal-adrenocortical axis in rats. Endocrinology 86:202–206

Phifer RF, Orth DN, Spicer S (1974) Specific demonstration of the human hypophyseal adrenocortico-melanotropic (ACTH-MSH) cell. J Clin Endocrinol Metab 39:684–692

Poirier G, Labrie F, Barden N, Lemaire S (1972) Thyrotropin-releasing hormone receptor: its partial purification from bovine anterior pituitary gland and its close association with adenyl cyclase. FEBS Lett 20:283–286

Ratner A (1970) Stimulation of luteinizing hormone release in vitro by dibutyryl cyclic AMP and theophylline. Life Sci 9:1221–1226

Ratner A, Wilson MC, Srivastava L, Peake GT (1974) Stimulatory effects of prostaglandin E_1 on rat anterior pituitary cyclic AMP and luteinizing hormone release. Prostaglandins 5:165–167

Raymond V, Beaulieu M, Labrie F (1978) Potent antidopaminergic activity of estradiol at the pituitary level on prolactin release. Science 200:1173–1175

Raymond V, Lépine J, Lissitzky JC, Côté J, Labrie F (1979) Parallel release of ACTH, β-endorphin, α-MSH and β-MSH-like immunoreactivities in rat anterior pituitary cells in culture. Mol Cell Endocrinol 16:113–122

Reeves JR, Séguin C, Lefebvre FA, Kelly PA, Labrie F (1980) Similar LHRH binding sites in the rat anterior pituitary and ovary. Proc Natl Acad Sci USA 77:5567–5571

Rigler GL, Peake GT, Ratner A (1978) Effect of luteinizing hormone releasing hormone on accumulation of pituitary cyclic AMP and GMP in vitro. J Endocrinol 76:367–372

Roberts JL, Herbert E (1977) Characterization of a common precursor to corticotropin and beta-lipotropin: cell-free synthesis of the precursor and identification of corticotropin peptides in the molecule. Proc Natl Acad Sci USA 74:4826–4830

Rose JC, Conklin PM (1978) TSH and ACTH secretion and cyclic adenosine 3′,5′-monophosphate content following stimulation with TRH or lysine vasopressin in vitro: suppression by thyroxine and dexamethasone (40239). Proc Soc Exp Biol 158:524–529

Samli MH, Geschwind LL (1968) Some effects of energy-transfer inhibitors and of Ca^{++}-free and K^{+}-enhanced media on the release of luteinizing hormone (LH) from the rat pituitary gland in vitro. Endocrinology 82:225–231

Sato T, Hirono M, Juyjo T, Iseka T, Taya K, Igarashi M (1975) Direct action of prostaglandins on rat pituitary. Endocrinology 96:45–49

Scarpa A, Baldassare J, Inesi G (1972) The effect of calcium ionophores on fragmented sacroplasmic reticulum. J Gen Physiol 60:735–749

Schally AV, Arimura A, Bowers CY, Kastin AJ, Sawano AS, Redding TW (1968) Hypothalamic neurohormones regulating anterior pituitary function. Recent Prog Horm Res 24:497–588

Schally AV, Dupont A, Arimura A, Redding TW, Linthicum GL (1975) Isolation of porcine GH-release inhibiting hormone. Fed Proc Fed Am Soc Exp Biol 34:584–586

Schally AV, Coy DH, Meyers CA (1978) Hypothalamic regulatory hormones. Ann Rev Biochem 47:89–128

Schlender KK, Wei SH, Villar-Palassi C (1969) VDP-glucose: glycogen alpha-4-glucosyltransferase I kinase activity of purified muscle protein kinase. Cyclic nucleotide specificity. Biochim Biophys Acta 191:272–278

Schofield JG (1967) Measurement of growth hormone released by ox anterior pituitary slices in vitro. Biochem J 103:331–341

Schofield JG (1970) Prostaglandin E_1 and the release of growth hormone in vitro. Nature 228:179–180

Shaar CJ, Clemens JA (1974) The role of catecholamines in the release of anterior pituitary prolactin in vitro. Endocrinology 95:1202–1212

Sheterline P, Schofield JG (1975) Endogenous phosphorylation and dephosphorylation of microtubule-associated proteins isolated from bovine anterior pituitary. FEBS Lett 56:297–302

Spence JW, Sheppard MS, Kraicer J (1980) Release of growth hormone from purified somatotrophs: interrelation between CA^{2+} and adenosine 3′5′-monophosphate. Endocrinology 106:764–769

Spona J (1973) LHRH interaction with the pituitary plasma membrane. FEBS Lett 34:24–26

Spona J (1975) LHRH sensitive adenylate cyclase in isolated plasma membranes of rat adenohypophyses. Endocrinol Exp (Bratisl) 9:27–33

Steiner AL, Peake GJ, Utiger RD, Karl IE, Kipnis DM (1970) Hypothalamic stimulation of growth hormone and thyrotropin release in vitro and pituitary 3′,5′-adenosine cyclic monophosphate. Endocrinology 86:1354–1360

Strittmatter WJ, Davies JN, Lefkowitz RJ (1977a) Alpha-adrenergic receptor in rat parotid cells 1. Correlation of L-tritiated dehydroergocryptine binding and catecholamine stimulated potassium efflux. J Biol Chem 252:5472–5477

Strittmatter WJ, Davies WJ, Lefkowtiz RJ (1977b) Alpha-adrenergic receptor in rat parotid cells. II. Desensitization of receptor binding sites and potassium release. J Biol Chem 252:5478–5482

Sundberg DK, Fawcett CP, McCann SM (1976) The involvement of cyclic 3′,5′-cyclic AMP in the release of hormones from the anterior pituitary in vitro. Proc Soc Exp Biol Med 151:149–154

Swerdloff RS, Odell WD (1968) Feedback control of male gonadotropin secretion. Lancet 2:683–687

Swerdloff RW, Walsh PC, Odell WD (1970) Control of LH and FSH secretion in the male: evidence that aromatization of androgens to estradiol is not required for inhibition of gonadotropin secretion. Steroids 20:13–22

Takahara J, Arimura A, Schally AV (1974) Suppression of prolactin release by a purified porcine PIF preparation and catecholamines infused into a rat hypophyseal portal vessel. Endocrinology 95:462–465

Tal E, Friedman S (1978) Correlation between 3′,5′-cyclic AMP levels and thyrotropin in separated rat pituitary thyrotropin cells. Experientia 34:1286–1288

Tal E, Szabo M, Burke G (1974) TRH and prostaglandin action on rat anterior pituitary: dissociation between cyclic AMP levels and TSH release. Prostaglandins 5:175–182

Theoleyre M, Berault A, Garnier J, Jutisz M (1976) Binding of LHRH to pituitary plasma membranes and the problem of adenylate cyclase stimulation. Mol Cell Endocrinol 5:365–377

Titeler M, List S, Seeman P (1980) High affinity dopamine receptors (D_3) in rat brain. Commun Psychopharmacol 3:411–420

Tsafriri A, Koch Y, Lindner HR (1973) Ovulation rate and serum LH levels in rats treated with indomethacin or prostaglandin E_2. Prostaglandins 3:461–467

Vale W, Guillemin R (1967) Potassium-induced stimulation of thyrotropin release in vitro. Requirement for presence of calcium and inhibition by thyroxine. Experientia 23:855–857

Vale W, Rivier C (1976) Regulation of ACTH secretion by anterior pituitary cells in culture. Fed Proc 35:2209–2214

Vale W, Rivier J (1977) Substances modulating the secretion of ACTH by cultured anterior pituitary cells. Fed Proc 36:2094–2099

Vale W, Burgus R, Guillemin R (1967) Presence of calcium ions as a requisite for the in vitro stimulation of TSH release by hypothalamic TRF. Experientia 23:853–855

Vale W, Grant G, Amoss M, Blackwell R, Guillemin R (1972) Culture of enzymatically dispersed pituitary cells: functional validation of a method. J Clin Endocrinol Metab 91:562–572

Vale W, Rivier C, Yang L, Minick S, Gillemin R (1978) Effects of purified hypothalamic corticotropin-releasing factor and other substances on the secretion of adrenocorticotropin and β-endorphin like immunoactivities in vitro. Endocrinology 103:1910–1915

Vale W, Spiess C, Rivier C, Rivier J (1981) Characterization of a 41-residue ovine hypothalamic peptide that stimulates secretion of corticotropin and β-endorphin. Science 2213:1394

Wagner TO, Adams TE, Nett TM (1979) GnRH interactions with anterior pituitary. I. Determination of the affinity and number of receptors for GnRH in ovine anterior pituitary. Biol Reprod 20:140–149
Waisman DM, Singh TJ, Wang JH (1978) The modulator-dependent protein kinase. A multi-functional protein kinase activable by the Ca^{2+}-dependent modulator protein of the cyclic nucleotide system. J Biol Chem 253:3387–3390
Wakabayashi K, Kamberi IA, McCann SM (1969) In vitro response of the rat pituitary to gonadotrophin-releasing factors and to ions. Endocrinology 85:1046–1056
Wakabayashi K, Date Y, Tamaoki B (1973) On the mechanism of action of luteinizing hormone-releasing factor and prolactin release inhibiting factor. Endocrinology 92:698–704
Wilber JF, Seibel MJ (1973) Thyrotropin releasing hormone interactions with an anterior pituitary membrane receptor. Endocrinology 92:888–893
Wilber JF, Peake GT, Mariz I, Utiger RD, Daughaday WH (1968) Theophylline and epinephrine effect upon the secretion of growth hormone (GH) and thyrotropin (TSH) in vitro. Clin Res 16:277–280
Wilber JF, Peake GT, Utiger RD (1969) Thyrotropin release in vitro: stimulation by cyclic 3′,5′-adenosine monophosphate. Endocrinology 84:758–760
Williams LT, Mullikin D, Lefkowitz RJ (1978) Magnesium-dependence of agonist binding to adenylate cyclase-coupled hormone receptors. J Biol Chem 253:2984–2989
Wolfe DJ, Brostrom CO (1979) Properties and functions of the calcium-dependent regulator. Adv Cyclic Nucleotide Res 11:27–88
Yates FE, Maran JW (1974) In: Knobil E, Sawyer WH (eds) The pituitary gland and its neuroendocrine control, part 2. American Physiological Society, Washington, DC (Handbook of physiology, sect 1, vol IV, chap 36, pp 367–404)
Yen SSC, Tsai CC, Vandenberg G, Rebar R (1972) Gonadotropin dynamics in patients with gonadal dysgenesis: a model for the study of gonadotropin regulation. J Clin Endocrinol Metab 35:897–904
Zimmerman G, Gleischer N (1970) Role of calcium ions in the release of ACTH from rat pituitary tissue in vitro. Endocrinology 87:426–429
Zor U, Kaneko T, Schneider HPG, McCann SM, Field JB (1969) Stimulation of anterior pituitary adenyl cyclase activity and adenosine 3′,5′-cyclic phosphate by hypothalamic extract and prostaglandin E_1. Proc Natl Acad Sci USA 63:918–625
Zor U, Kaneko T, Schneider HPG, McCann SM, Field JB (1970) Further studies of stimulation of anterior pituitary cyclic adenosine 3′,5′-monophosphate formation by hypothalamic extract and prostaglandins. J Biol Chem 245:2883–2888

CHAPTER 28

The Role of Cyclic Nucleotides in the Thyroid Gland

S. D. Holmes and J. B. Field

Overview

In this review we have analyzed the available evidence concerning the action of thyroid-stimulating hormone (TSH) and the role cyclic AMP plays in mediating the intracellular effects of this hormone. The binding of TSH to thyroid plasma membranes, the coupling of binding to activation of adenylate cyclase and the role of gangliosides and phospholipids in these processes have been briefly reviewed. The stimulation of adenylate cyclase and cyclic AMP formation by TSH and the different regulatory mechanisms involved have been discussed in some detail. TSH rapidly activates protein kinase and maximal activation of the enzyme is achieved prior to maximal elevations of cyclic AMP. Protein kinase activities can be isolated from thyroid cytosol and membranes and some work has been undertaken to identify some of the substrates that are phosphorylated. TSH stimulates morphological and biochemical changes in the thyroid of which most can be mimicked by cyclic AMP or dibutyryl cyclic AMP. However, some processes, for example $^{32}PO_4$ incorporation into phospholipids, are independent of cyclic AMP and as yet no second messenger has been implicated in colloid exocytosis. Various control mechanisms have been elucidated in TSH stimulation of cyclic AMP of which some may be of physiological importance. Iodide and thyroid hormones have been postulated to exert a negative feedback on TSH-stimulated cyclic AMP formation and adrenergic agents through the α-adrenergic receptor can also inhibit TSH stimulation. Cholinergic agents may also play some inhibitory role but the exact nature of this action is not clear. Thyroid-stimulating immunoglobulins can raise thyroidal cyclic AMP levels but there are important differences in their mode of action compared to TSH. Adrenergic agents can also increase cyclic AMP levels by activation of β-receptors, and separate receptors have also been found for cholera toxin and prostaglandins. The way in which the action of TSH is controlled or terminated may be linked with the phenomenon of desensitization. For example, prior exposure of thyroid tissue to TSH results in refractoriness to further stimulation of the hormone via the adenylate cyclase-cyclic AMP system. Various loci have been implicated for this process. Lastly, the TSH stimulation and cyclic AMP levels in various thyroid diseases are examined and possible causes for the alterations are discussed.

A. Mechanism of Action of TSH

I. The TSH Receptor

1. Binding of TSH to Thyroid Plasma Membranes

The initial event in the action of TSH is binding to its specific receptor site(s) on the thyroid plasma membrane. Such receptors have been identified in preparations of thyroid slices, homogenates, cells and purified thyroid plasma membranes (MANLEY et al. 1972, 1974; AMIR et al. 1973; MEHDI et al. 1973; SMITH and HALL 1974a; W. MOORE and WOLFF 1974; VERRIER et al. 1974; KOTANI et al. 1975). Optimal conditions necessary for TSH binding have differed widely in the literature on points of pH, time, temperature and ionic strength of the buffer used. A number of reports have shown that the binding of TSH was maximal at a pH lower than physiological (W. MOORE and WOLFF 1974; TATE et al. 1975a; AMIR et al. 1976; YAMAMOTO and RAPOPORT 1978; PEKONEN and WEINTRAUB 1979). In contrast, reports of maximal binding at pH 7.4 have also appeared (MANLEY et al. 1974; KOTANI et al. 1975; TAKAHASHI et al. 1978). There has also been disagreement on the effect of temperature and salt concentration on TSH binding (see review FIELD 1975; KOTANI et al. 1975). A recent report of PEKONEN and WEINTRAUB (1979) demonstrated that under physiological incubation conditions (pH 7.4, 37 °C in the presence of 50 m*M* NaCl), although the total TSH binding was decreased, the amount of TSH causing 50% inhibition of tracer binding was 1000-fold lower than when pH, temperature and salt concentrations were those that permitted maximal binding.

There has been controversy as to whether there are one or two classes of TSH-binding sites (MANLEY and et al. 1972; AMIR et al. 1973; LISSITZKY et al. 1973; SMITH and HALL 1974b; VERRIER et al. 1974; KOTANI et al. 1975) and if negative cooperativity could also account for the non-linear Scatchard plots (DEMEYTS et al. 1973). The difference in reported number of binding sites could be reflected in the variable incubation conditions used, as PEKONEN and WEINTRAUB (1979) showed that using highly unphysiological conditions the Scatchard plots were linear, whereas with more physiological conditions the Scatchard plots were curvilinear. Detailed kinetic studies by POWELL-JONES et al. (1979) support the idea that two separate binding sites are present at physiological pH but only one low affinity site at pH 6. A wide range of high affinity K_a values from 10^{-8} to 10^{-12} *M* have been published (W. MOORE and WOLFF 1974; KOTANI et al. 1975; A. SATO et al. 1977; AZUKIZAWA et al. 1977; YAMAMOTO and RAPOPORT 1978). Most workers, however, have shown that the high affinity site has an apparent K_a of 10^{-9} to 10^{-10} *M* (SMITH and HALL 1974; VERRIER et al. 1974; TATE et al. 1975a; TAKAHASHI et al. 1978; PEKONEN and WEINTRAUB 1979). Similar differences also exist for the low affinity K_a but most values are of the order 10^{-6} to 10^{-7} *M* (MANLEY et al. 1972; W. MOORE and WOLFF 1974; KOTANI et al. 1975). The high affinity site probably reflects the biological TSH receptor because of its sensitivity to near physiological TSH concentrations (10^{-12} to 10^{-10} *M*). The role of the low affinity site is unclear since it is sensitive only to pharmacological TSH concentrations and predominates under unphysiological conditions (PEKONEN and WEINTRAUB 1979).

Disagreement also exists concerning the dissociation of bound labelled hormone after the addition of unlabelled TSH. Although some workers have found rapid, complete displacement (AMIR et al. 1973) other reports have shown that the dissociation is slow and not complete (MANLEY et al. 1972; VERRIER et al. 1974; KOTANI et al. 1975). The latter results correlate with the fact that TSH can persistently bind to beef thyroid slices, as measured by cyclic AMP generation (DERUBERTIS et al. 1975).

2. Characterization of the Receptor

TSH receptors have been extracted from thyroid tissue by treatment with Triton (MANLEY et al. 1974; DAWES et al. 1978) and lithium diiodosalicylate (TATE et al. 1975b). The TSH binding characteristics of the solubilized membrane receptors were found to be very similar to the particulate membrane receptors (TATE et al. 1975b, DAWES et al. 1978). MANLEY et al. (1974) found that guinea pig thyroid membranes contained two types of hormone-receptor complexes with molecular weights of 150,000 and 500,000. DAWES et al. (1978) reported only one receptor complex of molecular weight 50,000 while TATE et al. (1975b) found the solubilized receptors to be heterogenous with molecular weights ranging from 15,000 to 280,000. Trypsin digestion converted the high molecular weight components to a component with a molecular weight of 15,000–30,000. MEHDI et al. (1977) obtained similar values (15,000–275,000) with solubilized human TSH receptors. The apparent differences in the above reports probably reflects species difference and differences in the conditions used to extract and analyze the receptor preparations.

Gangliosides have been shown to inhibit ^{125}I-labelled TSH binding to TSH receptors. The order of efficacy of inhibition was $G_{D1b} > G_{T1} > G_{M1} > G_{M2} = G_{M3} > G_{D1a}$ (MULLIN et al. 1976a). A later report from this group (MULLIN et al. 1978) demonstrated that a ganglioside constituting only 0.015% of the total thyroid gangliosides was the most potent inhibitor of ^{125}I-TSH binding while G_{D1a}, the most abundant ganglioside, showed little ability to inhibit TSH binding. It is possible that gangliosides may be a component or contribute to the formation of the TSH receptor.

3. Coupling Process

It is believed that the initial association between TSH and receptor involves electrostatic interactions between positively charged residues on the TSH molecule and specifically orientated negatively charged residues within the receptor binding site (GROLLMAN et al. 1977). There is also evidence to suggest that gangliosides might be involved in the binding coupling process (TATE et al. 1975b; MELDOLESI et al. 1976, 1977; MULLIN et al. 1976a). It has been demonstrated that neuraminidase digestion of the solubilized TSH receptor prevented binding of TSH (TATE et al. 1975b). However, this might only be a property of the solubilized receptor as W. MOORE and FELDMAN (1976) did not demonstrate any change in TSH binding after bovine membranes were first incubated with neuraminidase. Gangliosides (see Sect. A.I.2) have also been reported to inhibit the binding of TSH (MULLIN et al. 1976a, 1978) to bovine thyroid plasma membranes. These gangliosides were also absent from a thyroid tumor which was unable to bind TSH or respond to it metabolically (MELDOLESI et al. 1976). Whether gangliosides are involved in the TSH binding or coupling process is a matter of controversy since other workers have failed to show any interaction of gangliosides with TSH binding or stimulation of cyclic AMP (HOLMES et al. 1980b).

Membrane phospholipids have been implicated in the binding and action of TSH. Treatment of membranes with phospholipase A results in an increased binding of TSH but inhibition of TSH stimulation of adenylate cyclase (W. MOORE and WOLFF 1974). Phosphatidylcholine and phosphatidylserine can partially restore TSH stimulation of adenylate cyclase activity in phospholipase treated membranes (YAMASHITA and FIELD 1973; YAMASHITA et al. 1976). By introducing fluorescent probes into purified human thyroid membranes, solubilized membrane proteins and TSH receptors, MEHDI et al. (1977) suggested that lipids modulate TSH-receptor interactions and that the TSH receptor proteins segregate in association with the phospholipid which is in the "fluid" phase. These results imply that phospholipids may be an integral part of the coupling mechanism that relates hormone binding to stimulation of adenylate cyclase activity.

Prostaglandins have been implicated as possible intermediates in the action of TSH on the adenylate cyclase-cAMP system (S. SATO et al. 1972; YU et al. 1972). However this role of prostaglandins seems unlikely as will be discussed in a later section (B.II.).

II. TSH and Adenylate Cyclase Activity

1. Correlation Between Binding of TSH and Activation of Adenylate Cyclase

TSH activation of adenylate cyclase in membrane preparations from bovine (KOTANI et al. 1975), porcine (VERRIER et al. 1977), guinea pig (MANLEY et al. 1974) and human (CARAYON et al. 1979) thyroids have been closely correlated with the receptor site occupancy by the hormone. The concentration of TSH required to obtain half-occupation of the receptor sites was similar to the concentration of the hormone that half-stimulated the enzyme, 1.8 to 6 n*M* (KOTANI et al. 1975; VERRIER et al. 1977; CARAYON et al. 1979). This evidence provides support for the involvement of the adenylate cyclase system in the action of TSH. However, other factors might be involved in regulating TSH binding and activation of adenylate cyclase. For example, GTP potentiates TSH stimulation of adenylate cyclases but either diminishes (KOTANI et al. 1975) or has no effect (W. MOORE and WOLFE 1974) on binding of the hormone. W. MOORE and WOLFF (1974) have reported other situations in which there is a discrepancy between TSH binding and activation of adenylate cyclase activity.

2. Time Course and Dose Response

TSH can stimulate adenylate cyclase activity within 30 s (PASTAN and KATZEN 1967; ZOR et al. 1969) and the stimulation is linear for up to 40 min (BECH and NISTRUP MADSEN 1978). Sensitivity to TSH has varied considerably, and the lowest detectable concentration of TSH able to stimulate adenylate cyclase activity that has been reported was 0.0125 mU/ml by BECH and NISTRUP MADSEN (1978) using non-toxic goitrous thyroid membranes. The concentration of TSH (approximately 10–200 mU/ml) required for maximal activation of adenylate cyclase has also been variable (ZOR et al. 1969; WOLFF and JONES 1971; ORGIAZZI et al. 1976a; BECH and NISTRUP MADSEN 1978). The discrepancy in the reports involved in measuring adenylate cyclase activity are probably related to species difference, methodology and the contamination of ATP with GTP, which can potentiate TSH action (KOTANI et al. 1975).

3. Regulation

The mechanism by which TSH activates adenylate cyclase is not completely known. Hormonal stimulation of adenylate cyclase requires GTP (RODBELL et al. 1971), a catalytic site for the conversion of MgATP to cyclic AMP, a regulatory site for divalent cations and a guanine nucleotide regulatory component (RODBELL 1978). The current theory of activation of adenylate cyclase is that the hormone can displace GDP bound to the guanine nucleotide binding protein permitting binding of GTP which then activates the catalytic component. The subsequent hydrolysis of GTP on the guanine nucleotide binding component reverts the system to the inactive form (ABRAMOWITZ et al. 1979). This mechanism is consistent with the observation of hormone stimulated GTPase activity (CASSEL et al. 1977). Mg^{2+} increased TSH activation of adenylate cyclase (W. MOORE and WOLFF 1974) and GTP was shown to potentiate TSH stimulation of the enzyme (W. MOORE and WOLFF 1974; S. SATO et al. 1974; KOTANI et al. 1975). Other ions that can stimulate thyroidal adenylate cyclase are F^- (W. MOORE and WOLFF 1974) and Mn^{2+} at low concentrations. (HABHAB et al. 1977). K^+ can increase the TSH stimulation of the enzyme while Ca^{2+}, Na^+ and Li^+ inhibit adenylate cyclase (W. MOORE and WOLFF 1974). ITP has also been shown to increase enzyme activity (WOLFF and COOK 1973). Besides these regulators other possible control mechanisms also exist, for example, iodide (see Sect. A.VI.1), prostaglandins (see Sect. B.III) and refractoriness (see Sect. C.II).

III. TSH and Cyclic AMP Formation

1. Cyclic AMP as the Intracellular Mediator of the Effects of TSH

The intracellular effects of many hormones are mediated by cyclic AMP and the general Sutherland model of hormone action is applicable to TSH and the thyroid. TSH should (1) activate adenylate cyclase and increase the intracellular level of cyclic AMP. (2) Agents that can enhance the cyclic AMP concentration of thyroid cells should mimic the action of TSH. (3) Agents that can decrease cyclic AMP levels should inhibit the action of TSH. The above criteria and evidence that cyclic AMP is indeed the intracellular mediator of many of the effects of TSH is reviewed by DUMONT (1971) and discussed in Section A.V.

2. Time Course and Dose Response

The kinetics of cyclic AMP accumulation in thyroid slices, lobes or cells after stimulation by TSH exhibit a relatively rapid rise to a plateau (10–30 min) after which

Table 1. Minimum TSH concentration required to stimulate various thyroid functions

Parameter	TSH μU/ml	Reference
Thyroid hormone release	5	CHAPMAN and MALAN (1975)
Cyclic AMP formation	5–10	RAPOPORT and ADAMS (1978)
Adenylate cyclase activity	12.5	BECH and NISTRUP MADSEN (1978)
^{131}I release	50	BROWN and MUNRO (1967)
^{32}P incorporation into phospholipids	500	FIELD et al. (1968)

The normal concentration of TSH is 0.6–4.2 μU/ml (HALL et al. 1971). In primary hypothyroidism the values are greatly in excess of this

the levels begin to decrease (KENDALL-TAYLOR 1972; VAN SANDE and DUMONT 1973; TAKASU et al. 1978). The decrease in cyclic AMP levels with the continued presence of TSH and a phosphodiesterase inhibitor has been associated with refractoriness (RAPOPORT 1976; see Sect. C.II). In general, compared to adenylate cyclase activation cyclic AMP accumulation is more sensitive to TSH (half maximal activation lower) and the amount of stimulation is also higher. RAPOPORT (1976) and RAPOPORT and ADAMS (1978) developed a bioassay for TSH using dog thyroid cells in culture and the measurement of cyclic AMP. The threshold of sensitivity to TSH was very low, significant stimulation observed at concentrations of 5–10 μU/ml. The differences in the time courses for cyclic AMP accumulation and the concentration of TSH required for maximal activation have varied in the literature. The reasons are multiple, but in part depend on the different rates of diffusion of TSH in slices, lobes or cells, tissue preparation and the marked sensitivity of one species compared to another. The limit of sensitivity to TSH stimulation of various parameters is exemplified in Table 1. (The values shown will vary from species to species.)

3. Regulation

The levels of cyclic AMP in vivo are mainly regulated by its synthesis (see Sect. A.II 3) and degradation by phosphodiesterase. Two phosphodiesterases exist in the thyroid, one with a low K_m and V_{max}, the other with a higher K_m and V_{max} (SZABO and BURKE 1972; NAGASAKA and HIDAKA 1976) of which probably the latter is of more physiological importance. Cyclic GMP has been demonstrated to increase cyclic AMP-dependent phosphodiesterase activity (ERNEUX et al. 1977) and may play an important role in regulating cyclic AMP levels. In several systems cyclic AMP and cyclic GMP concentrations are reciprocally related and the two nucleotides seem to exert opposite regulatory roles (GOLDBERG et al. 1973). The action of cyclic GMP is further discussed in Sect. A.VI.4. Other factors may also play an important role in controlling cyclic AMP levels; for example, iodide (Sect. A.VI.1), thyroid hormones (Sect. A.VI.2), adrenergic agonists (Sect. A.VI.3) and the development of refractoriness (Sect. C.II). The overall regulation of cyclic AMP is very complex and probably other factors in its control may yet be discovered.

IV. TSH and Protein Kinase Activity

1. Time Course and Dose Response

Current evidence suggests that intracellular effects of cyclic AMP are mediated by activation of protein kinases (Kuo and Greengard 1969) involving dissociation of the enzyme into catalytic and regulatory subunits (Tao et al. 1970; Corbin et al. 1972). Incubation of thyroid slices with TSH increased the protein kinase activity ratio (activity in the absence compared to that in the presence of exogenous cyclic AMP) within 1–3 min, the maximal increase being observed by 10 min (Spaulding and Burrow 1974; Field et al. 1975). Schumacher and Hilz (1978), utilizing thyrocytes isolated from bovine thyroid tissue, found slightly different kinetics in that activation of protein kinase reached maximal levels within 2–5 min after TSH addition.

Protein kinase activity was increased by as little as 0.05 mU/ml TSH in bovine thyrocytes (Schumacher and Hilz 1978) and 0.25 mU/ml in bovine thyroid slices (Field et al. 1975). Half maximal activation of protein kinase was induced by 0.1–0.2 mU/ml TSH (Schumacher and Hilz 1978) while maximal activation was achieved with approximately 1.0 mU/ml TSH (Field et al. 1975; Schumacher and Hilz 1978).

2. Correlation with Cyclic AMP Levels

There has been some discrepancy between cyclic AMP concentration and hormone response. For example, the minimal amount of TSH required to elicit colloid droplet formation does not significantly increase cyclic AMP levels (Williams 1972). This can be explained by the fact that, firstly, bound cyclic AMP correlates with protein kinase activity not total cyclic AMP (Schumacher and Hilz 1968). Secondly, small elevations of total cyclic AMP are sufficient to activate the protein kinase since TSH concentrations that half-maximally activate the enzyme are 20 times lower than those required for half-maximal accumulation of total cyclic AMP and maximal activation of protein kinase precedes maximal elevation of cyclic AMP (Schumacher and Hilz 1978).

3. Phosphoprotein Phosphatase

This phosphatase has been demonstrated in calf (Spaulding and Burrow 1975b) and rat (Huprikar et al. 1979) thyroid and could be a control mechanism for inactivating enzymes that have been phosphorylated. Protein kinase activity is elevated in rats that have received goitrogen (Delbauffe and Pavlovic-Hournac 1976) and depressed in rats that have received T_4 or hypophysectomy (Huprikar et al. 1979). Phosphoprotein phosphatase activity was shown to parallel that of protein kinase in the above experiments (Huprikar et al. 1979). This would provide indirect evidence that the phosphatase is regulated by TSH.

4. Possible Substrates to be Phosphorylated

Two to three peaks of protein kinase activity can be separated from thyroid cytosol by different procedures (Spaulding and Burrow 1972; Delbauffe et al. 1979).

DELBAUFFE et al. (1979) have also shown that the Type I and Type II kinase, which are cyclic AMP-dependent, have a differential sensitivity to TSH. The exact role of the different kinases in the thyroid is as yet unknown. Thyroid plasma membrane also contains cyclic AMP-dependent and cyclic AMP-independent protein kinase activities (ROQUES et al. 1975; SUZUKI and FIELD 1978), and some work has been undertaken to elucidate the nature of the protein substrates that are phosphorylated. GIRAUD et al. (1977) identified the ATP hydrolysing subunit of Na^+, K^+ ATPase, a glycoprotein related to an aggregation promoting factor and possibly contractile proteins as substrates. SUZUKI and FIELD (1978), using sodium dodecyl sulfate polyacrylamide gel electrophoresis of intact plasma membranes, demonstrated approximately 30 protein bands several of which were substrates for endogenous protein kinase. SPAULDING and SCHUBART (1978) studied the distribution of phosphate incorporated into acid soluble proteins and found that endogenous histones H_3 and H_1 had a delayed response to TSH and might be involved in the expression of genetic information, e.g., RNA polymerase activity. In contrast, a minor basic protein, A5, was phosphorylated after 10 min and might be responsible for some of the early effects of TSH (SPAULDING and SCHUBART 1978).

It is evident that not all the substrates for protein kinase have been identified and neither have the links between activation of the enzyme and morphological and metabolic activities of TSH.

V. Role of Cyclic AMP in Thyroid Metabolism

1. Colloid Endocytosis and Exocytosis

Reabsorption of thyroglobulin and hormone release occurs by endocytosis (NADLER et al. 1962; WOLLMAN et al. 1964; EKHOLM and SMEDS 1966). The predominant type of endocytosis seems to be phagocytosis; pseudopods formed by the apical plasma membrane protrude into the follicle lumen where they enclose portions of colloid which then appear in the follicle cells as colloid droplets. The process of pseudopod formation is very rapid. However, KETELBANT-BALASSE et al. (1976) showed that the rise in cyclic AMP levels in response to TSH precedes this effect. Indeed, most of the events associated with the TSH stimulation of colloid resorption and hormone secretion have been reproduced by the administration of cyclic AMP or dibutyryl cyclic AMP (PASTAN and WOLLMAN 1967; RODESCH et al. 1969). Microtubules (WILLIAMS and WOLFF 1970) and microfilaments (WILLIAMS and WOLFF 1971 a) have also been implicated in colloid droplet formation and thyroid hormone release as the TSH stimulation of this process is inhibited by colchicine (which inhibits microtuble function) and cytocholasin B (which interferes with microfilaments). These agents do not inhibit the TSH stimulation of cyclic AMP or glucose oxidation.

Newly synthesized thyroglobulin is transported through the apical region of the follicle cell enclosed in vesicles which empty into the follicle lumen where the thyroglobulin is stored (BJORKMAN and EKHOLM 1973). The effect of TSH on exocytosis has been shown to be recognizable within 5 min (EKHOLM et al. 1975). The mechanism by which TSH regulates the exocytosis of vesicles is not known.

2. Iodine Metabolism

TSH has been reported to have a biphasic effect on iodide transport, stimulation occurring after a lag period of several hours (HALMI et al. 1960; WILSON et al. 1968; KNOPP et al. 1970). Dibutyryl cyclic AMP can accurately reproduce this effect. However, there is some uncertainty regarding the role of cyclic AMP in this context as GRANNER and HALMI (1972) were unable to demonstrate a relationship between the iodide pump and adenylate cyclase activity.

The effects of TSH on organification and secretion of thyroid hormones and iodide are also mediated by activation of the adenylate cyclase-cyclic AMP system (AHN and ROSENBERG 1968; WILLIAMS and WOLFF 1971 b). In bovine thyroid cells (WILSON et al. 1968) and dog thyroid slices (AHN and ROSENBERG 1970) incubation with dibutyryl cyclic AMP stimulated ^{131}I incorporation into iodoproteins and iodothyronines. The release of thyroid hormones and iodide in vitro from a number of species has also been obtained with dibutyryl cyclic AMP and cyclic AMP (ENSOR and MUNRO 1969; ONAYA and SOLOMON 1970; TONOUE et al. 1970); similar results have been obtained in vivo (BASTOMSKY and MCKENZIE 1967; BURKE 1968). ENSOR and MUNRO (1969) also showed that maximally effective concentrations of TSH or cyclic AMP were not additive. It seems probable that cyclic AMP is intimately concerned with the processes of thyroid hormone synthesis and secretion.

3. Glucose Oxidation

Dibutyryl cyclic AMP increased glucose-l-^{14}C oxidation by dog thyroid slices (PASTAN 1966), had no effect on rat thyroid slices, and decreased glucose-1-^{14}C oxidation in beef thyroid slices (PASTAN and MACCHIA 1967). The last observation is consistent with the fact that low doses of TSH actually inhibit glucose-1-^{14}C oxidation in the thyroids of beef and man (MERLEVEDE et al. 1963; OTTEN and DUMONT 1972). However, MACCHIA et al. (1969) reported increased glucose-1-^{14}C oxidation on addition of cyclic AMP to beef thyroid homogenates. In dog thyroid slices cyclic AMP was found to be ineffective (BURKE 1968) but, in another study utilizing tissue from thyroid hormone pretreated dogs, stimulation of glucose-1-^{14}C oxidation was obtained with cyclic AMP (RODESCH et al. 1969). TSH can also augment glucose oxidation from glucose-6-^{14}C (FIELD et al. 1959) and can accelerate glucose metabolism via the Emden-Meyerhof pathway and Krebs cycle (FIELD et al. 1961; OTTEN and DUMONT 1972), only a small fraction of the glucose being metabolized via the pentose cycle (MERLEVEDE et al. 1963). As NADP is a cofactor essential for hexose monophosphate activity and TSH can increase the concentration of this pyridine nucleotide, TSH has been postulated to be the mechanism for the increased glucose-1-^{14}C oxidation (PASTAN et al. 1963). However, cyclic AMP could have a direct effect on NAD kinase (MACCHIA et al. 1969). Despite the areas of uncertainty in the literature, it does appear that the effects of TSH on glucose oxidation are mediated by cyclic AMP. The review of DUMONT (1971) also favors this view.

Dibutyryl cyclic AMP can increase lactate formation but not pyruvate oxidation suggesting that the former effect is also related to activation of the adenylate cyclase-cyclic AMP system (GILMAN and RALL 1968).

4. Nucleic Acid Metabolism

New RNA synthesis is required for many thyroidal responses to TSH, including new protein synthesis (SHERWIN and TONG 1976), colloid droplet formation (ECKHOLM and ELMQVIST 1968) and part of the iodide pump. TSH increased the V_{max} of the iodide transport system in isolated thyroid cells and this delayed effect was blocked by inhibitors of RNA and protein synthesis (KNOPP et al. 1970). The kinetics of the inhibitory effect suggested that TSH first induces the synthesis of a specific mRNA which later codes for transport protein. This effect can be reproduced by dibutyryl cyclic AMP (KNOPP et al. 1970).

ADIGA et al. (1971) reported that RNA polymerase activity was stimulated in nuclei isolated from dibutyryl cyclic AMP treated tissue. However, this was only indirect evidence of the involvement of cyclic AMP in nucleic acid metabolism as addition of dibutyryl cyclic AMP to isolated nuclei did not increase RNA polymerase activity (ADIGA et al. 1971). Dibutyryl cyclic AMP can also reproduce the effects of TSH on enhancing the incorporation of ^{14}C-labelled adenine and uridine into RNA (WILSON and WRIGHT 1970). These results suggest that TSH, acting through cyclic AMP, can stimulate RNA synthesis by activation of nuclear polymerase.

HALL and TUBMAN (1965) observed that TSH stimulated incorporation ^{14}C labelled formate, glycine and adenine into adenine moieties of RNA. Glucose could also reproduce this effect and together with TSH produced additive stimulatory effects. However, in the presence of ribose, additional TSH or glucose did not result in further stimulation. HALL and TUBMAN (1965) postulated that the TSH stimulation of RNA synthesis occurred through the increased availability of ribose for the production of nucleoside precursors. This mechanism cannot account for the incorporation of labelled uridine (WILSON and WRIGHT 1970) nor the increased ^{32}P-phosphate (KERKOF and TATA 1969) incorporation into RNA.

5. Protein Synthesis and Growth

The uptake of α-amino isobutyric acid and other amino acids as well as the incorporation of amino acids into protein by isolated thyroid cells was found to be stimulated by both TSH and dibutyryl cyclic AMP while other nucleotides had no effect (WILSON et al. 1968; ADIGA et al. 1971). In T_4-pretreated mice, daily injections of cyclic AMP resulted in an enhancement of injected ^3H-leucine incorporation into thyroid protein and increased thyroid protein content and weight (PISAREV et al. 1970). WOLFF and VARRONE (1969) have also shown that several methylxanthines (inhibitors of phosphodiesterase activity) can potentiate goitre formation in vivo. These results imply that the TSH induced elevation of cyclic AMP is correlated with increased protein synthesis and growth in the thyroid.

Studies utilizing human thyroid cells in culture have produced conflicting results on whether TSH stimulates growth. TSH reduced (WESTERMARK et al. 1979) or increased (WINAND and KOHN 1975) ^3H-thymidine incorporation into thyroid cells and cell cultures grown in the presence of TSH had a slower (WESTERMARK et al. 1979) or faster (WINAND and KOHN 1975) growth rate.

MATSUZAKI et al. (1978) have reported an involvement of polyamines with thyroid tissue growth. They demonstrated that polyamine synthesis and growth increased in a roughly parallel manner. TSH increases ornithine decarboxylase activity (FRIEDMAN et al. 1979), the regulatory enzyme of the polyamine biosynthetic pathway, which is regulated by cyclic AMP (ZUSMAN and BURROW 1975), providing further evidence for the involvement of the adenylate cyclase-cyclic AMP system in thyroid growth.

6. Phospholipid Metabolism

The actions of cyclic AMP and dibutyryl cyclic AMP have been tested on phospholipid synthesis but the results have been inconclusive. BURKE (1968) and KERKOF and TATA (1969) obtained some stimulation (approximately 50%) with dibutyryl cyclic AMP while the majority of other workers either found inconsistent (PASTAN and MACCHIA 1967) or no stimulation at all (PASTAN 1966; PASTAN and MACCHIA 1967; SCOTT et al. 1970). The above evidence indicates that the effects of TSH on ^{32}P incorporation into phospholipids is probably not mediated by cyclic AMP. There is also further indirect evidence. Firstly, adrenergic antagonists inhibited effects of TSH on adenylate cyclase activity but did not abolish the TSH stimulation of phospholipid synthesis (BURKE 1969; LEVEY et al. 1969). Secondly, there is dissociation of the effects of various prostaglandins (FIELD et al. 1971). PGA_1 inhibited phospholipid synthesis although it increased cyclic AMP levels. PGF_1 stimulated phospholipid synthesis but had no effect on cyclic AMP levels, and PGE_1 increased both cyclic AMP and phospholipid synthesis although the amount required for the latter effect was far greater than for the former. Lastly, cholera toxin can mimic TSH by its effects on increasing intracellular cyclic AMP; however, cholera toxin does not augment the incorporation of ^{32}P into phospholipids (MASHITER et al. 1973).

VI. Inhibitors of TSH-Stimulated Thyroidal Cyclic AMP Formation

1. Iodide

Iodide in excess is known to suppress several thyroidal activities, most of which are mediated through the adenylate cyclase-cyclic AMP system (NAGATAKI 1974; VAN SANDE et al. 1975b). The majority of reports have demonstrated that iodide alone had no effect on basal cyclic AMP or adenylate cyclase activity (VAN SANDE et al. 1975b; HASHIZUME et al. 1976; RAPOPORT et al. 1976; SADDOCK et al. 1978; SHERWIN 1978). However, POCHET et al. (1977) found inhibition of adenylate cyclase. Whether a high iodine diet (RAPOPORT et al. 1976), injections of iodide (HASHIZUME et al. 1976) or preincubation with iodide in vitro (VAN SANDE et al. 1975b; SHERWIN 1978) were used, inhibition of the TSH stimulation of cyclic AMP or adenylate cyclase was observed. Inherent in the inhibition in vitro was the necessity to preexpose the tissue to iodide before addition of TSH (VAN SANDE and DUMONT 1973; VAN SANDE et al. 1975b; SADDOCK et al. 1978). Only SHIMIZU and SHISHIBA (1975) and FRIEDMAN et al. (1977) were unable to demonstrate the inhibitory effect of iodide on ability of TSH to stimulate cyclic AMP formation or to activate adenylate cyclase, respectively, although an inhibition of the TSH stimulated colloid droplet formation was observed by SHIMIZU and SHISHIBA (1975). From experiments using perchlorate and methimazole, it was evident that iodide uptake and organification were essential for the expression of the inhibitory effect of iodide upon the adenylate cyclase system (VAN SANDE et al. 1975b; RAPOPORT et al. 1976). VAN SANDE et al. (1975b) proposed that iodide is oxidized to an unidentified compound which can then exert a negative feedback on cyclic AMP formation. Several hypothesis to account for the depression of cyclic AMP levels by iodide have been tested. Increased hydrolysis of cyclic AMP seems improbable because iodide does not effect phosphodiesterase activity (RAPOPORT et al. 1975; POCHET et al. 1977; SADDOCK et al. 1978). Attempts to determine if iodide has a direct inhibitory effect on the adenylate cyclase or if it specifically interferes with the stimulatory action of TSH have yielded conflicting results. PGE_1 stimulation of cyclic AMP has been reported to be unaffected (RAPOPORT et al. 1976) or inhibited (VAN SANDE et al. 1975b; HASHIZUME et al. 1976) in the presence of iodide. Similarly, fluoride stimulation of adenylate cyclase has been shown to be inhibited (POCHET et al. 1977) or unchanged (RAPOPORT et al. 1976) by iodide. Iodide or an organic form of iodine may effect TSH binding to its receptors thereby preventing stimulation of cyclic AMP formation; however iodine enrichment, either in vitro or in vivo did not affect the affinity or number of TSH binding sites (UCHIMURA et al. 1979).

Whether the inhibitory action of iodide is located on the adenylate cyclase or affects the coupling between hormone and enzyme remains to be further investigated.

2. Thyroid Hormones

Observations on the action of T_3 and T_4 on TSH stimulation of cyclic AMP accumulation have been conflicting. SHIMIZU and SHISHIBA (1975), RAPOPORT et al. (1976, 1977) and SHUMAN et al. (1976) found no effect of thyroid hormones in vitro while TAKASU et al. (1974) and FRIEDMAN et al. (1977) reported that addition of T_4 or T_3 together with TSH decreased the anticipated rise in adenylate cyclase activity or cyclic AMP formation. In vivo administration of T_3 or T_4 followed by an in vitro incubation with TSH also resulted in a decrease in the response to TSH (YU et al. 1976). Experiments performed entirely in vivo (GAFNI and GROSS 1975) also showed an inhibitory action of T_3 and T_4 on TSH induced cyclic AMP accumulation. The above results would appear to favor the existence of a short-loop negative feedback phenomena (FRIEDMAN et al. 1977). Since thyroid hormones have been shown to inhibit rather than augment thyroidal cyclic AMP phosphodiesterase activity (NAGASAKA and HIDAKA 1976) the inhibition of TSH induced cyclic AMP formation cannot be attributed to thyroid hormone induced enhancement of the degradative enzyme. However, as pharmacological concentrations of thyroid hormones were used in vitro to observe inhibition (SHIMIZU and SHISHIBA 1975; FRIEDMAN et al. 1977), this must raise some doubts as to the physiological importance of these observations. Also, as a result of the in vivo administration of T_3 or T_4 to animals with intact pituitaries (GAFNI and GROSS 1975; YU et al. 1976), this may suppress endogenous TSH secretion and thereby influence the subsequent cyclic AMP response to TSH, as was later confirmed in the work of Friedman et al. (1979). Although the effects of thyroid hormones on cyclic AMP formation are difficult to interpret because of the varied reports, the available evidence supports the concept of an inhibitory effect of thyroid hormones on various thyroid functions subsequent to cyclic AMP generation (SHIMIZU and SHISHIBA 1975; SHISHIBA et al. 1975; YU et al. 1976; FRIEDMAN et al. 1977).

3. Adrenergic Agonists

An alpha-adrenoceptor modulates the effects of TSH on various parameters of thyroid function. In canine thyroid slices, norepinephrine inhibits the stimulation by TSH of cyclic AMP formation following a 30 min incubation (YAMASHITA et al. 1977). Similarly, norepinephrine interfered with the ability of either PGE_1 or cholera toxin to enhance the formation of cyclic AMP (YAMASHITA et al. 1979). Phentolamine could also prevent the decline in cyclic AMP levels that followed the peak effect of TSH. Catecholamines have also been reported to inhibit both the TSH and dibutyryl cyclic AMP stimulated release of thyroid hormone in mouse thyroid lobes (MAAYAN et al. 1977). As with the cyclic AMP data, phentolamine could abolish this effect. Although catecholamines stimulate cyclic AMP levels via the beta-adrenoceptor (see Sect. B.III), the alpha-adrenoceptor appears to exert some inhibitory effect upon the synthesis of cyclic AMP.

4. Cholinergic Agonists

Acetylcholine and carbamylcholine increase thyroidal cyclic GMP levels by stimulating a muscarinic receptor (YAMASHITA and FIELD 1972b; VAN SANDE et al. 1975a, 1979; DECOSTER et al. 1976); neither compound augments the concentration of cyclic AMP. TSH does not effect cyclic GMP levels (YAMASHITA and FIELD 1972b; VAN SANDE et al. 1975a). The effects of carbamylcholine on cyclic GMP accumulation as well as the carbamylcholine-induced inhibition of TSH-stimulated cyclic AMP formation are suppressed in calcium-depleted thyroid slices (VAN SANDE et al. 1975a, 1979). The existence of cholinergic-sensitive cyclic GMP formation as well as cholinergic nerve terminals in some thyroids (MELANDER et al. 1974a) would be compatible with a negative cholinergic regulation of TSH stimulation. However, cholinergic agents also increase glucose oxidation (PASTAN et al. 1961), iodide organification (VAN SANDE et al. 1975a) and thyroid hormone release (ISHII et al. 1968). This provides evidence for a dual control system in which Ca^{2+} is essential for both processes. The role of cyclic GMP has not been elucidated in thyroid tissue but it appears to be a signal responding to changes in Ca^{2+} concentration (GOLDBERG et al. 1978). From immunofluorescence studies, FALLON et al. (1974) proposed (from its localization) that cyclic GMP may be involved in the iodination of thyroglobulin.

B. Other Stimulators of Thyroidal Cyclic AMP Formation

I. Thyroid-Stimulating Immunoglobulins

Various types of thyroid-stimulating immunoglobulins (TSI) have been detected in the serum of patients with Graves' disease and named according to the assay method of their detection. The first TSI's to be discovered were the long-acting thyroid-stimulator (LATS; ADAMS and PURVES 1956), named because of its delayed effect in the McKenzie bioassay (McKenzie 1958) and LATS-protector (LATS-P; Adams and Kennedy 1967) designated by its ability to block the binding of LATS to a specific human thyroid particulate fraction. On the basis of increased colloid droplet formation, Onaya et al. (1973) described the "human thyroid stimulator" and Smith and Hall (1974a, b) measured "thyroid stimulating immunoglobulins" with a competitive binding assay using TSH and human thyroid membranes. Orgiazzi et al. (1976a) described the "human thyroid adenyl cyclase stimulator" and McKenzie and Zakarija (1976) "thyroid-stimulating antibody" based on cyclic AMP measurement in human thyroid slices.

Stimulation of adenylate cyclase activity by TSI has been reported in human thyroid membrane preparations (Mukhtar et al. 1975; Orgiazzi et al. 1976a; Mehdi and Kriss 1978; Bech and Nistrup Madsen 1978, 1979) and by LATS in dog and beef thyroid homogenates (T. Kaneko et al. 1970; Levey and Pastan 1970). However, Holmes et al. (1978) and Wolff and Jones (1971) failed to detect any stimulatory effect of LATS and LATS-P on adenylate cyclase activity of human and beef thyroid membranes respectfully. It also appears that 60 min incubations are required to obtain consistent stimulation of adenylate cyclase (Bech and Nistrup Madsen 1978, 1979); in contrast with the more rapid action of TSH (see Sect. A.II.2). The stimulation of cyclic AMP formation by LATS (Yamashita and Field 1972a; Kendall-Taylor 1972) or TSI (McKenzie and Zakarija 1976) has been demonstrated in a variety of species, however, LATS-P is specific for the human thyroid. The measurement of cyclic AMP formation in thyroid slices appears to a very sensitive method for the detection of TSI (Zakarija and McKenzie 1978). However, in order to obtain maximal activation of thyroidal cyclic AMP formation in vitro by TSI an incubation time of 60 min or greater is required (Kendall-Taylor 1972; McKenzie and Zakarija 1976; Zakarija and McKenzie 1978; Holmes et al. 1978, 1979). The time course of action of TSI again shows a lag phase in contrast to TSH (see Sect. A.III.2). Nistrup Madsen and Bech (1979) showed that incubation of human thyroid homogenate with cortisol decreased the adenylate cyclase response to TSI whereas the TSH response was unchanged or increased. This result, together with the lag phase in activation by TSI, would appear to indicate that TSH and TSI activate adenylate cyclase via different mechanisms. However, the observations made on goitrous thyroid slices that submaximal concentrations of TSH and TSI were additive in their effects on cyclic AMP formation and the absence of additive effects with maximal concentrations of TSH (Holmes et al. 1978) are compatible with a common pathway of action. The current hypothesis regarding TSI is that they are antibodies to the TSH receptor (Smith et al. 1977; Schleusener et al. 1978). This is based on the fact that TSI and unlabelled TSH can displace ^{125}I-TSH from thyroid membranes in an analogous fashion (Smith and Hall 1974a; 1974b; Petersen et al. 1977). However, although initial reports found good correlation between TSI stimulation of adenylate cyclase activity and inhibition of ^{125}I-TSH binding (Smith and Hall 1974a; Mukhtar et al. 1975), more extensive studies by others have not substantiated this observation (McKenzie et al. 1978; Sugenoya et al. 1979).

Yamashita and Field (1972a) first reported inhibition by LATS of the TSH-induced stimulation of adenylate cyclase in bovine thyroid membranes. This effect was attributed to a conformational change in the membrane rather than specific interaction with the TSH receptor since it was non-competitive and both LATS and normal IgG also decreased glucagon stimulation of liver membrane adenylate cyclase (YAMASHITA and FIELD 1972a). This effect was later confirmed using TSI and human thyroid membrane preparations (HOLMES et al. 1978; NISTRUP MADSEN and BECH 1979). MUTO et al. (1980) raised antibodies against purified bovine thyroid plasma membranes and found an inhibitory effect of the immunized sera on TSH stimulation of adenylate cyclase which was also non-competitive. The immunized sera, by itself, stimulated adenylate cyclase activity in the thyroid plasma membranes. In addition, low concentrations of IgG from immunized sera enhanced while high concentrations inhibited ^{125}I-TSH binding. OCHI et al. (1979) have also found that although Graves' disease IgG could displace ^{125}I-TSH from purified thyroid membranes, unlabelled TSH could not displace ^{125}I-LATS. These results imply that the antibody is not binding to the TSH receptor but induces a conformational change in the plasma membrane which could activate adenylate cyclase and effect the binding of ^{125}I-TSH.

II. Prostaglandins

Many of the effects of TSH on the thyroid can be reproduced by prostaglandins. PGE_1 activates thyroid plasma membrane adenylate cyclase (WOLFF and JONES 1970; KOWALSKI et al. 1972; MASHITER et al. 1974) and generation of cyclic AMP (T. KANEKO et al. 1969; ZOR et al. 1969). Prostaglandins have been shown to stimulate glucose oxidation (ZOR et al. 1969), iodide organification (RODESCH et al. 1969), colloid droplet formation (DEKKER and FIELD 1970) as well as ^{131}I and thyroid hormone release (RODESCH et al. 1969), processes which appear to be mediated by cyclic AMP. The approximate order of potency of the prostaglandins in stimulating adenylate cyclase or cyclic AMP formation is $PGE_1 > PGE_2 > PGA_1 > PGB_1 > PGF_1$ (MASHITER and FIELD 1974). In general, the stimulation is less than that observed with TSH (FIELD et al. 1971).

S. SATO et al. (1972) suggested that prostaglandins were obligatory intermediates in TSH action, as prostaglandin antagonists could block both TSH and PGE_1 stimulation of adenylate cyclase. YU et al. (1972) further substantiated this theory by finding that TSH could increase cellular levels of prostaglandin. However, other reports in the literature are not consistent with this theory. Firstly, indomethacin, which inhibits prostaglandin synthesis, does not inhibit the ability of TSH to increase cyclic AMP levels (MASHITER et al. 1974) or adenylate cyclase activity (WOLFF and MOORE 1973; MASHITER et al. 1974). TSH can increase adenylate cyclase activity in thyroid membrane preparations that do not respond to prostaglandins (WOLFF and JONES 1971), and TSH and PGE_1 have additive effects on cyclic AMP formation (MASHITER et al. 1974). Furthermore, while BOEYNAEMS et al. (1979a) found that TSH had no effect on prostaglandin release, HAYE and JACQUEMIN (1977) demonstrated that although TSH could increase the levels of arachidonate this was not the limiting factor in prostaglandin biosynthesis. The suggestion that TSH and prostaglandins might share a common receptor (BURKE 1970; SATO et al. 1972) is also unlikely in view of the radioreceptor studies of M. MOORE and WOLFF (1973) and W. MOORE and WOLFF (1974) and KOTANI et al. (1975).

Boeynaems et al. (1979a) demonstrated that carbamylcholine and epinephrine can stimulate the release of prostaglandins from dog thyroid slices, probably through a muscarinic and an α-adrenergic receptor respectively. In the absence of exogenous Ca^{2+}, these stimulatory effects were inhibited. Iodide was found to specifically inhibit the carbamylcholine induced release of prostaglandins (Boeynaems et al. 1979b). However, the exact significance of this cholinergic action on the thyroid and the inhibition by iodide remain to be fully elucidated.

III. Adrenergic Agonists

Adrenergic innervation of the follicle cells has been demonstrated in a number of species (Melander et al. 1974c, 1975a) and would suggest the existence of an adrenergic control of thyroid metabolism (Melander et al. 1974a, 1974b). Catecholamines stimulate adenylate cyclase activity and cyclic AMP formation in thyroid tissue of a variety of species (Melander et al. 1974a, Marshall et al. 1975; Spaulding and Burrow 1975a; Aiyoshi et al. 1978) although Maayan et al. (1977) were unable to demonstrate epinephrine stimulation of cyclic AMP formation using mouse thyroid lobes. Adrenergic stimulation is less than that produced by TSH but is appreciably faster, reaching its maximum effect within one to two minutes (Spaulding and Burrow 1975a; Aiyoshi et al. 1978). The effect appears to be mediated through the β-adrenergic receptor (Marshall et al. 1975; Melander et al. 1975a; Spaulding and Burrow 1975a; Aiyoshi et al. 1978); however, some adrenergic effects have been inhibited by α-adrenergic antagonists (Ahn and Rosenberg 1970; Maayan and Ingbar 1970). Other cyclic AMP mediated processes are also stimulated by catecholamines, for example, colloid droplet formation (Melander et al. 1975b), thyroid hormone synthesis (Maayan and Ingbar 1968) and release (Melander 1970).

IV. Cholera Toxin

Cholera toxin increases cyclic AMP concentrations in thyroid slices but in contrast to the effect of TSH (see Sect. A.III.2) this action requires at least a 25 min incubation at 37 °C (Mashiter et al. 1973). Cholera toxin can also reproduce many of the cyclic AMP-mediated effects of TSH, e.g., glucose oxidation, iodide organification and colloid droplet formation (Mashiter et al. 1973; Van Sande et al. 1979). The B subunit of the toxin interacts with cell surface receptors which are believed to be G_{MI} gangliosides (Cuatrecasas 1973). This induces a conformational change in the toxin molecule which results in activation of the adenylate cyclase by the A subunit. It has been proposed that the action of the A subunit requires its translocation through the membrane (Gill 1976) thereby resulting in the lag period.

It has been proposed that TSH and cholera toxin have an analogous mode of action (Ledley et al. 1976, 1977; Mullin et al. 1976b). However, beside the delayed action of cholera toxin; many other characteristics and requirements of cholera toxin action on adenylate cyclase differ from those of TSH. Cholera toxin catalyses an NAD dependent enzymatic process involving ADP-ribosylation (Moss et al. 1977; Moss and Vaughan 1977) and there is no evidence to suggest that TSH activates adenylate cyclase through an NAD dependent mechanism (Moss et al. 1978). HOLMES et al. (1980b) demonstrated that cholera toxin bound to thyroid slices did not impair the subsequent stimulation of cyclic AMP by TSH. Although TSH increases ^{32}P incorporation into phospholipids, cholera toxin cannot reproduce this effect (MASHITER et al. 1973). TSH and cholera have additive effects on adenylate cyclase activity (HOLMES et al. 1980b) and their effects on cyclase can also be dissociated by cooling (VAN SANDE et al. 1979). These results bear strongly against the hypothesis that TSH and cholera toxin activate adenylate cyclase by similar mechanisms.

C. Desensitization – Characterization of the Phenomenon

I. Effects on Binding Process

In view of the persistent binding of TSH to plasma membranes (DERUBERTIS et al. 1975), the mechanism by which the actions of TSH are controlled or terminated is poorly understood. The development of refractoriness to hormonal stimulation after previous exposure to the hormone might be responsible for the physiologic regulation of the target cell sensitivity (RAFF 1976; KOLATA 1977; TELL et al. 1978). Previous exposure of thyroid slices (SHUMAN et al. 1976) or cells (Y. KANEKO 1976; RAPOPORT and ADAMS 1976) to TSH induces refractoriness to further stimulation by TSH. However, this desensitization was not associated with a change in the binding characteristics of TSH (RAPOPORT and ADAMS 1976; FIELD et al. 1977). This is in contrast to the results of HOLMES et al. (1980a) who demonstrated that rats exposed to chronically elevated endogenous TSH (induced by tapazole) for 4–5 weeks had half the number of thyroidal TSH binding sites compared to control rats and decreased biologic response to TSH. The difference in the above reports could reflect the different time of exposure to elevated TSH, hours in vitro (RAPOPORT and ADAMS 1976; FIELD et al. 1977) and 4–5 weeks in vivo, which might induce different regulatory mechanisms.

TSH receptors have also been identified in adipose tissue of a number of species (TENG et al. 1975; GILL et al. 1978a, b). In rats treated with tapazole, the increased endogenous TSH had no effect on the affinity constant, number of TSH binding sites or biologic effect of TSH in epididymal fat membranes (HOLMES et al. 1980a). These results would suggest that TSH receptors in thyroid and adipose tissue are independently regulated.

II. Effect on Cyclic AMP-Adenylate Cyclase System

In the thyroid, decreased sensitivity to TSH stimulation of the adenylate cyclase-cyclic AMP system as a consequence of prior exposure to TSH has been described using thyroid lobes from rats fed goitrogen (ZAKARIJA and MCKENZIE 1975, 1977; HOLMES et al. 1980a), thyroid slices (SHUMAN et al. 1976) or isolated thyroid cells (Y. KANEKO 1976; RAPOPORT and ADAMS 1976). Desentization of thyroid slices was stimulator specific since prior incubation with TSH did not modify the stimulation induced by PGE_1 (SHUMAN et al. 1976) or cholera toxin (HOLMES et al. 1980a) nor did PGE_1 incubation inhibit the subsequent stimulation by TSH (SHU-

MAN et al. 1976). The failure of TSH to stimulate adenylate cyclase activity in homogenates of thyroid slices previously incubated with TSH has been reported (SHUMAN et al. 1976). Desensitization does not appear to affect the catalytic activity of adenylate cyclase since NaF and PGE_1 responses were unaffected (SHUMAN et al. 1976). It also appears that the diminished cyclic AMP response to TSH was not due to increased phosphodiesterase activity (RAPOPORT and ADAMS 1976; SHUMAN et al. 1976). ZAKARIJA and MCKENZIE (1977) also measured phosphodiesterase activity in thyroid tissue from propylthiouracil (PTU) treated rats and found it to be increased. However, they also measured cyclic AMP in lobes taken directly from PTU and control rats and still found a 2-fold increase in the amount of cyclic AMP in the PTU compared to control rats. Such results would appear to indicate that the adenylate cyclase is stimulated to a greater extent than the phosphodiesterase (ZAKARIJA and MCKENZIE 1977).

III. Effect on Other Metabolic Parameters

Initial incubation of thyroid slices with TSH induces diminished responsiveness to the subsequent addition of the hormone when measuring protein kinase activity, glucose oxidation (FIELD et al. 1977), iodide organification (FIELD et al. 1979; HOLMES et al. 1980a), colloid droplet formation and thyroid hormone secretion (FIELD et al. 1979). Such refractoriness is also associated with a process thought not to be mediated by cyclic AMP (see Sect. A.V.6) ^{32}P incorporation into phospholipids (FIELD et al. 1977). During refractoriness the stimulation of glucose oxidation by PGE_1 and dibutyryl cyclic AMP was significantly diminished, as was the stimulation by acetylcholine of ^{32}P incorporation into phospholipids (FIELD et al. 1977). These results indicate that other metabolic sites beside activation of adenylate cyclase are responsible for the development of refractoriness. Furthermore, the stimulatory effects of dibutyryl cyclic AMP and PGE_1 on iodide organification were abolished in slices previously incubated with TSH (FIELD et al. 1979). However, HOMES et al. (1980a) showed that the dibutyryl cyclic AMP stimulation of iodide organification was unchanged in tapazole treated compared to control rats. The difference in these results could be due to the length of time and concentration of TSH that the thyroids were exposed to.

It has been shown that iodide, T_3 and T_4 (inhibitors of TSH stimulation of cyclic AMP, Sect. A.VI.) have no effect on the refractory process (SHUMAN et al. 1976; FIELD et al. 1979) but whether new protein synthesis is required remains unclear because of contradictory reports (RAPOPORT and ADAMS 1976; SHUMAN et al. 1976; FIELD et al. 1979). The actual significance of refractoriness to TSH stimulation remains unclear but could be of some physiologic importance in modulating the effects of TSH on the thyroid.

D. Clinical Aspects

I. Graves' Disease

The basal levels of cyclic AMP in thyroid tissue obtained from Graves' disease patients has been reported to be the same as normal tissue or nontoxic goitres

(KENDALL-TAYLOR 1973; ONAYA et al. 1973; FIELD et al. 1974; TAKASU et al. 1974, 1976; ORGIAZZI et al..1975; VALENTA 1976). HOLMES et al. (1978) did report significantly higher basal levels of cyclic AMP in thyrotoxic tissue compared to goitrous tissue; however, this could have resulted from expressing the data on the basis of per mg protein. FIELD et al. (1974) and TAKASU et al. (1974, 1976) showed that normal thyroid slices accumulated more cyclic AMP than did slices of thyrotoxic thyroids when incubated with the same concentration of TSH. KENDALL-TAYLOR (1973) and HOLMES et al. (1978) demonstrated that goitrous tissue slices were more responsive than slices from thyrotoxic thyroids when incubated with TSH. However, Field et al. (1974) and ORGIAZZI et al. (1975, 1976a) reported that the stimulation of adenylate cyclase by TSH was equally effective in membrane preparations from normal or Graves' disease tissue. There are two reports using cultured thyroid cells in which the adenylase cyclase activity in Graves' disease cells has a lower basal and elevated response to TSH when compared to normal, adenoma and goitrous tissue (WINAND and WADELEUX 1976; LEE et al. 1977). These results have been correlated with an abnormal ganglioside pattern in the Graves' disease membranes (LEE et al. 1977). The effect of TSH on ^{32}P incorporation into phospholipids of Graves' and normal thyroid slices was found to be the same (FIELD et al. 1974; SCHNEIDER 1974) as were protein kinase activities (ORGIAZZI et al. 1975). Graves' disease thyroids were less responsive to TSH when glucose oxidation was measured (FIELD et al. 1974).

The greater sensitivity to TSH of preparations of goitres and normal thyroid compared to Graves' tissue might result from the pre-operative treatment of Graves' diesease patients with antithyroid drugs and iodide (ONAYA et al. 1978). Binding studies (MUKHTAR et al. 1975; CARAYON et al. 1978) showed no difference in the affinity constant or number of TSH binding sites between Graves' or normal thyroid tissue.

II. Thyroid Nodules

1. Functioning Nodules

In a sample of 10 euthyroid autonomous adenomas, basal adenylate cyclase was higher but the response to TSH was not significantly different from normal tissue (TANINI et al. 1978). Both LARSEN et al. (1973) and TANINI et al. (1978) demonstrated increased basal adenylate cyclase activity in toxic adenomas; however, LARSEN et al. (1973) reported increased responsiveness to TSH (2 samples) in contrast to TANINI et al. (1978) who found that the TSH stimulation of adenylate cyclase was significantly decreased (6 samples). LARSEN et al. (1973) also reported that the adenomas responded to a much greater extent to TSH than the surrounding normal tissue when iodide organification was measured. The conflicting data may arise from the small number of tissue samples tested. This diseased tissue is not associated with a change in the affinity or number of TSH binding sites compared to normal tissue (CARAYON et al. 1978; KARLSSON and DAHLBERG 1979). These results suggest the possibility of a defect in the coupling mechanism between TSH and adenylate cyclase.

2. Non-Functioning Nodules

Thyroid nodules appear non-functional or "cold" on radioiodine scanning because of defective uptake of iodide, rather than absence of TSH responsiveness. Benign cold thyroid nodules have increased basal adenylate cyclase activity (DeRubertis et al. 1972; Orgiazzi et al. 1976b; Kalderon and Sheth 1978), glucose-1-^{14}C oxidation and ^{32}P incorporation into phospholipids in vitro (DeRubertis et al. 1972). These nodules also demonstrate increased TSH responsiveness measuring adenylate cyclase (DeRubertis et al. 1972; Orgiazzi et al. 1976b; Kalderon and Smith 1978) and ^{32}P incorporation (DeRubertis et al. 1972) and normal TSH responses when cyclic AMP, glucose-1-^{14}C oxidation (DeRubertis et al. 1972) and iodide organification were assessed (Field et al. 1973).

The elevated response of adenylate cyclase to TSH may be due to a change in the binding characteristics of the thyroid cell. However, no difference was noted in the affinity or binding capacity of TSH between non-functioning and normal thyroid tissue (Karlsson and Dahlberg 1969). In contrast Takahashi et al. (1978) demonstrated that cold adenomas had a decreased number of TSH receptors. This data is difficult to reconcile with the enhanced responsiveness of the adenylate cyclase system which could result from increased coupling between hormone and enzyme.

III. Thyroid Carcinoma

A number of reports have shown major biochemical differences between carcinomatous and normal thyroid tissue. Higher basal adenylate cyclase activity has been reported in carcinomatous compared to normal thyroid (Orgiazzi et al. 1977; Field et al. 1978) although this was not found in two undifferentiated carcinomas (Orgiazzi et al. 1977). In a small sample of carcinomas, Sand et al. (1976) observed higher (but not different) adenylate cyclase activities compared to normal. Basal levels of cyclic AMP are also elevated in thyroid carcinoma (Valenta 1976; Field et al. 1978; Thomas-Morvan 1978).

Besides the difference in the basal activities, the TSH stimulation of the above parameters was decreased in carcinomatous tissue. Although Field et al. (1978) demonstrated no change in the mean response to TSH measuring adenylate cyclase, some carcinomas did not respond to TSH at all. Sand et al. (1976) reported similar observations. However, the TSH stimulation of cyclic AMP formation was consistently lower in the carcinomas compared to normal thyroid tissue (Field et al. 1978; Thomas-Morvan 1978). The effect of TSH on intermediary metabolism from carcinomas showed decreased ^{32}P incorporation into phospholipids in response to TSH but no change in iodide organification or glucose oxidation (Field et al. 1978). In a study of 44 human thyroid cancers, TSH also had no effect on iodine metabolism in 46% of the cases (Thomas-Morvan et al. 1974).

The data available on TSH binding characteristics suggest there is no difference between normal and malignant tissue (Ichikawa et al. 1976; Clark and Castner 1979) although one of two papillary carcinomas studied did show reduced association constants for both low and high affinity receptors (Ichikawa et al. 1976). In three papillary and one follicular carcinoma, Takahashi et al. (1978) found a reduced number of receptors and in two medullary carcinomas the number of receptors were two orders of magnitude less than normal tissue. FIELD et al. (1978) found no difference in the binding of TSH to carcinomatous compared to surrounding normal tissue. However, there was not a good correlation between the binding of TSH and the stimulation of adenylate cyclase activity in either tissue. The reason for this discrepancy is not known (see Sect. A.II.1). It is not clear if carcinomatous tissue has a defect in the TSH binding capacity because of limited number of samples tested or whether the decreased responsiveness might (also) reside in the coupling and/or adenylate cyclase.

References

Abramowitz J, Iyengar R, Birnbaumer L (1979) Review: guanyl nucleotide regulation of hormonally-responsive adenylyl cyclases. Mol Cell Endocrinol 16:129–146

Adams DD, Kennedy TH (1967) Occurrence in thyrotoxicosis of a gamma globulin which protects LATS from neutralization by an extract of thyroid gland. J Clin Endocrinol Metab 27:173–177

Adams DD, Purves HD (1956) Abnormal responses in the assay of thyrotrophin. Proc Univ Otago Med Sch 34:11–12

Adiga PR, Murthy PVN, McKenzie JM (1971) Stimulation by thyrotropin, long-acting thyroid stimulator and dibutyryl 3′,5′-adenosine monophosphate of protein and ribonucleic acid synthesis and ribonucleic acid polymerase activities in porcine thyroid in vitro. Biochemistry 10:702–710

Ahn CS, Rosenberg IN (1968) Prompt stimulation of the organic binding of iodine in the thyroid by adenosine 3′,5′-phosphate in vivo. Proc Natl Acad Sci USA 60:830–835

Ahn CS, Rosenberg IN (1970) Iodine metabolism in thyroid slices: effects of TSH dibutyryl cyclic 3′,5′ AMP, NaF and prostaglandin E_1. Endocrinology 86:396–405

Aiyoshi Y, Yamashita K, Yamashita S, Ogata E (1978) Effects of norepinephrine on cyclic nucleotide levels in dog thyroid slices. Endocrinology 102:1527–1533

Amir SM, Carraway TF, Kohn LD, Winand R (1973) The binding of thyrotropin to isolated bovine thyroid plasma membranes. J Biol Chem 248:4092–4100

Amir SM, Goldfine ID, Ingbar SH (1976) Properties of the interaction between bovine thyrotropin and bovine thyroid plasma membranes. J Biol Chem 251:4693–4699

Azukizawa MG, Kurtzman G, Pekary AE, Hershman JM (1977) Comparison of the binding characteristics of bovine thyrotropin and human chorionic gonadotropin to thyroid plasma membranes. Endocrinology 101:1880–1889

Bastomsky CH, McKenzie JM (1967) Cyclic AMP: mediator of thyroid stimulation by thyrotropin. Am J Physiol 213:753–758

Bech K, Nistrup Madsen S (1978) Human thyroid adenylate cyclase in non-toxic goitre: sensitivity of TSH, fluoride and thyroid stimulating immunoglobulins. Clin Endocrinol 8:457–466

Bech K, Nistrup Madsen S (1979) adenylate cyclase stimulating immunoglobulins in thyroid diseases. Clin Endocrinol 11:47–58

Bjorkman U, Ekholm R (1973) Thyroglobulin synthesis and intracellular transport studied in bovine thyroid slices. J Ultrastruct Res 45:231–253

Boeynaems JM, Waelbroeck M, Dumont JE (1979a) Cholinergic and alpha-adrenergic stimulation of prostaglandin release by dog thyroid in vitro. Endocrinology 105:988–995

Boeynaems JM, Galand N, Dumont JE (1979b) Inhibition by iodide of the cholinergic stimulation of prostaglandin synthesis in dog thyroid. Endocrinology 105:996–1000

Brown J, Munro DS (1967) A new in vitro assay for thyroid-stimulating hormone. J Endocrinol 38:439–449

Burke G (1968) Effects of cyclic 3′,5′-adenosine monophosphate and dibutyryl cyclic 3′,5′-adenosine monophosphate on basal and stimulated thyroid function. J Clin Endocrinol Metab 28:1816–1823

Burke G (1969) Effects of adrenergic blocking agents on basal and stimulated thyroid function. Metabolism 18:961–967
Burke G (1970) Effects of prostaglandins on basal and stimulated thyroid function. Am J Physiol 218:1445–1452
Burke G (1973) Effects of thyrotropin and N_6, O_2-dibutyryl cyclic 3′,5′-adenosine monophosphate on prostaglandin levels in the thyroid. Prostaglandins 3:291–297
Carayon P, Guibot M, Jaquet PL, Lissitzky S (1978) Interaction de la TSH avec les membranes plasmiques de thyroides humaines normales et pathologiques. Ann Endocrinol (Paris) 39:57–58
Carayon P, Guibout M, Lissitzky S (1979) The interaction of radioiodinated thyrotropin with human plasma membranes from normal and diseased thyroid glands. Ann Endocrinol (Paris) 40:211–227
Cassel D, Levkovitz H, Selinger Z (1977) The regulatory GTPase cycle of turkey erthrocyte adenylate cyclase. J Cyclic Nucleotide Res 3:393–406
Chapman RS, Malan PG (1975) Thyroidal stimulation by thyrotrophin: differential release of tri-iodothyronine relative to thyroxine. J Endocrinol 65:17P
Clark OH, Castner BJ (1979) Thyrotropin receptors in normal and neoplastic human thyroid tissue. Surgery 85:624–630
Corbin JD, Brostrom CO, Alexander BL, Krebs EG (1972) Adenosine-3′,5′-monophosphate-dependent protein kinase from adipose tissue. J Biol Chem 247:3736–3743
Cuatrecasas P (1973) Interaction of vibrio cholerae enterotoxin with cell membranes. Biochemistry 12:3547–3558
Dawes PJD, Petersen VB Rees Smith B, Hall R (1978) Solubilization and partial characterization of human and porcine thyrotropin receptors. J Endocrinol 78:89–102
Decoster C, Van Sande J, Mockel J (1976) Role of cyclic GMP in thyroid metabolism. Arch Int Physiol Biochim 84:1061–1062
Dekker A, Field JB (1970) Correlation of effects of thyrotropin, prostaglandins and ions on glucose oxidation, cyclic AMP and colloid droplet formation in dog thyroid slices. Metabolism 19:453–464
Delbauffe D, Pavlovic-Hournac M (1976) Hormonal regulation of thyroidal protein phosphokinase activities. FEBS Lett 69:59–62
Delbauffe D, Ohayon R, Pavlovic-Hournac M (1979) Hormonal regulation of thyroidal protein phosphokinase activities – 2. Differential sensitivity of type-I and type-II cAMP-dependent enzymes to the treatment of rats with thyroxine. Mol Cell Endocrinol 14:141–155
DeMeyts P, Roth J, Neville DM Jr, Gavin JR, Lesniak MA (1973) Insulin interactions with its receptors: experimental evidence for negative cooperativity. Biochem Biophys Res Commun 55:154–161
DeRubertis F, Yamashita K, Dekker A, Larsen PR, Field JB (1972) Effects of thyroidstimulating hormone on adenylate cyclase activity and intermediary metabolism of "cold" thyroid nodules and normal human thyroid tissue. J Clin Invest 51:1109–1117
DeRubertis FR, Chayoth R, Zor U, Field JB (1975) Evidence for persistent binding of biologically active TSH to thyroid in vitro. Endocrinology 96:1579–1586
Dumont JE (1971) The action of thyrotropin on thyroid metabolism. Vitam Horm 29:287–412
Eckholm R, Elmqvist LG (1968) Inhibition of endocytosis in the thyroid follicle cell by actinomycin. Exp Cell Res 48:640–643
Ekholm R, Smeds S (1966) On dense bodies and droplets in the follicular cells of the guinea pig thyroid. J Ultrastruct Res 16:71–82
Ekholm R, Engstrom G, Ericson LE, Melander A (1975) Exocytosis of protein into the thyroid follicle lumen: an early effect of TSH. Endocrinology 97:337–346
Ensor JM, Munro DS (1969) A comparison of in vitro actions of TSH and cyclic AMP on the mouse thyroid gland. J Endocrinol 43:477–485
Erneux C, Van Sande J, Dumont J, Boeynaems J (1977) Cyclic nucleotide hydrolysis in the thyroid gland: general properties and key role in interrelation between concentration and cyclic AMP and cyclic GMP. Eur J Biochem 72:137–147

Fallon EF, Agrawal R, Furth E, Steiner AL (1974) Cyclic guanosine and adenosine 3′,5′-monophosphates in canine thyroid: localization by immunofluorescence. Science 184:1089–1091
Field JB (1975) Thyroid-stimulating hormone and cyclic 3′,5′-monophosphate in the regulation of thyroid gland function. Metabolism 24:381–393
Field JB, Pastan I, Johnson P, Herring B (1959) In vitro stimulation of the hexose monophosphate pathway in thyroid by thyroid stimulating hormone, Biochem Biophys Res Commun 1:284–287
Field JB, Pastan I, Herring B, Johnson P (1961) Studies in the mechanism of action of thyroid stimulating hormone on glucose oxidation. Biochim Biophys Acta 50:513–520
Field JB, Remer A, Bloom G, Kriss JR (1968) In vitro stimulation by long-acting thyroid stimulator of thyroid glucose oxidation and ^{32}P incorporation into phospholipids. J Clin Invest 47:1553–1560
Field JB, Dekker A, Zor U, Kaneko T (1971) In vitro effects of prostaglandins on thyroid gland metabolism. Ann NY Acad Sci 180:278–282
Field JB, Larsen PR, Yamashita K, Mashiter K, Dekker A (1973) Demonstration of iodide transport defect but normal iodide organification in non-functioning nodules of human thyroid glands. J Clin Invest 52:2404–2417
Field JB, Larsen PR, Yamashita K, Chayoth R (1974) Effect of TSH on iodine metabolism and intermediary metabolism in tissue from patients with Graves̀ disease. J Clin Endocrinol Metab 39:942–949
Field JB, Bloom G, Kerins ME, Chayoth R, Zor U (1975) Activation of protein kinase in thyroid slices by thyroid-stimulating hormone. J Biol Chem 250:4903–4910
Field JB, Bloom G, Chou CY, Kerins ME (1977) Inhibition of TSH stimulation of protein kinase, glucose oxidation and phospholipid synthesis in thyroid slices previously exposed to hormone. J Clin Invest 59:659–665
Field JB, Bloom G, Chou MCY et al. (1978) Effects of thyroid-stimulating hormone on human thyroid carcinoma and adjacent normal tissue. J Clin Endocrinol Metab 47:1052–1058
Field JB, Dekker A, Titus G, Kerins ME, Worden W, Frumess R (1979) In vitro and in vivo refractoriness to thyrotropin stimulation of iodine organification and thyroid hormone secretion. J Clin Invest 64:265–271
Friedman Y, Lang M, Burke G (1977) Inhibition of thyroid adenylate cyclase by thyroid hormone: a possible locus for short-loop negative feedback phenomenon. Endocrinology 101:858–868
Friedman Y, Lang M, Levasseur S, Burke G (1979) Demonstration of a tonic regulatory thyrotropin effect on thyroid function. Endocrinology 104:467–475
Gafni M, Gross J (1975) Effect of elevated doses of thyrotropin on mouse thyroid. Endocrinology 97:1486–1493
Gill DM (1976) The arrangement of subunits of cholera toxin. Biochemistry 15:1242–1248
Gill DL, Marshall NJ, Ekins RP (1978a) Binding of thyrotrophin to receptors in fat tissue. Mol Cell Endocrinol 10:89–102
Gill DL, Marshall NJ, Ekins RP (1978b) Characterization of thyrotrophin binding to specific receptors in human fat tissue. Mol Cell Endocrinol 12:41–51
Gillman AG, Rall TX (1968) The role of adenosine 3′,5′-phosphate in mediating effects of thyroid stimulating hormone on carbohydrate metabolism of bovine thyroid slices. J Biol Chem 243:5872–5881
Giraud A, Couraud F, Lissitsky S (1977) Thyrotropin-induced plasma membrane protein kinase modifications in porcine thyroid cells. Mol Cell Endocrinol 7:297–312
Goldberg N, O'Dea R, Haddox M (1973) Cyclic GMP and phosphodiesterases. Adv Cyclic Nucleotide Res 3:155–223
Goldberg ND, Graff G, Haddox MK, Stephenson JH, Glass DB, Moser ME (1978) Redox modulation of splenic cell soluble guanylate cyclase activity: activation by hydrophilic and hydrophobic oxidants represented by ascorbic acid and dehydroascorbic acids, fatty acid hydroperoxides and prostaglandin endoperoxides. Adv Cyclic Nucleotide Res 9:101–130

Granner DK, Halmi NS (1972) Lack of positive correlation between adenyl cyclase activity and iodide transport in rat thyroids. Endocrinology 91:409–414
Grollman EF, Lee G, Ambesi-Impiombato FS et al. (1977) Effects of thyrotropin on the thyroid cell membrane: hyperpolarization induced by hormone-receptor interaction. Proc Natl Acad Sci USA 74:2353–2356
Habhab O, Bhalla RC, Halmi NS (1977) Adenylate cyclase activity of normal and goitrous rat thyroid. Proc Soc Exp Biol Med 156:382–387
Hall R, Tubman J (1965) Further studies on effects of thyroid stimulating hormone on thyroid nucleotide biosynthesis. J Biol Chem 240:3132–3135
Hall R, Amos J, Ormston BJ (1971) Radioimmunoassay of human serum thyrotrophin. Br Med J 2:582–585
Halmi NS, Granner DK, Doughman DJ, Peters BH, Muller G (1960) Biphasic effect of TSH on thyroidal iodide collection in rats. Endocrinology 67:70–81
Hashizume K, Akasu F, Takazawa K, Endo W, Onaya T (1976) Inhibitory effect of acute administration of excess iodide on the formation of adenosine 3′,5′-monophosphate induced by thyrotropin in mouse thyroid lobes. Endocrinology 99:1463–1468
Haye B, Jacquemin C (1977) Incorporation of [^{14}C]arachidonate in pig thyroid lipids and prostaglandins. Biochim Biophys Acta 487:231–242
Holmes SD, Dirmikis SM, Martin TJ, Munro DS (1978) Effect of human thyroid stimulating hormone and immunoglobulins on adenylate cyclase activity and the accumulation of cyclic AMP in human thyroid membranes and slices. J Endocrinol 79:121–130
Holmes SD, Dirmikis SM, Martin TJ, Munro DS (1979) Evidence that both long-acting thyroid stimulator and long-acting thyroid stimulator-protector stimulate the human thyroid gland. J Endocrinol 80:215–221
Holmes SD, Gitlin J, Titus G, Field JB (1980a) Effect of increased circulating thyroid-stimulating hormone (TSH) on in vitro TSH stimulation of thyroid and adipose tissue. Endocrinology 106:1892–1899
Holmes SD, Titus G, Chou M, Field JB (1980b) Effects of TSH and cholera toxin on the thyroidal adenylate cyclase-cyclic AMP system. Endocrinology 107:2076–2081
Huprikar S, Lang M, Friedman Y, Burke G (1979) Parallel regulation of cyclic AMP-dependent protein kinase and phosphoprotein phosphatase in rat thyroid. FEBS Lett 99:167–171
Ichikawa T, Saito E, Abe Y, Homma M, Muraki T, Ito K (1976) Presence of TSH receptor in thyroid neoplasms. J Clin Endocrinol Metab 42:395–398
Ishii J, Shizume K, Okinaka S (1968) Effect of stimulation of the vagus nerve on the thyroid release of I^{131}-labelled hormones. Endocrinology 82:7–16
Kalderon AE, Sheth V (1978) Secretion and adenylate cyclase in thyroid nodules. Arch Pathol Lab Med 102:381–386
Kaneko T, Zor U, Field JB (1969) Thyroid-stimulating hormone and prostaglandin E_1 stimulation of cyclic 3′,5′-adenosine monophosphate in thyroid slices. Science 163:1062–1063
Kaneko T, Zor U, Field JB (1970) Stimulation of thyroid adenyl cyclase activity and cyclic AMP by LATS. Metabolism 19:430–438
Kaneko Y (1976) Cyclic AMP level of human thyroid cells in monolayer culture. TSH induced refractoriness to TSH action. Horm Metab Res 8:202–206
Karlsson FA, Dahlberg PA (1979) Human thyrotropin receptors are expressed independently of the state of thyroid hormone production in thyroid tissue. Horm Metab Res 11:399–403
Kendall-Taylor P (1972) Adenyl cyclase activity in the mouse thyroid gland. J Endocrinol 52:533–540
Kendall-Taylor P (1973) Effects of LATS and LATS-protector on human thyroid adenyl cyclase activity. Br Med J 3:72–75
Kerkof PR, Tata JR (1969) The subcellular distribution of ^{32}P-labelled phospholipids, ^{32}P-labelled ribonucleic acid and ^{125}I-labelled iodoprotein in pig thyroid slices. Biochem J 112:729–739
Ketelbant-Balasse P, Van Sande J, Neve P, Dumont JE (1976) Time sequence of 3′,5′-cyclic AMP accumulation and ultrastructural changes in dog thyroid slices after acute stimulation by TSH. Horm Metab Res 8:212–215

Knopp J, Stolc V, Tong W (1970) Evidence for the induction of iodide transport in bovine thyroid cells treated with thyroid-stimulating hormone or dibutyryl cyclic adenosine 3′,5′-monophosphate. J Biol Chem 245:4403–4408

Kolata G (1977) Hormone receptors: how are they regulated. Science 196:747–800

Kotani M, Kariya T, Field JB (1975) Studies of thyroid-stimulating hormone binding to bovine plasma membranes. Metabolism 24:959–971

Kowalski K, Sato S, Burke G (1972) Thyrotropin and prostaglandin E_2-responsive adenyl cyclase in thyroid plasma membranes. Prostaglandins 2:441–452

Kuo JF, Greengard P (1969) Cyclic nucleotide-dependent protein kinases. IV. Widespread occurrence of adenosine 3′,5′-monophosphate dependent protein kinase in various tissues and phyla of the animal kingdom. Proc Natl Acad Sci USA 64:1349–1355

Larsen PR, Yamshita K, Dekker A, Field JB (1973) Biochemical observations in functioning human thyroid adenomas. J Clin Endocrinol Metab 36:1009–1018

Ledley FD, Mullin BR, Lee G et al. (1976) Sequence similarity between cholera toxin and glycoprotein hormones: implications for structure activity relationship and mechanism of action. Biochem Biophys Res Commun 69:852–859

Ledley FD, Lee G, Kohn LD, Habig W-H, Hardgree MC (1977) Tetanus toxin interactions with thyroid plasma membranes. J Biol Chem 252:4049–4055

Lee G, Grollman EF, Aloj SM, Kohn LD, Winand RJ (1977) Abnormal adenylate cyclase activity and altered membrane gangliosides in thyroid cells from patients with Graves' disease. Biochem Biophys Res Commun 77:139–146

Levey GS, Pastan I (1970) Activation of thyroid adenyl cyclase by long-acting thyroid stimulator. Life Sci 9:67–73

Levey GS, Roth J, Pastan I (1969) Effect of propranolol and phentolamine on canine and bovine responses to TSH. Endocrinology 84:1009–1015

Lissitzky S, Fayet G, Verrier B, Hennen G, Jaquet P (1973) Thyroid stimulating hormone binding to cultured thyroid cells. FEBS Lett 29:20–24

Maayan ML, Ingbar SH (1968) Epinephrine: effect on uptake of iodine by dispersed cells of calf thyroid gland. Science 162:124–125

Maayan ML, Ingbar SH (1970) Effects of epinephrine on iodine and intermediary metabolism in isolated thyroid cells. Endocrinology 187:588–595

Maayan ML, Debons AF, Krimsky I, Volpert EM, From A, Dawry F, Siclari E (1977) Inhibition of thyrotropin- and dibutyryl cyclic AMP-induced secretion of thyroxine and triidothyronine by catecholamines. Endocrinology 101:284–291

Macchia V, Meldolesi MF, Maselli P (1969) Effect of cyclic 3′,5′-AMP on glucose metabolism in thyroid homogenates. Endocrinology 85:895–898

Manley SW, Bourke JW, Hawker RW (1972) Reversible binding of labelled and nonlabelled thyrotrophin by intact thyroid tissue in vitro. J Endocrinol 55:555–563

Manley SW, Bourke JR, Hawker RW (1974) The thyrotrophin receptor in guinea-pig thyroid homogenate: general properties. J Endocrinol 61:419–436

Marshall NJ, VonBocke S, Malan PG (1975) Studies on isoproterenol stimulation of adenyl cyclase in membrane preparations from bovine thyroid. Endocrinology 96:1520–1524

Mashiter K, Field JB (1974) The thyroid gland. In: Ramwell PW (ed) The prostaglandins, vol II. Plenum, New York, p 49

Mashiter K, Mashiter GD, Hauger RL, Field JB (1973) Effects of cholera and E. coli enterotoxin on cyclic adenosine 3′,5′-monophosphate levels and intermediary metabolism in the thyroid. Endocrinology 92:541–549

Mashiter K, Mashiter G, Field JB (1974) Effects of prostaglandin E_1, ethanol and TSH on the adenylate cyclase activity of beef thyroid membranes and cyclic AMP content of dog thyroid slices. Endocrinology 94:370–376

Matsuzaki S, Kakegawa T, Suzuki M, Hamana K (1978) Thyroid function and polyamines III. Changes in ornithine decarboxylase activity and polyamine contents in the rat thyroid during hyperplasia and involution. Endocrinol Jpn 25:129–139

McKenzie KM (1958) The bioassay of thyrotropin in serum. Endocrinology 63:372–382

McKenzie JM, Zakarija M (1976) A reconsideration of a thyroid stimulating immunoglobulin as the cause of hyperthyroidism in Graves' disease. J Clin Endocrinol Metab 42:778–781

McKenzie JM, Zakarija M, Sato A (1978) Humoral immunity in Graves' disease. Clin Endocrinol 7:31–45
Mehdi SQ, Kriss JP (1978) Preparation of radiolabelled thyroid-stimulating immunoglobulins (TSI) by recombining TSI heavy chains with ^{125}I-labelled light chains: direct evidence that the product binds to the membrane thyrotropin receptor and stimulates adenylate cyclase. Endocrinology 103:296–301
Mehdi SQ, Nussey SS, Gibbons CP, El Kabir DJ (1973) Binding of thyroid stimulators of human thyroid membranes. Biochem Soc Trans 1:1005–1006
Mehdi SQ, Nussey SS, Shindelman JE, Kriss JP (1977) The influence of lipid substitution on thyrotropin-receptor interactions in artificial vesicles. Endocrinology 101:1406–1412
Melander A (1970) Amines and mouse thyroid activity. Acta Endocrinol (Copenh) 65:371–384
Melander A, Ericson LE, Sundler F (1974a) Sympathetic regulation of thyroid hormone secretion. Life Sci 14:237–246
Melander A, Ericson LE, Sundler F, Ingbar SH (1974b) Sympathetic innervation of the mouse thyroid and its significance in thyroid hormone secretion. Endocrinology 94:959–966
Melander A, Ericson LE, Ljunggren JG et al. (1974c) Sympathetic innervation of the normal human thyroid J Clin Endocrinol Metab 39:713–718
Melander A, Sundler F, Westgren U (1975a) Sympathetic innervation of the mouse thyroid and its significance in thyroid hormone secretion. Endocrinology 96:102–106
Melander A, Ranklev E, Sundler F, Westgren U (1975b) Beta$_2$-adrenergic stimulation of thyroid hormone secretion. Endocrinology 97:332–336
Meldolesi MF, Fishman PH, Aloj SM, Kohn LD, Brady RO, (1976) Relationship of gangliosides to structure and function of TSH receptors-their absence on plasma membranes of a thyroid tumor defective in TSH receptor activity. Proc Natl Acad Sci USA 73:4060–4064
Meldolesi M, Fishman PH, Aloj SM et al. (1977) Separation of the glycoprotein and ganglioside components of TSH receptor activity in plasma membranes. Biochem Biophys Res Commun 75:581–588
Merlevede W, Weaver G, Landau BR (1963) Effects of thyrotropic hormone on carbohydrate metabolism in thyroid slices. J Clin Invest 42:1160–1171
Moore M, Wolff J (1973) Binding of prostaglandin E_1 to beef thyroid membranes. J Biol Chem 248:5705–5711
Moore WV, Feldman L (1976) Thyroid-stimulating hormone binding to beef thyroid membranes, role of N-acetylneuraminic acid. J Biol Chem 251:4247–4253
Moore WV, Wolff J (1974) Thyroid stimulating hormone binding to beef thyroid membranes. Relation to adenyl cyclase activity. J Biol Chem 249:6255–6263
Moss J, Vaughan M (1977) Mechanism of action of choleragen, evidence for ADP rebosyltransferase activity with arginine as an acceptor. J Biol Chem 252:2455–2457
Moss J, Osborne JC Jr, Fishman PH, Brewer HB Jr, Vaughan M, Brady RO (1977) Effect of gangliosides and substrate analogues on the hydrolysis of nicotinamide adenine dinucleotide by choleragen. Proc Natl Acad Sci USA 74:74–78
Moss J, Ross PS, Agosto G, Birken S, Canfield RE, Vaughan M (1978) Mechanism of action of choleragen and the glycopeptide hormones: is the nicotinamide adenine dinucleotide glycohydrolase activity observed in purified hormone preparations intrinsic to the hormone. Endocrinology 102:415–419
Mukhtar ED, Smith BR, Pyle GA, Hall R, Vice P (1975) Relation of thyroid-stimulating immunoglobulins to thyroid function and effects on surgery, radioiodine and antithyroid drugs. Lancet 1:713–715
Mullin BR, Fishman PH, Lee G, Aloj SM, Ledley FD, Winand RJ, Kohn LD, Brady RO (1976a) Thyrotropin-ganglioside interactions and their relationship to the structure and function of thyrotropin receptors. Proc Natl Acad Sci USA 73:842–846
Mullin BR, Aloj SM, Fishman PH, Lee G, Kohn LD, Brady RO (1976b) Cholera toxin interactions with thyrotropin receptors on thyroid plasma membranes. Proc Natl Acad Sci USA 73:1679–1683

Mullin BR, Pacuszka T, Lee G, Kohn LD, Brady RO, Fishman PH (1978) Thyroid gangliosides with high affinity for thyrotropin: potential role in thyroid regulation. Science 199:77–79
Muto H, Totsuka Y, Chou MCY, Field JB (1980) Effects of antibodies to bovine thyroid plasma membranes on in vitro basal and thyroid stimulating hormone stimulation of bovine thyroid adenylate cyclase. Endocrinology 107:707–713
Nadler NJ, Sarkar SK, Leblond CP (1962) Origin of intracellular colloid droplets in the rat thyroid. Endocrinology 71:120–129
Nagasaka A, Hidaka H (1976) Human thyroid cyclic nucleotide phosphodiesterase. Its characterization and the effect of several hormones on the activity. Biochim Biophys Acta 438:449–460
Nagataki S (1974) Effect of excess quantities of iodide. In: Greep RO (ed) Handbook of Physiology, vol III, sect 7. American Physiological Society, Washington, DC, p 329
Nistrup Madsen S, Bech K (1979) TSH and thyroid stimulating antibodies (TSAb) activate thyroid adenylate cyclase through different pathways. Acta Med Scand [Suppl] 624:35–42
Ochi Y, Hosoda S, Hachiya T, Yoshimura M, Miyazaki T, Kajita Y (1979) Studies on a receptor assay for an antibody to human thyroid plasma membrane. Acta Endocrinol (Copenh) 91:89–98
Onaya T, Solomon DH (1970) Stimulation by prostaglandin E_1 of endocytosis and glucose oxidation in canine thyroid slices. Endocrinology 86:423–426
Onaya T, Kotani M, Yamada T, Ochi Y (1973) New in vitro tests to detect the thyroid stimulator in sera from hyperthyroid patients by measuring colloid droplet formation and cyclic AMP in human thyroid slices. J Clin Endocrinol Metab 36:859–866
Onaya T, Miyakawa M, Makiuchi M, Furihata R (1978) Altered responsiveness to thyrotropin in thyroid slices of Graves' disease preoperatively treated with excess iodide. J Clin Endocrinol Metab 47:405–409
Orgiazzi J, Chopra IJ, Williams DE, Solomon DH (1975) Evidence for normal thyroidal adenyl cyclase, cyclic AMP-binding and protein-kinase activities in Graves' disease. J Clin Endocrinol Metab 40:248–255
Orgiazzi J, Williams DE, Chopra IJ, Solomon DH (1976a) Human thyroid adenyl cyclase-stimulating activity in immunoglobulin G of patients with Graves' disease. J Clin Endocrinol Metab 42:341–354
Orgiazzi J, Chopra IJ, Solomon DH, Williams DE (1976b) Activite adenylate cyclase des nodules thyroidiens froids. Ann Endocrinol (Paris) 37:107–108
Orgiazzi J, Munari Y, Rostagnat A, Dutrieux N, Mornex R (1977) Adenyl cyclase activity in thyroid carcinomas. Ann Radiol (Paris) 20:757–758
Otten J, Dumont JE (1972) Glucose metabolism in normal human thyroid tissue in vitro. Eur J Clin Invest 2:213–219
Pastan I (1966) The effect of dibutyryl cyclic 3′,5′-AMP on the thyroid. Biochem Biophys Res Commun 25:14–16
Pastan I, Katzen R (1967) Activation of adenyl cyclase in thyroid homogenates by thyroid stimulating hormone. Biochem Biophys Res Commun 29:792–798
Pastan I, Macchia V (1967) Mechanism of thyroid stimulating hormone action. Studies with dibutyryl 3′,5′-adenosine monophosphate and lecithinase C. J Biol Chem 242:5757–5761
Pastan I, Wollman SH (1967) Colloid droplet formation in dog thyroid in vitro. J Cell Biol 35:262–266
Pastan I, Herring B, Johnson P, Field JB (1961) Stimulation in vitro of glucose oxidation in thyroid by acetylcholine. J Biol Chem 236:340–342
Pastan I, Johnson P, Kendig E, Field JB (1963) Pyridine nucleotides in the thyroid. II. The effect of thyroid stimulating hormone, epinephrine, serotonin, acetylcholine, menadione and glucose concentration on the levels of TPN and TPNH. J Biol Chem 238:3366–3368
Pekonen F, Weintraub BD (1979) Thyrotropin receptors on bovine thyroid membranes: two types with different affinities and specificities. Endocrinology 105:352–359
Petersen VB, Dawes JD, Smith BR, Hall R (1977) The interaction of thyroid stimulating antibodies with solubilized human thyrotrophin receptors. FEBS Lett 83:63–67

Pisarev MV, DeGroot LJ, Wilber JF (1970) Cyclic AMP production of goiter. Endocrinology 87:339–342
Pochet R, Van Sande J, Erneux C, Dumont JE (1977) Inhibition of thyroid adenylate cyclase by iodide. FEBS Lett 83:33–36
Powell-Jones CHJ, Thomas CG Jr, Nayfeh SN (1979) Contribution of negative cooperativity to the thyrotropin-receptor interaction in normal human thyroid: kinetic evaluation. Proc Natl Acad Sci USA 76:705
Raff M (1976) Self regulation of membrane receptors. Nature 259:265–266
Rapoport B (1976) Dog thyroid cells in monolayer tissue culture: adenosine 3′,5′-cyclic monophosphate response to thyrotropic hormone. Endocrinology 98:1189–1197
Rapoport B, Adams J (1976) Induction of refractoriness to TSH stimulation in cultured thyroid cells. Dependence on new protein synthesis. J Biol Chem 251:6653–6661
Rapoport B, Adams RJ (1978) Bioassay of TSH using dog thyroid cells in monolayer culture. Metabolism 27:1732–1742
Rapoport B, West MN, Ingbar SH (1975) Inhibitory effect of dietary iodine on the thyroid adenylate cyclase response to thyrotrophin in the hypophysectomized rat. J Clin Invest 56:516–519
Rapoport B, West MN, Ingbar SH (1976) Mechanism of inhibition by iodine of thyroid adenylate cyclase response to thyrotropic hormone. Endocrinology 99:11–22
Rapoport B, Adams RJ, Rose M (1977) Cultured thyroid cell adenosine 3′,5′-cyclic monophosphate response to thyrotropin: loss and restoration of sensitivity to iodide inhibition. Endocrinology 100:755–764
Rodbell M (1978) The role of nucleotide regulatory components in the coupling of hormone receptors and adenylate cyclase. In: Folco G, Paoletti R (eds) Molecular biology and pharmacology of cyclic nucleotides. Elsevier North-Holland Biomedical, Amsterdam Oxford New York, p 1
Rodbell M, Birnbaumer L, Pohl SL, Krans HMJ (1971) The glucagon sensitive adenyl cyclase system in plasma membranes of rat liver. V. An obligatory role of guanyl nucleotides in glucagon action. J Biol Chem 246:1877–1882
Rodesch F, Neve P, Willems C, Dumont JE (1969) Stimulation of thyroid metabolism by thyrotropin, cyclic 3′,5′-AMP, dibutyryl cyclic 3′,5′-AMP and prostaglandin E_1. Eur J Biochem 8:26–32
Roques F, Tirard A, Lissitzky S (1975) Phosphorylation of purified thyroid plasma membranes incubated with ^{32}P-ATP. Mol Cell Endocrinol 2:303–316
Saddock C, Gafni M, Gross J (1978) Effect of iodide on the adenyl cyclase system of the mouse thyroid in vivo. Acta Endocrinol (Copenh) 88:517–527
Sand G, Jortay A, Pocket R, Dumont JE (1976) Adenylate cyclae and protein phosphokinase activities in human thyroid. Comparison of normal glands, hyperfunctioning nodules and carcinomas. Eur J Cancer 12:447–453
Sato S, Szabo M, Kowalski K, Burke G (1972) Role of prostaglandins in thyrotropin action on the thyroid. Endocrinology 90:343–356
Sato S, Yamada T, Furihata R, Makiuchi M (1974) Effect of guanyl nucleotides on the stimulation of adenyl cyclase activity in human thyroid plasma membranes by TSH and PGE_2. Biochim Biophys Acta 332:166–174
Sato A, Zakarija M, McKenzie J (1977) Characteristics of TSH binding to bovine thyroid plasma membranes and the influence of human IgG. Endocr Res Commun 4:95–113
Schleusener H, Kotulla P, Finke R, Soije H, Meinkold H, Adlokofer F, Wenzel KW (1978) Relationship between thyroid status and Graves' disease-specific immunoglobulins. J Clin Endocrinol 47:379–384
Schneider PB (1974) TSH stimulation of ^{32}P incorporation into phospholipids of thyroids from patients with Graves' disease. J Clin Endocrinol Metab 38:148–150
Schumacher M, Hilz H (1978) Protein-bound cAMP, total cAMP and protein kinase activation in isolated bovine thyrocytes. Biochem Biophys Res Commun 80:511–518
Scott TW, Freinkel N, Klein JH, Nitzan M (1970) Metabolism of phospholipids, neutral lipids and carbohydrates in dispersed porcine thyroid cells: comparative effects of pituitary thyrotropin and dibutyryl 3′,5′-adenosine monophosphate on the turnover of individual phospholipids in isolated cells and slices from pig thyroid. Endocrinology 87:754–863

Sherwin JR (1978) Iodide induced suppression of thyrotropin-stimulated adenosine 3',5'-monophosphate production in cat thyroid slices. Horm Res 9:271–278

Sherwin JR, Tong W (1976) Stimulatory actions of TSH and dibutyryl cAMP on transcription and translation in the regulation of thyroidal protein synthesis. Biochim Biophys Acta 425:502–510

Shimizu T, Shishiba Y (1975) Effect of triiodothyronine or iodide on the thyroidal secretion in vitro: inhibition of TSH- and dibutyryl cyclic AMP-induced endocytosis. Endocrinol Jpn 22:55–60

Shishiba Y, Takaishi M, Miyachi Y, Ozawa Y (1975) Alterations of thyroidal responsiveness to TSH under the influence of circulating thyroid hormone: Short feedback regulatory effect. Endocrinol Jpn 22:367–371

Shuman SJ, Zor U, Chayoth R, Field JB (1976) Exposure of thyroid slices to thyroid-stimulating hormone induces refractoriness of the cyclic AMP system to subsequent hormone stimulation. J Clin Invest 57:1132–1141

Smith BR, Hall R (1974a) Thyroid stimulating immunoglobulins in Graves' disease. Lancet 2:427–431

Smith BR, Hall R (1974b) Binding of thyroid stimulators to thyroid membranes. FEBS Lett 42:301–303

Smith BR, Pyle GA, Petersen VB, Hall R (1977) Interaction of thyroid-stimulating antibodies with the human thyrotrophin receptor. J Endocrinol 75:401–407

Spaulding SW, Burrow GN (1972) Several adenosine 3',5'-monophosphate dependent protein kinases in the thyroid. Endocrinology 91:1343–1349

Spaulding SW, Burrow GN (1974) TSH regulation of cyclic AMP-dependent protein kinase activity in the thyroid. Biochem Biophys Res Commun 59:386–391

Spaulding SW, Burrow GN (1975a) B-adrenergic stimulation of cyclic AMP and protein kinase activity in the thyroid. Nature 254:374–349

Spaulding SW, Burrow GN (1975b) Phosphoprotein phosphatase activity in the thyroid. Proc Soc Exp Biol Med 150:568–570

Spaulding SW, Schubart UK (1978) Time course of thyrotropin-dependent protein phosphorylation in thyroid slices. Endocrinology 103:2334–2341

Sugenoya A, Kidd A, Row VV, Volpe R (1979) Correlation between thyroid-displacing activity by immunoglobulins from patients with Graves' disease and other thyroid disorders. J Clin Endocrinol Metab 48:398–402

Suzuki S, Field JB (1978) Thyroid plasma membrane-associated protein kinases: properties and substrates of solubilized and insoluble enzymes. Endocrinology 103:1783–1793

Szabo M, Burke G (1972) Adenosine 3',5'-cyclic phosphate phosphodiesterase from bovine thyroid: isolation and properties of a partially purified soluble factor. Biochim Biophys Acta 284:208–219

Takahashi H, Jiang NS, Gorman CA, Lee CY (1978) Thyrotropin receptors in normal and pathological human thyroid tissue. J Clin Endocrinol Metab 47:870–876

Takasu N, Sato S, Tsukui T, Yamada T, Furihata R, Makiuchi M (1974) Inhibitory action of thyroid hormone on the activation of adenyl cyclase-cyclic AMP system by TSH in human thyroid tissue from euthyroid subjects and thyrotoxic patients. J Clin Endocrinol Metab 39:772–778

Takasu N, Sato S, Tsukui T, Yamada T, Miyakawa M, Makiuchi M, Furihata R (1976) Comparison of PGE_1 and TSH stimulation of cyclic AMP synthesis in thyroid tissue from euthyroid subjects and thyrotoxic patients. J Clin Endocrinol Metab 43:69–79

Takasu N, Charrier B, Mauchamp J, Lissitsky S (1978) Modulation of adenylate cyclase/cyclic AMP response by thyrotropin and prostaglandin E_2 in cultured thyroid cells. Eur J Biochem 90:131–138

Tanini A, Rotella C, Toccafondi R (1978) TSH-responsive adenylate cyclase activity in human thyroid adenomas. In: Folco G, Paoletti R (eds) Molecular biology and pharmacology of cyclic nucleotides. Elsevier/North-Holland Biomedical, Amsterdam Oxford New York, p 307

Tao M, Solas ML, Lipmann F (1970) Mechanism of activation by adenosine 3',5'-monophosphate of a protein phosphokinase from rabbit reticulocytes. Proc Natl Acad Sci USA 67:408–414

Tate RL, Schwartz HI, Holmes JM, Kohn LD (1975a) Thyrotropin receptors in thyroid plasma membranes. J Biol Chem 250:6509–6515
Tate RL, Holmes JM, Kohn LD (1975b) Characteristics of a solubilized TSH receptor from bovine thyroid plasma membranes. J Biol Chem 250:6527–6533
Tell GP, Haour F, Saez JM (1978) Hormonal regulation of membrane receptors and cell responsiveness: a review. Metabolism 27:1566–1592
Teng CS, Rees Smith B, Anderson J, Hall R (1975) Comparison of thyrotrophin receptors in membranes prepared from fat and thyroid tissue. Biochem Biophys Res Commun 66:836–841
Thomas-Morvan C (1978) Effect of TSH on cAMP and cGMP levels in thyroid cancers, adenomas and normal human thyroid tissue. Acta Endocrinol (Copenh) 87:106–113
Thomas-Morvan C, Nataf B, Tubiana M (1974) Thyroid proteins and hormone synthesis in human thyroid cancer. Acta Endocrinol (Copenh) 76:651–669
Tonoue T, Tong W, Stolc V (1970) TSH and dibutyryl-cyclic AMP stimulation of hormone release from rat thyroid glands in vitro. Endocrinology 86:271–277
Uchimura H, Amir SM, Ingbar SH (1979) Failure of organic iodine enrichment to influence the binding of bovine thyrotropin to rat thyroid tissue. Endocrinology 104:1207–1210
Valenta LJ (1976) Thyroid peroxide, thyroglobulin, cAMP and DNA in human thyroid. J Clin Endocrinol Metab 43:466–469
Van Sande J, Dumont JE (1973) Effect of thyrotropin, prostaglandin E_1 and iodide on cyclic 3′,5′-AMP concentration in dog thyroid slices. Biochim Biophys Acta 313:320–328
Van Sande J, Decoster C, Dumont JE (1975a) Control and role of cyclic GMP in the thyroid. Biochem Biophys Res Commun 62:168–175
Van Sande J, Grenier G, Willems C, Dumont JE (1975b) Inhibition by iodide of the activation of the thyroid cyclic 3′,5′-AMP system. Endocrinology 96:781–786
Van Sande J, Pochet R, Dumont JE (1979) Dissociation by cooling of hormone and cholera toxin activation of adenylate cyclase in intact cells. Biochim Biophys Acta 585:282–292
Verrier B, Fayet G, Lissitzky S (1974) Thyrotropin-binding properties of isolated thyroid cells and their purified plasma membranes. Eur J Biochem 42:355–365
Verrier B, Planells R, Lissitzky S (1977) Thyrotropin binding to and adenylate cyclase activity of porcine thyroid plasma membranes. Eur J Biochem 74:243–252
Westermark B, Karlsson FA, Walinder O (1979) Thyrotropin is not a growth factor for human thyroid cells in culture. Proc Natl Acad Sci USA 76:2022–2026
Williams JA (1972) Cyclic AMP formation and thyroid secretion by incubated mouse thyroid lobes. Endocrinology 91:1411–1417
Williams JA, Wolff J (1970) Possible role of microtubules in thyroid secretion. Proc Natl Acad Sci USA 67:1901–1908
Williams JA, Wolff J (1971a) Cytochalasin B inhibits thyroid secretion. Biochem Biophys Res Commun 44:422–427
Williams JA, Wolff J (1971b) Thyroid secretion in vitro: multiple actions of agents affecting secretions. Endocrinology 88:206–217
Wilson BD, Wright RL (1970) Mechanism of TSH action: effects of dibutyryl cyclic AMP on RNA synthesis in isolated thyroid cells. Biochem Biophys Res Commun 41:217–224
Wilson B, Raghupathy E, Tonoue T, Tong W (1968) TSH-like actions of dibutyryl cAMP in isolated bovine thyroid cells. Endocrinology 83:877–884
Winand RJ, Kohn LD (1975) TSH effects on thyroid cells in culture. J Biol Chem 250:6534–6540
Winand R, Wadeleux P (1976) Measurement of cyclic AMP in thyroid cell culture, from thyroids of patients with different thyroid disorders. Arch Int Physiol Biochim 84:1124–1126
Wolff J, Cook GH (1973) Activation of thyroid membrane adenylate cyclase by purine nucleotides. J Biol Chem 248:350–335
Wolff J, Jones AB (1970) Inhibition of hormone-sensitive adenyl cyclase by phenothiazines. Proc Natl Acad Sci USA 65:454–459
Wolff J, Jones AB (1971) The purification of bovine thyroid plasma membranes and the properties of membrane bound adenyl cyclase. J Biol Chem 246:3939–3947
Wolff J, Moore WV (1973) The effect of indomethacin on the response of thyroid tissue to thyrotropin. Biochem Biophys Res Commun 51:34–39

Wolff J, Varrone S (1969) The methylxanthines. A new class of goitrogens. Endocrinology 85:410–414

Wollman SH, Spicer SS, Burstone MS (1964) Localization of esterase and acid phosphatase in granules and colloid droplets in rat thyroid epithelium. J Cell Biol 21:191–201

Yamamoto M, Rapoport B (1978) Studies on the binding of radiolabeled thyrotropin to cultured human thyroid cells. Endocrinology 103:2011–2019

Yamashita K, Field JB (1972a) Effects of long-acting thyroid stimulator and thyrotropin stimulation of adenyl cyclase activity in thyroid plasma membranes. J Clin Invest 51:463–471

Yamashita K, Field JB (1972b) Elevation of cyclic GMP levels in dog thyroid slices caused by acetylcholine and sodium fluoride. J Biol Chem 247:7062–7066

Yamashita K, Field JB (1973) The role of phospholipids in TSH stimulation of adenylate cyclase in thyroid plasma membranes. Biochim Biophys Acta 304:686–692

Yamashita K, Oka H, Kaneko T, Ogata E (1976) Impairment and restoration of response to TSH in dog thyroid slices after treatment with phospholipase-A and Lubrol-PX. Horm Metab Res 8:47–50

Yamashita K, Yamashita S, Ogata E (1977) Regulation of cyclic AMP levels in canine thyroid slices by alpha-adrenergic action. Life Sci 21:607–612

Yamashita K, Yamashita S, Ogata E (1979) Alpha adrenergic interaction with stimulators of cyclic AMP concentrations in canine thyroid slices. Life Sci 24:563–570

Yu SC, Chang L, Burke G (1972) Thyrotropin increases prostaglandin levels in isolated thyroid cells. J Clin Invest 51:1038–1042

Yu S, Friedman Y, Richman R, Burke G (1976) Altered thyroidal responsivity to TSH induced by circulating thyroid hormones. J Clin Invest 57:754–755

Zakarija M, McKenzie J (1975) Cyclic AMP in the thyroid of the rat fed propylthiouracil: in vitro unresponsiveness to thyrotropin. Endocr Res Commun 2:419–429

Zakarija M, McKenzie J (1977) Effects of thyrotropin and thyroid hormones in vivo on thyroid responsiveness to thyrotropin in vitro. Endocr Res Commun 4:343–355

Zakarija M, McKenzie JM (1978) Zoological specificity of human thyroid-stimulating antibody. J Clin Endocrinol Metab 47:249–254

Zor U, Kaneko T, Lowe IP, Bloom G, Field JB (1969) Effect of thyroid-stimulating hormone and prostaglandins on thyroid adenyl cyclase activation and cyclic adenosine 3′:5′-monophosphate. J Biol Chem 244:5189–5192

Zusman DR, Burrow GN (1975) Thyroid-stimulating hormone regulation of ornithine decarboxylase activity in the thyroid. Endocrinology 97:1089–1095

CHAPTER 29

Parathyroid Hormone, Bone and Cyclic AMP*

P. Barrett and H. Rasmussen

Overview

In analyzing the question of whether or not cyclic AMP is a second messenger in the action of parathyroid hormone (PTH) on bone, a review of the available facts gives only a partial answer. The answer is both yes and no. Yes, cyclic AMP is a messenger in the action of parathyroid hormone. No, it is not the sole messenger mediating the effects of this hormone. A major difficulty in giving a more precise answer is that bone is a tissue in which two peptide hormones, PTH and calcitonin (CT), both cause an increase in the tissue content of cyclic AMP even though they induce dramatically different physiological responses. A major hurdle in understanding this apparent paradox is that bone is a heterogenous tissue containing at least three major functional cell types; osteoclasts, osteoblasts, and osteocytes. Physiological data indicates that both PTH and CT alter osteoclastic and osteocytic function, and that PTH, at least, alters osteoblastic function. The problem is further complicated by the fact that there are both immediate (early) and long term (late) effects of these hormones upon bone cell function, and bone cell number. Furthermore, since some studies are carried out in vivo in older animals, and others in fetal bone in tissue culture, the proportion of different cell types differs from one experimental system to another.

The present review focuses upon the early effects of these hormones. The basic facts are that both CT and PTH increase the cyclic AMP content of bone within minutes after their addition, and that particulate fractions from this tissue contain both PTH- and CT-dependent adenylate cyclases. In terms of cell types involved, the major effect of CT upon cyclic AMP metabolism appears to be exerted upon osteoclast-like cells and the major effect of PTH upon osteoblast-like cells, but it remains possible and even likely that PTH also stimulates adenylate cyclase in osteoclastlike cells.

The role of cyclic AMP as the messenger for the PTH-mediated activation of osteoclastic bone resorption is problematical. The strongest evidence in its support is the observation that infusion of dibutyl cyclic AMP or cyclic AMP will increase release of calium from bone. Conversely, pretreatment of animals with phosphodiesterase inhibitors does not enhance the effect of subsequently administered PTH. Likewise, PDE inhibitors do not enhance the resorptive ef-

* Supported by a grant from the National Institute for Arthritis (No. 721M 41 47754, No. 721M 41 47762)

fect of this hormone upon bone grown in tissue culture. Similarly, cholera toxin which greatly augments cyclic AMP production in bone *in vivo or in vitro does not* stimulate bone resorption but actually *inhibits* PTH-mediated resorption. Furthermore, structural analogs of PTH modified at the N-terminus, stimulate bone resorption even though they are incapable of activating adenylate cyclase.

The bulk of evidence favors the view that an increase in cyclic AMP within the osteoclast is neither a sufficient nor necessary feature of PTH-induced bone resorption. On the other hand, there is data that suggests that a rise in intracellular calcium ion concentration is of importance in this PTH-mediated response. These data are: (1) PTH stimulates calcium uptake into bone cells; (2) the magnitude of the resorptive effect of PTH depends upon extracellular calcium concentration; (3) Verapamil, a calcium-channel blocker, inhibits this effect of PTH; and (4) A 23187, a calcium ionophore, under appropriate circumstances increases bone resorption and induces several of the metabolic changes after PTH administration.

The most intriguing unresolved issue is the role of cyclic AMP in regulating osteoclast function. If a rise in cyclic AMP is one of the second messengers in the action of PTH on these cells, as well as being a second messenger for CT, then both hormones must cause the generation of additional messengers to account for their differing effects upon the function of these cells. In the case of PTH, this additional message may well be an increase in the cytosolic calcium ion concentration. In the case of CT it may well be a decrease in cytosolic calcium ion content either due to a direct effect of CT upon the intracellular distribution of calcium, or an indirect effect mediated by an action of CT upon cellular phosphate metabolism.

Resolution of this intriguing question, and answers to many others raised in this review await the development of methods for obtaining homogenous populations of functional bone cells, and/or refined cytochemical methods for analyzing the effects of these hormones upon specific cell types in the intact tissue.

A. Introduction

PTH is a single chain polypeptide secreted by the parathyroid glands. It consists of a single chain of 84 amino acid residues. PTH has two primary physiological functions: (1) the maintenance of the plasma calcium concentration; and (2) the regulation of bone remodeling. The regulation of plasma calcium by PTH is accomplished through its effects on calcium exchange in several organs. Either directly or indirectly, parathyroid hormone increases the renal retention of calcium, enhances intestinal calcium absorption, and accelerates net bone mineral mobilization. Taken together these effects of PTH cause enhanced entry of calcium into the general extracellular fluids and thereby raise the serum calcium concentration. The serum calcium concentration, in turn, regulates PTH secretion. A rise in serum calcium acts to inhibit secretion.

The regulation of the rate of bone turnover by parathyroid hormone occurs over a much longer time span and is accomplished by its effects in activating new bone remodeling units (RASMUSSEN and BORDIER 1974). In both endosteal and cortical bone the constant remodeling of bone takes place at discrete sites and the sequence of cellular events at any one site is always the same. The initial event is the activation of osteoprogenitor cells to preosteoclasts and then to osteoclasts. These latter are responsible for bone resorption. After 10–20 days the osteoclasts disappear, bone resorption ceases, and at the site are found mononuclear cells. At a subsequent time usually weeks, osteoblasts appear at these sites and initiate bone formation which is then followed by mineralization. Thus, the sequence (ARF) activation→resorption→formation is the temporal sequence at each site, and the balance between resorption and subsequent formation determines changes in net bone mass.

Parathyroid hormone acts at least in 2 sites in this sequence. It increases the rate of activation of new units, and it increases the activity of individual osteoclasts. It may also prolong the life time of osteoclasts. In addition, it eventually increases the number of osteoblasts, and may simultaneously suppress the activity of individual osteoblasts. Finally, it appears to act upon osteocytes (bone cells trapped within the bone matrix) and induce them to cause bone resorption.

The major effects of parathyroid hormone on bone relate either to the *short term* action of parathyroid hormone in controlling plasma calcium concentration, or to the *long term* effects of modulating skeletal homeostasis. Our focus here is to consider the evidence for cyclic AMP as an intracellular mediator of the effects of parathyroid hormone on bone. The bulk of experimental information pertaining to the role of cyclic AMP as an intracellular signal derives from experiments designed to study the effect of relatively brief exposure of bone tissue to parathyroid hormone. Hence, it must be kept in mind that conclusions drawn from this data will be most pertainent to our understanding of the more dramatic and rapidly occurring bone resorptive effects of parathyroid hormone. PARSONS has recently emphasized that in addition to duration of exposure, the dose of hormone is an important determinant of the bone's response to PTH. He has grouped the various actions of parathyroid hormone on bone in terms of these dose response characteristics. Anabolic effects of parathyroid hormone, i.e., those promoting bone formation and mineralization, are in general evoked by *continued* exposure to *low levels* of parathyroid hormone, or may appear only as a *delayed* response to the short term exposure to high dose levels (PARSONS 1976). Since the long term effects of low dose PTH administration upon cyclic AMP metabolism in bone have not been studied, only the role of cyclic AMP in the mediation of the short term, high dose effects of PTH on bone metabolism can be evaluated.

In conceptual terms, the notion of cyclic AMP as an intracellular mediator of parathyroid hormone action in skeletal tissue requires that certain fixed relationships exist (with respect to time of onset, dose, agonist specificity, directional coupling) between the hormone induced "resorptive" effect and the activation of adenyl cyclase. We will evaluate these relationships and consider some problems unique to bone and PTH physiology, including the cellular heterogeneity of bone and chemical heterogeneity of circulating PTH, which complicate the assessment of cyclic AMP as a cellular messenger of PTH in bone.

B. Cyclic AMP as Messenger in Bone

As in other tissues, the activation of the adenylate cyclase-cyclic AMP system in bone by parathyroid hormone occurs rapidly (CHASE et al. 1969; CHASE and AURBACH 1970) and precedes in time most of the induced changes in bone cell function. Exceptions to this time sequence are PTH induced alterations in membrane potential and calcium transport (MEARS 1971; DZIAK and STERN 1975). A 10-fold increase in the cyclic AMP content of calvaria can be detected within two minutes after the initiation of a PTH infusion in vivo, before any alteration in the plasma nucleotide level has occurred (NAGATA et al. 1975). In cultured bone cells, a detectable rise in intracellular cyclic AMP occurs as early as 2 min after hormone exposure (PECK et al. 1974a).

Physiological plasma levels of parathyroid hormone (1–84) are within the molar range of 10^{-13} to 10^{-11}. These estimates have been obtained by radioimmunoassay measurements in man (iPTH $\sim 5 \times 10^{-11}$ *M*) (ARNAUD et al. 1971; POTTS et al. 1971) and by calculation from known rates of hormonal clearance and measured rates of secretion (10^{-13}) (PARSONS and REIT 1974; PARSONS et al. 1973). If cyclic AMP is a mediator of the physiologic effects of PTH one would expect the linear part of the log dose response curve for either cyclase activation or cyclic AMP accumulation to fall within the range of hormone concentrations found in the circulation. In most bone cell and skeletal tissue preparations assayed, the linear part of the log dose response curve occurs between $10^{-9}-10^{-6}$ *M* (PARSONS et al. 1975; HEKKELMAN et al. 1975), i.e., 4–5 orders of magnitude greater than the plasma levels of PTH. Equally important is the discrepancy which exists between the dose effect profile of the adenyl cyclase cyclic AMP system and the dose effect profiles of the PTH-induced resorptive effects on bone found both in vivo and in vitro (PARSONS et al. 1975; HEKKELMAN et al. 1975; HERRMANN-ERLEE et al. 1978). In general, changes in bone cell metabolism characteristic of PTH-stimulated bone resorption are demonstrable at PTH concentrations which are ten to one hundred fold lower than those required to increase bone cell cyclic AMP levels (HERRMANN-ERLEE et al. 1978). This would suggest that the PTH-stimulated increase in citrate production, calcium release, phosphate release and histologic evidence of bone resorption proceed in the absence of a rise in cellular cyclic AMP.

Several investigators, using isolated bone cell preparations, have reported methods for pretreatment of cells which result in greater accumulation of cyclic AMP on subsequent challenge with PTH. Pretreatment of isolated bone cells with adenosine results in increased basal levels of cyclic AMP and greater sensitivity to parathyroid hormone stimulation. The effect of adenosine is rapid, readily reversible and, when present at a concentration of 500 μM, a 10-fold rise in cellular cyclic AMP can be elicited by PTH at a concentration of 1 ng/ml ($\sim 10^{-10}$ *M*) (PECK et al. 1974a). This concentration of PTH is without effect in the absence of adenosine. Glucocorticoid addition to fetal cells in *culture* has been shown to potentiate the cyclic AMP response to PTH two to four fold (CHEN and FELDMAN 1978; NG et al. 1979). This effect is glucocorticoid specific, dose dependent (with a half maximal effect at 1.3 n*M* dexamethasone) and involves the modulation of both adenylate cyclase and phosphodiesterase activity. This potentiation effect requires a latent period of at least 24 h. These latter studies suggest that glucocorticoids have a potentially important role in maintaining the responsiveness of the bone adenyl cyclase-cyclic AMP system to parathyroid hormone activation and have been interpreted by some as demonstrating a permissive effect of glucocorticoids in the action of PTH. However, comparisons between dose response curves for cyclase activation and resorptive responses have yet to be made in these systems. In this regard, it is noteworthy that significant metabolic responses to PTH can be detected at physiological doses (10^{-12}–10^{-13}) of parathyroid hormone in bone cell cultures that have been pretreated with prednisolone (WONG 1979b).

If cyclic AMP is an important mediator of PTH induced bone resorption, one would expect it to respond to PTH as a unique signal. In fact, the bone adenyl cyclase-cyclic AMP system can be stimulated by several agonists, i.e., PTH, prostaglandins, or calcitonin. From this lack of specificity and considering the extremely high doses of PTH needed to activate adenyl cyclase, one might suspect that PTH induced cyclase activation is not coupled to *its* biological effects but instead results from non-specific stimulation of receptors of other agonists for which it possesses limited affinity. Other data, however, indicates that calcitonin and prostaglandins act at receptor sites distinct from those involved with PTH action. CHASE and OBERT have shown that trypsin pretreatment selectively impairs PTH sensitive adenylate cyclase activity by 58% without modifying the response of the enzyme to calcitonin or prostaglandin E_2 (CHASE and OBERT 1975). Additionally, maximally effective doses of each agonist (PTH, PGE_2, calcitonin) result in additive increases in bone cell cyclic AMP (RODAN and RODAN 1974; JOHANNES et al. 1974; MARCUS and ORNER 1977). Finally, agents such as propranolol, indomethacin, aspirin and phenylbutazone can inhibit either the effect of salmon calcitonin (JOHANNES et al. 1974) or PGE_2 (MARCUS and ORNER 1977) but do not inhibit the response to PTH.

The observation that both parathyroid hormone and calcitonin are capable of increasing the concentration of cyclic AMP in bone is particularly difficult to reconcile with bone physiology since these hormones have opposing effects on many bone cell functions, most particularly, in terms of acute effects, PTH increases and CT decreases osteoclastic bone resorption. Bone, however, is a tissue made up of many cell types (osteoprogenitor cells, osteocytes, osteoblasts, osteoclasts, as well as possible preosteoblasts and preosteoclasts) each with distinct physiologic functions. It is currently not known whether these two hormones (PTH and CT) are acting at separate receptor sites on the same cell (this would necessitate an additional signal, other than cyclic AMP, to confer specificity), or whether these two hormones are acting at receptor sites on the membranes of different cell types. The question is not whether PTH and CT have actions on the same cell type, because it is clear from a variety of studies that this is true (MEARS 1971; RASMUSSEN and BORDIER 1974) but whether the adenyl cyclase coupled responses of these hormones occur within the same cell.

To distinguish between these two possibilities requires the development of homogeneous bone cell systems which can be independently challenged by each hormone. Recently experimental systems have been developed with this goal in mind, but the data generated from several laboratories does not as yet support a single conclusion. COHN and associates (LUBEN et al. 1976) have investigated the effect of parathyroid hormone and calcitonin on cyclic AMP levels in subcultured cell populations released from mouse calvaria by sequential enzymatic digestion. Cells that are released early have been provisionally identified as osteoclasts by their metabolic characteristics. Exposure of these cells to calcitonin (110 ng/ml) results in a 300% increase in their cyclic AMP content. These same cell cultures, however, respond equally well to a parathyroid hormone (200 ng/ml) challenge. Cells that are released later have been *functionally* identified as osteoblasts. These osteoblast-like cells respond to parathyroid hormone with a dramatic 1200% increase in their cyclic AMP content, but do not show any activation of the adenylate cyclase cyclic AMP system by calcitonin.

Other separation techniques have also made use of the anatomical distribution of bone cells in fetal rat calvaria. Calvaria stripped of their periostea, and bone cells dispersed from them are more enriched in cells which respond to PTH 1–34 (400% at 100 ng/ml) than are periosteal segments and periosteal cells (LUBEN et al. 1976).

In contrast, salmon calcitonin (2.5–25 ng/ml) induces a 50%–200% enhancement of the cyclic AMP levels in periosteal tissue but produces no detectable rise in cyclic AMP within calvaria cells (PECK et al. 1977). While periosteal tissue contains a large percentage of fibroblasts (PUZAS et al. 1979) this difference in adenyl cyclase responsiveness appears to be unrelated to their presence since skin fibroblasts cultured similarly are calcitonin insensitive. These distinctions suggest that the adenylate cyclase-cyclic AMP systems of various cell types may be selectively responsive to one agonist or the other but they are not absolute and appear to depend upon the assay conditions. Thus, differential hormone response varies with length of time of culture (PECK et al. 1977) and hormone concentration. SMITH and JOHNSTON (1974, 1975), using higher doses of agonists, (PTH 1–84 4 ug/ml, calcitonin 8 ug/ml) have reported a complete cross over of activities in calvaria stripped of their periostea. When assayed in the presence of EGTA and DMSO, a cyclase response in the periosteum could be evoked by both hormones. Since no technique to date has achieved the separation of morphologically distinct cell types, it seems premature to assign adenyl cyclase responses induced by these two hormones to separate or specific cell types within bone. Thus, from this type of an examination, it is not possible to determine if an additional signal may be necessary to confer specificity to the intracellular response to parathyroid hormone and calcitonin.

C. Heterogeneity of Circulating PTH

A final important question regarding the specificity of cyclic AMP as a mediator of PTH action on bone concerns which of the multiple molecular forms of circulating PTH is the principal agonist of the effects of PTH on bone. While PTH with an 84 amino acid sequence is the dominant hormonal form secreted by the parathyroid gland (HABENER et al. 1971), it is only one of the many forms of the hormone present in the circulation (BERSON and YALOW 1968). The enzymatic cleavage of PTH by peripheral tissues leads to the generation of several large metabolites (5,000–7,000 MW) and (3,000–4000 MW) (SEGRE et al. 1974, 1978; HRUSKA et al. 1975, 1978; NEUMAN et al. 1975a, b) which are either further degraded in situ or are returned to the circulation. The physiological significance of the peripheral metabolism of PTH is not yet understood. Amino terminal fragments of PTH greater than 28 amino acids in length have substantial biological activity in many different bioassay systems, i.e., chick hypercalcemic assay (PARSONS et al. 1975), rat renal adenyl cyclase assay (TREGEAR et al. 1973; ROSENBLATT et al. 1976, 1978), skeletal cyclic AMP accumulation (HERRMANN-ERLEE et al. 1978).

Recent data suggest that PTH 1–84 and PTH 1–34 may not be equivalent agonists in liver (MARTIN et al. 1976) and bone (MARTIN et al. 1978, 1979). This would suggest that the peripheral metabolism of PTH could be an important determinant of the action of PTH.

At present, there is some debate in the literature concerning the true agonist for bone. MARTIN et al. (1978) have been unable to detect an arterio-venus (A-V) difference of PTH by radioimmunoassay in an isolated tibial bone perfusion system, when PTH 1–84 is infused. In contrast, they have measured a 36% extraction ratio across the bone when PTH 1–34 is infused. Based on this data they have proposed that PTH 1–84 is not the true agonist for skeletal tissue. It is additionally noteworthy that in these studies the infusion of PTH 1–84 also failed to elicit the *expected* increase in cyclic AMP. Only a 50%–80% increase in perfusate cyclic AMP was measured compared to the 5-fold enhancement evoked by the infusion of PTH 1–34. In contrast, GOLTZMAN has demonstrated the potentiation of the adenyl cyclase-enzyme by 1–84 PTH in skeletal tissue prepared from rabbit calvaria to be equivalent on a molar basis to the synthetic PTH 1–34 analog, when assessed under conditions shown to prevent detectable hormone proteolysis (GOLTZMAN 1978). These data are in good agreement with data from similar studies measuring adenylate cyclase activity in renal cortical tissue (GOLTZMAN et al. 1976) and suggest that cleavage of PTH 1–84 is not required for cyclase activation in either tissue. Moreover, in rat calvarium, native PTH 1–84 demonstrates 30% more activity than its synthetic peptide 1–34 in enhancing cyclic AMP content. Parallelism of the long-dose response curves of these two agonists suggests a similar-mode of action (HERRMANN-ERLEE et al. 1978). These findings are supported by the studies of NEWMAN, who followed the distribution and metabolism of fully active labeled PTH 1–84 in bone tissue as a function of time after its injection in vivo in rat. chicken and dog. Diaphyses of femora and humeri dissected free of marrow, were demineralized, homogenized, and chromatographed under denaturing conditions (NEUMAN et al. 1975 a, b). Ten min after the injection of PTH 1–84, 50% of the hormone extracted by bone chromatographed as the intact 1–84 species. At 60 min, the percentage of the total radioactivity in bone that chromatographed as PTH 1–84 was reduced to 20%, a reduction consistent with evidence that skeletal tissue metabolizes PTH (FREITAG et al. 1979). Thus, at present, the bulk of experimental evidence indicates that PTH 1–84 is probably the true agonist in skeletal tissue.

D. Correlations Between Responses to PTH and Changes in cAMP

It is self-evident that establishment of a correlation between an induced change in cyclic AMP concentration and an induced change in bone cell function critically depends upon the sensitivity in measuring each event. In several tissues it is known that significant amounts of cyclic AMP are bound to intracellular receptor proteins (HARBON et al. 1976; DUFAU et al. 1977; KNIGHT 1975). The concentration of cyclic

AMP under basal conditions is within the range of 10^{-7} to 10^{-6} *M* if a uniform distribution within the cell is assumed (AURBACH and CHASE 1976), and this is in the same range as the K_m for cyclic AMP of several cyclic AMP dependent protein kinases. Hence, a small change in cyclic AMP concentration or cellular distribution may result in a significant change in enzyme activity. Recent studies have provided evidence for a single class of cyclic AMP binding sites in the cytosol of bone cells with an affinity of 5.9×10^{-8} *M* (MARCUS et al. 1979).

Incubation of intact bone cells with PTH results in a dose dependent depletion of unoccupied cyclic AMP binding sites and a rise in intracellular cyclic AMP. However, PTH dependent cyclic AMP binding site depletion reaches a plateau at an intracellular cyclic AMP concentration 50% below the maximum inducible level in this system. While receptor occupancy changes in response to the ambient concentration of cyclic AMP, their data would suggest critical fluctuations in binding site occupancy may occur with only modest changes in total intracellular cyclic AMP. Therefore, lack of a correlation between alterations in cellular cyclic AMP and alterations in bone cell function induced in response to PTH may not necessarily be evidence against AMP as an intracellular mediator.

Important evidence in support of cyclic AMP as an intracellular messenger of parathyroid hormone is the ability of exogenous cyclic AMP, Db cyclic AMP and theophylline to mimic the effects of parathyroid hormone on serum and urinary concentrations of calcium, phosphorus and hydroxyproline in the parathyroidectomized animal (WELLS and LLOYD 1967, 1969; RASMUSSEN et al. 1968).

I. Hypercalcemic Effect of PTH in vivo

Before considering this data in detail, several important aspects of bone physiology must be recalled. The mobilization of skeletal calcium via osteoclastic and osteocytic resorption is acknowledged as one of the principal means by which PTH elevates plasma calcium during long term hypersecretion (MUNSON et al. 1963; ARNAUD et al. 1967; HIRSCH and MUNSON 1969). However, minute to minute maintenance of plasma calcium does not appear to involve the breakdown of calcified bone matrix. This is clear in at least two experimental situations where the physiological and not the pharmacological effects of PTH have been investigated. In the adult rat, the immediate (0–2 h) decrease in plasma calcium following acute parathyroidectomy does not appear to be associated with a decrease in bone resorption since urinary hydroxyproline excretion remains unchanged (KALU et al. 1974). In the awake dog, during low dose PTH infusions (100 ng/kg), plasma calcium levels rise without any accompanying increase in plasma phosphate or urinary hydroxyproline excretion (PARSONS 1974). These facts do not exclude the participation of bone in the acute changes in plasma calcium, but suggest that resorption is not involved in controlling these changes. On theoretical grounds, NEUMAN has calculated (NEUMAN and RAMP 1971) that in the adult man a 10% rise in the calcium concentration of the ECF could be accomplished by a net transfer of only 0.3% of the surface mineral or 0.1% of the total bone mineral of the skeleton. A significant alteration in the concentration of plasma calcium (10%) can be effected by a miniscule change in the fluxes of calcium in and out of bone without invoking mechanisms of resorption or bone formation. In agreement with this are the experimental findings that the rise in serum calcium after parathyroid administration in the hamster (BIDDULPH and GALLIMORE 1974) and the fall in serum calcium after parathyroidectomy in the rat (KALU et al. 1974) could not be accounted for quantitatively by alterations in the rate of urinary calcium excretion. In both of these systems, bone was considered as important and of equal sensitivity to the kidney in regulating the acute changes (0–2 h) of plasma calcium (PARFITT 1979).

Single injections of theophylline (WELLS and LLOYD 1967) and Db-cyclic AMP (WELLS and LLOYD 1969) will retard the fall in serum calcium following acute parathyroidectomy and in the chronically parathyroidectomized animal, will cause a rise in serum calcium with a time course similar to that of PTH induced hypercalcemia. Bilateral nephrectomy does not alter this effect of theophylline suggesting that it does not depend upon a renal action for its effect. Moreover, pretreatment with theophylline enhances the hypercalcemic effect of Db-cyclic AMP which is itself antagonized by calcitonin, or imidazole which is in agreement with the known antagonism of these agents for the hypercalcemic effect of parathyroid hormone (MUNSON and HIRSCH 1968). However, while pretreatment with theophylline enhances the hypercalcemic effect of Db-cyclic AMP it does not potentiate the effect of a submaximal dose of PTH.

The hypercalcemic response to parathyroid hormone is coupled to a latent rise in urine calcium when the filtered load of calcium exceeds the maximum tubular reabsorptive capacity of the nephron. Simultaneous with this hypercalciuria is an increased excretion of hydroxyproline (RASMUSSEN et al. 1967) as calcium is mobilized from bone matrix (RASMUSSEN et al. 1968).

Infusions of Db-cyclic AMP lead to an immediate rise in the rate of urinary phosphate excretion followed by a delayed rise in the excretion of both urinary calcium and hydroxyproline (RASMUSSEN and TENENHOUSE 1968). These effects upon calcium and hydroxyproline mobilization from bone are blocked by CT administration in the same manner in which TCT blocks PTH induced effects. Additional specificity is suggested by the fact that infusions of closely related nucleotides (5′ AMP, 2′3′ AMP, 5′ GMP) do not induce similar changes in urinary electrolyte patterns. However, several discrepancies exist between the actions of PTH and Db-cyclic AMP.

During early infusion times (2–6 h) Db-cyclic AMP induces changes in Ca and phosphate fluxes similar to those induced by PTH quantitatively and qualitatively, but during later infusion times (greater than 18 h) Db-cyclic AMP is less effective than PTH in mobilizing calcium and hydroxyproline from bone. Moreover, theophylline does not potentiate the hypercalciuric and phosphaturic actions of submaximal doses of PTH, but is effective in augmenting these effects induced by Db-cyclic AMP. These data suggest that Db-cyclic AMP is a less potent stimulator of bone resorption than PTH. The effect of Db-cyclic may be mediated by a mechanism different than that controlled by PTH.

Following a brief intravenous infusion of parathyroid hormone in the parathyroidectomized rat, a marked and transient (30 min) increase in the plasma levels of cyclic AMP can be detected, before the rise in serum calcium is manifest (NAGATA et al. 1975). This influx of cyclic nucleotide into plasma is largely from bone. Calvarial cyclic AMP levels rise a dramatic 10 fold within two min before any change in plasma nucleotide levels can be detected. PTH induced changes in plasma nucleotide levels can be demonstrated in the parathyroidectomized-nephrectomized rat. Low dose infusions of parathyroid hormone, >0.05 U/100 g body wt., elevate the concentration of calcium in the plasma but are without effect in altering plasma levels of cyclic AMP or calvarial cyclic AMP content. Additionally, a rise in serum calcium evoked by the administration of higher submaximal doses of PTH i.p., or by EGTA induced endogenous PTH secretion can not be correlated with changes in cyclic nucleotide levels.

On the other hand, when high doses of PTH are infused, >10 U PTH/100 g body wt., a good quantitative correlation can be made between the effect of PTH on cyclic AMP metabolism and its effects on calcium mobilization. This coupling between enhanced production of cyclic AMP and calcium mobilization is not absolute.

Prior calcitonin treatment (NAGATA et al. 1975) and vitamin D-deficiency (KAKUTA et al. 1975) prevent the rise in serum calcium elicited by parathyroid hormone but do not modify the induced increases in the concentration of cyclic AMP in the plasma and bone compartments. However, like PTH, Db-cyclic AMP is without effect in inducing a hypercalcemic (RASMUSSEN et al. 1963) and a hypercalciuric response (RASMUSSEN and FEINBLATT 1971) in the D-deficient animal.

II. Demineralization Effect of PTH in vitro

A direct assessment of the short term demineralization response of skeletal tissue to parathyroid hormone has been studied in vitro in organ culture systems of calvaria or fetal limbs (RAISZ 1965a; KLEIN and RAISZ 1971; HERRMANN-ERLEE and MEER 1974). Assessment of PTH-induced demineralization has been made either by direct measurement of the change in the stable calcium concentration of the organ culture medium (HERRMANN-ERLEE and MEER 1974) or by the measurement of radioactive calcium released from isotopically prelabeled bone (KLEIN and RAISZ 1971). PTH causes a dose dependent acceleration of the rate of calcium and phosphate release from bone. This effect requires a latency period of 24 h (RAISZ 1976). Db-cyclic AMP and aminophylline do not reproduce the dose dependent effect of PTH on bone demineralization, but effect it in a biphasic way. Low concentrations (0.1–0.4 m*M*) of these agents induce a significant release of calcium and phosphate from bone, while higher concentrations (0.5 m*M*–1.0 m*M*) have the opposite effect, causing a significant uptake of calcium into bone (VAES 1968; HERRMANN-ERLEE and MEER 1974) or an inhibition or radiolabeled calcium release. No histological evidence of drug induced cell toxicity can be found at these higher doses of Db-cyclic AMP (HERRMANN-ERLEE and MEER 1974). The addition of Db-cyclic AMP and theophylline to cultures incubated with submaximal doses of PTH does not potentiate the demineralization response but instead results in a decrease in the release of calcium and phosphate from bone. This antagonistic effect of Db-cyclic AMP and aminophylline persists at all concentrations despite increased levels of cyclic AMP. These data would suggest that either maximally high levels of intracellular cyclic AMP or persistently high levels of intracellular cyclic AMP inhibit PTH induced demineralization. Consistent with this notion is the effect of cholera toxin on PTH induced calcium release from bone in culture (NAGATA et al. 1977). Cholera toxin, a potent stimulator of the adenylate cyclase enzyme in a variety of mammalian cells and membranes (FINKELSTEIN 1973; GILL 1975), causes a rise in cyclic AMP content of bone. This increase is of slower onset and of longer duration than that after PTH addition. Levels of cyclic AMP measured at 5–7 h after the addition of cholera toxin are comparable in magnitude to those found in the tissue exposed to PTH for 5 min. Cholera toxin itself does not cause the demineralization of calcium from bone and antagonizes the demineralizing effect to PTH.

Structural analogs of parathyroid hormone in which the amino terminus has been modified have been used in organ culture systems to investigate the coupling between the effect of parathyroid hormone on cellular cyclic AMP and its effect on bone demineralization. The activities of desamino-PTH (1–34), PTH (2–34), and PTH (3–34) in enhancing the cyclic AMP content of calvaria are a scant 10% of the activity of PTH (1–34) (HERRMANN-ERLEE et al. 1978). These analogs of PTH modified at the amino terminus have also been shown to have little effect in stimulating cyclic AMP production in the rat renal adenylate cyclase system (GOLTZMAN et al. 1975). In contrast, all of these fragments are active in inducing bone demineralization in organ culture. On a molar basis they are less potent agonists than PTH 1–34 or native PTH 1–84 in stimulating the release of calcium from bone but show significant activity at concentrations that produce esentially no increase in bone cell cyclic AMP. In addition, the slopes of their log dose response curves are similar to that of native PTH 1–84. The differential activity of these agents expressed in bone in organ culture supports previously made observations about the differential activity of PTH (2–34) in the renal cortical adenyl cyclase assay and in the in vivo chick hypercalcemic assay. Unlike the renal adenylate cyclase assay, this fragment (PTH 2–34) is 65% as active on a molar basis as native PTH 1–84 in vivo in inducing a rise in serum calcium in young challenged animals (PARSONS et al. 1975).

The differential activities displayed by these fragments in these two different bioassay systems was originally interpreted as indicating different structural requirements of the receptors for parathyroid hormone in kidney and bone; however, in light of their differential activities within a single tissue (bone) this explanation is not tenable. One might conclude from the bone organ culture data that there exist several classes of PTH receptors not all of which are coupled to the activation of adenyl cyclase. Thus, the structural requirements dictated by a receptor in the membrane would determine if the adenylate cyclase-cyclic AMP system were activated.

While these synthetic PTH analogs demonstrate little capacity to stimulate cyclic AMP production in bone and kidney, it is noteworthy that they can antagonize PTH-induced adenyl cyclase activation (GOLTZMAN et al. 1975). Furthermore, these analogs can inhibit specific binding of parathyroid hormone to renal cortical membranes (SEGRE et al. 1979). Moreover, desamino-ala-1PTH 1–34, which is virtually inactive in stimulating adenylate cyclase activity in canine renal membranes, will demonstrate partial agonist activity in the presence of Gpp(NH)p, the non-hydrolyzable analog of GTP (GOLTZMAN et al. 1978), producing 40% of the maximal stimulation of cyclase activity evoked by native PTH 1–84. Therefore, it appears that these analogs share some affinity for the same receptors as native PTH 1–84, that there is not a fixed linkage between hormone binding at these receptors and adenylate cyclase activation, and that in the absence of coupling between hormone binding and cyclase activation, parathyroid hormone fragments can nevertheless stimulate bone resorption.

III. Metabolic Effects of PTH in Bone

Demineralization is only one part of the bone resorptive response evoked by PTH. Several metabolic alterations in bone are also evoked by this hormone. These include increased lactic acid and citric acid production, increased glucose consumption and acid phosphatase activity, decreased collagen synthesis and alkaline phosphatase activity, and increased hyaluronate synthesis (RAISZ 1976). These alterations in bone cell function are an integral and important part of the action of parathyroid hormone on bone since the net removal of matrix, in addition to mineral, is required for bone remodeling and for the long term maintenance of serum calcium.

Of additional importance is the fact that these alterations of metabolic activity can be studied in isolated bone cell systems, where the correlation between cyclic AMP production and cell activation can be more readily evaluated at physiological doses of PTH and eventually in the absence of heterogeneous cell types. Furthermore, by examining a metabolic function characteristic of an individual bone cell type which is modulated by calcitonin and parathyroid hormone in opposing ways, it should be possible to determine if cyclic AMP is a unique or common intracellular message.

1. Glucose Metabolism

Unlike most tissues, bone exhibits an anaerobic pattern of glucose metabolism even in the presence of oxygen. Thus, rates of glucose utilization are higher and rates of oxygen consumption lower than those found in kidney or liver when measured on the basis of cell nitrogen or DNA (PECK and DIRKSEN 1966). As much as 60%–80% of the glucose utilized appears as lactic acid (COHN and FORSCHER 1962; NISBET et al. 1970). Approximately 85% of the glucose utilized goes via the Embden-Meyerhof pathway while 15% is utilized by the pentose shunt. Parathyroid hormone added to bone in culture markedly increases the consumption of glucose and the accumulation of citric and lactic acid. Whereas the amount of lactic acid accumulated/mole of glucose consumed is not altered in response to PTH, PTH treated calvaria accumulate more citrate/mole glucose consumed that control calvaria. This finding may reflect either a diversion of glycolytic products to citrate (NISBET et al. 1970) or an inhibition of citrate oxidation (LUBEN and COHN1976). Calvaria cultured under anoxic conditions also demonstrate increased rates of glucose consumption and lactate accumulation similar to levels attained with parathyroid hormone, but unlike PTH treated calvaria, citrate accumulation is not increased (NISBET et al. 1970). Moreover, it is difficult to reconcile concomitant increases in both citrate and lactate accumulation when PTH is without effect on the oxidation or production of other tricarboxylic acid intermediates and is without effect on altering oxygen consumption (WOLINSKY and COHN 1969) unless these effects are occuring within different bone cell types.

2. Lactate Production

Parathyroid hormone is not a unique hormonal potentiator of lactate flux in calvaria. Calcitonin and epinephrine are less active, but can reproduce this action of PTH on bone. Db-cyclic AMP and phosphodiesterase inhibitors (aminophylline and Ro 20–2926) increase lactate flux in a dose dependent and reversible manner. Unlike hormonal stimulation, however, stimulation by these agents requires their continued presence despite the fact that nucleotide levels are elevated to the same degree. While, on a molar basis, Db-cyclic AMP is less effective than PTH in stimulating lactate flux, it is effective in potentiating submaximal doses of parathyroid hormone (HEKKELMAN et al. 1975; HERRMANN-ERLEE and MEER 1974).

Structural analogs of PTH, desamino PTH 1–34, PTH 2–34, PTH 3–34, which weakly stimulate cyclic AMP production, weakly stimulate lactate flux (HERRMANN-ERLEE et al. 1978). While calcitonin (NISBET et al. 1970) and Verapamil (HERRMANN-ERLEE et al. 1977) are powerful inhibitors of PTH induced demineralization, they are without effect on PTH induced lactate accumulation.

It would appear, then, that PTH stimulated lactate accumulation is an adenylate cyclase coupled response which is not directly linked to bone demineralization.

3. Citrate Production

The previously mentioned ability of parathyroid hormone to enhance citrate production in bone has been studied by either measuring net citrate accumulation or the rate of decarboxylation of ^{14}C-citrate. Pretreatment of bone cells by exposure to Verapamil or calcitonin (HERRMANN-ERLEE et al. 1977; NISBET et al. 1970), inhibits the PTH induced accumulation of citrate without affecting the rise in intracellular cyclic AMP, demonstrating that these responses are dissociable. Moreover, if this effect of PTH is examined by measuring the rate of ^{14}C-citrate decarboxylation, calcitonin is not antagonist. On the other hand, PTH induced inhibition of $^{14}CO_2$ yield from ^{14}C-citrate can be duplicated by Db-cyclic AMP, despite the fact that other hormones or basic proteins are without effect (WOLINSKY and COHN 1969; CHU et al. 1971). The inhibition by PTH of $^{14}CO_2$ released is dose related and cannot be evoked with biologically inactive (oxidized) hormone. While the inhibition of $^{14}CO_2$ production represents a good in vitro bioassay system for parathyroid hormone it may not represent a direct effect of PTH on citrate decarboxylation. A decrease in $^{14}CO_2$ recovery would be expected if the specific activity of the labeled substrate pool were diluted. Since net accumulation of citrate is enhanced following a PTH challenge, decreased $^{14}CO_2$ production could indicate net synthesis of citrate. Moreover, this interpretation is consistent with the experimental observation that in isolated bone cells the effect of PTH on citrate decarboxylation is not immediate but requires several hours to develop (WONG et al. 1978). On the other hand, NAGATA and RASMUSSEN have provided substantial evidence for a direct inhibitory effect by PTH on isocitrate dehydrogenase activity in the kidney (NAGATA and RASMUSSEN 1968) based on measurements of the pattern of changes of the Krebs cycle intermediates following a PTH challenge in vivo. Comparable studies in bone have not been reported.

The effect of PTH on citrate accumulation in bone has been localized to bone cell subcultures that functionally behave as osteoblasts (LUBEN et al. 1976, 1977).

These cells make collagen, possess PTH sensitive alkaline phosphatase activity and do not enhance the rate of calcium and phosphorus release when layered on dead bone (COHN and WONG 1978).

Because these cell cultures show a cyclic AMP response to parathyroid hormone but not to calcitonin, they provide a valuable system in which to investigate the dependence of $^{14}CO_2$ production on intracellular cyclic AMP. However, since this PTH induced activity is not antagonized by calcitonin, they do not provide a system to investigate the specificity of cyclic AMP as an intracellular message.

In cultures of these osteoblast-like cells, PTH inhibits [^{14}C]-citrate decarboxylation in a dose dependent way within a concentration range of 10^{-7} *M* to 10^{-10} *M* PTH (WONG 1979a, b). At concentrations of medium calcium above 0.2 m*M*, Db-cyclic AMP at 10^{-4} *M* inhibits [^{14}C]-citrate decarboxylation as effectively as 2×10^{-8} *M* PTH. The potentiating effect of Db-cyclic AMP on a submaximal dose of PTH has not been reported nor have the effects of phosphodiesterase inhibitors been studied. However, in the absence of medium calcium, [^{14}C]-citrate decarboxylation is not inhibited, either by parathyroid hormone or Db-cyclic AMP, yet under these incubation conditions, parathyroid hormone enhances intracellular cyclic AMP as effectively as in the presence of 1.8 m*M* calcium. Furthermore, raising medium calcium from 0–5 m*M* incrementally inhibits [^{14}C]-citrate decarboxylation without enhancing intracellular cyclic AMP. A similar inhibition of [^{14}C]-citrate decarboxylation can be effected using $1{,}25(OH)_2D_3$, the most active metabolite of vitamin D (COHN and WONG 1978), in the absence of a change in cellular cyclic AMP.

It has been concluded by these authors that, as in the kidney so in the bone, calcium ion can reproduce the metabolic effects of parathyroid hormone in the absence of detectable changes in cellular AMP content.

4. Hyaluronate Synthesis

In organ cultures, the incorporation of [^{3}H]-glucosamine into hyaluronate during bone resorption has been used as another metabolic indicator of PTH activity. Parathyroid hormone produces a rapid, dose related increase in the incorporation of [^{3}H]-glucosamine into hyaluronate. This increase in labeling represents enhanced net synthesis not simply accelerated turnover (LUBEN et al. 1974). Parathyroid hormone stimulation of hyaluronate synthesis persists after PTH is removed from the incubation medium and is blocked by calcitonin, effects similar to that of PTH on mineral release (LUBEN and COHN 1976).

This action of parathyroid hormone has been localized to bone cells which in culture behave as osteoclasts. These cells have significant acid phosphatase activity and enhance the rate of release of Ca and phosphate when layered on dead bone. These activities are sensitive to stimulation by PTH. This later effect of PTH (200 ng/ml) is antagonized by calcitonin (110 ng/ml) as is PTH stimulated hyaluronate synthesis. Activities such as alkaline phosphatase, prolyl hydroxylase, and citrate oxidation are marginal in these cell cultures and are not sensitive to PTH inhibition (LUBEN et al. 1976, 1977). Unlike the functional osteoblast cultures, these subcultures respond to both parathyroid hormone and calcitonin with an equal potentiation (300% of control) of cellular cyclic AMP. However, because these cells in culture cannot be morphologically identified as osteoclasts, it is at present difficult to know if both of these hormones are in fact cyclic AMP agonists in the osteoclast. Since the rate of hyaluronate synthesis responds to both parathyroid hormone and calcitonin, in a homogeneous cell culture it should be possible to determine if cyclic AMP acts as a common signal for both hormones.

PTH stimulates hyaluronate synthesis in a dose dependent fashion within the range of 10^{-8} to 10^{-10} M (WONG 1979a, b). A near maximal effect is duplicated by Db-cyclic AMP at 10^{-4} M. Db-cyclic AMP is without effect in the absence of medium calcium, as is parathyroid hormone. However, under zero calcium conditions, parathyroid hormone enhancement of intracellular cyclic AMP is not impaired. In addition, hyaluronate synthesis can be stimulated by elevations in medium calcium in the absence of any detectable increase in bone cell cyclic AMP (WONG et al. 1978).

These data would again suggest that calcium is an important mediator of many PTH effects and that the generation of cyclic AMP alone is an insufficient signal to induce them.

5. Collagen Synthesis

Parathyroid hormone has an inhibitory effect on bone collagen synthesis. In vitro incorporation of [^{3}H]-proline into collagenase-digestible protein is inhibited by PTH, in a dose-dependent manner, at doses of PTH (100 ng/ml) which stimulate resorption in vitro. This inhibitory effect is specific for bone collagen. The incorporation of label into non-collagen protein or cartilage is unaltered by PTH. Moreover, this effect can be ascribed to an inhibition of synthesis and is not the result of changes in amino acid uptake, precursor pool size or degradation of newly synthesized collagen (DIETRICH et al. 1976). PTH has also been reported to cause a marked inhibition of collagen prolyl hydroxylase in bone cells (COHN and WONG 1978). Parathyroid hormone inhibition of collagen synthesis can be reproduced by concentration of Db-cyclic AMP (<0.3 mM) which are effective in promoting demineralization in vitro. PTH-inhibition of collagen synthesis is not antagonized by calcitonin at concentrations which inhibit PTH-induced calcium release.

These data would suggest that cyclic AMP may be involved in the mediation of this effect of PTH. Whether PTH-inhibition of collagen production occurs at the level of RNA synthesis or subsequent translational steps is unsolved.

6. RNA Synthesis

There is good evidence that PTH produces significant alteration in RNA metabolism in bone. The autoradiographic results of BINGHAM et al. (1969) demonstrated a specific decrease in the labeling of osteoblastic RNA in vivo following treatment of rabbits with PTH. In addition, suppression of the incorporation of ^{3}H-uridine into bulk RNA in vitro has been demonstrated in "osteoblastic cells" released from periosteum stripped calvaria (SMITH and JOHNSTON 1973).

In contrast to the inhibitory effect of parathyroid hormone on RNA synthesis in osteoblasts parathyroid hormone stimulates the labeling of RNA in mesenchymal cells and osteoclasts (BINGHAM et al. 1969) when administered in vivo. PTH causes a rapid (within 15 min) enhancement of the incorporation of radioactively labeled uridine into RNA precursor pools and into bulk RNA in isolated calvarial cells in vitro as well (PECK et al. 1974b). This in vitro effect has been observed at near physiological levels of parathyroid hormone (5–10 ng/ml). Neither oxidized hormone nor basic polypeptides are effective in enhancing the incorporation of labeled uridine, while PTH 1–34, the synthetic peptide fragment of PTH, is capable of replicating the effect. This effect of parathyroid hormone may involve cyclic AMP as a mediator since exogenous Db-cAMP and cyclic AMP increase the incorporation of labeled uridine into acid soluble and RNA fractions. Both the time course and the maximum level of stimulation of Db-cAMP and cyclic AMP action is similar to that of PTH and the effects of maximal concentrations of each agent are not additive, suggesting that the mechanism of action is similar. This action of parathyroid hormone may in fact be basic to the hypercalcemic effect of parathyroid hormone in vivo and is consistent with the observation that PTH causes a significant increase in the average size of the osteoclasts and their ruffled borders within 90 min of administration (HOLTROP et al. 1979). This action of parathyroid hormone may also explain the in vitro experimental observation that brief exposure to parathyroid hormone causes a prolonged demineralization response which is not dependent upon the continued presence of the hormone, and which can be blocked by simultaneous treatment with inhibitors of RNA synthesis (RAISZ 1965b).

E. Calcium As Messenger

In 1968, RASMUSSEN and TENNENHOUSE postulated that calcium ion, in conjunction with cyclic AMP, served as an intracellular message for the actions of parathyroid hormone. While this hypothesis was based largely on studies examining the actions of parathyroid hormone on renal gluconeogenesis, the authors emphasized at that time the overall importance of calcium as an intracellular signal for the induction of a response to parathyroid hormone in other target tissues.

In bone, it is not difficult to appreciate the existence of an additional hormone-induced regulator of cell function because of the complex interrelationships which exist between the primary bone hormones, parathyroid hormone, calcitonin and vitamin D.

We have previously discussed the necessity of an additional signal in mediating the action of calcitonin and parathyroid if these receptors are linked to cyclic AMP formation within the same cell. Additional support for a second intracellular messenger in mediating the resorptive actions of parathyroid hormone derives from the fact that $1,25(OH)_2D_3$, a steroid hormone whose receptor is located within the cell (BRUMBAUGH and HAUSSLER 1974), mimics the resorptive effects of parathyroid hormone on bone. While the renal biosynthesis of $1,25(OH)_2D_3$ is regulated by parathyroid hormone through both a cyclic AMP and ion-mediated pathway both in vitro (RASMUSSEN et al. 1972) and in vivo (HORIUCHI et al. 1977), $1,25(OH)_2D_3$ itself does not enhance either basal or PTH stimulated cyclic AMP levels in rat or mouse calvaria (HERRMANN-ERLEE and GAILLARD 1978; GEBAUER and FLEISCH 1978) or in separated bone cell subcultures (WONG et al. 1977). Yet, in bone organ culture $1,25(OH)_2D_3$ stimulates the release of calcium, the production of lactic and citric acid, enhances the synthesis of hyaluronate and causes qualitative changes in bone histology which are typical of changes induced by high doses of parathyroid hormone (RAISZ et al. 1972; STERN et al. 1975; HERRMANN-ERLEE and GAILLARD 1978; GEBAUER and FLEISCH 1978; WONG et al. 1977). Moreover, in vitamin D deficiency, parathyroid hormone remains a potent agonist of the adenylate cyclase-cyclic AMP system in bone but is without effect in vivo in inducing a rise in serum calcium (RASMUSSEN and FEINBLATT 1971; ARNAUD et al. 1966; KAKUTA et al. 1975). These complex interrelationships provide evidence that a common event in the activation of bone cells must be shared by these two dissimilar agonists, parathyroid hormone and $1,25(OH)_2D_3$.

The possibility that PTH-induced bone cell activation is additionally coupled to an alteration in intracellular calcium is supported by a variety of experimental evidence obtained in vivo and in vitro. After a single intravenous injection of parathyroid hormone, a transient decrease in serum calcium concentration can be measured as early as two minutes, and for as long as 20 min, before the hypercalcemic response to parathyroid hormone develops (RASMUSSEN and FEINBLATT 1971; PARSONS et al. 1971; PARSONS and ROBINSON 1971; BOELKINS et al. 1976). This transient hypocalcemia induced by PTH has been demonstrated in rats, chickens, cats, monkeys, and dogs (RASMUSSEN and FEINBLATT 1971; PARSONS et al. 1971; PARSONS and ROBINSON 1971; BOELKINS et al. 1976) and requires fully active parathyroid hormone (TASHJIAN et al. 1964). The nature of this ion shift has been studied in some detail by following changes in the specific activity of calcium in the blood and urine following PTH injection in animals previously labeled with Ca^{45} (RASMUSSEN and FEINBLATT 1971; PARSONS et al. 1971; PARSONS and ROBINSON 1971). These experiments indicate that parathyroid hormone causes a rapid loss of calcium from plasma and a preferential uptake of calcium into bone.

The effect of parathyroid hormone on bone cell calcium exchange has been studied directly in an isolated bone cell system (DZIAK and STERN 1975). PTH 1–34 (0.02 U/ml) increases calcium exchange by 40% within one minute after its addition in vitro to freshly isolated calvarial cells. This effect of PTH on calcium uptake cannot be reproduced on efflux, does not involve a change in total cellular calcium, and appears to be evoked by PTH 1–84, but with much less reproducibility (DZIAK and BRAND 1974). While these experiments cannot identify the responding cell type, because a heterogeneous cell preparation was used for these studies, they do establish that the flux of calcium into bone induced by PTH in vivo is into a cellular compartment. Calcium transport effects of PTH are not without precedent, and have been extensively studied in cultured monkey kidney cells where PTH induces its most dramatic changes in the rates and size of an exchangeable pool thought to be mitochondria (BORLE and UCHIKAWA 1968).

In bone, it appears that the effect of PTH on bone cell calcium transport is not a cyclic AMP mediated event. Neither exogenous cyclic AMP (10^{-7} to 10^{-6} *M*) nor Db-cyclic AMP (10^{-4} to 10^{-3} *M*) has any effect on bone cell calcium exchange. Addition of methylisobutylxanthine (0.1 m*M*) at a concentration which causes a 200% increase in cellular cyclic AMP is without effect on altering calcium transport. In addition, incubation at 4 °C inhibits the enhancement of cellular cyclic AMP evoked by parathyroid hormone; yet incubation at 4 °C magnifies the effect of parathyroid hormone on calcium transport, resulting in 127% increase in uptake (DZIAK and STERN 1975). These experiments indicate that the stimulation of calcium flux by PTH is an early response which is separate from parathyroid hormones activation of the adenylate-cyclase cyclic AMP system. The immediacy of this effect of parathyroid hormone is essential if an alteration in intracellular calcium is to serve as an initiator of cell response.

The possibility exists that in bone cells this response may be coupled to or result from a change in membrane potential. MEARS (1971) has recorded a stable depolarization ($-\Delta$ 8 mV) of the membrane potential of osteoclasts following parathyroid hormone treatment and a hyperpolarization ($+\Delta$ 7 mV) of the membrane potential after calcitonin addition. It is not known as yet if the stimulation of the rate of calcium exchange by PTH is secondary to this effect of parathyroid hormone on membrane potential (via a voltage dependent calcium channel). It seems likely that if the change in membrane potential and in calcium uptake are not coupled, but are indeed separable, they will both be important events in mediating the cellular actions of parathyroid hormone on bone.

The possible messenger role of calcium in PTH-mediated bone resorption has been explored by other methods. If calcium is given with an intravenous injection of parathyroid hormone, a transient hypercalcemia is induced which markedly enhances the subsequent osteolytic response to parathyroid hormone (PARSONS et al. 1973; DACKE and KENNY 1973). The ability of calcium to potentiate the subsequent response to PTH is the basis of the sensitivity of the chick hypercalcemic bioassay. This same phenomenon can be demonstrated in vitro in bone organ culture. Addition of Verapamil (0.02 m*M*), a calcium channel blocker in muscle and heart, markedly (60%) inhibits PTH (0.1 μ/ml) induced demineralization in mouse calvaria incubated under hypocalcemic (0.8 m*M*) conditions. This inhibition of PTH induced bone demineralization by Verapamil is not related to alterations in cyclic nucleotide levels and can be partially overcome by raising the ambient calcium concentration in the incubation medium, suggesting that the basis for this inhibition is reduced calcium flux into bone (HERRMANN-ERLEE et al. 1977).

While the available experimental evidence strongly supports the concept that calcium is a modifier of PTH induced demineralization, the role of calcium as an initiator of PTH induced mineral release is not clear. DZIAK and STERN (1976) have reported that the calcium ionophore, A 23187, at concentrations from 0.1–0.3 μg/ml, stimulates Ca^{45} release from prelabeled long bones, an effect which is antagonized by calcitonin. However, at these concentrations, A 23187 significantly enhanced (~50%) cyclic nucleotide levels. At higher concentrations (10 μg/ml), A 23187 had a general inhibitory effect on cell function, decreasing bone lactate production and cellular ATP. At concentrations of ionophore >3.0 mg/ml bone demineralization was not stimulated, nor was intracellular cyclic AMP enhanced. In contrast, IVEY et al. (1976) have reported that the ionophores A 23187 and X-5374 within a range of 1 μ*M* to 2 μ*M* did not stimulate 45 Ca release from bone in calvarial cultures. Moreover, A 23187 as well as X-5374 inhibited in a dose-dependent manner bone demineralization induced by submaximal doses of PTH in media of either high or low calcium. For the present, any conclusions concerning the specific effects of A 23187 on bone demineralization must be postponed since the authors (IVEY et al. 1976) themselves have acknowledged these differences, but could find no basis for the discrepancies.

The role of calcium in the inhibitory action of parathyroid hormone on collagen synthesis is also not well understood. Both A 23186 and Verapamil inhibit the in vitro formation of collagen and non-collagen protein (DIETRICH and PADDOCK 1979; DIETRICH and DUFFIELD 1979). Since A 23187 should increase intracellular calcium and Verapamil decrease intracellular calcium, it is impossible at this time to correlate the effects of these two agents on protein synthesis with their effects on intracellular calcium. However, the differential effect of Verapamil on collagen synthesis appears to be related to its effect on calcium flux, since the inhibition can be overcome by raising the medium calcium, whereas the inhibition induced by A 23187 is not affected by changes in medium calcium. Despite this apparent specificity, the inhibitory effect of Verapamil on collagen synthesis is more difficult to reconcile with the effects of parathyroid hormone on bone cell calcium, since PTH raises intracellular calcium.

Calcium appears to be an important modulator if not mediator of PTH action on citrate oxidation and hyaluronate synthesis. In the absence of parathyroid hormone, the elevation of medium calcium from 1.8–5.0 m*M* incrementally enhances hyaluronate synthesis and inhibits [^{14}C]-citrate decarboxylation, mimicking the time course of hormonal activation and the extent of the maximal responses evoked by PTH. These changes occur without an elevation of cellular nucleotide levels. When calcium is added to a PTH challenge of bone subcultures, the elicited responses are additive at submaximal doses of potentiator only. Moreover, in the absence of medium calcium, parathyroid hormone is without effect in altering these metabolic activities. Yet, despite these similarities, the stimulation of hyaluronate synthesis evoked by PTH and that evoked by calcium, differ in an important respect. The calcium induced increase is not sensitive to inhibition by calcitonin (WONG et al. 1978). Thus, it would appear that cyclic AMP alone is an insufficient mediator of the action of PTH but may function as a modulator of the responses induced by alterations in either extracellular or intracellular calcium elicited by PTH and/or CT.

References

Arnaud C, Rasmussen H, Anast C (1966) Further studies on the interrelationship between parathyroid hormone and vitamin D. J Clin Invest 45:1955–1964

Arnaud CD, Tenenhouse AM, Rasmussen H (1967) Parathyroid hormone. Annu Rev Physiol 29:349–372

Arnaud CD, Tsao HS, Littledike T (1971) Radioimmunoassay of human parathyroid hormones in serum. J Clin Invest 50:21–34

Aurbach GC, Chase LR (1976) Cyclic nucleotides and biochemical actions of parathyroid hormone and calcitonin. In: Aurbach GD (ed) Parathyroid gland. American Physiological Society, Washington, DC p 353–381 (Handbook of physiology, Endocrinology, vol VII, pp 353–381)

Berson SA, Yalow RS (1969) Immunochemical heterogeneity of parathyroid hormone in plasma. J Clin Endocrinol Metab 28:1037–1047

Biddulph DM, Gallimore LB (1974) Sensitivity of the kidney to parathyroid hormone and its relationship to serum calcium in the hamster. Endocrinology 94:1241–1246

Bingham PJ, Brazen IA, Owen M (1969) The effect of parathyroid extract on cellular activity and plasma calcium levels in vivo. J Endocrinol 45:387–400

Boelkins JN, Mazurkiewicz M, Mazar PE, Mueller WJ (1976) Changes in blood flow to bones during the hypocalcemic and hypercalcemic phases of the response to parathyroid hormone. Endocrinology 98:403–412

Borle AB, Uchikawa T (1978) Effects of parathyroid hormone on the distribution and transport of calcium in cultured kidney cells. Endocrinology 102:1725–1723
Brumbaugh PF, Haussler MR (1974) 1α25 Dihydroxycholecalciferol receptors in intestine. II. Temperature-dependent transfer of the hormone to chromatin via a specific cytosol receptor. J Biol Chem 249:1258–1262
Chase LR, Aurbach GD (1970) The effect of parathyroid hormone on the concentration of adenosine 3′-5′ monophosphate in skeletal tissue in vitro. J Biol Chem 245:1520–1526
Chase LR, Obert KA (1975) Selective proteolysis of the receptors for parathyroid hormone in skeletal tissue. Metabolism 24:1067–1071
Chase LR, Fedak SA, Aurbach GD (1969) Activation of skeletal adenyl cyclase by parathyroid hormone in vitro. Endocrinology 84:761–768
Chen TL, Feldman D (1978) Glucocorticoid potentiation of the adenosine 3′-5′ monophosphate response to parathyroid hormone in cultured rat bone cells. Endocrinology 102:589–596
Chu LL, MacGregor RR, Hamilton JW, Cohn DV (1971) A bioassay for parathyroid hormone based on hormonal inhibition of CO_2 production from citrate in mouse calvarium. Endocrinology 89:1425–1432
Cohn DV, Forschel BK (1962) Aerobic metabolism of glucose by bone. J Biol Chem 237:615–618
Cohn DV, Wong GL (1978) Isolated osteoclast- and osteoblast-like cells in culture. In: Copp DH, Talmage RV (eds) Endocrinology of calcium metabolism. Excerpta Medica, Amsterdam London New York
Dacke CG, Kenny A (1973) Avian bioassay method for parathyroid hormone. Endocrinology 92:463–470
Dietrich JW, Duffield R (1979) Effects of the calcium antagonists Verapamil on in vitro synthesis of skeletal collagen and non-collagen protein. Endocrinology 105:1168–1172
Dietrich JW, Paddock DN (1979) In vitro effects of ionophore A 23187 on skeletal collagen and non-collagen protein synthesis. Endocrinology 104:493–499
Dietrich JW, Canalis EM, Maina DM, Raisz LG (1976) Hormonal control of bone collagen synthesis in vitro: effects of parathyroid hormone and calcitonin. Endocrinology 98:943–949
Dufau ML, Tsuruhara T, Horner A, Podesta E, Catt KJ (1977) Intermediate role of adenosine 3′-5′ cyclic monophosphate and protein kinase during gonadotropin-induced steroidogenesis in testicular interstitial cells. Proc Natl Acad Sci 74:3419–3423
Dziak R, Brand JS (1974) Calcium transport in isolated bone cells. II. Calcium transport studies. J Cell Physiol 84:85–96
Dziak R, Stern PH (1975) Calcium-transport in isolated bone cells. III. Effect of parathyroid hormone and cyclic 3′5′ AMP. Endocrinology 97:1281–1284
Dziak R, Stern P (1976) Responses of fetal rat bone cells and bone organ cultures to the ionophore, A 23187. Calcif Tissue Res 22:137–147
Finkelstein RA (1973) Cholera. CRC Crit Rev Microbiol 2:553–623
Freitag JJ, Martin KJ, Conrades MB, Slatopolsky E (1979) Metabolism of parathyroid hormone by fetal rat calvaria. Endocrinology 104:510–516
Gebauer U, Fleisch H (1978) Effect of 1,25-dihydroxycholecalciferol on adenosine 3′-5′ cyclic monophosphate production in calvaria of mice. Calcif Tissue Res 25:223–225
Gill DM (1975) Involvement of nicotinamide adenine dinucleòtide in the action of cholera toxin in vitro. Proc Natl Acad Sci USA 72:2064–2068
Goltzman D (1978) Examination of the requirement for metabolism of parathyroid hormone in skeletal tissue before biological action. Endocrinology 102:1555–1562
Goltzman D, Peytremann A, Callahan E, Tregear GW, Potts JT (1975) Analysis of the requirements for parathyroid hormone action in renal membranes with the use of inhibitory analogues. J Biol Chem 250:3199–3203
Goltzman D, Peytremann A, Callahan EN, Segre GV, Potts JT (1976) Metabolism and biological activity of parathyroid hormone in renal cortical membranes. J Clin Invest 57:8–19
Goltzman D, Callahan EN, Tregear GW, Potts JT (1978) Influence of guanyl nucleotides on parathyroid hormone-stimulated adenyl cyclase in renal cortical membranes. Endocrinology 103:1352–1359

Habener JG, Powell D, Murray TM, Mayer GP, Potts JT (1971) Parathyroid hormone: secretion and metabolism in vivo. Proc Natl Acad Sci USA 68:2986–2991
Harbon SL, Khac DO, Vesin MF (1976) Cyclic AMP binding to intracellular receptor proteins in rat myometrium. Effects of epinephrine and prostaglandin E_1. Mol Cell Endocrinol 6:17–21
Hekkelman JW, Herrmann-Erlee MPM, Gaillard PJ (1975) Studies on the mechanism of parathyroid hormone action on embryonic bone in vitro. In: Talmadge R, Owens M, Parsons J (eds) Calcium regulating hormones. Excerpta Medica, Amsterdam London New York
Herrmann-Erlee MPM, Gaillard PJ (1978) The effects of 1,25 dihydroxycholecalciferol on embryonic bone in vitro: a biochemical and histological study. Calcif Tissue Res 25:111–118
Herrmann-Erlee MPM, Meer JD (1974) The effects of dibutyryl cyclic AMP, aminophylline and propranolol on PTE-induced bone resorption in vitro. Endocrinology 94:424–434
Herrmann-Erlee MPM, Gaillard PJ, Hekkelman JW, Nijweide PJ (1977) The effect of Verapamil on the action of parathyroid hormone on embryonic bone in vitro. Eur J Pharmacol 46:51–58
Herrmann-Erlee MPM, Gaillard PJ, Hekkelman JW (1978) Regulation of the response of embryonic bone to PTH and PTH fragments. A morphological and biochemical study. In: Copp DH, Talmage RV (eds) Endocrinology of calcium metabolism. Excerpta Medica, Amsterdam London New York
Hirsch PF, Munson PL (1969) Thyrocalcitonin. Physiol Rev 49:548–622
Holtrop ME, King GI, Cox KA, Reit B (1979) Time-related changes in the ultrastructure of osteoclasts after injection of parathyroid hormone in young rats. Calcif Tissue Int 27:129–135
Horiuchi N, Suda T, Takahashi H, Shimazawa E, Ogata E (1977) In vivo evidence for the intermediary role of 3′-5′cyclic AMP in parathyroid hormone-induced stimulation of 1α25 dihydroxyvitamin D_3 synthesis in rats. Endocrinology 101:969–974
Hruska KA, Kopelman R, Rutherford WE, Klahr S, Slatopolsky E (1975) Metabolism of immunoreactive parathyroid hormone in the dog: the role of the kidney and the effects of chronic renal disease. J Clin Invest 56:39–48
Hruska K, Martin K, Greenwalt A, Klahr S, Slatopolsky E (1978) Characterization of parathyroid hormone uptake, degradation and fragment production by liver and kidney. In: Copp DH, Talmage RV (eds) Endocrinology of calcium metabolism. Excerpta Medica Amsterdam London New York, pp 313–317
Ivey JL, Wright DR, Tashjian AH (1976) Bone resorption in organ culture; inhibition by the divalent cation ionophores A 23187 and X-537 A. J CLin Invest 58:1327–1338
Johannes N, Heersche M, Marcus R, Aurbach GD (1974) Calcitonin and the formation of 3′-5′AMP in bone and kidney. Endocrinology 94:241–247
Kakuta S, Suda T, Sasaki S, Kimura N, Nagata N (1975) Effects of parathyroid hormone on the accumulation of cyclic AMP in bone of vitamin D-deficient rats. Endocrinology 97:1288–1293
Kalu DN, Hadji-Georgopoulos A, Sarr MG, Solomon BA, Foster GV (1974) The role of parathyroid hormone in the maintenance of plasma calcium levels in rats. Endocrinology 95:1156–1165
Klein DC, Raisz LG (1971) The role of adenosine 3′-5′ monophosphate in the hormonal regulation of bone resorption: studies with cultured fetal bone. Endocrinology 89:818–826
Knight BL (1975) Adenosine 3′-5′ cyclic monophosphate-dependent protein kinase in brown fat from newborn rabbits. Biochem J 152:577–582
Luben RA, Cohn DV (1976) Effects of parathormone and calcitonin on citrate and hyaluronate metabolism in cultured bone. Endocrinology 98:413–419
Luben RA, Goggins JF, Raisz LG (1974) Stimulation by parathyroid hormone of bone hyaluronate synthesis in organ culture. Endocrinology 94:737–746
Luben RA, Wong GL, Cohn DV (1976) Biochemical characterization with parathormone and calcitonin of isolated bone cells: provisional identification of osteoclasts and osteoblasts. Endocrinology 99:526–533

Luben RA, Wong GL, Cohn DV (1977) Parathormone-stimulated resorption of devitalised bone by cultured osteoclast-type bone cells. Nature 265:629–630
Marcus R, Orner FB (1977) Cyclic AMP production in rat calvaria in vitro: interaction of prostaglandins with parathyroid hormone. Endocrinology 101:1570–1578
Marcus R, Arvensen G, Orner FB (1979) Fluctuation of adenosine 3′-5′ monophosphate-binding site occupancy as an index of hormone dependent adenosine 3′-5′ monophosphate formation in bone cells. Endocrinology 104:744–750
Martin K, Hruska D, Greenwalt A, Klahr S, Slatopolsky E (1976) Selective uptake of intact parathyroid hormone by the liver. Differences between hepatic and renal uptake. J Clin Invest 58:781–788
Martin KJ, Freitag JJ, Conrades MB, Hruska KA, Klarh S, Slatopolsky E (1978) Selective uptake of the synthetic amino terminal fragment of bovine parathyroid hormone by isolated perfused bone. J Clin Invest 62:256–261
Martin KJ, Hruska KA, Freitag JJ, Klahr S, Slatopolsky E (1979) The peripheral metabolism of parathyroid hormone. N Engl J Med 301:1092–1098
Mears DC (1971) Relationship between membrane potential and metabolic activity of osteoclasts. Endocrinology 88:1021–1028
Munson PL, Hirsch PF (1968) Discovery and pharmacologic evaluation of thyrocalcitonin. Am J Med 43:678–683
Munson PL, Hirsch PF, Tashjian AH (1963) Parathyroid gland. Annu Rev Physiol 75:325–360
Nagata N, Rasmussen H (1968) Parathyroid hormone and renal cell metabolism. Biochemistry 1:3728–3733
Nagata N, Sasaki M, Kimura N, Nakane K (1975) The hypercalcemic effect of parathyroid hormone and skeletal cyclic AMP. Endocrinology 96:725–731
Nagata N, Ono Y, Kimura N (1977) Inhibition by cholera toxin of parathyroid hormone-induced calcium release from bone in culture. Biochem Biophys Res Commun 78:819–826
Neuman WF, Ramp WK (1971) The concept of a bone membrane: some implications. In: Cellular mechanisms for calcium transfer and homeostasis. Academic Press, New York London
Neuman WF, Neuman MW, Sammon PJ, Simon W, Lane K (1975a) The metabolism of labeled parathyroid hormone. III. Studies in rat. Calcif Tissue Res 18:251–261
Neuman WF, Neuman MW, Lane K, Miller L, Sammon PJ (1975b) Metabolism of labeled parathyroid hormone. V. Collected biological studies. Calcif Tissue Res 18:271–287
Ng B, Hekkelman JW, Heersche JN (1979) The effect of cortisol on the adenosine 3′-5′ monophosphate response to parathyroid hormone of bone in vitro. Endocrinology 104:1130–1135
Nisbet JA, Helliwell S, Nordin BEC (1970) Relation of lactic and citric acid metabolism to bone resorption in tissue culture. Clin Orthop 28:220–230
Parfitt AM (1979) Equilibrium and disequilibrium hypercalcemia new light on an old concept. Metab Bone Dis Rel Res 1:279–293
Parsons JA (1976) Parathyroid physiology and the skeleton. In: Bourne GH (ed) Biochemistry and Physiology of Bone, vol IV. Academic Press, New York London
Parsons JA, Reit B (1974) Chronic response of dogs to parathyroid hormone infusion. Nature 250:254–257
Parsons JA, Robinson CJ (1971) Calcium shift into bone causing transient hypocalcemia after injection of parathyroid hormone. Nature 230:581–582
Parsons JA, Neer RM, Potts JT (1971) Initial fall of plasma calcium after intravenous injection of parathyroid hormone. Endocrinology 89:735–740
Parsons JA, Reit B, Robinson CJ (1973) A bioassay for parathyroid hormone using chicks. Endocrinology 92:454–462
Parsons JA, Rafferty B, Gray D et al. (1975) Pharmacology of parathyroid hormone and some of its fragments and analogues. In: Talmage R, Owen M, Parsons J (eds) Calcium regulating hormones. Excerpta Medica, Amsterdam London New York, pp 33–39
Peck WA, Dirksen TR (1966) The metabolism of bone tissue in vitro. Clin Orthop 24:243–265

Peck WA, Carpenter J, Messinger K (1974a) Cyclic 3′-5′ adenosine monophosphate in isolated bone cells. II. Responses to adenosine and parathyroid hormone. Endocrinology 94:148–153
Peck WA, Messinger K, Kimmich G, Carpenter J (1974b) Stimulation of uridine incorporation in isolated bone cells by parathyroid hormone and cyclic AMP. Endocrinology 95:289–297
Peck WA, Burks JK, Wilkins J, Rodan SB, Rodan GA (1977) Evidence for preferential effects of parathyroid hormone, calcitonin and adenosine on bone and periosteum. Endocrinology 100:1357–1364
Potts JT, Murray TM, Peacock M et al. (1971) Parathyroid hormone: sequence, synthesis, immunoassay studies. Am J Med 50:639–649
Puzas JE, Vignery A, Rasmussen H (1979) Isolation of specific bone cell types by free-flow electrophoresis. Calcif, Tissue Int 27:263–268
Raisz LG (1965a) Bone resorption in tissue culture. Factors influencing the response to parathyroid hormone. J Clin Invest 44:103–116
Raisz LG (1965b) Inhibition by actinomycin D on bone resorption induced by parathyroid hormone or vitamin D. Proc Soc Exp Biol Med 119:614–617
Raisz LG (1976) Mechanisms of bone resorption. In: Aurbach GD (ed) Parathyroid gland. American Physiological Society (Handbook of physiology, Endocrinology, vol VII)
Raisz LG, Trummel CL, Holick MF, DeLuca HF (1972) 1,25 Dihydroxycholecalciferol, a potent stimulator of bone resorption in tissue culture. Science 175:768–769
Rasmussen H, Bordier P (1974) The physiological and cellular basis of metabolic bone disease. Williams & Wilkins, Baltimore
Rasmussen H, Feinblatt J (1971) The relationship between the actions of vitamin-D, parathyroid hormone and calcitonin. Calcif Tissue Res 6:265–279
Rasmussen H, Tenenhouse A (1968) Cyclic adenosine monophosphate, Ca and membranes. PNAS 59:1364–1370
Rasmussen H, DeLuca H, Arnaud C, Hawker C, Von Stedingk M (1963) The relationship between vitamin D and parathyroid hormone. J Clin Invest 42:1940–1946
Rasmussen H, Anast C, Arnaud C (1967) Thyrocalcitonin, EGTA, and urinary electrolyte excretion. J Clin Invest 46:746–752
Rasmussen H, Pechet M, Fast D (1968) Effect of dibutyryl cyclic adenosine 3′-5′ monophosphate, theophylline and other nucleotides upon calcium and phosphate metabolism. J Clin Invest 47:1843–1850
Rasmussen H, Wong M, Bikle D, Goodman DBP (1972) Hormonal control of the renal conversion of 25-hydroxycholecalciferol to 1,25-dihydroxycholecalciferol. J Clin Invest 51:2502–2504
Rodan SB, Rodan GA (1974) The effect of parathyroid hormone and thyrocalcitonin on the accumulation of cyclic adenosine 3′-5′ monophosphate in freshly isolated bone cells. J Biol Chem 249:3068–3074
Rosenblatt M, Goltzman D, Keutmann H, Tregear GW, Potts JT (1976) Chemical and biological properties of synthetic, sulfur-free analogues of parathyroid hormone. J Biol Chem 251:159–164
Rosenblatt M, Segre GV, Tregear GW, Shepard GL, Tyler GA, Potts JT (1978) Human parathyroid hormone: synthesis and chemical, biological and immunological evaluation of the carboxyl-terminal region. Endocrinology 103:978–984
Segre GV, Niall HD, Habener JF, Potts JT (1974) Metabolism of parathyroid hormone, physiological and clinical significance. Am J Med 56:774–784
Segre GV, D'Amour P, Rosenblatt M, Potts JT (1978) Heterogeneity and metabolism of parathyroid hormone. In: Copp DH, Talmage RV (eds) Endocrinology of calcium metabolism. Excerpta Medica, Amsterdam London New York
Segre GV, Rosenblatt M, Reiner BL, Mahaffey JE, Potts JT (1979) Characterization of parathyroid hormone receptors in canine renal cortical plasma membranes using a radioiodinated sulfur-free hormone analogue. J Biol Chem 254:6980–6986
Smith DM, Johnston CC (1973) Studies of the metabolism of separated bone cells. I. Techniques of separation and identification. Calcif Tissue Res 11:56–69
Smith DM, Johnston CC (1974) Hormonal responsiveness of adenylate cyclase activity from separated bone cells. Endocrinology 95:130–139

Smith DM, Johnston CC (1975) Cyclic 3′-5′adenosine monophosphate levels in separated bone cells. Endocrinology 96:1261–1269

Stern PH, Trummel CL, Schnoes HK, DeLuca HF (1975) Bone resorbing activity of vitamin D metabolism and congeners in vitro: influence of hydroxyl substitutes in the A ring. Endocrinology 97:1552–1558

Tashjian AH, Ontjes DA, Munson PL (1964) Alkylation and oxidation of methionine in bovine parathyroid hormone: effects on hormonal activity and antigenicity. Biochemistry 3:1175–1182

Tregear GW, Reitschoten J, Greene E et al. (1973) Bovine parathyroid hormone: minimum chain length of synthetic peptide required for biological activity. Endocrinology 93:1349–1353

Vaes G (1968) Parathyroid hormone-like action of N^6-2′-0-dibutyryladenosine-3′,5′ (cyclic) monophosphate on bone explants in tissue culture. Nature 219:939–940

Wells H, Lloyd W (1967) Effects of theophylline on the serum calcium of rats after parathyroidectomy and administration of parathyroid hormone. Endocrinology 81:139–144

Wells H, Lloyd W (1969) Hypercalcemic and hypophosphatemic effects of dibutyryl cyclic AMP in rats after parathyroidectomy. Endocrinology 84:861–867

Wolinsky I, Cohn DV (1969) Oxygen uptake and $^{14}CO_2$ production from citrate and isocitrate by control and parathyroid hormone-treated bone maintained in tissue culture. Endocrinology 84:28–36

Wong GL (1979a) Induction of metabolic changes and down regulation of bovine parathyroid hormone-responsive adenylate cyclase are dissociable in isolated osteoclastic and osteoblastic bone cells. J Biol Chem 254:34–37

Wong GL (1979b) Basal activities and hormone responsiveness of osteoclast-like and osteoblast-like bone cells are regulated by glucocorticoids. J Biol Chem 254:6337–6340

Wong GL, Cohn DV (1975) Target cells in bone for parathormone and calcitonin are different: enrichment for each cell type by sequential digestion of mouse calvaria and selective adhesion to polymeric surfaces. Proc Nat Acad Sci USA 72:3167–3171

Wong GL, Luben R, Cohn DV (1977) 1,25 Dihydroxycholecalciferol and parathormone: effect on isolated osteoclast-like and osteoblast-like cells. Science 197:663–665

Wong GL, Kent GN, Ku KY, Cohn DV (1978) The interaction of parathyroid hormone and calcium on the hormone-regulated synthesis of hyaluronic acid and citrate decarboxylation in isolated bone cells. Endocrinology 103:2274–2282

CHAPTER 30

The Role of Cyclic Nucleotides and Calcium in Adrenocortical Function

B. L. Brown

Overview

The adrenal cortex is of mesodermal origin and develops from the coelomic epithelium. It surrounds the medulla, which is ectodermal in origin, and the whole is enclosed within a capsule. The cortex comprises three clearly definable zones of steroidogenically active cells: the zona glomerulosa, zona fasciculata and zona reticularis. As well as differing in microscopic appearance, the cell zones differ in the pattern of steroid secretion and in the responsiveness to various regulators. Thus, aldosterone is produced exclusively by the zona glomerulosa, whereas cortisol (in those species that produce it e.g. man) is synthesised exclusively by the zona fasciculata-reticularis. However, a number of steroids (notably corticosterone, deoxycorticosterone, 18-hydroxycorticosterone and 18-hydroxydeoxycorticosterone) are produced by both the zona glomerulosa and the zona fasciculata-reticularis regions. Recent studies have indicated a preferential output of deoxycorticosterone by zona reticularis cells as compared with zona fasciculata cells (Bell et al. 1979; see also J. Tait and Tait 1979 and J. Tait et al. 1980a for review).

Various cell preparations have been used in studies of the intracellular control mechanisms governing steroidogenesis. Whole adrenal cortex preparations, although containing a preponderance of zona fasciculata-reticularis cells, are clearly the least useful of all preparations for these studies. Preparations consisting mainly (90%–95%) of glomerulosa cells can be prepared by stripping the capsule (and associated cells) from the rat adrenal gland (Giroud et al. 1956). The tissue remaining (the decapsulated gland) comprises an approximately equal proportion of fasciculata and reticularis cells (J. Tait et al. 1980a). The cells in these tissue preparations may be dispersed and studied in suspension. Furthermore, the work of Tait and his colleagues (J. Tait et al. 1974, 1980a; Bell et al. 1979) has shown that it is possible to separate these cell types both by velocity sedimentation (J. Tait et al. 1974, 1980a, b; Bell et al. 1978) and by column filtration (McDougall et al. 1979; J. Tait et al. 1980a). Thus, a preparation of glomerulosa cells can be obtained (from capsular strippings) with minimal (less than 0.5%) contamination by fasciculata cells. Purified preparations of both fasciculata and reticularis cells can be obtained from decapsulated glands (Bell et al. 1979).

It has become clear, particularly from work using purified cell preparations, that the specificity of steroid secretion is determined by the nature of the stimulation (Haning et al. 1970; J. Tait et al. 1974). Thus, steroid output from zona glomerulosa cells is altered by adrenocorticotropic hormone (ACTH), angiotensin II, changes in K^+ concentration and, at least in the rat, by serotonin (J. Tait et al. 1974), whereas cells of the zona fasciculata region respond only to ACTH (and its analogues).

Over the years there have been a number of excellent reviews of the role of cyclic nucleotides in adrenal cortical function including recent ones by Halkerston (1975), Schulster et al. (1976), Saez et al. (1981) and J. Tait et al. (1980a).

This reviewer's intention is not to reiterate the history of this field but rather to consider in some detail the work subsequent to the comprehensive review by Halkerston (1975). For clarity it has been necessary on occasions to refer to work already included in that review. An attempt has been made to delineate the effects of regulatory substances on the individual zones of the gland. Clearly, this has not always been possible since mixed populations of cells have often been used in the studies cited. The problems asssociated with studies of intracellular events using heterogeneous tissue preparations are becoming increasingly realised. One can only hope that this trend continues.

A. Primary Interaction of Effectors with Adrenocortical Cells

I. ACTH Receptors

Adrenocorticotropin (ACTH) is synthesised as a 31,000 dalton precursor by the anterior pituitary gland. This 31 K precursor is also believed to be the precursor of the lipotropins, melanotropins and endorphins and has been designated proopiocortin. ACTH is chemically related to αMSH, βMSH and the lipotropins through a common heptapeptide sequence which in ACTH is residues 4–10.

Schulster and Schwyzer (1980) reviewed the effects of analogues and derivatives of ACTH and came to the following conclusions: a) discrete sequence of adjacent aminoacids are responsible for the different components of the total biological action, b) different target cells may be stimulated by different portions of the molecule and c) partial sequences can produce effects similar to those they elicit when contained in the complete molecule. All of the known biological actions of ACTH are exerted by the N-terminal portion, ACTH 1–24. This active sequence has been further sub-divided into a potentiator sequence (1–4) and message sequence (5–9) and an address sequence (11–23) for adrenal cortex steroidogenic receptors. The message sequence stimulates the steroidogenic response and the production of cyclic AMP (Schulster and Schwyzer 1980). As stated by Halkerston (1975) there is a considerable body of evidence supporting the premise that ACTH receptors are located on the outer plasma membrane surface. ACTH chemically linked to insoluble and inert polymers was effective in stimulating adrenal steroidogenesis in cell suspensions (Schimmer et al. 1968; Selinger and Civen 1971; Richardson and Schulster 1972). The size of the complexes apparently precluded entry into the cell, and it has been demonstrated that neither ACTH nor smaller peptides were released from the complexes during incubation. The majority of the studies on the binding of ACTH to plasma membrane receptors have employed iodinated peptide as the radioligand. The obvious reason for

Table 1

	$K_D(1)$	$K_D(2)$
LEFKOWITZ et al. (1970)	1.1×10^{-12} M	3.3×10^{-8} M
MCILHINNEY and SCHULSTER (1975)	2.5×10^{-10} M (3,000)[a]	1×10^{-8} M (30,000)[a]
YANAGIBASHI et al. (1978)	2.6×10^{-10} M (7,350)[a]	7.1×10^{-9} M (57,400)[a]

[a] Number of binding sites/cell

this is the considerably higher (2,000 Ci/mmole) specific activities attainable vis-a-vis tritiated ACTH (40 Ci/mmole). However, this approach is not devoid of attendant problems. It is now clear that the preparation of biologically active radioiodinated ACTH is considerably more difficult than originally believed. For example, LOWRY et al. (1973) showed that di-iodination at either Tyr^2 or Tyr^{23} caused significant (97% or 43%) reduction in biological potency as compared to unlabelled ACTH. Nevertheless, most workers have been careful to demonstrate that the iodinated peptide was the mono-iodinated form and was biologically active. This is clearly important since the relatively large iodine atom might be expected to alter the properties of the peptide and the iodination procedure may chemically modify various aminoacids (e.g. methionine oxidation) thus altering the biological activity of the hormone. When a relatively gentle procedure using lactoperoxidase for labelling ACTH to a specific activity greater than 2,000 Ci/mmole was used (MCILHINNEY and SCHULSTER 1975) binding sites of both high and low affinity were observed. Interestingly, the affinity constants they observed for the two types of binding sites are similar to those originally reported by LEFKOWITZ et al. (1970, 1971). The binding constants of these two orders of binding sites observed are shown in Table 1. Also shown in this table are the binding constants recently reported by YANAGIBASHI et al. (1978), showing remarkable agreement with the previous studies. Since mixed populations of cells were used for these studies, one alternative explanation might be that the binding sites for ACTH are not the same on the various cell types. MOYLE et al. (1973) in a study of the effects of the o-nitrophenyl sulphenyl derivative of ACTH (NPS-ACTH) also came to the conclusion that there may be two receptors for ACTH either on the same or different cell types. Other groups have not observed two orders of binding constants; only the low affinity site being detected (FINN et al. 1972; SAEZ et al. 1974; WAYS et al. 1976).

Nevertheless, it is reasonably clear that the binding sites for ACTH on adrenal membranes fulfill most of the criteria for true receptors. The ability of ACTH and its analogues to inhibit binding appears to parallel their effects in bioassays (SAEZ et al. 1975; WAYS and ONTJES 1979; WAYS et al. 1976). There is evidence for negative cooperativity in that ACTH itself increases the rate of dissociation (SAEZ et al. 1981). The rate of dissociation is also increased by GTP. YANAGIBASHI et al. (1978) also reported that the apparent dissociation constants derived from the effects of ACTH on Ca^{++} influx and steroidogenesis correlated well with the K_D of the high affinity receptor. Their conclusions from these studies was that the high affinity receptor was linked to Ca^{++} influx whereas the low affinity site was coupled to adenylate cyclase at supraphysiological ACTH concentrations. Previously,

MCILHINNEY and SCHULSTER (1975) also showed a correlation between occupancy of the high affinity binding sites and stimulation of steroidogenesis. They also suggested that the low affinity receptor appeared to be related to cyclic AMP production.

BONNAFOUS et al. (1977) reported that ACTH 1–24, ACTH 5–24, ACTH 6–24, and ACTH 7–24 stimulated adenylate cyclase activity in adrenal membranes. However, ACTH 5–24, 6–24, and 7–24 were all partial agonists, and ACTH 8–24 was inactive. High concentrations (10–250 μM) of ACTH 1–24, 5–24, 6–24, and 7–24 inhibited both stimulated and basal adenylate cyclase activity. They also reported that the adrenal adenylate cyclase was only slightly affected by Gpp(NH)p. Recently, it has been shown that ACTH 6–24 inhibited the actions of ACTH 1–39 and ACTH 5–24 to a different extent (BRISTOW et al. 1980). The concentration of ACTH 1–39 required to elicit an increase in cyclic AMP accumulation was within one order of magnitude to that required to stimulate steroidogenosis. However, for ACTH 5–24, cyclic AMP accumulation only occurred at peptide concentrations more than 100-fold higher than that required for stimulation of steroidogenesis. They proposed that ACTH 1–39 can act via either of two receptors and that binding to one elicits steroidogenesis through the mediation of cyclic AMP and that binding to the other receptor also elicits steroidogenesis without the mediation of cyclic AMP. The implications of these findings of receptor heterogeneity have been recently discussed by SCHULSTER and SCHWYZER (1980). They proposed a novel concept, "compartment guidance concept", to explain the various observations on the mode of action of ACTH. According to this hypothesis, cyclic AMP (either basal or stimulated concentrations) is necessary but insufficient to produce the effects, and other actions of ACTH are necessary to "guide cyclic AMP into the correct compartment for eliciting steroidogenesis and lipolysis".

There is evidence for the presence of "spare receptors" in adrenal cells. For example, at maximally effective (on steroidogenesis) concentrations of ACTH, cyclic AMP accumulation was less than 10% of maximum (MACKIE et al. 1972). Furthermore, studies on the binding of ^{125}I-ACTH to intact adrenal cells revealed that only about 12% of the cellular binding sites were filled when steroidogenesis was maximal.

II. Angiotensin Receptors

Receptors exhibiting a high affinity for angiotensin II have been found on glomerulosa cells (BRECHER et al. 1974; DOUGLAS et al. 1978a; CAPPONI and CATT 1979; see also review by REGOLI 1979). The relative affinities of analogues of the peptide correlate well with their biological activities (DOUGLAS et al. 1976; CATT et al. 1979). There is evidence that the circulating concentration of angiotensin II can have profound modulatory effects on its own receptors. In one study it was shown that infusion of angiotensin II into rats resulted in increases in both angiotensin II receptors and angiotensin-induced steroidogenic responses of the glomerulosa cells (HAUGER et al. 1978). Moreover, angiotensin II receptors are affected by changes in sodium and potassium intake (DOUGLAS and CATT 1976). The effect of sodium appears to be due largely to changes in the circulating concentration of angiotensin. Thus, decreased sodium intake leads to an increase in blood angiotensin levels and an increase in angiotensin II receptors and aldosterone secretion. In the short term, the effect of sodium deficiency was an increase in the affinity of the angiotensin II receptor, followed within a few days by an increase in the number of receptor sites (AGUILERA et al. 1978). CATT and co-workers have suggested that most of the effects of sodium deficiency on aldosterone secretion are mediated by changes in the circulating concentration of angiotensin II and the consequent increase in the sensitivity of the glomerulosa cell to the peptide (CATT et al. 1979). This effect of sodium deficiency could be blocked by the use of an inhibitor of converting enzyme to prevent the generation of angiotensin II (AGUILERA and CATT 1978), thus giving further support to the hypothesis that the effects of sodium are mediated by angiotensin levels. In contrast to the indirect effect of sodium intake, potassium appears to have a direct effect on the glomerulosa cell to increase the number and affinity of angiotensin II receptors (DOUGLAS and CATT 1976; CATT et al. 1979). The effect of nephrectomy on angiotensin II receptors is controversial. On the one hand, DOUGLAS and CATT (1976) reported that angiotensin II receptors in the rat adrenal were reduced after nephrectomy. However, it has been reported that nephrectomy resulted in increased binding of angiotensin II and that administration of angiotensin to nephrectomised rats caused a decrease in adrenal angiotensin binding (DEVYNCK et al. 1976; PERNOLLET et al. 1977). In their recent review, J. TAIT et al. (1980a) have suggested that the different preparations used by the two major groups might, at least in part, be the cause of the discrepant results.

AGUILERA et al. (1979) observed that the receptor binding capacity of rat glomerulosa cell membranes for both angiotensin II and angiotensin III (des-Asp^1-angiotensin II) was identical. Essentially similar results were obtained using dog zona glomerulosa cells (DOUGLAS et al. 1978b). The binding affinity for angiotensin III was lower than for angiotensin II, reflecting the lower sensitivity of the aldosterone response to angiotensin III. This difference in the binding affinities was less marked in the dog zona glomerulosa. They also found that there was considerable metabolism of angiotensin peptides by rat glomerulosa cells, with faster degradation of angiotensin III. They concluded that prior conversion of AII to AIII was not necessary for the action of the native peptide. It has also been reported that the binding of angiotensin II to its receptor in the zona glomerulosa cell membrane is not affected by the absence of calcium (FAKUNDING et al. 1979), and it was suggested that any calcium-dependent step in the mechanism of action of angiotensin had a post receptor locus.

B. Adrenocortical Adenylate Cyclase

GRAHAME-SMITH et al. (1967) first reported ACTH activation of adrenal adenylate cyclase. Others demonstrated that the enzyme was particulate (TAUNTON et al. 1969; KELLY and KORITZ 1971) and located in the plasma membrane (FINN et al. 1972). Since these initial reports there have been relatively few studies on this enzyme in the adrenal cortex. However, work with other systems has progressed considerably so that a number of general points can be made about this enzyme system.

As reviewed elsewhere, [see BIRNBAUMER and IYENGAR (1982)] the initial step in the process of adenylate cyclase activation is the specific and reversible interaction of the ligand with a receptor molecule on the plasma membrane of the target cell. Considerable evidence now exists for the concept that the receptor moiety and the catalytic site exist as separate entities. The nature of the link (or transducer) between these moieties has been the subject of intense experimentation in recent years. It is now clear that one component of this transduction mechanism is a nucleotide regulatory protein ("N") which binds guanine nucleotides. Binding of GTP to the regulatory protein transiently activates the catalytic activity of adenylate cyclase. The action of a GTPase causes hydrolysis of the bound GTP with subsequent inactivation of the adenylate cyclase. Analogues of GTP such as guanylyl imidodiphosphate, Gpp(NH)p, are poor substrates for the GTPase and they induce an almost irreversible activation of the enzyme. Cholera toxin appears to inhibit the activity of the GTPase and to cause the ADP-ribosylation of certain membrane proteins. Another factor which appears to enhance hormone-stimulated adenylate cyclase activity has been discovered recently. This factor, which is found in cytosol preparations, has not been fully characterised but appears to be a labile protein (possibly with associated phosphate groups) with a molecular weight of around 20,000 daltons (SANDERS et al. 1977; KATZ et al. 1978; EGAN et al. 1978; CRAWFORD et al. 1980).

I. Adrenocorticotropin

The adrenal adenylate cyclase ressembles the enzyme from other enkaryotic sources (for a review of adrenal adenylate cyclase see GLYNN et al. 1979). The adrenal enzyme is activated by GTP and Gpp(NH)p (LONDOS and RODBELL 1975; GLOSSMANN and GIPS 1975; GLYNN et al. 1978), and ACTH stimulated activity has been shown to be enhanced by GTP (GLOSSMANN and GIPS 1975; GLYNN et al. 1977; TELL et al. 1978). Activation by Gpp(NH)p is a slow process which, when complete, renders the enzyme insensitive to hormonal activation. This process can be competitively blocked by GTP (GLOSSMANN and GIPS 1975; GLYNN et al. 1978). GLYNN et al. (1977) observed that GTP (10 μM) had no significant effect on the concentration of ACTH 1–24 needed to half maximally stimulate the bovine adrenal enzyme although enzyme activity was enhanced at all hormone concentrations tested. The major effect of ACTH was to increase the rate of enzyme activation (GLYNN et al. 1978). Similarly, GLOSSMANN and STRUCK (1976) showed that Gpp(NH)p had little effect on the concentration of ACTH which half maximally stimulated the bovine enzyme. However, these investigators showed that this nucleotide caused a 20-fold decrease in the concentration of ACTH required to half maximally stimulate the enzyme from the adrenal cortex of the rat. Other differences between the rat and bovine enzymes are that about 10-fold higher concentrations of GTP are required to half maximally activate the bovine enzyme (LONDOS and RODBELL 1975; GLOSSMANN and GIPS 1975). Furthermore, the rat enzyme preparation is more sensitive to GTP after dialysis of the particulate fraction (LONDOS and RODBELL 1975) whereas the bovine enzyme is not (GLOSSMANN and GIPS 1976).

ACTH and GTP appear to act synergistically to reduce the requirement of adrenal adenylate cyclase for Mg^{++} (GLYNN et al. 1977). LONDOS and RODBELL (1975) showed that, in the presence of ACTH and GTP, high Mg^{++} concentrations (above 5 m*M*) inhibited the activity of the rat enzyme. A similar, although less pronounced, effect has been observed for the bovine enzyme (GLOSSMANN and GIPS 1975; GLYNN et al. 1977). There is also evidence to suggest that Mg^{++} (in the absence of any effect of exogenous nucleotide) is an activator of the adrenal enzyme (GLYNN et al. 1978).

Some ten years ago, LEFKOWITZ et al. (1970) first reported that EGTA abolished ACTH stimulated adenylate cyclase activity in mouse tumour preparations but had no effect on basal enzyme activity. Subsequently, GLOSSMANN and GIPS (1976) also observed inhibition of the activation of the bovine enzyme by EGTA. They also found that this effect could be reversed by readdition of Ca^{++}, Mn^{++}, Co^{++} or Sr^{++}. Recently, KATZ et al. (1981) reported that micromolar concentrations of free Ca^{++} were required for stimulation of the rat adrenal adenylate cyclase, and that other divalent cations (Mn^{++}, Co^{++} and Ba^{++}) could substitute for Ca^{++}. In the presence of 1 m*M* EGTA, 1 m*M* ATP and 5 m*M* $MgCl_2$, added Ca^{++} and Mn^{++} each increase ACTH stimulated activity in a dose dependent manner with maximal effects at 0.1–1.0 µ*M* free Ca^{++}, and 0.01–0.1 µ*M* free Mn^{++}. Furthermore, in the presence of Gpp(NH)p, increasing the cation concentration decreased the hormone concentration required for half-maximal stimulation. Higher concentrations of free Ca^{++} (above 10 µ*M*) inhibited basal and ACTH- or fluoride-stimulated enzyme activity. DAZORD et al. (1975) also found that high concentrations of Ca^{++} inhibited hormone stimulation. KATZ et al. (1980) concluded that the stimulatory effects of divalent cations on ACTH- and fluoride-sensitive adenylate cyclase suggested that the cations act at the nucleotide regulatory site to enhance coupling of hormone receptors to catalytic subunits. MAHAFFEE and ONTHES (1980) also came to the conclusion that Ca^{++} exerts its stimulatory effect at the level of the interaction of the nucleotide binding site with the enzyme. SAEZ et al. (1981) have interpreted these data as suggesting that Ca^{++} favours the reaction of guanine nucleotides with their binding site. They also suggest that Ca^{++} may accelerate the interaction between occupied receptors and the "N" unit.

II. Angiotensin

Studies at the beginning of the 1970's indicated that angiotensin had no effect on adenylate cyclase activity in bovine adrenals (GOODFRIEND and LIN 1970), in bovine fasciculata cells (PEYTREMANN et al. 1973) or in normal and tumour rat adrenals (SCHORR and NEY 1971). Subsequent studies (e.g., SHIMA et al. 1978) appear to have confirmed this view, although, as mentioned later, there is some evidence that angiotensin may alter cyclic AMP levels in some circumstances.

III. Cholera Toxin

HAKSAR et al. (1974) initially reported a stimulatory effect of cholera toxin on isolated rat adrenal cells which was enhanced after neuraminidase treatment of the cells. Subsequently, PALFREYMAN and SCHULSTER (1975) reported a correlation between stimulation of cyclic AMP accumulation and steroidogenesis in response to cholera toxin in intact cells.

GLOSSMANN and STRUCK (1977) showed that cholera toxin stimulated basal enzyme activity in bovine adrenal membranes and enhanced the maximal response to GTP. They also concluded from studies with the GTP analogues, Gpp(NH)p and GTPγS that cholera toxin either acted at the guanyl nucleotide regulatory site or that it affected GTP turnover. Although they were unable to observe any effect on GTP hydrolysis, it now seems clear that their results are compatible with the evidence from other systems that cholera toxin causes inhibition of GTPase activity (CASSEL and SELINGER 1977).

IV. Adenosine

Adrenal cortical membranes contain binding sites for adenosine. WOLFF and COOK (1977) working with cells of the Y1 adrenal tumour cells observed that adenosine stimulated the adenylate cyclase, that 2-chloroadenosine was equipotent with adenosine and that this stimulation was inhibited by theophylline. Thus, it appears that this effect is mediated through the so-called R-sites for adenosine action (LONDOS and WOLFF 1977). Subsequently, LONDOS and WOLFF (1977) reported that although low concentrations of adenosine stimulated the Y1 adenylate cyclase, higher concentrations were inhibitory suggesting that this tumour contained both R- and P-sites for adenosine. The concentration range over which adenosine exhibits these opposing effects is clearly different for different cells. Thus, GLYNN and COOPER (1978) reported that adenosine inhibited the adenylate cyclase in bovine adrenal membranes over the same concentration range that it stimulated the Y1 cyclase system. It was suggested that this inhibitory effect was mediated through P-sites.

C. Intracellular Cyclic Nucleotides and Calcium Ion

Perusal of the literature since 1975 reveals an increasing awareness of the problems involved in using mixed cell populations for the investigation of the relative roles of intracellular mediators in adrenal steroidogenesis. However, even in some of the studies attempting to differentiate between effects on zona glomerulosa or zona fasciculata-reticularis cells, the extent of the cross-contamination is not always clear. Furthermore, very few investigators have attempted to purify the various cell types; the major exception being TAIT and his co-workers (J. TAIT et al. 1974, 1980a; BELL et al. 1979; S. TAIT et al. 1974).

It is becoming increasingly difficult to consider cyclic AMP as the unique intracellular mediator. Recent studies in numerous other tissues have indicated that it may be facile to do so and it has become clear that the intracellular signalling systems may be complex and involve interrelationships between signals. The three major putative mediator signals, i.e. cyclic AMP/cyclic GMP/calcium ion, will therefore not be considered in isolation here but rather an attempt will be made to integrate the data into a coherent story.

I. Adrenocorticotropin

There is a wealth of evidence (see HALKERSTON 1975; SCHULSTER et al. 1976) indicating that under certain conditions ACTH stimulates the accumulation of cyclic AMP in adrenal tissue. However, the hypothesis that this nucleotide serves as an obligatory mediator of ACTH action has been increasingly questioned.

Many studies have shown that low concentrations of ACTH cause an increase in steroid production without detectable increases in cyclic AMP (see HALKERSTON 1975 for review; BEALL and SAYERS 1972; SHARMA et al. 1976; RAMACHANDRAN and MOYLE 1977; PERCHELLET et al. 1978; SAEZ et al. 1978, 1981). Various conclusions have been drawn regarding this dissociation including that the assay methods for cyclic AMP are too insensitive, that cyclic AMP is operationally compartmentalised or that cyclic AMP is not an obligatory mediator of steroidogenesis. It has also been suggested that cyclic GMP (SHARMA et al. 1974, 1976) or the cyclic AMP/cyclic GMP ratio (RUBIN et al. 1977) are important mediators of steroidogenesis.

In recent years a number of investigators have carefully re-examined the apparent discrepancy between the concentrations of ACTH required for stimulation of cyclic AMP and steroidogenesis. As discussed later in this chapter a good correlation exists between cortisol production and protein kinase activation in human adrenal cells in response to ACTH, to prostaglandin E_1 and to dibutyryl cyclic AMP (SAEZ et al. 1978, 1981). PODESTA et al. (1979) indicated that, in the presence of a low concentration of isobutyl methyl xanthine (IBMX), low doses of ACTH (in the region of $10^{-12}M$) caused a small rise in both extracellular and total intracellular cyclic AMP. At concentrations around the threshold for steroidogenesis, ACTH induced an increase in receptor-bound cyclic AMP which correlated well with steroid production, and which was not dependent on the presence of IBMX. There was a concomitant decrease in free cyclic AMP receptor sites (PODESTA et al. 1979). Essentially similar results were reported by SALA et al. (1979). They observed significant changes in extracellular cyclic AMP, receptor-bound cyclic AMP and free receptor sites at doses of ACTH as low as 10^{-12} M. These investigators concluded that, although the measurement of extracellular cyclic AMP (in the presence of a phosphodiesterase inhibitor) was a sensitive index of cyclic AMP production, the measurement of receptor bound cyclic AMP gives a more accurate measurement of active nucleotide concentrations (SALA et al. 1979). Recently, J. TAIT et al. (1980a) have critically assessed these reports and have reached the conclusion that the advantage of measuring bound rather than extracellular cyclic AMP to achieve good correlations is doubtful except perhaps from a conceptual view-point. J. TAIT et al. (1980a) have also challenged claims that the factor responsible for the good correlations of cyclic AMP and steroid production was the measurement of receptor bound cyclic AMP. They list the other important factors as being: (1) the use of a phosphodiesterase inhibitor at a critical concentration; (2) the use of shorter time intervals, and pre-incubation of the cells to provide more constant and lower basal conditions; and (3) the use of more sensitive assay methods for cyclic AMP. With regard to incubation times, it is clear that total cyclic AMP levels rise rapidly in response to ACTH (at those concentrations that are effective) and reach a peak 5–10 min after initiation of stimulation and then decline towards baseline values (ALBANO and BROWN 1974; RUBIN et al. 1977). Thus the dose-response relationships observed will be critically dependent on the incubation times chosen. Furthermore, the kinetics of cyclic AMP accumulation will be dependent on the presence or absence of phosphodiesterase inhibitors. J. Tait et al. (1980 a) also suggest that separation of cell types could contribute to better correlations between nucleotide and steroid outputs. They cite a study by Hyatt et al. (1980) which showed that, after velocity sedimentation, the purest preparation of zona fasciculata cells gave a greater maximal cyclic AMP response than unpurified adrenal cells, and they suggest that the use of such purified cell preparations could improve the correlations.

Early studies on the role of calcium in the mode of action of ACTH indicated that the binding of the peptide did not require calcium whereas activation of adenylate cyclase required an optimal concentration of the cation (see Halkerston 1975). Sayers et al. (1972) reported that increasing the extracellular calcium concentration from 0–7.65 mM increased the response of both corticosterone and cyclic AMP production. Farese and Prudente (1975) observed that, following calcium deprivation, the effect of readdition of calcium on steroidogenesis and cyclic AMP production was maximal at around 0.2 mM. Furthermore, a number of studies have shown that, in the absence of extracellular calcium, the steroidogenic response to exogenous cyclic AMP is reduced (Birmingham et al. 1960; Haksar and Peron 1973; Birmingham and Bartova 1973), indicating that the requirement for calcium in ACTH action was at more than one step. Farese and Prudente (1977) reported that incubation of adrenal sections for increasing periods of time in calcium-free media caused a progressive decrease in ACTH-induced steroidogenesis, protein synthesis and cyclic AMP accumulation. Moreover, in his review Halkerston (1975) presented the evidence which suggested that this calcium requirement is more critical for events preceding cyclic AMP formation.

More recently Shima et al. (1979 a), in a study of the effects of ACTH and calcium on cyclic AMP production by the decapsulated gland (i.e. fasciculata-reticularis cells) of the rat, observed that increasing concentrations of Ca^{++} enhanced the stimulation of cyclic AMP accumulation by ACTH. This effect was prevented by lanthanum but not by tetracaine or verapamil. In addition, high concentrations of calcium caused an increase in steroidogenesis. Steroid production was stimulated at doses of ACTH which did not cause a detectable rise in cyclic AMP. Thus, the primary action of ACTH was concluded to be increased mobilisation of calcium which stimulated steroidogenesis independently of the cyclic AMP system. (This hypothesis, however, may have to be re-examined in the light of the studies on receptor occupancy and extracellular cyclic AMP discussed earlier). These workers further suggested that higher concentrations of ACTH activate adenylate cyclase dependent on extracellular calcium. This is reminiscent of the studies mentioned earlier on binding, suggesting two orders of binding site for ACTH only one of which is related to cyclic AMP. Haksar et al. (1976) also found that lanthanum inhibited ACTH-stimulated cyclic AMP accumulation and steroidogenesis. They suggested that the effect of La^{+++} on corticosterone formation was almost entirely due to the inhibition of cyclic AMP formation since La^{+++} did not affect either the stimulation of steroidogenesis by dibutyryl cyclic AMP or the basal or glucose-stimulated conversion of steroid precursors to corticosterone. They also reported that La^{+++} inhibited the cyclic AMP formed in response to ACTH by almost 90% whereas the reduction in corticosterone was only 20%.

WARNER and CARCHMAN (1978) reported that Ruthenium red and methoxy-verapamil (calcium antagonists) and A 23187 (a cation ionophore) inhibit the ACTH- or cyclic AMP-induced steroidogenesis. ACTH-induced steroidogenesis was inhibited while the cyclic AMP-induced steroidogenesis was unaffected by EGTA. From this data they suggested that both the antagonist and the ionophore were affecting intracellular calcium which played a distinct role in steroidogenesis. However, LYMANGROVER and MARTIN (1978) reported that A 23187 stimulated corticosterone production from superfused rat adrenal cortical tissue was dependent on the presence of extracellular calcium. They also reported that threshold concentrations of ionophore potentiated the action of 1 mUnit of ACTH but not 10 mUnits.

LEIER and JUNGMANN (1973) observed that ACTH and dibutyryl cyclic AMP caused an increased uptake of $^{45}Ca^{++}$ into adrenal cells (although only after 90 min of incubation). YANAGIBASHI (1979) reported that Ca^{++} influx was induced by ACTH 1–24, the extent of the effect being dependent on the external calcium concentration. This effect was observed with a dose of ACTH (100 p*M*) which had no effect on cyclic AMP concentrations. However, JAANUS and RUBIN (1971) did not observe any increase in Ca^{++} uptake on ACTH stimulation. In a recent study, WILLIAMS et al. (1980) reported that ACTH (3×10^{-8} *M*) had no effect on efflux of $^{45}Ca^{++}$ from pre-loaded cells under conditions in which angiotensin II increased efflux from capsular cells. NEHER and MILANI (1976, 1978) reported that a suspension of colloidal Ca^{++} stimulated steroidogenesis in isolated rat adrenocortical cells in the absence of ACTH. More recently, this group has suggested that this effect of colloidal calcium may involve changes in cyclic AMP concentrations.

SHARMA and his colleagues in a series of investigations spanning several years have concluded that cyclic GMP, acting via cyclic GMP dependent protein kinase, is a physiological mediator of ACTH action on adrenal steroidogenesis (SHARMA et al. 1974, 1976; PERCHELLET et al. 1978; PERCHELLET and SHARMA 1977, 1979). They observed that low doses of ACTH, which did not cause detectable increases in cyclic AMP accumulation, increased cyclic GMP accumulation and steroidogenesis (SHARMA et al. 1974, 1976). They concluded that stimulation of steroidogenesis by low concentrations of ACTH (less than 5 μUnits) is mediated by cyclic GMP whereas at higher concentrations of ACTH the effect is mediated by cyclic AMP (SHARMA et al. 1974). The same group also reported that neither submaximal nor supramaximal doses of ACTH induced a rise in cyclic AMP in the first 30 min of incubation of isolated adrenal cells, whereas cyclic GMP accumulation was accompanied by an increase in phosphorylation and steroidogenesis (PERCHELLET et al. 1978). HARRINGTON et al. (1978) also reported that cyclic GMP concentrations in rat adrenal cells increased in a dose related manner in response to ACTH under conditions in which no changes in cyclic AMP were observed. These workers concluded that cyclic GMP rather than cyclic AMP mediates ACTH-stimulated steroidogenesis. In a more recent study, PERCHELLET and SHARMA (1979) reported that the increase in cyclic GMP accumulation and steroidogenesis, normally seen in response to ACTH, was not observed when the isolated rat adrenal zona fasciculata cells were incubated in a calcium-free medium. They also showed that calcium, in the absence of ACTH, did not stimulate cyclic GMP accumulation or steroidogenesis.

In contrast, RUBIN et al. (1977) reported that ACTH caused a decrease in cyclic GMP in bovine cortical cells in the first 5 min but that at 15–30 min this reverted to an increase. These investigators observed an increase in cyclic AMP at 5 min in response to ACTH. They observed that PGE_2 caused a rise in the concentration of both nucleotides but the increase in cyclic GMP preceeded that of cyclic AMP. They suggested that the regulation of steroidogenesis may be related to the relative amounts of these two cyclic nucleotides rather than the absolute concentrations.

A possible role for cyclic GMP as a mediator of ACTH action in the rat was also investigated by HAYASHI et al. (1979). They observed that low (1 p*M*) concentrations of ACTH elicited an increase in cyclic GMP production, but that higher concentrations (100 p*M*) had no effect. However, it appeared that the change in cyclic GMP was confined to the extracellular fraction. Furthermore, the change in cyclic GMP production was not apparent until at least 15 min of incubation. They concluded that this data, together with the findings that cyclic GMP derivatives were poor stimuli of steroidogenesis, indicated that cyclic GMP was unlikely to mediate the acute effects of ACTH.

WHITLEY et al. (1975) observed that when ACTH was injected intravenously into hypophysectomised rats and the adrenal cyclic nucleotide content measured 3 min later, there was a dose-dependent increase in cyclic AMP but a fall in cyclic GMP (between 0 and 0.2 mU ACTH).

RUBIN and LAYCHOCK (1978) have suggested that in those situations in which steroidogenesis is stimulated without an effect on cyclic AMP, such as stimulation by NPS-ACTH, a mechanism involving prostaglandin possibly via an effect of calcium on phospholipase A_2 may be operating.

It has been clear for some time that prostaglandins can enhance corticosteroidogenesis (e.g., FLACK and RAMWELL 1972; SARUTA and KAPLAN 1972; WARNER and RUBIN 1975; HONN and CHAVIN 1976). Aldosterone production is also increased by some prostaglandins (SARUTA and KAPLAN 1972; HONN and CHAVIN 1977). SARUTA and KAPLAN (1972) reported that the steroidogenic action of prostaglandins required extracellular calcium. They also reported an increase in cyclic AMP concentrations in response to PGA_1, $PGF_{1\alpha}$ and $PGF_{2\alpha}$. ROLLAND and CHAMBAZ (1977) found that PGA_1, PGE_2, and $PGF_{2\alpha}$ increased cholesterol side-chain cleavage in isolated adrenal mitochondria provided that calcium was present. In another study, it was reported that certain doses (10 μg/ml and 100 μg/ml) of PGA_1 and PGA_2 increased both cortisol and cyclic AMP output but that lower doses depressed both parameters (HONN and CHAVIN 1977). Moreover, a low dose of PGA_1 increased aldosterone output whereas higher doses depressed aldosterone biosynthesis. The B series prostaglandins appeared to have similar effects to the E series compounds, although only low doses of PGB_1 and PGB_2 stimulated aldosterone secretion (HONN and CHAVIN 1977).

DAZORD et al. (1974) observed that PGE_1 stimulated adenylate cyclase activity and that this stimulation was unaffected by the presence of chelating agents. A PGE_2-induced elevation in the concentration of both cyclic AMP and cyclic GMP in bovine adrenal cells was observed by RUBIN et al. (1977). These investigators also reported that the rise in cyclic GMP preceded the rise in cyclic AMP. In one study it was found that prostacyclin (PGI_2), which is formed from cyclic endoperoxides, was the most potent stimulator of steroidogenesis in isolated cat adrenal cells (ELLIS et al. 1978). Calcium deprivation only partially inhibited this effect of prostacyclin. Steroidogenesis was accompanied by an increase in the accumulation of intracellular cyclic AMP. SAEZ et al. (1978) reported that PGE_1 (like ACTH) induced a increase in cyclic AMP-dependent protein kinase activity in both normal and tumour human adrenal glands and that in one tumour in which the adenylate cyclase was unaffected by PGE_1, there was also no effect on protein kinase activity or steroidogenesis.

It has been shown that ACTH induces a calcium-dependent increase in phospholipase activity (LAYCHOCK et al. 1977a) and production and release of PGE_2 and $PGF_{2\alpha}$ (LAYCHOCK et al. 1977b; LAYCHOCK and RUBIN 1975, 1976; RUBIN and LAYCHOCK 1978). LAYCHOCK et al. (1977b) observed that an increase in $PGF_{2\alpha}$ release occurred on perifusion of cat adrenal glands with ACTH. This release declined to basal levels on removal of ACTH whereas steroidogenesis continued at a maximal rate for at least 30 min. Both ACTH and NPS-ACTH stimulated prostaglandin and steroid release, but NPS-ACTH had no measureable effect on cyclic AMP concentrations. Indomethacin, although abolishing the stimulated prostaglandin release, had little effect on steroidogenesis. Calcium deprivation blocked prostaglandin and steroid release induced by ACTH or NPS-ACTH but did not affect steroid release stimulated by monobutyryl cyclic AMP. They concluded that, although prostaglandins play a role in steroidogenesis, they do not appear to be obligatory mediators. RUBIN and LAYCHOCK (1978) have reported that pregnenolone did not augment prostaglandin release and have suggested that the action of ACTH on prostaglandin release would appear to be taking place at the cell membrane or at a step prior to the conversion of pregnenolone to corticosteroid.

SCHREY and RUBIN (1979) have presented further evidence for a role for phospholipase in the action of ACTH. They reported that ACTH caused an increase in the incorporation of [^{14}C]-arachidonic acid into phosphatidyl inositol within 2 min of incubation of cat adrenal cells. This effect was observed with low doses of ACTH (2 μUnits/ml) and the dose response paralleled that of cortisol secretion. The increased incorporation was dependent on the presence of extracellular Ca^{++} and could be mimicked by the calcium ionophore, A 23187. Substances known to inhibit phospholipase A_2 activity were also effective in inhibiting arachidonate incorporation into phosphatidyl inositol. Both ACTH and A 23187 also caused a loss of arachidonic from prelabelled phospholipids. They concluded that an early action of ACTH was a calcium dependent turnover of arachidonyl phosphatidyl inositol and that selective re-acylation of the lyso-phosphatidyl inositol followed rapidly. RUBIN and LAYCHOCK (1978) had previously suggested lysophospholipids may play a role in modulating adenylate cyclase activity and exocytosis. They further suggested that ACTH may have separate actions on adenylate cyclase and phospholipase A_2 which may be relevent to the previously mentioned findings of dual ACTH receptors. These workers also speculated on the possible modulatory role of the prostaglandins produced on activation of phospholipase by ACTH. They suggested that the prostaglandins may act as calcium ionophores or that they may modulate the level of the cyclic nucleotides within the cell.

A recent series of reports by Farese and his colleagues has focussed attention on the role of polyphosphoinositides in the control of adrenal steroidogenesis. Mitochondrial cholesterol side-chain cleavage is stimulated by polyphosphorylated phospholipids (Farese and Sabir 1979), thus mimicking the effect of ACTH on pregnenolone synthesis. Moreover, ACTH raises adrenal polyphosphoinositide concentrations (Farese et al. 1979). Administration of ACTH in vivo induced comparable increases in both corticosterone and polyphosphoinositide. Furthermore, cyclic AMP also increased polyphosphoinositide and corticosterone when added to adrenal sections, and these effects were dependent on the presence of calcium (Farese et al. 1980). This group had previously suggested that calcium may amplify the effects of ACTH on steroidogenesis (Farese and Prudente (1978). They also observed that adrenal cytosol contains an ACTH-induced steroidogenic factor which increases pregnenolone synthesis when added to adrenal mitochondria (Farese and Sabir 1980). The phospholipids, cardiolipin, diphosphoinositide and triphosphoinositide were found to be present in adrenal cytosol and the cyclic AMP- and ACTH-induced changes in adrenal cytosolic activity and polyphosphoinositide levels were abolished by cycloheximide (Farese and Sabir 1980; Farese et al. 1980). It has been established previously that cycloheximide and other protein synthesis inhibitors block the steroidogenic actions of ACTH and cyclic AMP (see Halkerston 1975) and it appeared that a cycloheximide-sensitive mediator of ACTH action may be a polyphosphoinositide. It has also been shown that the increases in polyphosphoinositides were accompanied by increases in phosphatidyl inositol and phosphatidic acid and that these changes were also blocked by cycloheximide (Farese et al. 1980). These investigators have suggested that the ACTH-stimulated rise of cyclic AMP leads to an increase in the phosphatidic acid-polyphosphoinositide cycle and that this cycle may be involved in the steroidogenic (and other) actions of ACTH (Farese et al. 1980).

ACTH also stimulates steroidogenesis in zona glomerulosa cells. Albano et al. (1974) reported that purification of zona glomerulosa cells from the capsular preparation resulted in a fall in the response of cyclic AMP to ACTH but that this peptide retained its ability to stimulate cyclic AMP production in this preparation. Fujita et al. (1979) also reported that ACTH stimulated cyclic AMP accumulation in purified zona glomerulosa cells. Fakunding et al. (1979) reported that aldosterone production by zona glomerulosa cells stimulated by ACTH was dependent on the extracellular Ca^{++} concentration. They showed that ACTH stimulated aldosterone and cyclic AMP production at all calcium concentrations tested and that the production of steroid was correlated with the increase in cyclic AMP accumulation. However, the dichotomy between the dose response relationships was apparent at all calcium concentrations. Reduction of extracellular Ca^{++} concentration resulted in an increase in the ACTH concentration required for halfmaximal stimulation of steroid and cyclic AMP production and in a reduction in the maximal output of aldosterone. They suggested that calcium is required for the coupling of the ACTH receptor with adenylate cyclase in the zona glomerulosa cell membrane as also suggested for the zona fasciculata. They also found steroid production stimulated by exogenous cyclic AMP, cholera toxin or serotonin was decreased as the Ca^{++} concentration was reduced but that the calcium concentration did not cause a decline in the concentration required for half-maximal concentration. They concluded that calcium had another action i.e. at an intracellular locus subsequent to the action of cyclic AMP. SHIMA et al. (1979b) reported that high concentrations of intracellular calcium potentiated the stimulatory action of ACTH on both cyclic AMP and aldosterone output. They also reported that tetracaine or verapamil inhibited the ACTH-stimulated aldosterone production without affecting cyclic AMP accumulation. In contrast, lanthanum reduced both aldosterone and cyclic AMP production.

II. Angiotensin

The zona glomerulosa, the site of aldosterone synthesis, functions independently of the other zones of the adrenal. As mentioned earlier, steroidogenesis in the zona glomerulosa is stimulated by a number of substances including ACTH, angiotensin II, increased extracellular K^+ and serotonin (J. TAIT et al. 1974). The intracellular mechanisms mediating the effect of angiotensin are surrounded with uncertainty. Although, there is some evidence that cyclic AMP accumulation in zona fasciculata cells is increased by angiotensin II (PEYTREMANN et al. 1973; ALBANO et al. 1974), it appears that this effect may have been due to an impurity present in the preparation of [Asn^1] angiotensin II (Hypertensin) since recent studies with pure Asn^1 and Asp^1 angiotensin II have shown that neither compound stimulates steroidogenesis in zona fasciculata cells (J. TAIT et al. 1981). However, SHIMA et al. (1978) reported that neither cyclic AMP levels nor corticosterone output was increased by angiotensin II in the decapsulated fraction of the gland. VALLOTTON et al. 1981) reported that pure angiotensin II (10^{-7} *M*) was without effect on cyclic AMP accumulation in bovine zona fasciculata cells. A similar lack of effect was observed in dog zona fasciculata cells (FUJITA et al. 1979). Furthermore, as stated earlier, angiotensin II appears to have no effect on adenylate cyclase activity in the adrenal (GOODFRIEND and LIN 1970; PEYTREMANN et al. 1973; SCHORR and NEY 1971; SHIMA et al. 1978).

Although it has been reported that high doses of Asn^1-angiotensin II (i.e. above 10^{-4} *M*) had an effect on increasing cyclic AMP accumulation in rat zona glomerulosa cells (ALBANO et al. 1974), it is probable that this effect was also due to the impurities in the angiotensin preparation used (J. TAIT et al. 1981). Most of the early studies indicated that changes in cyclic AMP concentration did not occur with doses lower than 10^{-4} *M* angiotensin II (SARUTA et al. 1972; PEYTREMANN et al. 1974; ALBANO et al. 1974). More recently, FUJITA et al. (1979) reported that cyclic AMP accumulation was not increased by a wide range of doses of Asp^1-angiotensin II (10^{-11} *M* to 10^{-5} *M*) in dog or rat capsular cells. Extracellular and receptor-bound cyclic AMP were also unaffected by angiotensin II or the analogue des-Asp^1-angiotensin II. The addition of the phosphodiesterase inhibitor (IBMX) did not alter the lack of stimulation of cyclic AMP production by the peptide. SHIMA et al. (1978) also reported that aldosterone production in capsular fractions was increased by angiotensin II (Hypertensin 10^{-5} *M*) without any effect on cyclic AMP concentrations. Furthermore, theophylline increased cyclic AMP accumulation but neither increased steroid production nor affected the stimulation due to angiotensin. It should be borne in mind, however, that theophylline has other actions than as a phosphodiesterase inhibitor and may be inhibiting protein synthesis. Increasing concentrations of calcium stimulated the production of both cyclic AMP and aldosterone; angiotensin II further increased this calcium-induced aldosterone production but was without effect on the calcium stimulated cyclic AMP accumulation. The calcium antagonists, tetracaine, verapamil and lanthanum inhibited both basal and angiotensin-stimulated aldosterone secretion. This study also indicated that phosphodiesterase activity was increased in slices of the capsular fraction that had been incubated with angiotensin II. They concluded that angiotensin acts on the glomerulosa cell to increase intracellular calcium and that this ionic alteration is involved in the control of steroidogenesis concomitant with an increase in cyclic nucleotide phosphodiesterase activity. CHIU and FREER (1979) reported that methoxyverapamil (10^{-4} *M*) blocked the steroidogenic response to angiotensin II (as well as to K^+ and ACTH). However, this treatment was less effective than simple removal of Ca^{++} from the incubation medium.

FAKUNDING et al. (1979) observed that only ACTH elicited a stimulation of cyclic AMP in zona glomerulosa cells. They also, like SHIMA et al. (1978), reported that angiotensin II failed to increase cyclic AMP levels in the presence of calcium. In fact a slight (but not significant) depression of cyclic AMP concentration was observed at the lower Ca^{++} concentrations; a finding consistent with the reported increase in phosphodiesterase activity (SHIMA et al. 1978). We have also observed a small but consistent decrease in cyclic AMP accumulation which is usually more pronounced at higher concentrations (10^{-7} *M* to 10^{-4} *M*) of angiotensin II (J. TAIT et al. 1980b). However, aldosterone output stimulated by angiotensin II was calcium dependent (FAKUNDING et al. 1979). Reduction of the extracellular calcium concentration diminished the maximum aldosterone response but did not result in a change of the concentration of angiotensin required for half-maximal stimulation of aldosterone production. These investigators concluded that this data, taken with the previously mentioned results indicating that calcium did not affect the binding of angiotensin II to zona glomerulosa cells and that calcium may act at a intracellular locus subsequent to the activation of cyclic AMP, suggested that angiotensin II required calcium at a point subsequent to the initial interaction. They suggested that the cellular response to angiotensin is more sensitive to calcium depletion than that mediated by ACTH or cyclic AMP, and that Ca^{++} plays a more critical role.

In recent studies TAIT and his colleagues have investigated the effect of stimulators of glomerulosa steroidogenesis on $^{45}Ca^{++}$ efflux from these cells (J. TAIT et al. 1980b; WILLIAMS et al. 1980). Using a superfusion apparatus they observed that $^{45}Ca^{++}$ efflux from preloaded cells was unaffected by serotonin (10^{-4} *M*), K^{++} (8.4 m*M* and 5.9 m*M*) and ACTH (3×10^{-8} *M*). However, Asp[1]-angiotensin II (10^{-9} *M* and 10^{-10} *M*) had a significant effect on $^{45}Ca^{++}$ efflux that was correlated with stimulation of steroidogenesis. Moreover, they observed that this effect was specific for glomerulosa cells. GOODFRIEND and ELLIOTT (1980) also reported that $^{45}Ca^{++}$ efflux was affected by angiotensin II.

In a recent study, BING and SCHULSTER (1978) reported that Asp-angiotensin II (2×10^{-10} *M* to 2×10^{-6} *M*) caused a significant increase in cyclic AMP accumulation in incubations of cells from capsular strippings of the rat adrenal. They also reported a good correlation between cyclic AMP content and steroid production over this range of angiotensin concentrations. Further, they showed a close agreement between decreases in cyclic AMP and aldosterone production in response to the angiotensin II antagonist, Sar[1], Ala[8]-angiotensin II. J. TAIT et al. (1980a) have discussed our re-examination of the incubation conditions used by BING and SCHULSTER (1978) and reported that an increase in cyclic AMP accumulation is still not observed with Asp[1]-angiotensin II stimulation.

The reasons underlying the discrepancy between the work of BING and SCHULSTER (1978) and the other investigators who have concluded that the effect of angiotensin is not mediated by cyclic AMP (SARUTA et al. 1972; PEYTREMANN et al. 1974; ALBANO et al. 1974; SHIMA et al. 1978; FUJITA et al. 1979; FAKUNDING et al. 1979; J. TAIT et al. 1980a, b) are unclear. It is true, however, that relatively high concentrations of peptide were employed in some of these studies (SARUTA et al. 1972; PEYTREMANN et al. 1974; ALBANO et al. 1974; SHIMA et al. 1978). Nevertheless, the concentrations used by FAKUNDING et al. (1979) of 10^{-8} M and J. TAIT et al. (1980b) of between 10^{-11} M and 10^{-6} M also did not result in any increase in cyclic AMP. It appears that under certain situations both cyclic AMP mediated and cyclic AMP independent mechanisms may function.

The possible role of cyclic GMP in the mode of action of angiotensin has been investigated. DOUGLAS et al. (1978b) reported that angiotensin II, angiotensin III, K^+ (15 mM) and ACTH had no effect on this nucleotide in dog glomerulosa cells. We observed a similar lack of effect of angiotensin II in rat glomerulosa cells (BELL et al. 1981).

Recent studies have indicated that angiotensin III (des Asp[1] angiotensin II) does not increase cyclic AMP accumulation (J. TAIT et al. 1980b; DOUGLAS et al. 1978b) but that it does increase $^{45}Ca^{++}$ efflux from glomerulosa cells with a lower potency, reflecting its effect on steroidogenesis (J. TAIT et al. 1980b).

III. Potassium

Small changes in the extracellular potassium ion concentration cause an increase in aldosterone (and corticosterone) production from the zona glomerulosa cell. Indeed, extracellular potassium is a necessary requirement for stimulation of aldosterone production. The possible role for intracellular K^+ in the control of steroidogenesis in glomerulosa cells has been reviewed recently by J. TAIT et al. (1980a). A number of investigators have reported changes in cyclic AMP concentrations in response to increases in K^+ concentration; from 5.2 mM to 9.2 mM (SARUTA et al. 1972); from 3 mM to 6 mM (BOYD et al. 1973); from 3.6 mM to 6.4 mM (ALBANO et al. 1974; S. TAIT et al. 1974). The latter workers also showed that fractionation of the capsular cells and hence virtual elimination of the fasciculata contamination did not affect the cyclic AMP response to increased K^+ concentration. They also reported that increasing the extracellular K^+ concentration from 3.6 mM to 5.9 mM resulted in a near maximal increase in corticosterone production without a significant change in cyclic AMP accumulation. At higher concentration of K^+ (8.4 mM) cyclic AMP levels were considerably higher although steroid production was only slightly increased (over the value at 5.9 mM). This effect of 8.4 mM K^+ was apparent at 40 min of incubation. However, other studies have reported that changes in K^+ concentration do not affect cyclic AMP accumulation. For example, FAKUNDING et al. (1979) observed that the addition of 14.5 mM K^+ to the incubation medium had no effect on cyclic AMP concentrations at any of the calcium concentrations tested. They concluded that K^+, like angiotensin, had an action which was critically dependent on calcium concentration. The studies of MACKIE et al. (1978) in which a significant effect on $^{45}Ca^{++}$ efflux was observed in zona glomerulosa cells incubated with increased extracellular K^+ concentrations, lends some support to this conclusion.

However, using a superfusion apparatus that reduced dead space and eliminated excessive adsorption of calcium, TAIT and co-workers have shown that increasing extracellular K^+ from 3.6 m*M* to either 5.9 m*M* or 8.4 m*M* had no effect on $^{45}Ca^{++}$ efflux from zona glomerulosa cells (J. TAIT et al. 1980b). It should be remembered that, under identical conditions, angiotensin II did affect Ca^{++} efflux.

It is of some interest that FUJITA et al. (1979) reported a lack of additivity between the steroid responses to K^+ and angiotensin II; they suggested that these agents might share a common mechanism of action on steroidogenesis. However, it should be borne in mind that these workers do not find an effect of K^+ on cyclic AMP accumulation whereas others do. Furthermore, TAIT and co-workers (S. TAIT et al. 1974b; J. TAIT and TAIT 1976) reported that steroid output stimulated maximally by cyclic AMP could be further increased by changes in K^+ concentration suggesting that both cyclic AMP dependent and cyclic AMP independent mechanisms may operate.

IV. Serotonin

Steroidogenesis in the rat zona glomerulosa is stimulated by serotonin (MULLER and ZIEGLER 1968; J. TAIT et al. 1974, 1980c). Indeed the maximum response to serotonin in purified glomerulosa cells is similar to that induced by ACTH, by increased K^+ and by angiotensin II. This response is inhibited by serotonin antagonists (AL-DUJAILI et al. 1980). Serotonin caused an increase in cyclic AMP accumulation in preparations of rat adrenal capsular cells (ALBANO et al. 1974; S. TAIT et al. 1974). However, at one dose (10^{-8} *M*) serotonin did not increase cyclic AMP accumulation whereas steroid output was virtually maximal. It would be interesting to see whether determination of extracellular or receptor-bound cyclic AMP abolished this dichotomy as discussed earlier for ACTH on zona fasciculata cells. FUJITA et al. (1979) also reported that serotonin (10^{-8} *M* to 10^{-5} *M*) increased cyclic AMP accumulation in rat capsular cells.

FAKUNDING et al. (1979) reported that the maximum response to serotonin was reduced when the extracellular Ca^{++} was lowered. However, J. TAIT et al. (1980b) reported that serotonin (10^{-4} *M*) had no effect on efflux of $^{45}Ca^{++}$ from preloaded glomerulosa cells.

D. Actions of Cyclic Nucleotides in the Adrenal Cortex

A primary effect of cyclic AMP is the activation of protein kinases. The adrenal cortex contains cyclic AMP-dependent protein kinase activity which is rapidly activated by ACTH. The dose-response curves, however, indicate that low, steroidogenic doses of ACTH, which fail to stimulate protein kinase activity (see

HALKERSTON 1975). These results have also been used to call into question the view that cyclic AMP is the sole and obligatory mediator of steroidogenesis in the adrenal. Nevertheless, it is clearly important to investigate the mechanism of action of cyclic nucleotides (and of calcium ion) for the insight such studies may provide into the relative roles of the putative intracellular mediators.

Consequently, a number of investigators have studied the role of protein kinases using various approaches, one of the most popular of which has been the use of tumour cells. A number of human adrenocortical tumours display a diminished or absent response to ACTH. In some cases this appears to be dependent on altered protein kinases. In one such tumour there appears to be an absence of one isoenzyme of protein kinase, the other protein kinase being unaffected by cyclic AMP (RIOU et al. 1977). SAEZ et al. (1978) studied the protein kinase activity of normal and malignant human adrenal tissue. They observed that high concentrations of ACTH completely activated the protein kinase of normal adrenal cells at 3 min [see also the similar results reported by RICHARDSON and SCHULSTER (1973) using rat adrenal cells]. At this time only a small increase in cyclic AMP was observed and there was no detectable increase in steroidogenesis. They suggested that activation of protein kinase requires only small increases in intracellular cyclic AMP (SAEZ et al. 1981). These investigators also observed a close-linked correlation between protein kinase activation and cortisol production at all doses of ACTH (10^{-11} *M* to 10^{-6} *M*), although the concentration of ACTH required for half maximal stimulation was lower for cortisol production than for protein kinase activation (SAEZ et al. 1978, 1981). Similar correlations were observed with PGE_1 and dibutyryl cyclic AMP (SAEZ et al. 1978). They concluded that cyclic AMP dependent protein kinase plays a major role in the control of steroidogenesis at low concentrations of ACTH. They also conclude that their results explain the dichotomy between steroid output and intracellular cyclic AMP accumulation. As discussed earlier, the studies on the effect of ACTH on receptor-bound and extracellular cyclic AMP led to a similar conclusion (PODESTA et al. 1979; SALA et al. 1979). SAEZ and his co-workers also reported that ACTH failed to stimulate either protein kinase activity or steroidogenesis in a tumour in which the adenylate cyclase was unresponsive to the hormone, although the tumour did respond to PGE_1 and to dibutyryl cyclic AMP. Another tumour, in which adenylate cyclase and protein kinase activities were unresponsive to prostaglandin, did respond to ACTH with increases in both protein kinase activity and steroidogenesis.

Similar conclusions were reached from the results of studies on mutants of the Y1 mouse adrenocortical tumour cell. It has been reported that protein kinase activity in mutants displaying an alteration in cyclic AMP dependent protein kinase closely paralleled the steroidogenic response in response to ACTH and cyclic AMP (SCHIMMER et al. 1977; RAE et al. 1979). In mutant cells with diminished adenylate cyclase responsiveness to ACTH, the hormone had little effect on steroidogenesis whereas the response to cyclic nucleotides was normal.

This view of the importance of protein kinase activity in regulating steroidogenesis is not supported by MOYLE et al. (1976) who found that nitrophenylsulphenyl-ACTH (NPS-ACTH), which inhibited the effect of ACTH on cyclic AMP accumulation, caused an increase in corticosteroidogenesis without affecting protein kinase activity. However, they also reported that very high doses of NPS-ACTH will stimulate protein kinase activity. SHARMA et al. (1976) reported that while millimolar concentrations of cyclic AMP and cyclic GMP stimulated both steroidogenesis and protein kinase in a dose dependent manner, lower (micromolar) concentrations caused protein kinase activation without affecting steroidogenesis. They also reported that ACTH stimulated steroidogenesis, cyclic GMP accumulation and protein kinase activity in the absence of any detectable rise in cyclic AMP accumulation. They came to the conclusion that not all of the cyclic nucleotide dependent protein kinase activities are necessarily involved in the steroidogenic response. These same investigators showed that neither cycloheximide nor actinomycin D affected the phosphorylation induced by ACTH, cyclic AMP or cyclic GMP suggesting that the inhibitory effect of these drugs on steroidogenesis is exerted at a step beyond protein phosphorylation.

SHARMA and his colleagues have also studied the role of protein kinase in a rat adrenocortical carcinoma. ACTH does not appear to stimulate cyclic AMP production, protein kinase activity or steroidogenesis in these cells. Millimolar concentrations of cyclic AMP and cyclic GMP activated protein kinase but, unlike in the normal cell, did not stimulate steroidogenesis suggesting that the tumour protein kinase may be unrelated to steroidogenesis in these cells (SHARMA et al. 1977a). Micromolar concentrations of cyclic AMP (but not cyclic GMP) appear to stimulate protein kinase activity in these cells (SHARMA et al. 1977a). The lack of effect of cyclic GMP on protein kinase led these workers to suggest that there may also be a defective cyclic GMP dependent protein kinase in these cells (SHARMA 1977a). Furthermore, the same group have reported that a defective cyclic AMP dependent protein kinase has been partially purified from adrenocortical carcinoma cells (SHARMA et al. 1977b). Although this protein specifically bound cyclic AMP it failed to phosphorylate exogenous substrate. They suggested that the lack of cyclic AMP dependent protein kinase activity may be responsible for the loss of cyclic AMP control of steroidogenesis in these tumour cells. It is now apparent that there are cyclic AMP-independent protein kinases in adrenal cells (COCHET et al. 1977a; MCPHERSON and RAMACHANDRAN 1980). There is also evidence that a cyclic AMP independent protein kinase is located on the external face of the plasma membrane (MCPHERSON and RAMACHANDRAN 1980) and that its activity is increased by ACTH.

Elucidation of the nature of endogenous substrates for protein kinases is still far from complete. It has been known for some time that cholesterol esterase can act as a substrate (TRZECIAK and BOYD 1974). More recent studies have shown that cyclic AMP-dependent protein kinase, cyclic AMP, ATP and magnesium ions are required for activation of cholesterol esterase (BECKETT and BOYD 1977; NAGHSHINEH et al. 1978). The time course of activation closely paralleled the time course of phosphorylation of the enzyme (BECKETT and BOYD 1977). The activation of cholesterol esterase upon incubation with ATP, cyclic AMP and magnesium ions and the cytosol fraction from bovine adrenal cortex was inhibited by protein kinase inhibitor. These workers also suggested that deactivation of cholesterol esterase involved dephosphorylation catalysed by a phosphoprotein phosphatase dependent on magnesium or calcium ions (BECKETT and BOYD 1977). In an investigation of the role of protein kinases in ACTH-induced steroidogenesis, HOFMANN et al. (1978) investigated the effect of protein kinase catalytic subunit on rat cholesterol sidechain cleavage. They came to the conclusion that acute stimulation by ACTH does not involve protein kinase mediated phosphorylation of this enzyme system. COCHET et al. (1977b) reported the presence, in adrenal particulate preparations, of an endogenous protein (or lipoprotein) substrate for both cyclic AMP-dependent and independent protein kinases. The biological significance of this substrate is not known.

E. Concluding Remarks

Undoubtedly, the considerable efforts made by numerous researchers over the past five years have led to a better understanding of the control of adrenal steroidogenesis. One of the shifts of opinion during this time has been a return to the view that cyclic AMP is a major mediator of ACTH action (probably on all zones of the adrenal cortex). This change has been brought about primarily through investigations on the various pools of cyclic nucleotides. However, it is unlikely that other intracellular messengers are not involved in some way. Clearly, calcium is necessary for ACTH action, but the loci of its effects, apart from at the level of adenylate cyclase and phospholipase A_2, have yet to be elucidated. Likewise, it is possible that cyclic GMP is also involved in the intracellular signalling system (perhaps especially at low concentrations of hormone), although evidence in this area remains somewhat controversial despite strenuous research effort. Other questions that remain unanswered include the nature of the intracellular substrates for protein kinases, the role of cyclic nucleotide-independent protein kinases and the involvement of prostaglandins and phospholipids (particularly the polyphosphoinositides) in the intracellular control mechanisms. The results of attempts to understand how these systems are integrated within the cell will make fascinating reading over the next few years.

On the whole, less is known about the mechanism of action of the various stimuli (apart from ACTH) of steroidogenesis in the zona glomerulosa. While there is some agreement that cyclic AMP is a mediator of the action of serotonin, the intracellular control mechanisms governing steroidogenesis stimulated by angiotensin and potassium are still somewhat controversial. The majority opinion appears to be that cyclic AMP is a major intracellular mediator of the effects of changes in the concentration of potassium ions but that the mediation of angiotensin action involves a cyclic AMP independent/calcium dependent mechanism. However, the lack of complete agreement in this area may indicate that this situation is not immutable but that other (including cyclic AMP-dependent) mechanisms may operate under certain circumstances. Indeed, the recent suggestion that cyclic AMP-dependent and calcium-dependent mechanisms may be alternative means to the same end warrants further investigation. It will be interesting to see if future work in this area supports this intriguing hypothesis. Other aspects which should be worth studying include the possible role of calmodulin and phospholipids especially polyphosphoinositides in the control of steroidogenesis in the zona glomerulosa.

Acknowledgements. I am grateful to Professor J. F. TAIT, F.R.S. and Mrs. S. A. S. TAIT, F. R. S. for their constructive critical comments during the writing of this review. I would also like to express my gratitude to Professor and Mrs. TAIT, and to Dr. J. M. SAEZ for allowing me to see their manuscripts prior to publication.

Work performed in the reviewer's laboratory and the collaborative studies with J. F. TAIT and S. A. S. TAIT were funded, to a large degree, by the Medical Research Council.

References

Aguilera G, Catt KJ (1978) Regulation of aldosterone secretion by the renin-angiotensin system during sodium restriction in rats. Proc Natl Sci USA 75:4057–4061

Aguilera G, Hauger RL, Catt KJ (1978) Control of aldosterone secretion during sodium restriction: adrenal receptor regulation and increased adrenal sensitivity to angiotensin II. Proc Natl Acad Sci USA 75:975–979

Aguilera G, Capponi A, Baukai A, Fujita K, Hauger R, Catt KJ (1979) Metabolism and biological activities of angiotensin II and des-Asp'-angiotensin II in isolated adrenal glumerulosa cells. Endocrinology 104:1279–1285

Albano JDM, Brown BL (1974) The distribution of adenosine 3′:5′ cyclic monophosphate between adrenal tissue and medium after stimulation with corticotropin. Trans Biochem Soc 2:412–415

Albano JDM, Brown BL, Ekins RP, Tait SAS, Tait JF (1974) The effects of potassium, 5-hydroxytryptamine, adrenocorticotrophin and angiotensin II on the concentration of adenosine 3′:5′-cyclic monophosphate in suspensions of dispersed rat adrenal zona glomerulosa and zona fasciculata cells. Biochem J 142:391–400

Al-Dujaili EAS, Boscaro M, Espiner EA, Edwards CRW (1980) In vitro and in vivo effects of indoleamines on aldosterone biosynthesis in the rat. Abstr Int Congr Endocrinol, Melbourne. Published by International Society of Endocrinology

Beall RJ, Sayers G (1972) Isolated adrenal cells: steroidogenesis and cyclic AMP accumulation in response to ACTH. Arch Biochem Biophys 148:70–76

Beckett GJ, Boyd GS (1977) Purification and control of bovine adrenal cortical cholesterol ester hydrolase and evidence for the activation of the enzyme by phosphorylation. Eur J Biochem 71:223–233

Bell JBG, Gould RP, Hyatt PJ, Tait JF, Tait SAS (1978) Properties of rat adrenal zona reticularis cells: preparation by gravitational sedimentation. J Endocrinol 77:25–41

Bell JBG, Tait JF, Tait SAS, Barnes GD and Brown BL (1981) Lack of effect of angiotensin on levels of cyclic AMP in isolated adrenal zona glomerulosa cells from the rat. Journal of Endocrinology 91:145–154

Bell JBG, Gould RP, Hyatt PJ, Tait JF, Tait SAS (1979) Properties of rat adrenal zona reticularis cells: production and stimulation of certain steroids. J Endocrinol 83:435–447

Bing RF, Schulster D (1978) Adenosine 3′,5′-cyclic monophosphate production and steroidogenesis by isolated rat adrenal glomerulosa cells. Effects of angiotensin II and Sar^1, ala^8-angiotensin II. Biochem J 176:39–45

Birmingham MK, Bartova A (1973) Effects of calcium and theophylline on ACTH- and dibutyryl cyclic AMP-stimulated steroidogenesis and glycolysis by intact mouse adrenal glands in vitro. Endocrinology 92:743–749

Birmingham MK, Kurlents E, Lane R, Muhlstock B, Traikov H (1960) Effects of calcium on the potassium and sodium content of rat adrenal glands, on the stimulation of steroid production by adenosine 3′:5′-monophosphate, and on the response of the adrenal to short contact with ACTH. Can J Biochem 38:1077–1085

Birnbaumer L, Iyengar R (1982) Coupling of receptors to adenylate cyclases. In: Nathanson JA, Kebabian JW (eds) Cyclic Nucleotides. Springer, Berlin Heidelberg New York (Handbook of experimental pharmacology, vol 58/I)

Bonnafous J-C, Fauchere J-L, Schwyzer R (1977) Stimulation and inhibition of bovine adrenal cortex cell membrane adenylate cyclase by synthetic corticotropin fragments and the effects of 5′-guanylyl-imidodiphosphate. FEBS Lett 78:247–250

Boyd J, Mulrow PJ, Palmore WP, Silvo P (1973) Importance of potassium in the regulation of aldosterone production. Circ Res [Suppl] 1:39–45

Brecher PI, Pyun HY, Chobanian AV (1974) Studies on the angiotensin II receptor in the zona glomerulosa of the rat adrenal gland. Endocrinology 95:1026–1033

Bristow AF, Gleed C, Fauchere J-L, Schwyzer R, Schulster D (1980) Effects of ACTH (corticotropin) analogues on steroidogenesis and cyclic AMP in rat adrenocortical cells. Biochem J 186:599–603

Capponi AM, Catt KJ (1979) Angiotensin II receptors in adrenal cortex and uterus. Binding and activation properties of angiotensin analogues. J Biol Chem 254:5120–5127

Cassel D, Selinger Z (1977) Mechanism of adenylate cyclase activation by cholera toxin: inhibition of GTP hydrolysis at the regulatory site. Proc Natl Acad Sci USA 74:3307–3311

Catt KJ, Harwood JP, Aguilera G, Dufau ML (1979) Hormonal regulation of peptide receptors and target cell responses. Nature 280:109–116

Chiu AT, Freer RJ (1979) Angiotensin-induced steroidogenesis in rabbit adrenal: effects of pH and calcium. Mol Cell Endocrinol 13:159–166

Cochet C, Job D, Chambaz EM (1977a) Characterisation of a cyclic AMP-independent protein kinase in the bovine adrenal cortex. FEBS Lett 83:53–58

Cochet C, Job D, Chambaz EM (1977b) Characterisation of an endogenous substrate of protein kinase in the bovine adrenal cortex. FEBS Lett 83:59–62

Crawford A, MacNeil S, Amirrasooli H, Tomlinson S (1980) Properties of a factor in cytosol that enhances hormone-stimulated adenylate cyclase activity. Biochem J 188:401–407

Dazord A, Morera AM, Bertrand J, Saez JM (1974) Prostaglandin receptors in human and ovine adrenal glands: binding and stimulation of adenylate cyclase in subcellular preparations. Endocrinology 96:352–359

Dazord A, Gallet D, Saez JM (1975) Adenyl cyclase in rat, ovine and human adrenal preparation. Horm Metab Res 7:184–189

Devynck M-A, Rouzaire-Dubois B, Chevillotte E, Meyer P (1976) Variations in the number of uterine angiotensin receptors following changes in plasma angiotensin levels. Eur J Pharmacol 40:24–37

Douglas J, Catt KJ (1976) Regulation of angiotensin II receptors in rat adrenal cortex by dietary electrolytes. J Clin Invest 58:834–843

Douglas J, Saltman S, Fredlund P, Kondo T, Catt KJ (1976) Receptor binding of angiotensin II and antagonists. Correlation with aldosterone production by isolated canine adrenal glomerulosa cells. Circ Res [Suppl II] 38:108–111

Douglas J, Aguilera G, Kondo T, Catt KJ (1978a) Angiotensin II receptors and aldosterone production in rat adrenal glomerulosa cells. Endocrinology 102:685–696

Douglas J, Saltman S, Williams C, Bartley P, Kondo T, Catt K (1978b) An examination of possible mechanisms of angiotensin II-stimulated steroidogenesis. Endocr Res Commun 5:173–188

Egan JJ, Majeska RJ, Rodan GA (1978) Adenylate cyclase enhancing factor from rat osteosarcoma cytosol. Biochem Biophys Res Commun 80:176–182

Ellis EF, Shen JC, Schrey MP, Carchman RA, Rubin RP (1978) Prostacyclin: a potent stimulator of adrenal steroidogenesis. Prostaglandins 16:483–490

Fakunding JL, Chow R, Catt KJ (1979) The role of calcium in the stimulation of aldosterone production by adrenocorticotropin, angiotensin II, and potassium in isolated glomerulosa cells. Endocrinology 105:327–333

Farese RV, Prudente WJ (1977) Localisation of the metabolic processes affected by calcium during corticotropin action. Biochim Biophys Acta 497:386–395

Farese RV, Prudente WJ (1978) On the role of calcium in adrenocorticotropin-induced changes in mitochondrial pregnenolone synthesis. Endocrinology 103:1264–1271

Farese RV, Sabir AM (1979) Polyphosphorylated glycerolipids mimic adrenocorticotropin-induced stimulation of mitochondrial pregnenolone synthesis. Biochim Biophys Acta 575:299–304

Farese RV, Sabir AM (1980) Polyphosphoinositides: Stimulator of mitochondrial cholesterol side-chain cleavage and possible identification as an adrenocorticotropin-induced, cycloheximide sensitive, cytosolic, steroidogenic factor. Endocrinology 106:1869–1879

Farese RV, Sabir AM, Vandor SL (1979) Adrenocorticotropin acutely increases adrenal polyphosphoinositides. J Biol Chem 254:6842–6844

Farese RV, Sabir MA, Vandor SL, Larson RE (1980) The phosphatidate-polyphosphoinositide cycle: a new effector system for controlling steroidogenesis by ACTH and cyclic AMP. Clin Res 28:259A

Finn FM, Widnell CC, Hofmann K (1972) Localisation of an adrenocorticotropic hormone receptor on bovine adrenal cortical membranes. J Biol Chem 247:5695–5702

Flack JD, Ramwell PW (1972) A comparison of the effects of ACTH, cyclic AMP, dibutyryl cyclic AMP and PGE_2 on corticosteroidogenesis in vitro. Endocrinology 90:371–377

Fujita K, Aguilera G, Catt KJ (1979) The role of cyclic AMP in aldosterone production by isolated zona glomerulosa cells. J Biol Chem 254:8567–8574

Giroud CJP, Stachenko K, Venning EH (1956) Secretion of aldosterone by the zona glomerulosa of rat adrenal glands in vitro. Proc Soc Exp Biol Med 92:154–158

Glossmann H, Gips H (1975) Bovine adrenal cortex adenylate cyclase: properties of the particulate enzyme and effects of guanyl nucleotides. Naunyn Schmiedebergs Arch Pharmacol 289:77–97
Glossmann H, Gips H (1976) Adrenal cortex adenylate cyclase: is Ca^{++} involved in ACTH stimulation? Naunyn Schmiedbergs Arch Pharmacol 292:199–203
Glossmann H, Struck CJ (1976) Adrenal cortex adenylate cyclase. In vitro activity of ACTH fragments and analogues. Naunyn Schmiedebergs Arch Pharmacol 294:199–206
Glossmann H, Struck CJ (1977) Adrenal cortex adenylate cyclase. In vitro modification of the enzyme by cholera toxin. Naunyn Schmiedebergs Arch Pharmacol 299:175–185
Glynn P, Cooper DM (1978) Inhibition of bovine adrenocortical adenylate cyclase by adenosine. Biochim Biophys Acta 526:605–612
Glynn P, Cooper DM, Schulster D (1977) Modulation of the response of bovine adrenocortical adenylate cyclase to corticotropin. Biochem J 168:277–282
Glynn P, Cooper DM, Schulster D (1978) Activation of adenylate cyclase in bovine adrenal cortex membranes by magnesium ions, guanine nucleotides and corticotropin. Biochim Biophys Acta 524:474–478
Glynn P, Cooper DM, Schulster D (1979) The regulation of adenylate cyclase of the adrenal cortex. Mol Cell Endocrinol 13:159–166
Goodfriend TL, Elliott ME (1980) Angiotensin alters ^{45}Ca fluxes in bovine adrenal glomerulosa cells. Fed Proc 39:515
Goodfriend TL, Lin SY (1970) Receptors for angiotensin I and II. Circ Res [Suppl I] 26, 27:163–170
Grahame-Smith DG, Butcher RW, Ney RL, Sutherland EW (1967) Adenosine 3',5'-monophosphate as the intracellular mediator of the action of adrenocorticotropic hormone on the adrenal cortex. J Biol Chem 242:5535–5541
Haksar A, Peron FG (1973) The role of calcium in the steroidogenic response of rat adrenal cells to adrenocorticotropic hormone. Biochim Biophys Acta 313:363–371
Haksar A, Maudsley DV, Peron FG (1974) Neuraminidase treatment of adrenal cells increases their response to cholera enterotoxin. Nature 251:514–415
Haksar A, Maudsley DV, Peron FG, Bedigian E (1976) Lanthanum inhibition of ACTH-stimulated cyclic AMP and corticosterone synthesis in isolated rat adrenocortical cells. J Cell Biol 68:142–153
Halkerston IDK (1975) Cyclic AMP and adrenocortical function. Adv Cyclic Nucleotide Res 6:99–136
Haning R, Tait SAS, Tait JF (1970) In vitro effects of ACTH, angiotensins, serotonin and potassium on steroid output and conversion of corticosterone to aldosterone by isolated adrenal cells. Endocrinology 87:1147–1167
Harrington CA, Fenimore DC, Farmer RW (1978) Regulation of adrenocortical steroidogenesis by cyclic 3'-5'-guanosine monophosphate in isolated rat adrenal cells. Biochem Biophys Res Commun 85:55–61
Hauger RL, Aguilera G, Catt KJ (1978) Angiotensin II regulates its receptor sites in the adrenal glomerulosa zone. Nature 271:176–178
Hayashi K, Sala G, Catt K, Dufau ML (1979) Regulation of steroidogenesis by adrenocorticotropic hormone in isolated adrenal cells. The intermediate role of cyclic nucleotides. J Biol Chem 254:6678–6683
Hofmann K, Kim JJ, Finn FM (1978) The role of protein kinases in ACTH-stimulated steroidogenesis. Biochem Biophys Res Commun 84:1136–1143
Honn KV, Chavin W (1976) Prostaglandin modulation of the mechanism of ACTH action in the human adrenal. Biochim Biophys Res Commun 73:164–170
Honn KV, Chavin W (1977) Effects of A and B series prostaglandins on cAMP, cortisol and aldosterone production by the human adrenal. Biochem Biophys Res Commun 76:977–982
Hyatt PJ, Wale LW, Bell JBG, Tait JF, Tait SAS (1980) Adenosine 3':5'-cyclic monophosphate levels in purified rat zona fasciculata and reticularis cells and the effect of adrenocorticotrophic hormone. J Endocrinol 85:435–442
Jaanus SD, Rubin RP (1971) The effect of ACTH on calcium distribution in the perfused cat adrenal gland. J Physiol (Lond) 213:581–598

Katz MS, Kelly TM, Pineyro MA, Gregerman RI (1978) Activation of epinephrine and glucagon sensitive adenylate cyclases of rat liver by cytosol protein factors. J Cyclic Nucleotide Res 5:389–407
Katz MS, Catt KJ, Fakunding JL (1981) Activation of ACTH-sensitive rat adrenal adenylate cyclase by micromolar concentrations of divalent cations. Abstr 4th International Conference on Cyclic Nucleotides. Adv Cyclic Nucleotide Res 14, Abstr. No. WE. A4
Kelly LA, Koritz SB (1971) Bovine adrenal cortical adenyl cyclase and its stimulation by adrenocorticotropic hormone and NaF. Biochim Biophys Acta 237:141–155
Laychock SG, Rubin RP (1975) ACTH-induced prostaglandin biosynthesis from ^{3}H-arachidinic acid by adrenocortical cells. Prostaglandins 10:529–540
Laychock SG, Rubin RP (1976) Indomethacin-induced alterations in corticosteroid and prostaglandin release by isolated adrenocortical cells of the cat. Br J Pharmacol 57:273–278
Laychock SG, Franson RC, Weglicki WB, Rubin RB (1977a) Identification and partial characterisation of phospholipases in isolated adrenocortical cells: The effects of ACTH and calcium. Biochem J 164:753–756
Laychock SG, Warner W, Rubin RP (1977b) Further studies on the mechanisms controlling prostaglandin biosynthesis in the cat adrenal cortex: the role of calcium and cyclic AMP. Endocrinology 100:74–81
Lefkowitz RJ, Roth J, Pastan I (1970) ACTH receptors in the adrenal: specific binding of ACTH-^{125}I and its relation to adenyl cyclase. Proc Natl Acad Sci USA 65:745–752
Lefkowitz RJ, Roth J, Pastan I (1971) ACTH-receptor interaction in the adrenal: a model for the initial step in the action of hormones that stimulate adenyl cyclase. Ann NY Acad Sci 185:195–209
Leier DJ, Jungmann RA (1973) Adrenocorticotropic hormone and dibutyryl adenosine cyclic monophosphate-mediated Ca^{2+} uptake by rat adrenal glands. Biochim Biophys Acta 329:196–210
Londos C, Rodbell M (1975) Multiple inhibitory and activating effects of nucleotides and magnesium on adrenal adenylate cyclase. J Biol Chem 250:3459–3465
Londos C, Wolff J (1977) Two distinct adenosine-sensitive sites on adenylate cyclase. Proc Natl Acad Sci USA 74:5482–5486
Lowry PJ, McMartin C, Peters J (1973) Properties of simplified bioassay for adrenocorticotropic activity using the steroidogenic response of isolated adrenal cells. J Endocrinol 59:43–55
Lymangrover JR, Martin R (1978) Effects of ionophore A 23187 on in vitro rat adrenal corticosterone production. Life Sci 23:1193–1200
Mackie C, Richardson MC, Schulster D (1972) Kinetics and dose-response characteristics of adenosine 3′:5′ monophosphate production by isolated rat adrenal cells stimulated with adrenocorticotrophic hormone. FEBS Lett 23:345–348
Mackie C, Warren RL, Simpson ER (1978) Investigations into the role of calcium ions in the control of steroid production by isolated adrenal zona glomerulosa cells of the rat. J Endocrinol 77:119–127
Mahaffee DD, Ontjes DA (1980) The role of calcium in the control of adrenal adenylate cyclase. Enhancement of enzyme activation by guanyl-5′-yl-imidodiphosphate. J Biol Chem 255:1565–1571
McDougall JG, Williams BC, Hyatt PJ, Bell JBG, Tait JF, Tait SAS (1979) Purification of dispersed rat adrenal cells by column filtration. Proc R Soc Lond [Biol] 206:15–32
McIlhinney RAJ, Schulster D (1975) Studies on the binding of ^{125}I-labelled corticotrophin to isolated rat adrenocortical cells. J Endocrinol 65:175–184
McPherson MA, Ramachandran J (1980) Corticotropin stimulates cyclic nucleotide independent protein kinase activity of intact adrenocortical cells. Biochem Biophys Res Commun 94:1057–1065
Moyle WR, Kong YC, Ramachandran J (1973) Steroidogenesis and cyclic adenosine 3′,5′-monophosphate accumulation in rat adrenal cells. J Biol Chem 248:2409–2417
Moyle WR, MacDonald GJ, Garfink JE (1976) Role of histone kinases as mediators of corticotropin-induced steroidogenesis. Biochem J 160:1–9
Muller J, Ziegler WH (1968) Stimulation of aldosterone biosynthesis in vitro by serotonin. Acta, Endocrinol (Copenh) 59:23–35

Naghshineh S, Treadwell CR, Gallo LL, Vahouny GV (1978) Protein-kinase-mediated phosphorylation of a purified sterol ester hydrolase from bovine adrenal cortex. J Lipid Res 19:561–569

Neher R, Milani A (1976) Mode of action of peptide hormones. Clin Endocrinol (Oxf) [Suppl] 5:295–395

Neher R, Milani A (1978) Steroidogenesis in isolated adrenal cells: excitation by calcium. Mol Cell Endocrinol 9:243–253

Palfreyman JP, Schulster D (1975) On the mechanism of action of cholera toxin on isolated rat adrenocortical cells. Comparison with the effects of adrenocorticotrophin on steroidogenesis and cyclic AMP output. Biochim Biophys Acta 404:221–230

Perchellet JP, Sharma RK (1977) Metabolic regulation of steroidogenesis in isolated adrenocortical carcinoma cells. ACTH regulation of guanosine cyclic 3′,5′-monophosphate levels. Biochem Biophys Res Commun 78:676–683

Perchellet JP, Sharma RK (1979) Mediatory role of calcium and guanosine 3′,5′-monophosphate in adrenocorticotropin-induced steroidogenesis by adrenal cells. Science 203:1259–1261

Perchellet JP, Shanker G, Sharma RK (1978) Regulatory role of guanosine 3′,5′-monophosphate in adrenocorticotropin hormone-induced steroidogenesis. Science 199:311–312

Pernollet M-G, Devynck M-A, Mathews PG, Meyer P (1977) Post-nephrectomy changes in adrenal angiotensin II receptors in the rat: influence of exogenous angiotensin and a competitive inhibitor. Eur J Pharmacol 43:361–372

Peytremann A, Nicholson WE, Brown RD, Liddle GW, Hardman JG (1973) Comparative effects of angiotensin and ACTH on cyclic AMP and steroidogenesis in isolated bovine adrenal cells. J Clin Invest 52:835–842

Peytremann A, Brown RD, Nicholson WE, Island DP, Liddle GW, Hardman JG (1974) Regulation of aldosterone synthesis. Steroids 24:451–462

Podesta EJ, Milani A, Steffen H, Neher R (1979) Steroidogenesis in isolated adrenocortical cells. Correlation with receptor-bound adenosine 3′:5′-cyclic monophosphate. Biochem J 180:355–363

Rae PA, Gutmann NS, Tsao J, Schimmer BP (1979) Mutations in cyclic AMP-dependent protein kinase and corticotropin (ACTH)-sensitive adenylate cyclase affect adrenal steroidogenesis. Proc Natl Acad Sci USA 76:1896–1900

Ramachandran J, Moyle WR (1977) ACTH-activation of steroid release and correlation with adenylate cyclase activity. Proc Int Congr Endocrinol (5th) 1:520–525

Regoli D (1979) Receptors for angiotensin: a critical analysis. Can J Physiol Pharmacol 57:129–139

Richardson MC, Schulster D (1972) Corticosteroidogenesis in isolated adrenal cells. Effect of adrenocorticotrophic hormone, adenosine 3′:5′-monophosphate and 1–24 adrenocorticotrophic hormone diazotised to polyacrylamide. J Endocrinol 55:127–139

Richardson MC, Schulster D (1973) The role of protein kinase activation in the control of steroidogenesis by adrenocorticotrophic hormone in the adrenal cortex. Biochem J 136:993–998

Riou JP, Evain D, Perrin F, Saez JM (1977) Adenosine 3′5′-cyclic monophosphate-dependent protein kinase in human adrenocortical tumors. J Clin Endocrinol Metab 44:413–419

Rolland PH, Chambaz EM (1977) Effect of prostaglandins on steroidogenesis by bovine adrenal cortex mitochondria. Mol Cell Endocrinol 7:325–333

Rubin RP, Laychock SG (1978) Prostaglandins and calcium membrane interactions in secretory glands. Ann NY Acad Sci 307:377–390

Rubin RP, Laychock SG, End DW (1977) On the role of cyclic AMP and cyclic GMP in steroid production by bovine cortical cells. Biochim Biophys Acta 496:329–339

Saez JM, Morera AM, Dazord A, Bataille P (1974) Interaction of ACTH with its adrenal receptors: specific binding of ACTH 1–24, its o-nitrophenyl derivative and ACTH 11–24. J Steroid Biochem 5:925–933

Saez JM, Dazord A, Morera AM, Bataille P (1975) Interactions of ACTH with its adrenal receptors. Degradation of ACTH 1–24 and ACTH 11–24. J Biol Chem 250:1683–1689

Saez JM, Evain D, Gallet D (1978) Role of cyclic AMP and protein kinase on the steroidogenic action of ACTH, prostaglandin E_1, and dibutyryl cyclic AMP in normal adrenal cells and adrenal tumor cells from humans. J Cyclic Nucleotide Res 4:311–321

Saez JM, Morera A-M, Dazord A (1981) Mediators of the effects of ACTH on adrenal cells. Adv Cyclic Nucleotide Res 14:563–579

Sala GB, Hayashi K, Catt KJ, Dufau ML, (1979) Adrenocorticotropin action in isolated adrenal cells. The intermediate role of cyclic AMP in stimulation of corticosterone synthesis. J Biol Chem 254:3861–3865

Sanders RB, Thompson WJ, Robinson GA (1977) Epinephrine and glucagon stimulated cardiac adenylyl cyclase activity: regulation by endogenous factors. Biochim Biophys Acta 498:10–20

Saruta T, Kaplan NM, (1972) Adrenocortical steroidogenesis: the effects of prostaglandins. J Clin Invest 51:2246–2251

Saruta T, Cook R, Kaplan NM (1972) Adrenocortical steroidogenesis: studies on the mechanism of action of angiotensin and electrolytes. J Clin Invest 51:2239–2245

Sayers G, Beall RJ, Seelig S (1972) Isolated adrenal cells: adrenocorticotropic hormone, calcium, steroidogenesis and cyclic adenosine monophosphate. Science 175:1131–1133

Schimmer BP, Veda K, Sato GH (1968) Site of action of adrenocorticotropic hormone. Biochem Biophys Res Commun 32:806–810

Schimmer BP, Tsao J, Knapp M (1977) Isolation of mutant adrenocortical tumour cells resistant to cyclic nucleotides. Mol Cell Endocrinol 8:135–145

Schorr I, Ney RL (1971) Abnormal hormone-responses of an adrenocortical cancer adenyl cyclase. J Clin Invest 50:1295–1300

Schrey MP, Rubin RP (1979) Characterisation of a calcium-mediated activation of arachidonic acid turnover in adrenal phospholipids by corticotropin. J Biol Chem 254:11234–11241

Schulster D, Schwyzer R (1980) ACTH receptors. In: Schulster D, Levitzki A (eds) Cellular receptors for hormones and neurotransmitters. John Wiley and Sons, New York Chichester

Schulster D, Burstein S, Cooke BA (1976) Molecular endocrinology of the steroid hormones. John Wiley and Sons, New York Chichester

Selinger RCL, Civen M (1971) ACTH diazotised to agarose: effects on isolated adrenal cells. Biochem Biophys Res Commun 43:793–799

Sharma RK, Ahmed NK, Sutliff LS, Brush JS (1974) Metabolic regulation of steroidogenesis in isolated adrenal cells of the rat. ACTH regulation of cGMP and cAMP levels and steroidogenesis. FEBS Lett 45:107–110

Sharma RK, Ahmed NK, Shanker G (1976) Metabolic regulation of steroidogenesis in isolated adrenal cells of rat. Relationship of adrenocorticotropin-, adenosine 3′:5′-monophosphate – and guanosine 3′:5′-monophosphate-stimulated steroidogenesis with the activation of protein kinase. Eur J Biochem 70:427–433

Sharma RK, Shanker G, Ahmed NK (1977a) Metabolic regulation and relationship of endogenous protein kinase activity and steroidogenesis in isolated adrenocortical carcinoma cells of the rat. Cancer Res 37:472–475

Sharma RK, Shanker G, Ahrens H, Ahmed NK (1977b) Partial purification and characterisation of the defective cyclic adenosine 3′:5′-monophosphate binding protein kinase from adrenocortical carcinoma. Cancer Res 37:3297–2200

Shima S, Kawashima Y, Hirai M (1978) Studies on cyclic nucleotides in the adrenal gland. VIII. Effects of angiotensin on adenosine 3′,5′-monophosphate and steroidogenesis in the adrenal cortex. Endocrinology 103:1361–1367

Shima S, Kawashima Y, Hirai M (1979a) Studies on cyclic nucleotides in the adrenal gland. IX. Effects of ACTH on cyclic AMP and steroid production by the zona fasciculata-reticularis of the adrenal cortex. Acta Endocrinol (Copenh) 90:139–146

Shima S, Kawashima Y, Hirai M (1979b) Effects of ACTH and calcium on cyclic AMP production and steroid output by the zona glomerulosa of the adrenal cortex. Endocrinol Jpn 26:219–225

Tait JF, Tait SAS (1976) The effect of changes in potassium concentration on the maximal steroidogenic response of purified zona glomerulosa cells to angiotensin II. J Steroid Biochem 7:687–690

Tait JF, Tait SAS (1979) Recent perspectives on the history of the adrenal cortex. J Endocrinol 83:3P–24P
Tait JF, Tait SAS, Gould RP, Mee MSR (1974) The properties of adrenal zona glomerulosa cells after purification by gravitational sedimentation. Proc R Soc Lond [Biol] 185:375–407
Tait JF, Tait SAS, Bell JBG (1980a) Steroid hormone production by mammalian adrenocortical dispersed cells. Essays Biochem 16:99–174
Tait JF, Tait SAS, Bell JBG, Hyatt PJ, Williams BC (1980b) Further studies on the stimulation of rat adrenal capsular cells. Four types of responses. J Endocrinol 87:11–27.
Tait JF, Bell JBG, Hyatt PJ, Tait SAS, Williams BC (1981) Dispersed cells of the adrenal cortex. In: Proceedings international physiological society meeting, Budapest. Pergamon Press London. Adv Physiol Sci 13 (1981). Eds: E. Stark, G. B. Makara, Zs. Acs., E. Enderoczi.
Tait SAS, Tait JF, Gould RP, Brown BL, Albano JDM (1974). The preparation and use of purified and unpurified dispersed adrenal cells and a study of the relationship of their cAMP and steroid output. J Steroid Biochem 5:775–787
Taunton OD, Roth J, Pastan I (1969) Studies on the adrenocorticotropic hormone-activated adenyl cyclase of a functional adrenal tumor. J Biol Chem 244:247–253
Tell GP, Cathiard AM, Saez JM (1978) Guanosine triphosphate sensitive adenylate cyclase of adrenocorticotropic hormone and prostaglandin resistant adrenocortical tumours. Cancer Res 38:955–959
Trzeciak WH, Boyd GS (1974) Activation of cholesteryl esterase in bovine adrenal cortex. Eur J Biochem 46:201–207
Vallotton MB, Capponi AM, Grillet C, Knupfer AL, Hepp R, Khosla MC, Bumpus FM (1981) Characterisation on angiotensin receptors on bovine adrenal fasciculata cells. Proc Natl Acad Sci USA
Warner W, Carchman RA (1978) Effects of Ruthenium Red, A 23187 and D-600 on steroidogenesis in Y-1 cells. Biochim Biophys Acta 528:409–415
Warner W, Rubin RP (1975) Evidence for a possible prostaglandin link in ACTH-induced steroidogenesis. Prostaglandins 9:83–95
Ways DK, Ontjes DA (1979) Reversal of persistently stimulated steroidogenesis by GTP and an inhibitory adrenocorticotropin analogue in adrenal cells treated with adrenocorticotropin. Mol Pharmacol 15:271–286
Ways DK, Zimmermann CF, Ontjes DA (1976) Inhibition of adrenocorticotropin effects on adrenal cell membranes by synthetic adrenocorticotropin analogues: correlation of binding and adenylate cyclase activation. Mol Pharmacol 12:789–799
Whitley TH, Stowe NW, Ong S-H, Ney RL, Steiner AL (1975) Control and localisation of rat adrenal cyclic adenosine 3′5′ monophosphate. J Clin Invest 56:146–154
Williams BC, McDougall JG, Tait JF, Tait SAS, Zananiri FAF (1980) Calcium efflux from superfused isolated rat adrenal glomerulosa cells. Abstr Int Congr Endocrinol, Melbourne, No 655. Published by International Society of Endocrinology
Wolff J, Cook GH (1977) Activation of steroidogenesis and adenylate cyclase by adenosine in adrenal and Leydig tumor cells. J Biol Chem 252:687–693
Yanagibashi K (1979) Calcium ions as "second messenger" on corticoidogenic action of ACTH. Endocrinol Jpn 26:227–232
Yanagibashi K, Kamiya N, Lin G, Matsuba M (1978) Studies on adrenocorticotropic hormone receptor using isolated rat adrenocortical cells. Endocrinol Jpn 25:545–551

CHAPTER 31

A Role of Cyclic AMP in the Gastrointestinal Tract: Receptor Control of Hydrogen Ion Secretion by Mammalian Gastric Mucosa

W. J. THOMPSON, E. D. JACOBSON, and G. C. ROSENFELD

Overview

Isolated gastric parietal cells are reviewed as a method to elucidate the mechanisms involved in drug and hormone modulation of hydrogen ion production and secretion. General concepts of the regulation of gastric acid secretion are discussed. Recent data on the pharmacology of acid secretion in isolated parietal cells is emphasized with particular reference to receptor-secretagogue interactions, multiple second messenger production, and effected cellular pathways. The development of the major sequential and non-sequential hypotheses of acid secretagogue regulation are traced, as well as the positive and negative consequences of merging either hypothesis with the concept of intracellular second messenger production. The major findings with respect to cyclic AMP metabolism are summarized for several experimental preparations, including intact gastric mucosa, cell free systems, and isolated gastric glands. Studies on isolated parietal cells emphasize the interaction of cell function with cyclic nucleotide phosphodiesterase inhibition and adenylyl cyclase regulation. The authors conclude that the evidence supports the concept of separate parietal cell receptors for the acid secretagogues, acetylcholine and histamine. Cyclic AMP appears to be a second messenger pathway of cellular regulation for histamine, while calcium mobilization is a second messenger pathway for acetylcholine and histamine. A mechanism is presented in the form of a working hypothesis to explain the singular and potentiative effects of acetylcholine and histamine on acid secretion. The second messengers, calcium and cyclic AMP, are visualized as ultimate activators of the phosphorylation of key membrane phosphate acceptor proteins, but at different sites. Phosphorylation of the phosphate acceptors is postulated to be the result of the independent actions of calmodulin and cyclic AMP-dependent protein kinases. Thus, it is proposed that histamine and acetylcholine (and perhaps gastrin) may stimulate acid secretion independently and, in combination, potentiate secretion by promoting multiple levels of phosphorylation.

A. Introduction

THEORELL (1978) has recently coined the term "molecular physiology" to describe the current trend of using isolated oxyntic cell systems to study the regulation of hydrogen ion production and secretion in the stomach. Isolated cells offer a method to elucidate the complex relationships between membrane structure and function, cellular ion transport, and metabolic and mechanical forces modulated by hormones and drugs. In this review, it is our intention to: (1) discuss, in general, the regulation of hydrogen ion secretion, (2) examine recent data on the pharmacology of acid secretion in isolated mammalian parietal cell systems, and (3) emphasize the coupling of receptor interactions to second messenger production and molecular information transfer in parietal cells. This field has attracted much interest and comment and the reader is referred to other recent review articles on acid secretion, each with a different emphasis: biochemical (SACHS et al. 1977, 1978), physiological (STREWLER and ORLOFF 1977; SOLL and WALSH 1979), clinical (SOLL and GROSSMAN 1978; LEVINE 1977), and regulatory (RUOFF and SEWING 1977; ROSENFELD et al. 1980).

B. The Regulation and Pharmacology of Acid Secretion

An indispensible concept to understanding the actions of hormones and drugs is that of receptors, first formulated by Ehrlich and Langley (PARASCONDOLA 1980) at the turn of this century. Since gastric acid secretion is known to be regulated by at least three endogenous secretagogues, gastrin, acetylcholine, and histamine, the receptor concept (ARIENS and BELD 1977) provides a framework for pursuit of the molecular effects of these chemically diverse endocrine, neuroendocrine, and paracrine substances, respectively (Fig. 1). Which of these regulators is the most important physiologically is not fully understood. Based upon the purification of gastrin(s) by GREGORY and TRACY (1974) and the experiments of GROSSMAN et al. (1948), gastrin must be considered a major regulator of acid secretion. Questions still remain as to the physiological roles of histamine and acetylcholine.

Regulation of the function of the cells which produce gastric acid, namely the parietal cells (Fig. 2), appears to occur either through: (1) sequential secretagogue release such that only one interacts with the target cell, (2) separate, but interacting, cellular receptors for each secretagogue, or (3) separate cellular receptors for each secretagogue which act independently but whose pathways interact at a distant locus. If release is sequential, it is reasonable to entertain the notion that one of the secretagogues is a final common mediator through which all other external stimuli will act. This model was implicit in the proposal of BABKIN (1938) that vagal stimulation of acid secretion required secondary release of histamine, which is ubiquitously distributed in the tissues of the body, with particularly high concentrations located in the gastric mucosa near the highest density of parietal cells (LUNDELL 1974). MACINTOSH (1938) formulated the concept that histamine acted to mediate the actions of the other secretagogues. Subsequently, CODE (1965) championed this thesis. This final common mediator hypotheses gradually lost support, mainly because of arguments emphasizing the potency ratio of histamine to gastrin and cholinergic agents (1:100), the question of histamine release, and observations of maximal response as discussed by RANGACHARI (1978) and JOHNSON (1971).

The initial general description by DALE and LAIDLOW (1980) of the effects of histamine was extended by POPIELSKI (1920) who noted the ability of histamine to stimulate acid secretion. After the discovery of the classic antihistaminics by BOVET

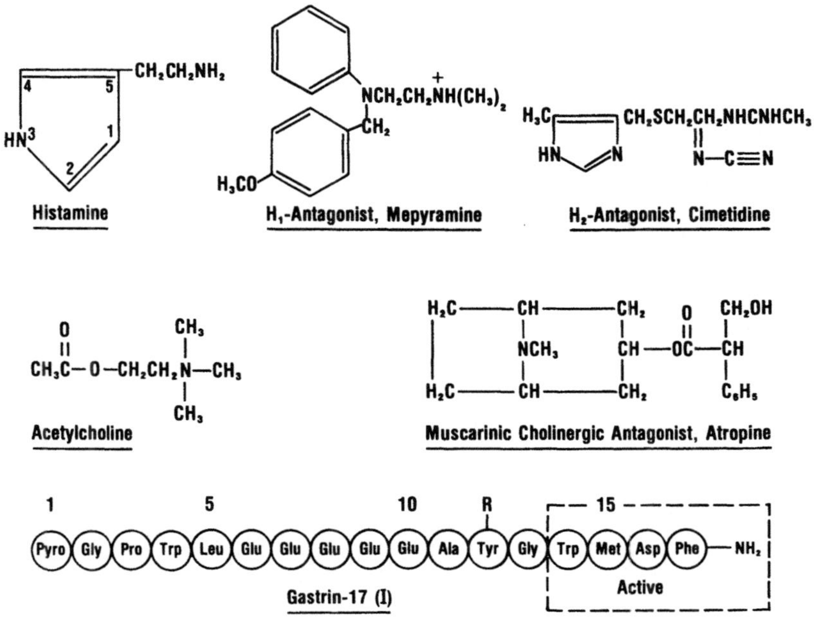

Fig. 1. Major endogenous acid secretagogues and pharmacological antagonists

and STAUB (1937), it was realized that at concentrations which were maximally effective on responses such as smooth muscle contraction, classified now as an H_1 type response (ASH and SCHILD 1966), these compounds did not inhibit the acid secretory response to histamine; this stimulatory property of histamine is classified now as an H_2 type response (BLACK et al. 1972). The synthesis of burimamide by Black and colleagues (BLACK et al. 1972, 1973) and later metiamide, cimetidine (BRIMBLECOMBE et al. 1975), ranitidine (RUOFF et al. 1979; BRADSHAW et al. 1979), and tiotidine (YELLIN et al. 1979) solidified the pharmacological definition of an H_2-type histaminic receptor classification. These drugs have no demonstrable H_2 agonist activity, and antagonize the actions of histamine on acid secretion by reversibly shifting the histamine dose-response curve to the right without altering its maximal effect. The H_2-receptor classification was also strengthened by the finding that analogues of histamine such as 4-methylhistamine and dimaprit have relatively specific H_2 agonist properties. The reader is referred to recent reviews by FELDMAN and RICHARDSON (1978) and BRIMBLECOMBE et al. (1978) for more complete information on H_2-receptor antagonists. It must be emphasized that H_2-histamine receptors are defined by response, not biochemical, criteria, although some support has been provided for H_1 and H_2 physical distinctions (OSBAND and MCCAFFREY 1979).

In addition to blocking histamine's effects, the H_2-receptor antagonists also were found to inhibit acid secretion induced by gastrin or acetylcholine, thus revitalizing the final common mediator hypothesis. The proposal that histamine mediates the effects of other endogenous stimuli on gastric acid secretion has two, as yet unproven, implications: first, that histamine is always released locally prior to onset of secretion; and, second, that the plasma membrane of parietal cells has only

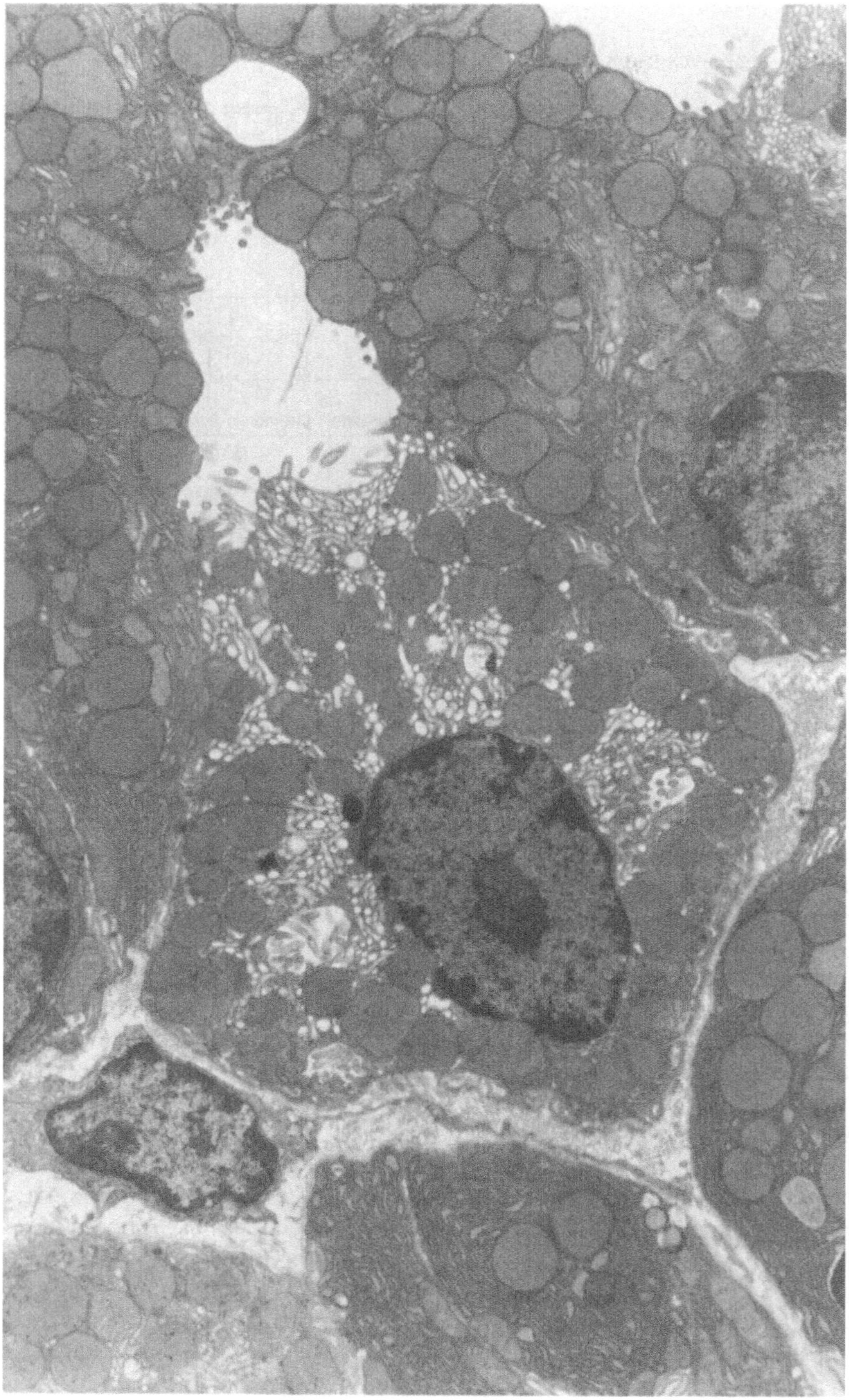

Fig. 2. Electron micrograph of rat gastric parietal cell (× 9,000)

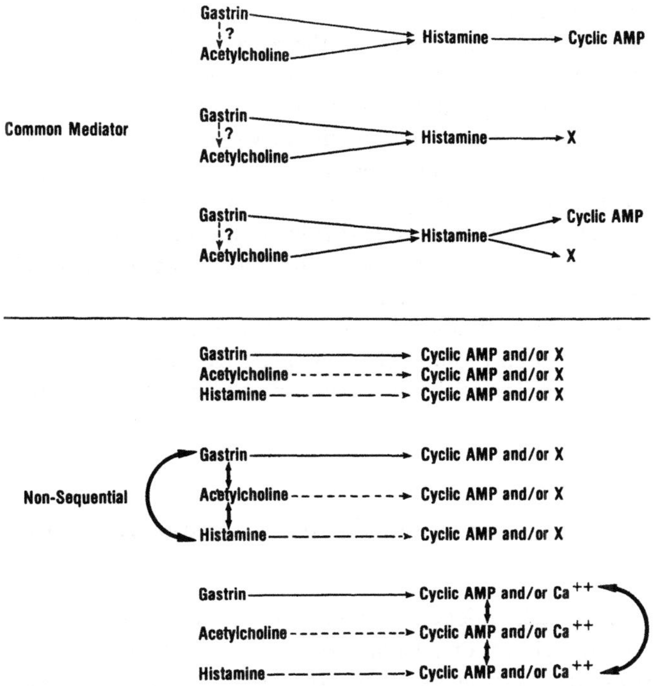

Fig. 3. Schematic representation of secretagogue action hypotheses. Upper portion represents common mediator type hypotheses where histamine is the only secretagogue which actually interacts with parietal cells. Lower portion represents non-sequential hypotheses where each secretagogue interacts with specific parietal cell receptors. The hypotheses are differentiated by no receptor interactions or pathway interactions, receptor interactions and no pathway interactions, or pathway interactions only

H_2-receptors and no functional receptors for other secretagogues. The latter postulate is especially critical to the theory of histamine as the final common mediator because prandial events are known to prompt endogenous release of gastrin and acetycholine, both of which stimulate acid secretion in dose dependent fashion. Furthermore, controversy persists since this hypothesis must explain the observation that the specific anticholinergic antagonist, atropine, reduces acid secretion induced by gastrin, histamine, as well as acetylcholine (FELDMAN and RICHARDSON 1978). In lieu of such data, GROSSMAN and KONTUREK (1974) proposed an alternate model in which parietal cells contain distinct receptors for histamine, gastrin, and acetylcholine, and secretagogue interaction of one receptor alters the properties of the other secretagogue receptors. In addition this model proposed that histamine was the major stimulant for acid secretion, its actions being modified by acetylcholine and gastrin. The concepts of spare receptors and percentage occupancy for maximal effect that have been useful in autonomic pharmacology and polypeptide hormone action have not been utilized in the case of acid secretagogues.

The coupling of either the final common mediator or the multiple receptor hypotheses to yet another hypothesis regarding regulation of acid secretion *within* the parietal cell has complicated matters further. Histamine, the first direct messenger, was proposed to act exclusively through the intracellular second messenger, cyclic

AMP (HARRIS and ALONSO 1965). This inherently attractive idea would simplify secretagogue regulation, particularly if the secretagogues were to act sequentially. However, until recently the testing of this hypotheses has shed little light on which secretagogue(s) actually regulate parietal cell function (JACOBSON and THOMPSON 1976). Figure 3 shows, in schematic form, the general pathways which might be involved in the coupling of either sequential or multiple receptor concepts to a second messenger hypothesis utilizing cyclic AMP or unknows such as calcium. In the sequential models histamine is the sole regulator interacting with parietal cells. Multiple pathway models require each secretagogue to interact with cells directly and are distinguished by receptor interactions or resultant second messenger pathway interactions. It is our view that only with the recent successful preparation of isolated gastric glands and parietal cells has progress been made with regard to the relationship between secretagogue receptor content and their involvement with cyclic AMP.

C. In vivo, in situ, and in vitro Gastric Studies of Cyclic AMP Metabolism

The role of cyclic nucleotides in the regulation of gastric acid secretion in systems other than isolated glands or cells has been extensively reviewed (RUOFF and SEWING 1977; SOLL and GROSSMAN 1978; SOLL and WALSH 1979; SACHS et al. 1978; THOMPSON and JACOBSON 1977). Tables 1–4 summarize the major conclusions of previously published studies in this field. The data in each table is subdivided according to species studied. The data which supports cyclic AMP as a necessary mediator of gastric acid secretion is shown in Tables 1 and 3 and the data which is against the role of cyclic AMP as a mediator is shown in Tables 2 and 4. Tables 1 and 2 compile studies conducted since mid-1975, the date of our previous comprehensive review of this literature (JACOBSON and THOMPSON 1976). Evidence obtained prior to that review is presented in Tables 3 and 4 and is included with the hope that it will prove useful to scholars interested in the older background information on this subject.

In our previous review of the literature (JACOBSON and THOMPSON 1976) we concluded that there were no convincing data for or against the postulates of HARRIS and ALONSO (1965) obtained from non-cellular gastric systems on the role of cyclic AMP in mediating secretagogue stimulation of acid secretion. Although some of our previous objections to the use of inadequate or outdated methodologies for the analyses of adenylyl cyclase, cyclic nucleotide quantity, and cyclic nucleotide phosphodiesterases have been overcome, and despite the sophistication of current methodology, more recent results have not been more definitive. For example, LEVINE (1977) and SCHWARTZEL et al. (1977) have commented that several studies on gastric cyclic nucleotide levels failed to complete even the simplist of controls to verify cyclic nucleotide hydrolysis by phosphodiesterase. We also note that many reports in this field have appeared in unreviewed, secondary literature (e.g., symposia) and in abstract form. Although such reports are not necessarily invalid and can have the effect of stimulating progress, this type of information should not be accepted as dogma.

Table 1. Recent evidence *favoring* cyclic nucleotides in acid secretagogues action

Rat	
	Histamine ↑ Adenylate cyclase activity (AC) [1]
	Histamine ↑ cAMP; blocked by H_2 antagonists [2]
	Pentagastrin ↑ AC [3]
	Pentagastrin ↑ cAMP; blocked by H_2 antagonists [4]
	Carbachol ↑ AC and cAMP [5]
	DbcAMP ↑ acid secretion; not blocked by H_2 antagonists [6]
	Cyclic AMP causes secretory ultrastructural changes in parietal cells [7]
	Cyclic AMP is localized histochemically to parietal cell areas [8]
	Histamine is localized histochemically to parietal cells [9]
	Ethanol ↑ cAMP and acid secretion [10]
	Halothane ↑ cAMP and acid secretion [11]
	Histamine, pentagastrin and cAMP ↑ carbonic anhydrase [12]
Mouse	
	DbcAMP ↑ acid secretion [13]
Guinea Pig	
	Histamine ↑ AC; blocked by H_1 and H_2 antagonists [14]
	Histamine ↑ cAMP [15]
	PDE inhibitors ↑ acid secretion [16]
	Prostaglandins ↑ AC; not blocked by H_1 and H_2 antagonists [17]
Rabbit	
	Histamine ↑ AC [18]
Dog	
	Histamine ↑ fundic AC, not antral AC; prostaglandins ↑ both [19]
	H_2 antagonists block AC by histamine, but not AC by prostaglandin [20]
	Polyphloretin blocks AC ↑ by prostaglandins, but not AC by histamine [21]
	H_2 not H_1 antagonists ↓ basal AC [22]
	Histamine ↑ cAMP [23]
	Arachidonic acid ↓ cAMP and acid secretion [24]
	Low concentrations of ethanol ↑ AC and cAMP [25]
Human	
	Histamine ↑ fundic, not antral AC; blocked by H_2 antagonists [26]
	$H_2 \gg H_1$ as antagonists of AC [27]
	Prostaglandins ↑ AC additive to histamine; no H_2 block [28]
	Epinephrine ↑ AC additive to histamine; no H_2 block [29]
	Ethanol (5%) ↑ AC and mucosal cAMP [30]

[1] Nafrady and Wollemann (1977); Salganik (1977). [2] Sewing and Ruoff (1977); Puurunen et al. (1978). [3] Nafrady and Wollemann (1977). [4] Sewing and Ruoff (1977); Sewing et al. (1976). [5] Sewing and Ruoff (1975). [6] Main and Pearce (1978); Watanabe et al. (1977); Bunce et al. (1976). [7] Salganik et al. (1976). [8] Katsumata and Glick (1975). [9] Salganik et al. (1976); Cross (1977). [10] Puurunen and Karppanen (1975); Puurunen et al. (1977). [11] Geumei and Danhof (1978). [12] Salganik et al. (1976). [13] Wan (1976); Ekblad et al. (1978). [14] Thompson and Jacobson (1977); Perrier and Griessen (1976); Ruoff et al. (1979); Dousa et al. (1979); Wollin et al. (1976); Anttila et al. (1976); Anttila and Westerman (1976). [15] Puurunen et al. (1978); Canfield et al. (1977). [16] Canfield et al. (1976, 1977, 1978a). [17] Perrier and Griessen (1976); Dousa et al. (1979); Wollin et al. (1976). [18] Katsumata and Yagi (1976). [19] Tao et al. (1976); Dozois et al. (1977, 1978); Dozois and Dousa (1977). [20] Dozois et al. (1977); Dozois and Dousa (1977). [21] Dozois and Dousa (1977); Dozois et al. (1978). [22] Ruoff and Sewing (1976). [23] Dozois et al. (1978). [24] Konturek et al. (1979). [25] Puurunen et al. (1976). [26] Simon and Kather (1977a, b, c, d); Simon et al. (1977, 1978b). [27] Simon and Kather (1977d, 1978a, b, 1979b); Simon et al. (1977, 1978a). [28] Simon et al. (1978b). [29] Simon and Kather (1977c); Simon et al. (1977). [30] Karppanen et al. (1976). AC = adenylyl cyclase, PDE = cyclic nucleotide phosphodiesterase

Table 2. Recent evidence *against* cyclic nucleotides in acid secretagogue action

Rat
AC ↑ by prostaglandin E_1, secretin and epinephrine, but not by histamine, pentagastrin and carbachol [1]
Cyclic AMP ↑ by epinephrine, isoproterenol and salicylates [2]
Protein kinase ↓ by pentagastrin and by H_2 antagonist [3]
Carbachol more potent than histamine to ↑ cAMP [4]
Guinea Pig
AC ↑ by prostaglandins, but not carbachol or pentagastrin [5]
Cyclic AMP content not ↑ by pentagastrin or bethanechol [6]
H_1 and H_2 antagonists equipotent of histamine ↑ AC [7]
Rabbit
AC not ↑ by tetragastrin [8]
Dog
AC ↑ by prostaglandins, not by histamine, pentagastrin or carbachol [9]
Cyclic AMP ↑ by prostaglandins, not histamine, pentagastrin, or bethanechol [10]
Theophylline ↑ cAMP, but not acid secretion [11]
20% ethanol ↓ acid secretion but not cAMP [12]
Human
Fundic AC ↑ by prostaglandins, VIP, and epinephrine [13]
Fundic or luminal cAMP content not ↑ by histamine, betazole or pentagastrin nor by hypersecretory diseases [14]
Acid secretion due to histamine or pentagastric not ↑ by methylxanthines [15]

[1] THOMPSON et al. (1977a, b). [2] MITZNEGG et al. (1977); RUOFF (1977a, b). [3] CAPOBIANCO et al. (1977). [4] RUOFF and SEWING (1975a, 1977). [5] PERRIER and GRIESSEN (1976); THOMPSON and JACOBSON (1977); ANTTILA et al. (1976). [6] CANFIELD et al. (1978b); KARPPANEN et al. (1974). [7] ANTTILA et al. (1976). [8] KATSUMATA and YAGI (1976). [9] JACOBSON and THOMPSON (1976); TAO et al. (1976); DOZOIS and DOUSA (1977); DOZOIS et al. (1978); COOKE et al. (1974). [10] TAO et al. (1976); TAGUE et al. (1977); DOZOIS et al. (1978); CHAUDHURY and JACOBSON (1978); KONTUREK et al. (1979); TALEV (1976); TALEV et al. (1978); THURSTON et al. (1976). [11] COOKE et al. (1974); LEVINE et al. (1978). [12] TAGUE and SHANBOUR (1977). [13] SIMON and KATHER (1977c, d, 1978a, b, c, 1979a); SIMON et al. (1977, 1978a). [14] TALEV (1976); BOWER et al. (1974a, b); LEVINE et al. (1977). [15] COOKE et al. (1974)

I. Exogenous Administration and Intact Mucosa

The restrictions imposed by using in vivo stomach preparations are the limited viability and cellular heterogeneity of such tissue, and the difficulty in distinguishing between direct and indirect effects of exogenously administered agents. LEVINE (1977) has conducted extensive, controlled studies using this approach and has concluded that secretagogues increase the quantity but not the concentration of cyclic nucleotides in gastric juice. He suggested that no cellular cyclic nucleotide correlation was obvious from the analyses of gastric juice. THURSTON et al. (1979) was also unable to demonstrate changes in canine mucosal cyclic AMP following histamine or acetylcholine, but they did detect small changes in cyclic GMP. RUOFF and SEWING (1975a) showed that all secretagogues increased rat mucosal cyclic AMP, and metiamide, but not atropine, inhibited the small increases caused by administration of histamine or the active peptide of gastrin, pentagastrin. Using an in vivo canine gastric chamber, BOWEN et al. (1975) extended their previous findings which showed that dibutyryl cyclic AMP failed to initiate acid secretion in the

Table 3. Previous evidence *favoring* cyclic nucleotides in acid secretagogue action

Rat
Histamine ↑ AC [1]
Histamine ↑ mucosal cAMP [2]
Gastrin ↑ AC and mucosal cAMP [3]
Carbachol ↑ mucosal cAMP [4]
DbcAMP ↑ acid secretion [5]
Cyclic AMP ↑ acid secretion [6]
Theophylline ↑ acid secretion [7]
Adrenalectomy ↓ acid secretion and mucosal cAMP [8]
Guinea Pig
Histamine ↑ AC [9]
Histamine ↑ mucosal cAMP [10]
Theophylline ↑ acid secretion [11]
Rabbit
Histamine ↑ AC [12]
Acid secretion ↑ by cAMP, dbcAMP, theophylline [13]
Dog
Histamine ↑ AC [14]
Histamine and theophylline ↑ luminal cAMP [15]
Pentagastrin ↑ AC [16]
Methylxanthines augment secretagogue responses [17]
Human
Histamine and betazole ↑ luminal cAMP [18]
Caffeine ↑ acid secretion [19]
Theophylline augments secretagogue responses [20]

[1] Bersimbaev et al. (1972). [2] Narumi and Maki (1973a); Domschke et al. (1973a, b); Ruoff and Sewing (1973). [3] Bersimbaev et al. (1972); Narumi and Maki (1973b); Ruoff and Sewing (1973); Salganik et al. (1971, 1972, 1973); Holian et al. (1973); Domschke et al. (1972). [4] Narumi and Maki (1973b); Ruoff and Sewing (1973). [5] Namuri and Maki (1973a, b); Salganik et al. (1972); Jawaharlal and Berti (1972); Main and Whittle (1972), 1974); Niada and Prino (1973); Whittle and Main (1972). [6] Salganik et al. (1972); Ramwell and Shaw (1968). [7] Miederer et al. (1973). [8] Domschke et al. (1972). [9] Perrier and Laster (1969, 1970); Dousa and Code (1973, 1974); Wollin et al. (1974, 1975a, b). [10] Wollin et al. (1975a, b). [11] Spencer (1974). [12] Sung et al. (1973). [13] Fromm et al. (1975). [14] Spenney and Hirschowitz (1972). [15] Bieck et al. (1973). [16] Spenny and Hirschowitz (1972). [17] Robertson et al. (1950); Bieck et al. (1973); Gabrys et al. (1973). [18] Bieck et al. (1973); Bower et al. (1974a, b); Levine and Washington (1973). [19] Robertson et al. (1950); Debas et al. (1971). [20] Mertz (1969)

dog. However, these investigators found that dibutyryl cyclic AMP increased acid secretion in the presence of submaximal doses of histamine and suggested the appealing possibility of a modulatory role for cyclic AMP. Of technical import is the report by Ruoff and Sewing (1977) indicating that postmortem changes in gastric mucosal cyclic nucleotides can occur unless limited by microwave irradiation. In toto (Tables 1–4), the evidence from the in vivo administration of exogenous agents is inconclusive regarding the direct role of cyclic AMP or cyclic GMP in secretagogue induced acid secretion.

Preparations of isolated mucosa and organs minimize potential effects of secretagogue induced release of neural and humoral factors in the whole animal, but do not obviate the difficulty imposed by the inherent cellular heterogeneity of the target tissue. Histamine and dibutyryl cyclic AMP were shown to increase acid out-

Table 4. Previous evidence *against* cyclic nucleotides in acid secretagogue action

Rat
Histamine does not ↑ mucosal cAMP [1]
Pentagastrin in does not ↑ AC [2]
Pentagastrin does not ↑ mucosal cAMP [3]
Carbachol does not ↑ mucosal cAMP [4]
Prostaglandins, glucagon secretion and isoproterenol ↑ AC [5]
Cyclic AMP does not ↑ acid secretion [6]
Guinea Pig
Pentagastrin does not ↑ AC [7]
Histamine and pentagastric do not ↑ mucosal cAMP [8]
Prostaglandins ↑ AC [9]
Rabbit
Pentagastin and urecholine do not ↑ AC [10]
Histamine, pentagastrin and urecholine do not ↑ mucosal cAMP [11]
Dog
Histamine does not ↑ AC [12]
Histamine does not ↑ mucosal cAMP [13]
Pentagastrin does not ↑ cAMP [14]
Theophylline and papaverine do not ↑ acid secretion [15]
Cyclic AMP does not initiate acid secretion [16]
Human
Pentagastrin does not ↑ mucosal cAMP or acid secretion [17]
Hypergastrinemia produces no ↑ in mucosal or luminal cAMP [18]

[1] KARPPANEN et al. (1973a, b); NARUMI and MAKI (1973a, b). [2] BERSIMBAEV et al. (1971, 1972); RUOFF and SEWING (1975b); HOLIAN et al. (1973). [3] KARPPANEN et al. (1973a, b). [4] NARUMI and MAKI (1973b). [5] THOMPSON et al. (1977b). [6] MAIN and WHITTLE (1974); TAFT and SESSIONS (1972a, b). [7] PERRIER and LASTER (1969, 1970). [8] KARPPANEN et al. (1973a, b); KARPPANEN and WESTERMANN (1973). [9] PERRIER and LASTER (1969, 1970); WOLLIN et al. (1974, 1975a, b). [10] SUNG et al. (1973); THOMPSON et al. (1977b). [11] AMER (1974). [12] SUNG et al. (1973); MAO et al. (1972). [13] BIECK et al. (1973); MAO et al. (1973). [14] MAO et al. (1973). [15] ROBERTSON et al. (1950); BIECK et al. (1973); MAO et al. (1972). [16] BOWEN et al. (1975); LEVINE and WILSON (1971); LEVINE et al. (1967a, b). [17] DOMSCHKE et al. (1974); BOWER et al. (1973, 1974a). [18] DOMSCHKE et al. (1974); LEVINE (1974)

put from isolated guinea pig gastric mucosa (SJOSTRAND et al. 1978). However, the long latent period of three hours to onset of secretion suggests serious technical problems with the preparation. Using piglet gastric mucosa, EKBLAD et al. (1978) showed a rapid increase in cyclic AMP content following histamine. This increase coincided with a decrease in tissue resistance and an increase in hydrogen ion secretion. By 15 min cyclic AMP levels had substantially declined while the changes in resistance and acid secretion persisted. In either isolated rat mucosa (MAIN and PEARCE 1977, 1978) or whole immature rat and guinea pig stomachs (BUNCE et al. 1976; HOLTON and SPENCER 1976), histamine, pentagastrin, acetylcholine, theophylline and dibutyryl cyclic AMP were clearly shown to increase acid secretion. An important finding was that histamine H_2-receptor antagonists blocked the response to histamine, but not that to dibutyryl cyclic AMP. Increased cyclic AMP levels in isolated guinea pig stomach prompted by inhibition of phosphodiesterase was also shown to be associated with increased acid secretion (CANFIELD et al. 1978a, b). However, CHEW and HERSEY (1978), on the basis of results obtained using chambered bullfrog gastric mucosa, as well as tissue slices, concluded that there is a lack of quantitative correlation between cyclic AMP levels and rates of acid secretion, and that histamine (and other secretagogues) act by some mechanism that does not include cyclic AMP. In the main, therefore, the results obtained using isolated organs and mucosae (Tables 1–4) have shed little light, except by tenuous association, on the relationship between the action of histamine and cAMP.

II. Cell Free Systems

The investigation of the response of adenylyl cyclase activity in cell free gastric mucosal particulate preparations from various mammalian species has tended to reflect the inordinate complexity of this enzyme system. The treatment afforded adenylyl cyclase enzymology has, at times, been cavalier; this is unfortunate in view of the critical importance of this topic to any discussion of acid secretagogue action mediated by cyclic AMP production. Furthermore, only histamine among the three major acid secretagogues has been demonstrated by documented studies to be an activator of this enzyme system. These studies have utilized crude particulate preparations from fundic mucosa of the dog (RUOFF and SEWING 1976; DOZOIS et al. 1977, 1978), guinea pig (ANTILLA et al. 1976; PERRIER and GRIESSEN 1976; WOLLIN et al. 1976; DOUSA et al. 1979), rabbit (SUNG et al. 1973), and human (see authors SIMON, KATHER, RUOFF, and SEWING 1976–1979). No methodologically sound data have been obtained showing that rat mucosal adenylyl cyclase is activated by histamine, despite a systematic search for such an effect (THOMPSON et al. 1977a). The adenylyl cyclase system of rat parietal cells is, also activated by histamine, but this effect of histamine can only be observed using carefully controlled conditions and isolated parietal cells (THOMPSON et al. 1980; ROSENFELD et al. 1980).

A summary of the results of studies on histamine activation of adenylyl cyclase in cell free gastric mucosa (Tables 1–4) reveals that: (1) maximal activation of "basal" activities (approximately 10–40 pmoles/min/mg of fresh particulate preparations from each of several species) required a histamine concentration near 100 μM; (2) the EC_{50} for histamine approximated 20 μM; (3) histamine analogues active as secretagogues, such as 4-methyl-histamine, dimaprit, N^{α}-methyl-histamine, and N^{α}, N^{α}-dimethylhistamine, also activated adenylyl cyclase, but none with higher apparent affinity than histamine; (4) histamine analogues with little or no activity as acid secretagogues such as 2-methyl-histamine and 2-(2-pyridyl) ethylamine either did not affect or weakly activated the enzyme; (5) histamine activation was inhibited by both H_2-type antagonists such as metiamide, burimimide, and cimetidine and H_1 type antagonists such as mepyramine, tripelennamine, dimethindine, and chlorpheniramine. H_1 and H_2 antagonists both appear to be competitive inhibitors of histamine activated adenylyl cyclase. The relative IC_{50}'s of the two classes of antagonists appear to differ by a factor of 20- to 50-fold; the H_2 agents being of higher potency with apparent K_i's in the low micromolar range. With respect to histamine antagonist specificity, TEPPERMAN et al (1979) have reemphasized the limitations of using the acid secretory response to define receptor specificity and antagonist potency in terms of H_1 and H_2 systems. In fact, adenylyl cyclase inhibition by H_1-antagonists is quite consistent with in situ and isolated cell response findings *(vida infra)*. Another explanation is the possibility that the act of breaking the cell alters receptor configuration such that the adenylyl cyclase system can not discriminate between classes of antagonists. Although few studies have fully characterized the pharmacology of histaminic activation of mucosal adenylyl cyclase (ANTTILA and WESTERMANN 1976; THOMPSON and JACOBSON 1977; PERRIER and GRIESSEN 1976; ROSENFELD et al. 1980), the collective data suggest that histamine acts via an H_2-receptor system coupled to adenylyl cyclase.

Although we recognize that no accumulation of negative findings provides final proof, existing data simply do not implicate cyclic AMP in the cellular actions of either gastrin or acetylcholine. In our view, no data obtained with cell-free preparations as reported in the primary literature demonstrate that (penta)gastrin or acetylcholine or its analogues modulate adenylyl cyclase activity. To the contrary, in vivo inhibitors of acid secretion, such as beta-adrenergic agents, prostaglandins, and polypeptide hormones of the secretin family, were found to stimulate cell-free mucosal adenylyl cyclase in several species, including the rat (THOMPSON et al. 1977b), guinea pig (WOLLIN et al. 1976; ROSENFELD et al. 1976), and human (SIMON and KATHER 1979a, b). Although data obtained with guinea pig mucosa were interpreted to suggest that inhibitors of acid secretion act upon different cellular adenylyl cyclases from those influenced by histamine (WOLLIN et al. 1976), the conclusion was based upon additivity and distribution studies. We have previously discussed the difficulty of interpreting this type of study (THOMPSON et al. 1977c). A comparative study in which the sensitivities of adenyl cyclase to inhibitors and stimulators of acid secretion were tested, in similarly prepared and treated mucosal tissues from several species, served to underscore the problem of variability in species response (THOMPSON and JACOBSON 1977).

Although the interpretation of results from cell-free measurement of adenylyl cyclase activity is facilitated by the apparent absence of neural and humoral factors, membrane heterogeneity is severely limiting and the release of inhibitors is a definite possibility. Also, one has to approach negative findings cautiously because of the nature of the adenylyl cyclase system. It is an enzyme system which protends the classic structure-function relationship of membrane bound enzyme systems. The catalytic component of the system which is responsible for catalyzing the conversion of ATP to cyclic AMP and PP_i in the presence of Mg^{++} is but one of three major subunits contained entirely in membrane bilayers (ABRAMOWITZ et al. 1979). The other two components are the hormone receptor which is the site of hormone binding and the guanyl nucleotide regulatory component (G). The G subunit serves to bind GTP and influence, first, the "coupling" of the hormone-receptor complex in the outer portion of the membrane bilayer with the catalytic subunit on its inner portion and, second, the binding of the hormone to the receptor subunit.

GTPase activity is also associated with adenylyl cyclase catalytic activity and one hypothesis suggests that the GTPase is, in fact, the G regulatory component which serves to regulate by a hydrolytic cycle and the formation of inactive GDP-enzyme (ABRAMOWITZ et al. 1979). Guinea pig (ANTTILA et al. 1976), rat (THOMPSON et al. 1977a), and human (SIMON and KATHER 1977d) mucosal adenylyl cyclases have been shown to be affected by guanyl nucleotide derivatives such as 5′-guanyl diphosphoimide (Gpp(NH)p), a GTP analogue resistant to hydrolysis.

GTPase activity of cell membranes is in enormous excess of that which affects adenylyl cyclase, and it is not unexpected that cell membrane proteins with submicromolar affinities for GDP are saturated with GDP when isolated. Therefore, GDP dissociation and GTP binding are important factors in the coupling of the secretagogue occupied receptor with adenylyl cyclase catalytic subunits.

Hormonal association and dissociation, GTP binding and hydrolysis, subunit lateral diffusion and association add a time and temperature dimension (hysteresis) to the analysis of adenylyl cyclase. Such parameters have recently been studied in isolated rat parietal cells (THOMPSON et al. 1978; ROSENFELD et al. 1980; BEARER et al. 1979, 1980) and are important factors in the activation of adenylyl cyclase by histamine, beta-adrenergic agents, and secretin, but not with cholinergic, gastrin or prostaglandin effectors. Given these complexities of the adenylyl cyclase system it is not surprising that analyses of its activity in homogenates and in particulate fractions of mucosal scrapings reflect the influences of species variability, mechanical disruption, temperature, protease activity, sulfhydryl and lipid oxidation, nucleotide metabolism, divalent cation binding, membrane composition, or even covalent modification. Any one or more of these variables could have produced either positive or negative results with various effectors in cell free systems as have been reported in the literature.

III. Isolated Gastric Glands

BERGLINDH and OBRINK (1976) have successfully achieved the isolation of gastric glands from rabbit mucosa and have used this preparation to study secretagogue effects. The gland preparation, which is composed of at least four cell types, eliminates the influences of systemic factors, as well as that of contaminating surface epithelial cells. The matter of cellular heterogeneity, however, is still prominent and precludes definitive interpretation of cyclic nucleotide studies. Apparently, glands can also be isolated from human mucosa (FELLENIUS et al. 1979). Although no reports have appeared which attempt to link effector responses directly with cyclic nucleotide metabolism, several indirect pieces of information make this association likely (BERGLINDH et al. 1976; BERGLINDH 1977a, b, c).

Using oxygen consumption; an indirect measure of H^+ ion production, ^{14}C-aminopyrine accumulation in acid compartments; and morphological changes as measures of parietal cell response, the glands were shown to be stimulated by histamine (EC_{50} 4 μM), carbachol, and cyclic AMP or dibutyryl cyclic AMP, but not by pentagastrin or gastrin. Dibutyryl cyclic AMP gave the highest maximal response. For oxygen consumption, maximal concentrations of dibutyryl cyclic AMP and histamine showed similar time courses, each with linear increases between 5 and 10 min when a steady state ensued. Dose-response curves with carbachol could not be obtained since cholinergic activation was transient, lasting 15–20 min, before returning to basal values or below basal values in studies of aminopyrine accumulation. Burimamide (24 μM) and atropine (1 μM) blocked, respectively, the effect of histamine (1–100 μM) and carbachol (100 μM) on O_2 consumption. Burimamide did not effect the carbachol response, but atropine (100 μM) did have some effect on histamine (4 μM) stimulated O_2 consumption. Dibutyryl cyclic AMP responses were unaffected by either blocking agent. H_1-antagonist studies may need additional clarification primarily because of the failure to show dose-response relationships for carbachol and the use of extraordinarily high concentrations of antagonists.

Aminophylline enhanced O_2 consumption in response to histamine both by decreasing histamine's ED_{50} to 0.2 μM and increasing the maximum response. No effect of aminophylline on carbamylcholine-induced increase in O_2 consumption was observed. Thus, aminophylline, which is presumed to inhibit cyclic AMP phosphodiesterase, was secretagogue selective, suggesting different mechanisms of cellular stimulation. However, these pathways must converge since the combinations of histamine or dibutyryl cyclic AMP with carbamylcholine showed increased maximal responses (potentiation). The mechanistic implications of these studies seem to substantiate some of the conclusions drawn from analyses of adenylyl cyclase in cell-free systems, namely, that histamine utilizes pathways involving cyclic AMP metabolism, carbachol acts by another pathway, and gastrin remains inactive.

With respect to the major hypotheses of secretagogue action, it is our view that the studies with isolated gastric glands do not support, and probably refute, the hypothesis that histamine is the final common mediator of all secretagogue action. The lack of effect of (penta)gastrin, however, also does not support the proposal that parietal cells have receptors for all three secretagogues, although negative results do not necessarily refute the hypothesis. It is possible that receptors for gastrin were destroyed during gland preparation and/or that the hormone may have been degraded, bound, sequestered, or otherwise prevented from reaching its site of action. It might also be argued that gastrin acts by releasing histamine, which was ineffective due to dilution; however, the final common mediator hypothesis then would require that the action of carbamylcholine be via histamine release, an effect apparently not influenced by dilution. However, the effect of carbachol was not blocked by the H_2-antagonist, burimamide. In any case, no present hypothesis appears adequate to explain these results.

From results obtained by measuring gastric mucosal or juice cyclic nucleotide content or adenylyl cyclase activity after administration of agents in vivo or in situ as well as their addition to intact tissues and cell free systems, it appears that definitive data on the role of cyclic nucleotide in gastric secretion can be approached only with isolated and purified parietal cells. Definitive data mean to the authors that one could conclude: (1) histamine, gastrin, and/or acetylcholine cause a reproducible, dose-dependent, increase in *parietal cell* adenylyl and/or guanylyl cyclase activity (not that of other mucosal cells) which is inhibited specifically by secretagogue antagonists; (2) histamine, gastrin, and/or acetylcholine cause a reproducible, dose-dependent increase in cyclic AMP and/or cyclic GMP which is also inhibited specifically by secretagogue antagonists and influenced by putative inhibitors of cyclic nucleotide phosphodiesterase; and (3) exogenously administered cyclic nucleotides or their analogues mimic the effects of the secretagogues on acid secretion. These, of course, represent the minimal criteria of SUTHERLAND and ROBISON (ROBISON et al. 1971) for showing the mediation of hormonal control of a cellular response by cyclic AMP. These rather stringent demands, although not absolutely necessary *to implicate* cyclic AMP in secretagogue action, are certainly required *to define* the mechanism of action of these agents in the regulation of hydrogen ion production and secretion. Thus, resolution of the mechanisms of action of gastric acid secretagogues at the molecular, pharmacological and biochemical level requires the study of isolated parietal cells.

D. Isolated Gastric Parietal cells

I. Cell Preparations

Methodologies have been developed to isolate parietal cells from the gastric mucosa of dog (SCHOLES et al. 1976; SOLL 1978a; MAJOR and Scholes 1978), rat (SONNENBERG et al. 1978; LEWIN et al. 1974, 1976; KUROKAWA et al. 1975; THOMPSON et al. 1980; ECKNAUER et al. 1980), guinea pig (BATZRI and GARDNER 1978a, b) mouse (ITO et al. 1977), and rabbit (GLICK 1974). These procedures are in addition to those previously available for more easily obtained cells of amphibian mucosa (BLUM et al. 1971; WIEBELHAUS et al. 1974; FORTE et al. 1972). The availability of isolated cells has led to the advent of molecular physiology and pharmacology of acid secretion. At the outset of this discussion we are obliged to report that no single parietal cell preparation is yet available that satisfies all necessary physiological, pharmacological, and biochemical criteria. Nevertheless, isolated cells are beginning to contribute to our understanding of parietal cell function and control, and it is clear that much more information will be forthcoming.

Isolated, viable cells have several advantages as an in vivo model for secretagogue action, enabling the direct study of: (1) membrane receptors, structure, and enzymes specific to parietal cells; (2) metabolic parameters including cyclic nucleotides and energy substrates and their regulation by hormones and drugs; and (3) cell specific functions without influences from other cell types, but with the capability of reconstituting these influences. Furthermore, this preparation permits precise control of the cellular environment, as well as having the capacity for better statistics, sampling, and reproductibility than are available with intact mucosa, thereby improving detection, discrimination, and analysis of responses between experimental and control cells. Finally, with isolated cells it is possible to develop short and long term culture, somatic cell hybridization, and cell fusions. The disadvantages of using isolated cells include the possibility of damage during preparation, the loss of endogenous cell influences, the loss of polarity and symmetry between serosa and lumen, a limiting quantity of cells for certain biochemical studies, and a dependence upon indirect methods for measuring acid secretion.

Parietal cells are the largest cells in the gastric mucosa (12–25 μ) and have a very distinctive morphology (Fig. 2). With mouse parietal cells serving as a reference for mammalian systems, morphological changes of the smooth endoplasmic reticulum in the parietal cells are intimately linked to acid secretion (ITO and WINCHESTER 1963; HELANDER and HIRSCHOWITZ 1974; ITO et al. 1977). Canaliculi are thought to be formed from the fusion of tubulovesicular structures. Upon secretagogue stimulation, tubulovesicles decrease, canalicular space increases, and microvilli in the canaliculi become more numerous. SACHS et al. (1979) have recently documented that the surfaces of these structures are sites of acid secretion in gastric glands. It has been suggested that one role of cyclic AMP is to regulate these morphological changes (FORTE et al. 1977), processes not dependent upon protein synthesis. However, in amphibian cells, active acid secretion, such as that induced by theophylline, is not required to produce canalicular morphological modification (CARLISLE et al. 1978). The mitochondrial content of parietal cells is so high compared to other mucosal cell types that their enzymes are used for cellular identity. The characteristic acidophilic cycloplasm of parietal cells has been demonstrated using numerous staining procedures (WATTEL and GEUZE 1977; SOLL 1978a). HELANDER (1977) has summarized earlier studies in the rat mucosa to calculate that the 10 cm^2 of the 0.4 mm thick, acid-secreting portion of the stomach contains approximately 60×10^6 parietal cells, each near 1,500 μ^3 size. The surface area of the canalicular membrane secreting acid was calculated to possess an astounding 780 cm^2 which would be expected to increase by 3- to 10-fold under maximal stimulating conditions.

Parietal cells show a non-uniform distribution throughout the body of the stomach and are found in the isthmus, neck, and base of the gastric glands (CROSS 1977). These cells show a correlation between their mass and animal body weight and age (BRALOW and KOMAROV 1962). Because of this distribution, the first step in parietal cell isolation procedures is an enzymatic digestion of the surface epithelial cells with collagenase or non-specific proteases. The next step in isolation, usually in the presence of divalent cation chelators, is one of dispersal to achieve individual cells. Finally, parietal cells are purified (or more accurately enriched) by methods which take advantage of their characteristic density, mass, and/or size. Such separations are conducted with linear sucrose (LEWIN et al. 1974), albumin (ROMRELL et al. 1975), or Ficoll density gradients (MAJOR and SCHOLES 1978); Ficoll/sucrose (THOMPSON et al. 1980) or PERCOLL discontinuous gradients (DIAL et al. 1980); low speed centrifugation (LEWIN et al. 1976; SCHOLES et al. 1976; SONNEBERG et al. 1978; BATZRI and GARDNER 1978a); or counter-flow centrifugation in cell culture media (SOLL 1978a).

II. Parietal Cell Responses and Cyclic Nucleotide Metabolism

It is presumptuous to draw definitive conclusions on the role of cyclic AMP in responses to acid secretagogues in isolated cells because any summary statements require the synthesis of results obtained on cells isolated from different species and by different procedures. Comparison studies have not been studied from the same view-point in any laboratory. In a recent review of evidence obtained with isolated cells (ROSENFELD et al. 1980), we concluded that histamine interacts with the parietal cell H_2 type receptor system to activate adenylyl cyclase and stimulate the accumulation of cellular cyclic AMP, which then mediates an increase in acid secretion. This conclusion was based upon the following: (1) SCHOLES et al. (1976), SOLL (1978a, b), SOLL and WOLLIN (1979) using canine parietal cells; BATZRI and GARDNER (1978b, 1979) using guinea pig cells; and Sonnenberg et al. (1978), LEWIN et al. (1976) and ROSENFELD et al. (1980) using rat cells demonstrated a histamine induced increase in the cellular accumulation of cyclic AMP. Where determined, the ED_{50}'s for histamine were in the low micromolar range. Responses to histamine were inhibited by H_1- and H_2-receptor blockers (BATZRI and GARDNER 1979). The H_2-receptor antagonists had 10-fold higher inhibitory potencies than H_1-receptor antagonists. Basal cyclic AMP levels in all studies were remarkably similar, 0.5–2 pmol cyclic AMP/10^6 cells, and most measurements were obtained with reliable radioimmunoassay procedures. Putative cyclic AMP phosphodiesterase inhibitors such as isobutylmethyl xanthine, theophylline, or ICI 63,197 were generally required, and each markedly enhanced histamine induced cyclic AMP accumulation. (2) A complete series of histaminic agonists had similar ED_{50}'s for both aminopyrine accumulation and adenylyl cyclase stimulation in highly enriched rat parietal cells. Similarly, the K_i's for H_2-receptor antagonists showed complete agreement for adenylyl cyclase and aminopyrine responses (DIAL et al. 1979, 1980; BEARER et al. 1980; ROSENFELD et al. 1980); (3) In the presence of suboptimal concentrations of isobutylmethylxanthine there was an excellent correlation in isolated canine parietal cells between histamine stimulated cyclic AMP accumulation and O_2 consumption (SOLL 1978 a). Incomplete studies indicated that aminopyrine accumulation correlated less well with cyclic AMP accumulation, although in those studies aminopyrine responses were shown to be more sensitive to cyclic nucleotide phosphodiesterase inhibitors, suggesting that the kinetics of cyclic AMP formation relative to degradation need more detailed investigation; (4) preliminary antagonist binding data suggested the presence of H_2-receptors in rat parietal cell particulate fractions (ROSENFELD et al. 1980); and (5) dibutyryl cyclic AMP mimicked the effect of histamine and isobutylmethylxanthine on O_2 consumption, K^+ uptake, and aminopyrine accumulation in several studies.

In isolated parietal cell systems no evidence has been obtained that cholinergic agonists or gastrin act to modify cyclic nucleotide metabolism. In rat parietal cells, adenylyl cyclase activity was unaffected by carbachol or gastrin in the presence or absence of guanine nucleotides (THOMPSON et al. 1980; BEARER et al. 1980). Studies of cyclic AMP content in guinea pig (BATZRI and GARDNER 1978 b) or dog parietal cells (SOLL and WOLLIN 1979) were also negative with respect to these agents. In-addition, gastrin and carbachol did not increase the accumulation of cyclic AMP in the presence of histamine and isobutylmethylxanthine in isolated cells.

Each of the findings listed above can be criticized. Experiments on cyclic AMP levels in canine cells are suspect because of inadequate cell purity (50%), and lack of either time-course analyses of drug responses or documentation of agonist and antagonist dose-response relationships. Published reports of guinea pig and canine parietal cell preparations have not utilized established morphological criteria for parietal cell identity, but rather have relied heavily on biochemical analyses for characterization. Cells from guinea pig and rat mucosa have not been characterized using O_2 consumption as an index of function. Interestingly, the basal rates of O_2 consumption in all cell preparations are rather similar (5 μ mol/10^6 cells/hr). Adenylyl cyclase studies are lacking in all but rat parietal cells.

There is also the interesting paradox of increased cyclic AMP levels in guinea pig and canine cells induced by prostaglandins, potent in vivo inhibitors of acid secretion. In canine cell populations, prostaglandin responses were diminished in the purer parietal cells preparations (MAJOR and SCHOLES 1978; WOLLIN et al. 1979), although increased purity did not appear to resolve the issue in the 70–80% pure guinea pig preparations. An unexplained result reported by BATZRI and GARDNER (1978 a) was that dibutyryl cyclic AMP altered the influx of potassium, a response not modified by histamine. Prostaglandins do not activate rat parietal cell adenylyl cyclase supporting an indirect mode of action of these agents on acid secretion as proposed by DOUSA and DOZOIS (1977). Secretin, also an inhibitor of acid secretion, increased cyclic AMP in isolated canine cells (WOLLIN et al. 1979). This was thought to occur primarily in chief cell contaminants, but remains to be fully studied since secretin activated rat parietal cell adenylyl cyclase (BEARER et al. 1979; THOMPSON et al. 1978). Isolated parietal cells from mouse and rabbit mucosa have not been studied with respect to nucleotide and secretagogue stimulated responses.

1. Cyclic Nucleotide Phosphodiesterase Inhibitors

The dependence upon cyclic nucleotide phosphodiesterase inhibitors in order to observe histamine responses, as well as cyclic AMP accumulation in isolated parietal cells, requires comment. While all the inhibitors used (isobutylmethylxanthine, Ro-76398, theophylline, and ICI 63,197) have multiple actions (including effects on calcium transport, ATP depletion, membrane structure, and adenylyl cyclase), their only common mode of action is inhibition of cyclic nucleotide phosphodiesterase activity. Some support for the latter as their mechanism of action in gastric secretion stems from their similar relative potencies as activators of aminopyrine accumulation and as competitive inhibitors of the purified, high affinity, relatively cyclic AMP specific form of cyclic AMP phosphodiesterase (theophylline RO-76398 = ICI 63,197 < MIX isobutylmethylxanthine vs 180 μM, 9 μM, 4 μM, and 9 M, respectively; EPSTEIN et al. 1981). Direct studies of the cyclic nucleotide phosphodiesterase system in isolated parietal cells have not been reported, although our preliminary studies have shown the presence of low affinity, calmodulin sensitive and high affinity enzyme forms, characteristic phosphodiesterase forms observed in other mammalian tissues (THOMPSON and STRADA 1978).

Indirect evidence suggests that methylxanthine inhibition of cyclic nucleotide phosphodiesterase is necessary to elicit responses to histamine in intact parietal cells. First, BATZRI and GARDNER (1978b), SOLL and WOLLIN (1979), SCHOLES et al. (1976), and SONNENBERG et al. (1978), each measured an increase in cyclic AMP levels in the presence of these agents alone. Second, uncharacteristic time courses were obtained in both guinea pig and rat cells for histamine induced accumulation of cyclic AMP in the presence of theophylline. In each system, in the presence of 5 or 10 mM theophylline, histamine-stimulated cyclic AMP accumulation increased linearly until about 10 min and then remained constant throughout the duration of incubation (30 min). In most cell systems, even in the presence of phosphodiesterase inhibitors, a decrease in cyclic AMP to near basal levels is observed shortly after the rapid activation of adenylyl cyclase and cyclic AMP accumulation by agonist receptor occupation. Therefore, the level of cyclic AMP reflects a steady state governed by adenylyl cyclase synthesis from ATP, high affinity cyclic AMP phosphodiesterase hydrolysis to 5′-AMP (the K_m of the low affinity enzyme form in all systems studied thus far is too high to account for any basal hydrolysis), high affinity binding (e.g., the R subunit of protein kinase), and in some cases, cyclic nucleotide efflux. Upon stimulation adenylyl cyclase rapidly proceeds to a desensitized state (no longer activatable) and cyclic AMP phosphodiesterase hydrolyzes cyclic AMP.

Reported basal cyclic AMP content in parietal cells approximates 0.25 pmol/10^6 cells. With an intracellular water volume estimated to be 1.2 µl/10^6 cells (unpublished calculations), we estimate the cellular concentration of cyclic AMP to be

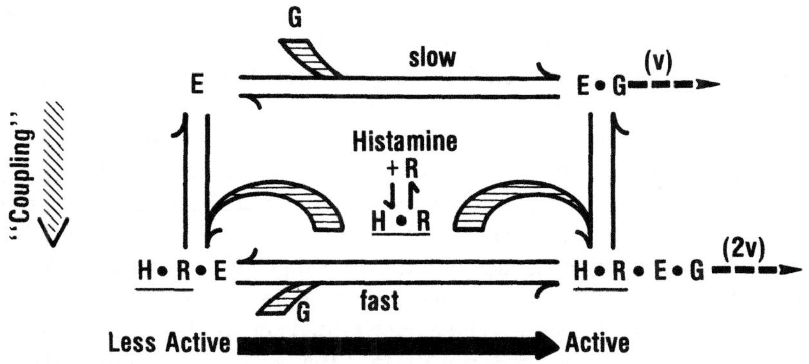

Fig. 4. Schematic representation of rat parietal cell adenylyl cyclase activation by histamine. The catalytic subunit is represented by *E*, guanine nucleotide binding site by *G*, and the H_2 receptor by *R*. The G subunit binds to E in the presence of *GTP* to partially activate catalysis *V*. Full activation is obtained by "*coupling*" of *E.G* with the active form of the histamine occupied receptor *H.R 2V*. *H.R* binding to *E* in the absence of *GTP* or *G* does not activate the enzyme, but facilitates the rate of *GTP* activation *2V*. The active form of *G* is considered to sequentially dissociate *GDP* and bind *GTP*, after which hydrolysis and the release of phosphate restores the inactive *GDP* bound form

approximately 0.2 μ*M* or about one-sixth the apparent K_m of high affinity cyclic AMP phosphodiesterase of mammalian tissues (THOMPSON and STRADA 1978). Perhaps fortuitously, the basal rate of rat parietal cell adenylyl cyclase is near 0.2 pmol/min/10^6 cells as measured under optimal conditions (THOMPSON et al. 1980). It would appear from these calculations that for histamine to cause net synthesis of cyclic AMP in parietal cells, cyclic AMP phosphodiesterase must be inhibited either by normal endogenous controls or pharmacological intervention. If not, cyclic AMP, which is initially at levels well below the K_m of the enzyme, would simply be hydrolyzed at a faster rate following increased secretagogue induced synthesis. There are several physical, kinetic, and covalent regulatory mechanisms for cyclic nucleotide phosphodiesterases which serve as controls in this system (THOMPSON and STRADA 1978). Thus, it seems reasonable to suggest that H_2-receptors are linked not only to adenylyl cyclase, but perhaps also to high affinity phosphodiesterase. From published histamine time-response curves alone, it is not possible to deduce if adenylyl cyclase becomes desensitized (tachphylaxis) after stimulation by histamine. A factor which needs additional study is the relatively low intrinsic activity of histamine as an agonist when compared to adrenergic and polypeptide effectors and what effect this might have on cyclic AMP synthesis and/or degradation.

2. Adenylyl Cyclase

Studies on histaminic activation of adenylyl cyclase have been limited to rat parietal cells (THOMPSON et al. 1978, 1981; BEARER et al. 1981; ROSENFELD et al. 1980). A kinetic model of our findings is illustrated in Fig. 4. Parietal cell adenylyl cyclase conforms to the blue print more extensively studied in other tissues as referred to in Sect. C.II above. Histamine activation of parietal cell adenylyl cyclase by an H_2-receptor system is virtually dependent upon guanine nucleotide cofactor.

Activation by Gpp(NH)p and/or histamine shows hysteretic modifications of catalysis with first order rate dependence suggestive of an enzyme-like "coupling" process between histamine occupied receptor sites, GTP occupied guanine nucleotide regulatory sites, and the catalytic site.

Gpp(NH)p, an analog of GTP which is less easily hydrolyzed, increases "basal" adenylyl cyclase activity to a level intermediate between that of histamine plus Gpp(NH)p and basal activity. Fully active enzyme was observed only in the presence of histamine and Gpp(NH)p. Incubation with histamine alone did not cause activation; however, the subsequent addition of Gpp(NH)p allowed the fully active enzyme to be expressed in less time than required previously. The enzyme activity reached a truly "activated state", since the elevated activity persisted after washing the system free of histamine and Gpp(NH)p. After washing, the activated state was not reversed by the subsequent addition of histamine, cimetidine, or GTP alone, but was partially reversed by adding histamine plus GTP. Therefore, parietal cell adenylyl cyclase activation depends upon H_2-receptor occupancy and receptor activation, GDP dissociation and GTP association with the nucleotide binding unit, and the interaction of these subunits of the enzyme system with the catalytic subunit. Presumably, the process is normally reversed by GTP hydrolysis, hormone dissociation, and receptor desensitization and further processing. Using Gpp(NH)p to study histamine activation, an activated state is observed due to the lack of GTP hydrolysis and an accumulation of active catalytic subunits.

E. Recapitulation and Speculation

With the advent of isolated cell systems, the age of "molecular physiology" of gastric secretion is just beginning. Certainly, methodologies for cell isolation need technical improvement, and additional functional indexes are required. The data obtained from all gastric systems seem to indicate that, in parietal cells, cyclic AMP acts as a second messenger for histamine, but not for acetylcholine or gastrin. Studies with isolated systems have shown an acid secretory response of parietal cells, depending upon the species studied, to all three acid secretagogues, but histamine requires the concomitant inhibition of cyclic nucleotide phosphodiesterase. An H_2-receptor system has been defined for histamine. Biochemical and pharmacological studies have clearly identified muscarinic cholinergic receptors in isolated cells (ROSENFELD et al. 1978; ECKNAUER et al. 1979, 1980). Acid secretory responses to gastrin require substantiation in species other than the dog. Interestingly, full gastrin responses were observed only in the presence of histamine and methylxanthines. Thus, it would appear that the final common mediator hypothesis proposed for histamine and the proposal of a singular role of cyclic nucleotide as the mediator of all secretagogue action are not adequate.

I. Second Messengers for Acetylcholine and Gastrin: Relationship to Cyclic Nucleotides and Histamine

If cyclic AMP is not the second messenger mediating the cellular actions of acetylcholine and gastrin, are there other second messengers and, if so, at which biochemical locus in parietal cells do these secretagogues act? KASBEKAR (1974) has suggested that intracellular calcium is involved in secretagogue regulation of acid secretion, and the regulatory role of serum calcium has been suspect for some time (e.g., WARD et al. 1964). Although this postulate did not include cholinergic agents, results obtained from studies of isolated gastric glands and parietal cells suggest that calcium may be an intracellular second messenger for acetylcholine as observed in other systems (PUTNEY 1978, 1979; SCHEELE and HAYMOVITS 1979). Calcium apparently is also necessary for histamine and cholinergic induced responses in isolated rat parietal cells (G.C. ROSENFELD, personal communication). Additionally, MAIN and PEARCE (1978) have shown calcium modulation of all secretagogue actions in isolated rat gastric mucosa.

SOLL and WALSH (1979) have recently emphasized the interdependence of secretagogue regulation of parietal cells consistent with the multiple receptor hypotheses of GROSSMAN and KONTUREK (1974). SOLL (1978 b) has proposed a working hypothesis based on studies of partially purified canine parietal cells which differs from that of GROSSMAN and KONTUREK in that no interactions between secretagogue receptors are hypothesized. In his view, each secretagogue acts on separate receptors on the parietal cell; cholinergic and histaminergic antagonists being specific for each class of agonist. The conflicting findings of apparent non-specific antagonist inhibition documented by in vivo studies (e.g. PARSONS 1977) are visualized as a function of the tonic or phasic release of local histamine and acetylcholine which potentiate secretion. The antagonists act as specific blockers at the level of the parietal cell, but appear to be non-specific due to the inhibition of the potentiated response caused by the endogenous secretagogues. In SOLL's model no mechanisms for secretagogue potentiation were proposed. In our opinion either maximal responses achieved with each secretagogue or their relative affinities require careful and extensive analyses with respect to dose and time variables particularly when involving more then one drug or hormone, and sufficient analysis has not yet been obtained. GARDNER et al. (1978) have discussed how potentiation might explain seemingly paradoxical in vivo inhibitory effects by apparently specific antagonists, such as atropine and cimetidine, of different classes of acid secretagogues. Potentiation of secretagogue responses as measured by O_2 consumption in canine parietal cells was not dramatic, lacked detailed dose time analyses, and was generally only additive (SOLL 1978 b). Thus, more studies are needed in isolated cells to define this working hypothesis.

One difficulty in unraveling the role of secretagogues in the regulation of parietal cell function is that the biochemical and cellular events in the production and transport of H^+ by the secretory membrane are complex and not completely understood. Of special significance has been the recent definition and characterization of a gastric, K^+-adenosine triphosphatase (SACHS et al. 1978, 1979). The enzyme, which has been localized to the acid secreting membrane, appears to provide for H^+ translocation with concomitant K^+ influx. In other tissues, calcium mobilization is associated with receptor- and voltage-dependent K^+ permeability (PUTNEY 1979). Future experiments will be needed to define the relationships, if any, that exist between cyclic AMP and/or calcium and the H^+ for K^+ exchange mechanisms.

Our view is that secretagogue interactions reflect cellular interactions of the pathways regulated by receptor-initiated second messenger production. Cyclic

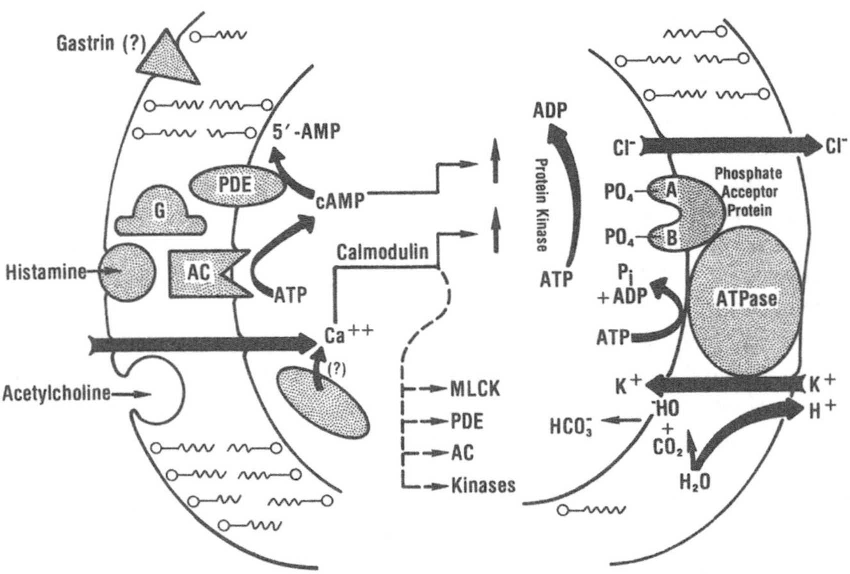

Fig. 5. Multiple Pathway Hypothesis of Acid Secretagogue Receptor Regulation. The acid secretagogues, histamine and acetylcholine, are schematically hypothesized to act individually to modulate the same effect, acid secretion via K^+-ATPase, or to act together to potentiate the effect of each utilizing different pathways with the same end point. Multiple levels of phosphorylation of a phosphate acceptor system which is linked to an ATPase and K^+ for H^+ exchange may occur via a protein kinase that is both cyclic AMP dependent and calmodulin dependent. Acetylcholine binds to a muscarinic cholinergic receptor linked to calcium channels which stimulates calmodulin binding and kinase activation. Histamine binding to an H_2-receptor in the presence of *GTP* activates coupling to adenylyl cyclase **AC** and/or possibly high affinity cyclic AMP phosphodiesterase *PDE* to produce cyclic AMP and also cause protein kinase activation. Additional calcium-calmodulin binding could result in the coordinated effects of activation of myosin light chain kinase *MLCK* and morphological changes associated with acid secretion, feedback regulation of adenylyl cyclase and low affinity cyclic AMP phosphodiesterase, and energy substrate mobilization by phosphorylase kinase or lipase stimulations

AMP-dependent phosphorylation by protein kinases is one of the accepted modes for regulation of metabolic processes and cell structure and might be expected to be involved in parietal cell function. Recently, the phosphate acceptor protein of cardiac sarcoplasmic reticulum, phospholamban, has been shown to contain separate sites, one regulated by cyclic AMP-dependent protein kinase and the second by calmodulin-independent protein kinase (LEPEUCH et al. 1979). Calmodulin, originally discovered as a cyclic AMP phosphodiesterase activator, is a ubiquitous calcium binding protein which, in the presence of calcium, binds to and modifies a variety of enzymes (WOLFF and BROSTROM 1979) including calcium-dependent ATPase. Additionally, intestinal cells show cyclic nucleotide dependent membrane phosphorylations (SHLATZ et al. 1978, 1979).

Our hypothesis incorporating these findings to secretagogue regulation of parietal cell hydrogen ion production is shown schematically below (Fig. 5). We suggest that acid secretagogues act through specific receptors on parietal cells. Acetylcholine and histamine both involve the mobilization of calcium from intracellular and/or extracellular sites, but histamine alone increases cyclic AMP. Both second messengers, calcium and cyclic AMP, ultimately activate phosphorylation of a key membrane phosphate acceptor protein, but at different sites, which results in activation of K^+-ATPase and acid secretion. Therefore, histamine can stimulate independently or its effects can be potentiated by acetylcholine, or perhaps by gastrin, by promoting multiple levels of phosphorylation to modify the rate of acid secretion. The calcium second messenger system through calmodulin could also result in coordinate activation of enzymes such as myosin light chain kinase for morphological modifications, feedback regulation of adenylyl cyclase and cyclic AMP phosphodiesterase, and energy substrate mobilization to support acid secretion. It will be interesting to further define the secretory process since H^+ secretion is dependent upon Cl^- ion, as well as attendent Cl^- for HCO_3 exchange on the nutrient side (HELANDER 1977).

Acknowledgements. The authors wish to thank Mrs. LAURA JACOBSON for her expertise in library science which proved invaluable to us. Our appreciations as well go to Mrs. SHIRLEY WASHINGTON and CATHYANN DIXON for secretarial aid.

References

Abramowitz J, Iyengar R, Birnbaumer L (1979) Guanyl nucleotide regulation of hormonally-responsive adenylyl cyclases. Mol Cell Endocrinol 16:129–246

Amer MS (1974) Cyclic GMP and gastric acid secretion. Am J Dig Dis 19:71–73

Anttila P, Westermann E (1976) Effects of cimetidine on adenylate cyclase activity of guinea pig gastric mucosa stimulated of histamine, sodium fluoride and 5′-guanylylimidodiphosphate. Naunyn Schmiedebergs Arch Pharmacol 294:209–211

Anttila P, Lucke C, Westermann E (1976) Stimulation of adenylate cyclase of guinea pig gastric mucosa by histamine, sodium fluoride and 5′-guanylylimidodiphosphate and inhibition by histamine H_1- and H_2-receptor antagonists in vitro. Naunyn Schmiedebergs Arch Pharmacol 296:31–36

Ariens EJ, Beld AJ (1977) The receptor concept in evolution. Biochem Pharmacol 26:913–918

Ash ASF, Schild HO (1966) Receptors mediating some actions of histamine. Br J Pharmacol 27:427–439

Babkin BP (1938) The abnormal functioning of the gastric secretory mechanism as a possible factor in the pathogenesis of peptic ulter. Can Med Assoc J 38:421–429

Batzri S, Gardner JD (1978a) Cellular cyclic AMP in dispersed mucosal cells from guinea pig stomach. Biochim Biophys Acta 541:181–189

Batzri S, Gardner JD (1978b) Potassium transport in dispersed mucosal cells from guinea pig stomach. Biochim Biophys Acta 508:328–338

Batzri S, Gardner JD (1979) Action of histamine on cyclic AMP in guinea pig gastric cells: inhibition by H_1- and H_2-receptor antagonists. Mol Pharmacol 16:406–416

Bearer CF, Chang LK, Rosenfeld GC, Thompson WJ (1979) Interactions of acid secretagogues with adenylyl cyclase of rat gastric parietal cells. Fed Proc 38:596

Bearer CF, Chang LK, Rosenfeld GC, Thompson WJ (1981) Histamine stimulation of rat gastric parietal cell adenylyl cyclase: modulation by guanine nucleotides. Biochim Biophys Acta 207:325–336

Berglindh T (1977a) Absolute dependence in chloride for acid secretion in isolated gastric glands. Gastroenterology 73:874–880

Berglindh T (1977b) Effects of common inhibitors of gastric acid secretion on secretagogue-induced respiration and aminopyrine accumulation in isolated gastric glands. Biochim Biophys Acta 464:217–233

Berglindh T (1977c) Potentiation by carbachol and aminophylline of histamine-and db-cAMP induced parietal cell activity in isolated gastric glands. Acta Physiol Scand 99:75–84

Berglindh T, Obrink KJ (1976) A method for preparing isolated glands from the rabbit gastric mucosa. Acta Physiol Scand 96:150–159

Berglindh T, Helander HF, Obrink J (1976) Effects of secretagogues on oxygen consumption aminopyrine accumulation and morphology in isolated gastric glands. Acta Physiol Scand 97:401–414

Bersimbaev RI, Argutinskaya SV, Salganik RI (1971) The stimulating action of gastrin pentapeptide and histamine on adenylyl cyclase activity in rat stomach. Experientia 27:1389–1390

Bersimbaev RI, Argutinskaya SV, Salganik RI (1972) Effect of pentagastrin and histamine on adenyl cyclase activity in the rat stomach. Biokhimiia 37:792–796

Bieck PR, Oates JA, Robinson GA, Adkins RB (1973) Cyclic AMP in the regulation of gastric secretion in dogs and humans. Am J Physiol 224:158–164

Black JW, Duncan WAM, Durant CJ, Ganellin CR, Parsons ME (1972) Definition and antagonism of histamine H_2-receptors. Nature 236:385–390

Black JW, Duncan WAM, Emmet JC, Ganellin CR, Hesselbo T, Parsons ME, Wyllie JH (1973) Metiamide-an orally active histamine H_2-receptor antagonist. Agents and Actions 3:133–137

Blum AL, Shah GT, Wiebehaus VD, Brennan FT, Helander HF, Ceballos R, Sachs G (1971) Pronase method for isolation of viable cells from *Necturus* gastric mucosa. Gastroenterology 61:189–200

Bovet D, Staub AM (1937) Action protectrice des éthers phénoliques au cours de l'intoxication histaminique. CR Sor Biol (Paris) 124:547–551

Bowen JC, Pawlik W, Kuo YM, Williams DW, Shanbour LL, Jacobson ED (1975) Modulation of stimulated acid secretion by dibutyryl cyclic AMP in the dog stomach. Gastroenterology 69:285–288

Bower R, Sode J, Lukash W, Lipschutz W (1973) Cyclic nucleotides in pentagastrin stimulated human gastric acid secretion. Clin Res 21:961

Bower RH, Sode J, Lipschutz W (1974a) Cyclic GMP and gastric acid secretion. Am J Dig Dis 19:582

Bower R, Sode J, Lukash W, Lipshutz W (1974b) Plasma and gastric juice cyclic guanosine monophosphate following betazole stimulation in man. Clin Res 22:19A

Bower RH, Sode J, Lipshutz WH (1977) Cyclic adenosine monophosphate and human gastric acid secretion. Am J Dig Dis 22:705–711

Bradshaw J, Brittain RT, Clitherow JW, Daly MJ, Jack D, Price BJ, Stables R (1979) Ranitidine: a new potent, selective histamine H_2-receptor antagonist. Br J Pharmacol 66:464P

Bralow SP, Komarov SA (1962) Parietal cell mass and distribution in stomachs of Wistar rats. Am J Physiol 203:550–552

Brimblecombe RW, Duncan WAM, Durant CJ, Emmet JC, Ganellin CR, Parsons ME (1975) Cimetidine-a non thiorea H_2-receptor antagonist. J Int Med Res 3:86–92

Brimblecome RW, Duncan WAM, Durant GJ, Emmet JC, Ganellin CR, Leslie GB, Parsons MW (1978) Characterization and development of cimetidine as a histamine H_2-receptor antagonist. Gastroenterology 74:339–347

Bunce KT, Parsons ME, Rollings NA (1976) The effect of metiamide on acid secretion stimulated by gastrin, acetylcholine and dibutyryl cyclic adenosine 3′,5′-monophosphate in the isolated whole stomach of the rat. B J Pharmacol 58:149–156

Canfield SP, Curwain BP, Spencer J (1976) A quantitative relationship between acid secretion and mucosal 3,5-cyclic AMP in the isolated guinea pig stomach. J Physiol (Lond) 260:61–62P

Canfield SP, Curwain BP, Spencer J (1977) A possible role for cyclic adenosine 3′,5′-monophosphate in the regulation of acid secretion in the isolated stomach of guinea pig. Br J Pharmacol 56:327–332

Canfield SP, Curwain BP, Spencer J (1978a) Acid secretion and cyclic nucleotide content of the guinea pig isolated stomach in the presence of the ionophore A 23187. Acta Hepatagastroenterol (Stuttg) 25:155–157

Canfield SP, Curwain BP, Phillips JO, Price G (1978b) Acid secretion without changes in mucosal cyclic nucleotides in the guinea pig stomach. J Physiol (Lond) 272:52–53P

Capobianco JO, Mollison KW, Lee Y-H, Hung PP (1977) Correlation between gastrin protein kinase and secretion in the pylorus ligated rat. Biochem Pharmacol 26:991–994
Carlisle KS, Chew CS, Hersey SJ (1978) Ultrastructural changes and cyclic AMP in frog oxyntic cells. J Cell Biol 76:31–42
Chaudhury TK, Jacobson ED (1978) Prostaglandin cytoprotection of gastric mucosa. Gastroenterology 74:58–63
Chew CS, Hersey SJ (1978) Dissociation between oxyntic cell cAMP formation and HCl secretion in bullfrog gastric mucosa. Am J Physiol 235:E 140–E 149
Code CF (1965) Histamine and gastric secretion: a later look. Fed Proc 24:1311–1321
Cooke AR, Chvasta TE, Granner DK (1974) Histamine, pentagastrin, methyl xanthines and adenyl cyclase activity in acid secretion. Proc Soc Exp Biol Med 147:674–678
Cross SAM (1977) Localization of histamine and histamine H_2-receptor antagonists in the gastric mucosa. Histochem J 9:619–644
Dale HH, Laidlow PP (1910) The physiological action of β-iminazolylethylamin. J Physiol (Lond) 41:318–344
Debas HT (1977) Regulation of gastric acid secretion. Fed Proc 36:1933–1937
Debas HT, Cohen MM, Holubitsky IB, Harrison RC (1971) Caffeine stimulated acid and pepsin secretion: Dose-response studies. Scand J Gastroenterol 6:453–457
Dial EJ, Thompson WJ, Rosenfeld GC (1979) Characterization of the histamine response of isolated rat parietal cells using ^{14}C-aminopyrine. Physiologist 22:29
Dial E, Thompson WJ, Rosenfeld GC (1981) Isolated parietal cells: histamine response and pharmacology. J Pharmacol Exp Ther 219:585–590
Domschke W, Domschke S, Classen M, Demling IL (1972) Glucocorticoids and gastric secretion: the role of cyclic adenosine-3′,5′-monophosphate. Gastroenterology 63:252–256
Domschke W, Domschke S, Classen M, Demling L (1973a) Histamine, cyclic 3′,5′-AMP and gastrin acid secretion in rats. Acta Hepatogastroenterol (Stuttg) 20:181–182
Domschke W, Domschke S, Classen M, Demling L (1973b) Histamine and cyclic 3′,5′-AMP in gastrin acid secretion. Nature 241:454–455
Domschke W, Domschke S, Rosch W, Classen M, Demling L (1974) Failure of pentagastrin to stimulate cyclic AMP accumulation in human gastric mucosa. Scand J Gastroenterol 9:467–471
Dousa TP, Code CF (1973) Stimulation of cyclic AMP formation in guinea pig gastric mucosa by histamine and N methylhistamine and their blockade by metiamide. In: Wood CJ, Simkins MA (eds) International symposium on H_2-receptor antagonists. pp 331–340
Dousa TP, Code CF (1974) Effect of histamine and its methyl derivatives on cyclic AMP metabolism in gastric mucosa and its blockade by an H_2 receptor antagonist. J Clin Invest 53:334–337
Dousa TP, Dozois RR (1977) Interrelationships between histamine, prostaglandins, and cyclic AMP in gastric secretion: a hypothesis. Gastroenterology 73:904–912
Dousa TP, Hui YSF, Northrup TE (1979) Inhibition of histamine-sensitive adenylate cyclase from the guinea pig gastric mucosa by noliniun bromide. Biochem Pharmacol 28:343–344
Dozois RR, Dousa TP (1977) Interactions of prostaglandin E_2 (PGE_2) and its methylated analogue with dog fundic gastric mucosa (FGM) adenylate cyclase (AC). Clin Res 25:309A
Dozois RR, Wollin A, Rettmann RD, Dousa TP (1977) Effect of histamine on canine gastric mucosal adenylate cyclase. Am J Physiol 232:E35–E38
Dozois RR, Kim JK, Dousa TP (1978) Interaction of prostaglandins with canine gastrin mucosal adenylate cyclase-cyclic AMP system. Am J Physiol 235:E546–E551
Ecknauer R, Thompson WJ, Johnson JR, Rosenfeld GC (1979) Isolated parietal cells: cholinergic pharmacology and function. Fed Proc 38:884
Ecknauer R, Thompson WJ, Johnson LR, Rosenfeld GC (1980) Isolated parietal cells: [^{3}H]QNB binding to putative cholinergic receptors. Am J Physiol 239:G204–G209
Ekblad EBM, Machen TE, Licko V, Rutten MJ (1978) Histamine, cyclic AMP, and secretory response of piglet gastric mucosa. Acta Physiol Scand [Special Suppl] p 69–80

Epstein PM, Strada SJ, Sarada K, Thompson WJ (1981) Catalytic and kinetic properties of purified high affinity cyclic AMP phosphodiesterase from dog kidney. Arch Biochem Biophys (in press)

Feldman M, Richardson CT (1978) Histamine H_2-receptor antagonists. Adv Intern Med 23:1–24

Fellenius E, Elander B, Wallmark B, Haglund U, Ave L (1979) Studies on acid secretory mechanism and drug action in isolated gastric glands from man. In: Hormone receptors in digestion and nutrition. 355–360

Forte JG, Ray TK, Poulter JL (1972) A method for preparing oxyntic cells from frog gastric mucosa. J Appl Physiol 32:714–717

Forte TM, Machen TE, Forte JG (1977) Ultrastructural changes in oxyntic cells associated with secretory function: a membrane-recycling hypothesis. Gastroenterology 73:941–955

Fromm D, Schwartz JH, Quijano R (1975) Effects of cyclic adenosine 3′,5′-monophosphate and related agents on acid secretion by isolated rabbit gastric mucosa. Gastroenterology 69:453–462

Gabrys BF, Nyhus LM, Van Meter SW, Bombeck CT (1973) The effect of aminophylline on pentagastrin-induced gastric secretion in the dog. Am J Dig Dis 18:563–566

Gardner JD, Jackson MJ, Batzri S, Jensen RT (1978) Potential mechanisms of interaction among secretagogues. Gastroenterology 74:348–354

Geumei A, Danhof I (1978) Hydrochloric acid and cyclic 3′,5′-adenosine monophosphate content of rodent gastric juice after halothane administration. Pharmacology 16:24–246

Glick DM (1974) Stimulation chloride transport by isolated parietal cells. Biochem Pharmacol 23:3283–3288

Gregory RA, Tracy HJ (1964) The constitution and properties of two gastrins extracted from hog antral mucosa. Gut 5:103–117

Grossman MI, Konturek SJ (1974) Inhibition of acid secretion in dog by metiamide a histamine antagonist acting on H_2-receptors. Gastroenterology 66:517–521

Grossman MI, Robertston CR, Ivy AC (1948) Proof of a hormonal mechanism for gastric secretion. Am J Physiol 153:1–9

Harris JB, Alonso D (1965) Stimulation of the gastric mucosa by adenosine-3′,5′-monophosphate. Fed Proc 24:1368–1376

Helander HF (1977) An attempt to correlate functional and morphological data for the gastric parietal cells. Gastroenterology 73:956–957

Helander HF, Hirschowitz BI (1974) Quantitative ultrastructural studies on inhibited and on partly stimulated gastrin parietal cells. Gastroenterology 67:447–451

Holian O, Nyhus M, Bombeck CT (1973) The effect of pentagastrin on adenylyl cyclase. Gastroenterology 64:746

Holton P, Spencer J (1976) Acid secretion by guinea-pig isolated stomach. J Physiol (Lond) 255:465–479

Ito S, Winchester RJ (1963) The fine structure of the gastrin mucosa in the bat. J Cell Biol 16:541–477

Ito S, Munro DR, Schofield GC (1977) Morphology of the isolated mouse oxyntic cell and some physiological parameters. Gastroenterology 73:887–898

Jacobson ED, Thompson WJ (1976) Cyclic and gastric secretion: the illusive second messenger. Adv Cyclic Nucleotide Res 7:199–224

Jawaharlal K, Berti F (1972) Effects of dibutyryl cyclic AMP and a new cyclic nucleotide on gastric acid secretion in the rat. Pharmacol Res Commun 4:143–149

Johnson LR (1971) Control of gastric secretion: no room for histamine? Gastroenterology 61:106–118

Karppanen HO, Westermann E (1973) Increased production of cyclic AMP in gastric tissue by stimulation of histamine$_2$(H_2) receptors. Naunyn Schmiedebergs Arch Pharmacol 279:83–87

Karppanen HO, Neuvonen PI, Westermann E (1973 a) Effect of some gastric stimulants on the production of cyclic AMP in minced gastric tissue. In: Proceedings of the Deutsche Pharmakologische Gesellschaft, Berlin Heidelberg New York, p R35

Karppanen HO, Neuvonen PJ, Westermann E (1973 b) Effect of some gastric stimulants on the production of cyclic AMP in minced gastric tissue. Naunyn Schmiedebergs Arch Pharmacol [Suppl] 277:R35
Karppanen HO, Neuvonen PJ, Bieck PR, Westermann E (1974) Effect of histamine, pentagastrin and theophylline on the production of cyclic AMP in isolated gastric tissue of the guinea pig. Naunyn Schmiedebergs Arch Pharmacol 284:14–23
Karppanen H, Puurunen J, Kairaluoma M, Larmi T (1976) Effects of ethyl alcohol on the adenosine 3′,5′-monophosphate system of the human gastrin mucosa. Scand J Gastroenterol 11:605–607
Kasbekar DK (1974) Calcium-secretagogue interactions in the stimulation of gastric acid secretion. Proc Soc Exp Biol Med 145:234–239
Katsumata Y, Glick D (1975) Effects of drugs influencing gastric secretion on the quantitative histological distribution of cyclic adenosine 3′,5′-monophosphate in the rat stomach. Gastroenterology 69:409–415
Katsumata Y, Yagi K (1976) Distribution of adenyl cyclase sensitive to histamine in rabbit gastric mucosa. Biochem Pharmacol 25:603–604
Konturek SJ, Mikos E, Pawlik W, Walus K (1979) Direct inhibition of gastric secretion and mucosal blood flow by arachidonic acid. J Physiol (Lond) 286:15–28
Kurokawa Y, Saito S, Kanamaru R, Sato T, Sato H (1975) Separation of gastric mucosal cells of rat with proteolytic enzymes, pronase, and trypsin, with special reference to the collection, morphology, and viability of the generative cells. Tohonu J Exp Med 116:241–252
LePeuch CJ, Haiech J, Demaille JG (1979) Concerted regulation of cardiac sarcoplasmic reticulum calcium transport by cyclic adenosine monophosphate dependent and calcium-calmodulin-dependent phosphorylation. Biochemistry 18:5150–5156
Levine RA (1974) Source of gastric juice cyclic adenosine monophosphate (cAMP) in pernicious anemia. J Clin Invest 53:45 a
Levine RA (1977) Role of cyclic nucleotides in gastrointestinal diseases. In: Volicer L (ed) Clinical aspects of cyclic nucleotide, chap 8. Spectrum, New York, pp 229–261
Levine RA, Washington A (1973) Increased cyclic AMP production in human gastrin juice in response to secretagogues. Gastroenterology 64:863
Levine RA, Wilson DE (1971) The role of cyclic AMP in gastric secretion. Ann NY Acad Sci 185:363–375
Levine RA, Cafferata EP, McNally EF (1967 a) Inhibitory effect of adenosine 3′,5′-monophosphate on gastric secretion and gastrointestinal motility in vivo. Recent Adv Gasterenterol 1:408–410
Levine RA, Cafferata EP, McNally EF (1967 b) Inhibitory effect of adenosine 3′,5′-monophosphate on gastric secretion and gastrointestinal motility in vivo. 3rd World Congr Gastroenterol 1:408–410
Levine RA, Schwartzel EH, Bachman S, Talev JN (1977) Gastric cyclic nucleotide concentrations in health and disease. Gastroenterology 73:737–745
Levine RA, Schwartzel EH, Bachman S, Talev JN (1978) Effects of secretagogues and theophylline and canine gastric mucosal cyclic nucleotides. J Lab Clin Med 92:813–821
Lewin M, Cheret AM, Soumarmon A, Girodet J (1974) Méthode pour l'isolement et le tri des cellules de la muquease fundique du rat. Biol Gastroenterol 7:139–144
Lewin M, Cheret AM, Soumarmon A, Girodet J, Ghesquier D, Grelac F, Bonfils S (1976) Isolated cells and a highly enriched population of parietal cells from rat gastric mucosa for the study of H^+ secretion mechanism. In: Case RM, Goebell H (eds) Stimulus-secretion coupling in the gastrointestinal tract. University park Press, Baltimore, pp 371–375
Lundell L (1974) Histamine metabolism of the gastric mucosa following antrectomy. J Physiol (Lond) 241:437–451
MacIntosh FC (1938) Histamine as a normal stimulant of gastric secretion. J Exp Physiol 28:87–98
Main IHM, Pearce JB (1977) Histamine output from the rat isolated gastric mucosa during acid secretion stimulated by pentagastrin, methacoline and dibutyryl cyclic adenosine 3′,5′-monophosphate. Br J Pharmacol 61:461P

Main IHM, Pearce JB (1978) Effects of calcium on acid secretion from the rat isolated gastric mucosa during stimulation with histamine, pentagastrin, methacholine and dibutyryl cyclic adenosine-3′,5′-monophosphate. Br J Pharmacol 64:359–368
Main IHM, Whittle BJR (1972) The relationship between rat gastric mucosal blood flow and acid secretion during oral or intravenous administration of prostaglandins and dibutyryl cyclic AMP. Adv Bioasci 9:271–275
Main IHM, Whittle BJR (1974) Prostaglandin E_2 and the stimulation of rat gastric acid secretion by dibutyryl cyclic 3′,5′-AMP. Eur J Pharmacol 26:204–211
Major JS, Scholes P (1978) The localization of a histamine H_2-receptor adenylate cyclase system in canine parietal cell and its inhibition by prostaglandins. Agents Actions 8/4:324–331
Mao CC, Shanbour LL, Hodgins DS, Jacobson ED (1972) Adenosine 3′,5′-monophosphate (cyclic AMP) and secretion in the canine stomach. Gastroenterology 63:427–438
Mao CC, Jacobson ED, Shanbour LL (1973) Mucosal cyclic AMP and secretion in the dog stomach. Am J Physiol 225:893–896
Mertz DP (1969) Effect of theophylline on acid secretion stimulated human gastric mucosa. Experientia 25:269–270
Miederer SE, Kaess H, Stadelmann O (1973) Contribution on the problem of the liberation of gastrin by methylxanthines. Klin Wochenschr 51:42–44
Mitznegg P, Estler C-J, Loew FW, van Seil J (1977) Effect of salicylates on cyclic AMP in isolated rat gastric mucosa. Acta Hepatogastroenterol (Stuttg) 24:372–376
Nafrady J, Wollemann M (1977) Direct stimulatory action of pentagastrin on the adenylate cyclase of rat stomach mucosa. Biochem Pharmacol 26:2083–2085
Narumi S, Maki Y (1973a) Possible role of cyclic AMP in gastric acid secretion in rat. Activation of carbonic anhydrase. Biochim Biophys Acta 311:90–97
Narumi S, Maki Y (1973b) The role of cyclic AMP in the gastrin acid secretion of rats. Jpn J Pharmacol 23:93
Niada R, Prino G (1973) Effect of a sulphated glycopeptide on rat gastric acid secretion stimulated by histamine, bethanechol, pentagastrin and dibutyryl cyclic AMP. Br J Pharmacol 48:550–552
Osband M, McCaffrey R (1979) Solubilization, separation, and partial characterization of histamine H_1 and H_2 receptors from calf thymocyte membranes. J Biol Chem 254:9970–9972
Parascandola J (1980) Origins of receptor theory. Trends Pharmacol Sci 1(7):189–192
Parsons ME (1977) The antagonism of histamine H_2-receptors in vitro and in vivo with particular reference to the actions of cimetidine. In: Proceedings of the second international symposium on histamine H_2-receptor antagonists, chap 2. Excerpta Medica, Amsterdam London New York, pp 13–23
Perrier CV, Griessen M (1976) Action of H_1 and H_2 inhibitors on the response of histamine sensitive adenylyl cyclase from guinea pig mucosa. Eur J Clin Invest 6:113–120
Perrier CV, Laster L (1969) Adenyl cyclase activity of guinea-pig gastric mucosa (Abstr) Clin Res 17:596
Perrier CV, Laster L (1970) Adenyl cyclase activity of guinea pig gastric mucosa: stimulation by histamine and prostaglandins. J Clin Invest 49:73a
Popielski L (1920) Imidazolylathylamin und die Organextrakte I. Pfluegers Arch 178:214–236
Putney JW Jr (1978) Role of calcium in the actions of agents affecting membrane permeability. In: Weiss GB (ed) Calcium in drug action. Plenum, New York, pp 173–194
Putney JW Jr (1979) Stimulus-permeability coupling: role of calcium in the receptor regulation of membrane permeability. Pharmacol Rev 30:209–245
Puurunen J, Karppanen H (1975) Effects of ethanol on gastric acid secretion and gastric mucosal cyclic AMP in the rat. Life Sci 16:1513–1520
Puurunen J, Karppanen H, Kairaluoma M, Lahmi T (1976) Effects of ethanol on the cyclic AMP system of the dog gastric mucosa. Eur J Pharmacol 38:275–279
Puurunen J, Hiltunen K, Karppanen H (1977) Ethanol-induced changes in gastric mucosal content AMP and ATP in the rat. Eur J Pharmacol 42:85–89

Puurunen J, Lucke L, Schwabe U (1978) Effect of the phosphodiesterase inhibitor AK 62711 on gastric secretion and gastric mucosal cyclic AMP. Naunyn Schmiedebergs Arch Pharmacol 304:69–75
Ramwell PW, Shaw JE (1968) Prostaglandin inhibition of gastric secretion. J Physiol (Lond) 195:34–36
Rangachari PK (1978) Histamine as the final common mediator: a view from the fence. Acta Physiol Scand [Special Suppl] pp 209–218
Robertson CR, Rossiere CE, Blickenstaff D, Grossman MI (1950) The potentiating action of certain xanthine derivatives on gastric acid secretory responses in the dog. J Pharmacol Exp Ther 99:362–365
Robison GA, Butcher RW, Sutherland EW (1971) Cyclic AMP. Academic Press, New York London
Romrell LJ, Coppe MR, Munro DR, Ito S (1975) Isolation and separation of highly enriched fractions of viable mouse gastric cells by velocity sedimentation. J Cell Biol 65:428–438
Rosenfeld G, Jacobson ED, Thompson WJ (1976) Re-evaluation of the role of cyclic AMP in histamine-induced gastric acid secretion. Gastroenterology 70:832–835
Rosenfeld GC, Ecknauer R, Johnson LR, Thompson WJ (1978) Purified gastric mucosal parietal cells: demonstration of (^{3}H)QNB binding to cholinergic receptors. In: Proceedings of the 7th international congress of pharmacology. Paris, Pergamon Press, Ltd, p 132
Rosenfeld GC, Strada SJ, Dial EJ, Bearer CF, Thompson WJ (1980) Histamine, cyclic nucleotides, and gastric parietal cell secretion. Adv Cyclic Nucleotide Res 12:255–265
Ruoff H-J (1977a) Cyclic AMP and cyclic GMP in the rat gastric mucosa. Naunyn Schmiedebergs Arch Pharmacol 298:167–173
Ruoff H-J (1977b) Rat gastric mucosal cAMP and cGMP after adrenergic stimulation and blockade. Eur J Pharmacol 44:349–354
Ruoff H-J, Sewing K-F (1973) Cyclic adenosine 3′,5′-monophosphate (cyclic AMP) in the rat gastric mucosa after pentagastrin, histamine and carbachol. Acta Hepatogastroenterol (Stuttg) 20:172–173
Ruoff H-J, Sewing K-F (1975a) Influence of atropine, metiamide and vagotomy on cAMP of resting and stimulated gastric mucosa. Eur J Pharmacol 32:227–232
Ruoff H-J, Sewing K-F (1975b) Adenylate cyclase and phosphodiesterase in the rat gastric mucosa after starvation, feeding and pentagastrin. Naunyn Schmiedebergs Arch Pharmacol 288:147–153
Ruoff H-J, Sewing K-F (1976) Adenylate cyclase of the dog gastric mucosa: stimulation by histamine and inhibition by metiamide. Naunyn Schmiedebergs Arch Pharmacol 294:207–208
Ruoff HJ, Sewing K-F (1977) Cyclic nucleotides and gastrin acid secretion. In: Cramer H, Schultz J (eds) Cyclic 3′,5′-nucleotides: mechanisms of action, chap 9. John Wiley and Sons, New York Chichester, pp 147–159
Ruoff H-J, Gladziwa U, Sewing K-F (1979) The new H_2-receptor antagonist renatidine as a potent inhibitor of gastric mucosal adenylate cyclase. Gastroenterology 76:1230
Sachs G, Spenney JG, Rehm WS (1977) Gastric secretion. Int Rev Physiol 12:127–171
Sachs G, Spenney JG, Lewin M (1978) H^+ transport: regulation and mechanism in gastric mucosa and membrane vesicles. Physiol Rev 58:106–173
Sachs G, Rabon E, Helander HF, Ito S, Dibona DR, Saccomani G, Berglindh T (1979) Role of K^+ in parietal cell biology. In: Hormone receptors in Digestion and Nutrition. 327–336
Salganik RI (1977) Role of cyclic 3′,5′-AMP′-dependent phosphorylation of membrane proteins in the activation of oxyntic cells. Gastroenterology 73:920
Salganik RI, Argutinskaya SV, Bersimbaev RI (1971) Induction of transcription in the stimulating action of a gastrin pentapeptide on gastric acid secretion. Experientia 27:53
Salganik RI, Argutinskaya SV, Bersimbaev RI (1972) The stimulating action of gastrin pentapeptide, histamine and cyclic adenosine 3′,5′-monophosphate on carbonic anhydrase in rat stomach. Experientia 28:1190–1191

Salganik RI, Argutinskaya SV, Bersimbaev RI, Zimonina TV (1973) Effect of pentagastrin, histamine and cyclic 3',5'-AMP on carboanhydrase activity in rat stomach mucosa. Biokhimiia 38:174–177
Salganik RI, Bersimbaer RI, Argutinskaya SV, Kiseleva EV, Khristolyubora NB, Deribas VI (1976) Integration of biochemical functions of different cells of rat gastric mucosa for hydrochloric acid secretion. Mol Cell Biochem 12:181–191
Scheele G, Haymovits A (1979) Cholinergic and peptide-stimulated discharge of secretory protein in guinea pig pancreatic lobules. J Biol Chem 254:10346–10353
Scholes P, Cooper A, Jones D, Major J, Walters M, Wilde C (1976) Characterization of an adenylate cyclase system sensitive to histamine H_2-receptor excitation in cells from dog gastric mucosa. Agents Actions 6:677–682
Scholes P, Lee J, Major J, Walters M (1979) Prostaglandin and histamine effects on cyclic AMP levels in parietal cells. In: Yellin TO (ed) Histamine receptors. Spectrum, New York, pp 285–297
Schwartzel EH, Bachman S, Levine RA (1977) Cyclic nucleotide activity in gastrointestinal tissues and fluids. Anal Biochem 78:395–405
Sewing K-F, Ruoff H-J (1975) Gastric mucosal protein biosynthesis in relation to cAMP levels and adenylate cyclase activity. Naunyn Schmiedebergs Arch Pharmacol 287:R49
Sewing K-F, Ruoff H-J (1977) Effect of secretory stimulants and inhibitors on gastric mucosal cAMP. Mater Med Pol 2:98–100
Sewing K-F, Ruoff H-J, Ekerdt R (1976) Discussion paper on protein synthesis and the cyclic AMP system in the resting and stimulated gastric mucosa of rats. In: Case RM, Goebell H (eds) Stimulus secretion coupling in the gastrointestinal tract. University Park Press, Baltimore, pp 193–195
Shlatz LJ, Kimberg DV, Cattieu KA (1978) Cyclic nucleotide dependent phosphorylation of rat intestinal microvillus and basal-lateral membrane proteins by an endogenous protein kinase. Gastroenterology 75:838–846
Shlatz LJ, Kimberg DV, Cattieu KA (1979) Phosphorylation of specific rat intestinal microvillus and basal-lateral membrane proteins by cyclic nucleotides. Gastroenterology 76:293–298
Simon B, Kather H (1977a) Inhibition of histamine-sensitive adenylate cyclase of human mucosa by cimetidine. Leber Magen Darm 6:383–385
Simon B, Kather H (1977b) Histamine-sensitive adenylate cyclase in fundic gastric mucosa. Am J Dig Dis 22:746–747
Simon B, Kather H (1977c) Adenylate cyclase of human gastric mucosa. Stimulation of enzyme activity by histamine and catecholamines. Digestion 16:175–179
Simon B, Kather H (1977d) Histamine-sensitive adenylate cyclase of human gastrin mucosa. Gastroenterology 73:429–431
Simon B, Kather H (1978a) Distribution of prostaglandin-sensitive adenylate cyclase in human upper gastrointestinal tract. Digestion 17:264–267
Simon B, Kather H (1978b) Adenylate cyclase of human gastric mucosa. Stimulation by prostaglandins. Res Exp Med (Berl) 173:113–117
Simon B, Kather H (1978c) Activation of human adenylate cyclase in the upper gastrointestinal tract by vasoactive intestinal polypeptide. Gastroenterology 74:722–725
Simon B, Kather H (1979a) Modulation of human gastric mucosal adenylate cyclase activity by prostacyclin. Digestion 19:137–139
Simon B, Kather H (1979b) Prostaglandin-sensitive adenylate cyclase in human gastric mucosa. Inhibition by nonsteroid anti-inflammatory agents. Pharmacology 19 2:96–103
Simon B, Czygan P, Frohling W, Kather H (1977) Topographical studies on histamine – and adrenaline – sensitive adenylate cyclases in gastric and duodenal mucosal of human beings. Digestion 16:185–188
Simon B, Kather H, Kommerell B (1978a) Effects of prostaglandins and their methylated analogues upon human adenylate cyclase in the upper gastrointestinal tract. Digestion 17:547–553
Simon B, Kather H, Kommerell B (1978b) Histamine-sensitive adenylate cyclase of human gastric mucosa. A model for H_2-receptor excitation. Br J Pharmacol 5:277–278
Sjostrand E, Ryberg B, Olbe L (1978) Stimulation and inhibition of acid secretion in the isolated guinea pig gastric mucosa. Acta Physiol Scand [Special Suppl] pp 181–185

Soll AH (1978a) The actions of secretagogues on oxygen uptake by isolated mammalian parietal cells. J Clin Invest 61:370–380
Soll AH (1978b) The interaction of histamine with gastrin and carbamylcholine on oxygen uptake by isolated mammalian parietal cells. J Clin Invest 61:381–389
Soll AH, Grossman MI (1978) Cellular mechanisms in acid secretion. Annu Rev Med 29:495–507
Soll AH, Walsh JH (1979) Regulation of gastric acid secretion. Annu Rev Physiol 41:35–53
Soll AH, Wollin A (1979) Histamine and cyclic AMP in isolated canine parietal cells. Am J Physiol 237(5):E444–450
Sonnenberg A, Hunziker W, Koelz HR, Fisher JA, Blum AL (1978) Stimulation of endogenous cyclic AMP (cAMP) in isolated gastric cells by histamine and prostaglandin. Acta Physiol Scand [Suppl] July:307–317
Spencer J (1974) Gastric secretion in the isolated stomach of the guinea pig J Physiol (Lond) 237:1–3
Spenney JG, Hirschowitz BI (1972) Characterization of gastric cell membrane. Fed Proc 31:828
Strewler GJ, Orloff J (1977) Role of cyclic nucleotides in the transport of water and electrolytes. Adv Cyclic Nucleotide Res 8:311–361
Sung GP, Jenkins BC, Racey Burns L, Hackney V, Spenny JG, Sachs G, Wiebelhaus VD (1973) Adenyl and guanyl cyclase in rabbit gastric mucosa. Am J Physiol 225:1359–1363
Taft RC, Sessions JT Jr (1972a) Inhibition of gastric acid secretion by dibutyryl cyclic adenosine 3′,5′-monophosphate (Db-cAMP). Clin Res 20:43
Taft RC, Sessions JT Jr (1972b) Inhibition of gastric acid secretion by dibutyryl cyclic adenosine 3′,5′-monophosphate (Db-cAMP). Gastroenterology 62:820
Tague LL, Shanbour LL (1977) Effects of ethanol on bicarbonate-stimulated ATPase, ATP, and cyclic AMP in canine gastric mucosa. Proc Soc Exp Biol Med 154:37–40
Tague LL, Amer MS, Jacobson ED (1977) Histamine, cyclic AMP and gastric secretion in the dog. Am J Dig Dis 22:13–15
Talev JN (1976) Cyclic GMP and cyclic AMP in stimulated human and canine gastric mucosa and juice. Evidence against their regulatory role in gastric acid secretion. Gastroenterology 70:940
Tao P, Holian O, Wilson DE (1976) Histamine and prostaglandin interactions with the cyclic AMP system during canine gastric secretion. Gastroenterology 70:941
Theorell T (1978) Reasons and trends in gastric research. Acta Physiol Scand [Special Suppl] pp 11–18
Tepperman BL, Jacobson ED, Rosenfeld GC (1979) Histamine H_2-receptors in the gastric mucosa: role in acid secretion. Life Sci 24:2301–2308
Thompson WJ, Jacobson ED (1977) Comparison of the effects of secretory stimulants and inhibitors on gastric mucosal adenylyl cyclases of various species. Proc Soc Exp Biol Med 154:377–381
Thompson WJ, Strada SJ (1978) Hormonal regulation of cyclic nucleotide phosphodiesterase. Receptors Horm Action 3:553–577
Thompson WJ, Chang LK, Jacobson ED (1977a) Rat gastric mucosal adenylyl cyclase. Gastroenterology 72:244–250
Thompson WJ, Chang LK, Rosenfeld GC, Jacobson ED (1977b) Activation of rat gastric mucosal adenylyl cyclase by secretory inhibitors. Gastroenterology 72:251–254
Thompson WJ, Rosenfeld GC, Jacobson ED (1977c) Adenylyl cyclase and gastric acid secretion. Fed Proc 36:1938–1941
Thompson WJ, Ferkany JW, Chang LK, Jacobson ED, Rosenfeld GC (1978): Guanine nucleotide dependent histamine activation of adenylyl cyclase in purified gastric parietal cells. Adv Cyclic Nucleotide Res 9:737
Thompson WJ, Chang LK, Rosenfeld GC (1981) Histamine regulation of adenylyl cyclase of enriched rat gastric parietal cells. Am J Physiol 240:G76–G84
Thurston D, Tao P, Wilson DE (1976) Relationships between cyclic nucleotides and prostaglandin action in canine gastric secretion. Clin Res 24:538A
Thurston D, Tao P, Wilson DE (1979) Cyclic nucleotides and the regulation of canine gastric acid secretion. Dig Dis Sci 24:257–264

Wan BYC (1976) Effects of dibutyryl cyclic AMP and phosphodiesterase inhibitors on acid secretion by mouse stomach in vitro. Br J Pharmacol 56:357–358p
Ward JT, Adesola AO, Welbourn RB (1964) The parathyroids, calcium, and gastric acid secretion in man and the dog. Gut 5:173–183
Watanabe K, Watanabe HY, Goto Y, Kariya Y (1977) Measurement of gastric acid secretion in isolated gastric mucosa of the rat: Effects of secretagogues and inhibitors including cyclic adenosine monophosphate related agents and an H_2 receptor antagonist. Chem Pharm Bull (Tokyo) 25:1934–1940
Wattel W, Geuze JJ (1977) Ultrastructural and carbohydrate histochemical studies on the differentiation and renewal of mucosal cells in the rat gastric fundus. Cell Tissue Res 176:445–462
Wiebelhaus VD, Blum AL, Sachs G (1974) Isolation of oxyntic cells. Methods Enzymol 32:707–717
Wolff DJ, Brostrom CO (1979) Properties and functions of the calcium dependent regulator protein. Adv Cyclic Nucleotide Res 11:27–88
Wollin A, Code CF, Dousa TP (1974) Evidence for separate histamine and prostaglandin sensitive adenylate cyclases (AC) in guinea pig gastric mucosa (GM). Clin Res 22:606A
Wollin A, Code CF, Dousa TP (1975a) Interaction of histamine and prostaglandins with adenylate cyclase and cyclic AMP phosphodiesterase from guinea pig gastric mucosa. Clin Res 23:206A
Wollin A, Barnes LD, Hui YS, Dousa TP (1975b) Activation of protein kinase in the guinea pig fundic gastric mucosa by histamine. CURE, preprint No 81
Wollin A, Code CF, Dousa TP (1976) Interaction of prostaglandins and histamine with enzymes of cyclic AMP metabolism from guinea pig gastric mucosa. J Clin Invest 57:1548–1553
Wollin A, Soll AH, Samloff M (1979) Actions of histamine, secretion, and PGE_2 on cyclic AMP production by isolated canine fundic mucosal cells. Am J Physiol 237(5):E437–443
Yellin TO, Buck SH, Gilman DJ, Jones DF, Waidleworth JM (1979) ICI 125, 211: a new gastric antisecretory agent acting on histamine H_2-receptors. Life Sci 25:2001–2009

CHAPTER 32

The Role of Cyclic Nucleotides in the Vasculature

D. H. NAMM

Overview

The role of cyclic AMP and GMP in the vasculature is reviewed with reference to contractile state, adrenergic receptors, occurrence and function in endothelial and smooth muscle cells, vascular disease and cellular sites of action. An attempt has been made to interpret the often conflicting and fragmented reports in order to summarize the present state of knowledge of this field. Evidence is presented supporting the thesis that, in vascular muscle, cyclic AMP is a mediator of β-adrenergic relaxation. The evidence is less complete for the involvement of cyclic AMP with other mediators of vascular muscle relaxation. Cyclic GMP also appears less likely to be a mediator or determinant of adaptive responses of vascular smooth muscle. The occurrence and possible function of cyclic nucleotides in vascular endothelial cells is discussed. The knowledge of hormonal control of this vascular cell type is in its infancy and thus far our understanding of the role of cyclic nucleotides is at a speculative stage. Studies which attempt to correlate cyclic AMP concentration in arterial tissue of hypertensive or arteriosclerotic animals with the altered vascular state of these disease are reviewed. These reports raise the possibility that cyclic nucleotide metabolism may be altered in such disease states. The site and biochemical mechanism(s) of action of cyclic AMP within vascular smooth muscle are discussed, with particular emphasis on the possible action of the nucleotide on calcium ion translocation.

A. Introduction

The state of the art on the role of cyclic nucleotides in vascular function has matured considerably from the time of my last assessment (NAMM and LEADER 1976). The controversy that existed then and the recognition of the need for more comprehensive and controlled studies has stimulated new and substantial solutions to some basic problems. In this report I will emphasize these positive achievements of the past 4–5 years rather than try to provide a catalog of all of the work done to date in this area. For those who desire a chronicle of vascular cyclic nucleotide research from its origins, I refer them to the excellent comprehensive summary of KRAMER and HARDMAN (1980). I have also excluded reviewing those contributions involving specifically the enzymology of the vascular cyclase-phosphodiesterase-protein kinase system. This area has not yet proven to offer knowledge unique to the vascular system or its function and is covered in detail in a general manner in Vol. 58/I on the *Biochemistry of Cyclic Nucleotides*.

B. The Role of Cyclic Nucleotides in Vascular Smooth Muscle Contractility

By the mid-1970's, considerable evidence of a circumstantial nature had been amassed to implicate cyclic AMP as a mediator for vascular relaxation and cyclic GMP for vascular contraction. At that time we cautioned against total acceptance of this Ying-Yang concept since some of the experimental support for it displayed shortcomings which derived, in part, from the strong bias to prove the hypothesis correct. Since that time, a few laboratories have performed more carefully designed studies with standardized techniques. In attempting to correlate contractile state to cyclic nucleotides, these studies have given more attention to factors such as time-course of response and dose-effect relationships which reduce inherent bias and provide reliable data.

The role of cyclic GMP in vascular contraction was addressed in a systematic manner in recent years in the laboratory of DIAMOND (DIAMOND and BLISARD 1976; DIAMOND 1978). This group showed that carbachol, an agent which is known to elevate the cyclic GMP content of a number of non-vascular tissues, was indeed capable of raising the concentration of this nucleotide in canine femoral arteries. However, these arteries did not contract when this biochemical phenomenon occurred. Phenylephrine, on the other hand, contracted these arteries with no change in cyclic GMP levels. Another finding which was inconsistent with a role of cyclic GMP as a mediator of vascular contraction was that nitroglycerin caused a 16-fold elevation of cyclic GMP and a substantial relaxant response in these arteries. It is my opinion that these results, which dissociate the cyclic GMP content of arterial preparations from their contractile state, give sufficient cause for serious doubt of the hypothesis that this nucleotide may be the second messenger of contractile hormones and neurotransmitters in the vasculature. It is interesting that evolving from the above evidence has come the suggestion that cyclic GMP might, instead, mediate vascular relaxation, a concept that would at least explain the relaxing effects of the nitrates on arterial and other muscle. SCHULTZ et al. (1979) have tested this notion for the vasculature and have shown that, indeed, cyclic GMP analogs relax isolated arterial strips at fairly low concentrations. This rather indirect supporting evidence must be tempered by the possibility that the added cyclic GMP may have altered vascular cyclic AMP content (through inhibition of phosphodiesterase) and by the observation of DIAMOND and BLISARD (1976) that carbachol can increase cyclic GMP in a phenylephrine-contracted artery with no reduction in its contractile state. Presently, the evidence would seem to support the hypothesis that cyclic GMP is not a mediator of changes in vascular tone but that its concentration may be modified in the vasculature coincident with alterations in tone, possibly by the known comodulator role of calcium ion in both phenomena (CLYMAN 1978).

The hypothesis that cyclic AMP mediates vascular relaxation has also been seriously tested and challenged in the past 4–5 years. The most strongly supported aspect of this hypothesis remains that the vascular relaxation as a result of β-adrenergic stimulation is mediated by increases in vascular smooth muscle cell cyclic AMP. The association between β-relaxation and cyclic AMP has been documented according to all 4 original Sutherland criteria and has been neither expanded upon nor challenged by any recent work (with perhaps the exception of receptor specificity – see below). Several workers have instead confirmed the close association of the rise in cyclic AMP content to the onset, duration and extent of relaxation of arteries to isoproterenol. What is still lacking is the elucidation of the casual link between cyclic AMP and the relaxation phenomena. While the cyclic AMP-relaxation hypothesis for β-adrenergic mediation has weathered the recent times well, the more general concept that cyclic AMP may underlie most other vascular relaxant responses has been seriously challenged by several experimental results. Adenosine, a potent relaxant of certain vascular beds, has been a likely candidate for mediation by cyclic AMP, as it elevates the content of the nucleotide in nonvascular tissue. KUKOVETZ et al. (1978) have provided extensive evidence that the relaxation of coronary arteries by adenosine is accompanied by increases in that tissue's content of cyclic AMP which occurs as a result of the nucleoside's stimulant action on adenylate cyclase. They found that the extent of the changes in cyclic AMP is consistent with a mediator role in the relaxant response. However, in direct contrast to the above findings, HERLIHY et al. (1976) were unable to show any significant changes in cyclic AMP levels in coronary arteries at relaxant concentrations of adenosine. These divergent results cannot be readily explained and suggest some basic methodological problem which, until resolved, must cause reservation in acceptance of the role of cyclic AMP in the vascular action of adenosine. Similarly, PGI_2, a potent stimulant of platelet adenylate cyclase and a potent vasodilator, was recently shown to cause a diminution of the cyclic AMP content of isolated coronary strips in association with a marked relaxant effect (SCHÖR and RÖSEN 1979). In this same category of inconsistency of the cyclic AMP change with relaxant events is the finding that papaverine has been shown by one lab (DIAMOND 1979) to relax isolated arteries with no change in the tissue content of cyclic AMP, while DEMPSEY-WAELDELE and STOCLET (1977) have demonstrated a small but significant elevation in cyclic AMP during papaverine-induced relaxation. Other vascular relaxant responses which have recently been shown not to be associated with increases in vascular cyclic AMP include those induced by elevations in potassium ion, (NGUYEN-DUONG et al. 1975), hyperosmolarity (LJUNG et al. 1975), and nitroglycerine, (DIAMOND and BLISARD 1976).

These several experiments, which appear to dissociate cyclic nucleotide alteration from vascular contractile changes, fail to support a unifying theory of vascular contractile control through the modification of endogenous cyclic nucleotide levels. Proponents of such a general theory argue that the experimental results that dissociate the two phenomena may be due to an inability to measure the cyclic AMP or cyclic GMP content of the physiologically-active pool or compartment. This is a valid proposal, supported by some data, and must be considered in the current evaluation of the hypothesis. However, I believe it is fair to say that in the last few years the simplistic idea that cyclic nucleotide levels are primary modulators of contractile events in vascular muscle has received more criticism than support. This should be viewed as a positive event since we definitely known more about this area than we did 4 years ago, even if it is only that we were wrong or overly simplistic about many of our ideas.

C. Adrenergic Receptor Modulation of Vascular Cyclic Nucleotides

There is general agreement in the literature that cyclic AMP is elevated in vascular tissue in response to β-adrenergic stimulants. Recent work has shown this to be the case not only in the vascular smooth muscle cell, the predominant cell type of the resistance vessels, but also in the endothelium of the arterial intima and of cerebral capillaries. In broken cell preparation of both cat pial vessels and microvessels, NATHANSON and GLASER (1979) demonstrated that adenylate cyclase was stimulated by isoproterenol, an affect blocked by propranolol and not phentolamine. Similarly, HERBST et al. (1979) have shown that norepinephrine increases cyclic AMP in intact brain microvessels; a phenomenon blocked selectively by β and not α-adrenergic antagonists. In studies on vascular endothelial and in intact arterial preparations SEIDEL et al. (1975) and DIAMOND and BLISARD (1976) have demonstrated that phenylephrine, a predominantly α-agonist is without effect on the cellular cyclic AMP content. These results in several preparations of the two major vascular cell types indicate that the α-adrenergic receptor does not appear to be directly linked to the vascular cyclic AMP system. The receptor mediating the arterial cyclic AMP increase caused by isoproterenol would appear to be distinct from the cardiac β-receptor since the latter but not the former can be blocked by practolol (LOCKWOOD and PHORNCHIRASILP 1977). This observation is consistent with the subclassification of β-receptors based on selective antagonism proposed by LANDS et al. (1967).

D. Cyclic Nucleotides and the Vascular Endothelium

With the advent of techniques to isolate and study the biochemistry of vascular endothelial cells recently, it appears that this cell type has a hormonally-sensitive cyclic nucleotide system. This information has dual importance. It implies that the physiological function of this vascular cell type may be under hormonal or neurotransmitter control through this mediator role of the cyclase system. Also, it raises once more the importance of recognizing the problem of studying cyclic nucleotide changes in intact arterial segments which are heterogenous in cell types. If one is studying vascular contractility and cyclic AMP in an arterial segment it may be important to isolate only the medial layers by removing not only adventitial fibroblast and lipocytes but the intimal endothelium as well. The contribution of the endothelial cell layer to be total cyclic nucleotide content depends very much on the artery under study. Since the arterial intima is comprised of only one cell layer, the thicker arteries are predominantly smooth muscle sources.

As was indicated previously, capillaries from brain vessels contain hormonally-sensitive cyclase activity. Endothelial cells from rabbit aorta isolated and maintained in culture also respond to hormones by changes in cyclic AMP and GMP (BUONASSISI and VENTER 1976). Cyclic GMP and cyclic AMP content of these cultured endothelial cells is increased by norepinephrine, acetylcholine, serotonin and phenylephrine. Histamine and angiotensin II elevate cyclic GMP only. Histamine has also been shown to activate capillary adenylate cyclase (JOO et al. 1975). At this time is not clear what physiological function these cyclic nucleotide responses to hormones may subserve in these cells. In the brain, capillaries may be under direct control by neural elements and thereby have their functions regulated by the effects of norepinephrine, (HERBST et al. 1979). Pinocytosis of macromolecules and their transport across capillary endothelium is increased by dibutyryl cyclic AMP (JOO et al. 1975).

E. Cyclic Nucleotides and Vascular Disease

In 1976, AMER suggested that hypertension was associated with elevated arterial ratios of cyclic GMP to cyclic AMP (see review by NAMM and LEADER 1976). While this association has not been directly challenged experimentally, its relevance to the cause of altered arterial reactivity seems today to be less meaningful. This is due to the dissociation of cyclic GMP from vascular responsiveness, as has been already discussed. More credible is the possibility that the hypertensive defect lies in the vascular cyclic AMP system alone. Diminished vascular cyclic AMP content has been consistently reported in genetically hypertensive rats (RAMANATHAN and SHIBATA 1974; SANDS et al. 1976), although the degree of hypertension has not directly correlated with cyclic AMP content. In addition, it should be cautioned that the cyclic AMP content, in these studies, was expressed in terms of wet weight or total arterial protein of arterial segments. Both of these measures may rise substantially in the hypertensive state with no increase in cellularity, the result being an apparent but not real diminution in cyclic nucleotide content per cell. It has always been my contention that nucleotide levels be expressed on some more meaningful cellular basis, e.g. DNA content. Thus, I still am less than fully convinced that there is a real, physiologically important decrement in arterial smooth muscle cellular cyclic AMP content in experimental hypertension. BHALLA et al. (1978 a) have recently presented evidence which suggests that the effects of cyclic AMP on Ca^{++} sequestration by arterial microsomes are altered in hypertension. They showed, in hypertensive animals, an impaired ability of cyclic AMP to cause phosphorylation of microsomal protein, suggesting a defect in the cyclic AMP-dependent protein kinase. The study of calcium ion movements within the vascular smooth muscle cell and their modification by cyclic AMP is replete with controversy and unresolved technical problems (see below). The question of this site being involved in hypertension should be clarified by overcoming the technical problems.

Recently, there have been several reports of altered cyclic AMP content in arteries from animals on an atherosclerotic diet (high cholesterol). AUGUSTYN and ZIEGLER (1975) reported elevation in cyclic AMP in lesioned areas of arteries from rabbits fed a cholesterol diet. In a similar study, SHIMAMOTO et al. (1976) report a transient increase followed by a profound decrease in arterial cyclic AMP in atherosclerotic rabbits. SINGER and BRODIE (1978) compared cyclic AMP content of aorta and coronary artery from two strains of pigeons with markedly different susceptibility to spontaneous atherosclerosis. They found that the strain resistant to the disease had one-half the cyclic AMP of the susceptible strain. JURUKOVA and BOSHKOV (1977) reported a decrease in both aortic cyclic AMP and adenylate cyclase in rats on an atherogenic diet.

Thus, we have no clear picture of whether cyclic AMP is elevated or reduced in atherosclerotic lesions. It must be remembered that atherosclerosis is a progressive disease, that the nature of the arterial pathology changes considerably with time, and that the extent and type of involvement is different for different vascular beds and in different animal species. In attempts to characterize changes in cyclic nucleotide metabolism in this disease process, more attention needs to be given to the timing of the sampling of the tissue, the morphological nature of the arterial pathology (e.g. cellular proliferation, lipid inclusion, necrosis) and on what basis the content of nucleotide is expressed. Here, content per μg of DNA seems imperative.

F. The Effect of Cyclic AMP on Calcium Ion Movements in Vascular Muscle Cells

One of the most active areas of vascular research concerning the cyclic nucleotides has been the examination of calcium transport and sequestration by subcellular fragments. The generation of new data has considerably amplified the original observations of BAUDOUIN-LEGROS and MEYER (1973) but, as yet, falls short of actually identifying a site of regulation of the vascular contractile response by the cyclic nucleotide. This is undoubtedly partially due to the fact that these studies have preceded or at best paralleled the development of technology to adequately isolate and define subcellular fractions or arterial tissue.

Reports have appeared over the past 4 years which have attempted to answer three questions: (1) Does cyclic AMP or cyclic GMP alter the rate or extent of calcium ion uptake by the sarcoplasmic reticulum of the vascular smooth muscle cell? (2). Is there a cyclic nucleotide-dependent phosphorylation of the membranes of the sarcoplasmic reticulum (SR) and is this phenomenon related to any change in calcium ion transport? (3). Is the protein kinase that catalyzes phosphorylation of the vascular sarcoplasmic reticulum endogenous to this structure or does the cytosolic enzyme mediate the phosphate transfer from ATP to the membrane protein?

ALLEN (1977) and SANDS et al. (1977) were unable to demonstrate any influence of cyclic AMP on calcium uptake by aortic microsomes. In the latter study, no effect could be observed with cyclic AMP even when exogenous protein kinase or phosphorylase kinase was added. FITZPATRICK and SZENTIVANYI (1977) and THORENS and HAEUSLER (1978) likewise were unable to demonstrate an effect of the cyclic nucleotides alone on calcium uptake into fragments of SR from rabbit aorta. However, both groups were able to show that both cyclic AMP and GMP enhanced calcium uptake when an exogenous protein kinase was present. These workers proposed that calcium translocation may be regulated by cyclic nucleotides through their influence on cytosolic protein kinases. BHALLA et al. (1978b) have reported that the addition of cyclic AMP to rat aortic microsomes results in their phosphorylation by stimulation of an endogenous protein kinase and that this is associated with increased calcium ion uptake. Added protein kinase, while further enhancing microsomal phosphorylation by ATP, did not substantially affect the cyclic AMP-augmentation of calcium uptake. Thus, these studies support the concept that the nucleotide regulates a kinase resident in the SR membrane which modulates membrane calcium pumping. These studies suggest, also, that phosphorylation via an external kinase may not be specifically linked to the calcium pump site.

It would seem that we have no consistent answers at this time to the important question raised by the studies done to date. Perhaps the solutions to the question concerning cyclic nucleotides will come only after we have a better understanding of the biochemistry and physiology of the SR system in vascular smooth muscle. There are as yet basic problems associated with criteria for its isolation and purification, the characteristic of calcium binding, and the relevance it might have to the contractility of the smooth muscle cell. Until these problems are resolved, the ambiguous and conflicting results of the effects of cyclic nucleotide on this system have to be viewed with caution.

G. Conclusion

Our current understanding of the role of cyclic nucleotides in the vasculature has been substantially augmented by the work of the past 4–5 years. The more recent reports have confirmed earlier doubts that contractility is primarily determined by cyclic nucleotide levels but has strengthened the notion that cyclic AMP is a mediator of β-adrenergic dilatory responses and therefore may be physiologically important in triggering the vascular responses to circulating epinephrine and β-adrenergic drugs. The presumptive role of cyclic nucleotides in arterial and capillary endothelium is a very exciting development in this area and warrants further work *vis a vis* permeability and pinocytotic functions of this cell type. There exist substantial conflicts and ambiguities in the area of the effects of cyclic nucleotides in intracellular translocation of calcium, and their role, if any, in hypertension and atherosclerosis. Part of these experimental conflicts are undoubtedly due to the difficulty in working with a tissue of heterogeneous cellular type. Also, there is the consistent lack of attention to the quantification of nucleotide content based on cellularity. The rapidity with which this tissue responds to various stimuli to produce new medial smooth muscle cells and elaborate extracellular protein in disease states should be of greater concern to workers in this area and normalization of data to DNA content of arteries should be adopted for all biochemical results.

References

Allen JC (1977) Ca^{++}-binding properties of canine aortic microsomes: lack of effect of cyclic AMP. Blood Vessels 14:91–104

Augustyn JM, Ziegler FD (1975) Endogenous cyclic adenosine monophosphate in tissue of rabbits fed an atherogenic diet. Science 187:449–450

Baudouin-Legros M, Meyer P (1973) Effects of antiotensin, catecholamines and cyclic AMP on calcium storage in aortic microsomes. Br J Pharmacol 47:377–383

Bhalla RC, Webb RC, Singh D, Ashley T, Brock T (1978a) Calcium fluxes, calcium binding and adenosine cyclic 3′,5′-monophosphate-dependent protein kinase activity in the aorta of spontaneously hypertensive and Kyoto Wistar normotensive rats. Mol Pharmacol 14:468–477

Bhalla RC, Clinton Webb R, Singh D, Brock T (1978b) Role of cyclic AMP in rat aortic microsomal phosphorylation and calcium uptake. Am J Physiol 234:H505–H514

Buonassisi V, Venter JC (1976) Hormone and neurotransmitter receptors in an established vascular endothelial cell line. Proc Natl Acad Sci USA 73:1612–1616

Clyman RI (1978) Regulation of cyclic nucleotide metabolism in the human umbilical artery. Prostaglandin Thromboxane Res 4:175–183

Dempsey-Waeldele F, Stoclet J-C (1977) Effects of papaverine on cyclic nucleotide levels in the isolated rat aorta. Eur J Pharmacol 46:63–66

Diamond J (1978) Role of cyclic AMP in control of smooth muscle contraction. Cyclic Nucleotide Res 9:327–340
Diamond J, Blisard KS (1976) Effects of stimulant and relaxant drugs on tension and cyclic nucleotide levels in canine femoral artery. Mol Pharmacol 12:688–692
Fitzpatrick DF, Szentivanyi A (1977) Stimulation of calcium uptake into aortic microsomes by cyclic AMP and cyclic AMP-dependent protein kinase. Arch Pharm (Weinheim) 298:255–275
Herbst TJ, Raichle ME, Ferrendelli JA (1979) β-adrenergic regulation of adenosine 3′,5′-monophosphate concentration in brain microvessels. Science 240:330–332
Herlihy JT, Beckman EL, Berne RM, Rubio R (1976) Adenosine relaxation of isolated vascular smooth muscle. Am J Physiol 230:1239–1243
Joó F, Rakonczay Z, Wollemann M (1975) cAMP-mediated regulation of the permeability in the brain capillaries. Experientia 31:582–584
Jurokova Z, Boshkov B (1977) Cyclic adenosine monophosphate system in experimental atherosclerosis. Prog Biochem Pharmacol 14:268–270
Kramer GL, Hardman JG (1980) Cyclic nucleotides and blood vessel contraction. In: The cardiovascular system II. American Physiological Society, Washington, DC (Handbook of Physiology) ed: Bohr DF, Somlyo AP, and Sparks HV 2:179–204
Kukovetz WR, Poch G, Holzmann S, Wurm A, Rinner I (1978) Role of cyclic nucleotides in adenosine-mediated regulation of coronary blood flow. Cyclic Nucleotide Res 9:397–402
Lands AM, Arnold A, McAuliff JP, Luduena FP, Brown TG (1967) Differentiation of receptor systems activated by sympathomimetic amines. Nature 214:597–598
Ljung B, Isaksson O, Johansson B (1975) Levels of cyclic AMP and electrical events during inhibition of contractile activity in vascular smooth muscle. Acta Physiol Scand 94:154–166
Lockwood R, Phornchirasilp S (1977) Selective block of cardiovascular adenylate cyclase activation in vivo. J Pharm Pharmacol 29:184–186
Namm DH, Leader JP (1976) Occurrence and function of cyclic nucleotides in blood vessels. Blood Vessels 13:24–47
Nathanson JA, Glaser GH (1979) Identification of β-adrenergic-sensitive adenylate cyclase in intracranial blood vessels. Nature 278:567–569
Nguyen-Duong H, Brecht K, Gebert G (1975) Cyclic AMP and the potassium-induced vasodilation. Pfluegers Arch 356:3–8
Ramanathan S, Shibata S (1974) Cyclic AMP blood vessels of spontaneous hypertensive rat. Blood Vessels 11:31–318
Sands H, Sinclair D, Mascali J (1976) Cyclic AMP and protein kinase in the spontaneously hypertensive rat aorta and tissue-culture aortic smooth muscle cells. Blood Vessels 13:361–373
Sands H, Mascali J, Paietta E (1977) Determination of calcium transport and phosphoprotein phosphatase activity in microsomes from respiratory and vascular smooth muscle. Biochim Biophys Acta 500:222–234
Schör K, Rösen P (1979) Prostacyclin (PGI_2) decreases the cyclic AMP level in coronary arteries. Arch Pharm (Weinheim) 306:101–103
Schultz KD, Bohme E, Kreye VA, Schultz G (1979) Relaxation of hormonally stimulated smooth muscle tissue by the 8-bromo derivative of cyclic GMP. Arch Pharm (Weinheim) 306:1–9
Seidel CL, Schnarr RL, Sparks HV (1975) Coronary artery cyclic AMP content during adrenergic receptor stimulation. Am J Physiol 229:265–269
Shimamoto T, Kidaka H, Moriya K, Kobayshi M, Takahashi T, Numano F (1976) Hyperreactive arterial endothelial cells: a clue for the treatment of atherosclerosis. Ann NY Acad 275:266–285
Singer AL, Brodie AF (1978) Cyclic AMP metabolism in pigeon arteries: comparison of atherosclerotic-resistant and -susceptible strains. J Mol Cell Cardiol 10:347–361
Thorens S, Haeusler G (1978) Effects of adenosine 3′:5′-monophosphate and guanosine 3′:5′-monophosphate on calcium uptake and phosphorylation in membrane fractions of vascular smooth muscle. Biochim Biophys Acta 512:415–428

CHAPTER 33

The Role of Cyclic Nucleotides in the Pineal Gland

M. Zatz

Overview

Several features of the biochemistry and physiology of the rat pineal gland make it a useful system for the investigation of the roles of cyclic nucleotides. The gland converts information concerning environmental lighting into variations in the synthesis and secretion of its hormone, melatonin. A number of the anatomical and biochemical elements in this sequence have been identified and can be measured or manipulated separately. The enzyme serotonin N-acetyltransferase (SNAT), plays a critical role in the synthesis of melatonin. The activity of this enzyme is controlled by the neurotransmitter norepinephrine, which is released by the sympathetic nerves innervating the gland. β-Adrenergic stimulation markedly increases the activity of SNAT by a mechanism which normally requires both RNA and protein synthesis. This induction is mediated by activation of adenylate cyclase and, presumably, of protein kinase. There is also a circadian rhythm in hormone synthesis which is reflected in each of the components of the system. This rhythm permits the investigation of variations in β-adrenergic receptors, cyclic AMP levels, adenylate cyclase, phosphodiesterase, protein kinase, and SNAT activity in a physiological context. The regulation of these elements, and of cyclic GMP, in the rat pineal gland, are described.

A. Introduction

The rat pineal gland is a neuroendocrine transducer. Information concerning environmental lighting reaches the gland through its sympathetic innervation and controls a hormonal output, the synthesis and secretion of melatonin. Cyclic nucleotides, particularly cyclic AMP, play a central role in this transduction. A number of the steps between the environmental input and hormonal output can be measured and manipulated independently. This enables us to consider the regulation of and by cyclic nucleotides in their physiologic context.

The rat pineal gland itself is rather small (1 mg wet weight) and lies nestled between the cerebral hemispheres (Wurtman et al. 1968). Its location allows for rapid removal and its small size allows for the use of simple organ culture techniques. Although physically within the cranium, it is functionally outside the blood-brain barrier and accessible to pharmacological agents in vivo (Axelrod 1974). A critical anatomical feature of the rat pineal is its innervation. The rat pineal gland is innervated exclusively by sympathetic nerves originating in the superior cervical ganglia

(Kappers 1960). This allows for the examination of denervated glands after bilateral ganglionectomy and the application of the extensive information available concerning catecholamine neurotransmitters.

I. Synthesis of Melatonin

The pineal gland synthesizes and secretes melatonin. This indoleamine has a number of potent physiological effects. In amphibians, it regulates skin color. In birds, it regulates circadian rhythms (Menaker et al. 1978). In mammals, it mediates the effects of light on reproductive cycles and maturation. Its role in man remains uncertain. However, recent developments in assay techniques have generated an upsurge in the investigation of melatonin, its regulation and effects, in man and other animals (Reppert and Klein 1980). The physiology of melatonin has been reviewed elsewhere (Wurtman and Moskowitz 1977; Reiter 1978; Reppert and Klein 1980).

The elucidation of the structure of melatonin (Lerner et al. 1958) and, shortly afterward, of the enzymes and cofactors involved in its synthesis (Weissbach et al. 1960; Axelrod and Weissbach 1961) initiated the modern era in pineal research. The key intermediate in the synthesis is serotonin (5-hydroxytryptamine), whose concentration is particularly high in the pineal (Giarman and Day 1959). This compound is formed from tryptophan by the successive actions of tryptophan hydroxylase and l-aromatic amino acid decarboxylase (Snyder and Axelrod 1964). In the pineal, serotonin can be N-acetylated by serotonin N-acetyltransferase using acetyl CoA (Weissbach et al. 1960). The N-acetylserotonin that is formed is then O-methylated by hydroxyindole-O-methyltransferase (Axelrod and Weissbach 1961) to form 5-methoxy-N-acetyltryptamine, which is melatonin. The regulation of the enzyme serotonin N-acetyltransferase (SNAT) appears to be the pivotal step in the regulation of melatonin synthesis, and SNAT, in turn, is regulated by cyclic AMP (Klein and Weller 1973).

II. Circadian Rhythms in Pineal Indoleamines

Environmental lighting and the daily light-dark cycle have profound effects on melatonin and its precursors. Under ordinary light-dark cycles, melatonin synthesis is enhanced at night. Each of melatonin's precursors also shows a diurnal cycle. Quay first described the diurnal rhythm in serotonin levels in 1963. Levels of this precursor are high during the day and fall during the night. Subsequently, the rhythms in the levels of N-acetylserotonin (Klein and Weller 1972a) and melatonin (Lynch 1971) were found. Levels of these compounds are low during the day and rise at night.

These diurnal changes are regulated by environmental light. Constant light suppresses the diurnal changes – the indoleamines remain at their daytime levels (Snyder et al. 1965). If the normal lighting schedule is reversed, the rhythm of the pineal gradually shifts and becomes consistent with the new lighting schedule (Snyder et al. 1967). However, the pineal's rhythm is not simply a response to environmental cycles of light and darkness. When rats are kept in continuous darkness, or blinded, the rhythms persist (Snyder et al. 1965). Indoleamine metabolism con-

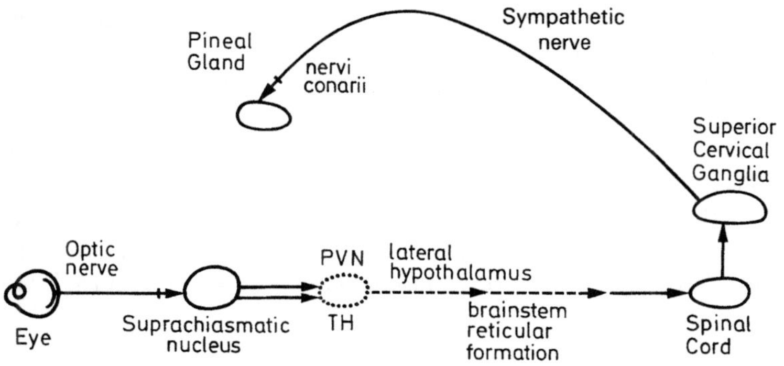

Fig. 1. A schematic diagram of the anatomical pathway regulating the rat pineal gland. *RH*, tract, retinohypothalamic tract; *PVN*, periventricular nucleus; *TH*, tuberal hypothalamic area

tinues to rise and fall as it does in a light-dark cycle, but with a period slightly longer than 24 h. Thus, the circadian rhythms in the pineal are generated by an endogenous oscillator but are regulated by an inhibitory effect of environmental lighting.

In mammals, information concerning environmental lighting must come through the eyes. In contrast, the pineals of amphibians and birds are directly photosensitive (MENAKER et al. 1978). The anatomical pathway involved in light's effects on the rat pineal follows a circuitous neuronal route that passes through the hypothalamus and spinal cord (MOORE and KLEIN 1974) (Fig. 1). Visual information is carried by a special pathway to the suprachiasmatic nucleus of the hypothalamus (MOORE and EICHLER 1976). It may be that the oscillator which generates circadian rhythmicity resides in the suprachiasmatic nucleus (RUSAK and ZUCKER 1979). Lesions in the nucleus abolish all circadian rhythms, not just that of pineal function. In the rat pineal, indoleamine metabolism after such lesions remains at its daytime level.

III. Neuroendocrine Transduction

The sympathetic nerves from the superior cervical ganglia provide the final pathway by which the circadian oscillator drives the rat pineal gland. In the rat, these nerves are the pineal's sole source of innervation (KAPPERS 1960). Denervation of the gland by bilateral ganglionectomy (SNYDER et al. 1965) or decentralization, by cutting the preganglionic fibers from the spinal cord to the ganglia (SNYDER and AXELROD 1965), abolishes the gland's circadian rhythms. Thus, the circadian rhythms in pineal metabolism are driven by a cyclical variation in the rate of sympathetic stimulation. There is an increased firing of these nerves in darkness (TAYLOR and WILSON 1970) and an increased turnover of neurotransmitter in the gland at night (BROWNSTEIN and AXELROD 1974). Artificial stimulation of the sympathetic nerves mimics the nocturnal changes in the gland (VOLKMAN and HELLER 1971). Continuous exposure to light abolishes the diurnal rhythms (as do denervation and decentralization) by reducing the adrenergic stimulation of the gland.

The neurotransmitter norepinephrine mediates the effects of sympathetic stimulation on the rat pineal. The sympathetic nerve endings in the gland contain and release norepinephrine. Addition of norepinephrine caused a marked increase in the formation of melatonin by rat pineal glands in organ culture (AXELROD et al. 1969). This effect was prevented by propranolol, a β-adrenergic blocking agent, but not by α-adrenergic blocking agents (WURTMAN et al. 1971). Injection of isoproterenol, a β-adrenergic agonist, in vivo, produced a fall in serotonin levels and a rise in levels of N-acetylserotonin (BROWNSTEIN et al. 1973a, b). These findings indicated that the nocturnal increase in pineal indoleamine metabolism is caused by the stimulation of β-adrenergic receptors by the sympathetic neurotransmitter norepinephrine. The key to the cycle in indoleamine levels is the diurnal variation in β-adrenergic stimulation.

B. Induction of Serotonin N-Acetyltransferase (SNAT) Activity by Beta-Adrenergic Stimulation

Which step in the biosynthetic pathway is regulated by the β-adrenergic receptor? Addition of norepinephrine to pineals in culture caused a sharp increase in the activity of serotonin N-acetyltransferase (SNAT), while there was only a small increase in hydroxyindole-O-methyltransferase activity (KLEIN and BERG 1970). In the intact animal, there is a marked elevation (about 50-fold) in the activity of SNAT during the night (KLEIN and WELLER 1970) and only a small (about 2-fold) increase in hydroxyindole-O-methyltransferase activity (AXELROD et al. 1965). This physiologic elevation in SNAT can be prevented by prior treatment with reserpine (which depletes the nerve endings of neurotransmitter), or by propranolol (which blocks the β-adrenergic receptors) (DEGUCHI and AXELROD 1972b). Injection of isoproterenol during the daytime stimulates the β-adrenergic receptors and markedly increases SNAT activity in vivo (DEGUCHI and AXELROD 1972a). Propranolol can block the effect of isoproterenol. Both the nocturnal rise in SNAT activity and the rise in SNAT activity caused by isoproterenol are followed by a fall in the concentrations of serotonin, the enzyme's substrate, and an increase in N-acetylserotonin, the enzyme's product (BROWNSTEIN et al. 1973a, b). The rhythm in SNAT activity persists in continuous darkness and is abolished by light or superior cervical ganglionectomy (KLEIN et al. 1971). These findings clearly indicated that the regulation of SNAT activity is the pivotal component in the pineal's circadian rhythms and in their control by the β-adrenergic receptor (KLEIN and WELLER 1973).

The increase of SNAT activity following β-adrenergic stimulation appears to be due to induction of the enzyme. Enzyme activity after pharmacological stimulation shows a lag of about an hour before it starts to rise. There is a similar lag between lights out and the nocturnal increase in activity. Inhibition of protein synthesis by cycloheximide blocks the nocturnal rise or the increase caused by isoproterenol in vivo or in vitro. Actinomycin D can also block the increase in activity, as will be described below.

Detailed studies of the regulation of SNAT activity and of its induction have been hampered by the lability of the enzyme. It is therefore uncertain as to whether the protein synthesis required is that of the holoenzyme or of an activator. Active enzyme has not yet been purified because the activity is rapidly lost in cell free systems. The enzyme can be stabilized, however by its substrate acetyl CoA, or by certain other sulfhydryl containing compounds, which permits it to be assayed conveniently in pineal homogenates (BINKLEY et al. 1976). Inactivation seems to depend upon disulfide exchange and may be reversed by treatment with dithiothreitol. D.C. KLEIN and his co-workers (personal communication) have been using this property to try to stabilize and purify the enzyme by affinity chromatography.

I. Roles of Cyclic AMP

Cyclic AMP mediates the effects of β-adrenergic stimulation on SNAT activity in the rat pineal gland. Although an increase in cyclic AMP levels preceding the nocturnal rise in SNAT activity has not yet been demonstrated (ROMERO et al. 1975b), there is a rapid increase in pineal cyclic AMP after stimulation by β-adrenergic agonists in vivo (DEGUCHI 1973) or in vitro (STRADA et al. 1972). Both the elevation in cyclic AMP levels and in SNAT activity are blocked by propranolol. Theophylline, which inhibits the destruction of cyclic AMP, potentiates the elevation in cyclic AMP levels and in SNAT activity caused by norepinephrine (STRADA et al. 1972). Cholera toxin (MINNEMAN and IVERSEN 1976a) which irreversibly activates adenylate cyclase, and dibutyryl cyclic AMP (KLEIN et al. 1970; DEGUCHI and AXELROD 1973b), which mimics cyclic AMP, are also quite effective in inducing SNAT activity in vitro.

The presence of catecholamine-stimulated adenylate cyclase activity in pineal homogenates was demonstrated even before the β-adrenergic stimulation of SNAT activity had been recognized (WEISS and COSTA 1967, 1968a). Comparison of the effects of various sympathomimetic agonists and antagonists showed that the adenylate cyclase is coupled to a β-adrenergic receptor. Other hormones, which act on adenylate cyclase in other tissues, are not effective in the rat pineal. The presence of phosphodiesterases in pineal homogenates was also demonstrated (WEISS and COSTA 1968b). Thus, all of the Sutherland criteria for determining whether cyclic AMP mediates the effect of a hormone have been met for the β-adrenergic stimulation of SNAT activity in the rat pineal.

Experiments assessing the effects of β-adrenergic stimulation and cyclic AMP on SNAT activity under various conditions suggest three roles for cyclic AMP (Fig. 2). The first action of cyclic AMP is to maintain SNAT in an active form. At night, when SNAT activity is high, injection of cycloheximide causes a "slow" decline in SNAT activity ($t_{1/2} \sim$h). This presumably reflects proteolytic degradation of the enzyme. In contrast, exposure of rats to light during the night causes a precipitous fall in SNAT activity ($t_{1/2} < 5$ min) (KLEIN AND WELLER 1972b; DEGUCHI and AXELROD 1972b). Injection of isoproterenol before the rats were exposed to light prevented the fall in enzyme activity. Pharmacologically, injection of propranolol during the night has a similar effect to that of light. In vitro, propranolol can rapidly reduce SNAT activity in pineal cells which have been preincubated in isoproterenol (PARFITT et al. 1976). Levels of cyclic AMP fall just before the fall in SNAT activity in such experiments (KLEIN et al. 1978). Addition of dibutyryl cyclic AMP shortly before propranolol can prevent this effect. Thus, some level of continued β-adrenergic stimulation (or cyclic AMP) is required to maintain the SNAT in an active form. If stimulation is reduced below this level, there is a rapid

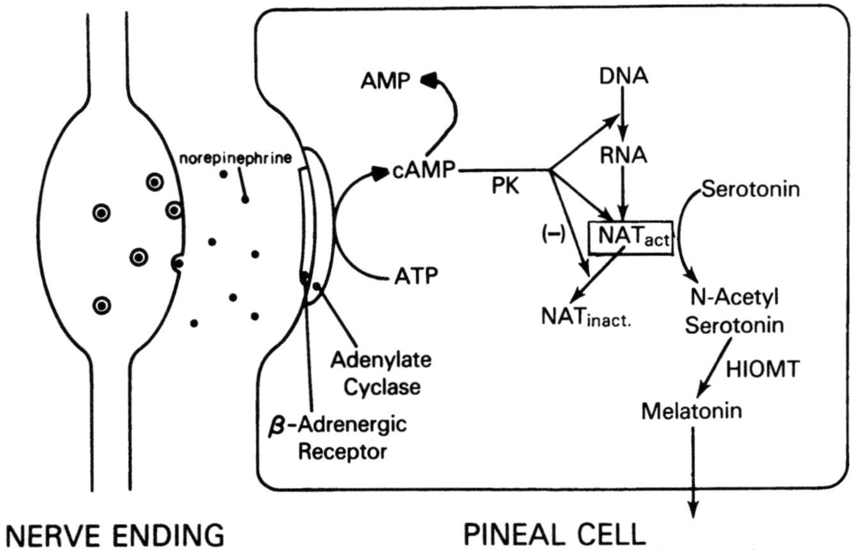

Fig. 2. A schematic diagram of the biochemical pathway regulating the synthesis of melatonin. *PK*, cyclic AMP-dependent protein kinase; NAT_{act}, active serotonin N-acetyltransferase; NAT_{inact}, inactive serotonin N-acetyltransferase; *HIOMT*, hydroxyindole-O-methyltransferase

fall in SNAT activity, perhaps due to disagregation or inactivation of the enzyme. There is some evidence that such inactivation may involve disulfide exchange (D. C. Klein, personal communication). Whatever its mechanism, this inactivation appears to be irreversible. Although SNAT activity can be rapidly reinduced in pineals from animals exposed briefly to light at night, reinduction requires de novo protein synthesis (Romero et al. 1975 a).

The second and third components of cyclic AMP's actions on SNAT are concerned with protein synthesis. Apparently, the stimulation of both transcription and translation are required for the nocturnal induction of SNAT activity. Both actinomycin D (Romero et al. 1975 a) and cycloheximide (Deguchi and Axelrod 1972 b) block the nocturnal increase in SNAT activity or the induction of the enzyme caused by injection of isoproterenol during the day. The requirement for RNA synthesis is related to the lag seen before SNAT activity begins to rise after β-adrenergic stimulation (Romero and Axelrod 1975). In cultured glands taken from animals at the end of the day, actinomycin D blocks the induction of SNAT by isoproterenol. This occurs if the transcription blocker is added before or during the lag period, but not if it is added after the lag period (Zatz et al. 1976 b). However, in glands taken at midnight, from animals whose nocturnal enzyme activity was reduced by exposure to light, reinduction caused by isoproterenol showed virtually no lag period and no inhibition by actinomycin D (Table 1) (Romero et al. 1975 a). Thus, the lag period reflects a period of RNA synthesis, presumably of messenger RNA. In the reinduction at midnight, a full complement of RNA, synthesized during the initial nocturnal induction, remains available for translation upon β-adrenergic stimulation. During the latter half of the night the complement of RNA available for the reinduction of SNAT activity falls, so that by morning,

Table 1. Effect of light and actinomycin D on the induction of pineal N-acetyltransferase activity by isoproterenol

Treatment	N-acetyltransferase (pmoles/pineal per 10 min ± SE)	
	Induction after 18 h light	Reinduction at midnight after 20 min light
	At 1 h	
Isoproterenol	100 ± 20	1,380 ± 120
Isoproterenol plus actinomycin D	40 ± 10	1,030 ± 80
	At 3 h	
Isoproterenol	980 ± 100	1,140 ± 160
Isoproterenol plus actinomycin D	150 ± 40	890 ± 140

At midnight, animals that had been exposed to 6 h of darkness were brought into a lighted room and injected with actinomycin D (5 mg/kg, i.p.) or vehicle. Simultaneously, animals exposed to light for 18 h were injected with actinomycin D or vehicle. After 20 min, all animals were injected with (−)-isoproterenol (+)-bitartrate (5 mg/kg, s.c.). Groups were killed 1 and 3 h after isoproterenol injection and their pineal glands assayed for N-acetyltransferase activity. (Adapted from ROMERO et al. 1975a)

and certainly by the next night, transcription is again required to increase SNAT activity. This rise and fall of presumptive messenger RNA parallels that of SNAT activity during the night. The synthesis of this RNA appears to be stimulated by activation of the β-adrenergic receptor, acting via cyclic AMP. Induction of SNAT in response to dibutyryl cyclic AMP shows the same variation in lag (ZATZ et al. 1976a) and in inhibition by actinomycin D (ROMERO et al. 1975a) as it does in response to isoproterenol.

Rat pineal glands with low SNAT activity do not increase their enzyme activity in organ culture without exogenous stimulation. Addition of cycloheximide blocks induction by β-adrenergic stimulation or by dibutyryl cyclic AMP regardless of the history of the glands. This suggests that a translational step is always required for induction of SNAT activity by β-adrenergic stimulation. Thus, cyclic AMP appears to increase SNAT activity by promoting its transcription, translation, and maintenance in an active form.

Despite the requirement for ongoing transcription and translation during the nocturnal or pharmacologically stimulated induction of SNAT activity, a general increase in RNA or protein synthesis caused by β-adrenergic stimulation has not been observed (MORRISSEY and LOVENBERG 1978a, b). Furthermore, although it is parsimonious to speak of the induction of SNAT itself, the peptide involved in the nocturnal increase in SNAT activity has not been characterized.

The only known mechanism for the action of cyclic AMP in eukaryotic cells is through the activation of protein kinase. The pineal gland is rich in cyclic AMP-dependent kinase (FONTANA and LOVENBERG 1971). If protein kinase is involved in the induction of SNAT, its activity should be increased by exposure of intact cells to agents which induce SNAT. This was demonstrated for isoproterenol (ZATZ and O'DEA 1976) and cholera toxin (ZATZ 1977). In addition, it has been shown that incubation of glands with isoproterenol promotes the phosphorylation of a specific nuclear protein with a molecular weight of about 34,000 (WINTERS et al. 1977). The increased phosphorylation occurred mainly during the early, actinomycin D-sensitive, phase of induction when the necessary RNA would be synthesized. These data are consistent with a role for cyclic AMP-dependent protein kinase in the induction of SNAT activity. However, evidence for critical intermediate steps, such as the translocation of the kinase, has not been obtained (see JOHNSON, Vol. 1).

Current understanding of the steps that lead to the nocturnal increase in melatonin synthesis are summarized in Fig. 2. The entire sequence is initiated by an increased rate of neurotransmitter release from the sympathetic nerve endings. Norepinephrine interacts with the β-adrenergic receptor, stimulating adenylate cyclase and increasing the production of cyclic AMP. Cyclic AMP, in turn, induces an increase in SNAT activity, perhaps through activation of protein kinase. The increased SNAT activity ultimately results in increased production and secretion of melatonin. In the intact animal, light reduces the release of norepinephrine from the sympathetic nerve endings and "turns off" the gland.

II. Regulation of Sensitivity to Stimulation

The rat pineal gland is driven by the cycles of β-adrenergic stimulation that impinge upon it. Left to itself, the gland remains quiescent. When stimulated, by its nerve or by pharmacologic agonists, the pineal always responds with the induction of SNAT activity. However, the characteristics and magnitude of the response vary depending on the history of the gland. In general, the responsiveness of the gland is an inverse function of the extent and duration of its previous exposure to agonists. A period of increased stimulation leads to a decreased response to subsequent stimulation. Conversely, a period of decreased stimulation leads to increased sensitivity. Since the gland undergoes alternate periods of stimulation and quiescence in vivo, and these can be modified by environmental lighting, the rat pineal provides a physiologic model for the regulation of sensitivity.

Glands taken from rats after a period of light exposure are more sensitive to isoproterenol than are glands taken from animals at the end of their dark period (ROMERO and AXELROD 1974, 1975). There is an increased potency of isoproterenol and an increase in the maximum SNAT activity attained, in the supersensitive glands (Fig. 3). Other procedures which increase or diminish the stimulation of the gland also produce appropriate changes in sensitivity to subsequent stimulation. Exposure to isoproterenol itself reduces the response to subsequent administration of isoproterenol (DEGUCHI and AXELROD 1973a; ROMERO and AXELROD 1975). Reduction of stimulation by denervation, reserpine, or 6-hydroxydopamine increases the response to subsequent exogenous stimulation (DEGUCHI and AXELROD 1973a, b; STRADA and WEISS 1974).

The basis of the changes in responsiveness of the pineal gland to β-adrenergic stimulation may reside in mechanisms regulating any of the components or steps involved in the induction of SNAT. As it happens, there appear to be multiple sites involved in the regulation of the pineal's responsiveness. Each of the elements involved in cyclic AMP metabolism, viz. the β-adrenergic receptors, adenylate cyclase, phosphodiesterase, and cyclic AMP-dependent protein kinase, changes as a consequence of enhanced or diminished stimulation and contributes to the overall regulation of the gland's sensitivity.

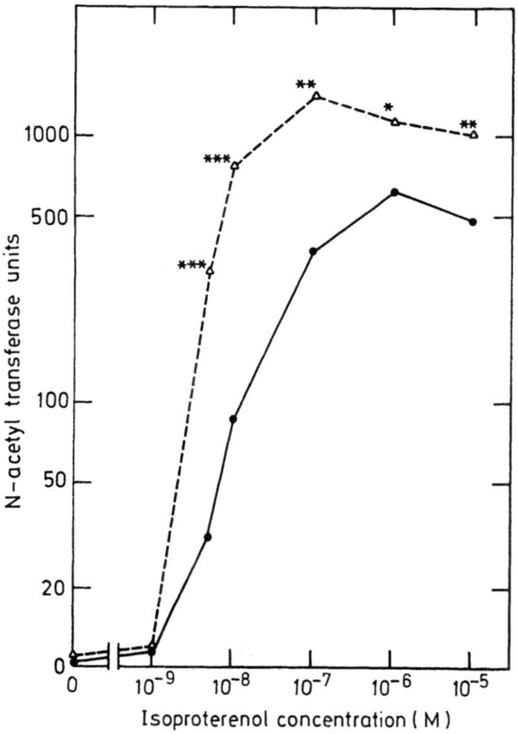

Fig. 3. Diurnal change in sensitivity of rat pineal N-acetyltransferase to induction by L-isoproterenol in organ culture. Pineals obtained from animals killed at the end of the light period (△) or at the end of the dark period (●) were incubated in the presence of various concentrations of L-isoproterenol for 10 h. Glands were homogenized and assayed for N-acetyltransferase; units are pmol/gland per 10 min. Note ordinate is shown in log scale. (Adapted from ROMERO and AXELROD 1974)

1. Accumulation of Cyclic AMP

The accumulation of cyclic AMP within the pineal has been used as an indicator of the gland's initial response to β-adrenergic stimulation. Pharmacologic stimulation quickly increases cyclic AMP levels in vivo (DEGUCHI 1973; DEGUCHI and AXELROD 1973 a; STRADA and WEISS 1974). However, the magnitude of the acute increase is much lower in the pineals of animals injected in the morning than in the pineals of animals injected at the end of the day (ROMERO and AXELROD 1975; ROMERO et al. 1975 b) (Fig. 4). This is because of the sympathetic stimulation of the pineal which occurs physiologically during the night but not during the day. Pharmacologic stimulation also reduces the acute response to subsequent stimulation. Two hours after injection of isoproterenol, the acute response of cyclic AMP levels to a second dose of agonist is diminished 85% in comparison with the response in untreated animals (OLESHANSKY and NEFF 1975a). Conversely, reduction of sympathetic stimulation following denervation (bilateral superior cervical ganglionectomy) (STRADA and WEISS 1974) or depletion of neurotransmitter (reserpine treatment) (DEGUCHI and AXELROD 1973 a) caused a doubling in the acute response of cyclic AMP to β-adrenergic stimulation. The physiologic responses of the pineal

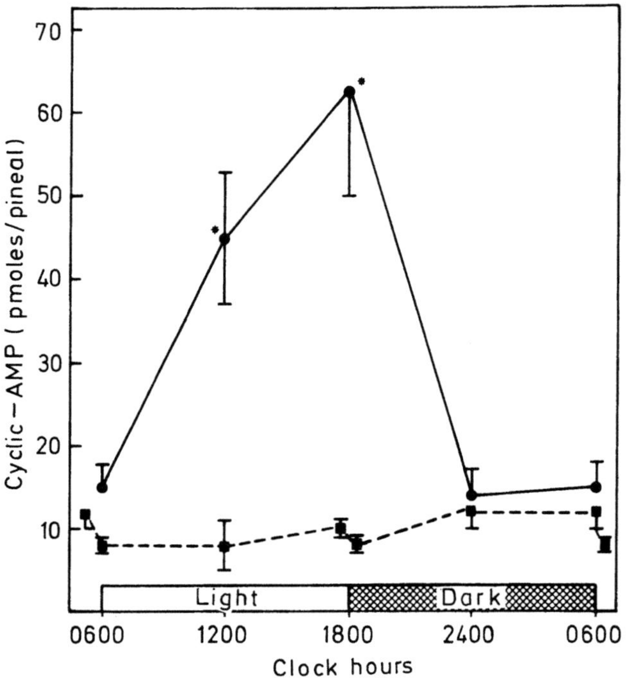

Fig. 4. Diurnal variation in the accumulation of cyclic AMP after isoproterenol administration in the rat pineal gland. At the various times indicated, rats were injected with saline (■) or L-isoproterenol-bitartrate (●) (5 mg/kg) and pineal cyclic AMP levels were measured 10 min later. (Adapted from ROMERO et al. 1975b)

are preserved when the gland is explanted into organ culture (STRADA et al. 1972). Decreased or increased stimulation of the gland *prior to culture* causes an increase or decrease in the acute response of cyclic AMP to pharmacologic stimulation in culture. Enhanced responses occur following periods of diminished stimulation caused by denervation, reserpine, or exposure to light (DEGUCHI and AXELROD 1973a; STRADA and WEISS 1974; KEBABIAN et al. 1975).

For the most part, changes in the capacity of the pineal to accumulate cyclic AMP correlate with changes in the gland's ability to induce SNAT activity. One exception is that the pineal appears maximally subsensitive with respect to cyclic AMP accumulation in the middle of the night (ROMERO et al. 1975b). This is also the time of highest phosphodiesterase activity (MINNEMAN and IVERSEN 1976b). However, under these conditions, the reinduction of SNAT activity (by isoproterenol after brief exposure of the animals to light) is not subsensitive (J. A. ROMERO and M. ZATZ, unpublished work). This may be related to the gland's unique resistance to inhibition by actinomycin D under these conditions. At midnight, the reduced accumulation of cyclic AMP may be sufficient to stimulate the translation which is required. Since transcription as well as translation is required under all other conditions the diurnal changes in sensitivity observed may reflect the regulation of the transcriptional steps which are usually required for an increase in SNAT activity.

a) Receptor and Adenylate Cyclase

The first step in the action of catecholamines on the pinealocytes is the binding of agonist to the β-adrenergic receptors. In order to assess the role of the β-adrenergic binding sites in the regulation of sensitivity, the characteristics of binding of ^{3}H-dihydroalprenolol to pineal membranes were investigated (ZATZ et al. 1976a). ^{3}H-Dihydroalprenolol is a potent β-adrenergic receptor antagonist labelled to high specific activity. It was introduced for the study of β-adrenergic binding sites by LEFKOWITZ et al. (1974). Specific binding of ^{3}H-dihydroalprenolol to pineal membranes was rapid, reversible, and saturable. It displayed a high affinity for the ligand and a finite, low concentration of binding sites. Assessment of specific binding in the presence of various concentrations of nonradioactive agonists or antagonists generated competition curves which reflected the potency of these agents in binding to the β-adrenergic receptors (ZATZ et al. 1976a). Such experiments demonstrated that the binding sites were stereospecific and that the order of potency for various agonists was that which would be expected if the binding sites reflected the physiologic β-adrenergic receptors. Since incubations were performed in crude homogenates, the effects of GTP were not explored.

The adenylate cyclase activity in pineal homogenates provided a tool with which to assess the binding sites. The coupling of the β-adrenergic receptors to adenylate cyclase is maintained in homogenates of rat pineal (WEISS and COSTA 1968a). The affinity constants determined from the effects of various concentrations of agonists on the adenylate cyclase corresponded closely to the affinity constants determined from competition curves using ^{3}H-dihydroalprenolol binding (ZATZ et al. 1976a). Thus, the specific binding sites for ^{3}H-dihydroprenolol reflected the binding sites regulating adenylate cyclase activity in the rat pineal.

In comparing the properties of the β-adrenergic receptor in supersensitive and subsensitive glands (KEBABIAN et al. 1975), more β-adrenergic binding sites were found in the homogenates of supersensitive glands. Glands taken from animals exposed to light for 24 h had about 70% more binding sites than did glands taken from animals at the end of their 12 h dark period (Fig. 5). These binding sites showed a diurnal cycle in their number, increasing with the rats' exposure to light and decreasing with their exposure to darkness (ROMERO et al. 1975b). There was also a light-dark difference in the adenylate cyclase activity (KEBABIAN et al. 1975). Supersensitive glands contained more basal and hormone-sensitive adenylate cyclase activity (Fig. 5). A similar increase in adenylate cyclase activity had previously been shown in homogenates of denervated glands (WEISS and COSTA 1967). Injection of isoproterenol mimicked the effect of darkness in reducing the number of receptor binding sites and the activity of catecholamine-sensitive adenylate cyclase (KEBABIAN et al. 1975). These data suggested that the effect of darkness on the β-adrenergic receptor sites and on the adenylate cyclase activity were due to the increased β-adrenergic stimulation of the pinealocytes during the night.

The changes observed in receptor binding sites and in adenylate cyclase activity appeared to be changes in "V_{max}." There were no significant differences in the apparent affinity of agonists or antagonists for the binding sites, nor in the potency of their effects on the adenylate cyclase, between supersensitive and subsensitive glands. Thus, the changes in the potency of isoproterenol in inducing SNAT activity, which are observed with changes in sensitivity, were not accounted for.

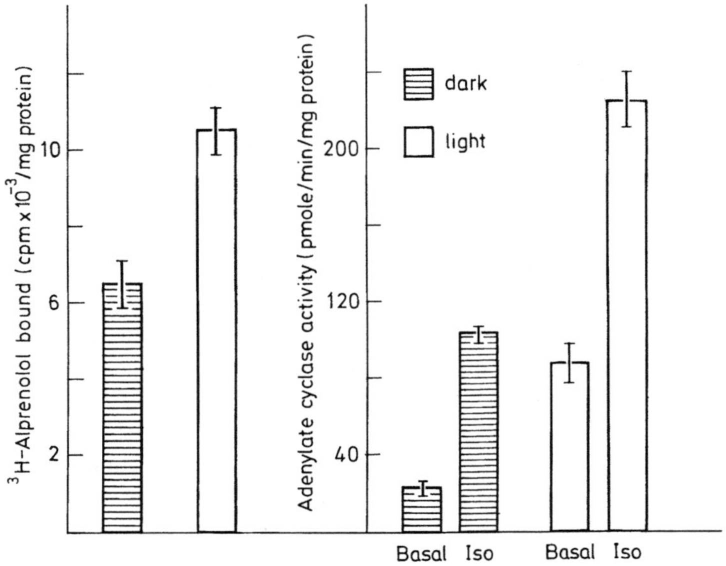

Fig. 5. Effect of environmental lighting on specific binding of ^{3}H-dihydroalprenolol and on adenylate cyclase activity. Specific binding of ^{3}H-dihydroalprenolol, using concentrations that provided near-maximal binding, was determined in homogenates of glands taken from animals exposed to continuous light for 24 h or from animals exposed to their usual 12 h darkness. Basal and isoproterenol stimulated adenylate cyclase activity were also determined in such homogenates. (Adapted from KEBABIAN et al. 1975)

Nonetheless, the correlations observed suggested that the β-adrenergic binding sites participate in the regulation of pineal sensitivity. Increased adrenergic stimulation, caused by the nocturnal release of norepinephrine or by the experimental injection of isoproterenol, reduces the number of β-adrenergic binding sites and causes subsensitivity. The reduced number of binding sites in subsensitive glands may limit the response of adenylate cyclase and ultimately the extent of SNAT induction.

An interesting recent investigation of β-adrenergic receptors in aged rats (GREENBERG and WEISS 1978) showed that old animals had fewer available β-adrenergic receptors in their brains and pineal glands. This appeared to be due to a failure to "resensitize." The pineal receptors did not increase with exposure to light as did those of younger animals. These data suggested a defect in the regulation of sensitivity in aged animals.

Despite the correlations between the β-adrenergic binding sites and adenylate cyclase activity, the changes observed in the binding sites cannot fully account for the changes in adenylate cyclase activity or the changes in sensitivity. There must be additional changes beyond the binding sites. The pineal can be stimulated and SNAT activity induced by agents that bypass the β-adrenergic receptors. Nevertheless, the gland displays supersensitivity and subsensitivity to these agents.

One such agent is cholera toxin. Cholera toxin activates pineal adenylate cyclase and causes the accumulation of cyclic AMP and the induction of SNAT

Table 2. Effects of cholera toxin on supersensitive and subsensitive rat pineal glands

	SNAT Activity (pmol/10 min/gland)		Cyclic AMP (pmol/gland)		Adenylate Cyclase Activity (pmol/mg protein/min)	
	Control	Toxin	Control	Toxin	Control	Toxin
12 h dark	<20	237±33	16±3	25±4	30±6.5	111± 4
24 h light	<20	572±84	19±2	60±4	45±8	155±12

Pineal glands were removed from rats which had been exposed to darkness for 12 h or to light for 24 h. They were preincubated in Krebs-Ringer-glucose (control) or in Krebs-Ringer-glucose containing 50–100 μg/ml cholera toxin (toxin) for 15 min. Glands were transferred to enriched media and incubated further. Serotonin N-acetyltransferase (SNAT) activity was assayed in groups of 12 individual glands after 8 h. Cyclic AMP accumulation and adenylate cyclase activity ("basal") were assayed, in groups of 4 homogenates, after 2 h (Adapted from ZATZ 1977)

(MINNEMAN and IVERSEN 1976a). Although it does not interact with the β-adrenergic receptors, denervated pineals and glands taken from animals exposed to light for 24 h are as supersensitive to the action of cholera toxin as they are to the action of isoproterenol (ZATZ 1977). Supersensitivity and subsensitivity were observed with respect to the induction of SNAT, the accumulation of cyclic AMP, and the activation of adenylate cyclase (Table 2).

Another agent which activates adenylate cyclase by a mechanism which bypasses the β-adrenergic receptor is the fluoride ion. Homogenates of pineals from light-exposed animals showed greater fluoride-stimulated adenylate cyclase activity than did homogenates of glands taken from animals at the end of the night (ZATZ 1977). A similar increase had been shown previously in denervated glands (WEISS and COSTA 1967). These data indicate that there must be changes in the adenylate cyclase as well as in the β-adrenergic binding sites with changes in sensitivity.

b) Phosphodiesterase

The extent of cyclic AMP accumulation is regulated by the rate of its degradation as well as by the rate of its synthesis. Phosphodiesterase activity increases after stimulation by isoproterenol (OLESHANSKY and NEFF 1975b) or cholera toxin (MINNEMAN and IVERSEN 1976a). These changes seem to be mediated by cyclic AMP and require ongoing protein synthesis. A more rapid destruction of cyclic AMP would reduce the tissue level of cyclic AMP achieved after stimulation. Thus, changes in phosphodiesterase also contribute to the regulation of sensitivity. There is also a diurnal cycle in phosphodiesterase activity, which is high at midnight and low at midday (MINNEMAN and IVERSEN 1976b). However, this diurnal cycle does not match the diurnal cycle in the sensitivity of SNAT to induction. Also, denervated pineals did not show the reduction in phosphodiesterase activity (MINNEMAN and IVERSEN 1976b) which would be expected if changes in phosphodiesterase contributed to their supersentivity. Thus, changes in phosphodiesterase activity appear to contribute to some, but not all, forms of sensitivity change.

Table 3. Stimulation of pineal protein kinase activity by exposure of glands to cholera toxin or isoproterenol in organ culture

	Protein Kinase Activity (nmoles ^{32}P incorporated/mg protein/10 min)			
	Experiment 1		Experiment 2	
	Control	Toxin	Control	Isoproterenol
12 h dark	1.3 ± 0.07	1.8 ± 0.1	2.1 ± 0.1	2.6 ± 0.3
24 h light	2.2 ± 0.2	4.6 ± 0.4	3.4 ± 0.1	4.3 ± 0.3

Pineal glands were removed from rats which had been exposed to darkness for 12 h or to light for 24 h. In the experiment with cholera toxin, groups of 5 glands were preincubated for 15 min in the presence or absence of 100 μg/ml cholera toxin and transferred to enriched media. After 2 h, pineal protein kinase activity was assayed in supernatants from individual glands. In the experiment with isoproterenol, groups of 7 glands were placed in organ culture containing 0.1 μ*M* 1-isoproterenol or in control medium. After 20 min incubation, glands were assayed for protein kinase activity. Activities shown are in the absence of added cyclic AMP (Adapted from ZATZ 1977 and ZATZ and O'DEA 1976)

2. Cyclic AMP-Dependent Protein Kinase

The mechanisms which regulate cyclic AMP accumulation, taken together, also cannot fully account for the regulation of the pineal's sensitivity to β-adrenergic stimulation. Dibutyryl cyclic AMP, which mimics the actions of cyclic AMP but is resistant to degradation by phosphodiesterase, is an effective inducer of SNAT activity (KLEIN et al. 1970). This agent bypasses the steps involved in regulating cyclic AMP levels. Yet the pineal gland displays supersensitivity and subsensitivity to its actions (ROMERO and AXELROD 1975). Thus, there is a variation in the effectiveness, as well as in the accumulation, of cyclic AMP which is involved in the regulation of sensitivity.

Evidence consistent with a role for cyclic-AMP dependent protein kinase in the induction of SNAT was summarized above. The greater accumulation of cyclic AMP seen after stimulation of supersensitive glands would be expected to give a greater stimulation of protein kinase activity in supersensitive than in subsensitive glands (Table 3). This was found to be the case (ZATZ and O'DEA 1976). There was a greater increase in "basal" protein kinase activity (without added cyclic AMP) in response to isoproterenol (in vivo or in organ culture), and also to cholera toxin (in organ culture), in the supersensitive glands (Table 3). This kind of difference in protein kinase activity would not be sufficient to implicate protein kinase in the regulation of sensitivity.

There was, however, also a change in cyclic AMP-dependent protein kinase activity which could not be accounted for by the changes in cyclic AMP accumulation. In the presence of maximally effective concentrations of cyclic AMP (added), or after treatment with dibutyryl cyclic AMP, there was more protein kinase activity in the supersensitive than in the subsensitive glands (ZATZ and O'DEA 1976). This difference appeared to be primarily an increased "V_{max}". Both basal and cyclic-AMP stimulated protein kinase activity were increased (Fig. 6). There was no significant change in apparent affinity for ATP, histone, or cyclic AMP. Super-

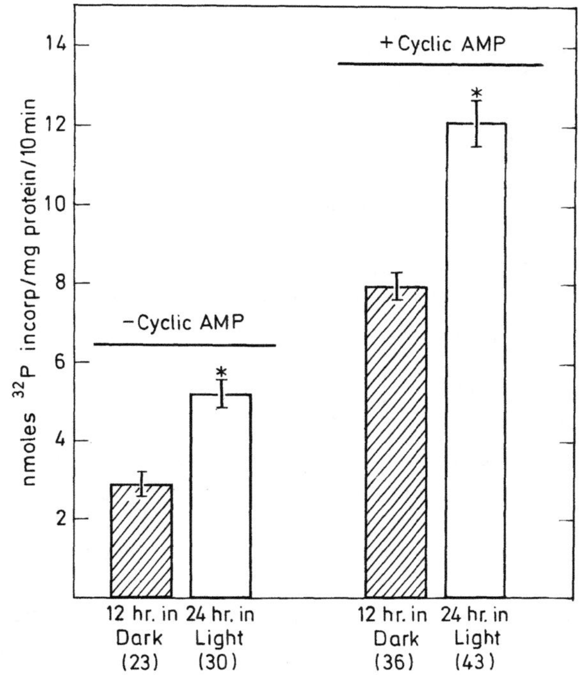

Fig. 6. Effect of light and darkness on pineal protein kinase activity. Pineal supernatants obtained from animals exposed to light for 24 h or from animals killed at the end of their normal 12 h dark period were compared. Protein kinase activity was assayed in the presence and absence of added cyclic AMP. (Adapted from ZATZ and O'DEA 1976)

sensitive glands obtained after treatment of rats with reserpine, or after denervation, also showed a 50–100% increase in soluble cyclic AMP-dependent protein kinase activity. These data may account for the changes in sensitivity to dibutyryl cyclic AMP. Changes in cyclic AMP-dependent protein kinase may modulate the effectiveness of cyclic AMP, making a given concentration of cyclic AMP more effective in the supersensitive glands.

Thus, the overall sensitivity of the rat pineal to β-adrenergic stimulation appears to be regulated at multiple sites. Indeed, each of the steps in the induction of SNAT seems to participate. Supersensitive glands appear to have more β-adrenergic binding sites, more catecholamine-sensitive adenylate cyclase activity, less phosphodiesterase activity, and more cyclic AMP-dependent protein kinase activity than do subsensitive glands.

C. Cyclic GMP

It has been proposed that intracellular cyclic GMP may complement or counteract the effects of cyclic AMP (GOLDBERG and HADDOX 1977). Cyclic GMP might, therefore, be expected to inhibit pineal indoleamine metabolism. Indeed, high concentrations of potassium both inhibit SNAT induction (PARFITT et al. 1975) and increase cyclic GMP levels (O'DEA and ZATZ 1976). However, in the absence of nerve endings, potassium still inhibits induction but does not increase cyclic GMP. Also, although an experiment suggesting inhibition of SNAT by the addition of dibutyryl cyclic GMP has been reported (WILKINSON 1976), we have been unable to demonstrate an effect of exogenous cyclic GMP or its analogues on SNAT induction. Various concentrations of dibutyryl cyclic GMP (or 8-bromo-cyclic GMP) failed to affect enzyme induction by various concentrations of isoproterenol, or dibutyryl cyclic AMP, in either supersensitive or subsensitive glands (R. F. O'DEA and M. ZATZ, unpublished work). Nor was a clear diurnal variation in cyclic GMP levels, or in their response to stimulation, demonstrable.

Nonetheless, cyclic GMP itself is responsive to stimulation of the rat pineal. Exposure of explanted glands to norepinephrine or to depolarizing concentrations of potassium increases cyclic GMP levels (O'DEA and ZATZ 1976). The phosphodiesterase inhibitor, isobutylmethylxanthine, potentiates the effects of stimulation (ZATZ and O'DEA 1977). Cyclic AMP levels are also increased under these conditions. However, the regulation of cyclic AMP and cyclic GMP levels differ. Stimulation of cyclic GMP by norepinephrine is not mediated by the β-adrenergic receptor. Isoproterenol is less effective in increasing cyclic GMP than is norepinephrine. Cyclic GMP response to norepinephrine can be blocked by α-adrenergic antagonists. The exact nature of the "receptor" mediating the increase in cyclic GMP levels remains ambiguous, however. Guanylate cyclase may not be directly coupled to receptors. As in other systems, pineal guanylate cyclase in homogenates is not responsive to hormonal stimulation. The influx of extracellular calcium may provide an intermediate step in the stimulation of guanylate cyclase activity by neurotransmitter or depolarization. In the rat pineal, as in other systems, the increases in cyclic GMP levels caused by potassium or norepinephrine both require extracellular calcium (SCHULTZ et al. 1973).

The requirement for extracellular calcium suggested an association between the stimulation of cyclic GMP and the release of neurotransmitter. Some evidence has been presented implicating cyclic GMP in the α-adrenergic regulation of presynaptic function in the pineal (PELAYO et al. 1977, 1978). Cyclic GMP itself is released by the gland in parallel with the release of norepinephrine. Electrical field stimulation, veratridine, or high concentrations of potassium caused a calcium-dependent efflux of cyclic GMP (ZATZ and WEINSTOCK 1978; O'DEA et al. 1978; ZATZ and O'DEA, 1977). This efflux can be blocked by probenecid, a drug which interferes with the transport of organic acids across membranes (O'DEA, et al., 1978).

All of the agents which can increase pineal cyclic AMP were found to be virtually ineffective in denervated glands. In view of the apparent requirement for intact nerve endings and calcium, the response of cyclic GMP was interpreted as being presynaptic. Nonetheless, the activity of guanylate cyclase (using manganese in cell-free homogenates), was not reduced in denervated glands (STRADA et al. 1976). Recent experiments by KLEIN et al. (1981) have provided the basis for an exciting reinterpretation of these results. KLEIN et al., restored the response of denervated glands in vivo by daily injections of norepinephrine, demonstrating that the response is postsynaptic. They also showed that long-term (7-days) exposure to constant light could mimic the effect of denervation, and that resumption of a daily light-dark cycle could (after 2 weeks) restore the gland's initial responsiveness. Thus, the daily sympathetic stimulation of the rat pineal appears to have a tonic sensitizing effect on the gland in terms of cyclic GMP. The cyclic GMP response is lost over a period of days after denervation as the gland desensitizes. In contrast, the cyclic AMP response is enhanced after denervation, as is well known. KLEIN et al. term the combination of these effects "seesaw signal processing." The regulation of the responsiveness of cyclic AMP and cyclic GMP by previous stimulation differs in the direction, the time course, and the receptor involved. This discovery has intriguing implications for the regulation of cellular responses involving cyclic nucleotides.

References

Axelrod J (1974) The pineal gland: a neurochemical transducer. Science 184:1341–1348

Axelrod J, Weissbach H (1961) Purification and properties of hydroxyindole-O-methyltransferase. J Biol Chem 236:211–213

Axelrod J, Wurtman RJ, Snyder SH (1965) Control of hydroxyindole-O-methyltransferase activity in the rat pineal gland by environmental lighting. J Biol Chem 240:949–954

Axelrod J, Shein HM, Wurtman RL (1969) Stimulation of ^{14}C-melatonin synthesis from ^{14}C-tryptophan by noradrenaline in rat pineal in organ culture. Proc Natl Acad Sci USA 62:544–549

Binkley S, Klein DC, Weller JL (1976) Pineal serotonin N-acetyltransferase activity: protection of stimulated activity by acetyl CoA and related compounds. J Neurochem 26:51–55

Brownstein MJ, Axelrod J (1974) Pineal gland: a 24-h rhythm in norepinephrine turnover. Science 184:163–165

Brownstein MJ, Saavedra JM, Axelrod J (1973a) Control of pineal N-acetylserotonin by a beta-adrenergic receptor. Mol Pharmacol 9:605–611

Brownstein MJ, Holz R, Axelrod J (1973b) The regulation of pineal serotonin by a β-adrenergic receptor. J Pharmacol Exp Ther 186:109–113

Deguchi T (1973) Role of the beta adrenergic receptor in the elevation of adenosine cyclic 3′,5′-monophosphate and induction of serotonin N-acetyltransferase in rat pineal glands. Mol Pharmacol 9:184–190

Deguchi T, Axelrod J (1972a) Induction and superinduction of serotonin N-acetyltransferase by adrenergic drugs and denervation in the rat pineal. Proc Natl Acad Sci USA 69:2208–2211

Deguchi T, Axelrod J (1972b) Control of circadian change of serotonin N-acetyltransferase in pineal organ by the β-adrenergic receptor. Proc Natl Acad Sci USA 69:2547–2550

Deguchi T, Axelrod J (1973a) Supersensitivity and subsensitivity of the β-adrenergic receptor in pineal gland regulated by catecholamine transmitter. Proc Natl Acad Sci USA 70:2411–2414

Deguchi T, Axelrod J (1973b) Superinduction of serotonin N-acetyltransferase and supersensitivity of adenylate cyclase to catecholamine in denervated pineal gland. Mol Pharmacol 9:612–618

Fontana JA, Lovenberg W (1971) A cyclic AMP-dependent protein kinase of the bovine pineal gland. Proc Natl Acad Sci USA 68:2787–2790

Giarman NJ, Day M (1959) Presence of biogenic amines in the bovine pineal body. Biochem Pharmacol 1:235–237

Goldberg ND, Haddox MK (1977) Cyclic GMP metabolism and involvement in biological regulation. Annu Rev Biochem 46:823–896

Greenberg LH, Weiss B (1978) β-Adrenergic receptors in aged rat brain: reduced number and capacity of pineal gland to develop supersensitivity. Science 201:61–63

Johnson EM (1982) Nuclear protein phosphorylation and the regulation of gene expression. In: Nathanson JA, Kebabian JW (eds) Cyclic nucleotides. Springer, Berlin Heidelberg New York (Handbook fo experimental pharmacology, vol 58/I)

Kappers JA (1960) The development, topographical relations and innervation of the epiphysis cerebri in the albino rat. Z Zellforsch Mikrosk Anat 52:163–215

Kebabian JW, Zatz M, Romero JA, Axelrod J (1975) Rapid changes in rat pineal β-adrenergic receptor: alterations in ^{3}H-alprenolol binding and adenylate cyclase. Proc Natl Acad Sci USA 72:3735–3739

Klein DC, Berg GR (1970) Pineal gland: stimulation of melatonin production by norepinephrine involves cyclic AMP-mediated stimulation of N-acetyltransferase. Adv Biochem Psychopharmacol 3:241–263

Klein DC, Weller J (1970) Indole metabolism in the pineal gland: a circadian rhythm in N-acetyltransferase. Science 169:1093–1095

Klein DC, Weller J (1972a) The role of N-acetylserotonin in the regulation of melatonin production (Abstr). Excerpta Med Int Congr Ser 256:52

Klein DC, Weller J (1972b) Rapid light-induced decrease in pineal serotonin N-acetyltransferase activity. Science 177:532–533

Klein DC, Weller J (1973) Adrenergic adenosine 3′,5′-monophosphate regulation of serotonin N-acetyltransferase activity and the temporal relationship of serotonin N-acetyltransferase activity to synthesis of ^{3}H-N-acetylserotonin and ^{3}H-melatonin in cultured rat pineal. J Pharmacol Exp Ther 186:516–527

Klein DC, Berg GR, Weller J (1970) Melatonin synthesis: adenosine 3′,5′-monophosphate and norepinephrine stimulate N-acetyltransferase. Science 168:979–980

Klein DC, Weller JL, Moore RY (1971) Melatonin metabolism: neural regulation of pineal serotonin N-acetyltransferase activity. Proc Natl Acad Sci USA 68:3107–3110

Klein DC, Buda M, Kapoor CL, Krishna G (1978) Pineal serotonin N-acetyltransferase activity: an abrupt decrease in cyclic AMP may be the signal for "turn off". Science 199:309–311

Klein DC, Auerbach DA, Weller JL (1981) Seesaw signal processing in pineal cells: Homologous sensitization of adrenergic stimulation of cyclic GMP accompanies homologous desensitization of β-adrenergic stimulation of cyclic AMP. Proc Natl Acad Sci USA 78:4625–4629

Lefkowitz RJ, Mukherjee C, Coverstone M, Caron MG (1974) Stereospecific ^{3}H-alprenolol binding sites, β-adrenergic receptors, and adenylate cyclase. Biochem Biophys Res Commun 60:703–709

Lerner AB, Case JB, Takahashi Y, Lee TH, Mori W (1958) Isolation of melatonin, the pineal gland factor that lightens melanocytes. J Am Chem Soc 80:2587

Lynch HJ (1971) Diurnal oscillations in pineal melatonin content. Life Sci 10:791–795

Menaker M, Takahashi JS, Eskin A (1978) The physiology of circadian pacemakers. Annu Rev Physiol 40:501–526

Minneman KP, Iversen LL (1976a) Cholera toxin induces pineal enzymes in culture. Science 192:803–805

Minneman KP, Iversen LL (1976b) Diurnal rhythm in rat pineal cyclic nucleotide phosphodiesterase activity. Nature 260:59–61

Moore RY, Eichler VB (1976) Central neural mechanisms in diurnal rhythm regulation and neuroendocrine responses to light. Psychoneuroendocrinology 1:265–279

Moore RY, Klein DC (1974) Visual pathways and central neural control of a circadian rhythm in pineal serotonin N-acetyltransferase activity. Brain Res 71:17–33

Morrissey JJ, Lovenberg W (1978a) Protein synthesis in pineal gland during serotonin N-acetyltransferase induction. Arch Biochem Biophys 191:1–7

Morrissey JJ, Lovenberg W (1978b) Synthesis of RNA in the pineal gland during N-acetyltransferase induction. Biochem Pharmacol 27:551–555

O'Dea RF, Zatz M (1976) Catecholamine-stimulated cyclic GMP accumulation in the rat pineal: Apparent presynaptic site of action. Proc Natl Acad Sci USA 73:3398–3402

O'Dea RF, Gagnon C, Zatz M (1978) Regulation of cyclic GMP in the rat pineal and posterior pituitary glands. J Neurochem 31:733–738

Oleshansky MA, Neff NH (1975a) On the mechanism of tolerance to isoproterenol-induced accumulation of cAMP in rat pineal in vivo. Life Sci 17:1429–1432

Oleshansky MA, Neff NH (1975b) Rat pineal adenosine cyclic 3′,5′-monophosphate phosphodiesterase activity: modulation in vivo by a β-adrenergic receptor. Mol Pharmacol 11:552–557

Parfitt A, Weller JL, Sakai KK, Marks BH, Klein DC (1975) Blockade by ouabain or elevated potassium ion concentration of the adrenergic and adenosine cyclic 3′,5′-monophosphate-induced stimulation of pineal serotonin N-acetyltransferase activity. Mol Pharmacol 11:241–255
Parfitt A, Weller J, Klein DC (1976) β-adrenergic blockers decrease adrenergically stimulated N-acetyltransferase activity in pineal glands in organ culture. Neuropharmacology 15:353–358
Pelayo F, Dubocovich ML, Langer SZ (1977) Regulation of noradrenaline release in the rat pineal through a negative feedback mechanism mediated by presynaptic alpha-adrenoceptors. Eur J Pharmacol 45:317–318
Pelayo F, Dubocovich ML, Langer SZ (1978) Possible role of cyclic nucleotides in regulation of noradrenaline release from rat pineal through presynaptic adrenoceptors. Nature 274:76–78
Quay WB (1963) Circadian rhythm in rat pineal serotonin and its modulation by estrous cycle and photoperiod. Gen Comp Endocrinol 3:473–479
Reiter RJ (ed) (1978) The pineal and reproduction. Prog Reprod Biol 4
Reppert SM, Klein DC (1980) Mammalian pineal gland: basic and clinical aspects. In: Mota M (ed) Endocrine functions of the brain. Raven, New York
Romero JA, Axelrod J (1974) Pineal β-adrenergic receptor: diurnal variation in sensitivity. Science 184:1091–1092
Romero JA, Axelrod J (1975) Regulation of sensitivity to β-adrenergic stimulation in induction of pineal N-acetyltransferase. Proc Natl Acad Sci USA 72:1661–1665
Romero JA, Zatz M, Axelrod J (1975a) β-adrenergic stimulation of pineal N-acetyltransferase: adenosine 3′,5′-cyclic monophosphate stimulates both RNA and protein synthesis. Proc Natl Acad Sci USA 72:2107–2111
Romero JA, Zatz M, Kebabian JW, Axelrod J (1975b) Circadian cycles in binding of ^{3}H-alprenolol to β-adrenergic receptor sites in pineal. Nature 258:435–436
Rusak B, Zucker I (1979) Neural regulation of circadian rhythms. Physiol Rev 59:449–526
Schultz G, Hardman JG, Schultz K, Baird CE, Sutherland EW (1973) The importance of calcium ions for the regulation of guanosine 3′,5′ cyclic monophosphate levels. Proc Natl Acad Sci USA 70:3889–3893
Snyder SH, Axelrod J (1964) A sensitive assay for 5-hydroxytryptophan decarboxylase. Biochem Pharmacol 13:805–806
Snyder SH, Axelrod J (1965) Circadian rhythm in pineal serotonin: effect of monoamine oxidase inhibition and reserpine. Science 149:542–544
Snyder SH, Zweig M, Axelrod J, Fischer JE (1965) Control of the circadian rhythm in serotonin content of the rat pineal gland. Proc Natl Acad Sci USA 53:301–305
Snyder SH, Axelrod J, Zweig M (1967) Circadian rhythm in the serotonin content of the rat pineal gland: regulating factors. J Pharmacol Exp Ther 158:206–213
Strada SJ, Weiss B (1974) Increased response to catecholamines of the cyclic AMP system of rat pineal gland induced by decreased sympathetic activity. Arch Biochem Biophys 160:197–204
Strada S, Klein DC, Weller J, Weiss B (1972) Norepinephrine stimulation of cyclic adenosine monophosphate in cultured pineal glands. Endocrinology 90:1470–1475
Strada SJ, Kirkegaard L, Thompson WJ (1976) Studies of rat pineal gland guanylate cyclase. Neuropharmacology 15:261–266
Taylor AN, Wilson RW (1970) Electrophysiological evidence for the action of light on the pineal gland in the rat. Experientia 26:267–269
Volkman PH, Heller A (1971) Pineal N-acetyltransferase: effect of sympathetic stimulation. Science 173:839–840
Weiss B, Costa E (1967) Adenyl cyclase activity in rat pineal gland: effects of chronic denervation and norepinephrine. Science 156:1750–1752
Weiss B, Costa E (1968a) Selective stimulation of adenyl cyclase activity in rat pineal by pharmacologically active catecholamines. J Pharmacol Exp Ther 161:310–319
Weiss B, Costa E (1968b) Regional and subcellular distribution of adenyl cyclase and 3′,5′-cyclic nucleotide phosphodiesterase in brain and pineal gland. Biochem Pharmacol 17:2107–2116

Weissbach H, Redfield BG, Axelrod J (1960) Biosynthesis of melatonin: enzymic conversion of serotonin to N-acetylserotonin. Biochim Biophys Acta 43:352–353
Wilkinson M (1976) Inhibition of the noradrenergic induction of pineal N-acetyltransferase by dibutyryl cyclic guanosine monophosphate and by ionophore X-537A. Neurosci Lett 2:29–33
Winters KE, Morrissey JJ, Loos PJ, Lovenberg W (1977) Pineal protein phosphorylation during serotonin N-acetyltransferase induction. Proc Natl Acad Sci USA 74:1928–1931
Wurtman RJ, Moskowitz MA (1977) The pineal organ. N Engl J Med 296:1329–1333, 1383–1386
Wurtman RJ, Axelrod J, Kelly D (1968) The pineal. Academic Press, New York London
Wurtman RJ, Shein HM, Larin F (1971) Mediation by β-adrenergic receptors of effect of norepinephrine on pineal synthesis of ^{14}C-serotonin and ^{14}C-melatonin. J Neurochem 18:1683–1687
Zatz M (1977) Effects of cholera toxin on supersensitive and subsensitive rat pineal glands: regulation of sensitivity at multiple sites. Life Sci 21:1267–1276
Zatz M, O'Dea RF (1976) Regulation of protein kinase in rat pineal: increased V_{max} in supersensitive glands. J Cyclic Nucleotide Res 2:427–439
Zatz M, O'Dea RF (1977) Efflux of cyclic nucleotides from rat pineal: release of cyclic GMP from sympathetic nerve endings. Science 197:174–176
Zatz M, Weinstock M (1978) Electric field stimulation releases norepinephrine and cyclic GMP from the rat pineal gland. Life Sci 22:767–772
Zatz M, Kebabian JW, Romero JA, Lefkowitz RJ, Axelrod J (1976a) Pineal β-adrenergic receptor: correlation of binding of ^{3}H-alprenolol with stimulation of adenylate cyclase. J Pharmacol Exp Ther 196:714–722
Zatz M, Romero JA, Axelrod J (1976b) Diurnal variation in requirement for RNA synthesis in the induction of pineal N-acetyltransferase. Biochem Pharmacol 25:903–906

CHAPTER 34

The Role of Cyclic Nucleotides in Epithelium

E. A. DUELL and J. J. VOORHEES

Overview

The skin is composed of two separate compartments, the epidermis which lacks a direct nerve or blood supply and is stratified into four different layers, and the dermis which contains a direct blood supply and is innervated. The basal lamina separates these two components. The epidermal portion of the skin has been utilized in most of the studies discussed in this review. The epidermal cells adjacent to the basal lamina are the only keratinocytes that undergo cell division in normal tissue. The other three layers undergo terminal differentiation.

A defect in the cyclic nucleotide system has been suggested as an important element in proliferative skin diseases such as psoriasis and atopy. Various enzymes involved in cyclic nucleotide metabolism have been investigated in both normal and psoriasis tissues. Most of the data presented concerns the cyclic nucleotide system in normal epidermis.

The receptors that interact with adenylate cyclase have been further investigated. The beta-adrenergic receptor appears to be β_2 in nature based upon the following data: salbutamol increases the levels of cyclic AMP; this increase is blocked by the antagonist butoxamine but not by practolol; isoproterenol is more effective than norepinephrine in increasing the cyclic AMP levels. Binding studies with labeled hydroxybenzylpindolol indicate that most of the binding with adult tissue is non-specific and that the binding to neonatal tissue is specific but the receptor appears to be uncoupled from adenylate cyclase.

Histamine receptor appears to be H_2 in nature since metiamide is effective in blocking the histamine-induced increase in cyclic AMP. Adenosine and adenine nucleotides elevate the levels of cyclic AMP in epidermal slices. The increase is blocked by theophylline but the increase is augmented by non-methyl xanthine phosphodiesterase (PDE) inhibitors. Adenosine also elevates the cyclic AMP levels in cultured epidermal basal cells.

PGE_2 increases the levels of cyclic AMP in the epidermis. The PGE_2 receptor has been implicated as the binding site for tetradecanoyl phorbol acetate (TPA) which induces hyperplasia in the epidermis. Indomethacin prevents TPA from inducing proliferation but this block is reversed by the application of PGE_2. TPA increases the levels of cyclic GMP in the epidermis and may give rise to transitory decreases in cyclic AMP.

Papaverine inhibits both cyclic AMP and cyclic GMP PDE but Ro 20-1724 inhibits only cyclic AMP hydrolysis. The modulator protein is present in the epidermis and increases PDE activity but the amount of modulator protein does not change with alterations in proliferative rate.

The most recent information has been in the data obtained from the cell culture systems. Increases in cyclic AMP in neonatal primary epidermal cultures of mouse or man, whether grown on plastic or 3T3 feeder layers, stimulate proliferation and differentiation of the cells. In contrast, an increase in cyclic AMP appears to inhibit proliferation of adult epidermal cells whether the cells are guinea pig in origin and grown on plastic or mouse, or human origin and grown on collagen gels or human explant cultures. The addition of cyclic AMP (and its derivatives) or compounds that elevate cyclic AMP (e.g. cholera toxin, epinephrine, and adenine nucleotides) to the adult cells in culture appear to inhibit proliferation and in some cases stimulate differentiation at concentrations that stimulate proliferation in the neonatal cultures.

The cyclic nucleotide levels in diseased tissues are still somewhat controversial but other approaches indicate that the altered cyclic nucleotide metabolism plays a role in epidermal proliferation and differentiation as indicated by the observations that compounds that elevate cyclic AMP levels improve the lesions while adrenergic antagonists aggravate the disease or induce proliferation in uninvolved tissues.

A. Introduction

The skin is composed of two separate compartments, the avascular, noninnervated epidermis and the innervated, vascular dermis. The basal lamina separates these two compartments. The epidermis is composed primarily of keratinocytes. The layer of epidermal cells adjacent to the basal lamina is the only population of keratinocytes that undergo cell division in nondiseased states and the cells within this layer are called basal cells. Once the epidermal cells leave the basal lamina area, the cells begin the process of terminal differentiation and form the spinous and granular layers of the epidermis. Keratohyalin granules, the differentiation product of the epidermis, are most prominent in the granular layer. The outermost layer, the stratum corneum, is composed of dead cells that lack normal cell organelles such as the nucleus and mitochondria. These cells provide the barrier function of the skin. The epidermal portion of the skin provides an excellent system for investigating the role of the cyclic nucleotides in the control of proliferation and differentiation (see also FREIDMAN, this volume).

B. Metabolism of Cyclic Nucleotides in Normal Skin

During the early 1970's, adenylate cyclase and the adenosine 3′,5′ cyclic monophosphate (cyclic AMP) system in the skin were investigated in several laboratories (MIER and URSELMANN 1970; MARKS and REBIEN 1972; DUELL et al. 1971; POWELL et al. 1971). VOORHEES and DUELL (1971) suggested that a defect in the cyclic AMP system might occur in proliferative epidermal diseases such as psoriasis. Most of the data obtained to data concerns the epidermal component of the skin (dermis is excluded) but in some instances whole skin has been used and thus makes extrapolation to only the epidermis more difficult.

The status of adenylate cyclase, guanylate cyclase, cyclic nucleotide phosphodiesterases and cyclic AMP-dependent protein kinases in epidermis or intact skin obtained from normal individuals and psoriatic patients were reviewed by VOORHEES et al. (1974a). The information contained in this review concentrates on the more recent data with special emphasis on the use of the primary epidermal cell cultures as models for assessing the effects of the cyclic nucleotides in the epidermis.

I. Adenylate Cyclase and Associated Receptors

A particulate fraction obtained from mouse or rat epidermis was used in early investigations to evaluate the types of receptors that interacted with adenylate cyclase. To reduce the possible loss of stimulation due to membrane disruption, epidermal tissue slices obtained from pig or mouse skin have been used to re-investigate the types of receptors that are present on the cell membrane of the epidermis.

1. Beta-Adrenergic Receptor

The beta adrenergic receptor was the first receptor shown to be present in the epidermis (MARKS and REBIEN 1972, DUELL et al. 1971). In mouse epidermis, the β-receptor appears to be of the β_2 subtype based on the following data: (1) salbutanol (10^{-5} to $10^{-3}M$) increased the levels of cyclic AMP to a maximum of 5-fold after 5 min of incubation. (2) Butoxamine but not practolol prevented this increase. (3) Isoproterenol (10^{-7} to $10^{-5}M$) was more effective than norepinephrine (10^{-5} to $10^{-3}M$) in inducing the increase in cyclic AMP (DUELL 1980a).

Preliminary investigations of the specificity of the binding of [^{125}I]-iodohydroxy-benzylpindolol to membrane fractions from mouse skin indicated a very high level (70%) of background or nonspecific binding in the adult tissue (SOLANKI and MURRAY 1978). Neonatal mouse skin has more specific [^{125}I]-iodohydroxybenzylpindolol binding sites than does adult skin; however, the neonatal skin has a much lower responsiveness to β-adrenergic agonists as measured by changes in the level of cyclic AMP. This indicates that the low responsiveness of neonatal skin to β-adrenergic agonists is not due to a lack of receptors but probably reflects the absence of a completely coupled β-adrenoceptor-adenylate cyclase system.

2. Histamine Receptor

A histamine receptor occurs in the epidermis of the pig. Incubation of pig epidermal slices with histamine (0.2 mM) resulted in a 4-fold increase in the cyclic AMP levels; the K_a for histamine was $6 \times 10^{-5}M$ (IIZUKA et al. 1976b). The receptor appears to be type H_2 since the histamine effect of the increase in cAMP can be blocked by the addition of metiamide to the tissue. Other antihistaminic compounds, particularly acetophanazine and promethazine, are almost as effective. The significance of the histamine receptor in the epidermis is not known since the epidermis would rarely be exposed to these high levels of histamine.

3. Adenosine Receptor

Adenosine or 5′ AMP increase the levels of cyclic AMP in epidermal slices of mouse, pig or human skin (IIZUKA et al. 1976a; DUELL 1980b). The apparent K_a of 0.16 m*M* was obtained for 5′AMP (IIZUKA et al. 1976a). A dose-response relationship was obtained with 5×10^{-4} to $10^{-2}M$ adenosine and increases in the cyclic AMP levels in the epidermis (DUELL 1980b). The increase in cyclic AMP induced by adenosine was blocked by 1 m*M* theophylline and was augmented by the non-methyl xanthine cyclic nucleotide phosphodiesterase inhibitors such as 0.1 m*M* papaverine or 0.05 m*M* Ro 20-1724. The addition of $5 \times 10^{-3}M$ adenosine to a primary culture of neonatal mouse basal cells resulted in a 2-fold increase in cyclic AMP concentrations (DUELL 1980b). The increase in cyclic AMP after the exposure to adenosine or adenine nucleotides and the inhibition of this increase by theophilline indicate that the epidermis probably has an adenosine receptor similar to the receptor found in other tissues.

4. Prostaglandin E_2 Receptor

The levels of prostaglandin E_2 and prostaglandin $F_2{}^{\alpha}$ are altered in psoriasis lesions (HAMMARSTRÖM et al. 1975). The epidermis responds to prostaglandins of the E series with an increase in the cyclic AMP level (VOORHEES et al. 1974a; ASO et al. 1975; ADACHI et al. 1975). The maximal response of the epidermis to prostaglandin is much smaller than that obtained with epinephrine, adenosine or histamine and may indicate that prostaglandins are a less important regulator of cyclic AMP than these other compounds.

The prostaglandin E receptor in the epidermis may be involved in the increase in epidermal cell proliferation caused by the tumor promoter, tetradecanoyl phorbol acetate (TPA). The in vivo treatment of mice with indomethacin (an inhibitor of prostaglandin synthesis) one hour prior to the application of TPA prevented the TPA-induced proliferation (FÜRSTENBERGER and MARKS 1978). Proliferation could be restored by the application of PGE_2 to the indomethacin-treated animals. Cyclic nucleotide levels were not measured in this study; therefore, the involvement of a cyclic AMP system in triggering of the proliferative event can only be inferred.

Controversy does exist as to whether TPA treatment has any effect on the level of cyclic AMP in the epidermis. The initial investigations of GRIMM and MARKS (1974) indicated that an increase in cyclic AMP levels occurred approximately 30 min and 30 h after the single in vivo application of 30 nmoles of TPA. The mice became refractory to the injections of isoproterenol (no increase in the levels of cyclic AMP) within 2 h of application of TPA and required 3 days for recovery. Others have attributed the change in the cyclic AMP levels to ischemic effects produced in the skin that were blocked by the application of TPA (MUFSON et al. 1977; MURRAY et al. 1977). GARTE and BELMAN (1978) and BELMAN et al. (1978) have investigated the single and multiple application of TPA to mice; multiple treatments which are required for the induction of tumors produced a small but consistent decrease in the levels of cyclic AMP and a 5- to 10-fold increase in the cyclic GMP levels in the epidermis (GARTE and BELMAN 1978). A single application of TPA did not effect cyclic AMP levels but did produce a transient increase in cyclic GMP. The possible cause and effect relationship between TPA application, the formation of PGE_1 or PGE_2, the alterations in the levels of cyclic AMP or cyclic GMP, and the induction of tumors or hyperplasia will require considerable additional investigations before a definitive statement can be made.

II. Guanylate Cyclase

MARKS (1973) observed that guanylate cyclase was present in the soluble fraction of the epidermis obtained from mice and that the levels of cyclic GMP could not be altered by a series of hormones. No consistent increases in the cyclic GMP levels could be obtained by C. MARCELO (personal communication) when a variety of compounds known to effect guanylate cyclase (such as derivatives of acetylcholine, nitric oxide and arachidonic acid) were added to epidermal slices in vitro. IIZUKA et al. (1979) reported that a slight increase in cyclic GMP may occur with the addition of 1 m*M* histamine; this is consistent with the original observations of VOORHEES et al. (1974b). In the future, the tissue slice preparation may yield more information concerning guanylate cyclase and its role in epidermal homeostasis.

III. Cyclic Nucleotide Phosphodiesterases

The early detection and characterization of cyclic nucleotide phosphodiesterases (PDE) was reviewed by VOORHEES et al. (1974a). Additional investigations have shown that mouse epidermis contains a modulator protein that is calcium dependent and activiates the PDE from mouse epidermis (MURRAY and ROGERS 1978). The level of modulator protein does not vary with the proliferative rates of the tissue. The effectiveness of several drugs as PDE inhibitors was investigated using human epidermal slices (RUSIN et al. 1978). Papaverine ($5 \times 10^{-4} M$) was very effective in preventing the hydrolysis of either cyclic AMP or cyclic GMP; RO 20-1724 ($5 \times 10^{-4} M$, 4-(3-butoxy-4-methoxy benzyl)-2-imidazolidione) was effective only in preventing the hydrolysis of cyclic AMP.

C. Effects of Cyclic Nucleotides on Cells in Culture

Rapid progress has been made in the last five years in the primary culturing of epidermal basal cells from mouse, guinea pig and man. Several variations in the techniques have been employed which permit an evaluation of the effects of the cyclic nucleotides on epidermis or dermis and the extrapolation of these results to possible in vivo control mechanisms.

I. Growth of Primary Epidermal Cultures on Plastic

1. Adult Guinea Pig Ear

The procedures for obtaining adult guinea pig ear epidermal cell cultures are similar to those of REGNIER et al. (1973). The addition of $10^{-3} M$ dibutyryl cyclic AMP to the cultures for 6 days increased incorporation of amino acids such as histidine, cystine and arginine (amino acids involved in keratohyalin synthesis) into cellular protein and increased the number of multilayered units (as determined by light and electron microscopy) (DELESCLUSE et al. 1976). Staining the cultures with Rodamine B gave further indications that differentiation had been enhanced by the addition of dibutyryl cyclic AMP. Earlier the inhibition of growth had been reported on these same types of cultures following the addition of cyclic AMP or compounds capable of elevating the levels of cyclic AMP, i.e. isoproterenol PGE_2, papaverine and theophylline (DELESCLUSE et al. 1974).

The changes in the cyclic AMP or cyclic GMP levels in these cultures in response to the addition of various prostaglandins have been studies (WILKINSON and ORENBERG 1979). PGD_2 (5 μM) was most effective (a 4-fold increase) in elevating the levels of cyclic AMP while 5 μM $PGF_{2\alpha}$ was most effective in elevating the levels of cyclic GMP after 60 min of incubation. The effects on growth or differentiation were not determined in this study. Thus, in the adult guinea pig ear system, an elevation in the levels of cyclic AMP appear to be associated with an increased degree of differentiation and a decreased rate of proliferation.

2. Neonatal Mouse

FUSENIG and WORST (1975) published a method for obtaining high yields of epidermal basal cells with 85–95% viability and approximately a 50% plating efficiency. The epidermal cultures are essentially free from fibroblasts due to Ficoll density gradient centrifugation. The monolayer cultures of epidermal cells contain cell surface, tissue specific antigens. The cells differentiate and can be maintained in culture for at least 2 weeks.

A similar method reported by MARCELO et al. (1978) yielded epidermal cells with slightly higher plating efficiencies and a longer life in culture. The rate of proliferation was assessed via tritiated thymidine incorporation into DNA; differentiation was assessed by the Kreyberg stain for keratinized cell products. The addition of dibutyryl cyclic AMP (10^{-3} to $10^{-5} M$) to the cultures for 4 days increased the proliferative rate of cells in culture (MARCELO 1979). The addition of 8-bromo cyclic AMP (10^{-3} to $10^{-5} M$) produced a dose- and time-dependent increase in the proliferative rate of the cells. The 8-bromo cyclic AMP ($10^{-3} M$) markedly increased the level of cyclic AMP within the cells. After exposure to cholera toxin (50 pg/ml to 1 μg/ml) for 5 days, a marked stimulation in proliferation occurred. The levels of cyclic AMP were elevated approximately 8- to 10-fold at the time points assayed. Thus the neonatal cultures respond to elevations in cyclic AMP via stimulation of proliferation. In contrast, 8-bromo cyclic GMP (10^{-6} to $10^{-8} M$) had no effect on the proliferative rate of the cultures.

The 8-bromo cyclic AMP addition produced a marked increase in Kreyberg stainable material particularly in the upper layers of the cultures. The addition of 8-bromo cyclic GMP to the cultures produced thickened layers, and dense fibrils occurred in the lower layers. Thus, the addition of 8-bromo cyclic GMP did alter the differentiation of the cultures which appeared somewhat abnormal compared to intact skin.

II. Growth of Primary Epidermal Cultures on Collagen Gels

Adult primary epidermal cell cultures, except for those obtained from guinea pig ear, require collagen gels for growth (KARASEK 1975). Primary cultures of adult human keratinocytes have been obtained by LIU and KARASEK (1978). Collagen coated plastic or glass dishes and the addition of $4 \times 10^{-4} M$ L-serine are required to produce larger number of cells for an extended period of time.

The adult primary cultures were utilized to investigate the effects of 8-bromo cyclic AMP on proliferation and differentiation (MARCELO and DUELL 1979). 8-Bromo cyclic AMP (10^{-3} and to $10^{-6} M$) decreased the incorporation of tritiated thymidine into DNA. The addition of cholera toxin (50 mg or 1 µg/ml) to the cultures resulted in an early stimulation of incorporation of tritiated thymidine into DNA; after 6 days this effect was lost. The divergent response of the adult cultures to two different agents that elevate the cyclic AMP levels in the cells presents interesting problems with interpretation and requires investigation into the mechanisms by which cyclic AMP exerts its effects.

III. Growth of Primary Epidermal Cultures on 3T3 Feeder Layers

Epidermal basal cells obtained from human foreskins were plated on lethally-irradiated 3T3 cells (RHEINWALD and GREEN 1975). The addition of cholera toxin (10^{-9} to $10^{-2} M$) stimulated proliferation of the cells, as judged by the staining characteristics of the cultures with rhodanile blue (GREEN 1978). Dibutyryl cyclic AMP (10^{-4} or $3 \times 10^{-4} M$) also increased colony size in the cultures but was much less effective than the cholera toxin. Other compounds that can effect the cyclic AMP levels, such as isoproterenol (10^{-5}, $10^{-6} M$) or methyl isobutyl xanthine ($3 \times 10^{-5} M$), also stimulated the growth of the cultures. The foreskin cultures grew very poorly in the absence of 3T3 cells. The addition of conditioned medium from fibroblasts plus cholera toxin improved the growth of the cultures but could not effectively replace the 3T3 feeder layer.

IV. Outgrowths of Epidermal Cells From Explants

Compounds known to increase cyclic AMP levels in the epidermis were tested for effects on proliferation of the outgrowths of epidermal basal cells from adult human explant cultures. In most cases, the number of mitoses per 1,000 cells was used to determine the effect of the compound on proliferation. HARPER et al. (1974a) showed that cyclic AMP, dibutyryl cyclic AMP, and adenine nucleotides, at a concentrations of 10^{-4} to $10^{-3} M$, inhibited mitosis 50–60%. Adenine and the guanine-, cytosine-, or uridine-nucleotides did not inhibit mitosis. Other compounds such as epinephrine ($4.5 \times 10^{-6} M$), isoproterenol ($10^{-6} M$) and histamine ($10^{-6} M$) inhibited mitosis 50–70% in the epidermal outgrowth obtained from either normal skin or psoriasis lesions (HARPER et al. 1974b). The data obtained from the explant cultures indicate that proliferation of adult epidermis is inhibited by compounds that are capable of increasing the levels of cyclic AMP.

D. Cyclic Nucleotide Metabolism in Diseased Skin

The two most common non-malignant, proliferative diseases of the skin are psoriasis and atopic dermatitis. An alteration in the cyclic nucleotide system was suggested as a factor in the pathology of psoriasis (VOORHEES and DUELL 1971). Atopic dermatitis (the cutaneous portion of atopic abnormalities) may be a disease involving the beta adrenergic receptor, based on SZENTIVANYI's (1968) original suggestion that asthma may result from such receptor abnormalities in the respiratory system. A review of the information implicating alterations cyclic AMP and cyclic GMP systems with psoriasis was presented in 1975 (VOORHEES et al.; HALPRIN et al.) and a review of atopic dermatitis and cyclic nucleotides was discussed in 1977 (DUELL and VOORHEES).

I. Cyclic Nucleotide Levels in Psoriasis

The data remain somewhat contradictory with respect to the alterations in the levels of cyclic AMP in psoriasis versus normal epidermis (VOORHEES et al. 1972; HALPRIN et al. 1975). Two recent reports have re-evaluated the situation with somewhat opposing results. MARCELO et al. (1979) reported on results obtained from 34 normal individuals and 28 psoriasis patients using the radioimmunoassay to determine the cyclic nucleotide levels. The cyclic AMP levels in involved and uninvolved psoriasis epidermis were lower than in normal epidermis. The cyclic GMP levels were higher in the lesional psoriasis areas in comparison to normals or uninvolved psoriasis epidermis. The data of WADSKOV et al. (1979) were obtained from 10 psoriasis patients. A decrease in the cyclic AMP levels in the involved areas was obtained in comparison to the uninvolved areas. There appears to be no consistent increase or decrease in the levels of cyclic AMP if one compares the involved versus uninvolved area with normal epidermis. This may be due in part to the technical problems associated with the sampling of the tissue.

Another approach has been to isolate epidermal cells by a short trypsinization procedure and to incubate the cells in culture medium (GOMMANS et al. 1979). The epidermal cells isolated from psoriasis lesions shows a slight but statistically significant decrease in the resting levels of cyclic AMP in comparison to the cells isolated from normal individuals. The question of the actual cyclic AMP levels in vivo will probably never be resolved with present technology. An investigation of the enzymes and the mechanism by which cyclic AMP exerts its effects will probably be more fruitful.

II. Data Supporting an Altered Cyclic Nucleotide System in Psoriasis

A greatly diminished response of lesional epidermis to β-adrenergic activation has been demonstrated (YOSHIKAWA et al. 1975). On the other hand, an increase in cyclic AMP levels in both involved and uninvolved skin from psoriasis patients in response to the addition of histamine or adenosine has been reported (IIZUKA et al. 1978). Similar results were obtained by GOMMANS et al. (1979) when isolated cells were incubated with histamine or epinephrine. Thus, the β-adrenergic systems appear to be malfunctioning in psoriasis and may contribute to the disease process.

Other data that implicate an altered cyclic nucleotide system in psoriasis come from indirect evidence obtained by treating the diseased tissue with agents that are known to alter the levels of cyclic AMP under in vitro conditions. Papaverine (STAWISKI et al. 1975) or Ro 20-1724 (STAWISKI et al. 1979), when applied topically to lesional areas, improved the lesions to a greater extent than control cream. Less impressive results were obtained with the systemic administration of aminophylline or dyphylline; fifty percent of the treated patients improved (IANCU et al. 1979).

Agents that are known to interfere with the β-adrenergic system can potentiate the severity of the disease (SØNDERGAARD et al. 1976). Practolol, a β_1-antagonist, induces psoriasiform lesions and aggravates the disease in psoriatic patients to such an extent that the patients become refractory to conventional forms of therapy. The β-adrenergic antagonists, propranolol, increases the rate of proliferation in uninvolved areas (WILEY and WEINSTEIN 1979). Forty-eight hours after the intradermal injection of propranolol, psoriasis patients showed a three fold increase in the number of labeled cells in uninvolved areas when compared to epidermis of normal individuals. Other perturbations of the epidermal system, such as saline injection, also increase the proliferative rate, but to a lesser extent. Thus, circumstantial data would suggest that cyclic nucleotide metabolism is an important component in psoriasis.

III. Cyclic Nucleotide System in Atopic Dermatitis

Progress in the area of cyclic nucleotide metabolism and atopic dermatitis has been minimal since the last review of this area (DUELL and VOORHEES 1977). As previously described, activation of adenylate cyclase by epinephrine, as measured in a limited number of patients, appeared to be normal. This was true also of the cyclic AMP phosphodiesterase activity. On the other hand, the activity of cyclic AMP-dependent protein kinases from atopic patients was stimulated only 29% by cyclic AMP compared to 130% for normal epidermal samples (KUMAR et al. 1975). Further investigation of atopic dermatitis will be necessary before the importance of the cyclic nucleotides can be assessed.

References

Adachi K, Yoshikawa K, Halprin KM, Levine V (1975) Prostaglandins and cyclic AMP in epidermis. Br J Dermatol 92:381–388

Aso K, Orenberg EK, Farber EM (1975) Reduced epidermal cyclic AMP accumulation following prostaglandin stimulation: its possible role in pathophysiology of psoriasis. J Invest Dermatol 65:375–378

Belman S, Troll W, Garte S (1978) Effect of phorbol myristate acetate on cyclic nucleotide levels in mouse epidermis. Cancer Res 38:2978–2982

Delescluse C, Colburn NH, Duell EA, Voorhees JJ (1974) Cyclic AMP-elevating agents inhibit proliferation of keratinizing guinea pig epidermal cells. Differentiation 2:343–350

Delescluse C, Fukuyama K, Epstein WL (1976) Dibutyryl cyclic AMP-induced differentiation of epidermal cells in tissue culture. J Invest Dermatol 66:8–13

Duell EA (1980a) Identification of a beta$_2$-adrenergic receptor in mammalian epidermis. Biochem Pharmacol 29:97–101

Duell EA (1980b) Adenosine induced alterations in the adenosine 3′,5′-monophosphate levels in mammalian epidermis. Mol Pharmacol 18:49–52

Duell EA, Voorhees JJ (1977) Cyclic nucleotides and skin disorders. In: Cramer H, Schultz J (eds) Cyclic 3′,5′-nucleotides: mechanisms of action. John Wiley and Sons, New York Chichester, pp 367–379

Duell EA, Voorhees JJ, Kelsey WH, Hayes E (1971) Isoproterenol-sensitive adenyl cyclase in a particulate fraction of epidermis. Arch Dermatol 104:601–610

Fürstenberger G, Marks F (1978) Indomethacin inhibition of cell proliferation induced by the phorbolester TPA is reversed by prostaglandin E_2 in mouse epidermis in vivo. Biochem Biophys Res Commun 84:1103–1111

Fusenig NE, Worst PK (1975) Mouse epidermal cell cultures. II. Isolation, characterization and cultivation of epidermal cells from perinatal mouse skin. Exp Cell Res 93:443–457

Garte SJ, Belman S (1978) Effects of multiple phorbol myristate acetate treatments on cyclic nucleotide levels in mouse epidermis. Biochem Biophys Res Commun 84:489–494

Gommans JM, Bergers M, Van Erp PE, Van Den Hurk J, Van De Kerkhof P, Meier PD, Roelfzema H (1979) Studies on the plasma membrane of normal and psoriatic keratinocytes 2. Cyclic AMP and its response to hormonal stimulation. Br J Dermatol 101:413–419

Green H (1978) Cyclic AMP in relation to proliferation of the epidermal cell: a new view. Cell 15:801–811

Grimm W, Marks F (1974) Effect of tumor-promoting phorbol esters on the normal and the isoproterenol-elevated level of adenosine 3′,5′-cyclic monophosphate in mouse epidermis in vivo. Cancer Res 34:3128–3134

Halprin KM, Adachi K, Yoshikawa K, Levine V, Mui M, Hsia S (1975) Cyclic AMP and psoriasis. J Invest Dermatol 65:170–178

Hammarström S, Hamberg M, Samuelsson B, Duell E, Stawiski M, Voorhees J (1975) Increased concentrations of nonesterified arachidonic acid, 12L-hydroxy-5,8,10,14-eicosatetraenoic acid, prostaglandin E, and prostaglandin $F_{2\alpha}$ in epidermis of psoriasis. Proc Natl Acad Sci USA 72:5130–5134

Harper R, Flaxman A, Chopra D (1974a) Effect of pharmacological agents on human keratinocyte mitosis in vitro. I. Inhibition by adenine nucleotides. Proc Soc Exp Biol Med 146:1032–1036

Harper R, Flaxman B, Chopra D (1974b) Mitotic response of normal and psoriatic keratinocytes in vitro to compounds known to affect intracellular cyclic AMP. J Invest Dermatol 62:384–387

Iancu L, Shneur A, Cohen H (1979) Trials with xanthine derivatives in systemic treatment of psoriasis. Dermatologica 159:55–61

Iizuka H, Adachi K, Halprin K, Levine V (1976a) Adenosine and adenine nucleotides stimulation of skin (epidermal) adenylate cyclase. Biochim Biophys Acta 444:685–693

Iizuka H, Adachi K, Halprin K, Levine V (1976b) Histamine (H_2) receptor-adenylate cyclase system in pig skin (epidermis). Biochim Biophys Acta 437:150–157

Iizuka H, Adachi K, Halprin K, Levine V (1978) Cyclic AMP accumulation in psoriatic skin: differential responses to histamine, AMP, and epinephrine by the uninvolved and involved epidermis. J Invest Dermatol 70:250–253

Iizuka H, Adachi K, Aoyagi T, Halprin K, Levine V (1979) Cyclic GMP system in epidermis. II. Histamine stimulates cyclic GMP formation. J Invest Dermatol 73:313–316

Karasek M (1975) In vitro growth and maturation of epithelial cells from postembryonic skin. J Invest Dermatol 65:60–66

Kumar J, Solomon L, Schreckenberger A, Cobb J (1975) An evaluation of adenosine 3′,5′-cyclic monophosphate-dependent protein kinase activity in atopic dermatitis. J Invest Dermatol 65:522–524

Liu S, Karasek M (1978) Isolation and growth of adult human epidermal keratinocytes in cell culture. J Invest Dermatol 71:157–162

Marcelo C (1979) Differential effects of cAMP and cGMP on in vitro epidermal cell growth. Exp Cell Res 120:201–210

Marcelo C, Duell E (1979) Cyclic AMP stimulates and inhibits adult human epidermal cell growth. J Invest Dermatol 72:279

Marcelo C, Kim YG, Kaine J, Voorhees J (1978) Stratification, specialization, and proliferation of primary keratinocyte cultures. Evidence of a functioning in vitro epidermal cell system. J Cell Biol 79:356–370

Marcelo C, Duell E, Stawiski M, Anderson T, Voorhees J (1979) Cyclic nucleotide levels in psoriatic and normal keratomed epidermis. J Invest Dermatol 72:20–24

Marks F (1973) The second messenger system of mouse epidermis. III. Guanyl cyclase. Biochim Biophys Acta 309:349–356

Marks F, Rebien W (1972) The second messenger system of mouse epidermis. 1. Properties and β-adrenergic activation of adenylate cyclase in vitro. Biochim Biophys Acta 284:556–567

Mier P, Urselmann E (1970) The adenyl cyclase of skin. I. Measurement and properties. Br J Dermatol 83:359–363

Mufson R, Simsiman R, Boutwell R (1977) The effect of the phorbol ester tumor promoters on the basal and catecholamine-stimulated levels of cyclic adenosine 3′:5′-monophosphate in mouse skin and epidermis in vivo. Cancer Res 37:665–669

Murray A, Rogers A (1978) Calcium-dependent protein modulator of cyclic nucleotide phosphodiesterases from mouse epidermis. Biochem J 176:727–732

Murray AW, Solanki V, Verma AK (1977) Accumulation of cyclic adenosine 3′,5′-monophosphate in adult and newborn mouse skin: response to ischemia and isoproterenol. J Invest Dermatol 68:125–127

Powell JA, Duell EA, Voorhees JJ (1971) Beta-adrenergic stimulation of endogenous epidermal cyclic AMP formation. Arch Dermatol 104:359–365

Regnier M, Delescluse C, Prunieras M (1973) Studies on guinea pig skin cell cultures. I. Separate cultures of keratinocytes and dermal fibroblasts. Acta Derm Venereol (Stockh) 53:241–247

Rheinwald JG, Green H (1975) Serial cultivation of strains of human epidermal keratinocytes: the formation of keratinizing colonies from single cells. Cell 6:331–343

Rusin L, Duell E, Voorhees J (1978) Papaverine and Ro 20-1724 inhibit cyclic nucleotide phosphodiesterase activity and increase cyclic AMP levels in psoriatic epidermis in vitro. J Invest Dermatol 71:154–156

Solanki V, Murray A (1978) The β-adrenergic receptor of newborn mouse skin. J Invest Dermatol 71:344–346

Søndergaard J, Wadskov S, Jensen H, Mikkelsen H (1976) Aggravation of psoriasis and occurrence of psoriasiform cutaneous eruptions induced by practolol (eraldin). Acta Derm Venereol (Stockh) 56:239–243

Stawiski M, Powell J, Lang P, Schork A, Duell E, Voorhees J (1975) Papaverine: its effects on cyclic AMP in vitro and psoriasis in vivo. J Invest Dermatol 64:124–127

Stawiski M, Rusin L, Burns T, Weinstein G, Voorhees J (1979) Ro 20-1724: An agent that significantly improves psoriatic lesions in double-blind clinical trials. J Invest Dermatol 73:261–263

Szentivanyi A (1968) The beta-adenergic theory of the atopic abnormality in bronchial asthma. J Allergy 42:203–232

Voorhees J, Duell E (1971) Psoriasis as a possible defect of the adenyl cyclase-cyclic AMP cascade. Arch Dermatol 104:352–358

Voorhees J, Duell E, Bass L, Powell J, Harrell R (1972) Decreased cyclic AMP in the epidermis of lesions of psoriasis. Arch Dermatol 105:695–701

Voorhees J, Duell E, Stawiski M, Harrell R (1974a) Cyclic nucleotide metabolism in normal and proliferating epidermis. Cyclic Nucleotide Res 4:117–162

Voorhees J, Colburn N, Stawiski M, Duell E, Haddox M, Goldberg N (1974b) Imbalanced cyclic AMP and cyclic GMP levels in the rapidly dividing, incompletely differentiated epidermis of psoriasis. In: Clarkson B, Baserga R (eds) Control of proliferation in animal cells, vol 1. Cold Spring Harbor Laboratory, Cold Spring Harbor, NY, pp 635–648

Voorhees J, Marcelo C, Duell E (1975) Cyclic AMP, cyclic GMP, and glucocorticoids as potential metabolic regulators of epidermal proliferation and differentiation. J Invest Dermatol 65:179–190

Wadskov S, Kassis V, Søndergaard J (1979) Cyclic AMP and psoriasis once more. Acta Derm Venereol (Stockh) 59:525–527

Wiley H, Weinstein G (1979) Abnormal proliferation of uninvolved psoriatic epidermis: differential induction by saline, propranolol, and tape stripping in vivo. J Invest Dermatol 73:545–547

Wilkinson D, Orenberg E (1979) Effect of prostaglandins on cyclic nucleotide levels in cultured keratinocytes. Prostaglandins 17:419–429

Yoshikawa K, Adachi K, Halprin K, Levine V (1975) On the lack of response to catecholamine stimulation by the adenyl cyclase system in psoriatic lesions. Br J Dermatol 92:619–624

CHAPTER 35

The Role of Cyclic Nucleotides in Platelets

D. C. B. MILLS

Overview

Cyclic AMP in blood platelets is regulated by several endogenous factors and can also be influenced by drugs. Elevation of platelet cAMP, either by inhibition of phosphodiesterase or by stimulation of adenylate cyclase, leads to the suppression of their responsiveness to stimulation, and their participation in haemostatic and thrombotic processes is reduced.

Platelet adenylate cyclase is regulated by specific receptors for prostaglandins I_2 and D_2, for adenosine ("P"- and "R"-type receptors) and for ADP and catecholamines, (α and β). PGI_2, PGE_1, PGD_2 adenosine and β-adrenergic agonists stimulate adenylate cyclase activity; ADP and α-adrenergic agonists inhibit the enzyme. Both receptor-mediated stimulation and inhibition are influenced by intracellular guanine nucleotides. The enzyme is also stimulated by histamine, cholera toxin and fluoride ion. Adenosine, acting on an intracellular "P" receptor, proaggregatory prostaglandins and endoperoxides inhibit the enzyme.

Platelets have three cyclic nucleotide phosphodiesterases, one relatively specific for cAMP (FI), one for cGMP (FIII) and a nonspecific, low affinity enzyme (FII). They differ in their physical characteristics, and in their susceptibility to inhibition by a variety of drugs.

Two cAMP-dependent protein kinases (type I and type II) have been detected, and an increase in platelet cAMP is associated with the phosphorylation of two membrane proteins, and with an increased ability of membrane vesicles to accumulate calcium. Many of the effects of cAMP may be mediated by the consequent reduction in intracellular free calcium ions.

Platelets have a powerful guanylate cyclase which, in contrast to the adenylate cyclase, is not membrane bound. The cGMP level in platelets is rapidly elevated during aggregation, and also when guanylate cyclase is stimulated by a variety of drugs, including inhibitors of aggregation (azide, nitroprusside), aggregating agents (fatty acids, calcium ionophore) and some compounds having no detectable effect on aggregation (ascorbic acid).

Elevation of cGMP level is a consequence rather than a cause of aggregation, and the function of this nucleotide remains a mystery.

Abnormalities of cAMP metabolism have been recognised in some conditions, Bartter's syndrome, essential thrombocythemia and acute thrombosis, in which platelet haemostatic function is abnormal, as well as others in which no functional abnormally has been detected. It is possible that the adenylate cyclase system of platelets may have a useful role as an indicator of events occurring in the brain or in other inaccessible organs.

A. Introduction

I. Natural History of Platelets

The basic biochemistry, physiology and morphology of the blood platelet have been reviewed by HOLMSEN et al. (1979), MARCUS and ZUCKER (1965), MUSTARD and PACKHAM (1970), WHITE (1979) and by ZUCKER (1980). Platelets circulate as small cells, lacking a nucleus, that are formed by the splitting off of cytoplasmic fragments from their parent cell, the megakaryocyte. Human blood contains from 150,000–450,000 platelets per microliter, or $0.7–2.5 \times 10^{12}$ in the total blood volume. The average volume of a human platelet is 7fl, so the total volume of the circulating platelets is between 5 and 20 ml/70 kg. The platelet survives in the blood stream for 5–10 days, until it is removed by the reticuloendothelial system. The main function of platelets is to provide the bulk of the haemostatic plug, the major initial defense against bleeding from injured blood vessels, particularly those in the middle range of size. Formation of the haemostatic plug is accomplished by the platelet's ability to undergo an extremely rapid transition from its normal, mutually repellent state to a condition in which it adheres avidly to other platelets and also to other surfaces, and by the catalytic effect that activated platelets have on the plasma coagulation mechanism.

II. Aggregation and Secretion

The aggregation of platelets can be induced by a large number of physiological stimuli, among which some of the more important are thrombin, ADP and collagen fibers. Other physiological aggregating agents, reviewed by MILLS and MACFARLANE (1976), include catecholamines, antigen/antibody complexes, fatty acids, prostaglandin endoperoxides and thromboxanes, serotonin, vasopressin and also PAF ("platelet activating factor", PAF-acether, 1-0-alkyl-2-acetyl glycerol-3-phosphoryl choline), a novel phospholipid produced by stimulated leukocytes (DEMOPOULOS et al. 1980) and by platelets (VARGAFTIG et al. 1981). Dog platelets are aggregated by cholinergic agents acting on a muscarinic receptor, and pig platelets are aggregated by prostaglandin E_2. Aggregation can also be induced by unphysiological agents including flouride ion, triethyl tin, methyl mercury and phorbol myrisate acetate. Aggregation is regarded as an active process for the platelet, and is inhibited by disruption of energy metabolism, by simultaneous blockade of glycolysis and respiration. A distinct process, agglutination, that does not require the metabolic machinery of the cell, occurs in the presence of coagulation factor VIII and the antibiotic, ristocetin.

The platelets themselves, when stimulated to aggregate, can release aggregating agents. These agents are either formed *de novo* (i.e. thromboxane A_2) or released from specific storage organelles (i.e. ADP). In human platelets, ADP is stored along with 5-hydroxytryptamine and calcium ion in the "dense bodies" which closely resemble enterochromaffin- and adrenal medullary chromaffin granules. The platelets may also secrete lysosomal enzymes, and a variety of factors, mostly protein in nature, that are stored together in organelles known as alpha-granules. These factors include proteins that are immunologically specific to the platelet

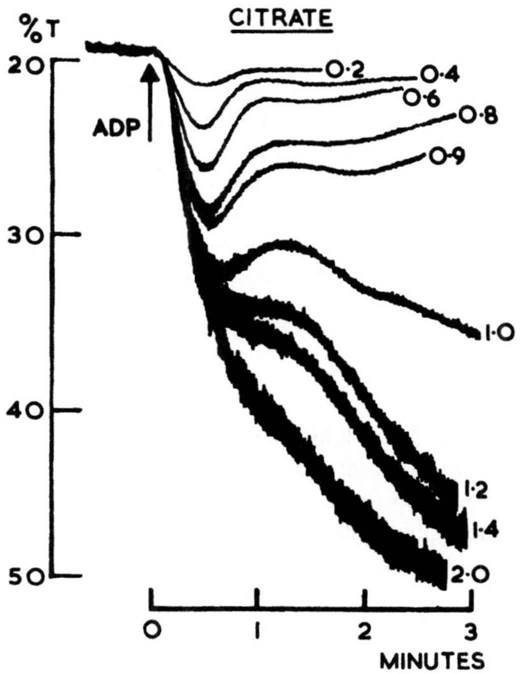

Fig. 1. Platelet aggregation recorded turbidometrically in human platelet rich plasma, prepared by centrifuging blood freshly drawn into 1/9th volume of 3.8% sodium citrate. A family of aggregation curves were traced and are shown superimposed to the point of addition of ADP *(arrow)*. The concentration (in μ*M*) of ADP used is given besides each trace. The second wave of aggregation is associated with the release of stored nucleotides and serotonin, and with the formation of prostaglandins, endoperoxides and thromboxane A_2. (From MILLS and ROBERTS 1965)

("platelet factor 4" and beta-thromboglobulin), agents that increase vascular permeability and others that stimulate growth and proliferation of smooth muscle cells in culture.

III. Changes During Activation

The nature of the change in the platelet membrane responsible for the transition from the "normal" to the "sticky" state is not well understood. Several aggregating agents induce the appearance on the membrane of specific binding sites for fibrinogen. Certain of the membrane glycoproteins – specifically GPIIb and GPIII – comprising the glycocalyx, or outer fuzzy coat of the cell, may be involved in a lectin-receptor like interaction with other membrane components, possibly even involving bound fibrinogen.

A complex reorganization, involving both cytoskeletal and contractile elements of the platelet, takes place during activation. Aggregation is usually accompanied by a "shape change"; within 5–10 s of exposure to an aggregating agent, the platelets lose the disc form that they have in the circulation, and throw out a variety of blebs and filamentous pseudopods. This process is associated with the loss of a marginal bundle of microtubules, and the appearance of a network of actin filaments oriented along the long axes of the pseudopods. The intracellular organelles coalesce towards the center of the cell, and the contents of the dense bodies are discharged by exocytosis into invaginated channels that communicate with the extracellular space. ATP consumption, glycolysis, glycogenoysis, phosphoinositol turnover and oxygen comsumption are all stimulated. The trigger for all of these processes is widely believed to be an increase in the cytoplasmic concentration of Ca2+, either by entry from the extracellular medium, or by the redistribution of one or more internally sequestered pools (DETWILER et al. 1978; FEINSTEIN et al. 1981).

IV. Effects on Coagulation

As well as providing building blocks for plug formation, activated platelets contribute in several ways to the initiation of coagulation, the process leading to the conversion of fibrinogen to fibrin, which is necessary to bind and stabilize the otherwise impermanent haemostatic plug. The activity generated on the surfaces of activated platelets – known as platelet factor 3 (PF3) – involves the release from the α-granules of factor Va, and its binding to the membrane in such a way as to form a specific site where factor Xa and factor II (prothrombin) can interact to form thrombin at a greatly accelerated rate. Platelets are also believed to contribute to the early or "contact" phase of coagulation, again providing surface binding sites where reactions involving several components can take place.

V. Clot Retraction

Platelets are necessary for the occurrence of the test tube phenomenon of clot retraction. This is an active process by which serum is expressed from a blood clot by the contraction of actomyosin filaments in extended pseudopods that have become attached to the fibrin network. The relation of clot retraction to physiological processes is not clearly demonstrated, but it may be involved in wound healing and in the organization and resolution of thrombi.

B. Adenylate Cyclase

I. Introduction

MARCUS and ZUCKER (1965) reported that cyclic AMP and its dibutryl derivative (DBcAMP) inhibit platelet aggregation. ARDLIE et al. (1967) showed that aggregation is inhibited by phosphodiesterase inhibitors of the methyl xanthine type, and first suggested that cyclic AMP might have a role in the regulation of platelet function. In 1969, the *annus mirabilis* for this subject, several groups reported that cyclic AMP metabolism in platelets is influenced by both aggregating agents and antagonists of aggregation, and that platelet cyclic AMP levels profoundly modify platelet behaviour in the test tube (ABDULLA 1969; MARQUIS et al. 1969; ROBISON et al. 1969; SALZMAN and NERI 1969; VIGDAHL et al. 1969; WOLFE and SHULMAN 1969; ZIEVE and GREENOUGH 1969). These discoveries have been reviewed by HASLAM and TAYLOR (1971 b), SALZMAN (1972, 1973), SALZMAN and WESENBERGER (1972), BOUSSER (1973), HASLAM (1973) and WEISSENBERG (1973). The unifying hypothesis put forward by SALZMAN (SALZMAN et al. 1970; SALZMAN and LEVINE 1971; SALZMAN 1972), proposed that aggregating agents and inhibitors of aggregation both act through changing cAMP levels, with increases leading to inhibition and decreases to activation. Powerful evidence, largely accumulated by HASLAM and his colleagues, has shown that for most agents, a reduction of platelet cAMP is neither necessary nor sufficient to induce or to potentiate aggregation (HASLAM et al. 1978 b). The association between an increase in cAMP and inhibition of platelet reactivity has been confirmed in a wide variety of situations, and has been established as one of the most clearly authenticated of all of the second messenger functions of cAMP.

II. Prostaglandins

1. Effects on Aggregation and on Cyclic AMP

The inhibition of platelet aggregation by prostaglandin E_1 (PGE_1) was first described by KLOEZE (1966) and subsequently confirmed by several authors (for a comprehensive review see SMITH and MACFARLANE 1974). PGE_1 stimulates adenylate cyclase and increases the intracellular level of cAMP. Other prostaglandins having similar effects to PGE_1 include PGE_2 (ROBISON et al. 1971; KLOEZE 1967, 1969; SHIO et al. 1972; MCDONALD and STEWART 1973, 1974), PGD_2 and PGD_1 (SMITH et al. 1974; MILLS and MACFARLANE 1974; NISHIZAWA et al. 1975), 6-keto-PGE_1 (WONG et al. 1979, 1980) and PGI_2, also known as prostacyclin (TATESON et al. 1977; GORMAN et al. 1977; BEST et al. 1977). $PGF_{1\alpha}$, $PGF_{2\alpha}$ and 6-keto-$PGF_{1\alpha}$, the principal product of the spontaneous decomposition of PGI_2, were all much less active. PGE_2 has a biphasic action: at concentrations higher than 1 μM, it stimulates cyclic AMP accumulation and inhibits aggregation, at lower concentrations it inhibits the cyclase and potentiates aggregation (SALZMAN 1972; SHIO et al. 1972; MACINTYRE and GORDON 1975).

Platelets stimulated by PGE_1 or PGI_2 make cAMP at a substantial rate, estimated at 2.5 nmoles, or 5%–6% of the cell's metabolically active ATP, per platelet per minute (MILLS 1975). This does not appreciably deplete the ATP pool, even when oxidative phosphorylation is blocked by antimycin A, as no change in the adenylate energy charge occurred unless glycolysis was inhibited by deoxy-D-glucose. HASHIMOTO et al. (1975) interpreted their observation, as pointing to a close association between cAMP and ATP formed by mitochondrial respiration.

In intact platelets, PGI_2 is 10- to 30-fold more potent than PGE_1, both as an inhibitor of aggregation (WHITTLE et al. 1978) and as a stimulator of adenylate cyclase (TATESON et al. 1977), with about 3-fold higher intrinsic activity; this difference in intrinsic activity is not evident when the activity of adenylate cyclase is measured in platelet membrane fragments (GORMAN et al. 1977), and it was very much reduced when the initial rates of cyclic AMP accúmulation were measured in intact cells (MILLS and MACFARLANE 1980). It appears to be largely a consequence of the shorter duration of action of PGE_1 compared with PGI_2 and PGD_2. After exposure to PGE_1 the peak levels of intracellular cyclic AMP are reached within 20–40 s (BALL et al. 1970; MILLS and SMITH 1972; HARWOOD et al. 1972; HASLAM and

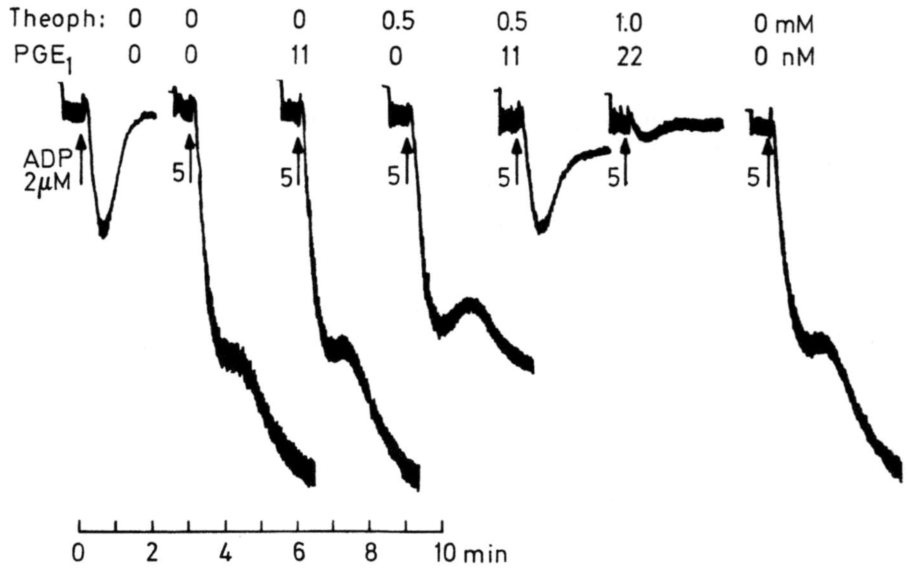

Fig. 2. Potentiation of the anti-aggregating effect of PGE_1 by theophylline (From MILLS et al. 1970)

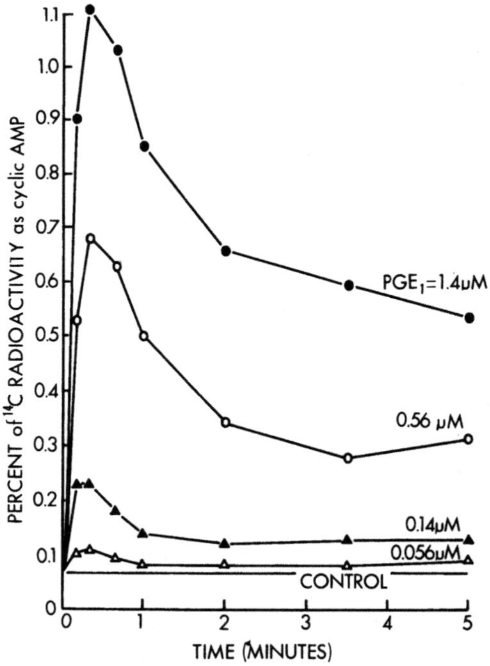

Fig. 3. Stimulation of cAMP formation by PGE_1, Platelet nucleotides were labelled by incubating platelet rich plasma with [^{14}C] adenine. Concentrations of PGE_1 used are given beside each curve. The ratio of the peak to the sustained level is independent of the PGE_1 concentration. (From MILLS and SMITH 1972)

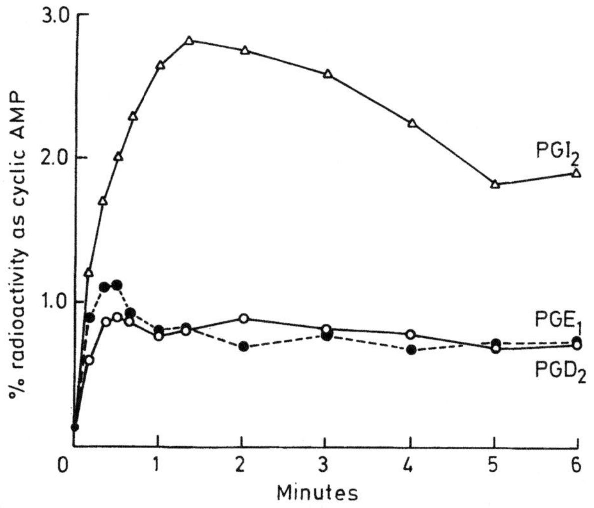

Fig. 4. Progress curve for cAMP accumulation after exposure to different prostaglandins. Initial rates after PGE_1 and PGI_2 are similar, while the rate for PGD_2 is lower. Response to PGE_1 rapidly reverses. (MILLS and MACFARLANE, unpublished work)

LYNHAM 1972; HONEGGER et al. 1975). By 60 s, the cyclic AMP levels may have fallen to between 60% and 30% of this peak. With PGI_2, the peak levels are reached later, and are maintained for longer times. PGE_2 potentiates the aggregating activity of prostaglandin endoperoxides (WEISS et al. 1976) and reduces the inhibitory effect of PGE_1, PGI_2 and PGD_2 on platelet aggregation (ANDERSON et al. 1980). MILLS and MACFARLANE (1980) have observed an inhibitory component of the action PGE_2 and PGE_1 on adenylate cyclase which may account for the difference in the time course between PGE_1 and PGI_2.

Several aggregation-promoting prostaglandins antagonise the stimulation of cyclic AMP accumulation by PGE_1. The endoperoxide intermediates of prostaglandin formation, PGG_2 and PGH_2 (GORMAN 1975; MILLER and GORMAN 976; SALZMAN 1977; CLAESSON and MALMSTEN 1977) and thromboxane A_2 (TxA_2) (MILLER et al. 1977; GORMAN 1979) as well as their stable synthetic analogues, all have this action, which GORMAN et al. (1979) have shown is independent of the release of the much stronger inhibitor, ADP. Neither MILLS and MACFARLANE (1977) nor BEST et al. (1979b) found any inhibitory activity of U44069 and U46619, the epoxymethano analogues of PGH_2, on cAMP formation stimulated by PGE_1, when the analogues were added after the PGE_1; though both inhibit when added first. As PGE_1 inhibits the response to both itself and PGD_2 and PGI_2, PGE_1 may have an inhibitory action through the same mechanism as the endoperoxides. This inhibitory effect is normally outweighed by its stimulation of the cyclase. The inhibitory component of the action of PGE_2 may involve a similar mechanism, and a delayed inhibitory effect of PGE_1 could account for the difference in the time course of cyclic AMP accumulation noted above (MILLS and MACFARLANE 1980).

The inhibitory effect of TxA_2 is inhibited by TMB-8 (8-N,N-dimethylaminooctyl 3,4,5-trimethoxybenzoate), an antagonist of several intracellular actions of calcium ions (GORMAN 1979), suggesting that calcium may be important in regulating adenylate cyclase activity (see RASMUSSEN and GOODMAN 1977). RODAN and FEINSTEIN (1976) showed that calcium inhibits the adenylate cyclase of platelet membranes with $K_i = 16\ \mu M$, and that A 23187, a divalent cationophore, inhibits the increase in cAMP caused by PGE_1 in intact cells. This latter effect, however, may have been due to the release of intracellular ADP.

SINHA and COLMAN (1979, 1980) have shown that platelet cAMP levels are raised on exposure to PGE_1 covalently linked to hexyl agarose. No release of the bound prostaglandin could be detected, though plasma treated with the insolubilized prostaglandin was also able to inhibit aggregation, apparently by a mechanism independent of cAMP.

2. Receptors for Prostaglandins

Platelet receptors for prostaglandins have been recently reviewed by MACINTYRE (1981). Specific receptors for PGI_2, PGE_1, PGE_2 and PGD_2 mediating the stimulation of adenylate cyclase activity have been identified by measuring the binding of appropriate radioligands to platelet membranes or to intact cells. GORMAN (1974) showed that PGE_1 and PGE_2 bind to the same site. The binding isotherms for PGI_2 and PGE_1 give curvilinear Scatchard plots which have been interpreted as indicating two classes of binding sites with different affinities. The high affinity binding ($K_d = 10^{-8}\ M$) of PGI_2 involves less than 100 sites per cell (SIEGL et al. 1979a; SHAFER et al. 1979) and is seen with platelets of several different species (SCHILLINGER and PRIOR 1980). With PGD_2, COOPER and AHERN (1979) found a single class of 210 sites/cell with $K_d = 53\ nM$ while SIEGL et al. (1979b) found 760 sites/cell and $K_d = 412\ nM$. The relative order of potency of different prostaglandins as competitors for binding strongly suggests that PGE_1, PGE_2 and PGI_2 all interact with the same receptor, and that PGD_2 has a specific and distinct receptor of its own. Both receptors appear to control the same catalytic unit, as maximal concentrations of PGE_1 and PGD_2 do not have additive effects (MILLS and MACFARLANE 1974). Indirect evidence for distinct D and I(E) receptors comes from several sources. PGD_2 has markedly different effects upon platelets of different species (SMITH et al. 1974), while PGE_1 and PGI_2 affect platelets from all species to a similar extent (WHITTLE et al. 1978). In certain human diseases, a similarly specific loss of response to PGD_2 has been reported (COOPER 1979a; COOPER et al. 1978b); furthermore, drugs related to polyphloretin phosphate selectively antagonise the effects of PGD_2 (MACINTYRE and GORDON 1977; WESTWICK and WEBB 1978). Finally COOPER (1979b), COOPER et al. (1979) and MILLER and GORMAN (1979) have shown that PGD_2 can selectively desensitize its own receptor without affecting the response to PGE_1 or PGI_2. It is not clear from the published data whether selective desensitization of the I(E) receptor has been demonstrated.

3. Physiological Significance

The importance of naturally occurring prostaglandins for the regulation of platelet function has been discussed by MONCADA and VANE (1979). SMITH et al. (1976) have shown that platelets stimulated by aggregating agents form PGD_2 in small amounts along with PGE_2 and $PGF_{2\alpha}$. This may account for increased cAMP levels found in platelets treated with thrombin (DROLLER and WOLFE 1972; BRUNO et al. 1974; DROLLER 1976) and may represent a negative feedback control mechanism limiting the propagation of a platelet thrombus. It has been proposed that PGI_2, which is synthesized by vascular endothelial cells, may regulate the behaviour of platelets in the circulation (VANE and MONCADA 1980); MARCUS et al. (1980) have shown that aspirin-treated human cultured endothelial cells present with thrombin-stimulated platelets reduce the amounts of TxB_2 that are formed. MONCADA and KORBUT (1978) have suggested that the antithrombotic action of dipyridamole, a weak inhibitor of PDE in vitro, could be due to potentiation of the effects of endogenous circulating PGI_2. Attempts to confirm the presence of PGI_2 in the circulation of normal animals have shown that these levels are very low (SMITH et al. 1978). STEER et al. (1980) could detect no effect of an anti-PGI_2 antibody on ADP-induced aggregation of human platelets in platelets rich plasma prepared and used within 3 min of venepuncture. HASLAM and MCCLENAGHAN (1980), using a sensitive assay based on the detection of small increases in cAMP in washed rabbit platelets labelled with tritiated adenine, found resting levels of PGI_2-like activity in rabbit plasma equivalent to 0.5–0.7 pmoles/ml. This level was too low to influence platelet aggregation, suggesting that PGI_2 might only be effective in areas close to its site of production.

BUNTING et al. (1976) have shown that endoperoxides (PGG_2 and PGH_2) synthesized by platelets may act as the substrate for the endothelial enzyme that generates PGI_2, and MARCUS et al. (1980) have shown that aspirin-treated human cultured endothelial cells present with thrombin-stimulated platelets reduce the amounts of TxB_2 that are formed and inhibit the aggregation, possibly by "stealing" endoperoxides produced by the platelets and converting them to PGI_2. On the other hand, HORNSTRA et al. (1979) found no difference in the amount of PGI_2 formed by aortic segments incubated with platelets from normal or from essential fatty acid deficient rats. NEEDLEMAN et al. (1980) found no evidence for the release of endoperoxides from thrombin-stimulated platelets unless formation of thromboxanes was inhibited by imidazole. They suggested that inhibition of thromboxane synthesis would be expected to be more effective than inhibition of cyclooxygenase in regulating platelet reactivity in vivo.

III. Adenosine

1. Inhibition of Aggregation and Stimulation of Adenylate Cyclase

Adenosine was originally found to inhibit platelet aggregation by BORN and CROSS (1963) who proposed that it acts competitively by blocking the interaction of ADP with a specific receptor. However, this mechanism was difficult to reconcile with several observations: Adenosine blocks aggregation induced by agonists other than ADP; and the maximum effect of adenosine is not immediate. MILLS and SMITH (1971) showed that adenosine and 2-chloroadenosine stimulate the accumulation of cyclic AMP and that their effects are enhanced by phosphodiesterase inhibitors of the pyrimidopyrimidine type. These compounds also inhibit the transport of adenosine into cells (HORCH et al. 1970), suggesting an extracellular site of action for adenosine. This was confirmed by HASLAM and ROSSON (1975) using p-nitrobenzylthioguanosine (NBTG), an inhibitor of adenosine transport that does not

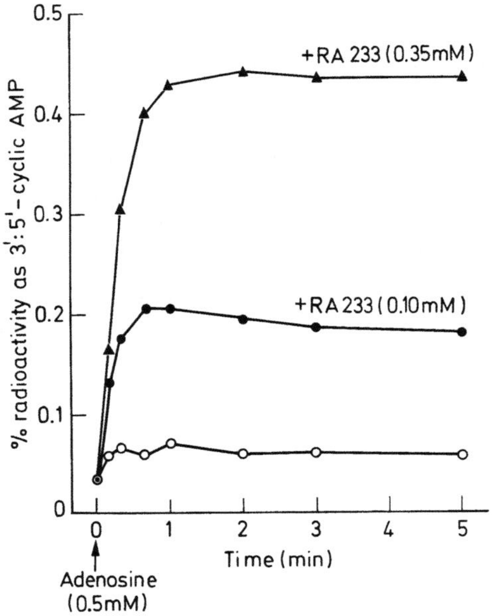

Fig. 5. Stimulation of cAMP formation by adenosine. The small effect is greatly augmented in the presence of RA 233, which both inhibits phosphodiesterase and blocks adenosine uptake into the cells, thereby preventing the inhibitory component of its action

affect phosphodiesterase. Adenosine stimulates adenylate cyclase in platelet lysates (HASLAM and LYNHAM 1972; JAKOBS et al. 1979) and its effects are inhibited competitively by the methylxanthine phosphodiesterase inhibitors, theophylline, caffeine and isobutylmethyl xanthine (SCHAUMANN et al. 1970; HASLAM 1973; JOHNSON et al. 1979).

Rat platelets are less readily inhibited by adenosine than are rabbit or human platelets (CUTHBERTSON and MILLS 1963) and show a smaller increase in cAMP than do human platelets (MICHEL et al. 1976).

2. Inhibition of Adenylate Cyclase

HASLAM and ROSSON (1975) found a biphasic effect of adenosine on the adenylate cyclase of intact platelets, stimulating at low concentrations (up to 40 μ*M*) and inhibiting at higher concentrations. The inhibitory effect was blocked by NBTG, suggesting an intracellular action. This is supported by HASLAM et al. (1978c) who have observed inhibition of adenylate cyclase in platelet lysates by 2′-deoxyadenosine 3′-monophosphate, a compound which does not readily cross cell membranes, and which does not block the inhibitory effect of PGE_1 on platelet aggregation. LONDOS and WOLFF (1977) tested a range of adenosine analogues as stimulators or inhibitors of the platelet membrane enzyme. Compounds substituted in the 2- position (2-chloro-, 2-methyl-, 2-amino-) were stimulators, as were some N^6 substituted derivatives (N^6-methyl-, N^6-phenylisopropyl-), while compounds substituted in the ribose ring (2′,5′-dideoxyadenosine (DDA), 9-*β*-d-xylofuranosyl adenine, 3′-deoxyadenosine) were inhibitors, as was 9-(tetrahydro-2-furyl adenine (SQ 22536) (HARRIS et al. 1979). These compounds inhibit both stimulation of cyclic AMP accumulation induced by PGE_1, and inhibition of platelet aggregation, reinforcing the conclusion that cAMP is the intracellular mediator of the inhibition of aggregation by PGE_1 (HASLAM 1978). On the other hand, neither SQ 22536 nor DDA induce aggregation, nor do they potentiate aggregation induced by ADP or by arginine vasopressin, collagen or arachidinate (HASLAM et al. 1978 b), though SQ 22536 slightly enhances aggregation induced by PGG_2 (SALZMAN 1977, 1978) or by the PGG_2 analogues, U 44069 and azo-PGH_2 (SALZMAN et al. 1979). This argues against the possibility that a reduction in the basal level of cyclic AMP is involved in the induction of aggregation (HASLAM et al. 1978 a, 1979 a).

Inhibition of adenylate cyclase by adenosine, DDA or SQ 22536 was non-competitive with respect to the substrate, Mg-ATP. Inhibition and stimulation of the cyclase by adenosine occurred in the presence of Gpp(NH)p and was associated with an increased affinity for Mg^{2+} (JAKOBS et al. 1979). A mechanism proposed for this inhibition by JOHNSON et al. (1979) invokes diversion of the enzyme to a slower path by enhanced Mg^{2+} binding.

3. Receptors for Adenosine

The platelet fits well into the scheme proposed for the classification of adenosine receptors into "P", for purine, and "R", for ribose (LONDOS and WOLFF 1977). The P site has a high specificity for the purine ring, is intracellular, and causes inhibition. The R site is relatively unspecific for the purine, accepting modifications of N^6 and C^2, but does not tolerate modification of the ribose. It is extracellular and causes stimulation. Neither AMP nor the unnatural L-enantiomorphic form of adenosine are able to stimulate this receptor (CUSACK et al. 1979). The structural specificity of the platelet "R" adenosine receptor can be deduced from the activities of a large number of analogues that have been tested as inhibitors of platelet aggregation, comprehensively reviewed by HASLAM and CUSACK (1981).

IV. Catecholamines

1. Effects on Platelet Aggregation

The α-adrenergic agonists, epinephrine and norepinephrine, when added to human patients at concentrations between 1 and 10 μ*M* cause primary aggregation (O'BRIEN 1963) and the release of stored nucleotides and serotonin – the platelet release reaction associated with secondary aggregation (MILLS et al. 1968); furthermore, they potentiate the actions of other aggregating agents (ARDLIE et al. 1966), even in species in which they do not induce aggregation (DODDS et al. 1978). Epinephrine and norepinephrine are of similar potency and isoproterenol is a weak inhibitor. The α-effects are blocked by phentolamine and by dihydroergotamine, but not by the β-blocker propranolol, and only weakly by the alkylating type of α-antagonist i.e. phenoxybenzamine (MILLS and ROBERTS 1967). These observations demonstrate that the pro-aggregatory effect of catecholamines is mediated by an α-adrenoceptor with a specificity somewhat different from the alpha-adrenoceptor of catecholaminergic neurones. Differentiation of the presynaptic (α_1) from the postsynaptic (α_2) receptor prompted the reexamination of the platelet response.

Although most of the newer α-adrenergic agonists do not induce aggregation, even of human platelets, several of them e.g. clonidine, lofexidine and phenylephrine, enhance aggregation by ADP and other agents (GRANT and SCRUTTON 1979; HSU et al. 1979). Some of these drugs are partial agonists; they also inhibit the effects of epinephrine (JAKOBS 1978b; LASCH and JACOBS 1979). Aggregation induced by catecholamines in inhibited strongly by yohimbine but not by prazosin (NEWMAN et al. 1978). Taken with the evidence that there is only a single type of receptor identifiable by agonist binding, these observations indicate that aggregation is mediated predominantly by interaction with an α_2 receptor with some unique properties. However, GRANT and SCRUTTON (1980) have shown that the predominantly α_1 agonist, methoxamine, potentiates aggregation and that this effect is blocked by the α_1 antagonist, prazosin. This suggests that there may be perhaps a small fraction of receptors of the postsynaptic type on platelets.

2. Effects on Cyclic AMP

PGE_1-stimulated adenylate cyclase is inhibited by epinephrine both in platelet lysates (ZIEVE and GREENOUGH 1969; JAKOBS et al. 1978a; STEER and WOOD 1979) and in intact platelets (ROBISON et al. 1969; MARQUIS et al. 1970; COLE et al. 1971; HASLAM and TAYLOR 1971a; MILLS and SMITH 1971; MOSCOWITZ et al. 1971; HARWOOD et al. 1972). The agonist and antagonist specificity of the receptor that mediates this effect is similar to that of the aggregation receptor (JAKOBS 1978b), and it is reasonable to assume, for the time being, that the two receptors are identical. Pig platelets, for which epinephrine is neither an aggregating agent nor a potentiator of aggregation, have an adenylate cyclase that is not inhibited by epinephrine (Jakobs et al. 1978a). Epinephrine inhibits human platelet adenylate cyclase stimulated by adenosine and by fluoride as well as the unstimulated activity (JAKOBS et al. 1976). Epinephrine inhibits adenylate cyclase by decreasing its V_{max} without affecting its affinity for the substrate, Mg-ATP, or for the activator Mg^{2+} (JAKOBS et al. 1978c). As well as being blocked by the α-adrenergic antagonist phentolamine, these effects of epinephrine were enhanced by β-blockers (HASLAM and TAYLOR 1971a; HASLAM 1975; JAKOBS et al. 1978b), indicating that epinephrine also interacts with a β-receptor that stimulates adenylate cyclase. ABDULLA (1969) described the stimulation of adenylate cyclase by isoproterenol and both the inhibition of aggregation and accumulation of cAMP in intact cells are enhanced by the presence of phosphodiesterase inhibitors (MILLS et al. 1970; MILLS and SMITH 1971). HASLAM and TAYLOR (1971a) have shown that epinephrine raises platelet cyclic AMP in the presence of phentolamine. JAKOBS et al. (1978b) showed that the β-receptor of platelets differs from β-receptors described in other tissues, as it is not stimulated by some typical β_2 agonists (i.e. orciprenaline) and is not blocked by β_1 antagonists like practolol. The balance between α- and β-effects of catecholamines varies between species. YU and LATOUR (1977) have reported that in rats epinephrine inhibits aggregation, an effect that is blocked by propranolol and is enhanced by phentolamine.

3. Catecholamine Receptors

α-adrenoceptors have been identified by the binding of radiolabeled α-blockers including dihydroergocryptine (KAFKA et al. 1977; ALEXANDER et al. 1978; NEWMAN et al. 1978), dihydroergonine (JAKOBS and RAUSCHEK 1978) and phentolamine (STEER et al. 1979). The binding of these ligands is rapid and reversible. Both α-adrenergic agonists and antagonists compete with the radiolabeled ligand for the binding sites; their order of potency agrees well with their effects on aggregation and on adenylate cyclase. At saturation, platelet membranes specifically bind between 100 and 200 fmoles of radiolabeled ligand per mg protein, which is equivalent to about 100–300 receptors on each platelet, depending on the assumptions made. Binding to intact platelets gives similar results (NEWMAN et al. 1978). Displacement of dihydroergocryptine binding by prazosin and by yohimbine has been used to differentiate between α_1 and α_2 receptors, and by this criterion the platelet receptors are exclusively of the α_2 type (HOFFMAN et al. 1979). The affinity of binding of α-adrenergic agonists was increased 4-fold by 1.25 mM Mg^{2+} and decreased 10-fold by 100 mM NaCl (TSAI and LEFKOWITZ 1978). The binding affinity for the antagonist ligand was not affected, and a good correlation was found between the effects of 100 mM NaCl on the ability of different agonists to displace antagonist binding, and their intrinsic activities as inhibitors of PGE_1-stimulated adenylate cyclase. Similar agonist-specific effects have been observed with guanine nucleotides (see below B.VIII).

The use of the specific α_2 antagonist, yohimbine, as the radioligand has the advantage over the nonspecific antagonists that it is less subject to non-specific, non displaceable binding than is, for example, dihydroergocryptine (MACFARLANE et al. 1981). MOTULSKY et al. (1980) found 207 ± 41 binding sites for yohimbine per platelet. Displacement by epinephrine of the binding of yohimbine to platelet membranes was decreased by magnesium and sodium and by GTP.

Early studies of the binding of α-adrenergic agonists to platelets have identified a large number of binding sites bearing little relation to the sites identified by antagonist binding (VAINER 1977; MCMILLAN et al. 1979). More recently, SHATTIL et al. (1981) have studied the binding of the partial agonist, clonidine, to platelet membranes: binding was increased by magnesium and reduced by GTP. HOFFMAN et al. (1980) have measured the binding of tritiated epinephrine to human platelet membranes. Binding was displaced by yohimbine and by phentolamine; prazosin was much less effective, and propranolol was without effect. This is consistent with the conclusion that, at 5 nM, epinephrine binds exclusively to a receptor of the α_2 type. Displacement of the binding of dihydroergocryptine was interpreted as supporting the proposal that the α_2 receptor exists in a high and a low affinity form, 55% of the receptors being in the high affinity state.

ROBERTS et al. (1979) found that the treatment of rabbits with estrogen caused a 40% reduction in the number of binding sites for dihydroergocryptine on the membranes of their platelets while the binding to uterine smooth muscle cell membrane was increased four-fold. Down regulation of the platelet a receptor after exposure of intact platelets to epinephrine has been demonstrated by COOPER et al. (1978a).

V. ADP

1. Aggregation and Cyclic AMP Effects

Like the α-adrenergic agonists, ADP both induces platelet aggregation and inhibits PGE_1-stimulated adenylate cyclase activity in intact platelets. A growing body of

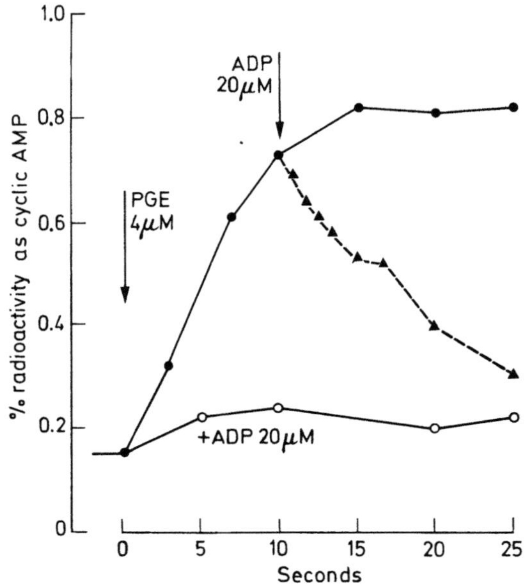

Fig. 6. Rapid reversal by ADP of the stimulation of cAMP accumulation by PGE_1. The response to PGE_1 in the presence of ADP is shown by the open circles, and in its absence by filled circles. When ADP was added 10 s after PGE_1 *(filled triangles)* cAMP accumulation abruptly reverses. (From MACFARLANE and MILLS 1981)

evidence points to the likelihood that these different effects of ADP are mediated by distinct receptors (MILLS 1979).

In intact platelets, ADP causes a rapid and almost complete inhibition of the adenylate cyclase activity stimulated by PGE_1 (COLE et al. 1971; MILLS and SMITH 1972), by PGD_2 (MILLS and MACFARLANE 1974) or by adenosine (HASLAM 1973). The concentrations required to inhibit adenylate cyclase (0.3–1 μ*M*) are similar to the concentrations causing aggregation. ATP, a specific, competitive inhibitor of the aggregating effect of ADP, also inhibits its effect on cyclic AMP (MACFARLANE and MILLS 1975). As ADP does not penetrate the cell membrane, it must be assumed to interact with a receptor on the outside of the membrane. The effect of ADP is very rapid, producing maximal inhibition of the rate of cAMP accumulation in intact cells within 1 s and with an activation (Hill) constant close to unity (MACFARLANE and MILLS 1981), while the reversal of this effect by ATP occurs within 2 s. The structural specificity of the receptor that mediates the inhibition of adenylate cyclase is very similar to that of the receptor through which ADP induces aggregation (HASLAM and CUSACK (1981). The most active analogs are those in which the purine ring is substituted in the 2-position. Other naturally occurring nucleoside diphosphates are inactive. Of the compounds that have been tested in this laboratory, 2 fluoro-, 2 chloro-, 2 azido-, 2 n-butylthio- and 2 methylthio-ADP are all aggregating agents and inhibitors of PGE_1-stimulated cAMP accumulation. There is, however, a considerable variation in the potency ratio for the two effects between the different analogues. 2 Methylthio-ADP, the most active inhibitor of cAMP accummulations, is 200-fold more active than ADP, while as an aggregating agent it is only 10-fold more active (MACFARLANE et al. 1979). The inhibitory effect of ADP and its analogues on cAMP synthesis is blocked by thiol reagents including N-ethylmaleimide (MILLS and SMITH 1972), cytochalasin A (MILLS and MACFARLANE 1975) and by p-mercuribenzenesulphonate (MILLS 1974). This last reagent, which penetrates only slowly through cell membranes, also inhibits ADP-induced platelet aggregation, but it does not inhibit the shape change that proceeds aggregation induced by ADP. Another analogue of ADP, 5′p-fluorosulphonylbenzoyl adenosine (FSBA), an inhibitor of ADP-induced platelet aggregation and shape-change, does not block the effect of ADP on cAMP (COLMAN et al. 1980).

2. Inhibition of Adenylate Cyclase

Early attempts failed to detect any inhibition by ADP of the adenylate cyclase of platelet homogenates except at high concentrations of ADP which could compete with substrate ATP (SALZMAN and LEVINE 1971; BARBER 1976). ADP, either released from the broken cells or formed from ATP by the action of endogenous ATP'ases, could have interfered with these experiments. With a purified preparation of platelet membranes and using the ATP'ase resistant analogue App(NH)p as substrate, COOPER and RODBELL (1979) demonstrated inhibition of both basal and PGE_1-stimulated adenylate cyclase by ADP and by ADP-βS, which both caused maximal inhibition of 27% at 10 μM in the presence of GTP. With a crude preparation of platelet particles, MELLWIG and JACOB (1980) showed that ADP inhibits both basal and PGE_1-stimulated activities by 40%–50%, but higher concentrations (up to 300 μM) were needed for the maximal effect. When GTP was replaced by the stable analogue, guanosine 5′-O-(3-thiotriphosphate), the inhibitory effect of ADP disappeared.

3. Platelet Receptors for ADP

Specific binding sites have been identified on platelet membranes by NACHMAN and FERRIS (1974) and by ADLER and HANDIN (1979). These sites are distinct from nucleotide diphosphate kinase, but have not been functionally identified as receptors. Intact platelets exhibit specific, saturable and displaceable binding of the ADP analogues 2 azido-ADP and 2 methylthio-ADP; the binding affinity of either compound closely parallels its activity as an inhibitor of cAMP accumulation (MACFARLANE and MILLS 1977; MACFARLANE et al. 1979, 1982). Each platelet has 500–1000 non-interactive binding sites. Binding is inhibited by MBS but not by FSBA. This suggests that the observed binding is to receptors that control cAMP metabolism, and that a different mechanism is involved in the initiation of aggregation. Attempts to covalently label the ADP receptor with the photoactivatable analogue agido-ADP were unsuccessful.

VI. Other Agents

The synthesis of cAMP by platelet membranes is stimulated by cholera toxin (MELLWIG and JACOBS 1980; JACOBS and SCHULTZ 1980) and by the fluoride anion (ZIEVE and GREENOUGH 1969; WOLFE and SHULMAN 1969; MCDONALD 1970), and is inhibited by thrombin and by serotonin (Zieve and Greenough 1969). Membranes from platelets treated with thrombin had lost most of their adenylate cyclase activity (Brodie et al. 1972) though Mills (1974) found that intact platelets treated with thrombin and then washed responded normally to PGE_1 with an increase in cAMP. Hughes and Insel (1980) found that cholera toxin was unable to stimulate adenylate cyclase in intact platelets.

Klysner et al. (1980) have reported that cAMP formation in platelets is stimulated by histamine acting specifically through an H2 receptor; the effect was blocked by cimetadine but not by H1 antagonists or α-adrenergic antagonists.

cAMP metabolism in platelets is influenced by a variety of physical stimuli. Chilling increases cAMP (Zappia et al. 1976). Stirring, centrifugation and gel filtration lower the level of cAMP (Salzman et al. 1976), possibly as a consequence of the release of intracellular ADP.

Cyclic AMP and adenylate cyclase activity measured by Lammernant-Guillmare et al. (1977) in platelets stored in ACD anticoagulant did not change over two days.

Heparin inhibits the PGE_1-stimulated adenylate cyclase of platelet homogenates (Reches et al. 1979) and reduces the inhibitory effect of PGE_1. By a different mechanism, heparin directly neutralizes the effect of PGI_2, (Saba et al. 1979) possibly by accelerating its spontaneous hydrolysis.

VII. Subcellular Localization of CydicAMP

Platelet nucleotides are distributed between two compartments, the metabolically inert and active fractions (Holmsen et al. 1979). DaPrada et al. (1972) found that cAMP was highly enriched in a granule fraction isolated from platelet lysates on a sucrose density gradient, but did not report any effects of hormones. The possibility that labelled cAMP might behave differently when the nucleotide pool was labelled by adenosine rather than with adenine, has been raised by Salzman (1972) and by Dechavanne and Lagarge (1974). These differences were not confirmed by Haslam (1975), and may be explained by the direct effects of adenosine on the cyclase (Sect. B.III). Cutler et al. (1978) found that in glutaraldehyde-fixed platelets, using a cytochemical technique, adenylate cyclase was predominantly localized in the membranes of the dense tubular system, rather than in the plasma membrane. This was attributed to a greater degree of inactivation of the plasma membrane enzyme by the fixative.

VIII. Effects of Guanine Nucleotides

A requirement for GTP for the hormonal regulation of platelet adenylate cyclase was first noted by Krishna et al. (1972), who used App(NH)p instead of ATP, as the substrate for the enzyme assay. Stimulation by PGE_1 did not occur unless small amounts of GTP were added. The maximal effect of GTP was seen at a concentration of 100 μM; higher concentrations of GTP were less effective. GTP enhanced both basal activity and PGE_1-stimulated enzyme, but inhibited F^--stimulated enzyme activity. Jakobs et al. (1978c) have shown that the inhibitory effect of epinephrine also requires the presence of GTP; the maximal effect occured at a concentration of 10 μ*M*. Other nucleotides including dGTP, GDP, ITP and UTP could replace GTP, but these compounds were less potent (STEER and WOOD 1979). In the presence of 100 μ*M* GTP, epinephrine inhibited basal cyclase by 50% and PGE_1-stimulated activity by 28%, and its action was immediate. The relatively stable GTP analogues Gpp(NH)p, Gpp(CH_2)p and GTPγS caused a progressive, irreversible stimulation of the enzyme; in the presence of these activators, epinephrine no longer inhibited enzyme activation and GTP became an inhibitor. GTP also enhanced the stimulation of platelet membrane adenylate cyclase by cholera toxin (MELLWIG and JAKOBS 1980): this effect was completely blocked by 10 μ*M* epinephrine (JAKOBS 1978c; JAKOBS and SCHULTZ 1979). These observations have been explained in terms of a model in which the active enzyme is described as a complex between the catalytic unit, a regulatory unit and GTP. The formation of the complex is favoured by stimulatory hormones and its degradation, through hydrolysis of GTP, by inhibitory hormones. GORMAN et al. (1976) found that the inhibitory effect of prostaglandin endoperoxides on prostaglandin-stimulated cyclase was antagonised by GTP and by its stable analogs.

Using ATP as the substrate, STEER and WOOD (1979) found little effect of GTP on the basal activity of a particulate fraction prepared from lysed platelets by centrifuging at 8700 g. PGE_1-stimulated the activity of this preparation in the absence of added GTP, though GTP increased the stimulation slightly. Inhibition of the adenylate cyclase activity of this preparation by epinephrine required the addition of GTP. The basal activity was increased by Gpp(NH)p and other stable GTP analogues; the rate of activation was increased by PGE_1 but was unaffected by epinephrine. These experiments suggest that the platelet has two distinct GTP binding sites, one associated with the stimulatory effect of PGE_1 and the other with the inhibitory effect of epinephrine. A preparation of adenylate cyclase from dog platelet membranes described by LONGNECKER et al. (1980) was stimulated by PGE_1 without the need for added GTP. The inhibitory effect of ADP on the platelet cyclase is also increased by GTP, and does not occur when the enzyme is activated by stable GTP analogues (MELLWIG and JAKOBS 1980).

The displacement of radiolabelled α-adrenergic antagonists from their binding sites on platelet membranes is also influenced by guanine nucleotides (TSAI and LEFKOWITZ 1979; STEER et al. 1979; MICHEL et al. 1980). The apparent affinity of epinephrine for the α-adrenergic site was reduced 10-fold in the presence of 4–10 μ*M* GTP, though the binding affinity of the antagonist was unchanged. The stable analogue Gpp(NH)p was as active as GTP; the effect was greatest in the presence of 6 m*M* Mg^{2+}. The ability of GTP to reduce the binding affinity of an α-adrenergic agonist or partial agonist was closely correlated with the intrinsic activity of the compound as an inhibitor of adenylate cyclase (TSAI and LEFKOWITZ 1979). These authors have proposed a dynamic receptor model for the α-adrenergic inhibition of platelet adenylate cyclase, based on similarities with the β-adrenergic stimulation of the enzyme in avian erythrocytes. According to this scheme, the initially formed, low affinity agonist-receptor complex is converted to a high affinity form in the presence of Mg^{2+} and a regulatory component of the cyclase. GTP causes the dissociation of the agonist-receptor complex and conversion of the enzyme to the activated (or inhibited) form. Hydrolysis of GTP to GDP and Pi then returns the enzyme to the unactivated state. This model is supported by the ob-

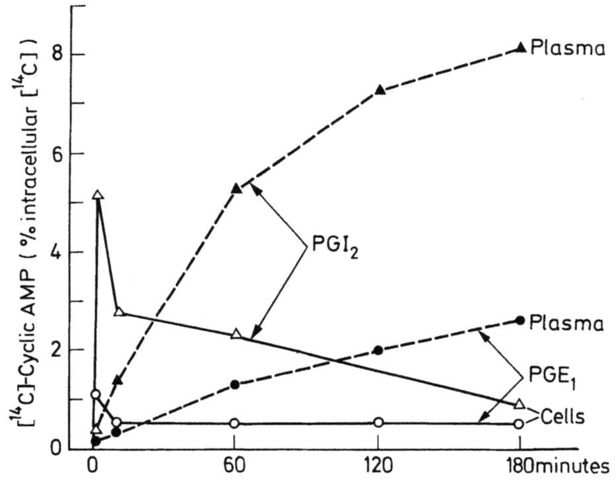

Fig. 7. Cyclic AMP accumulation in platelet rich plasma during extended incubation with PGE_1 or PGI_2. After an initial peak of intracellular radioactivity, the cAMP content of the platelets falls slowly, while cAMP continues to accumulate in the plasma, where it is not susceptible to that action of intracellular phosphodiesterase

servations of HOFFMAN et al. (1979) discussed above (Sect. B.IV.3); it suggests that the binding of prostaglandins and of ADP to platelet membranes may also be regulated by GTP.

C. Phosphodiesterase

I. Effects of Inhibitors

Inhibition of platelet aggregation by methylxanthines, including theophylline and caffeine, was described by ARDLIE et al. (1967) who suggested that these drugs could inhibit platelet functions by increasing the levels of cAMP. Papaverine inhibits aggregation and potentiates the inhibitory effect of adenosine (MARKWARDT et al. 1967), and is a strong inhibitor of platelet phosphodiesterase (MARKWARDT and HOFFMAN 1970). Phosphodiesterase inhibitors potentiate the effects of PGE_1, adenosine and isoproterenol on both aggregation and cAMP accumulation (MILLS et al. 1970; MILLS and SMITH 1971) and of PGI_2 (JORGENSEN et al. 1979). VIGDAHL et al. (1971) compared the activities of several phosphodiesterase inhibitors on a partly purified platelet enzyme. K_i values for competitive inhibition by papaverine (5μ*M*), dipyridamole (17 μ*M*), theophylline (0.8 m*M*) and caffeine (7 m*M*) were in good agreement with the relative activities of these compounds as aggregation inhibitors.

Phosphodiesterase from platelets is inhibited by several inhibitors of platelet aggregation, including adenosine (HORLINGTON and WATSON 1970) and 2-chloroadenosine (ASANO et al. 1977) and by PGE_1 (AMER and MARQUIS 1972). It is likely that stimulation of adenylate cyclase is the more significant action of these drugs, as adenosine does not have to enter the cell to inhibit aggregation, and PGE_1 causes only a transient increase in cAMP compared to the effects of PGD_2 and PGI_2 (Sect. B.II.1).

Table 1. Properties of the cyclic nucleotide phosphodiesterases from human platelets

	FI	FII	FIII
K_m for cAMP (μM)	500	40	0.35
K_m for cGMP (μM)	0.5	40	0.15
K_i for cAMP (μM)[a]	490	21	0.25
K_i for cGMP (μM)[b]		40	0.16
K_i for papaverine (μM)[b]	0.7	2.1	0.27
K_i for EG626 (μM)	43	9.5	1.0
Inhibition by 100 μM arachidonate	98%[a]	99%[a] 98%[b]	62%[b]
Inactivation by 30′ at 30	37%	32%	91%
Inactivation by 3 × Freeze/thaw	98%	52%	65%
Approximate Mr on Sepharose 6B	240,000	240,000	180,000
Migration rate on DEAE-cellulose	Fast	Medium	Slow
Sedimentation coefficient	8.9S	8.9S	4.6S

[a] With cGMP as substrate
[b] With cAMP as substrate. Data taken from HIDAKA et al. (1976a) and ASANO et al. (1977)

II. Properties of the Enzymes

Two forms of cAMP phosphodiesterase were described by SONG and CHEUNG (1971) and by AMER and MARQUIS (1972) and AMER and MAYNOL (1973); phosphodiesterase I was found in the soluble fraction, and phosphodiesterase II was partly soluble and partly associated with membranes. The activity of phosphodiesterase II, the higher affinity enzyme, was increased by epinephrine and reduced by PGE_1. A high and a low affinity phosphodiesterase were separated by PICHARD et al. (1973) by starch gel electrophoresis: the low affinity enzyme (Km 0.5 mM) was inhibited by dipyridamole, aminophylline and 6-mercaptopurine, but not by nortryptyline, an inhibitor of phosphodiesterase from brain (PICHARD et al. 1972). SMITH and MILLS (1971) found that human platelet phosphodiesterase was all soluble, and was more sensitive to inhibition by dipyridamole and its analogues RA 233 and RA 433 than were the enzymes from rabbit brain or bovine heart. Human platelet phosphodiesterase was not inhibited by KCN or by iodoacetamide (WANG et al. 1978) or by N-ethylmaleimide (MILLS 1974).

A third phosphodiesterase (FIII), relatively specific for cGMP, was identified by HIDAKA et al. (1974) and HIDAKA and ASANO (1976a): its properties are compared with those of the high (FI) and low (FII) affinity cAMP phosphodiesterases in Table 1. All three enzyme activities were inhibited by arachidonate and by other polyunsaturated fatty acids (HIROSE et al. 1978). This was not due to the formation of oxidation products, as neither soy bean lipoxidase nor thiol reducing agents influenced the inhibition.

III. Release from Platelets

Phosphodiesterase activity in heparin-anticoagulated rat plasma was very low when prepared from freshly drawn blood, but the enzyme activity increased if the blood was left standing for 1 h (PATTERSON et al. 1975). This probably reflects the release of phosphodiesterase from platelets. HIDAKA and ASANO (1976b) showed that phosphodiesterase is released from rat and from human platelets when they are stimulated either with thrombin or with the cationophore, A 23187. Of the three forms of phosphodiesterase identified in rat platelets, only two, a cAMP specific enzyme (MW 280,000) and a cGMP specific enzyme (MW 260,000) were released. A second cAMP specific enzyme (MW 180,000) was retained. Stimulation with A 23187 caused the release of about 80% of the total cAMP and cGMP phosphodiesterase activity in 10 min. Stimulation with thrombin caused a slower release, of about 40% in 30 min. Release of phosphodiesterase was closely associated with the uptake of Ca^{2+} ions from the medium.

IV. Regulatory Role of Phosphodiesterase

AMER and MARQUIS (1972) have reported that ADP and epinephrine increase the activity of high affinity cAMP phosphodiesterase. PICHARD and KAPLAN (1975) noted that dibutyryl cAMP increased the proportion of platelet phosphodiesterase that sedimented rapidly through a sucrose density gradient, and suggested that this represents an allosteric regulation mechanism. Because ADP and epinephrine decrease cAMP accumulation even in the presence of phosphodiesterase inhibitors, their effect on phosphodiesterase appears to be of lesser physiological consequence than their ability to inhibit adenylate cyclase.

V. Uses of Phosphodiesterase Inhibitors in Thrombosis

Dipyridamole (Persantine), a drug that was originaly introduced as a coronary vasodilator and which has anti thrombotic actions in a number of experimental conditions, is an inhibitor of platelet phosphodiesterase, though it is also a weak inhibitor of the arachidonate cyclooxygenase (BEST et al. 1979a). The drugs RA 233 and RA 433, which differ from dipyridamole in the nature of the substituents on the pyrimidopyrimide nucleus, are more active as inhibitors of platelet phosphodiesterase (SMITH and MILLS 1971; ROZENBERG and WALKER 1973; McELROY and PHILP 1976), but have proved too toxic for human use. MANNUCCI and PARETI (1974) found that dipyridamole increased the inhibitory effect on platelet aggregation (measured in platelet rich plasma) of dibutyryl cAMP infused into volunteers; in hypercholesterolemic rabbits, DEMBINSKA-KIEC et al. (1979a, b) found that dipyridamole reduced platelet cAMP levels and increased the severity of the arterial lesions produced by a cholesterol-rich diet. This effect was associated with a reduction in platelet ATP levels, possibly as a result of the powerful inhibition of adenosine uptake caused by this drug (SUBBARAO et al. 1977). MONCADA and KORBUT (1978) have shown that in rabbits its effect depends on potentiating the action of circulating endogenous prostacyclin. Whether this is also true for humans is uncertain, but the use of drugs that selectively inhibit platelet phosphodiesterase as antithrombotic agents is an attractive possibility for the pharmacological regulation of platelet aggregation in conditions disposing toward thrombosis (AMER and McKINNEY 1973).

D. Effects of Cyclic AMP on Platelet Function

I. Direct Effects

Cyclic AMP stimulates phosphofructokinase activity in platelet lysates (AKKERMAN et al. 1974) but increased levels of platelet cAMP are associated with inhibition of thrombin-stimulated glycolysis and glycogenolysis (WOLFE and SHULMAN 1979; ZIEVE and SCHMUCKLER 1971; SCHNEIDER 1974) and with a reduction in the liberation of arachidonate from phospholipids during exposure to aggregating agents (MINKES et al. 1977), resulting in a reduction in the synthesis of prostaglandins, endoperoxides and thromboxanes (VARGAFTIG and GHIGNARD 1975; MALMSTEN et al. 1976; GERRARD et al. 1977; LINDGREN et al. 1979). These effects may be due to the removal of Ca^{2+} required for the action of phospholipase A_2 (LAPETINA et al. 1977) and for glycogenolysis (GEAR and SCHNEIDER 1975). SCHAFER et al. (1980) found that oxygen consumption and malondialdehyde production in response to arachidonic acid were inhibited by agents that increase cAMP. This effect, which occured only in the presence of extracellular albumin, suggests inhibition of the cyclooxygenase, but FITZPATRICK and GORMAN (1979) found that thromboxanes continue to be produced even when cAMP levels were raised sufficiently to block aggregation.

STEINER (1978) has observed that cAMP binds to a subunit of platelet tubulin, increasing its rate of polymerization on warming, and suggesting a direct effect on platelet microtubule assembly. BARNES et al. (1974) have reported that cAMP affects the orientation of platelets on a glass slide.

II. Protein Kinases

Inhibition of platelet aggregation after elevation of cyclic AMP levels by PGE_1 does not hear a simple relationship to the cAMP level at any one time (BALL et al. 1970; MCDONALD and STUART 1973). This is partly due to the ability of some aggregating agents to rapidly lower the level, but even when aggregation is induced by vasopressin, which does not itself change cAMP levels (HASLAM and TAYLOR 1971b), the inhibition observed more closely follows the cAMP level measured 15 s. before the time when the aggregation rate is measured (HASLAM 1975). This suggested that the effect of cAMP is indirect. There is increasingly strong evidence that it is mediated by stimulation of protein phosphorylation.

A cAMP-dependent protein kinase associated with platelet membranes was described by BOOYSE et al. (1973). This enzyme had a molecular weight of 86,000, and it could be dissociated by cAMP into a catalytic and a regulatory subunit (see BEAVO and HUMBRY, Vol. 1). The enzyme phosphorylated endogenous membrane proteins of molecular weights 45,000, 28,000, 18,500 and 11,100 (BOOYSE et al. 1967). BISHOP and ROZENBERG (1975) found protein kinase activity in both soluble and particulate fractions of platelets. STEINER (1975) found that platelet membranes incubated with γ-[^{32}P]-ATP incorporated the [^{32}P]-PO_4 into three discrete components of molecular weight 52,000, 31,000 and 20,000: phosphorylation of the 52,000 dalton material was cAMP-dependent. This enzyme activity was stimulated by cations in the order $Mn^{++} > Co^{++} > Mg^{++}$; Ca^{++} was inactive. The [^{32}P]-PO_4 was found in hydroxy amino acids, mainly serine. A kinase from the soluble fraction of platelet lysates has been purified 12-fold by KAULEN and GROSS (1964). This enzyme was Mg^{++}-dependent, inhibited by Ca^{++}, and stimulated 2- to 3-fold by 1 μM cAMP or cGMP. Platelet actomyosin was not a substrate. ASSAF (1976, 1977) has crystalized a protein kinase purified 90-fold from platelet lysates. HASLAM et al. (1980) have described two cAMP dependent protein kinases comparable to the type 1 and type 2 enzymes in other tissues.

KARIYA et al. (1979) found that pretreatment of platelets with PGE_1 increased the activity of protein kinase in lysates prepared subsequently; similar effects were seen with PGA_1, which does not influence platelet aggregation.

III. Phosphorylation of Endogenous Substrates

The metabolically active fraction of platelet nucleotides can be labelled by incubating the cells with $[^{32}P]$-PO_4 (HOLMSEN 1965). APITZ-CASTRO et al. (1976) and APITZ-CASTRO and DEMURICIANO (1978) found a high molecular weight component of the platelet membrane whose state of phosphorylation was increased by dibutyryl cAMP (DBcAMP). PGE_1 and DBcAMP increase the phosphorylation of two polypeptides of molecular weights 24,000 and 22,000, designated P 24 and P 22 (HASLAM et al. 1978 d, 1979 b). These are clearly distinct from two additional polypeptides of molecular weights 47,000 and 20,000 (designated P 47 and P 20) whose phosphorylation is stimulated by treatment of the platelets with thrombin (LYONS et al. 1975), collagen or the ionophore A 23187 (FOX et al. 1979). Both P 47 and P 20 are soluble proteins, and P 20 has been identified with the light chain of platelet myosin (ADELSTEIN et al. 1978; DANIEL et al. 1977). HATHAWAY et al. (1981) have shown that the myosin light chain kinase of human platelets is a substrate for the catalytic subunit of cAMP dependent protein kinase, and that phosphorylation of this enzyme reduces its activity. This suggests a possible mechanism for the inhibitory effect of cAMP on platelet contractile activity through the regulation of actomyosin by light chain phosphorylation.

Phosphorylation of P 47 and P 20 following treatment of platelets with aggregating agents is thought to be due to an increase in the concentration of cytosolic calcium ion, and is inhibited by increases in cAMP (HASLAM and LYNHAM 1978; HASLAM 1978), suggesting that cAMP acts to remove Ca^{++} from the cytosolic compartment. Platelet membrane vesicles accumulate Ca^{++} in the presence of oxalate and ATP (GRETTE 1963; STATLAND et al. 1969; ROBLEE et al. 1973), and this uptake is stimulated by the combination of cAMP and a soluble platelet extract containing protein kinase (KÄSER-GLANZMANN et al. 1977). FOX et al. (1979) found that P 24 and P 22 were associated with platelet membranes sedimenting at between 19,000 and 90,000xg and that the accumulation of Ca^{++} by this fraction was enhanced by pretreatment of the platelets with PGE_1 and was inhibited by pretreatment with A 23187. It is not clear whether this membrane fraction derives primarily from the platelet plasma membrane or from intracellular organelles.

Platelets contain the ubiquitous calcium dependent regulator protein, calmodulin (MUSZBECK et al. 1977), but its effects on aggregation are not clearly defined. RAO et al. (1980) showed that trifluoperazine, a powerful antagonist of calmodulin-dependent reactions, has little effect on aggregation unless very high concentrations are used.

E. Cyclic GMP

I. Properties of Platelet Guanylate Cyclase

Platelets contain guanylate cyclase in large amounts. ADAMS and HASLAM (1978) found a specific activity for this enzyme of 0.5 pmoles/min/mg protein when platelets lysed by freezing and thawing were assayed at 30° in the presence of 4 m*M* $MnCl_2$. Others have found between 0.04 and 0.8 pmoles/min/mg in a variety of assay systems (BOHME et al. 1974; BARBER 1976; RODAN and FEINSTEIN 1976; GLASS et al. 1977a). The rather large range of values may reflect the influence of a number of factors that control the activity of this enzyme. Its activity spontaneously increased on standing (BOHME et al. 1974; GLASS et al. 1977a) by a process that was prevented by thiol reducing reagents. Nonionic detergents including Triton X100 and Lubrol PX stimulated activity (ADAMS and HASLAM 1978) as did various unsaturated fatty acids (BARBER 1976; HIDAKA and ASANO 1977). GLASS et al. (1977b) found that polyunsaturated fatty acids were most effective, and saturated fatty acids were inactive. ADAMS and HASLAM (1978) found that arachidonic and oleic acids were equally effective. HIDAKA and ASANO (1977) found that the stimulation of platelet guanylate cyclase, purified by DEAE-cellulose chromatography, by fatty acids was enhanced by the addition of lipoxidase. This was attributed to oxidation of susceptible sulfhydryl groups on guanylate cyclase. The enzyme activity was also stimulated by phospholipase A2, phosphatidyl choline and peroxides of arachidonic and linolenic acids. ASANO and HIDAKA (1977) describe the purification of guanylate cyclase to a specific activity of 3.1 nmoles/min/mg; this was increased 4-fold by arachidonic acid peroxide, and both the basal and stimulated activity were strongly inhibited by 1 m*M* ATP. From its elution behaviour on Sepharose 2B, the molecular weight was 180,000.

Platelet guanylate cyclase is a soluble enzyme. Small amounts of the enzyme with similar properties were found by RODAN and FEINSTEIN (1976) in a pariculate fraction but can be accounted for by contamination with cytoplasm (ADAMS and HASLAM 1978). The enzyme was stimulated by azide, nitrite and nitroprusside ions and by N-methyl-N′-nitro-N-nitrosoguanidine (WEISS et al. 1978) The pattern of activation by various factors found by ADAMS and HASLAM (1978) is quite complex, and the effects of preincubation, of detergents, fatty acids and azide ion depend upon the order of their addition. The greatest stimulation occurred with azide, but was reduced by prior treatment with Lubrol PX.

II. Control of Cyclic GMP Levels in Intact Platelets

Values for the resting cGMP level in the range 0.3–4 pmoles/10^8 platelets have been reported by numerous authors (BOHME and JAKOBS 1973; AGARWAL and STEINER 1976; GLASS et al. 1977b; SCHOEPFLIN et al. 1978; BEST et al. 1979b), with most results falling in the range 1–2 pmoles/10^8 platelets. The activity of guanylate cyclase in resting platelets is probably very low, due to the inhibitory effect of ATP, whose intracellular concentration is high (MILLS and THOMAS 1969; HOLMSEN et al. 1979). The difficulty of accurately measuring these low levels in the small tissue samples available and the presence of extracellular cGMP in platelet rich plasma led HASLAM and MCGLENAGHAN (1974) to introduce a prelabelling technique by which the intracellular guanine nucleotides are labelled by incubation of the cells with tritiated guanine. This has facilitated the investigation of the regulation of cGMP metabolism in intact cells. Considerable interest was originally aroused by observations that platelet cGMP levels were raised by aggregating agents including ADP (HASLAM 1975; HASLAM et al. 1978a), serotonin (AGARWAL and STEINER 1976; SCHOEPFLIN et al. 1977), collagen (HASLAM and MCGLENAGHAN 1974; CHIANG et al. 1975; HASLAM et al. 1975) and arachidonic acid (DAVIES et al. 1976). These results raised the possibility that cGMP might be a mediator of the aggregation process. In dog platelets, which are aggregated by cholinergic agents (CHUANG et al. 1974), both acetylcholine and carbamylcholine increased platelet cGMP levels, provided that calcium ions were present in the extracellular medium (HASLAM and SAY 1975; HASLAM 1975). Early observations of an increase in cGMP during aggregation induced by epinephrine (WHITE et al. 1973; JAKOBS et al. 1974) proved to be due to the ascorbic acid used as a preservative in the epinephrine solutions (GOLDBERG et al. 1975). Ascorbic acid neither induces aggregation nor enhances aggregation by other agents; this casts doubt on the association of cGMP with aggregation. An association between cGMP levels and the release reaction was suggested by the effects of cytochalasin B, which at low concentrations (1–5 μg/ml) increased both serotonin release and cGMP formation in response to collagen (HASLAM et al. 1975). Many experiments point to the conclusion that cGMP increases occur as a result of platelet aggregation rather than as part of the causal mechanism. The increases in cGMP with ADP or arachidonate were seen only if the platelet suspension was stirred, allowing aggregation to occur (HASLAM et al. 1978a). The increase in cGMP with collagen was inhibited by aspirin (HASLAM and MCGLENAGHAN 1974), which inhibits the formation of endoperoxides and thromboxanes. Although the stable PGG_2 analogues, U 44069 and U 46619, which aggregate platelets and cause the release of ADP, raised cGMP levels (BEST et al. 1979b), this effect was inhibited by the combination of creatine phosphate and creatine kinase, which removes released ADP (HASLAM et al. 1978a). Neither MILLER and GORMAN (1976) nor CLAESSON and MALMSTEN (1977) found an increase in cGMP in platelets exposed to the naturally occurring endoperoxide, PGG_2. Finally, HASLAM et al. (1978a) showed that ADP increased platelet cGMP levels during primary, reversible aggregation, when no endoperoxides are formed.

Cyclic GMP levels in platelets are increased by several drugs that inhibit aggregation including azide ion, nitrosoguanidines and nitroprusside. WEISS et al. (1978) found that the release of serotonin induced by thrombin was unaffected by either these drugs or by cGMP, 8-bromo-cGMP, or by dibutyryl cGMP. Indeed, according to CHIANG et al. (1976), cGMP and dibutyryl cGMP enhance aggregation and release of serotonin induced by epinephrine and collagen. They do not affect aggregation induced by ADP (CLAESSON and MALMSTEN 1977), and 8-bromo-cGMP is a strong inhibitor of aggregation and serotonin release induced by ADP (PARETI et al. 1978; HASLAM et al. 1980). These results are difficult to rationalize within a simple framework, and suggest that the involvement of cGMP in platelet functions is far from being completely understood. The effects of cGMP could be mediated by a cGMP-dependent protein kinase identified in platelet membranes by HAMET and COQUIL (1978).

F. Changes in Cyclic AMP Metabolism in Disease

The primary function of the platelet is the maintenance of haemostasis through the formation of the haemostatic plug. Consequently, most of the early interest in clinical abnormalities of cAMP metabolism in platelets was directed to conditions in which platelet function was known or suspected to be abnormal, i.e. in bleeding disorders and in conditions associated with thrombosis. It now seems likely that the platelet may be a useful indicator for functional abnormalities in other, less accessible organs such as the brain.

Thrombosis is associated with elevated levels of plasma lipids including cholesterol. Abnormalities of cAMP metabolism have been described in platelets whose cholesterol content was increased by prolonged incubation with cholesterol-rich liposomes. These platelets are abnormally sensitive to aggregation induced by epinephrine, but the number and affinity of α-adrenergic binding sites was unchanged (INSEL et al. 1978). Platelet cAMP was increased, but basal, PGE_1-, and fluoride-stimulated adenylate cyclase activity in lysates were all reduced (SINHA et al. 1977).

Aggregation by epinephrine is reduced in a variety of myeloproliferative disorders. In such conditions a reduction of adenylate cyclase activity (EGORAVA et al. 1978) and of epinephrine binding (VAINER and BUSSEL 1979) have been reported. KAYWIN et al. (1978) found a 50% reduction of binding sites for dihydroergocryptine in two patients with essential thrombocytosis and reduced responsiveness to adrenaline. Two other patients had normal numbers of binding sites and normal responsiveness. COOPER et al. (1978) have demonstrated, in 20 of 30 patients with essential thrombocytosis, a defect in the response of platelet adenylate cyclase to PGD_2 and a reduction in the number of PGD_2 binding sites. Five patients with reactive thrombocytosis had normal responsiveness. A specific reduction in the cyclase response to PGD_2 was also seen by COOPER (1979a) in 9 of 20 patients with acute thrombosis, and MEHTA and MEHTA (1980) have observed a reduced response to PGI_2 in 10 patients during episodes of angina pectoris.

PGE_1 and cAMP were both reduced on the third day after operation in patients undergoing surgery (LIGARDE and DECHAVANNE 1975) compared to their own preoperative levels. Neither measurement was correlated with the occurrence of venous thrombosis. YAMAZAKI et al. (1978) found no difference in the phosphodiesterases for cAMP or cGMP in patients with atherosclerosis when compared to healthy controls or to miscellaneous convalescent patients.

Patients being treated for heroin addiction with methadone showed a significant increase in PGE_1-stimulated adenylate cyclase during methadone withdrawal; the increase was correlated with the severity of the withdrawal symptoms (PANDEY et al. 1980). This raises the interesting question of whether the platelet has opiate receptors, as suggested by the findings of GRYGLEWSKI et al. (1979). RECHES et al. (1980) found no evidence for a modulating action of morphine on adenylate cyclase in platelet membranes, or the control of cAMP metabolism in intact cells. Further, they detected no specific binding of radiolabelled etorphine, a morphine receptor ligand, to platelet membranes.

Defective platelet aggregation, associated with a 2- to 4-fold elevation of the cAMP content of platelet rich plasma, occurs in Bartter's syndrome (STOFF et al. 1979), in which prostaglandin synthesis is abnormally high. Plasma from these patients increased cAMP levels in normal platelets. Both the aggregation defect and the platelet cAMP levels were corrected by treatment with inhibitors of prostaglandin synthesis.

SAMUEL et al. (1975) have reported that patients with cystic fibrosis, and their relatives have reduced inhibition of platelet aggregation by PGE_1.

Lithium carbonate, in concentration that are used in the treatment of affective disorders, reduces the stimulation of adenylate cyclase by PGE_1. A reduction by lithium of the inhibitory effect of epinephrine was seen by MURPHY et al. (1973) but not by WANG et al. (1974a). Patients suffering from moderately severe depression responded normally to PGE_1 and to epinephrine (WANG et al. 1974b; SCOTT et al. 1979).

ROTROSEN et al. (1978) found that platelets from schizophrenic patients are relatively unresponsive to PGE_1. This was confirmed for male but not for female patients by KAFKA et al. (1979). The number of α-adrenergic binding sites was higher in the men than in the women, but the patients were the same as controls of the same sex.

HAMET et al. (1978) have observed an increase in the formation of cAMP in platelets of spontaneously hypertensive rats stimulated by PGE_1, when compared to controls of the same age. The hypertensive rats also showed a lower increase in cAMP after exposure to epinephrine.

Possibly relevant to cAMP metabolism is the observation of ABDULLAH and HAMADAN (1975) that platelet lysates form PGE_1 from labelled eicosatrienoic acid when stimulated by high concentrations (100–450 μM) of ADP. This effect was decreased in 20 schizophrenic patients but was normal in depressed and manic patients. Platelets contain more PGE_1 than PGE_2 (LAGARDE et al. 1979) despite the relatively greater proportion of arachadonic acid, the precursor or 2-type PG's, than of eicosatrienoic acid in platelet membrane phospholipids. Increased production of E-type PG's has been seen in diabetes mellitus, a disease that strongly predisposes to thrombosis (HALUSHKA et al. 1977).

The investigation of cAMP metabolism in disease is still at early stage, but it has already made important contributions to the understanding of some pathological processes, including some that are not primarily associated with abnormalities of haemostasis. The platelet may prove to be a useful reporter of events and conditions occurring in inaccessible regions of the body.

References

Abdulla YH (1969) β-adrenergic receptors in human platelets. J Atherosclerosis Res 9:171–177

Abdulla YH, Hamadah K (1975) Effects of ADP on PGE_1-formation in blood platelets from patients with depression mania and schizophrenia. Br J Psychiatry 127:591–595

Adams AF, Haslam RJ (1978) Factors affecting the activity of guanylate cyclase in lysates of human blood patelets. Biochem J 174:23–35

Adelstein RL, Conti MA, Barylko B (1978) The role of myosin phosphorylation in regulating actin-myosin interaction in human blood platelets. Thromb Haemost 40:241–244

Adler JR, Handin RI (1979) Solubilization and characterization of a platelet membrane ADP-binding protein. J Biol Chem 254:3866–3872

Agarwal KC, Steiner M (1976) Effect of serotonin on cyclic nucleotides of human platelets. Biochem Biophys. Res Commun 69:962–969

Akkerman JWN, Gorter G, Sixma JJ, Stahl GEJ (1979) Influence of sulphate on effect of ADP, 3′,5′-cyclic AMP and citrate on human platelet phosphofructokinase activity. Int J Biochem 5:853–857

Alexander RW, Cooper B, Handin RI (1978) Characterization of human platelet alpha adrenergic receptor – correlation of (^{3}H) dihydroergocryptine binding with aggregation and adenylate cyclase inhibition. J Clin Invest 61:1136–1144

Amer M, Marquis NR (1972) The effect of prostaglandins, epinephrine and aspirin on cAMP phosphodiesterase activity of human blood platelets and their aggregation. In: Prostaglandins in cellular biology. Plenum Press, New York London, pp 93–105

Amer MS, Maynol RF (1973) Studies with phosphodiesterase III. Two forms of the enzyme from human blood platelets. Biochim Biophys Acta 309:149–156

Amer MS, McKinney GR (1973) Possibilities for drug development based on the cyclic AMP system. Life Sci 13:753–767

Anderson NH, Eggerman TL, Harker LA, Wilson CHD (1980) On the multiplicity of platelet prostaglandin receptors. I. Evaluation of competitive antagonism by aggregometry. Prostaglandins 19:711–755

Apitz-Castro R, DeMurciano A (1978) Modulation of platelet responsiveness through selective phosphorylation of plasma membrane proteins. Biochim Biophys Acta 544:529–539

Apitz-Castro R, Ramirez E, Maignon R, DeMurciano A, Ribbi A (1976) Plasma membrane phosphorylation by endogenous phosphate donors in human blood platelets. Selectivity of the action of cyclic AMP. Biochim Biophys Acta 455:371–382

Ardlie NG, Glew G, Schwartz CJ (1966) Influence of catecholamines on nucleotide-induced platelet aggregation. Nature 212:415–416

Ardlie NG, Glew G, Schultz BG, Schwartz CJ (1967) Inhibition and reversal of platelet aggregation by methyl xanthines. Thromb Diath Haemorrh 18:670–673

Asano T, Hidaka H (1977) Purification of guanylate cyclase from human platelets and the effect of arachidonic acid peroxide. Biochem Biophys Res Commun 78:910–918

Asano T, Ochai Y, Hidaka H (1977) Selective inhibition of separated forms of human platelet cyclic nucleotide phosphodiesterase by platelet aggregation inhibitors. Mol Pharmacol 13:400–406

Assaf SF (1976) Cyclic AMP mediated phosphorylation reactions in the regulation of blood platelet aggregation. Int J Biochem 7:535–540

Assaf SF (1977) Human platelet protein kinases reaction with platelet membranes and cytoplasmic enzymes and crystalization of a cyclic AMP-dependent protein kinase. Ann NY Acad Sci 283:159–174

Ball G, Brereton GG, Fulwood M, Ireland DM, Yates P (1970) Effect of prostaglandin E_1 alone or in combination with theophylline or aspirin on collagen induced platelet aggregation and on platelet nucleotides including adenosine 3′,5′ monophosphate. Biochem J 102:709–718

Barber AJ (1976). Cyclic nucleotides and platelet aggregation. Effect of aggregating agents on the activity of cyclic nucleotide metabolizing enzymes. Biochim Biophys Acta 444:579–595

Barnes FS, Gamow E, Burns A, deBoisfleury A (1974) Directional effects of cyclic AMP on platelets. Clin Sci Mol Med 46:307–309

Best LC, Martin TJ, Russell RGG, Preston FE (1977) Prostacyclin increases cyclic AMP levels and adenylate cyclase activity in platelets. Nature 267:850–851

Best LC, McGuire MB, Jones PBB, Holland TK, Martin TJ, Preston FE, Segal DS, Russell RGG (1979a) Mode of action of dipyridamole on human platelets. Thromb Res 16:367–379

Best LC, McGuire MB, Martin TJ, Preston FE, Russell RGG (1979b) Effects of epoxymethano analogs of prostaglandin endoperoxides on aggregation, on release of 3′,5′-cyclic AMP and cyclic GMP in human platelets. Biochim Biophys Acta 583:344–351

Bishop GA, Rosenberg MC (1975) The effect of ADP, calcium and some inhibitors of platelet aggregation on protein phosphokinases from human blood platelets. Biochim Biophys Acta 385:112–119

Bohme E, Jakobs KH (1973) Guanosine 3:5-monophosphate in human platelets. IRC Int Res Com Sys 1:30

Bohme E, Jung R, Mechler I (1974) Guanylate cyclase in human platelets. Methods Enzymol 38C:199–202
Booyse FM, Marr J, Young DC, Guiliani D, Rafelson ME (1967) Adenosine cyclic 3′,5′-monophosphate-dependent protein kinase from human platelets. Biochim Biophys Acta 422:60–72
Booyse FM, Guiliani D, Marr JJ, Rafelson ME (1973) Cyclic adenosine 3′,5′-monophosphate dependent protein kinase of human platelets: membrane phosphorylation and regulation of platelet function. Ser Haematol 6:351–366
Born GVR, Cross MJ (1963) Inhibition of the aggregation of blood platelets by substances related to adenosine diphosphate. J Physiol 166:29–30 P
Bousser M-G (1973) Prostaglandin E_1 and platelets. Biomedicine 1:95–102
Brodie GN, Baenziger NL, Chase LR, Majerus PW (1972) The effects of thrombin on adenylate cyclase activity and a membrane protein from human platelets. J Clin Invest 51:81–88
Bruno JJ, Taylor LA, Droller MJ (1974) Effects of prostaglandin E_2 on human platelet adenylate cyclase and aggregation. Nature 251:721–723
Bunting S, Gryglewski R, Moncada S, Vane JR (1976) Arterial walls generate from prostaglandin endoperoxides a substance (prostaglandin X) which relaxes strips of mesenteric and coeliac arteries and inhibits platelet aggregation. Prostaglandins 12:897–913
Chiang TM, Beachey EH, Kang AH (1975) Interaction of a chick skin collagen fragment (αl-CB 5) with human platelets. J Biol Chem 250:6916–6922
Chiang TM, Dixit SN, Kang AH (1976) Effect of 3′,5′-guanosine monophosphate on human platelet function. J Lab Clin Med 88:215–221
Chuang HYK, Shermer RW, Mason RG (1974) Acetylcholine-induced release reaction of canine platelets. Res Commun Chem Pathol Pharmacol 7:330–346
Claesson H-E, Malmsten C (1977) On the relationship of prostaglandin endoperoxide G_2 and cyclic nucleotides in platelet function. Eur J Biochem 76:277–284
Cole B, Robison GA, Hartmann RC (1971) Studies on the role of cyclic AMP in platelet function. Ann NY Acad Sci 185:477–487
Colman RW, Figures WR, Colman RF, Morinelli TA, Niewiarowski S, Mills DCB (1980) Identification of two distinct adenosine diphosphate receptors in human platelets. Trans Am Soc Phys 93:305–316
Cooper B (1979 a) Diminished platelet adenylate cyclase activation by prostaglandin D_2 in acute thrombosis. Blood 54:694–693
Cooper B (1979 b) Agonist regulation of the human platelet D_2 receptor. Life Sci 25:1361–1368
Cooper B, Ahern D (1979) Characterization of the platelet prostaglandin D_2 receptor. J Clin Invest 64:586–590
Cooper B, Handin RI, Young LH, Alexander RW (1978 a) Agonist regulation of the human platelet α-adrenergic receptor. Nature 274:703–706
Cooper B, Shafer AI, Puchalsky D, Handin RI (1978 b) Platelet resistance to prostaglandin D_2 in patients with myeloproliferative disorders. Blood 52:618–626
Cooper B, Schaffer AI, Puchalsky D, Handin RI (1979) Desensitization of prostaglandin activated platelet adenylate cyclase. Prostaglandins 17:561–571
Cooper DMF, Rodbell M (1979) ADP is a potent inhibitor of human platelet plasma membrane adenylate cyclase. Nature 282:517–518
Cusack NJ, Hickman ME, Born GVR (1979) Effects of D and L enantiomers of adenosine, AMP, ADP and their 2-azido-analogues on human platelets. Proc R Soc Lond [Biol] 206:139–144
Cuthbertson WFJ, Mills DCB (1963) Some factors influencing platelet clumping. J Physiol 169:9 P
Cutler L, Rodan G, Feinstein MB (1978) Cytochemical localization of adenylate cyclase and of calcium ion, magnesium ion activated ATP'ase in the dense tubular system of human blood platelets. Biochim Biophys Acta 542:357–371
Daniel JL, Holmsen H, Adelstein RS (1977) Thrombin-stimulated myosin phosphorylation in intact platelets and its possible involvement in secretion. Thromb Haemost 38:984–989

DaPrada M, Burckhard WP, Pletscher A (1972) Cyclic AMP of blood platelets: accumulation in organelles storing 5 hydroxytryptamine and ATP. Experientia 72:845
Davies T, Davidson MML, McGlenaghan MD, Saye A, Haslam RJ (1976) Factors affecting platelet cyclic GMP levels during aggregation induced by collagen and by arachidonic acid. Thromb Res 9:387–405
Dechavanne M, Lagarde M (1974) Mise en evidence de deux compartements d'AMP cyclique dans des suspensions de plaquettes humaines. Pathol Biol 22:17–21
Dembinska-Kiec A, Rucker W, Schonhofer PS (1979a) Effect of dipyridamole in experimental atherosclerosis. Action on PGI_2, platelet aggregation and atherosclerotic plaque formation. Atherosclerosis 33:315–327
Dembinska-Kiec A, Rucker W, Schonhofer PS (1979b) Effects of dipyridamole in vivo on ATP and cAMP content in platelets and arterial walls and on atherosclerotic plaque formation. Arch Pharmacol 309:59–64
Demopoulos CA, Pinkard RN, Hanahan DJ (1979) Platelet activating factor. Evidence for 1-0-alkyl-2-acetyl-sn-glycerol-3-phosphoryl choline as the active component (a new class of lipid chemical mediators). J Biol Chem 254:9355–9358
Detwiler TC, Charo IF, Feinman RD (1978) Evidence that calcium regulates platelet function. Thromb Haemost 40:207–211
Diesseroth A, Wolfe SM, Shulman NR (1970) Platelet phosphorylase activity in the presence of activators an inhibitors of aggregation. Biochem Biophys Res Commun 39:551–557
Dodds WJ (1978) Platelet function in animals: species specificities. In: DeGaetano G, Garattini S (eds) Platelets: A multidisciplinary approach. Raven Press, New York, pp 45–59
Droller MJ (1976) Thrombin-induced platelet prostaglandin production and a possible intrinsic modulation of platelet function. Scand J Haematol 17:167–178
Droller MJ, Wolfe SM (1972) Thrombin induced increase in intracellular cyclic 3',5'adenosine monophosphate in human platelets. J Clin Invest 51:3094–3103
Egorava VA, Belyaeva ZN, Blinova MN (1978) Activity of adenyl cyclase from platelets in some blood systemic impairments. Vopr Med Khim 24:28
Feinstein MB, Rodan GA, Cutler LS (1981) Cyclic AMP and calcium in platelet function. In: Gordon JL (ed) Platelets in biology and pathology, vol 2. Elsevier/North Holland, Amsterdam, pp 437–472
Fitzpatrick FA, Gorman RR (1979) Regulatory role of cyclic adenosine 3',5'-monophosphate on platelet cyclooxygenase and platelet function. Biochim Biophys Acta 582:44–58
Fox JEB, Say AK, Haslam RJ (1979) Subcellular distribution of the different platelet proteins phosphorylated on exposure to ionophore A 23187 or to prostaglandin E_1. Possible role of a membrane phosphopolypeptide in the regulation of calcium ion transport. Biochem J 184:651–661
Gear ARL, Schneider W (1975) Control of platelet glycogenolysis by calcium. Biochim Biophys Acta 392:111–120
Gerrard JM, Peller JD, Krick TP, White JG (1977) Cyclic AMP and platelet prostaglandin synthesis. Prostaglandins 14:39–50
Glass DB, Frey W 2nd, Carr DW, Goldberg ND (1977a) Stimulation of human platelet guanylate cyclase by fatty acids. J Biol Chem 252:1279–1285
Glass DB, Gerrard JM, Townsend D, Carr DW, White JG, Goldberg ND (1977b) The involvement of prostaglandin endoperoxide formation in the elevation of cyclic GMP levels during platelet aggregation. J Cyclic Nucleotide Res 3:37–44
Goldberg ND, Haddox MK, Nicol SE, Glass DB, Sanford CH, Kuehl FA Jr, Stensen RE (1975) Biologic regulation through opposing influences of cyclic GMP and cyclic AMP: the Yin Yang hypothesis. Adv Cyclic Nucleotide Res 5:307–330
Gorman RR (1974) Specific PGE_1 and PGE_2 binding sites on platelet membranes. Prostaglandins 6:542
Gorman RR (1975) Prostaglandin endoperoxides: possible new regulators of cyclic nucleotide metabolism. J Cyclic Nucleotide Res 1:1–9
Gorman RR (1979) Modulation of human platelet function by prostacyclin and thromboxane B2. Fed Proc 38:83–87

Gorman RR, Hamberg M, Samuelsson B (1976) Antagonism of the prostaglandin endoperoxide inhibition of hormone-stimulated a denylate cyclase by guanosine triphosphate and 5′guanylylimmidodiphosphate. Biochim Biophys Acta 444:596–603

Gorman RR, Bunting S, Miller O (1977) Modulation of human platelet adenylate cyclase by prostacyclin. Prostaglandins 13:377–388

Gorman RR, Wierenga W, Miller OV (1979) Independence of the cyclic AMP-lowering activity of thromboxane A_2 from the platelet release reaction. Biochim Biophys Acta 572:95–104

Grant JA, Scrutton MC (1979) Novel alpha$_2$-adrenoceptors primarily responsible for inducing human platelet aggregation. Nature 277:659–661

Grant JA, Scrutton MC (1980) Interactions of selective α-adrenoceptor agonists and antagonists with human and rabbit platelets. Br J Pharmacol 71:121–124

Grette K (1963) Relaxing factor in extracts of human platelets and its function in the cells. Nature 198:488–489

Gryglewski RJ, Szczeklik A, Krysztof B (1975) Morphine antagonises prostaglandin E1-mediated inhibition of human platelet aggregation. Nature 256:5–57

Halushka PV, Lurie D, Colwell JA (1977) Increased synthesis of prostaglandin E-like material by platelets from patients with diabetes melitus. N Engl J Med 297:1306–1310

Hamet P, Coquil JF (1978) Cyclic GMP binding and cyclic GMP phosphodiesterase in rat platelets. J Cyclic Nucleotide Res 4:281–290

Hamet P, Fraysse J, Franks DJ (1978) Cyclic nucleotides and aggregation in platelets of spontaneously hypertensive rats. Circ Res 43:583–591

Harris DN, Asaad MM, Phillips MB, Goldenberg HJ, Antonaccio MJ (1979) Inhibition of adenylate cyclase in human blood platelets by 9-substituted adenine derivatives. J Cyclic Nucleotide Res 5:125–134

Harwood JP, Moskowitz J, Krishna GG (1972) Dynamic interaction of prostaglandin and norepinephrine in the formation of adenosine 3′5′monophosphate in human and rabbit platelets. Biochim Biophys Acta 261:444–456

Hashimoto S, Shibata S, Kobayashi B (1975) Dependence of platelet adenylate cyclase system on oxidative phosphorylation. Thromb Diath Haemorrh 34:42–49

Haslam RJ (1973) Interactions of the pharmacological receptors of blood platelets with adenylate cyclase. Ser Haematol 6:333–350

Haslam RJ (1975) Role of cyclic nucleotides in platelet function. Ciba Found Symp 35:121–151

Haslam RJ (1978) Cyclic nucleotides in platelet function. In: Day HJ, Holmsen H, Zucker MB (eds) Platelet function testing. DHEW Publication (NIH) 78-1087, pp 487–503

Haslam RJ, Cusack NJ (1981) Blood platelet receptors for ADP and adenosine. In: Burnstock G (ed) Receptors and recognition, series B, vol 9: Purinergic receptors. Chapman & Hall, London

Haslam RJ, Lynham J (1972) Activation and inhibition of blood platelet adenylate cyclase by adenosine or by 2-chloroadenosine. Life Sci 11(II):1143–1154

Haslam RJ, Lynham J (1977) Relationship between phosphorylation of blood platelet proteins and secretion of platelet granule constituents. I. Effects of different aggregating agents. Biochem Biophys Res Commun 77:714–722

Haslam RJ, Lynham J (1978) Relationship between phosphorylation of blood platelet proteins and secretion of platelet granule contents. II. Effects of different inhibitors. Thromb Res 12:619–628

Haslam RJ, McGlenaghan MD (1974) Effects of collagen and of aspirin on the concentration of guanosine 3′:5′-cyclic monophosphate in human blood platelets: measurement by a prelabelling technique. Biochem J 138:317–320

Haslam RJ, McGlenaghan MD (1981) Measurement of circulating prostacyclin. Nature 292:364–366

Haslam RJ, Rosson GM (1975) Effects of adenosine on levels of adenosine cyclic 3′,5′-monophosphate in human blood platelets in relation to adenosine incorporation and platelet aggregation. Mol Pharmacol 11:528–544

Haslam RJ, Say A (1975) Effects of acetylcholine and carbachol on cyclic GMP levels in dog platelets ion relation to platelet function: role of extracellular Ca^{2+} ions. Fed Proc 34:231

Haslam RJ, Taylor A (1971a) Effects of catecholamines on the formation of adenosine 3′:5′-cyclic monophosphate in human blood platelets. Biochem J 125:377–379
Haslam RJ, Taylor A (1971b) Role of cyclic 3′5′ adenosine monophosphate on platelet aggregation. In: Caen JP (ed) Platelet aggregation. Masson, Paris, pp 85–93
Haslam RJ, Davidson MML, McClenagham MD (1975) Cytochalasin B, the blood platelet release reaction and cyclic GMP. Nature 253:455–457
Haslam RJ, McGlenaghan MD, Adams A (1975) Depression of cyclic GMP levels in blood platelets by acetylsalicylic acid (ASA) and related drugs. Adv Cyclic Nucleotide Res 5:821
Haslam RJ, Davidson MML, Davies T, Lynham JA, McGlenaghan MD (1978a) Regulation of blood platelet function by cyclic nucleotides. Adv Cyclic Nucleotide Res 9:533–552
Haslam RJ, Davidson MML, Desjardins JV (1978b) Inhibition of adenylate cyclase by adenosine analogues in preparations of broken and intact human platelets. Evidence for the unidirectional control of platelet function by cyclic AMP. Biochem J 176:83–95
Haslam RJ, Davidson MML, Desjardins JV, Fox J, Lynham J (1978c) Factors affecting the formation and actions of cyclic AMP in blood platelets. Adv Pharmacol Ther 4:75–85
Haslam RJ, Davidson MML, Fox J, Lynham J (1978d) Cyclic nucleotides in platelet function. Thromb Haemost 40:232–240
Haslam RJ, Davidson MML, Lemmex BWG, Desjardins JV, McCarry BE (1979a) Adenosine receptors of the blood platelet: interactions with adenylate cyclase. In: Baer HP, Drummond GI (eds) Physiological and regulatory functions of adenosine and adenine nucleotides. Raven Press, New York, pp 189–204
Haslam RJ, Lynham J, Fox J (1979b) Effects of collagen, ionophore A 23187 and prostaglandin E1 on the phosphorylation of specific proteins in blood platelets. Biochem J 178:397–406
Haslam RJ, Salama SE, Fox JEB, Lynham JA, Davidson MML (1980) Roles of cyclic nucleotides and of protein phosphorylation in the regulation of platelet function. In: Rotman A, Meyer FA, Gitler C, Silberberg A (eds) Platelets: Cellular Response Mechanism and their Biological Significance. Wiley, Chichester, pp 213–231
Hathaway DR, Eaton CR, Adelstein RS (1981) Regulation of human platelet myosin light chain kinase by the catalytic subunit of cyclic AMP-dependent protein kinase. Nature 291:252–254
Hidaka H, Asano T (1976a) Human Blood platelet 3′:5′-cyclic nucleotides phosphodiesterase. Isolation of low Km and high Km phosphodiesterase. Biochim Biophys Acta 429:485–497
Hidaka H, Asano T (1976b) Platelet cyclic 3′:5′-nucleotide phosphodiesterase released by thrombin and calcium ionophore. J Biol Chem 251:7508–7516
Hidaka H, Asano T (1977) Stimulation of human platelet guanylate cyclase by unsaturated fatty acid peroxides. Proc Natl Acad Sci USA 74:3657–3661
Hidaka H, Asano T, Shibuya M, Shimamoto T (1974) Cyclic GMP phosphodiesterase of human blood platelets and its inhibitors. Thromb Diath Haemorrh [Suppl] 60:321–327
Hirose S, Asano T, Hidaka H (1978) Effects of unsaturated fatty acids on separated forms of human platelet cyclic nucleotide phosphodiesterase. Thromb Res 12:701–706
Hoffman BB, LeDean A, Wood CL, Schocken DD, Lefkowitz RJ (1979) Alpha-adrenergic receptor subtypes: quantitative assessment by ligand binding. Life Sci 24:1739–1746
Hoffman BB, Michel T, Mulliken-Kilpatrick D, Lefkowitz RJ, Tolbert MEM, Filman H, Fain JN (1980) Agonist versus antagonist binding to a adrenergic receptors. Proc Natl Acad Sci USA 77:4569–4573
Holmsen H (1965) Incorporation of ^{32}P into platelet acid soluble organophosphates and their chromatographic identification. Scand J Clin Lab Invest 17:230–242
Holmsen H, Smith JB, Daniel JL, Holme S, Bills ,TK (1979) Platelet biochemistry. In: Schmidt RM (ed) CRC Handbook Series in Clinical Laboratory Science, vol 1. pp 273–312
Honegger H, Trimmer R, Bally P (1975) Rise and fall of the cAMP content in human blood platelets after stimulation of their adenyl cyclase with prostaglandin E_1. Experientia 31:729
Horch U, Kadatz R, Kopitar Z, Weisenberger H (1970) Pharmacology of dipyridamole and its derivatives. Thromb Diath Haemorh [Suppl] 42:253–266

Horlington M, Watson PA (1970) Inhibition of 3'5' cyclic AMP phosphodiesterase by some platelet aggregation inhibitors. Biochem Pharmacol 19:955–956

Hornstra G, Haddeman E, Don JA (1979) Blood platelets do not provide endoperoxides for vascular prostacyclin synthesis. Nature 279:66–68

Hsu CY, Knapp DR, Halushka PV (1979) The effects of alpha adrenergic agents on human platelet aggregation. J Pharmacol Exp Ther 28:36–37

Hughes RJ, Insel PA (1980) Regulation of cyclic AMP levels in human platelets. Fed Proc 39:424

Insel PA, Nirenberg P, Turnbull J, Shattil SJ (1978) Relationships between membrane cholesterol, α-adrenergic receptors, and platelet function. Biochemistry 17:5269–5274

Jakobs KH (1978 a) Inhibition of platelet adenylate cyclase by α-adrenergic agents. In: Falco G, Paoletti R (eds) Molecular biology and pharmacology of cyclic nucleotides: Proceedings of the NATO Advanced Study Institute on Cyclic Nucleotides. Elsevier/North Holland, New York

Jakobs KH (1978 b) Synthetic α-adrenergic agonists are potent α-adrenergic blockers in human platelets. Nature 274:819–820

Jakobs KH (1978 c) GTP-dependent inhibition of platelet adenylate cyclase by a adrenergic agents. In: Krause EG et al. (ed) Cyclic nucleotides and protein phosphorylation in cell regulation: Proc 12th FEBS Meeting. Pergamon, Oxford, pp 11–19

Jakobs KH, Rauschek R (1978) (^{3}H) Dihydroergonine binding to α-adrenergic receptors in human platelets. Klin Wochenschr [Suppl 1] 56:139–145

Jakobs KH, Schultz G (1979) Different inhibitory effects of adrenaline on platelet adenylate cyclase E.C. 4.6.1.1 in the presence of GTP plus cholera toxin and stable GTP analogs. Naunyn Schmiedebergs Arch Pharmacol 310:121–128

Jakobs KH, Bohme E, Mocikat S (1974) Cyclic GMP formation in human platelets. Naunyn Schmiedebergs Arch Pharmacol [Suppl] 282:R 40

Jakobs KH, Saur W, Schultz G (1976) Reduction of adenylate cyclase activity of human platelets by the alpha adrenergic component of epinephrine. J Cyclic Nucleotide Res 2:381–392

Jakobs KH, Sauer W, Schultz G (1978 a) Metal and metal-ATP interactions with human platelet adenylate cyclase: effects of alpha adrenergic inhibition. Mol Pharmacol 14:1073–1078

Jakobs KH, Saur W, Schultz G (1978 b) Characterisation of α- and β-adrenergic receptors linked to human platelet adenylate cyclase. Naunyn Schmiedebergs Arch Pharmacol 302:285–291

Jakobs KH, Saur W, Schultz G (1978 c) Inhibition of platelet adenylate cyclase by epinephrine requires GTP. FEBS Lett 85:167–170

Jakobs KH, Saur W, Johnson RA (1979) Regulation of platelet adenylate cyclase by adenosine. Biochim Biophys Acta 583:409–421

Johnson RA, Saur W, Jakobs KH (1979) Effects of prostaglandin E_1 and adenosine on metal and metal-ATP kinetics of platelet adenylate cyclase. J Biol Chem 234:1095–1101

Jorgensen KA, Dyerberg J, Stofferson E (1979) PGI_2 and the effect of phosphodiesterase inhibitors on platelet function. Pharmacol Res Commun 11:605–615

Kafka MS, Tallman JF, Smith CC, Costa JL (1977) Alpha adrenergic receptors on human platelets. Life Sci 21:1429–1438

Kafka MS, VanKammen DP, Bunney WE Jr (1979) Reduced cyclic AMP production in the blood platelets from schizophrenic patients. Am J Psychiatry 136:685–687

Kariya T, Kume S, Tanabe A, Kaneko T, Yamanaka M, Oda T (1979) Effects of PGE_1 on protein kinase activity and endogenous phosphorylation of intact human platelets. Biochem Pharmacol 28:2747–2751

Kaser-Glanzmann R, Jacabova M, George JN, Luscher EF (1977) Stimulation of calcium uptake in platelet membrane vesicles by adenosine 3',5'-cyclic monophosphate and protein kinase. Biochim Biophys Acta 466:429–440

Kaulen HD, Gross R (1964) Purification and properties of a soluble cyclic AMP dependent protein kinase of human platelets. Hoppe Seylers Z Physiol Chem 355:471–480

Kaywin P, McDonough M, Insel PA, Shattil SJ (1978) Platelet function in essential thrombocythemia. N Engl J Med 299:505–509

Kloeze J (1966) Influence of prostaglandins on platelet aggregation and platelet adhesiveness. In: Bergstrom S, Samuelsson B (eds) Proc II Nobel Symposium Interscience, London, pp 241–252

Kloeze J (1969) Relationship between chemical structure and platelet aggregation activity of prostaglandins. Biochim Biophys Acta 187:285–292

Klysner R, Geisler A, Hansen KW, Stahlskov P, Norn S (1980) Histamine H2 receptor-mediated cyclic AMP formation in human platelets. Acta Pharmacol Toxicol 47:1–4

Krishna G, Harwood JP, Barber AJ, Jamieson GA (1972) Requirement for guanosine triphosphate in the prostaglandin activation of adenylate cyclase of platelet membranes. J Biol Chem 247:2253–2254

Lagard M, Dechavanne M (1975) Etude de taux d'AMP cyclique (AMPc) et de prostaglandine E_1 (PGE_1) dans les plaquettes sanguines, avant et au cours des thromboses veineuses post-operatoires. Biomedicine 23:374–377

Lagard M, Dechavanne M, Rigaud M, Durand J (1979) Basal level of human platelet prostaglandins. PGE_1 is more elevated than PGE_2. Prostaglandins 17:685–705

Lammernant-Guillemare E, Corcelle-Cerf F, Lammernant J (1977) Cyclic 3′,5′-adenosine monophosphate level and adenylate cyclase activity in human blood platelets during storage in ACD solution. Blut 34:329–330

Lapetina EG, Schmitges CJ, Chandrabose K, Cuatrecasas P (1977) Cyclic adenosine 3′,5′-monophosphate and prostacyclin inhibit membrane phospholipase activity in platelets. Biochem Biophys Res Commun 76:828–835

Lasch P, Jakobs KH (1979) Agonistic and antagonistic effects of various α-adrenergic agonists in human platelets. Naunyn Schmiedebergs Arch Pharmacol 306:119–125

Lindgren JA, Claesson HE, Kindahl H, Hammerstrom S (1979) Effects of adenosine 3′:5′-monophosphate and platelet aggregation on thromboxane biosynthesis in human platelets. FEBS Lett 98:247–250

Londos C, Wolff J (1977) Two distinct adenosine sensitive sites on adenylate cyclase. Proc Natl Acad Sci USA 74:5482–5486

Longnecker GL, Koaciewicz LJ, Palmer SJ, Palmer GC (1980) Prostaglandin stimulation of canine platelet adenylate cyclase. Thromb Res 19:119–124

Lyons RM, Stanford N, Majerus PW (1975) Thrombin-induced protein phosphorylation in human platelets. J Clin Invest 56:924–936

Macfarlane DE, Mills DCB (1975) The effects of ATP on platelets: evidence against the central role of released ADP in primary aggregation. Blood 46:309–320

Macfarlane DE, Mills DCB (1977) The number and nature of ADP receptors on human blood platelets determined with a photoaffinity label. Thromb Haemost 38:241

Macfarlane DE, Mills DCB (1981) Inhibition by ADP of prostaglandin induced accumulation of cyclic AMP in intact human platelets. J Cyclic Nucleotide Res 7:1–11

Macfarlane DE, Stump DC (1981) Selective binding of ^3H yohimbine to the α_2-receptor of intact platelets – comparison with ^3H dihydroergocryptine binding. Thromb Haemost 46:24

Macfarlane DE, Srivastava PC, Mills DCB (1979) 2 Methylthioadenosine 5′-diphosphate, a high affinity probe for ADP receptors on the human platelet. Thromb Haemost 42:182

MacIntyre DE (1981) Platelet prostaglandin receptors. In: Gordon JL (ed) Platelets in biology and pathology, vol 2. Elsevier/North Holland, Amsterdam pp 211–247

MacIntyre DE, Gordon JL (1975) Calcium-dependent stimulation of platelet aggregation by PGE_2. Nature 258:337–339

MacIntyre DE, Gordon JL (1977) Discrimination between platelet prostaglandin receptors with a specific antagonist of bisenoic prostaglandins. Thromb Res 11:705–713

Maguire HM, Penglis-Caredes F, Gough GR (1974) Effects of the 3′5′-cyclic phosphates of 2-methylthioadenosine, 2-chloroadenosine and adenosine on platelet aggregation. Experientia 30:922–92454

Malmsten C, Granstrom E, Samuelsson B (1976) Cyclic AMP inhibits synthesis of prostaglandin endoperoxides (PGG_2) in human platelets. Biochim Biophys Acta 68:569–576

Mannucci PM, Pareti FI (1974) Platelet functions after intravenous administration in man of cyclic AMP and related drugs. J Lab Clin Med 84:828–838

Marcus AJ, Zucker MB (1965) The physiology of blood platelets. Grune & Stratton, New York

Markwardt F, Hoffmann A (1970) Effects of papaverine derivatives on cyclic AMP phosphodiesterase of human platelets. Biochem Pharmacol 19:2519–2520

Markwardt F, Barthel W, Glusa E, Hoffmann A (1967) Untersuchungen über den Einfluß von Papaverin auf Reaktionen der Blutplättchen. Naunyn Schmiedebergs Arch Pharmacol 257:420–431
Marquis NR, Vigdahl RL, Tavormina PA (1969) Platelet aggregation 1. Regulation by cyclic AMP and prostaglandin E_1. Biochem Biophys Res Commun 36:965–972
Marquis NR, Becker JA, Vigdahl RL (1970) Platelet aggregation 3. An epinephrine induced decrease in cyclic AMP synthesis. Biochem Biophys Res Commun 79:783–789
McDonald JW (1970) Lymphocyte and platelet adenylate cyclase. Can J Biochem 49:316–319
McDonald JW, Stuart RK (1973) Regulation of cyclic AMP levels and aggregation in human platelets by prostaglandin E_1. J Lab Clin Med 81:838–849
McDonald JW, Stuart RK (1974) Interaction of prostaglandins E_1 and E_2 in regulation of cyclic AMP and aggregation in human platelets: evidence for a common prostaglandin receptor. J Lab Clin Med 84:111–121
McElroy FA, Philp RB (1976) Relative potencies of dipyridamole and related agents as inhibitors of cyclic nucleotide phosphodiesterases: possible explanation of mechanism of inhibition of platelet function. Life Sci 17:1479–1490
McMillan R, Bakich MJ, Yelenofsky RJ (1979) The adrenaline binding site on human platelets. Br J Haematol 41:597–604
Mehta P, Mehta J (1980) Platelet function studies in coronary heart disease VIII. Decreased platelet sensitivity to prostacyclin in patients with myocardial ischaemia. Thromb Res 18:273–277
Mellwig KP, Jakobs KH (1980) Inhibition of platelet adenylate cyclase by ADP. Thromb Res 18:7–17
Michel H, Caen JP, Born GVR, Miller R, D'Auriac GA, Meyer P (1976) Relation between the inhibition of aggregation and the concentration of cAMP in human and rat platelets. Br J Haematol 33:27–38
Michel T, Hoffman BB, Lefkowitz RJ (1980) Differential regulation of the α-adrenergic receptor by Na and guanine nucleotides. Nature 288:709–711
Miller OV, Gorman RR (1976) Modulation of platelet cyclic nucleotide content by PGE_1 and the prostaglandin endoperoxide PGG_2. J Cyclic Nucleotide Res 2:79–87
Miller OV, Gorman RR (1979) Evidence for distinct prostaglandin I_2 and D_2 receptors in human platelets. J Pharmacol Exp Ther 210:134–140
Miller OV, Johnson RA, Gorman RR (1977) Inhibition of PGE_1-stimulated cyclic AMP accumulation in human platelets by thromboxane A_2. Prostaglandins 13:599–609
Mills DCB (1974) Factors influencing the adenylate cyclase system in human platelets. In: Sherry S, Scriabine A (eds) Platelets and thrombosis. University Park Press, Baltimore, pp 45–67
Mills DCB (1975) Initial biochemical responses of platelets to stimulation. Ciba Found Symp 35:153–167
Mills DCB (1979) The regulation of adenylate cyclase activity in human platelets. In: Mann KG, Taylor FB (eds) The regulation of coagulation. Elsevier/North Holland, New York, pp 419–427
Mills DCB, Macfarlane DE (1974) Stimulation of human platelet adenylate cyclase by prostaglandin D_2. Thromb Res 5:401–412
Mills DCB, Macfarlane DE (1975) Cytochalasins: effects on platelet aggregation, adenylate cyclase and membrane transport processes. Thromb Diath Haemorrh 34:917
Mills DCB, Macfarlane DE (1976) Platelet receptors. In: Gordon JL (ed) Platelets in biology and pathology. Elsevier, Amsterdam, pp 159–202
Mills DCB, Macfarlane DE (1977) Prostaglandins and platelet adenylate cyclase. In: Silver MJ, Smith JB, Kocsis JJ (eds) Prostaglandins in hematology. Spectrum, Fellbach, pp 219–233
Mills DCB, Macfarlane DE (1980) An inhibitory effect of prostaglandin E_1 (PGE_1) and prostaglandin-like aggregating agents on platelet cyclic AMP accumulation, Proc 18th Int. Congr. Hematol. Montreal
Mills DCB, Roberts GCK (1967a) Membrane active drugs and the aggregation of human blood platelets. Nature 213:35–38
Mills DCB, Roberts GCK (1967) Effects of adrenaline on human blood platelets. J Physiol 193:443–453

Mills DCB, Smith JB (1971) The influence on platelet aggregation of drugs that affect the accumulation of adenosine 3′:5′-cyclic monophosphate in platelets. Biochem J 121:185–196

Mills DCB, Smith JB (1972) The control of platelet responsiveness by agents that influence cyclic AMP metabolism. Ann NY Acad Sci 201:391–399

Mills DCB, Thomas DP (1969) Blood platelet nucleotides in man and other species. Nature 222:991–992

Mills DCB, Robb IA, Roberts GCK (1968) The release of nucleotides, 5-hydroxytryptamine and enzymes from human blood platelets during aggregation. J Physiol 195:715–729

Mills DCB, Smith JB, Born GVR (1970) Pharmacology of platelet aggregation inhibition. In: Mammen EF, Anderson GF, Barnhart MI (eds) Platelet adhesion and aggregation in thrombosis: Countermeasures. Schattauer, Stuttgart, pp 165–184

Minkes M, Stanford N, Chi MMY, Roth GJ, Raz A, Needleman P, Majerus PW (1977) Cyclic adenosine 3′5′-monophosphate inhibits availability of arachidonate to prostaglandin synthetase in human platelet suspensions. J Clin Invest 59:449–454

Mitchell JRA, Sharp AA (1964) Platelet clumping in vitro. Br J Haematol 10:78–93

Moake JL, Cimo PL, Widner P, Peterson DM, Gum JR (1977) Effects of prostaglandins, derivatives of cyclic 3′:5′-AMP, theophylline, cholinergic agents and colchicine on clot retraction in dilute platelet rich plasma and gel-separated platelet test systems. Thromb Diath Haemorrh 38:420–428

Moncada S, Korbut R (1978) Dipyridamole and other phosphodiesterase inhibitors act as antithrombotic agents by potentiating endogenous prostacyclin. Lancet I:1286–1287

Moncada S, Vane JR (1979) Pharmacology and endogenous roles of prostaglandin endoperoxides, thromboxanes and prostacyclin. Pharmacol Rev 30:293–331

Moskowitz J, Harwood JP, Reid WD, Krishna G (1971) The interaction of norepinephrine and prostaglandin E_1 on the adenylate cyclase of human and rabbit blood platelets. Biochim Biophys Acta 230:279–285

Motulsky HJ, Shattil SA, Insel PA (1980) Characterization of α^2-adrenergic receptors on human platelets using [^{3}H]yohimbine. Biochem Biophys Res Commun 97:1562–1570

Murer EH (1971a) Compounds known to effect the adenosine monophosphate level in blood platelets: effects on thrombin-induced clot retraction and platelet release. Biochim Biophys Acta 237:310–315

Murer EH (1971b) Effect of prostaglandin E_1 on clot retraction. Nature 229:112–113

Murphy D, Donnelly C, Moskowitz J (1973) Inhibition by lithium of PGE_1 and norepinephrine effects on cyclic AMP production in human platelets. Clin Pharmacol Ther 14:810–814

Mustard JF, Packham MA (1970) Factor influencing platelet function: adhesion, release and aggregation. Pharmacol Rev 22:97–187

Mustard JF, Kinlough-Rathbone RL, Packham M (1980) Prostaglandins and platelets. Annu Rev Med 31:89–96

Needleman P, Wyche A, Raz A (1979) Platelet and blood vessel arachidonate metabolism and interactions. J Clin Invest 63:345–349

Newman KD, Williams LT, Bishopric NH, Lefkowitz RJ (1978) Identification of alpha-adrenergic receptors in human platelets by (^{3}H)dihydroergocryptine binding. J Clin Invest 61:395–402

Nishizawa EE, Miller WL, Gorman RR, Bundy GL, Svensson J, Hamberg M (1975) Prostaglandin D_2 as a potential antithrombotic agent. Prostaglandins 9:109–121

O'Brien JR (1963) Some effects of adrenaline and antiadrenaline compounds on platelets in vitro and in vivo. Nature 200:763–764

Pandey GN, DeLeon-Jones FA, Inwang ET, Davies JM (1980) Effects of acute methadone withdrawal on prostaglandin E-stimulated ^{3}H cyclic adenosine monophosphate accumulation in human platelets. J Lab Clin Med 27:607–611

Pareti FI, Carrera D, Mannucci L, Mannucci PM (1978) Effect on platelet functions of derivatives of cyclic nucleotides. Thromb Haemost 39:404–410

Patterson WD, Hardman JG, Sutherland EW (1975) Hydrolysis of guanosine and adenosine 3′,5′-monophosphate by rat blood. Biochim Biophys Acta 384:159–167

Pichard A-L, Kaplan JC (1975) Effect of N^6,2′0-dibutyryl cyclic AMP upon the interconvertible forms of cyclic AMP phosphodiesterase from human platelets. Biochem Biophys Res Commun 64:342–346
Pichard A-L, Hanoune J, Kaplan JC (1972) Human brain and platelet cyclic adenosine 3′,5′-monophosphate phosphodiesterases: different response to drugs. Biochim Biophys Acta 279:217–220
Pichard A-L, Hanoune J, Kaplan JC (1973) Multiple forms of cyclic AMP phosphodiesterase from human blood platelets 1. Kinetic and electrophoretic characterization of two molecular species. Biochim Biophys Acta 315:370–377
Rasmussen H, Goodman DBP (1977) Relationships between calcium and cyclic nucleotides in cell activation. Physiol Rev 57:421–509
Reches A, Eldor A, Vogel Z, Solomon Y (1980) Do human platelets have opiate receptors? Nature 288:382–383
Roberts JM, Goldfein RD, Tsuchiya AM, Insel PA (1979) Estrogen treatment decreases adrenergic binding sites on rabbit platelets. Endocrinology 104:722–728
Robison GA, Arnold A, Hartmann RC (1969) Divergent effects of epinephrine and prostaglandin E_1 on the level of cyclic AMP in human blood platelets. Pharmacol Res Commun 1:325–332
Robison GA, Cole B, Arnold A, Hartmann RC (1971) Effects of prostaglandins on function and cyclic AMP levels of human platelets. Ann NY Acad Sci 180:324–331
Roblee LS, Shepro D, Belamarich FA (1973) Calcium uptake and associated adenosine triphosphatase activity of isolated platelet membranes. J Gen Physiol 61:462–481
Rodan GA, Feinstein MB (1976) Interrelationships between Ca^{2+} and adenylate and guanylate cyclases in the control of platelet secretion and aggregation. Proc Natl Acad Sci USA 73:1829–1833
Rotrosen J, Miller A, Mandio D, Traficante L, Gershon S (1978) Reduced PGE_1 stimulated cyclic AMP accumulation in platelets from schizophrenics. Life Sci 23:1989–1996
Rozenberg MC, Walker CM (1973) The effect of pyrimidine compounds on the potentiation of adenosine inhibition of aggregation, on adenosine phosphorylation and on phosphodiesterase activity of blood platelets. Biochem J 24:409–418
Saba HI, Saba SR, Blackburn CA, Hartmann RC, Mason RG (1979) Heparin neutralization of PGI_2: effects upon platelets. Science 205:499–501
Salzman EW (1972) Cyclic AMP and platelet function. N Engl J Med 286:358–363
Salzman EW (1973) Prostaglandins in the function of blood platelets. In: Baulieu E (ed) Les prostaglandines. INSERM, Paris, pp. 331–343
Salzman EW (1977) Interrelation of prostaglandin endoperoxide PGG_2 and cyclic 3′,5′-adenosine monophosphate in human blood platelets. Biochim Biophys Acta 499:48–60
Salzman EW (1978) Platelets, prostaglandins and cyclic nucleotides. In: DeGaetano G, Garrattini S (eds) Platelets: a multidisciplinary approach. Raven Press, New York, pp 227–238
Salzman EW, Levine L (1971) Cyclic 3′,5′-adenosine monophosphate in human blood platelets 2. Effect of N^6-2′o-dibutyryl cyclic 3′,5′-adenosine monophosphate on human platelet function. J Clin Invest 50:131–141
Salzman EW, Neri LL (1969) Cyclic 3′,5′-adenosine monophosphate in human blood platelets. Nature 224:609–610
Salzman EW, Weisenberger H (1972) Role of cyclic AMP in platelet function. Adv Cyclic Nucleotide Res 1:231–247
Salzman EW, Rubino EB, Sims RV (1970) Cyclic 3′,5′-adenosine monophosphate in human platelets 3. The role of cyclic AMP in platelet aggregation. Ser Haematol 3:100–113
Salzman EW, Lindon JN, Rodvien R (1976) Cyclic AMP in human blood platelets: relation to platelet prostaglandin synthesis induced by centrifugation or surface contact. J Cyclic Nucleotide Res 2:25–37
Salzman EW, MacIntyre DE, Steer ML, Gordon JL (1979) Effect on platelet activity of inhibition of adenylate cyclase. Thromb Res 13:1089–1101
Samuels CE, Robinson PG, Elliot RB (1975) Decreased inhibition of platelet aggregation by prostaglandin E_1 in children with cystic fibrosis and their parents. Prostaglandins 10:617–621

Schafer AI, Cooper B, O'Hara D, Handin RI (1979) Identification of platelet receptors for prostaglandin E_2 and D_2. J Biol Chem 254:2914–2917
Schafer AI, Levine S, Handin RI (1980) Regulation of platelet arachidonic acid oxidation by cyclic AMP. Blood 56:853–858
Schaumann W, Juhran W, Dietmann K (1970) Antagonism of theophylline to circulatory effects of adenosine. Arzneim 20:372–377
Schillinger E, Prior G (1980) Prostaglandin I_2 receptors in a particulate fraction of platelets of different species. Biochem Pharmacol 29:2297–2299
Schneider WHG (1974) Regulation of energy metabolism in human platelets by cyclic AMP. In: Baldini MG, Ebbe S (eds) Platelets: production, function, transfusion and storage. Grune & Stratton, New York, pp 177–186
Schoepflin GS, Pickett W, Austen KF, Goetzl EJ (1977) Evaluation of the cyclic GMP concentration in human platelets by sodium ascorbate and 5-hydroxytryptamine. J Cyclic Nucleotide Res 3:355–356
Schoepflin GS, Goetzl EJ, Austen KF (1978) The predominant contribution of platelets to baseline and ascorbate-stimulated increments in cyclic GMP in human mononuclear leucocytes. Cell Immunol 35:330–339
Scott M, Reading HW, Loudon JB (1979) Studies of human blood platelets in affective disorders. Psychopharmacology (Berlin) 60:131–135
Shattil SJ, McDonough M, Turnbull J, Insel PA (1981) Characterization of alpha-adrenergic receptor in human platelets using ^3H clonidine. Mol Pharmacol 19:179–183
Shio H, Ramwell PW, Jessup SJ (1972) Prostaglandin E_2: effects on aggregation, shape change and cyclic AMP of rat platelets. Prostaglandins 1:29–36
Siegl AM, Smith JB, Silver MJ, Nicolaou KC, Ahern D (1979a) Selective binding sites for (^3H) prostacyclin on platelets. J Clin Invest 63:215–220
Siegl AM, Smith JB, Silver MJ (1979b) Specific binding sites for prostaglandin D_2 on human platelets. Biochem Biophys Res Commun 90:291–296
Sinha AK, Colman RW (1978) Prostaglandin E_1 inhibits platelet aggregation by a pathway independent of adenosine 3′,5′-monophosphate. Science 200:202–203
Sinha AK, Colman RW (1980) Persistence of increased platelet cyclic AMP induced by prostaglandin E_1 after removal of the hormone. Proc Natl Acad Sci USA 77:2946–2950
Sinha AK, Shattil SJ, Colman RW (1977) Cyclic AMP metabolism in cholesterol-rich platelets. J Biol Chem 252:3310–3314
Smith JB, Macfarlane DE (1974) Platelets. In: Ramwell PW (ed) The prostaglandins, vol 2. Plenum, New York, pp 293–343
Smith JB, Mills DCB (1971) Inhibition of adenosine 3′:5′-cyclic monophosphate phosphodiesterase. Biochem J 120:20 P
Smith JB, Silver MJ, Ingerman CM, Kocsis JJ (1974) Prostaglandin D_2 inhibits the aggregation of the human platelets. Thromb Res 5:291–299
Smith JB, Ingerman CM, Silver MJ (1976) Formation of prostaglandin D_2 during endoperoxide-induced platelet aggregation. Thromb Res 9:413–418
Smith JB, Ogletree ML, Lefer AM, Nicolaou KC (1978) Antibodies with antagonise the effect of prostacyclin. Nature 274:64–65
Song S-Y, Cheung WY (1971) Cyclic 3′5′-nucleotide phosphodiesterase. Properties of the enzyme of human blood platelets. Biochim Biophys Acta 242:593–605
Statland BE, Heagan BM, White JG (1969) Uptake of calcium by platelet relaxing factor. Nature 223:521–522
Steer ML, Wood A (1979) Regulation of human platelet adenylate cyclase by epinephrine, prostaglandin E_1 and guanine nucleotides. J Biol Chem 254:10791–10797
Steer ML, Khorana J, Galgoci B (1979) Quantitation and characterization of human platelet alpha adrenergic receptors using (^3H) phentolamine Mol Pharmacol 16:719–728
Steer ML, MacIntyre DE, Levine L, Salzman EW (1980) Is prostacyclin a physiologically important circulating antiplatelet agent? Nature 283:194–195
Steiner M (1975) Endogenous phosphorylation of platelet membrane proteins. Arch Biochem Biophys 171:245–254
Steiner M (1978) 3′,5′-cyclic AMP binds to and promotes polymerization of platelet tubulin. Nature 272:834–835

Stoff JB, Stemmerman M, Steer M, Salzman EW, Brown RS (1980) A defect in platelet aggregation in Bartter's syndrome. Am J Med 68:171–180
Subbarao K, Rucinski B, Niewiarowski S (1977) Effect of dipyridamole on adenosine uptake by human platelets and ADP-induced platelet aggregation. Biochem Pharmacol 26:906–907
Tateson JE, Moncada S, Vane JR (1977) Effects of prostacyclin (PGX) on cyclic AMP concentrations in human platelets. Prostaglandins 13:387–397
Taylor PM, Heppinstall S (1978) Cyclic nucleotide phosphodiesterase activity and the platelet release reaction. Thromb Haemost 39:550–555
Taylor RG, Lewis JC, Rudell LL, Biddulph DM (1979) Low density lipoprotein modulation of cAMP in avian thrombocytes. Thromb Res 14:799–804
Tsai BS, Lefkowitz RJ (1978) Agonist-specific effects of monovalent and divalent cations on adenylate cyclase-coupled alpha receptors in rabbit platelets. Mol Pharmacol 14:540–548
Tsai BS, Lefkowitz RJ (1979) Agonist-specific effects of guanine nucleotides on alpha adrenergic receptors in human platelets. Mol Pharmacol 16:61–68
Vainer H (1977) ^{14}C-epinephrine interaction with platelet membrane binding sites. Cell Structure Function 2:267–280
Vainer H, Bussel A (1979) Decreased number of binding sites for [^{14}C]-epinephrine on human platelet membranes in chronic myeloid leukemia. IRCS Med Sci 7:47
Vane JR, Moncada S (1980) Prostacyclin. Blood cells and vessel walls: functional interactions. Ciba Found Symp 71:79–97
Vargaftig BB, Chignard M (1975) Substances that increase the cAMP content prevent platelet aggregation and the concurrent release of pharmacologically active substances evoked by arachidonic acid. Agents Actions 5:137–144
Vargaftig BB, Chignard M, Benveniste J, Lefort J, Wal F (1981) Background and present status of research on platelet activating factor (PAF-acether). Ann NY Acad Sci USA 370:119–137
Vigdahl RL, Marquis NR, Tavormina PA (1969) Platelet aggregation 2. Adenyl cyclase, prostaglandin E_1 and calcium. Biochem Biophys Res Commun 37:409–415
Vigdahl RM, Mongin J Jr, Marquis NR (1971) Platelet aggregation 4. Platelet phosphodiesterase and its inhibition by vasodilators. Biochem Biophys Res Commun 42:1088–1094
Wang TY, Hussey CV, Garancis JC (1977) Effects of dibutyryl cyclic adenosine monophosphate and prostaglandin E_1 on platelet aggregation and shape change. Am J Clin Pathol 67:362–367
Wang TY, Hussey CV, Sasse EA, Fabian JE (1978) Human platelet aggregation and cAMP system. cAMP level, adenyl cyclase, phosphodiesterase. Ann Clin Lab Sci 8:403–412
Wang Y-C, Pandey GN, Mendels J, Frazer A (1974a) Effects of lithium on prostaglandin E_1 stimulate adenylate cyclase of human platelets. Biochem Pharmacol 23:845–855
Wang Y-C, Pandey GN, Mendels J, Frazer A (1974b) Platelet adenylate cyclase response in depression: implications for a receptor defect. Psychopharmacologia 36:291–300
Weisenberger H (1973) Cyclic AMP and platelet function. In: Gerlach E, Moser K, Deutsch E, Wilmanns W (eds) Erythrocytes, thrombocytes and leucocytes. Thieme, Stuttgart, pp 327–333
Weiss A, Baenziger NL, Atkinson JP (1978) Platelet release reaction and intracellular cyclic GMP. Blood 52:524–531
Westwick J, Webb H (1978) Selective antagonism of prostaglandin (PG) E_1, PGD_2 and prostacyclin (PGI_2) on human and rabbit platelets by di-4-phloretin phosphate (DPP). Thromb Res 12:973–978
White JG (1979) Current concepts of platelet structure. Am J Clin Pathol 71:363–378
White JG, Goldberg ND, Estensen RD, Haddox MK, Rao GHR (1973) Rapid increase in platelet cyclic 3′,5′-guanosine monophosphate (cGMP) levels in association with irreversible aggregation, deganulation and secretion. J Clin Invest 52:89a
Whittle BJR, Moncada S, Vane JR (1978) Comparison of the effects of prostacyclin (PGI_2), prostaglandin E_1 and D_2 on platelet aggregation in different species. Prostaglandins 16:373–388
Wolfe SM, Shulman NR (1969) Adenyl cyclase activity in human platelets. Biochem Biophys Res Commun 35:265–272

Wolfe SM, Shulman NR (1970) Inhibition of platelet energy metabolism and release reaction by PGE_1, theophylline and cAMP. Biochem Biophys Res Commun 41:128–134
Wong PY-K, McGiff JC, Sun FF, Lee WH (1979) 6-Keto prostaglandin E_1 inhibits the aggregation of human platelets. Eur J Pharmacol 60:245–248
Wong PY-K, Malik KU, Desiderio DM, McGiff JC, Sun FF (1980) Hepatic metabolism of prostacyclin (PGI_2) in the rabbit. Formation of a potent novel inhibitor of platelet aggregation. Biochem Biophys Res Commun 93:486–494
Yamazaki H, Motomiya T, Mashimo N, Asano T, Hidaka H (1978) Platelet aggregation and cyclic nucleotide phosphodiesterase activity in atherosclerotic patients. Thromb Haemost 39:158–166
Yu SK, Latour JG (1977) Potentiation by α and inhibition by β adrenergic stimulation of rat platelet aggregation: a comparative study with human and rabbit platelets. Thromb Haemost 37:413–422
Zappia GC, Steiner M, Ando Y, Baldini M (1976) Effect of chilling on platelet adenosine 3′:5′-monophosphate and adenylate cyclase activity. Transfusion 16:122–129
Zieve PD, Greenough WB 3rd (1969) Adenyl cyclase in human platelets: activity and responsiveness. Biochem Biophys Res Commun 35:462–466
Zieve PD, Schmuckler M (1971) The effect of cyclic AMP on glycogenolysis and glycolysis in human platelets. Biochem Biophys Acta 252:280–284
Zucker MB (1980) The functioning of blood platelets. Sci Am 242:86–103

CHAPTER 36

Cyclic Nucleotides in the Immune Response

H. J. WEDNER

Overview

Cyclic AMP and cyclic GMP have been implicated as serving modulatory roles in a variety of immune functions. These include the activation of lymphocytes by both mitogenic lectins and antigens, the maturation of lymphocytes into antibody producing B cells or helper, suppressor and effector T cells, the production of specific antibody, and the action of a variety of cytotoxic T cells. In many of these studies the general rule has been that an increase in intracellular cyclic AMP concentration inhibits a particular immune response while an increase in intracellular GMP augments the response. However, as more data have emerged, this hypothesis has frequently not held true. To a large extent, studies of cyclic nucleotide action in the immune response have been compromised because of the marked complexity associated with immune function. That is, five or six individual cell types and as many soluble mediators may interact to produce a cellular or humoral immune response. As a result, investigations have indicated that cyclic AMP and cyclic GMP may enhance, inhibit or have no effect on the immune response, depending upon the timing of the stimulation by these nucleotides and upon the system being tested. Even in simplier systems, controversy has arisen; thus, data indicating a significant role for both cyclic AMP and cyclic GMP in lymphocyte activation, growth and development have been presented. In some instances, differences in experimental results have been interpreted as resulting from an examination of different lymphocyte subpopulations, while in others it has been proposed that a given cyclic nucleotide may have multiple effects on lymphocyte function due to intracellular compartmentalization of the nucleotide. Thus, although it is clear that cyclic nucleotides play an important mediator or modulatory roles at various stages in the immune response, the exact nature of cyclic nucleotide action remains to be elucidated.

A. Introduction

The analysis of the role of cyclic nucleotides in the immune response is not as straightforward as that seen in other cell systems. The induction of an immune response, either humoral or cell mediated, involves intimate cooperation among a large variety of cell types, both lymphoid and nonlymphoid. Some of these interactions augment the response (helper functions), while others tend to inhibit the response (suppressor function). Thus, the production on an antibody to a foreign protein, for example, is the end result of (1) macrophage processing of the antigen,

(2) presentation of the processed antigen to both T and B cells, interaction of B and several subsets of T cells (helper, suppressor, and possibly inducer T cells), (3) growth and maturation of the stimulated B cell population, and (4) production of detectable quantities of immunoglobulin directed against the original antigen.

From this brief description it is obvious that the effects of cyclic AMP or cyclic GMP on one particular cell type can have profound influence on the ultimate outcome of an immune response, and that depending upon the end point utilized, the effect of alterations in cyclic nucleotide levels may suppress or augment the response. Indeed, the actual role of cyclic AMP or cyclic GMP as modulators may, in fact, be opposite to that suggested by the end point measured. For example, if cyclic AMP serves as a stimulatory influence for the suppressor T cell, then addition of cyclic AMP or adenylate cyclase agonists at an appropriate time during the response would serve to increase suppression and decrease antibody production or the generation of effector T cells. In this instance one would be tempted to state that cyclic AMP was an inhibitor of the immune response. While in an overall sense this is true, in the biochemical sense the role of cyclic AMP was to mediate or modulate the function of the suppressor T cell. By this criterion cyclic AMP would be anything but an inhibitor.

For this reason much of the early work on cyclic AMP and cyclic GMP action in relationship to the immune response is very difficult to access (see PARKER et al. 1974; WEDNER and PARKER 1976). In many of these studies, particularly those performed in vivo, it was possible, depending upon the timing, to demonstrate that cyclic AMP, dibutyryl cyclic AMP, or agonists which elevated cyclic AMP (such as β-adrenergic agonists, prostaglandins, polynucleotides or cholera toxin) could augment, inhibit, or have no effect on an immune response depending upon (1) the type of antigen utilized, (2) the timing of the addition of cyclic AMP elevating agents (i.e. prior to antigen, after antigen, etc.), or (3) the end point assayed. We are now aware that these results were most probably the result of differential effects of these agents on each of the different cells involved in the immune response. Since these cells become functional at different times during the response, the addition of cyclic AMP or cyclic GMP or their agonists would be expected to have differing effects depending upon the time added.

For this reason many investigators have felt that the examination of cyclic AMP or cyclic GMP action in vivo, or in mixed cell populations in vitro, yield results which are difficult if not impossible to assess, and have looked to simpler systems to investigate the role of cyclic nucleotides in the immune response. One approach has been to investigate the enzymes involved in cyclic nucleotide generation, destruction, and action in lymphoid cells, with the hope of demonstrating differences in differing cell subsets. Another has been to examine the role of cyclic AMP or cyclic GMP in lymphocyte activation, the primary process of cell growth which underlies any immune response. The hope has been that this process, while still extremely complex, would provide some information on one critical portion of the immune response. In other cases, simpler in vitro systems have evolved in which individual areas which make up an immune response have been examined.

In this review, I will concentrate on these "simpler" systems, since these studies are the easiest to interpret. Studies of in vivo and in vitro antibody synthesis have been reviewed (PARKER et al. 1974; PARKER 1979) and the reader is referred to these.

B. Components of the Cyclic Nucleotide System in Lymphoid Tissue

I. Cyclic Nucleotide Levels

Since the majority of studies on the role of cyclic nucleotides in immune function has involved manipulation of lymphoid cells with subsequent assay of intracellular cyclic AMP or cyclic GMP, accurate measurement of the levels of these nucleotides has been extremely important. Utilizing human peripheral blood lymphocytes, early work demonstrated a significant variation in the resting levels of cyclic AMP from individual to individual (SMITH et al. 1971 a, b). It had originally been assumed that the variability in base line cyclic AMP levels, which ranged from approximately 2 pM/10^7 cells to >40 pM/10^7 cells, was simply a reflection of inherent biologic variability and of the metabolic status of the individuals who had donated the lymphocytes. Subsequently, work has been done to examine this variability in some detail.

Since the majority of the above studies had been done using heparinized blood, the role of heparin was first examined as a contributing factor in the variability (ATKINSON et al. 1977). Early studies from this laboratory demonstrated that incubation of lymphocytes with heparin tended to increase levels of intracellular cyclic AMP, with a progressive fall with time when the heparin was washed from the lymphocytes. Subsequent work demonstrated that a similar phenomenon was not seen with preservative-free heparin, suggesting that the preservative, benzyl alcohol, was responsible for the increase in intracellular cyclic AMP. Further studies demonstrated that a variety of aliphatic and aromatic alcohols were capable of a similar phenomenon (ATKINSON et al. 1977). This suggested at least one plausible explanation for the variability in the baseline cyclic AMP levels. However, when preservative-free heparin was substituted for the benzyl alcohol containing heparin preparation, the variability in baseline levels remained. Two other explanations for this phenomenon have appeared.

The first derives from observations that phagocytic stimuli, such as latex particles, are capable of inducing increases in intracellular cyclic AMP in lymphocytes (ATKINSON et al. 1975). Such particles are not phagocytized by the cells but merely bind to the surface. Using an immunocytochemical technique (WEDNER et al. 1972) it was demonstrated that the increase in intracellular cyclic AMP seen in these cells is local and appears only at the areas of the plasma membrane adjacent to the bound phagocytic particles (ATKINSON et al. 1975). Since many studies using lymphoid tissue are performed in the presence of either fetal calf serum or bovine serum albumin, both of which may contain significant amounts of large protein aggregates, these might serve as an appropriate phagocytic stimulus, and may be responsible in part for the observed differences in intracellular cyclic AMP levels in lymphocytes.

Another and perhaps more important phenomenon has recently emerged. Lymphocytes, when assayed immediately after withdrawal from individuals, contain relatively high levels of cyclic AMP. During the course of purification of lymphocytes by isopycnic centrifugation (EISEN et al. 1972) and incubation of lymphocytes either in physiologic saline or more complex media, there is a progressive fall in the levels of intracellular cyclic AMP (GOFFSTEIN et al. 1980). The decrease is seen in virtually 100% of individuals tested, and can be seen when cyclic AMP is assayed by radioimmunoassay or by the immunocytochemical technique. In many instances the decrease in intracellular cyclic AMP may be as much as 80–90% of the total intracellular cyclic AMP measured in lymphocytes immediately withdrawn from individual patients. Although it is not clear why this decrease in intracellular cyclic AMP occurs, recent studies have demonstrated that it is secondary to a decrease in adenylate cyclase activity rather than to an increase in phosphodiesterase activity (J. P. ATKINSON and H. J. WEDNER, unpublished data).

Because of the above noted variability, it is not clear at the present time what the normal resting level of cyclic AMP in situ is. However, most evidence suggests that the resting levels in the circulation are probably relatively high and that the levels seen in cells following purification and incubation are probably artificially low. The incubation of purified lymphocytes (with low levels of cyclic AMP) in human serum or plasma does not increase cyclic AMP Levels as one might expect if a serum factor were present which maintained the relatively high levels in situ (GOFTSTEIN et al. 1980).

It is important to point out that a similar fall in the intracellular levels of cyclic GMP does not occur (GOFTSTEIN et al. 1980). These levels remain constant for periods of six to eight hours after removal of the lymphocytes and during their purification. On the other hand, there has been some significant disagreement among groups of investigators on the methods for measuring intracellular cyclic GMP levels. In early studies (SMITH et al. 1971 a), cyclic GMP was measured by radioimmunoassay on cell extracts without attempts to purify the cyclic GMP prior to assay. Subsequent work from several laboratories (GOLDBERG and HADDOX 1977; COFFEY et al. 1979) has suggested that under these circumstances cyclic GMP cannot be accurately measured, and elaborate schemes for purification of this cyclic nucleotide on neutral alumina or Dowex columns have been proposed. However, other laboratories have found that these maneuvers may not be necessary and do not alter the levels of intracellular cyclic GMP. In additions, there are significant losses in nucleotide during purification which must be adjusted for (ATKINSON et al. 1978). Whether purification is undertaken or not, care must be taken to demonstrate that the measured level of cyclic GMP in lymphoid tissue accurately reflects real levels. This can generally be done by the addition of an internal standard (i.e., small amounts of cyclic GMP eiter unlabeled or radiolabeled) to extracts of lymphoid tissue and by the demonstration that the immunoreactive cyclic GMP is fully destroyed by cyclic nucleotide phosphodiesterase.

II. Adenylate Cyclase and Guanylate Cyclase

Adenylate cyclase has been measured in a variety of lymphoid cells including human peripheral blood lymphocytes and lymphocyte subpopulations (POLGAR et al. 1973; MONAHAN et al. 1975; POLGAR et al. 1977), human tonsilar tissue, and mouse spleen cells (MENAHAN et al. 1976). In all cases, adenylate cyclase has been demonstrated to be a membrane-bound enzyme like that found in numerous other tissues. A discussion of the subcellular localization of adenylate cyclase is included in the section on lymphocyte activation (below) and need not be dealt with further here.

However, a number of groups have examined differences in total adenylate cyclase activity in various lymphocyte subpopulations. This is of some importance since there are significant differences in the resting levels of cyclic AMP between T lymphocytes and B lymphocytes (BACH 1975; NIAUDET et al. 1976). Work by MENDELSOHN and NORDBERG (1979) has demonstrated that there are significant differences in adenylate cyclase levels between human B and T cells, with B cells having significantly higher levels, by a factor of 3 to 5, than do T cells, confirming previous work by several groups (POLGAR et al. 1973; MONAHAN et al. 1975; POLGAR et al. 1977). Similar studies have also been carried out in malignant lymphoid tissues, and, in general, malignant cells tend to have significantly lower levels of adenylate cyclase similar to those found in T lymphocytes (MENDELSOHN and NORDBERG 1979). Other workers have examined adenylate cyclase levels in mouse T and B lymphocytes (MENAHAN et al. 1976). The results of these studies have been similar to those described in human peripheral blood lymphocytes, in that mouse T cells have significantly lower levels of adenylate cyclase than do mouse B cells. Moreover, when these subpopulations of lymphocytes are stimulated with a variety of adenylate cyclase agonists, such as β-adrenergic agents or prostaglandins, the net stimulation of B cells has been consistently higher than the stimulation of T cells when measured either as an absolute increase in intracellular cyclic AMP or when expressed as a stimulation ratio.

Guanylate cyclase levels have also been assayed in lymphoid tissue (COFFEY et al. 1981). In contrast to adenylate cyclase, guanylate cyclase exists in both a soluble and particulate form with the majority of the enzyme in human lymphocytes being found in the soluble fraction. Early studies of guanylate cyclase activity were compromised by the lack of agents which were capable of stimulating this enzyme either in the intact cell or in broken cell preparations. Careful studies have suggested that many agents which were capable of stimulating guanylate cyclase activity in other cell systems did not stimulate the enzyme in lymphoid tissue. More recently, however, a number of laboratories have demonstrated agents which do actively stimulate guanylate cyclase. These agents have included sodium nitroprusside, a number of nitroso guanidine compounds, and ascorbic acid. In addition to this, at least one group has demonstrated an increase in guanylate cyclase activity in association with activation of lymphocytes. This will be discussed in some detail below (COFFEY et al. 1981). Although the extensive work that has been performed on adenylate cyclase in lymphoid tissue has not been duplicated on guanylate cyclase, preliminary studies from one laboratory have shown that the T/B cell differences seen in adenylate cyclase discussed above do not seem to be present with guanylate cyclase (J.P. ATKINSON and H.J. WEDNER, unpublished data).

III. Phosphodiesterase

Cyclic nucleotide phosphodiesterase has been examined in lymphocytes from a variety of species, with the majority of work being done on human peripheral blood lymphocytes and mouse splenic lymphocytes. Weiss and his co-workers have studied mouse spleen cell phosphodiesterase extensively (HAIT and WEISS 1976, 1977). Briefly this group has demonstrated that phosphodiesterase activity is present in both and B and T lymphocytes. In general, the overall level of phosphodiesterase tends to be higher in the T lymphocyte group than in the B lymphocyte group and may contribute to the lower basal levels of cyclic AMP found in the T lymphocyte subpopulation. In similar fashion, mouse leukemia cells also have elevated phosphodiesterase levels. A similar phenomenon has been seen in human leukemic lymphocytes (SCHER et al. 1976). Using a gel electrophoretic technique they have been able to demonstrate multiple forms of cyclic nucleotide phosphodiesterase in both B and T lymphocytes. These forms differ significantly in their kinetic properties and in their preference or lack of preference for either cyclic AMP or cyclic GMP. This group has also demonstrated that addition of calmodulin to phosphodiesterase extracted from mouse lymphocytes has little or no effect on the activity. However, when extracts of mouse lymphocytes are added to other phosphodiesterase preparations these are stimulated in appropriate fashion demonstrating that calmodulin is present in these preparations. This suggests that, at least as extracted, the phosphodiesterase is fully activated.

As with many other aspects of cyclic nucleotide metabolism in human peripheral blood lymphocytes, there has been some degree of controversy concerning cyclic nucleotide phosphodiesterase activity in these cells. LAGARDE and COLOBERT (1972) first demonstrated phosphodiesterase activity in human lymphocytes. They characterized two cyclic AMP hydrolytic activities. A "low K_m" enzyme ($K_m \simeq$ 2 μm) and a "high K_m" enzyme ($K_m \simeq$ 50–70 μm). In contrast, THOMPSON and his co-workers (THOMPSON et al. 1976; EPSTEIN et al. 1976) suggested that highly purified human peripheral blood lymphocytes disrupted by Dounce homogenization contained a single phosphodiesterase activity which was capable of hydrolyzing only cyclic AMP. The kinetics of this enzyme were those of a "low K_m (K_m= 0.75 μ*M*) enzyme and the activity was approximately 10-fold lower than that previously described. There was no activity which might have been considered a "high K_m" cyclic AMP enzyme, nor were these workers able to demonstrate enzyme activity capable of hydrolyzing cyclic GMP. These workers suggested that the cyclic AMP and cyclic GMP activities previously described were the result of contamination of the lymphocyte preparations by other elements, most notably platelets. They subsequently demonstrated that lymphocytes activated with mitogenic lectins rapidly acquired cyclic GMP hydrolytic activity (EPSTEIN et al. 1976) and suggested that this represented an important step in lymphocyte activation.

At least one study differs from those of THOMPSON and co-workers. WEDNER et al. (1979) disrupted lymphocytes by Dounce homogenization, and showed that lymphocytes prepared by this method had a single kinetic activity with an apparent K_m of approximately 1.5–2 μ*M* for cyclic AMP. There was no "high K_m" phosphodiesterase activity in these cells and little or no cyclic GMP hydrolytic activity was seen. If the lymphocytes were disrupted by sonication or if the Dounce preparation was further disrupted either by sonication or by incubation with nonionic detergents such as Triton X-100, then cyclic GMP hydrolytic activity and a "high K_m" cyclic AMP hydrolytic activity both appeared. The preparations utilized in this study were largely depleted of other cellular elements such as monocytes and platelets, indicating that the activity was inherent to the lymphocyte. Moreover, lymphocyte phosphodiesterase was shown to be electrophoretically different from that in platelets, excluding even the minor platelet contaminations as a contributor. This data suggested that in the intact lymphocyte the cyclic GMP and high K_m cyclic AMP hydrolytic activities were functionally segregated and could be released only by strong disruptive forces such as sonication. It also suggested that these enzymes, although present, were not accessible to exogenously added cyclic nucleotides and therefore were not measured in the cyclic nucleotide phosphodiesterase assay. Thus, it appears that the phosphodiesterase system, like the adenylate cyclase and protein kinase systems to be discussed below, shows a significant degree of compartmentalization within the human lymphocyte. That cyclic GMP phosphodiesterase activity is not released by homogenization in resting cells and is released in activated cells is intriguing and merits further study.

Data have also been presented demonstrating that the human peripheral blood lymphocyte, like the mouse lymphocyte, contains calmodulin activity (WEDNER, 1980). In the intact human lymphocyte, phosphodiesterase appears to be fully active and unresponsive to calmodulin stimulation. However, one can alter the system using the sulfhydryl binding agent diamide (diazine dicarboxylic acid bis[N,N′ dimethylamide]) and demonstrate that at least under these artificial circumstances calmodulin is capable of augmenting human lymphocyte phosphodiesterase activity.

IV. Protein Kinase Activity

Protein kinase activity in lymphocytic tissues has been examined by a number of groups in a variety of species most notably in human peripheral blood lymphocytes, mouse lymphocytes and pig lymphocytes. Earlier studies were concerned mainly with a description of the number and specificity of soluble protein kinases and the differentiation between cyclic nucleotide-dependent and cyclic nucleotide-independent enzymes. CROSS and ORD (1970) studied histone phosphorylation in lymphocytes incubated with mitogenic agents and demonstrated that there was an increase in histone phosphorylation associated with the activation process. They suggested that this was putative evidence for the presence of one or more species of protein kinase. No attempt was made in this study to demonstrate whether the kinase activity isolated was dependent upon cyclic nucleotides. MURRAY and his co-workers (1974) described a cyclic AMP-dependent protein kinase activity in human peripheral blood lymphocytes which was found in the soluble fraction. A number of other workers have utilized a variety of separation techniques to fractionate protein kinase activity. For example, PIRAS and co-workers (1977) utilizing a 10,000 G supernatant of purified human peripheral blood lymphocytes and DEAE-cellulose chromatography, were able to show six fractions of protein kinase activity, three of which preferentially phosphorylated casein while the other three phosphorylated histone proteins. In addition, they were able to demonstrate two casein kinases in the nuclear fraction. Of the six non-nuclear fractions which were described, only one, designated SH2, was stimulated by cyclic nucleotides. This fraction responded identically to cyclic GMP and cyclic AMP. Interestingly, another fraction which appeared later from the column was stimulated significantly by a combination of cyclic AMP and GTP.

MURRAY, KEMP and their co-workers (MURRAY et al. 1972; KEMP et al. 1975) have also studied the soluble protein kinase activity from human peripheral blood lymphocytes. They were able to resolve four kinase activities by DEAE cellulose chromatography. These included two histone kinases, one of which was cyclic AMP-dependent, and two casein kinases, neither of which was responsive to cyclic AMP. FARAGO et al. (1974) also demonstrated histone kinase activity in nuclei from human tonsillar lymphocytes. In their hands this kinase activity was not cyclic AMP-dependent, although nuclear histone kinase activity which is stimulated by cyclic AMP has been described in a number of other cell systems (KISH and KLEINSMITH 1974; RIKANS and RUDDON 1973; CASTAGNA et al. 1975). In a more recent study, HORENSTEIN et a. (1976) studied protein kinase activity in lymphocytes activated by phytohemagglutinin. They examined kinase activity in a 10,000 X G "supernatant fraction" and a "nuclear pellet." At 70 h there was a 3–4 fold increase in kinase activity in the soluble fraction and an 8–10 fold increase in the nuclear fraction. Kinase activity was studied using only exogenous substrates and cyclic AMP sensitivity was not examined. In a more extensive study, KIMPEL et al. (1976) studied protein kinase activity in human lymphocytes activated by PHA. Kinase activity was separated into Type I and Type II by DEAE-cellulose chromatography. Both Type I and Type II activity were present in resting lymphocytes and there was a marked increase in Type I activity at four h following additions of mitogen. KLIMPEL et al. suggested that this increase played an important role in the activation sequence. Similar column chromatographic separation of protein kinase activity has been obtained by a number of other groups in a variety of lymphocyte supernatants. In most cases two or three protein kinases which are stimulated by cyclic AMP have been described.

CHAPLIN and co-workers (CHAPLIN et al. 1979a, b) have examined protein kinase activity in unstimulated human peripheral blood lymphocytes and have attempted to characterize the kinase activity on the basis of its subcellular localization as well as its preference for various artificial protein substrates. These studies are described in significant detail in the succeeding sections.

V. Phosphoprotein Phosphatase

Little work has been done on phosphoprotein phosphatase activity in lymphocytes. Preliminary experiments (WEDNER, unpublished data) examined the ability of subcellular fractions of human peripheral blood lymphocytes to remove phosphate groups from phosphorylated histone protein. These studies demonstrated that there are high levels of phosphoprotein phosphatase activity in all fractions, including the 100,000 XG supernatant, mitochondrial, microsomal, and a fraction enriched in plasma membrane. The highest specific activity was found in the soluble supernatant. The enzyme activity has not been further characterized except to demonstrate that it is possible to inhibit these activities using a combination of sodium floride and sodium pyrophosphate (CHAPLIN et al. 1980). This ability is extremely important since studies of protein phosphorylation, particularly those involving gel electrophoresis to be described below require that phosphoprotein phosphatase activity be largely inhibited.

VI. Summary

It is clear that lymphocytes possess all of the biochemical machinery which is found in other cell types described in this Volume for the production, action and destruction of cyclic AMP and cyclic GMP. However, the activity of the components of this system varies significantly not only from species to species, but from lymphocyte subpopulation to lymphocyte subpopulation. It is important to point out that studies of cyclic nucleotide metabolism in subpopulations of lymphocytes from any species have only recently begun, and that the majority of studies which have been reported above were done on mixtures of B and T cells. Moreover, recent work has suggested that both B and T cells can be subdivided into other functional subsets (e.g. helper T cells, suppressor T cells, cytotoxic T cells) and identification of differences in enzyme activity in these smaller subsets of lymphocytes has not yet begun.

C. Lymphocyte Activation

I. Biochemical Changes in Activated Lymphocytes

a) Introduction

Lymphocyte activation is the biochemical process whereby cells resting in G_0 are induced into G_1 and progress through the cellular growth stages culminating in the synthesis of new DNA and one or more rounds of cell division. Both B and T lymphocytes have on their surface receptors which are capable of interacting with antigens. Those cells which bind antigen are activated, undergo cell division, and ultimately differentiate into a variety of immunologically mature cell types. The small number of cells which respond to any given antigen has, however, limited the type of biochemical studies which can be performed on antigen driven systems. For this reason, biochemical studies on lymphocyte activation have generally used a number of agents which are capable of activating all or a proportion of the lymphocytes (for review see WEDNER and PARKER 1976). The plant lectins, concanavalin A (con A) and phytohemagglutinin (PHA), are legume-derived proteins or glycoproteins which interact with sugar moieties on cell surface glycoproteins and activate primarily T lymphocytes. Anti-immunoglobulins, anti $\beta2$, microglobulin, and staph protein A interact with immunoglobulins presented on the surface of B lymphocytes and induce activation in these cells. Pokeweed mitogen and bacterial lipopolyccharide (LPS) also are mitogenic for B lymphocytes, although the mechanism of their interaction with these cells is not clear. All of these agents are believed to interact with structures within or near the cell surface, and induce lymphocyte activation in a manner which is analogous to antigens.

A large number of biochemical alterations have been described which occur at some point in the sequence from mitogen binding to cell division. For convenience we have divided these into those associated with the plasma membrane, the cytoplasm and the nucleus (PARKER et al. 1974; WEDNER and PARKER 1976).

b) Plasma Membrane-Related Events

Plasma membrane-related events include activation of adenylate or guanylate cyclase, increases in the efflux and influx of K^+ with a marked increase in the turnover of this ion, increases in the active or faciliated transport of Ca^{++}, amino acids, glucose, and ultimately of nucleosides, increases in the turnover of phosphate in phospholipids, and alterations in the structure of the microfilament-microtubule network attached to or lying just below the plasma membrane (EDELMAN 1976). Several of these plasma membrane related events have been suggested as the trigger for the activation sequence. Each of these changes occurs within minutes following the binding of lectin to the surface of the lymphocytes, with a gradual increase in the magnitude of the change over the next 6–8 h and in many cases maintenance of the high levels of activity over the next several days.

c) Cytoplasmic Changes

These include an alteration in the status of polyribosomes to the active from the inactive form (COOPER at al. 1975). This change can be detected within 60 min of lectin binding and is quite prominent a four hours following the initiation of activation. Increased incorporation of labeled amino acids into protein is detectable after 120 min but an increase in net protein synthesis cannot be detected for approximately 12 h. In addition, the activity of a number of enzymes for intermediary metabolism is increased, with increases in glucose utilization, pyruvate and lactate production, and fatty acid synthesis detectable within two to three hours of activation.

d) Nuclear Changes

Nuclear changes begin very rapidly following the addition of lectin to lymphocytes. Within 30 min there is an increase in the incorporation of radiolabeled phosphate and pyruvate into histones and acidic proteins, and changes in the thiol content of histones. There are modest increases in the incorporation of radiolabeled uridine into RNA within 30 min with much larger changes seen at 24–48 h. At 20 h there is an increase in the incorporation of radiolabeled thymidine into DNA with the maximum increase seen at 72 h.

e) Summary

The list of biochemical alterations given above, while by no means complete, does indicate the multiplicity of intracellular systems which are affected during the activation process. Thus, any biochemical signal which is proposed as the initiator for lymphocyte activation must provide sufficient diversity to account for these changes. In addition, it is now clear that there are a large number of chemical agents secreted by lymphocytes, monocytes and other cell types which are capable of modulating the response of the lymphocyte population (OPPENHEIM and ROSENSTREICH 1976). Thus, if one proposes a single biochemical alteration which transmits the message for lymphocyte activation it must be capable of integrating all of the signals which play upon the lymphocyte.

Four separate plasma membrane-related events have been most prominently suggested as the trigger which transmits the signal for the G_0-G_1 step. These are increases in intracellular cyclic nucleotides (WEDNER and PARKER 1976), increases in K^+ turnover (SEGAL and LICHTMAN 1976), increases in Ca^{++} influx (PARKER 1974), and alterations in microtubles or microfilaments (YAHARA and EDELMAN 1975). Each of these might possess the necessary characteristics to serve as the intracellular mediator of the activation signal. Each of these alterations appears to be relatively transient, however, and there are several lines of evidence which indicate that these early biochemical alterations are critical.

First, the work of SELL and SHEPPARD (1974) demonstrated that when lymphocytes are incubated with con A for four hours, and then the con A is removed with α-methyl manoside, there is marked inhibition of subsequent DNA synthesis. However, if these same cells are then incubated with PHA, the peak of DNA synthesis is earlier than in control lymphocytes with PHA alone, indicating that an early step had occurred which allowed the con A treated cells to progress to DNA synthesis more rapidly. Second, work by CHAPLIN and WEDNER (1978) indicated that the sulphydryl oxidizing agent, diamide (diazine dicarboxylic acid bis [N,N′ dimethyl amide]), totally inhibits lymphocyte activation only when added during the first 10–30 min following the addition of lectin. After this time, diamide is much less effective, indicating that a critical biochemical step occurs during this early time period. These studies indicate that there are critical events which occur rapidly following the binding of lectin to the surface of the lymphocyte.

II. Measurement of Lymphocyte Activation

Early events which occur during lymphocyte activation are generally correlated with the late events, particularly DNA or RNA synthesis; however, in some instances early events may occur in the absence of new DNA synthesis or cell division (COLLAVO et al. 1976). This does not indicate that these early events are unimportant, since a second inhibitory stimulus may abort the response before DNA synthesis occurs. An example of such a situation occurs with stimulation of lymphocytes with wheat germ agglutinin (GORDON et al. 1980; UDEY et al. 1980).

In general, lymphocyte activation is measured by the incorporation of radiolabeled precursors into newly formed DNA or RNA. A considerable volume of literature indicates that this is a valid indication that activation has taken place. However, recent evidence from our laboratory and others indicates that this method may not accurately reflect changes in lymphocyte activation when one compares two different cell populations or when comparing the same population incubated with different agents (BUCKLEY and WEDNER 1977). Thus, for example, changes in thymidine incorporation may be due to alteration in either the size or the specific activity of the thymidine pool.

An alternate method of looking at new DNA synthesis is to use lymphocytes which have been made permeable by the cold osmotic shock technique of BERGER and JOHNSON (1976). BUCKLEY and WEDNER (1978) have adapted this technique to both human and mouse lymphocytes and have shown that the permeable lymphocytes are capable of synthesizing new DNA when supplied with ATP and the four deoxyribose nucleotide triphosphates. The DNA synthesis is semiconservative as judged by cesium chloride density gradient centrifugation in the presence of bromo-deoxyuridine. In human lymphocytes, the DNA synthesis correlated well with activation measured by each of the other parameters described above. This technique, which eliminates the problems of pool size and specific activity, and can be accurately used as a measure of lymphocyte activation.

III. Alterations in Cyclic Nucleotides in Lectin Activated Lymphocytes

The changes in cyclic AMP or cyclic GMP in lectin-activated lymphocytes have been recently reviewed (PARKER et al. 1974; WEDNER and PARKER 1976; also see below). Briefly, early experiments (SMITH et al. 1971 a, b) demonstrated small but consistent and statistically significant increases in cyclic AMP in human peripheral blood lymphocytes incubated with PHA or con A. This group has confirmed these results in over 1,000 experiments using a variety of activation agents (WEDNER and PARKER 1976) and this work has been confirmed by a number of groups (KRISHNARA and TALWAR 1973; WEBB et al. 1974; WINCHURCH and ACTOR 1972). Other groups, however, have been unable to demonstrate increases in cyclic AMP (DERUBERTIS and ZENSER 1976; HADDEN et al. 1972), or have noted increases in cyclic AMP with both mitogenic and nonmitogenic lectins, suggesting that the effect may be unrelated to the activation signal (BURLESON and SAGE 1976). In contrast, HADDEN et al. (1972), and SCHUMM et al. (1974) have noted large increases in cyclic GMP in human lymphocytes in response to mitogens (see below) while others have been unable to confirm these results (WEDNER et al. 1975; Atkinson et al. 1978).

Because of the dichotomy of cyclic AMP action, i.e. mitogens increased intracellular cyclic AMP while other agents which increased intracellular cyclic AMP inhibited lectin induced activation, it was suggested that cyclic AMP might be compartmentalized within the lymphocyte with cyclic AMP localized in one part of the cell inducing activation while that in another inhibiting the activation process (WEDNER et al. 1975). To examine this question further an immunofluorescent technique to localize bound intracellular cyclic AMP (WEDNER et al. 1972; STEINER et al. 1976) was used, and consistent differences between various stimulators of adenylate cyclase was demonstrated (WEDNER et al. 1975). When lymphocytes were incubated with PHA, the increased fluorescence was noted only in patches within or near the plasma membrane. In contrast, PGE_1 caused increased fluorescence within the entire cytoplasm, and isoproterenol induced increases both in the cytoplasm and the cell nucleus (WEDNER et al. 1975). This data indicates that there is segregation of cyclic AMP within the human lymphocyte, since time course studies demonstrated that the patterns seen were not the result of diffusion of cyclic AMP from the external plasma membrane to other intracellular sites and suggested that there were intracellular adenylate cyclases which responded to PGE_1 and isoproterenol. These results have been confirmed using isolated subcellular fractions from human peripheral blood lymphocytes as described below.

IV. Adenylate Cyclase Activity in Isolated Subcellular Fractions From Human Peripheral Blood Lymphocytes

To further evaluate the compartmentalization of cyclic nucleotides in human peripheral blood lymphocytes, WEDNER and co-workers examined adenylate cyclase activity in subcellular fractions from human peripheral blood lymphocytes. Subcellular fractions were prepared by two methods: (1) centrifugation through a discontinuous sucrose density gradient yielding a fraction enriched in plasma membranes and a fraction enriched in mitochondria and microsomes (SNIDER and PARKER 1977; CHAPLIN et al. 1979 b), and (2) agitation of lymphocytes with Triton

X100 in 0.25 *M* sucrose containing 3.3 m*M* Ca^{++} followed by centrifugation through 2.25 *M* sucrose containing 3.3 m*M* Ca^{++}, at 105,000 X G to yield pure nuclei (WEDNER and PARKER 1977). Adenylate cyclase was assayed in the plasma membrane, microsomes, and mitochondria by radioimmunoassay (STEINER et al. 1972). Each of the preparations contained fluoride-stimulatable adenylate cyclase activity. The microsomes and mitochondria were stimulated by PGE_1 while the plasma membrane was unreactive to this agent. PHA stimulated the plasma membrane cyclase but not the other two fractions (SNIDER and PARKER 1977).

The nuclei, on the other hand, accumulated cyclic AMP in the presence of fluoride and exogenous ATP. Isoproterenol also stimulated cyclic AMP accumulation; however ATP was not necessary for cyclic AMP generation suggesting that the isoproterenol-sensitive cyclase used ATP generated within the nucleus as the substrate. PHA or PGE_1 had no effect. The nuclear adenylate cyclase activity was inhibited by Mg^{++} and stimulated by Mn^{++} and CA^{++} in contrast to the other subcellular fractions which were stimulated by Mg^{++} and inhibited by Ca^{++} (WEDNER and PARKER 1977). This data, which entirely confirmed the results of the studies using the immunocytochemical technique to localize cyclic AMP, demonstrated that there are multiple adenylate cyclase enzymes within the human peripheral blood lymphocytes which differ in their spatial presentation within the cell, their divalent cation requirements, and their responsiveness to known adenylate cyclase stimulators. Together, these studies suggest that cyclic AMP generated by a plasma membrane bound adenylate cyclase responsive to mitogenic agents is bound locally and may be responsible for the activation signal. Other agents stimulate the accumulation in other parts of the cell of cyclic AMP which may be inhibitory.

V. Cyclic AMP Binding to Lymphocyte Plasma Membranes

A corollary of the compartmentalization model proposed for the role of cyclic AMP in lectin activated lymphocytes (WEDNER et al. 1975) is that cyclic AMP generated at the plasma membrane must be rapidly bound to the plasma membrane where it exerts its effect or is destroyed by phosphodiesterase before it reaches other cellular compartments. To examine this question directly WEDNER and co-workers examined the binding of [^{3}H] cyclic AMP to plasma membranes isolated from human peripheral blood lymphocytes by the method of SNIDER and PARKER (1977). Plasma membranes contained high affinity binding sites with a K_d of 1.8×10^{-8} *M* and a total binding capacity of 2.66 picomoles/mg protein. The total number of binding sites was comparable to that seen in other cells, for example, approximately 5 pmole/mg protein in human red blood cell membranes (HALEY 1975). Other experiments demonstrated that if lymphocytes were incubated with agents which increase intracellular cyclic AMP and then rapidly chilled, little of the cyclic AMP bound would be lost during the time necessary to purify plasma membranes and examine the binding of [^{3}H] cyclic AMP. Cyclic AMP binding to plasma membrane was performed using lymphocytes incubated for 10 min at 37 °C with either 0.1 *M* NaCl (control), 3 µg/ml of con A or 30 µg/ml con A. Scatchard analysis revealed that the number of free binding sites decreased from 2.89 pmole/mg protein in control lymphocytes to 1.78 pmole per mg in the lymphocytes incubated with

30 μg/ml con A, 3 μg/ml con A gave an intermediate value. These data demonstrated that cyclic AMP generated at the plasma membrane in con A treated cells is rapidly bound to the plasma membrane, confirming the immunohistochemical data and providing support for the model of cyclic AMP action discussed above (H. J. WEDNER submitted for publication).

VI. Protein Phosphorylation in Intact Lymphocytes

In addition to studies of protein kinase activity described above, protein phosphorylation has been studied in lymphocytes preincubated with [^{32}P] phosphoric acid to label endogenous ATP pools and then incubated for short periods of time with a variety of activation agents or with N^6 monobutyryl cyclic AMP (MbcAMP), (WEDNER and PARKER 1976; CHAPLIN et al. 1979). The phosphorylated proteins were extracted and examined by SDS polyacrylamide gel electrophoresis (PAGE). In early studies, lymphocytes incubated with mitogenic agents or MbcAMP were disrupted in low ionic strength buffer and subjected to PAGE on 5.6% acrylamide gels. In these studies (WEDNER and PARKER 1976), lymphocytes incubated with MbcAMP showed an increase in phosphorylation in a large number of proteins ranging in MW from 10,000 to 90,000. Lymphocytes incubated with PHA showed a rise which was identical both in magnitude and pattern to that seen with MbcAMP. Cyclic GMP or 8 bromo cyclic GMP had no effect on protein phosphorylation (WEDNER and PARKER 1976). This data suggested that the increase in phosphorylation in PHA treated cells was the result of activation of a cyclic AMP dependent protein kinase or kinases. In a more recent study (CHAPLIN et al. 1980), lymphocytes were disrupted in a buffer system designed to inhibit protein kinase activity, phosphoprotein phosphatase activity, and proteolysis. Under these conditions, the overall increase in protein phosphorylation previously described was confirmed. However, the appearance of a 65,000 molecular weight protein which was uniquely phosphorylated in lymphocytes incubated with mitogenic lectins was noted. This protein was found in the soluble fraction and was not sensitive to MbcAMP or agents which raise intracellular cyclic AMP, such as isoproterenol or prostaglandin E (CHAPLIN et al. 1980a).

In the studies described above, unique phosphorylation of any protein in the particulate fraction was not seen, most probably due to the complexity of this fraction. However, when the particulate fraction was disrupted in 1% Nonidet-P40 (NP-40) and subjected to DEAE cellulose chromatography using a step gradient of NaCl, four particulate proteins which are phosphorylated in the presence of mitogenic concentrations of con A or PNA were noted – two of these proteins are large (MW 130–180X 10^3) and two in the range MW 35–45X 10^3 (H. J. WEDNER, unpublished data).

VII. Protein Kinase Activity in Lymphocyte Plasma Membranes

In addition to studies of overall protein kinase activity described above, protein kinase activity in plasma membranes and other subcellular fractions from lymphocytes has been examined (CHAPLIN et al. 1979a, b, 1980). These studies measured both exogenous and endogenous protein substrates. Each of the fractions tested, plasma membrane, microsomes or mitochondria, was capable of phosphorylating both endogenous substrates and three exogenous substrates (mixed histones, protamine and casein). Phosphorylation of endogenous substrates was also examined using two dimensional gel electrophoresis (O'FARREL 1975). Four to six proteins unique to the plasma membrane fraction were phosphorylated in the presence of cyclic AMP (CHAPLIN et al. 1979b).

In other experiments utilizing cellular fractions of human lymphocytes, CHAPLIN et al. (1979a) have demonstrated that the soluble cyclic AMP dependent kinase present is a Type I enzyme. This is interesting in light of the studies of KLIMPEL et al. (1976), we showed that there was an increase in Type I kinase activity in activated lymphocytes which begins four hours following addition of mitogen. How this increase relates to the very early activation events is not clear.

VIII. Summary

It is clear that the cyclic AMP system in the lymphocyte is quite complex. The evidence presented above suggests that adenylate cyclase, the generated cyclic AMP and cyclic AMP dependent protein kinase activity are highly compartmentalized in the lymphocyte. WEDNER and co-workers (1975) have utilized this complexity to formulate a model in which cyclic AMP is generated in response to mitogenic stimulate. The cyclic AMP is bound to the plasma membrane in this region of the cell and results in the phosphorylation of one or more plasma membrane associated protein substrates via a bound protein cyclic AMP dependent protein kinase, these substrates are then capable of initiating the activation sequence (WEDNER and PARKER 1975; CHAPLIN et al. 1979a, b, 1980). While this hypothesis is as yet largely untested, it is consistant with the compartmentalization described above, and provides a mechanism for diverse actions of cyclic AMP in lymphocyte function.

D. Cyclic GMP in Lymphocyte Activation

The role of cyclic GMP in lymphocyte activation has been an extremely controversial one. Early work on cyclic GMP and lymphocytes stimulated with PHA or Con A suggested that there were no alterations in the level of this nucleotide (C.W. PARKER, personal communication). HADDEN and co-workers (1972) re-examined the effect of PHA and Con A on intracellular cyclic GMP concentrations in human peripheral blood lymphocytes. The demonstrated multi-fold (up to 50 X) increases in intracellular cyclic GMP in lymphocytes incubated with optimal mitogenic doses of these lectins. In the same study they showed minimal or no increase in intracellular cyclic AMP when highly purified PHA or Con A were utilized. They suggested that the increase in cyclic AMP was related to the agglutinating power of these two lectins rather than their ability to stimulate lymphocyte proliferation. In further studies, HADDEN and co-workers (HADDEN et al. 1976) utilized succinylated Con A (a dimeric rather than tetrameric molecule) and demonstrated that this agent was also capable of increasing the levels of intracellular cyclic GMP at mitogenic concentrations. In contrast to tetrameric Con A, succinylated Con A showed no high dose inhibition while tetrameric Con A was inhibitory at higher concentrations. The increase in cyclic GMP for both tetrameric and dimeric Con A paralleled the stimulation of DNA synthesis in that succinylated Con A showed no high dose inhibition of DNA synthesis while tetrameric Con A had a definite prozone effect. In this same study COFFEY et al. noted increases in intracellular cyclic AMP with tetrameric Con A but not succinylated Con A and only at relatively high doses which would be in the high dose inhibitory area. They suggested that the increase in cyclic AMP may, in fact, represent a negative signal and be responsible for the high dose inhibition seen with native Con A. In further studies this group has measured increases in cyclic GMP with PHA, Con A, succinylated Con A, and the divalent cation ionophore A 23187. They have shown increases in cyclic AMP with Con A and the ionophore but have been unable to demonstrate significant increases in intracellular cyclic AMP with either PHA or succinylated Con A (COFFEY et al. 1977). The data on cyclic GMP has been confirmed by a number of laboratories utilizing human peripheral blood lymphocytes stimulated with PHA, Con A, the calcium ionophore A 23187 and pokeweed mitogen, mouse spleen cells stimulated with bacterial lypopolysaccharide, sheep red blood cells, sodium periodate as well as mitogenic lectins, guinea pig spleen cells stimulated with sodium periodate, rat spleen cells, peripheral blood lymphocytes, thymus stimulated with sheep red blood cells and mitogenic lectins. (The reader is referred to HADDEN et al. 1979 for a complete review of these studies.)

In contrast to this work, other groups have been unable to demonstrate increases in lymphocyte intracellular cyclic GMP following mitogenic stimulation (PARKER et al. 1974; WEDNER et al. 1975; WATSON 1976; BURLESON and SAGE 1976; ATKINSON et al. 1978). These latter studies have been criticized either for the use of relatively impure populations of lymphocytes or because no attempt was made to purify the extracted cyclic GMP prior to its analysis by radioimmunoassay. However, ATKINSON et al. (1978) attempted to clarify the discrepancy by mimicking the experiments of HADDEN's group as closely as possible. In these studies, cyclic GMP was assayed without further purification and following purification on one, two or three columns sequentially. This study demonstrated that there was no increase in intracellular cyclic GMP in lectin-stimulated human peripheral blood lymphocytes and that the purification of cyclic GMP did not alter this result. In addition, it was demonstrated that increases in cyclic GMP were noted with a variety of guanylate cyclase agonists such as sodium nitroprusside, the nitrosoguanidine compound, NNMG, or L ascorbic acid (ATKINSON et al. 1978). The discrepancy between these two groups remains to be clarified.

In attempts to clarify the role of cyclic GMP in lymphocyte proliferation a number of groups have examined the effects of exogenously added cyclic GMP, 8-bromo-cyclic GMP, or putative guanylate cyclase agonists on lymphocyte proliferation. In general, these studies have been relatively disappointing. Addition of cyclic GMP or 8-bromo-cyclic GMP to human peripheral blood lymphocytes does not induce a proliferative response (WEDNER et al. 1976), and in human peripheral blood lymphocyte addition of acetylcholine, which increases intracellular cyclic GMP in some hands, but not in others, does not induce a proliferative response. ATKINSON et al. (1978) incubated human peripheral blood lymphocytes with the known guanylate cyclase agonists, sodium nitroprusside, NNMG and ascorbic acid. Only sodium nitroprusside was able to augment the proliferative response induced by PHA or Con A, but was not solely mitogenic in of itself. However, the dose-response curve for augmentation of the proliferative response and elevation of the intracellular cyclic GMP were discordant, suggesting that in this instance sodium nitroprusside was acting by some other mechanism.

Two groups have reported induction of proliferation by cyclic GMP or 8-bromo-cyclic GMP in mouse splenic cells (DIAMANSTEIN and ULMER 1975; DERUBERTIS and ZENSER 1976). However, there is some evidence to suggest that the action of cyclic GMP in this instance was indirect and resulted from the elaboration of a mitogenic factor (leukocyte activating factor, LAF) from mouse macrophages which indirectly induced proliferation in the lymphocyte population.

Guanylate cyclase activity has also been examined in mitogen stimulated human peripheral blood lymphocytes (COFFEY et al. 1981). These workers demonstrated that preincubation of human peripheral blood lymphocytes with mitogenic doses of PHA and Con A in the presence of Ca^{++} was reflected by an increase in guanylate cyclase activity in lymphocytes disrupted in the absence of calcium but in the presence of Mn^{++}. The increase in guanylate cyclase activity was inhibited by dithioerythrotol and by inhibitors of the lipoxygenase but not the cyclooxygenase pathway of arachidonic acid metabolism. These authors suggested that stimulation of mitogenesis was the result of the action of mitogens to stimulate the production of hydroxy or hydroperoxy fatty acids which indirectly stimulate guanylate cyclase and result in a proliferative response.

E. Cyclic Nucleotides in Lymphocyte-Mediated Cytotoxicity

Lymphocytes, either sensitized or unsensitized, have been shown to interact with and destroy a variety of cell types. These include foreign cells (allograph rejection) as well as foreign tumor cells or in some cases endogenously-derived tumor cells. The type of killing has been divided into several categories, these include natural killer cell activity (NK, SCMC-spontaneous cell mediated cytolysis), lymphocyte mediated cytotoxicity (LMC) and antibody-dependent cellular cytotoxicity (ADCC). The first requires no prior sensitization of the lymphocytes while the later two categories represent sensitization either of a cell mediated or humoral response. Of these types, the most extensively studied has been lymphocyte cytotoxicity directed against tumor cell targets using lymphocytes from previously sensitized animals. Early work by HENNEY and LICHTENSTEIN (1971) utilizing isoproterenol and/or theophylline suggested that cyclic AMP was an inhibitory influence in cytolysis. However, in these studies it was not clear whether the effect of these agents was on the target cell or the killer T lymphocyte. STROM and his co-workers extended these observations using a variety of agents (for review see STROM and CARPENTER 1980). They demonstrated that a variety of adenylate cyclase agonists were capable of inhibiting cell mediated cytolysis, and they were able to show that the effect was directly upon the killer T lymphocyte and not on the target cell. Interestingly, they were able to show that lymphocytes incubated with cholera toxin (which required approximately 180 min to elevate intracellular cyclic AMP) were still cytotoxic within one hour after incubation, at time at which intracellular cyclic AMP levels remained low, but were unable to destroy target cells after the elevation of intracellular cyclic AMP had occurred. Since some studies, particularly those of GOLDBERG and HADDOX (1977) have suggested opposing action of cyclic AMP and cyclic GMP, STROM and co-workers examined the effect of putative guanylate cyclase activators on cell-mediated cytolysis. Utilizing low doses of acetylcholine (10^{-11} to 10^{-13} *M*), they found significant augmentation of lymphocyte-mediated cytotoxicity. They were able to block this effect using atropine but not inhibitors of nicotinic cholinergic receptors. They suggested that the effect of acetylcholine was via its ability to stimulate increases in intracellular cyclic GMP. They also showed that imidazole, which has been reported to inhibit cyclic GMP phosphodiesterase but not cyclic AMP phosphodiesterase, was also effective in augmenting cell-mediated cytolysis.

This same group has also examined antibody-dependent cellular cytotoxicity in a similar system (GAROVOY et al. 1975). The studies performed were similar to those described for lymphocyte mediated cytotoxicity and the results were comparable in that cyclic AMP, phosphodiesterase inhibitors, or adenylate cyclase agonists inhibited the response while acetylcholine augmented the response. Thus, this action on both cell-mediated cytotoxicity and antibody-dependent cytotoxicity is consistent with the hypothesis that, in general, artificial elevation of intracellular cyclic AMP inhibits lymphocyte activities while elevation of cyclic GMP is stimulatory. It should be pointed out that in the majority of these systems it has been difficult, if not impossible, to measure increases in either cyclic AMP or cyclic GMP during killer target cell interactions, which makes the analysis of the exact role of these cyclic nucleotides in the natural function of these cells difficult to assess. Many of these difficulties appear to be largely technical and result from the fact that inhomogenous populations of cells are being used and that, in many cases, it is difficult to dissect changes in the killer cell population from those in the target cell. One would anticipate, however, that these difficulties are not insoluble and data concerning changes in cyclic nucleotide levels in this system should be forthcoming.

F. Cyclic AMP in Proliferating Thymocytes

Cyclic AMP may also play a role in the proliferation of a subpopulation of thymus lymphocytes (WHITFIELD et al. 1974). These cells, called RR (rapidly responding), are not actively dividing but can be induced to begin the cell cycle by brief exposure to high Ca^{++} concentrations (1.5 m*M* or above). The initiation of the DNA synthetic process is extremely rapid with [^{3}H] thymidine incorporation seen within one to two hours. WHITFIELD and MACMANUS and their collegues (for review see WHITFIELD 1979) have shown that the brief exposure to Ca^{++} results in a large burst of intracellular cyclic AMP. The Ca^{++} response can be mimicked by exogenous cyclic AMP or by adenylate cyclase agonists such as PGE_1. In addition PGE_1 stimulated the increase in DNA synthesis more rapidly, suggesting that the Ca^{2+} step has been bypassed. These workers (WHITFIELD et ål. 1979) speculated that Ca^{++} entering thymocytes interacts with calmodulin which then stimulates adenylate cyclase directly or via some intermediate such as a cyclic AMP independant protein kinase. The increase in cyclic AMP leads to the release of a Type II cyclic AMP dependant protein kinase which initiates DNA synthesis.

It is interesting to note that cyclic GMP also is capable of initiating DNA synthesis in these same cells. The effect of cyclic GMP is seen at low concentrations and high concentrations but not at the intermediate concentrations. At the concentrations at which cyclic GMP is effective there is a concomitant increase in cyclic AMP and the authors suggest this is the mode of cyclic GMP action.

It should be noted that this system is not analogous to the mitogen activated lymphocytes discussed above. The Ca^{++}-activated cells are believed to be fixed at the G_1-S interface and DNA synthesis begins within one hour. In the resting small lymphocyte, the block is at the G_0 stage and DNA synthesis does not begin for 24 h or more. It is interesting to note that one group (WANG et al. 1978) has found that there is a burst of cyclic AMP in lectin-stimulated mouse spleen cells. This occurs at a time when the G_1-S interface is being bridged and it is possible that the increase in intracellular cyclic AMP is important at this stage in the cycle. This observation would seem to provide some credence for the importance of cyclic AMP in initiation of DNA synthesis.

On the other hand, WAKSMAN and his collegues (WAGSHAL et al. 1978, JEGASOTHY et al. 1976, 1978) have identified a soluble mediator, IDS (inhibitor of DNA synthesis), which, if present, binds to receptors on lymphocytes which are present on the cell surface at 18–24 h. This then inhibits the progression of these cells into S phase and prevents DNA synthesis. WAKSMAN's group has some evidence that IDS increases intracellular cyclic AMP and has suggested that this elevation is its mode of action. Thus, we are again confronted with apparently opposing aspects of cyclic AMP action in the lymphocyte. This may represent another example of compartmentalization of cyclic nucleotide action, or may be the result of differing actions of cyclic AMP on lymphocyte subsets.

G. Conclusions

Work to date has indicated that lymphoid cells contain the enzymatic machinery for the generation, action, and destruction of both cyclic AMP and cyclic GMP. The relative activities of these enzymes, however, differs among the lymphocyte subsets which have been examined. The functional significance of these differences remains obscure, and will require a comparison of the levels of the individual nucleotides with functional counterparts in well defined systems.

The data reviewed here have dealt largely with systems were cell-cell and cell-soluble mediator interactions have been kept to a minimum. These studies would seem to offer the best hope of elucidating the function of cyclic AMP and cyclic GMP in each segment of the immune response. It is doubtful that more complex systems, such as in vivo immune responses, will yield easily interpretable data until simpler systems are worked out.

This is not to indicate that the prospects for understanding the role of cyclic AMP or cyclic GMP is hopeless. Elegant systems using antigen specific continuously growing cell lines of both B and T cell origin are now becoming available and should yield significant new information. In addition, many of the soluble mediators involved in the immune response are being produced in large quantity using hybridoma techniques. Pure preparations of these agents should be available and the examination of the effect of these agents on isolated subsets of lymphocytes will yield valuable data on the role of cyclic AMP and cyclic GMP in cell-mediator interactions. Utilizing these newer techniques should allow a better knowledge of the role of cyclic nucleotides in individual segments of the immune response and allow one to piece together the overall role of these nucleotides in immune reactivity.

Acknowledgements: The author would like to thank Ms. MAMIE TOMICH, Ms. NANCY GRIMSHAW and Mrs. RUTH NOBLE for excellent help in preparing the manuscript. Some of the work reported here was supported by Grant I RO AI/CA 18281-01 ALY 01 from the National Institute of Allergy and Infectious Diseases.

References

Atkinson JP, Sullivan TJ, Kelly JM, Parker CW (1977) Stimulation by alcohols of cAMP metabolism in human lymphocytes. J Clin Invest 60:284–294

Atkinson JP, Kelly JP, Weiss A, Wedner HJ, Parker CW (1978) Enhanced intracellular cGMP concentrations and lectin induced lymphocyte transformation. J Immunol 121:2282–2291

Bach MA (1975) Differences in cyclic AMP changes after stimulation by prostaglandins and isoproterenol in lymphocyte subpopulations. J Clin Invest 55:1074–1081

Berger NA, Johnson ES (1976) Studies of DNA synthesis in permeabilized mouse L cells in DNA synthesis and its regulation. Goulian M, Hanawalt P (eds) Benjamin, Inc, Menlo Park, CA., pp 719–721

Buckley PJ, Wedner HJ (1977) Variation in DNA and RNA synthetic responses during activation of lymphocytes from inbred strains of mice. J Immunol 119:9–18

Buckley PJ, Wedner HJ (1978) Measurements of the DNA synthetic capacity of activated lymphocytes: Nucleotide triphosphate incorporation by permeabilized cells. J Immunol 120:1930–1940

Burleson DG, Sage HJ (1976) Effects of lectins on the levels of cAMP and cGMP in guinea pig lymphocytes: early responses of lymph node cells to mitogenic non-mitogenic lectins. J Immunol 116:696–703

Castagna M, Palmer WK, Walsh DA (1975) Nuclear protein-kinase activity inperfused rat liver stimulated with dibutyryl-adenosine cyclic 3′,5′-monophosphate. Eur J Biochem 55:192–199

Chaplin DD, Wedner HJ (1978) Inhibition of lectin-induced lymphocyte activation by diamide and other sulfhydryl reagents. Cell Immunol 36:303–311

Chaplin DD, Wedner HJ, Parker CW (1979 a) Protein phosphorylation in human peripheral blood lymphocytes. I. Subcellular distribution and partial characterization of adenosine 3′,5′-monophosphate-dependent protein kinase and protein phosphorylation in human peripheral blood lymphocytes. Biochem J 182:525–536

Chaplin DD, Wedner HJ, Parker CW (1979 b) Protein phosphorylation in human peripheral blood lymphocytes. II. Phosphorylation of endogenous plasma membrane and cytoplasmic proteins. Biochem J 182:537–546

Chaplin DD, Wedner HJ, Parker CW (1980) Protein phosphorylation in human peripheral blood lymphocytes: Mitogen-induced increased in protein phosphorylation in intact lymphocytes. J Immunol 124:2390–2398

Coffey RG, Hadden EM, Hadden JW (1977) Evidence for cyclic GMP and calcium mediation of lymphocyte activation by mitogens. J Immunol 119:1387–1394

Coffey RG, Hadden EM, Hadden JW (1981) Phytohemagglutinin stimulation of guanylate cyclase in human lymphocytes. J Biol Chem 256:4418

Collavo D, Biasi G, Colomball A (1976) Generation of cytotoxic cells in absence of blastogenesis by mouse cells in mixed culture. Eur J Immunol 6:612–618

Cooper HL, Berger SL, Brauerman R (1975) Free ribosomes in physiologically nondividing cells. Human peripheral lymphocytes. J Biol Chem 251:4891–4900

Cross ME, Ord MG (1970) Changes in the phosphorylation and thiol content of histones in phytohemagglutinin-stimulated lymphocytes. Biochem J 118:191–193

DeRubertis FR, Zenser T (1976) Activation of murine lymphocytes by cyclic guanosine 3′,5′-monophosphate: specificity and role in mitogen activity. Biochem Biophys Acta 428:91–103
Diamanstein T, Ulmer A (1975) Regulation of DNA synthesis by guanosine 5′-diphosphate cyclic guanosine-3′,5′-monophosphate and cyclic adenosine-3′,5′-monophosphate in mouse lymphoid cells. Exp Cell Res 93:309–314
Edelman GM (1976) Surface modulation in cell recognition and cell growth. Science 192:218–226
Eisen SA, Wedner HJ, Parker CW (1972) Isolation of pure human peripheral blood T-lymphocytes using nylon wool columns. Immunol Commun 1:571–577
Epstein PM, Hersh EM, Thompson WJ (1976) Comparison of cyclic nucleotide phosphodiesterase of cultured and isolated lymphoid cells. Fed Proc 35:511
Farago A, Antoni F, Fabian F (1974) Histone kinases and cyclic AMP-binding capacity of nuclei of human tonsillar lymphocytes. Biochim Biophys Acta 370:459–467
Goldberg ND, Haddox MK (1977) Cyclic GMP metabolism and involvement in biological regulation. Ann Rev Biochem 46:823–896
Goffstein BJ, Gordon LK, Wedner HJ, Atkinson JP (1980) cAMP concentrations in human peripheral blood lymphocytes: Changes in association with cell purification. J Lab Clin Med 96:1002–1014
Gordon LK, Hamill B, Parker CW (1980) The activation of blast transformation and DNA synthesis in human peripheral blood lymphocytes by wheat germ agglutinin. J Immunol 125:814–819
Hadden JW, Coffey RG, Ananthakrishnan R, Hadden EM (1979) Cyclic nucleotide and calcium in lymphocyte regulation and activation. Ann New York Academy of Sciences, pp 241–254
Hadden JW, Hadden EM, Haddox MK, Goldberg ND (1972) Guanosine 3′,5′-cyclic monophosphate: a possible intracellular mediator of mitogenic influences in lymphocytes. Pro Natl Acad Sci USA 69:3024–3027
Hadden JW, Hadden EM, Sadlik JR, Coffey RG (1976) Effects of concanavalin A and a succinylated derivative on lymphocyte proliferation and cyclic nucleotide levels. Proc Natl Acad Sci USA 73:1717–1721
Hadden JW, Johnson EM, Hadden EM, Coffey RG, Johnson LD (1975) In: Rosenthal AS (ed) Immune recognition. Academic Press, New York, pp 359–389
Hait WN, Weiss B (1976) Increased cyclic nucleotide phosphodiesterase activity in leukaemic lymphocytes. Nature 259:321–323
Hait WN, Weiss B (1977) Characteristics of the cyclic nucleotide phosphodiesterase of normal and leukemic lymphocytes. Biochim Biophys Acta 497:86–100
Haley BE (1975) Photoaffinity labeling of adenosine 3′,5′-cyclic monophosphate binding sites of human red cell membranes. Biochemistry 14:3852–3857
Henney CS, Lichtenstein LM (1971) The role of cyclic AMP in the cytolytic activity of lymphocytes. J Immunol 107:610–612
Horenstein et al. (1976) Protein phosphokinase activities of resting and proliferating human lymphocytes. Changes upon phytohemagglutinin stimulation are in acute lymphoblastic leukemia cells. Exp Cell Res 101:260–266
Jegasothy BV, Pacher AR, Waksman BH (1976) Cytokine inhibition of DNA synthesis: effect on cyclic adenosine monophosphate in lymphocytes. Science 193:1260–1262
Jegasothy BV, Namba Y, Waksman BH (1978) Regulatory substances produced by lymphocytes VII IDS (inhibitor of DNA synthesis) inhibits stimulated lymphocyte proliferation by activation of membrane adenylate cyclase at a restriction point in late G_1. Immunochemistry 15:551–555
Juhl H, Esmann V (1979) Purification and properties of cAMP dependent and independent histone kinases from human leukocytes. Mol Cell Biochem 26:3–18
Kemp BE, Froscio M, Rogers A, Murray AW (1975) Multitude protein kinases from human lymphocyte: identification enzymes phosphorylating exogenous histone and casein. Biochem J 145:241–249
Kish VM, Kleinsmith LJ (1974) Nuclear protein kinases: evidence for their heterogeneity, tissue specificity, substrate specificity and differentiate responses to cyclic adenosine 3′,5′-monophosphate. J Biol Chem 249:750–760

Klimpel GR, Byos CV, Russel DH, Lucas DO (1976) Cyclic-AMP-dependent protein kinase activation and the induction of ornithine decarboxylase during lymphocyte mitogenesis. J Immunol 123:817–824
Krishnaraj R, Talwar GP (1973) Role of cyclic AMP in mitogen induced transformation of human peripheral leukocytes. J Immunol 111:1010–1017
Lagarde A, Colobert L (1972) Cyclic 3′,5′-AMP phosphodiesterase of human blood lymphocytes. Biochim Biophys Acta 276:444–453
MacManus JP, Whitfield JF, Boynton AL, Rixon RH (1975) Role of cyclic nucleotides and calcium in the positive control of cell proliferation. Adv Cyclic Nuc Res 5:719–734
Menahan LA, Kemp RG (1976) Cyclic 3′,5′adenosine monophosphate phosphodiesterase in the thymus of normal and leukemic mice. J Cyclic Nucleotide Res 2:417–425
Mendelsohn J, Nordberg J (1979) Adenylate cyclase in thymus-derived and bone marrow-derived lymphocytes from normal donors and patients with chronic lymphocytic leukemia. J Clin Invest 63:1124–1132
Monahan TM, Marchand NW, Fritz RR, Abell CW (1975) Cyclic adenosine 3′,5′-monophosphate levels and activities of related enzymes in normal and leukemic lymphocytes. Cancer Res 35:2540–2547
Murray AW, Froscio M, Kemp BE (1972) Histone phosphatase and cyclic nucleotide stimulated protein kinase from human lymphocytes. Biochem J 129:995–1002
Murray AW, Froscio M, Rogers A (1974) Dissociation of rabbit muscle cyclic AMP dependent protein kinase into catalytic and regulatory subunits by p-chloromercuribenzoate and methylmercuric. FEBS Letters 48:238–240
Niaudet PG, Beaurain, Bach MA (1976) Differences in effect of isoproterenol stimulation on levels of cyclic AMP in human B and T lymphocytes. Eur J Immunol 6:834–836
O'Farrell PH (1975) High resolution 2-dimensional electrophoresis of proteins. J Biol Chem 250:4007–4021
Oppenheim JJ, Rosenstreich DL (1976) In Progress in Allergy. Signals regulating in vitro activation of lymphocytes, pp 65–194
Parker CW (1974) Correlation between mitogenicity and stimulation of calcium uptake in human lymphocytes. Biochem Biophys Res Commun 61:1180–1186
Parker CW (1979) Role of cyclic nucleotides in regulating lymphocytes. Annals New York Academy Science 332:255–261
Parker CW, Sillivan TJ, Wedner HJ (1974) In Advances in Cyclic Nucleotide research. Cyclic AMP and the immune response. Greengard P, Robinson A (eds) Raven Press, New York, 4:1–79
Piras MM, Horenstein A, Piras R (1977) Identification of multiple protein kinases in normal human lymphocytes. Enzyme 22:219–229
Polgar P, Vera JC, Kelley PR, Rutenberg AM (1973) Adenylate cyclase activity in normal and leukemic human leukocytes as determined by a radioimmunoassay for cyclic AMP. Biochim Biophys Acta 297:378–383
Polgar P, Vera JC, Rutenberg AM (1977) An altered response to cyclic AMP stimulation hormones in intact human leukemic lymphocytes (39701). Proc Soc Exp Biol Med 154:493–495
Rikans LE, Ruddon RW (1973) The role of 3′,5′-cyclic AMP in the control of nuclear protein kinase activity. Biochim Biophys Res Comm 54:387–394
Scher NS, Quagliata F, Malathi VG, Faig D, Melton A, Silber R (1976) Cyclic adenosine 3′,5′-monophosphate phosphodiesterase activity in normal and chronic lymphocytic leukemia lymphocytes. Cancer Res 36:3958–3962
Schumm DE, Morris HP, Webb TE (1974) Early biochemical changes in phytohemagglutenin-stimulated peripheral blood lymphocytes from normal and tumor bearing rats. Eur J Cancer 10:107–113
Segel GB, Lichtman MA, Hollander MM, Gordon BR, Klemperer MR (1976) Human lymphocyte potassium content during the initiation of phytohemagglutinin-induced mitogenesis. J Cell Physiol 88:43–48
Sell S, Sheppard HW 81974) Studies on rabbit lymphocytes in vitro: kinetics of reversible Con A stimulation and restimulation of blast transformation after blocking with anti-Con A. Exp Cell Res 84:153–158

Smith JW, Steiner AL, Newberry WM, Parker CW (1971 a) Cyclic adenosine 3′,5′-monophosphate in human lymphocytes. Alterations after phytohemagglutinin stimulation. J Clin Invest 50:432–441

Smith JW, Steiner AL, Parker CW (1971 b) Human lymphocyte metabolism. J Clin Invest 50:442–448

Snider DR, Parker CW (1977) Adenylate cyclase activity in lymphocyte subcellular fractions. Characterization of non-nuclear adenylate cyclase. Biochem J 162:473–482

Steiner AL, Ong S, Wedner HJ (1976) Cyclic nucleotide immunochemistry. Adv Cyclic Nucleotide Res 7:115–155

Steiner AL, Parker CW, Kipnis DM (1972) Radioimmunoassay for cyclic nucleotides. I. Preparation of antibodies and iodinated cyclic nucleotides. J Biol Chem 247:1106–1113

Strom TB, Carpenter CB (1980) Cyclic nucleotides in immunosuppression – neuroendocrine pharmacologic manipulation and in vivo immunoregulation of immunity acting via second messenger systems. Transplantation Proceedings 12:304–310

Thompson WJ, Ross CP, Pledger WJ, Strada SJ, Banner RL, Hersh EM (1976) Cyclic adenosine 3′,5′-monophosphate phosphodiesterase distinct forms in human lymphocytes and monocytes. J Biol Chem 251:4922

Udey MC, Chaplin DD, Wedner HJ, Parker CW (1980) Early activation events in lectin-stimulated human lymphocytes. Evidence that wheat germ agglutinin and mitogenic lectins cause similar early changes in lymphocyte metabolism. J Immunol 125:1544–1550

Wagshal AB, Jegasothy BV, Waksman BH (1978) Regulatory substances produced by lymphocytes IV cell cycle specificity of inhibitor of DNA synthesis. J Exp Med 147:171–181

Wang T, Sheppard JR, Foker JE (1978) Rise and fall of cyclic AMP required for onset of lymphocyte DNA synthesis. Science 201:155–157

Watson J (1976) The involvement of cyclic nucleotide metabolism in the initiation of lymphocyte proliferation induced by mitogens. J Immunol 117:1656–1663

Webb DR, Stites DP, Perlman JD, Austin KR, Fudenberg HH (1974) Control of mitogen-induced lymphocyte activation. Clin Immunol Immunopath 2:322–332

Wedner HJ (1980) The effect of diamide on cyclic AMP levels and cyclic nucleotide phosphodiesterase in human peripheral blood lymphocytes. Biochim Biophys Acta 628:407–481

Wedner HJ, Chan BY, Parker CS, Parker CW (1979) Cyclic nucleotide phosphodiesterase activity in human peripheral blood lymphocytes and monocytes. J Immunol 123:725–732

Wedner HJ, Dankner R, Parker CW (1975) Cyclic GMP and lectin induced lymphocyte activation. J Immunol 115:1682–1687

Wedner HJ, Hoffer BJ, Battenberg R, Steiner AL, Parker CW (1972) A method for detecting intracellular cyclic adenosine monophosphate by immunofluorescence. J Histochem and Cytochem 20:293–295

Wedner HJ, Parker CW (1975) Protein phosphorylation in human peripheral lymphocytes – stimulation by phytohemagglutinin and N^6 monobutryl cyclic AMP. Biochem Biophys Res Comm 62:808–815

Wedner HJ, Parker CW (1976) Lymphocyte activation. In: Kallos P, Waksman BH, de-Weck A (eds) Progress in Allergy. S. Karger, Basel, 20:195–300

Wedner HJ, Parker CW (1977) Adenylate cyclase activity in lymphocyte subcellular fractions. Biochem J 162:483–491

Whitfield JF, Boynton AL, MacManus JP, Sikorska M (1979) The regulation of cell proliferation by calcium and cyclic AMP. Molecular and Cellular Biochemistry 27:155–179

Whitfield JF, MacManus JP, Boynton AL, Gillan DJ, Isaacs RJ (1974) Concanavalin A and the initiation of thymic lymphoblast DNA synthesis and proliferation by calcium-dependent increase in cyclic GMP level. J Cell Physiol 84:455–458

Winchurch R, Actor P (1972) The effects of an immunoenhancing bacterial product on the adenyl cyclase activity of mouse spleen cells. J Immunol 108:1305–1311

Yahara I, Edelman GM ((1975) Modulation of lymphocyte receptor mobility by concanavalin A and colchicine. Ann NY Acad Sci 253:455–469

CHAPTER 37

The Role of Cyclic Nucleotides in Invertebrates

C. J. LINGLE, E. MARDER, and J. A. NATHANSON

Overview

This chapter presents data supporting a possible role for cyclic nucleotides in neurotransmitter- and hormone-mediated events in invertebrates. Although a large number of studies are described, emphasis is placed on those preparations in which both physiological and biochemical data are available. Among the major topics treated are: (1) the effects of biogenic amines, calcium and cyclic nuleotides on secretory processes in insect salivary glands; (2) the "neuromodulatory" effects of serotonin and cyclic nucleotides in relatively long-term changes in synaptic efficacy, including heterosynaptic facilitation and behavioral sensitization; (3) the possible involvement of cyclic nucleotides in voltage-dependent amine responses; and (4) the role of cyclic AMP in mediating the neurogenic control of light emission in photogenic tissue. The above topics as well as others are organized and presented according to the hormone or transmitter mediating the various physiological processes. These hormones and transmitters include serotonin, octopamine, dopamine, and certain peptides.

A. Introduction

In many invertebrate as well as vertebrate tissues, neurotransmitters and hormones are released from one site and interact with specific receptors on target tissues, thereby initiating specific physiological responses. This review will focus on those invertebrate preparations in which there is reasonable evidence implicating cyclic nucleotide mechanisms in neurotransmitter or hormone-mediated physiological responses. It is not intended to be a comprehensive discussion of cyclic nucleotide biochemistry nor will it attempt a detailed description of neurotransmitter or hormone-activated membrane conductances and physiological responses. Instead, it will emphasize the questions and problems associated with trying to state, with certainty, that a given physiological response results from a receptor-activated nucleotide cyclase stimulation. Certain subjects, such as light-activated cyclic nucleotide responses (in retina) and the role of cyclic nucleotides in development, are discussed elsewhere in this volume (see chapters by FARBER and MCMAHON).

In many of the preparations to be described below, one is forced to rely upon pharmacology alone to establish whether the receptor responsible for a given hormone- or neurotransmitter-elicited cyclic nucleotide change is the same receptor as that responsible for eliciting the physiological response. To do so properly requires a fairly extensive pharmacological profile of both the biochemistry and physiology of the preparation, something which, too often, is lacking in invertebrate cyclic nucleotide research.

Another frequently encountered problem is the question of whether the pharmacological agents used in a particular study are interacting competitively with the natural receptor binding site or are exerting non-specific or non-receptor-related effects. While it may not be difficult to establish whether pharmacological agents are competitive or not (with the receptor) when performing biochemical experiments, it is much more difficult to do so when looking at physiological responses. For example, in physiological experiments it is often unknown whether a given agent is a receptor blocker or an ion channel blocker (or both). This is of some concern in the following review, since pharmacological data are frequently used by authors to suggest that a given receptor-associated response may be cyclic nucleotide-mediated. Accordingly, the reader should be aware that such comparisons may be meaningless, since it is often unknown how the pharmacological agents interact with the preparation in vivo. As such data becomes available in the future, many of the correlations described below will be strengthened; others will be weakened.

Another concern in many studies is the problem posed by the presence of multiple receptors and multiple physiological responses activated simultaneously by a single neurotransmitter or hormone. In a large number of invertebrate preparations, physiological (particularly electrophysiological) data demonstrate more than one response to a given agonist, while biochemical experiments characterizing the receptor do not indicate the same degree of physiological heterogeneity. Presumably, such heterogeneity of responses in vivo may be due to post-receptor related mechanisms; i.e., different cyclic nucleotide-activated protein kinases, different protein substrates, etc. Also, some receptors may be non-nucleotide cyclase-associated in some instances and coupled to a cyclase in other instances. In such cases it is conceivable that the pharmacological characteristics of the receptor might not differ in the two instances. (This situation would be somewhat different from what we know of the dopamine receptor in vertebrates, in which the adenylate cyclase-enhancing D_1-receptor differs pharmacologically from the non-cyclase-enhancing-D_2-receptor.) Hopefully, carefully coordinated biochemical, pharmacological and physiological experiments will provide future resolution to the above questions.

B. Serotonin-Cyclic Nucleotide Interactions

This section will examine the evidence that supports an involvement of cyclic nucleotides in serotonin-mediated physiological processes. Before proceeding, it may be useful to outline some questions which should be addressed when evaluating each of the preparations discussed below. These same questions are applicable, also, to the various other hormones and neurotransmitters discussed in later sections.

(1) For each preparation, how many pharmacologically distinguishable serotonin receptors are present in the tissue being studied?

(2) If there is more than one receptor, which receptor mediates which physiological response, how many of each type are there, and what are their relative tissue distributions?

(3) If a nucleotide cyclase is present, does the receptor(s) responsible for activating the enzyme correspond to that (those) mediating any of the physiological responses?

(4) Can the electrophysiological correlates of any of the physiological responses be mimicked by intracellular injection of cyclic nucleotides or potentiated by phosphodiesterase inhibitors?

(5) Does cyclic nucleotide-dependent phosphorylation of a particular protein(s) occur in the preparation, and, if so, can the phosphorylated product be implicated in the electrophysiological correlates of serotonin action?

I. Molluscs

The transmitter action of serotonin in molluscs is well-established (GERSCHENFELD 1973; KEHOE and MARDER 1976). Serotonin-containing neurons have been identified (COTTRELL and POWELL 1971; COTTRELL 1977; PENTREATH and COTTRELL 1974; WEINREICH et al. 1973); the intracellular metabolism, packaging, and transport of serotonin have been studied (GOLDMAN and SCHWARTZ 1974, 1977; GOLDBERG et al. 1976, 1978; Goldman et al. 1976; SCHWARTZ et al. 1979; SHKOLNIK and SCHWARTZ 1980; AMBRON et al. 1980); and serotonin release by identified neurons has been demonstrated (GERSCHENFELD et al. 1978). Physiological responses to serotonin are found on neurons in molluscan central ganglia (STEFANI and GERSCHENFELD 1969; GERSCHENFELD and PAUPARDIN-TRITSCH 1974; PELLMAR and WILSON 1977) and on other target tissues including catch muscle (TWAROG 1976), heart (WELSH 1971; HIGGINS 1977; WILKENS and GREENBERG 1972), and other muscles (WEISS et al. 1975; LLOYD 1980a, b).

Electrophysiological studies have demonstrated that serotonin can activate a number of different physiological responses (GERSCHENFELD and PAUPARDIN-TRITSCH 1974; PELLMAR and WILSON 1977). These physiological responses include increases in Na^+ conductance, Cl^- conductance, and K^+ conductance; decreases in K^+ conductance and Na^+/K^+ conductance (GERSCHENFELD and PAUPARDIN-TRITSCH 1974). Additionally, in some cells, serotonin elicits an inward current which is evident only at depolarized membrane potentials (PELLMAR and WILSON 1977; PELLMAR and CARPENTER 1979; PELLMAR 1980; DETERRE et al. 1981), can influence heterosynaptic facilitation (SHIMAHARA and TAUC 1975, 1977), and has been implicated in behavioral sensitization (BRUNELLI et al. 1976; KLEIN and KANDEL 1978, 1980). Although, when first reported, these effects seemed to be disparate, recent work (see below) allows us to suggest that these phenomena may all be explicable according to a single mechanism.

Among the various preparations which have been studied, those involving peripheral tissues have the advantage of being relatively homogeneous; unfortunately they often present difficulties for sophisticated electrophysiological studies. Molluscan ganglia are thought of as the proverbial "simple system" and are relatively tractable to sophisticated electrophysiological studies and single cell biochemical analyses. The most recent work on these preparations (DRUMMOND et al.

1980a, b, c; CASTELLUCCI et al. 1980; KACZMAREK et al. 1980; DETERRE et al. 1981) provides new and convincing lines of evidence for the involvement of cyclic nucleotides in *some* of the physiological responses to serotonin shown in these ganglia.

1. Nerve Tissue

a) Biochemical Background

One of the earliest studies in this area was that of CEDAR and SCHWARTZ (1972), who demonstrated that a 5 min application of serotonin (usually at 2×10^{-4} *M*) to intact *Aplysia* ganglia in vitro resulted in increased accumulation of cyclic AMP. Typical increases in ganglionic cyclic AMP of about 8-fold occurred after such treatment, with a K_a for serotonin of about 6×10^{-6} *M*. These authors were unable to demonstrate serotonin-stimulated adenylate cyclase activity in tissue homogenates, and saw no appreciable inhibition by LSD (5×10^{-4} *M*) or methysergide (3×10^{-4} *M*) of the serotonin-stimulated increase in cyclic AMP accumulation. Subsequently, LEVITAN et al. (1974), incubated *Aplysia* ganglia for 10 min in 10^{-4} *M* serotonin and found about a 6-fold increase in cyclic AMP levels. Methysergide (10^{-3} *M*) reduced the effectiveness of this increase. Similar values for serotonin-stimulated increases in cyclic AMP levels have been reported in bag cells (KACZMAREK et al. 1978).

The first demonstration of serotonin-activated adenylate cyclase in molluscan membrane fractions was that of LEVITAN (1978), who reported a small but significant stimulation by 2×10^{-5} *M* serotonin of adenylate cyclase activity in particulate cell fractions from single neurons. This stimulation was blocked by 10^{-6} *M* LSD. DRUMMOND et al. (1980a) measured adenylate cyclase activity in membrane fractions from *Aplysia* ganglia, heart, and muscle and found that in all regions the enzyme showed a K_a for serotonin activation of about 1–2 micromolar. This affinity of serotonin is similar to that reported by NATHANSON and GREENGARD (1974) for serotonin-sensitive adenylate cyclase in cockroach ganglia (see below).

DRUMMOND et al. (1980b) have recently carried out a more extensive characterization of serotonin-sensitive adenylate cyclase in *Helix*. In particulate fractions of the circumesophageal ganglia, serotonin ($K_a = 1.65 \times 10^{-6}$ *M*), but not dopamine, stimulated enzyme activity. Of a number of serotonin-like agents tested, only the N-methyl and N-N-dimethyl derivatives of serotonin (and, to a lesser extent, 5-methoxytryptamine) were as potent as serotonin. Tryptamine, 5-methoxytryptamine, and 6-hydroxytryptamine were partial agonists which elicited maximal responses between 20 and 65% of that produced by serotonin. d-LSD was a competitive antagonist of serotonin stimulation, with a calculated K_i of 10 n*M*. Unlike previous results obtained in *Aplysia* (DRUMMOND et al. 1980a) or cockroach (NATHANSON and GREENGARD 1974) ganglia, LSD did not act as a partial serotonin agonist in *Helix*. Other ergot derivatives, including ergotamine ($K_i = 47$ n*M*) and dihydroergocryptine ($K_i = 97$ n*M*) were also potent antagonists, as were the neuroleptics, d-butaclamol ($K_i = 21$ n*M*) and cis-flupenthixol ($K_i = 100$ n*M*).

LEVITAN and BARONDES (1974) and LEVITAN et al. (1974) reported that incubations of *Aplysia* abdominal ganglia with high serotonin concentrations produced, after many hours, a "specific" phosphorylation of a 120,000 dalton protein.

In particulate preparations of the same ganglion, cyclic AMP stimulated the phosphorylation of a similar protein (BANDLE and LEVITAN 1977). More recently, in similar experiments, PARIS et al. (1980) have reported that serotonin stimulates the phosphorylation of a protein with an apparent molecular weight of about 137,000 daltons.

These biochemical studies suggest the existence of a serotonin receptor capable of activating adenylate cyclase activity. DRUMMOND et al. (1978, 1980a, b) have compared serotonin-inhibited [^{3}H]-LSD binding with serotonin-activated adenylate cyclase activity in *Helix* and *Aplysia*, and, on the basis of similar kinetic data, have suggested that the two methods are in fact measuring the same class of serotonin receptors. This is somewhat puzzling because although the rapid conductance increase responses to iontophoretic serotonin applications on cells of *Helix* and *Aplysia* ganglia are blocked by LSD (GERSCHENFELD and PAUPARDIN-TRITSCH 1974), there is little if any evidence that these rapid responses are mediated via a cyclic nucleotide reaction. It is possible that the actual number of receptor sites responsible for the serotonin-induced rapid conductance increases is very much smaller than those responsible for the adenylate cyclase activation. Alternatively, it is possible that the action of LSD on these physiological responses in non-competitive, so that the receptors involved might not be labelled in a LSD binding study, but would be "biochemically silent". Either way, it is important to bear in mind that because the electrophysiological responses to serotonin in these tissues are complex, it may not be easy to correlate the available biochemical and physiological data.

b) Involvement of Cyclic AMP in Serotonin-Elicited Physiological Responses

Recent evidence suggests that serotonin's effects on some molluscan neurons may occur through a cyclic AMP-mediated decrease of a voltage-sensitive K^+ conductance which permits more Ca^{++} to enter presynaptic cells, thus leading to increased neurotransmitter release. This increased transmitter release has significant consequences for at least one important behavior in the mollusc. As will be described below, elucidation of this phenomenon has been complicated by the inherent difficulties, under many experimental conditions, in distinguishing between increases in inward currents and decreases in outward currents.

Heterosynaptic facilitation occurs when the monosynaptic connection between two neurons is enhanced after the firing of action potentials in a third neuron (KANDEL and TAUC 1965; SHIMAHARA and TAUC 1975). SHIMAHARA and TAUC (1975) showed that iontophoretic serotonin applications to the neuropile area of *Aplysia* ganglia mimicked the effects of heterosynaptic facilitation at a specific synapse. Their interpretation was that serotonin was liberated by a third neuron, causing an increase in the amount of transmitter released from presynaptic nerve terminals. LSD blocked the effects of the heterosynaptic pathway, as well as those of serotonin. SHIMAHARA and TAUC (1976, 1977) identified a neuron capable of producing heterosynaptic facilitation and attempted to establish whether cyclic nucleotides were involved in this effect by applying dibutyryl cyclic AMP and theophylline to the neuropile region of the ganglion. They were able to mimic the effects of serotonin with dibutyryl cyclic AMP and to potentiate the effects with theophylline. These authors suggested that serotonin acts on the nerve terminal to enhance Ca^{++} entry into the nerve ending, thereby causing more transmitter release.

The gill-withdrawal reflex in *Aplysia* is an attractive preparation for the study of the cellular mechanisms underlying habituation and sensitization, synaptic phenomena which have been employed extensively in the study of long-term changes in neuronal function (KANDEL 1979). CASTELLUCCI and KANDEL (1976) argued that sensitization of the gill-withdrawal reflex is produced by an increase in the amount of transmitter released by the presynaptic sensory neurons, resulting in larger excitatory postsynaptic potentials (EPSPs) in the motor neurons. BRUNELLI et al. (1976) found that serotonin (applied in the bath) increased the amplitude of the monosynaptic EPSP from sensory neurons to motor neurons. This effect of serotonin was blocked by cinanserin, but not by LSD or methysergide. In other studies, BRUNELLI et al. (1976) injected cyclic AMP directly into the sensory cell body and found that the nucleotide mimicked the effects of serotonin on the amplitude of the EPSP recorded in the motor neurons.

KLEIN and KANDEL (1978) showed that when the K^+ conductance of the sensory cell body was blocked with tetraethylammonium (TEA), serotonin increased the duration of the plateau of the action potential, as did isobutylmethylxanthine (IBMX) and intracellular injections of cyclic AMP. These workers suggested that the prolongation of the action potential would lead to increased Ca^{++} influx and thus to more neurotransmitter release.

In 1977, PELLMAR and WILSON first described a serotonin response which is activated only when the membrane is depolarized to about -20 mV (PELLMAR and WILSON 1977; PELLMAR and CARPENTER 1979, 1980). This voltage-dependent response is quite slow, lasting 1–4 min, with a time-to-peak of about 10–20 s. Because of its time course and unconventional nature, PELLMAR (1980) investigated the possibility that cyclic nucleotides were mediating this current. PELLMAR (1980) found that direct intracellular injections of cyclic AMP mimicked the serotonin response in time course and in voltage sensitivity, although the effects of 5′-AMP and other cyclic AMP analogs were not reported. Intracellular injection of three different phosphodiesterase inhibitors, theophylline, IBMX, and RO-20-1724, had the paradoxical effect of reducing the current produced both by serotonin and by direct cyclic AMP injection.

More recently, DETERRE et al. (1981) found that the voltage-dependent serotonin-evoked inward current could be mimicked with intracellular injections of cyclic AMP and that this effect could be potentiated with IBMX. Adenylate cyclase activity in homogenates from these neurons was stimulated 87% by 10^{-5} *M* serotonin. In an attempt to discover the ionic mechanism for this voltage-sensitive serotonin response, these authors performed a number of ion replacement and intracellular injection studies and concluded that the response is likely due to a decrease in a voltage-sensitive and Ca^{++}-sensitive K^+ conductance.

These experiments complement recent physiological, biophysical, and biochemical experiments on the role of serotonin in behavioral sensitization in the gill-withdrawal response in *Aplysia*. HAWKINS and colleagues (HAWKINS 1981; HAWKINS et al. 1981a, b; BAILEY et al. 1981) have identified neurons capable of producing behavioral sensitization and have provided evidence that the cells are serotonergic. KLEIN and KANDEL (1980) were able, by voltage-clamping the sensory cells, to provide evidence that serotonin decreases a voltage-sensitive K^+ conductance, thus prolonging the time during which Ca^{++} enters the cell and enhancing neurotransmitter release. CASTELLUCCI et al. (1980) injected purified catalytic subunit of cyclic AMP-dependent protein kinase into sensory cells. They found that catalytic subunit injections mimicked the effects of serotonin on the facilitating pathway, broadening the Ca^{++} action potential, decreasing the input conductance, and increasing transmitter release These data, together with the parallel studies of KACZMAREK et al. (1980), who showed that injection of catalytic subunit into *Aplysia* bag cells increased the duration of a Ca^{++} spike, strongly support the argument that these membrane conductances are under cyclic nucleotide control.

In summary, these recent data suggest that behavioral sensitization in the gill-withdrawal reflex of *Aplysia* is due to a heterosynaptic pathway mediated by identified serotonergic neurons. The neurally released serotonin appears to act, via a cyclic AMP-mediated mechanism, to decrease a voltage-sensitive K^+ conductance, thus causing an increase in the Ca^{++} concentration in the presynaptic terminals producing, in turn, an increase in transmitter release. The ongoing experimental investigations of the above sequence of events constitute a promising area of current research on cyclic nucleotides in invertebrates. Additional biochemical and physiological experiments will be necessary to confirm and to refine the conclusions suggested by these data.

Other recent studies in *Aplysia* have concerned the possible role of cyclic nucleotides in the bursting behavior of certain neurons. R 15 is an endogenously active neuron in the abdominal ganglion which shows spontaneous oscillations of membrane potential in the absence of synaptic or hormonal activity. When serotonin is applied to R 15, the neuron hyperpolarizes and its endogenous bursting activity is terminated (DRUMMOND et al. 1980c). This serotonin-produced hyperpolarization is associated with an increase in K^+ conductance and is mimicked by intracellular injections of cyclic AMP analogues (DRUMMOND et al. 1980c; LEVITAN and NORMAN 1980). In addition, biochemical studies of serotonin-activated adenylate cyclase in the abdominal ganglion indicate that the pharmacological characteristics of this enzyme are similar to those of the serotonin-mediated physiological response (DRUMMOND et al. 1980a). These studies suggest that the hyperpolarizing increase in K^+ conductance may result from a serotonin-activated cyclic AMP accumulation. This contrasts with the serotonin-stimulated *decrease* in voltage-sensitive K^+ conductance seen in the process of behavioral sensitization (above) (KLEIN and KANDEL 1980; CASTELLUCCI 1980; DETERRE et al. 1981). Further studies will be necessary to determine whether serotonin-stimulated adenylate cyclase triggers different physiological responses in different cells or whether these apparently discrepant effects result from a common mechanism, such as an increase in intracellular Ca^{++}.

2. Heart

Molluscan hearts are sensitive to low concentrations of serotonin (WELSH 1971; LOVELAND 1963; LIEBESWAR et al. 1975; KOESTER et al. 1973; IRISAWA et al. 1972; WILKENS and GREENBERG 1972), and, in most cases, the reported action of serotonin is cardioacceleratory. Evidence that serotonin is the actual endogenous neurally-released excitatory transmitter has been presented by LOVELAND (1963) in studies of *Mercenaria* heart. In *Aplysia*, MAYERI et al. (1974) have identified a heart excitor motor neuron (RBHE) which causes slow depolarizing potentials in the heart muscle. LIEBESWAR et al. (1975) showed that serotonin application mimics the effects of RBHE stimulation, and that, by biochemical criteria, the RBHE motor neuron is serotonergic.

A number of groups, working on various molluscan heart preparations, have attempted to determine whether a serotonin-activated adenylate cyclase is implicated in the above physiological effects. WOLLEMANN and S-ROZSA (1975) reported the presence of a serotonin-activated adenylate cyclase (10-fold stimulation by 10^{-6} *M* serotonin) in cell-free particulate fractions from the ventricles of *Helix* and *Anodonata*. However, in order to show amine stimulation, these authors had to deplete the tissue of endogenous biogenic amines by pretreatment with reserpine. Similar data have been obtained from *Mercenaria* hearts (HIGGINS 1974; HIGGINS et al. 1978), both in homogenates and intact tissue slices. In these latter exeriments, the K_a for serotonin activation was about 10^{-7} *M*, somewhat lower than reported elsewhere. Methysergide (10^{-5} *M*) was reported to be effective in preventing serotonin-activation of the enzyme.

MANDELBAUM et al. (1979) have investigated the possibility that cyclic nucleotides mediate the excitatory serotonergic input in *Aplysia* heart. They found that whole hearts accumulated cyclic AMP after serotonin applications, and that the region of the atrioventricular valves showed significantly greater activity than other portions of the heart. The dose-dependent cyclic AMP accumulation was as much as 400-fold above control levels at 10^{-4} *M* serotonin. These authors found that perfusion of the heart with 2.5×10^{-4} *M* 8-bromo cyclic AMP or RO-20-1724 caused an increase in heart rate. Although MANDELBAUM et al. (1979) did not attempt a pharmacological comparison of the serotonin receptor mediating the cyclic AMP accumulation with that mediating the physiological response, KEBABIAN et al. (1979), also studying *Aplysia* heart muscle, found that 10^{-5} *M* bromo-LSD and lisuride were quite effective in inhibiting serotonin-activated increases in cyclic AMP and that fluphenazine and lergotrile were reasonably effective at 10^{-4} *M*. In physiological studies, LIEBESWAR et al. (1975) reported that the effects of serotonin and the effects of stimulation of the RBHE neuron were partially blocked by methysergide and bromo-LSD, but were most effectively blocked by cinanserin. Unfortunately, the effects of this latter antagonist on the serotonin-activated increase in cyclic AMP in heart muscle are not known. Therefore, at the present time, it is unclear whether the serotonin receptors mediating the cyclic AMP changes and the physiological response are the same.

3. Gill

Although currently there is no clear indication that serotonin is a neurotransmitter in gill muscles, PERETZ and ESTES (1974) have provided fluorescence histochemical evidence that serotonin is present in this tissue. Furthermore, KEBABIAN et al. (1979) have shown that serotonin stimulates the accumulation of cyclic AMP in the *Aplysia* gill, even when synaptic transmission is blocked with high Mg^{++}-containing saline (suggesting that serotonin is interacting with adenylate cyclase directly).

In these latter experiments, half-maximal stimulation of cyclic AMP levels was produced by 5×10^{-5} *M* serotonin. Additivity studies showed that the serotonin effect was separable from dopamine stimulation of cyclic AMP levels in the same tissue (see Sect. D.I on dopamine), although a considerable number of dopamine and serotonin agonists and antagonists failed to distinguish completely between the serotonin and dopamine receptors (as measured by stimulation of cyclic AMP levels in intact tissue). In related experiments, GENTLEMAN and MANSOUR (1977) studied the effects of serotonin on cyclic AMP accumulation and adenylate cyclase activity in intact and particulate fractions from *Abalone* gill. These experiments are difficult to compare with those above since only high serotonin concentrations were tested and the observed stimulation was significantly less than that reported by others.

4. Buccal Muscles

The accessory radula closer muscle of the buccal mass of *Aplysia* is innervated by at least two identified cholinergic motor neurons, B 15 and B 16 (COHEN et al. 1978). Additionally, this muscle receives branches from the metacerebral giant neuron (WEISS et al. 1978a), which is serotonergic (WEINREICH et al. 1973; GOLDMAN and SCHWARTZ 1974; GERSCHENFELD et al. 1978). WEISS et al. (1975, 1978a) have described a "neuromodulatory" effect of firing the metacerebral giant cell on tension developed in the accessory radula muscle elicited by stimulating the cholinergic motor neurons, B 15 and B 16. They report that only a small amount of tension results from B 15 and B 16 stimulation alone, but after the metacerebral cell is fired (or after serotonin application) the motor neurons produce more tension in the muscle. These results raise several questions: (1) Do metacerebral giant cell stimulation and serotonin application affect the terminals of the motor neurons, the muscle itself, or both? (2) If there is more than one site of action of serotonin, are the serotonin receptors the same? (3) Are cyclic nucleotides implicated in any of these effects? (4) Are there discrete conductance changes responsible for the effects? (5) Do the serotonin receptors mediating these effects on muscle resemble those found in the nervous system and elsewhere?

Partial answers to some of these questions are provided by WEISS et al. (1978a, b, 1979) who argue that there are at least two separable effects of metacerebral stimulation of the muscle, one (possibly the major one) being an alteration of the excitation-contraction coupling system, the other being an enhancement in the amplitude of the intracellularly-recorded excitatory junctional potential (EJP). The strongest argument in favor of a direct effect on the muscle excitation-contraction coupling mechanism was the finding that metacerebral giant cell stimulation enhanced the amplitude of contractions produced by direct electrical stimulation of the muscle or by direct application of acetylcholine (the excitatory transmitter released by the motor neurons).

Similar data are presented by KOBAYASHI and MUNEOKA (1980) working on the muscles of *Rapana thomasiana*. KOBAYASHI and MUNEOKA (1980) found that low serotonin concentrations enhanced nerve-evoked contractions in the radula contractor muscle, and also enhanced the contractions produced by direct electrical stimulation of the muscle, in the presence of high concentrations of cholinergic blocking agents. Again, the interpretation is that at least part of the neuromodulatory effect of serotonin is due to a direct effect on the muscle fiber's contractile functions. Neither of the above groups addresses the issue of whether the enhancements in EJP amplitudes which are sometimes observed are due to a serotonin-mediated increase in transmitter release or to a direct effect on muscle current-voltage relationships.

WEISS et al. (1978 b, 1979) further attempt to answer the question of whether cyclic nucleotides mediate these serotonergic neuromodulatory effects. They report that serotonin causes a 250- to 300-percent increase in cyclic AMP accumulation in intact buccal muscles with a half-maximal stimulation at about 3.5×10^{-6} *M*. Measurements of serotonin-stimulated adenylate cyclase activity in crude membrane fractions from the same muscle resulted in a K_a in about the same range, but with much less stimulation than that seen in intact tissue and much less than that reported by DRUMMOND et al. (1980 a). The reason for this discrepancy may be that DRUMMOND et al. assayed adenylate cyclase activity in the presence of added GTP, while WEISS et al. did not. In other experiments demonstrating the physiological relevance of the above biochemical studies, WEISS et al. (1978 b, 1979) have shown that electrical activity in the serotonin-containing metacerebral giant cell (which is thought to be responsible for the serotonin-activated neuromodulatory effects in this preparation) causes dramatic increases in cyclic AMP accumulation in the buccal muscles.

WEISS et al. (1979) also report that the cyclic nucleotide analogs, 8-bromo cyclic AMP and 8-parachlorophenylthio cyclic AMP, mimic the effect of serotonin in enhancing the amplitude of the muscle contractions. Since (unlike serotonin) the analogs also caused decrements in the amplitude of intracellularly recorded EJPs, the authors feel that the alteration in EJP amplitude may not be the primary site of serotonin's action. Harder to explain were the effects of the methyl xanthines, which diminished both EJPs and muscle contractile responses. The phosphodiesterase inhibitor, RO 20-1724, did produce some potentiation of the effects of metacerebral giant cell stimulation.

In summary, these data provide some, but certainly not complete, evidence that serotonin-activated adenylate cyclase may be involved in some of the physiological effects of metacerebral giant cell stimulation. Missing, still, are detailed pharmacological analyses of both the serotonin receptor mediating the activation of adenylate cyclase in this muscle, and of the receptor producing the physiological effects. Also missing, although undoubtedly very difficult to obtain due to the small size and electrical coupling of the muscle fibers, are physiological experiments to characterize further the presynaptic and postsynaptic effects, if any, of serotonin on specific membrane conductances.

5. Catch Muscles

"Catch" muscles in molluscs maintain tension for long periods of time in the absence of an active state, and with little expenditure of energy (TWAROG 1976). Serotonin is most likely the neurotransmitter released by the nerves which terminate the catch tension, and exogenous applications of very low serotonin concentrations (10^{-10} to 5×10^{-8} *M*) produce muscle relaxation (TWAROG 1954, 1976;

TWAROG and COLE 1972). COLE and TWAROG (1972) attempted to determine if these actions of serotonin were mimicked by cyclic AMP or by treatments likely to increase intracellular concentrations of cyclic AMP. They found that adding cyclic AMP to the bath was without effect, although in some preparations relaxation was produced by dibutyryl cyclic AMP. High theophylline concentrations produced relaxation, and short treatments with NaF enhanced serotonin-induced relaxations. Recently, KOHLER and LINDL (1980) characterized a serotonin-activated accumulation of cyclic AMP in the anterior byssus retractor muscle of *Mytilus* (the same as that studied by TWAROG and COLE). Their dose-response curves show a 30-fold increase in cyclic AMP levels after serotonin applications, with half-maximal stimulation at about 10^{-6} *M*. Thus, the physiological effects of serotonin are maximal at much lower doses than are the effects on cyclic AMP levels, and without additional pharmacological, physiological, and biochemical data it is difficult to know if the relaxation of catch tension is mediated via a cyclic nucleotide mechanism.

II. Insects

Beyond the extensive work by BERRIDGE and others on the role of serotonin and serotonin-sensitive adenylate cyclase in the fluid secretion process in blowfly salivary glands, much less is known concerning the role of serotonin and cyclic nucleotides in other insect tissues. Because of this, most of the following discussion will deal with the blowfly salivary gland. The remainder of the section will discuss the possible role of cyclic nucleotides in other physiological processes mediated by serotonin. These include: stimulation of fluid secretion by Malphigian tubules (MADDRELL et al. 1971), the acceleration of heartbeat (COLLIN and MILLER 1977), the acceleration of a myogenic rhythm in a locust skeletal muscle (EVANS and O'SHEA 1978), and possible involvement in the release of hormones from the *corpora cardiaca* (SAMARANAYAKA 1976). Because some of the effects of serotonin in insects occur at low concentrations in organs not known to receive serotonergic innervation, certain primary functions of serotonin may be mediated neurohormonally (see BERRIDGE 1972). However, as yet, there is no direct evidence for a source of humorally secreted serotonin in insects.

1. Salivary Gland

The salivary glands of the blowfly, *Calliphora erythrocephalus*, have been used to analyze the involvement of both cyclic AMP and calcium in the activation by serotonin of fluid secretion (reviewed by BERRIDGE and PRINCE 1972a, b; RASMUSSEN and GOODMAN 1977; see also BERRIDGE, this volume). Each gland consists of a single homogeneous cell layer arranged in a tubular structure surrounding a central lumen. The tissue is non-innervated and thought to be controlled by neurohumoral influences (OCHSMAN and BERRIDGE 1970). The secretory portion of the gland secretes a KCl solution, isotonic with the cellular contents, through the apical membrane into the lumen of the tubule. Serotonin applied to the basal membrane increases the rate of fluid secretion into the lumen. The system has been used to examine the pharmacology of the serotonin-activated secretory response (BER-

RIDGE 1972; BERRIDGE and PRINCE 1974), the nature of the permeability changes across both the apical and basal membranes during the action of serotonin (BERRIDGE and PRINCE 1971, 1972c; PRINCE and BERRIDGE 1972; BERRIDGE et al. 1975a), the involvement of both cyclic AMP and calcium in the serotonin-activated secretory and electrical changes (BERRIDGE and PATEL 1968; PRINCE and BERRIDGE 1973; BERRIDGE 1970; PRINCE et al. 1972), and, more recently, the involvement of membrane phospholipids in serotonin-activated calcium fluxes (FAIN and BERRIDGE 1979; BERRIDGE and FAIN (1979).

a) Serotonin-Activated Fluid Secretion

Fluid secretion into the lumen is activated by concentrations of serotonin over the range of 10^{-11} to 5×10^{-8} M with 50% activation at 10^{-10} M (BERRIDGE and PATEL 1968; BERRIDGE 1972). A secretion-producing principle isolated from the blowfly brain has been identified as serotonin, suggesting that it is the natural activator of secretion (BERRIDGE and PATEL 1968). Application of serotonin produces an increase in fluid secretion which reaches a maximal rate within 1 min and is maintained for the duration of the serotonin application (BERRIDGE 1970). Removal of serotonin results in a decrease in fluid secretion to control levels within two to three minutes. The responses are stable for hours.

Alterations of the serotonin molecule have led to the suggestion that the integrity of the quaternary nitrogen is essential for receptor activation, while the hydrophobic indole ring and 5-hydroxyl moieties are involved in positioning and stabilizing the molecule in a site that enables the charged nitrogen to activate the receptor (BERRIDGE 1972). Molecules lacking the hydroxyl group or with alterations in the indole ring are as effective as serotonin in activating maximal rates of secretion, although less potent. Alterations in the quaternary nitrogen prevent activation of secretion. LSD shows mixed agonist properties, activating at low concentrations rates of secretion similar to serotonin-activated maximal secretion rates. The onset of LSD-activated secretion is slower than the onset of serotonin-activated secretion, although LSD, when applied as a short pulse, produces a more prolonged activation of secretion than does serotonin. The response to LSD can be diminished in duration by exposure to serotonin or tryptamine during washout of LSD. This has led to the suggestion that the higher apparent affinity of LSD results from its hydrophobic interactions which maintain the LSD molecule in a position for repeated receptor activation.

Phenylethylamine and dopamine also activate fluid secretion with a maximal rate similar to serotonin, although the action of these amines occurs over the range of 10^{-5} to 10^{-3} M (BERRIDGE 1972). The lower potency of these amines is thought to reflect a low affinity for the serotonin receptor, arising from a reduced affinity for the hydrophobic sites near the receptor. However, the possibility should be considered that other amines may regulate other cellular processes within the salivary glands, and may be capable of activating fluid secretion through alternative routes. For example, the salivary gland of the cockroach and some other insects (see Sect. D.II below) appears to receive dopaminergic innervation (HOUSE et al. 1973; BLAND et al. 1973; FRY et al. 1974; KLEMM 1972; ROBERTSON 1975), and there is evidence that, in these glands, both serotonin and dopamine activate secretion through distinct receptors (BOWSER-RILEY et al. 1978). Although the blowfly salivary gland is not innervated, the argument for the presence of a single class of serotonin receptors would be strengthened by a demonstration that antagonists of the serotonin-activated fluid secretion, e.g., gramine, also block the responses to other amines, and that adenylate cyclase activation by serotonin can be distinguished from activation of cyclases by other amines.

b) Involvement of Cyclic AMP in Serotonin-Activated Fluid Secretion

Serotonin increases the cyclic AMP level of intact salivary glands with a time course closely paralleling the time course of serotonin-activated increases in fluid secretion (PRINCE et al. 1972). No increases in cyclic GMP have been observed. Both LSD and serotonin at 10 n*M* produce a similar activation of adenylate cyclase in the salivary gland (BERRIDGE and PRINCE 1974). The effects of other amines and the pharmacological characteristics of the serotonin-activated cyclic AMP increases have not been examined in detail.

Both cyclic AMP and theophylline increase fluid secretion in intact salivary glands; furthermore, theophylline lowers the threshold concentration of serotonin-activated secretion (BERRIDGE 1970). Ten m*M* cyclic AMP induces a rate of secretion identical to the maximal rates that occur in response to serotonin and with a similar time course of activation. The high concentration of cyclic AMP required to elicit fluid secretion is presumably due to the limited permeability of the basal membrane to cyclic AMP. A variety of cyclic AMP derivatives have also been tested for their ability to activate fluid secretion (BERRIDGE 1973). The integrity of the ribose and phosphate regions of the molecule appear to be essential for activation of fluid secretion. Compounds with modifications of the base region, such as cyclic tubercidin 3′,5′-monophosphate and cyclic uridine 3′,5′-monophosphate, are as effective as cyclic AMP. One agent with phosphate modification, adenosine 3′,5′-phosphorothioate, was found to inhibit cyclic AMP activation of secretion. This agent also inhibited serotonin-activated fluid secretion, providing support for the involvement of serotonin-stimulated increases in cyclic AMP in the activation of fluid secretion.

c) Physiological Mechanisms Underlying Fluid Secretion

If electrodes are positioned on opposite sides of the single cell layer of the salivary gland, a transepithelial potential of about +15 mV is recorded, lumen positive. An additional recording electrode positioned within a single salivary gland cell allows measurement of potential differences across both the basal and apical membranes of the cell. The potential across the basal membrane is about −45 mV while the apical membrane potential is about −60 mV (BERRIDGE et al. 1975a). The potential across the basal membrane is dependent on potassium concentration (BERRIDGE et al. 1976), while the basis for the apical membrane potential has not been fully determined, although it is thought to rest near the chloride equilibrium potential.

Exposure of the basal side of the epithelium to serotonin (10^{-8} *M*) causes the transepithelial potential to become more negative (to about 0 mV) within 10 s (BERRIDGE et al. 1975a). During prolonged serotonin application (longer than

1 min) the transepithelial potential is maintained at this plateau for the duration of the serotonin application. Upon removal of the serotonin, the potential returns to the control level. Short applications of serotonin yield a different result. The initial negativity is following during the washout of serotonin by a transient positive potential before returning to normal.

These transepithelial potentials have been correlated with changes in the basal and apical membrane potentials (PRINCE and BERRIDGE 1972; BERRIDGE et al. 1975a). The basal membrane undergoes a small 5–10 mV hyperpolarization during the application of serotonin. On the other hand, the apical membrane is apparently responsible for the bulk of the changes in the total transepithelial potential. During prolonged serotonin application, the apical membrane is depolarized to about −30 mV. Short serotonin application yields a biphasic potential response, a transient depolarization followed by a hyperpolarization.

These potential changes that occur in response to serotonin application have been correlated with cellular conductance changes (BERRIDGE et al. 1975a). The basal membrane undergoes an increase in conductance during the hyperpolarizations to serotonin, while the depolarization across the apical membrane is also correlated with a large conductance increase. The hyperpolarizing change in apical membrane potential following short serotonin pulses does not seem to be associated with a conductance change, and is thought to be indicative of the activity of a potassium pump.

d) Electrical Effects of Cyclic AMP

Although cyclic AMP mimics the effects of serotonin in activating fluid secretion, differences exist in their effects on the electrical changes in the epithelial membranes (BERRIDGE and PRINCE 1971; PRINCE and BERRIDGE 1972). Application of cyclic AMP to the salivary glands produces only a slowly developing positivity of the transepithelial potential. This has been shown to correspond to, first, a small hyperpolarization of the basal membrane similar to that observed in response to serotonin, and, second, to a large (>20 mV) hyperpolarization of the apical membrane. These membrane potential effects persist for the duration of cyclic AMP application. Theophylline also mimics the effects of cyclic AMP application but with a slower time course of action. The effects of cyclic AMP on the apical membrane differ markedly from the depolarization that occurs during prolonged serotonin application. However, the cyclic AMP-induced hyperpolarization is similar to the response of the apical membrane that occurs when either calcium or chloride ions are omitted from the bath saline during serotonin application. As yet, these membrane potential responses to cyclic AMP have not been correlated with cyclic AMP-induced conductance changes, but have been assumed to be identical to portions of the serotonin-mediated conductance changes. The results suggest that part of the electrical effects produced by serotonin occur independently of increases in intracellular cyclic AMP. However, the hyperpolarization of the apical membrane following short application of serotonin may involve a cyclic AMP-mediated effect. This is supported by the demonstration that theophylline enhances the hyperpolarizing phase of the serotonin-activated potential changes in the apical membrane (BERRIDGE and PRINCE 1971).

e) Model of Serotonin Action

BERRIDGE and co-workers have proposed the following model to explain the above phenomena (BERRIDGE et al. 1975a). Serotonin is thought to activate two processes, (1) an increased influx of calcium into the salivary gland cells, and (2) an increase in intracellular cyclic AMP through activation of an adenylate cyclase. It has been proposed that the increase in intracellular calcium produces an increase in the passive chloride permeability of both the basal and apical membranes, and a slight increase in potassium permeability of the basal membrane. The increase in intracellular cyclic AMP is thought to activate release of calcium from intracellular stores and to activate a potassium pump in the apical membrane.

The precision of the above model depends upon assumptions concerning the time sequence of the various permeability and pump events occurring in the two membranes. At present, the detailed parameters of this sequence are little understood but are certainly influenced by the interaction of changing concentrations of both calcium and cyclic AMP.

f) Role of Calcium

Following the initial removal of calcium from the bathing medium, serotonin produces a transient activation of fluid secretion which gradually diminishes to resting levels over 15–60 min (PRINCE et al. 1972; PRINCE and BERRIDGE 1972). This slow decay presumably reflects the depletion of calcium from intracellular stores and possibly the inability of the potassium pump to maintain activity without anion permeability increases. Measurement of the epithelial potentials during the absence of calcium indicates that prolonged application of serotonin activates only a transient depolarization of the apical membrane (corresponding to activation of anion permeability from residual calcium) following by a maintained hyperpolarization during the remainder of the serotonin application. These results implicate calcium in both the maintenance of fluid secretion and in the depolarizing phase of the membrane potential changes. However, a question is raised. If the hyperpolarization is indicative of ongoing pump activity and decreased intracellular chloride, why is fluid secretion inhibited? Apparently, under certain circumstances, cyclic AMP-activation of a potassium pump alone may be insufficient for the activation of fluid secretion, although fluid secretion can be activated in the absence of cyclic AMP increases (PRINCE et al. 1973; BERRIDGE et al. 1975b).

The calcium ionophore, A-23187, has been used to examine the possibility that part of the serotonin-activated responses are mediated by changes in intracellular calcium concentration independent of cyclic AMP alterations (PRINCE et al. 1973). Application of 10^{-6} M ionophore activates fluid secretion in the salivary gland, although the time course is lower than with serotonin application. Both the ionophore and serotonin produce an increase in calcium influx and efflux from the salivary gland. In addition, the ionophore produces a negativity of the transepithelial potential corresponding to the depolarizing phase of the apical membrane potential. These results are consistent with the involvement of increased calcium influx as an intermediary in activating the anion permeability involved in part of the action of serotonin. The ionophore produces no effect on cyclic AMP content of salivary glands, but inhibits the increases in cyclic AMP produced by serotonin. This is consistent with experiments in which the steady state level of cyclic AMP produced by serotonin in calcium-free salines exceed that formed with calcium present (PRINCE et al. 1972).

g) Overview of Blowfly Salivary Gland

The presence of two distinct, but interacting, serotonin-activated processes, both involved in fluid secretion, raises the question of whether the effects of serotonin are mediated by a single receptor site. At present, there is no direct evidence addressing this question. It has been shown that the dose-response relation for negative transepithelial potentials is the same as that for fluid secretion (BERRIDGE and PRINCE 1971). However, the negative potentials correspond only to the calcium-dependent portion of the serotonin-mediated action. In addition, there is no information concerning the pharmacological properties of the serotonin-activated physiological processes relative to the serotonin-activated adenylate cyclase activity.

Although the model proposed by BERRIDGE and his co-workers seems to explain adequately many aspects of their data, a few questions remain unexplained. For example, secretory activity is maintained in the absence of the postulated pump activity in at least two situations: first, during the application of a calcium ionophore, and second, during application of high potassium salines. During these situations, secretion is presumably induced by increases in intracellular calcium levels that activate anion permeability. Since pump activity is apparently not elevated during such secretory activity, it is clearly not required for secretion to occur. It would be interesting to know whether potassium remains the principal cation appearing in the lumen at such times. During normal activation of the secretion process, salivary glands transport calcium from the bathing medium into the lumen through the gland cells (BERRIDGE and LIPKE 1979). Either basal pump activity may be sufficient to maintain a reasonable level of fluid secretion or other cations may be transported into the lumen rapidly enough to maintain normal secretory rates.

A similar problem exists when secretion is inhibited either by removal of calcium or chloride. Under these conditions, both serotonin and cyclic AMP activate similar hyperpolarizations of the apical membrane which persist for the duration of the drug application. In contrast, the secretory rate falls to control levels, although the elevation in pump activity, as measured electrophysiologically, is maintained. If secretion fails due to depletion of anions available for movement into the lumen or because anion permeability is insufficient to follow cation movement into the lumen, it is not clear how pump activity could continue in the absence of any anion movement to maintain charge balance. It would appear that the elevation of pump activity may contribute only a small portion to the movement of ions into the lumen and to the enhanced secretory rates. This is curious in light of the elevation of secretion induced by cyclic AMP in the absence of significant increases in anion permeability. Certainly, the evidence summarized below supports a role for cyclic AMP in the regulation of the secretory process in blowfly salivary glands, but the nature of the nucleotide-mediated effects that occur independently of changes in cellular calcium metabolism are unclear.

In summary, (1) serotonin or exogenous cyclic AMP produce a similar activation of salivary gland fluid secretion. (2) Serotonin produces an increase in intracellular cyclic AMP with a time course that closely follows the time course of fluid secretion. The concentrations of serotonin required for elevation of cyclic AMP correspond to the concentrations required for fluid secretion. (3) Inhibition of cyclic AMP action by a nucleotide analog inhibits the action of serotonin. The mechanism of this inhibition is not known. (4) Theophylline enhances the activation of fluid secretion by low concentrations of serotonin and enhances certain components of the electrical action of serotonin that mimic the electrical effects of cyclic AMP. (5) Some of the effects of serotonin on salivary gland membrane potentials mimic those of cyclic AMP. Another portion of the action of serotonin can be attributed to increases in intracellular calcium through activation of calcium fluxes in the basal membrane. When the calcium-dependent portion of the serotonin action is blocked by removal of calcium or the omission of permeable anions from the bath, the electrical effects of serotonin on both apical and basal membranes exactly mimic the effects of cyclic AMP. However, under these conditions secretion is inhibited. The portion of the electrical effects thought to reflect anion permeability increases is mimicked by application of the calcium ionophore, A-23184. The homogeneity of the salivary gland epithelial tissue allows one to conclude that serotonin directly activates an adenylate cyclase in the salivary gland cells which is involved in the regulation of secretory activity. It is not clear that cyclic AMP increases are essential for activation of the fluid secretion process.

2. Nerve Tissue

Serotonin is known to be present in insect nerve tissue (KLEMM 1972; KLEMM and AXELSSON 1973; reviewed by PITMAN 1971), and a serotonin-sensitive adenylate cyclase has been identified (NATHANSON and GREENGARD 1973, 1974). This enzyme, which has been found in cockroach thoracic ganglia, can be distinguished from octopamine- and dopamine-sensitive cyclases by additivity and pharmacological experiments (NATHANSON and GREENGARD 1973, 1974). The K_a of the enzyme is about 6×10^{-7} *M*. The serotonin-sensitive enzyme is inhibited by d-LSD with a K_i of 5×10^{-9} *M*. At concentrations greater than 10^{-6} *M*, d-LSD, in the absence of serotonin, produces a stimulation of adenylate cyclase ($K_i > 4 \times 10^{-6}$ *M*) which exceeds maximal responses to serotonin. Bromo-LSD shows similar mixed antagonist-agonist activity, while cyproheptadine, which inhibits serotonin-sensitive cyclase activity with a K_i of 2×10^{-7} *M*, also reduces basal adenylate cyclase activity about 25% at 10^{-5} *M*. At low (antagonist) concentrations, neither LSD or BOL alter the maximal activation of the enzyme by serotonin, although the K_m's are shifted, suggesting a competitive type of inhibition. LSD was also observed to inhibit dopamine- and octopamine-sensitive cyclase activity, but at much higher concentrations (K_i greater than 10^{-5} *M*). Phentolamine also inhibited adenylate cyclase activity to serotonin ($K_i = 3 \times 10^{-6}$ *M*); to dopamine ($K_i = 2 \times 10^{-6}$ *M*), and octopamine ($K_i = 5 \times 10^{-7}$ *M*), indicating that phentolamine apparently does not very effectively discriminate among the different amine-sensitive cyclases.

At present, it is difficult to correlate the characteristics of the serotonin-sensitive adenylate cyclase from cockroach thoracic ganglia with the serotonergic effects described below in other insect tissues, since the pharmacology of the serotonin-activated physiological responses is frequently incomplete or hard to interpret in terms of a single receptor. On the other hand, in the blowfly salivary gland (above), for which the pharmacology of serotonin-activated secretion is fairly detailed, the pharmacology of the cyclase remains to be characterized. From what is known of the physiological effects of LSD in the salivary gland, it is possible that the salivary gland serotonin-sensitive cyclase may differ from that described in cockroach nervous tissue.

3. Muscle

In the semi-isolated heart of the cockroach, serotonin produces an increase in heart rate with 50% activation at about 5×10^{-7} *M* (COLLINS and MILLER 1977). Other amines also accelerate heart rate with the following order of potency: serotonin > synephrine > octopamine > tryptamine > dopamine > tyramine. 501C, a serotonergic peripheral antagonist in mammals, competitively inhibits responses to serotonin, while reducing responses to octopamine in a non-competitive manner, suggesting that separate receptors may be present for the two amines. No effect of prolonged applications of 10^{-5} *M* dibutyryl cyclic AMP or 10^{-4} *M* dibutyryl-cyclic GMP have been observed, although 10^{-3} *M* aminophylline transiently increases heart rate.

Similar to its effects on insect heart rate, serotonin accelerates the frequency of the myogenic rhythm in the locust extenser tibia muscle, with 50% activation of about 5×10^{-7} *M* (EVANS and O'SHEA 1978). This effect is blocked by gramine, a serotonin antagonist. In contrast to serotonin, octopamine reduces the frequency of the rhythm. However, when the primary effect of octopamine is blocked by phentolamine, an accelerating effect of octopamine, which is gramine-sensitive, can be observed. This latter effect occurs at octopamine concentrations less than 10^{-6} *M* and suggests that octopamine may be interacting with the serotonin response. As yet, there has been no report of a serotonin-sensitive adenylate cyclase in this tissue.

4. Malphigian Tubule

In the Malphigian tubules of both *Rhodnius* and *Carausius*, serotonin activates fluid secretion, with a 50% effective dose (EC_{50}) in *Rhodnius* of about 4×10^{-8} *M* (MADDRELL et al. 1971). The pharmacology of this activation shows substantial differences from the activation of fluid secretion in the blowfly salivary gland. Methyl- or methoxy-substitutions for the hydroxyl group or removal or placement of the hydroxyl-group at other ring positions creates a totally inactive molecule. 5-hydroxytryptophan (5-HTP) or 5-HTP-ethylester are also inactive. On the other hand, N-methylations or acetylation retains most of the secretory activity of the molecule.

In most cases, those agents which do not stimulate secretion inhibit the serotonin-activated secretion. This includes tryptamine, the hydroxyl substitutions, and 5-HTP ethyl ester. Bromo-LSD, tranylcypromine, iproniazid, and tyramine also inhibit fluid secretion, while lysergic acid is ineffective as either an agonist or antagonist. Indolealkylamines that antagonize the serotonin-induced secretion also block the secretion activated by an anti-diuretic hormone isolated from *corpora cardiaca* and brain.

In the Malphigian tubule, cyclic AMP also activates fluid secretion at rates similar to those activated by serotonin with an ED_{50} of 10^{-4} *M* in *Rhodnius* (MADDRELL et al. 1971). The threshold of the cyclic AMP effect is 10^{-4} *M* in *Carausius* and 4×10^{-5} *M* in *Rhodnius*. In *Carausius*, 10^{-4} *M* aminophylline produces a stimulation of secretion, while, in *Rhodnius*, high concentrations of aminophylline, theophylline, or caffeine are all without effect. Curiously, tryptamine, 5-methyltryptamine, tyramine, and bromo-LSD block cyclic AMP-activated fluid secretion at concentrations identical to those effective in antagonizing serotonin-activated secretion. It is difficult to reconcile these results with a direct action of serotonin on receptor-activated adenylate cyclase. The data point out the ambiguity that may result from pharmacological studies on "receptor-mediated" processes utilizing a parameter as indirect as fluid secretion in a non-homogeneous population of cells.

III. Crustacea

In the decapod Crustacea, a neurohormonal role for serotonin is more firmly established than in the insects, but the sites and mechanisms of action of circulating serotonin remain unclear. Although an additional neurotransmitter role for serotonin is likely, there is at present only indirect evidence for this (BERLIND 1977; FINGERMAN et al. 1981).

Serotonin is synthesized and stored in large amounts in the pericardial neurosecretory structures surrounding the decapod heart (MAYNARD and WELSH 1959; SULLIVAN et al. 1976, 1977). Calcium-dependent, neurally evoked release of serotonin from these neurosecretory structures has also been demonstrated (SULLIVAN 1978; see also LIVINGSTONE et al. 1981). Several potential sites of action of neurohormonally-released serotonin have been described, and in certain cases there is evidence for an involvement of cyclic AMP in the actions of serotonin. These sites include the cardiac ganglion (COOKE 1966; COOKE and HARTLINE 1975), heart muscle (BATTELLE and KRAVITZ 1978), and certain neuromuscular junctions from decapod limb muscles, particularly the opener muscle (DUDEL 1965; BATTELLE and KRAVITZ 1978; KRAVITZ et al. 1980). Additionally, there are some indications that serotonin may be involved in the control of release of peptide hormones from the eyestalks of decapods (FINGERMAN et al. 1974).

1. Heart

Since the initial reports of the presence of serotonin in pericardial neurosecretory structures (MAYNARD and WELSH 1959; COOKE and GOLDSTONE 1970), several studies have examined the effect of serotonin on crustacean heart preparations (COOKE 1966; BERLIND et al. 1970; FLOREY and RATHMAYER 1978; BATTELLE and KRAVITZ 1978; COOKE and HARTLINE 1975; LEMOS and BERLIND 1981). The primary effect of serotonin on isolated, perfused decapod hearts is to produce both an increase in frequency and amplitude of the heart beat (COOKE 1966; BATTELLE and KRAVITZ 1978; FLOREY and RATHMAYER 1978). These effects appear to result primarily from a direct action of serotonin on cardiac ganglion cells, rather than through effects on cardiac muscle fibers (COOKE 1966; COOKE and HARTLINE 1975). Two studies have attempted to address the possible involvement of cyclic nucleotides in these effects of serotonin.

In isolated heart preparations from the lobster, *Homarus americanus*, serotonin increases both the amplitude and frequency of cardiac contraction (BATTELLE and KRAVITZ 1978). At 10^{-6} *M*, a 60% increase in amplitude and a 46% increase in frequency have been reported. After a 5 min exposure to 0.1 m*M* IBMX, which causes a 20% increase in heart beat frequency, the level of cyclic AMP in heart muscle doubles. 5×10^{-7} *M* serotonin in the presence of IBMX increases cyclic AMP levels about 5-fold over IBMX controls.

Recently, LEMOS and BERLIND (1981) have compared the effects of serotonin, cyclic AMP, and pericardial organ extract (XPO) on parameters of cardiac ganglion activity. XPO contains inconsequential levels of amines and as such is thought to represent only the effects or pericardial organ peptide(s). Although XPO, serotonin, and cyclic AMP all produce an increase in the rate of bursting of isolated cardiac ganglia, XPO and cyclic AMP also increase the burst duration while serotonin decreases the burst duration. In addition, the application of phosphodiesterase inhibitors fails to potentiate the action of serotonin. On intact ganglia, XPO also produces a greater than 5-fold increase in cyclic AMP levels while serotonin (10^{-6} *M*) produces a greater than 2-fold increase. Since cyclic AMP application and pharmacological alterations in cyclic AMP levels more clearly mimic the effects of XPO than the effects of serotonin, and, since serotonin produces a smaller increase in cyclic AMP in the cardiac ganglion, these authors argue that cyclic AMP plays an important role in action of the XPO peptide, but little role in the effects of serotonin on the ganglion. Since separate pools of cyclic AMP within the ganglion may exert quite different effects on ganglion function, the possibility that some of the effects of serotonin are mediated by cyclic AMP certainly can not be excluded. In addition, in cardiac muscle, serotonin produces an over 4-fold increase in cyclic AMP levels, suggesting a direct action of serotonin on muscle fibers. As yet, no attempt has been made to characterize a serotonin-sensitive adenylate cyclase in decapod heart.

2. Limb Muscles

Crustacean limb muscles have also been examined as potential sites of action of neurohormonally serotonin. In *Homarus* opener muscle, serotonin produces an increase in the amplitude of nerve-evoked contractions and a prolonged contracture (BATTELLE and KRAVITZ 1978). In the crayfish, *Astacus*, a similar increase in nerve-evoked contractions of the opener muscle has also been observed, although no muscle contracture has been reported (FLOREY and RATHMAYER 1978). The enhancement of evoked contractions by serotonin probably results partly from an increase in transmitter release from the presynaptic terminal (DUDEL 1965; GLUSMAN and KRAVITZ 1978; KRAVITZ et al. 1980). In intact opener muscles, serotonin plus IBMX produce up to a 13-fold increase in cyclic AMP content over IBMX-treated controls, with an EC_{50} of about 5×10^{-8} *M* (BATTELLE and KRAVITZ 1978). IBMX, itself, produces a 2- to 3-fold increase in cyclic AMP content of the opener muscle. It is not clear what portion, if any, of the serotonin-induced increase in cyclic AMP occurs within presynaptic terminals. 10^{-7} *M* LSD blocks the stimulation due to 10^{-7} *M* serotonin, while 10^{-7} *M* LSD alone produces a 2-fold stimulation in cyclic AMP content. LSD is without effect on octopamine-produced elevations in cyclic AMP, suggesting that there may exist separate octopamine- and serotonin-sensitive adenylate cyclases in this muscle. However, there is as yet no direct evidence that the effects of serotonin on contractile properties result from an activation of the serotonin-sensitive adenylate cyclase.

3. Eyestalk (Hormone Release)

The release of red pigment dispersing hormone (RPDH) from the sinus gland of eyestalks of the fiddler crab, *Uca pugilator*, appears to be regulated by serotonin (RAO and FINGERMAN 1970; FINGERMAN and RAO 1970; FINGERMAN and FINGERMAN 1975). Serotonin induces dispersion of red pigment in the limbs of animals with intact eyestalks. Removal of eyestalks abolishes the effect of serotonin on pigment dispersion and serotonin produces no effect on isolated limbs. Whether serotonin mediates this effect as a hormone or a neurotransmitter is not known.

Dispersion or concentration of pigment also occurs when crabs are transferred from a white to a black background or vice versa. Red pigment undergoes a dispersion on transfer of an animal from a white to black background and concentrates when the animal is moved from black to white. The effects of serotonin antagonists and uptake blockers on the dispersion and concentration process have been examined (FINGERMAN et al. 1981). Both the agonist, LY 53857, and the uptake blockers, Fluvoxamine and Fluoxetine, facilitate the dispersion process in intact animals, but not in isolated limbs. This again supports the idea that serotonin plays a role in some step in the activation of release of the peptide hormone that produces pigment dispersion. Similar experiments discussed below implicate dopamine in the control of the hormone that produces pigment concentration.

Eyestalk extracts have also been shown to increase phosphorylase activity and to inhibit glycogen synthetase in decapod muscle tissue (KELLER 1965, 1966; RAMAMURTHI et al. 1968), and to produce glycogenolysis when injected into crayfish hemolymph (KELLER and ANDREW 1973). It is unclear whether these effects are mediated by the eyestalk hyperglycemic hormone (HGH) (KLEINHOLZ et al. 1967), or by serotonin. (Serotonin has been shown to directly increase phosphorylase activity in abdominal muscle (BAUCHAU and MENGEOT 1968).) A possible role of serotonin in activating release of HGH has also been suggested (KELLER and BEYER 1968).

Injection of cyclic AMP into limbs has also been shown to elevate blood glucose levels in both *Uca* and *Orconectes*, while 5′-AMP and adenosine are without effect. This action of cyclic AMP does not occur in animals without eyestalks, suggesting that a cyclic AMP-mediated process may be involved in controlling the release of HGH (SPINDLER et al. 1976). In these same studies, an attempt to demonstrate activation of abdominal muscle adenylate cyclase with eyestalk extracts was unsuccessful. Although it is possible that serotonin (and other amines) may play a significant role in regulation of blood sugar and metabolic state in peripheral muscles of the decapods, it is not at all clear to what extent the actions of serotonin may be mediated by effects on release of peptide hormones or by direct actions on the muscles themselves.

IV. Trematodes

1. Liver Fluke

A serotonin-sensitive cyclase occurs in the parasitic trematode, the liver fluke, *Fasciola hepatica* (MANSOUR et al. 1960). Serotonin is present in the fluke and its synthesis has been demonstrated in flukes bathed in 5-hydroxytryptophan (MANSOUR and STONE 1970). Serotonin and other indolealkylamines stimulate fluke motility, which is correlated with an increase in glucose uptake and lactic acid production (MANSOUR 1957, 1959; MANSOUR and LAGO 1958).

The activation of glycolysis by serotonin occurs in homogenates of flukes, indicating that the increases occurring in whole flukes are not secondary to increases in motor activity (MANSOUR and MANSOUR 1962). The activation of glycolysis by serotonin results from an increase in activity of phosphofructokinase (PFK) (MANSOUR and MANSOUR 1962; STONE and MANSOUR 1967). Serotonin also produces an increase in cyclic AMP levels in both whole flukes and in cell-free homogenates (MANSOUR et al. 1960; ABRAHAMS et al. 1976). The activation of PFK by serotonin in homogenates requires the presence of the particulate fraction containing serotonin-activated adenylate cyclase. Since cyclic AMP is as effective as serotonin in stimulating PFK activity in homogenates (STONE and MANSOUR 1967), the activation of PFK by serotonin appears to occur via stimulation of the adenylate cyclase with a probable subsequent activation of cyclic AMP-dependent protein kinase. Serotonin is without effect on the degradation of cyclic AMP, indicating that increases in cyclic AMP and PFK activity are not the result of an inhibition of phosphodiesterase activity (MANSOUR and MANSOUR 1977). Other biogenic amines, including dopamine, norepinephrine, epinephrine, and octopamine, produce no adenylate cyclase activation in homogenates (NORTHUP and MANSOUR 1978a), nor effects on fluke motility, suggesting that the adenylate cyclase is specifically serotonin-sensitive. The K_a of this enzyme is about 2×10^{-6} *M* in the presence of GTP (NORTHUP and MANSOUR 1978a).

Attempts to demonstrate a physiological role for the serotonin-activated cyclase beyond the activation of PFK have been less successful. Although the serotonin-sensitive cyclase shows some specific association with head regions of the fluke, suggesting a possible association with the anterior nerve ring, the specific cellular site of the serotonin-sensitive cyclase is unknown (ABRAHAMS et al. 1976). In the absence of this information, an attempt has been made to correlate aspects of the serotonin-activated metabolic effects and the effects on fluke motility (MANSOUR and STONE 1970; ABRAHAMS et al. 1976; NORTHUP and MANSOUR 1978a). Towards this end, kinetic studies of adenylate cyclase activation by serotonin in homogenates and its inhibition or activation by other indole agents has indicated that adenylate cyclase activation is mediated by a single class of sites (NORTHUP and MANSOUR 1978a). Bromo-LSD inhibits both the activation of motility and glycolysis by serotonin in intact flukes (MANSOUR 1959). In homogenates, bromo-LSD blocks the serotonin-activated adenylate cyclase and also reduces the basal level of adenylate cyclase. Other indolealkylamines show reasonable correlations in their ability to stimulate adenylate cyclase in homogenates and to increase fluke motility (NORTHUP and MANSOUR 1978a). However, experiments with d-LSD are less clear. In intact flukes, LSD activates fluke mobility as effectively as serotonin, and stimulates glucose uptake and lactic acid production (MANSOUR 1959). However, LSD (10^{-10} *M* to 10^{-3} *M*) apparently produces no significant increase in cyclic AMP levels in intact flukes (although it blocks serotonin-induced increases in cyclic AMP with an IC_{50} of 5×10^{-9} *M*) (ABRAHAMS et al. 1976). Despite this, PFK activity is increased markedly by LSD in intact flukes (MANSOUR and STONE 1970). Since LSD can produce about a 25% activation of adenylate cyclase activity relative to serotonin in homogenates, it is possible that some significant, but not detectable, stimulation of cyclic AMP accumulation by LSD occurs in whole flukes (NORTHUP and MANSOUR 1978a). Curiously, although LSD produces some activation of PFK in both intact flukes and whole homogenates, in particulate fractions, containing inactive PFK and adenylate cyclase, LSD produces no activation of PFK (MANSOUR and STONE 1970). No completely satisfactory explanation of these results has been offered, although one reason may lie in the dual agonist and antagonist effects of LSD on adenylate cyclase activity assayed in homogenates (NORTHUP and MANSOUR 1978a, b). Another possibility is that the activation of fluke motility by LSD may occur independently of an adenylate cyclase-mediated pathway. As a corollary, the activation by serotonin of adenylate cyclase and PFK might not be required for the increases in motility.

A cyclic AMP-dependent protein kinase has been found in homogenates with activity concentrated in the anterior end of the fluke (GENTLEMAN et al. 1976). Incubation of intact flukes with serotonin produces an increase in protein kinase activity in homogenates prepared subsequently, and this activation correlates with the serotonin-stimulated accumulation of endogenous cyclic AMP. LSD has been found to reduce the activation of protein kinase by serotonin.

2. Other Trematodes

Serotonin-activated increases in adenylate cyclase activity or cyclic AMP levels have also been reported in other trematode species (HIGASHI et al. 1973; MANSOUR and MANSOUR 1962) and in free-living flatworms, particularly the planaria, *Polycelis tenis*.

Early studies of adenylate cyclase in flatworm homogenates found no hormonal stimulation in the absence of GTP (FRANQUINET et al. 1976). However, in subsequent studies using the GTP analog, GMP-PNP, a serotonin sensitive adenylate cyclase was described with a K_a for serotonin of 4.5×10^{-8} *M* (FRANQUINET et al. 1978). Dopamine, epinephrine, and norepinephrine also produced some stimulation of adenylate cyclase, but this activity was not additive with the serotonin-sensitive activity. Methiothepin produced a dose-dependent inhibition of the serotonin-sensitive cyclase, but other anti-serotonergic agents were not examined. Fluphenazine, haloperidol, and propranolol inhibited basal cyclase activity more effectively than serotonin-sensitive activity. There was no significant difference in serotonin-sensitive cyclase from head, mid-region, or tail parts of the worms.

An examination of the histochemical localization of fluoride-stimulated adenylate cyclase activity during the regeneration of the turbellarian, *Dugesia lugubris*, has been reported (MORACZEWSKI and DUMA 1978). In nonregenerating animals, precipitates were located unevenly in patches on exterior surfaces of cell membranes or embedded in membranes. In regions of regenerating tissues, precipitates were also observed in association with perinuclear spaces and rough endoplasmic reticular cisternae. Unfortunately, the histochemical method used employed the precipitation of adenylate cyclase-released pyrophosphate by lead, a procedure which has considerable potential for producing staining artifacts (LEMAY and JARETT 1975; NATHANSON and BLOOM 1975).

C. Octopamine-Cyclic Nucleotide Interactions

Considerable evidence, described below, suggests that octopamine may function in invertebrates as a neurotransmitter as well as a neurohormone. In both roles, there is suggestive, but not conclusive, biochemical and pharmacological evidence that octopamine-stimulated cyclic AMP synthesis may be involved in mediating some of octopamine's actions.

I. Molluscs

1. Nerve Tissue

Octopamine has been identified in the cerebral, buccal, and pedal ganglia of *Aplysia* (SAAVEDRA et al. 1974; BROWNSTEIN et al. 1974; FARNHAM et al. 1978; MCCAMAN and MCCAMAN 1978), although the exact concentrations present are somewhat disputed (FARNHAM et al. 1978; MCCAMAN and MCCAMAN 1978). Octopamine does not appear to be present to a significant degree in *Aplysia* abdominal and pleural ganglia. Earlier experiments (SAAVEDRA et al. 1974) suggesting the presence of substantial concentrations of octopamine in individually dissected neurons from abdominal ganglia have not been substantiated by more recent studies of individual neurons from abdominal, buccal, and cerebral ganglia (FARNHAM et al. 1978; MCCAMAN and MCCAMAN 1978). Thus, the exact location of the octopamine in *Aplysia* ganglia is not yet clear. Electrophysiological studies do demonstrate specific responses to the microiontophoresis of octopamine onto neurons in these molluscan ganglia (CARPENTER and GAUBATZ 1974). Activation of such octopamine "receptors" most often results in membrane hyperpolarization mediated through an increase in membrane conductance, possibly to potassium. These same neurons have been reported to be much less responsive to norepinephrine, dopamine, and phenylethanolamine.

Octopamine has been reported, also, to cause hyperpolarization of neurons in the *Helix* brain (WALKER et al. 1972), and to cause both excitation and inhibition of identified neurons in the *Helix* subesophageal ganglion (BATTA et al. 1979). Although the inhibitory responses of the subesophageal neurons are mimicked by the catecholamines, the excitatory responses appear more specific for octopamine. Structure-activity relationships in these experiments showed that synephrine is the only amine as potent as octopamine. However, in contrast to its known potency in stimulating octopamine-sensitive adenylate cyclase in other invertebrates (see below), tyramine was much less effective in mimicking octopamine's effect on depolarization.

In *Aplysia* abdominal ganglia, phosphorylation of an 118,000 molecular weight protein has been reported to be enhanced following a several hour incubation in 0.1 m*M* octopamine (LEVITAN and BARONDES 1974; LEVITAN et al. 1974). This same dose of octopamine increases cyclic AMP levels in the ganglion. Simultaneous incubation with phentolamine, which was originally reported by NATHANSON and GREENGARD (1973, 1974) to inhibit activation of octopamine-sensitive adenylate cyclase in cockroach ganglia, blocks the octopamine-stimulated cyclic AMP accumulation in *Aplysia* and also prevents the octopamine-stimulated protein phosphorylation. Dibutyryl cyclic AMP mimics the effect of octopamine on specific protein phosphorylation, suggesting that octopamine may be acting through stimulation of an endogenous adenylate cyclase.

Localization studies within the *Aplysia* ganglion failed to find any specific octopamine-stimulated phosphorylation in large identified neurons, bag cell clusters, or nerve connectives; rather, most phosphorylation was in the remaining neuropil. Furthermore, subcellular fractionation of ganglion homogenates indicated an enrichment of specific protein phosphorylation in the crude mitochondrial fraction. These results suggest a possible synaptic localization of octopamine-stimulated, cyclic AMP-dependent protein phosphorylation.

2. Muscle

In the mollusc, *Tapes watlingi*, octopamine has been found to increase the amplitude of contraction of the spontaneously beating ventricle (DOUGAN and WADE 1978a, b). In this preparation, the relative agonist potencies of N-methyl-octopamine, alpha-methyl-octopamine, N-methyl-meta-octopamine, and several other analogs correlate reasonably well with the ability of these same amines to active octopamine-sensitive adenylate cyclase in the firefly light organ (NATHANSON and HUNNICUTT 1979b, unpublished work). Clozapine, a dibenzodiazepine antipsychotic drug, is a potent antagonist of octopamine in the *Tapes* ventricle; similarly, clozapine is a potent antagonist of the octopamine-sensitive adenylate cyclase in the firefly. On the other hand, metaclopramide and sulpiride, which also block octopamine's physiological effects in *Tapes* heart, are poor antagonists of octopamine-sensitive adenylate cyclase in the light organ. As yet, there has been no reported characterization of an octopamine-sensitive adenylate cyclase in this molluscan preparation.

In the gastropod, *Rapana thomasiana*, octopamine has been reported to enhance the twitch contraction of the radula protractor muscle (MUNEOKA and KOBAYASHI 1980) and to depress the twitch contraction of the radula retractor (KOBAYASHI and MUNEOKA 1980). Although both of these effects are blocked by phentolamine, there are as yet insufficient pharmacological data with which to draw any comparisons to the properties of octopamine-sensitive adenylate cyclase.

II. Insects

1. Photogenic Tissue

Current evidence suggests that octopamine may function as a transmitter in the neural control of light emission in the adult firefly *(Photuris* and *Photinus)* and in the firefly larva (glow worm) (see EVANS 1980a for review). The recent identification of a potent octopamine-sensitive adenylate cyclase in firefly light organs, together with physiological evidence (below), raises the possibility that cyclic AMP (or possibly pyrophosphate) may play a role in the triggering of light emission in these insects.

Anatomically, the adult light organ (or lantern) consists of rosettes of light emitting cells (or photocytes), each rosette surrounding a branched air tube (or tracheole) (BUCK 1947; BEAMS and ANDERSON 1955; KLUSS 1958). Fine structure studies indicate that the termination of each tracheole is surrounded by a specialized "end cell" in such a way that the end cell is interposed between the tracheole and photocyte (SMITH 1963; PETERSON and BUCK 1968; PETERSON 1970). Because microphotometric studies indicate that light emission begins near the centers of the rosettes, it is thought that the end or tracheolar cells may be important in flash initiation (BUCK 1947; HANSON et al. 1969). This presumptive localization appears consistent with fine structure studies which show the presence of afferent nerve endings which terminate between the tracheolar epithelium and the end cells. These nerve endings contain large, dense-core vesicles of a neurosecretory type, quite similar to those in other invertebrate neurons that are thought to be octopaminergic (HOYLE 1975; OERTEL et al. 1975; HOYLE et al. 1980). Light microscopic histochemical studies demonstrate that these nerve endings appear to come from axons arising in the terminal two abdominal ganglia which supply the lantern (HANSON 1962; T. A. CHRISTENSEN and A. D. CARLSON, personal communication). The large cell bodies of these axons are located dorsally near the midline; thus, they appear similar to the dorsal unpaired median (DUM) neurons identified in other insects as probably being octopaminergic (see below).

Electrical stimulation of the firefly abdominal nerve cord or the lantern nerves causes light emission in the lantern, and normal light flashing is preceded by a volley of nerve impulses in the lantern nerve (BUCK and CASE 1961; CASE and BUCK 1963; BUCK et al. 1963; CARLSON 1969). Biochemical studies indicate that the lantern contains octopamine (ROBERTSON and CARLSON 1976), and direct application of this amine (10^{-6} *M* to 10^{-4} *M*) to isolated lanterns causes light emission (SMALLEY 1965; CARLSON 1968a, b, 1972; BOROWITZ and KENNEDY 1968). This effect of octopamine is not blocked by reserpine or denervation, suggesting a postsynaptic site of action. Supporting the presence of aminergic nerve terminals which might be the source of the octopamine is the observation that the ability of amphetamine to elicit light emission is abolished by denervation or reserpine. The only other amine as potent as octopamine in eliciting light emission is its N-methylated derivative, synephrine. Norepinephrine, epinephrine, and tyramine are less potent, and isoproterenol and phenylephrine have little activity.

Recently, a potent and extremely active octopamine-sensitive adenylate cyclase has been identified in both adult and larval light organs (NATHANSON 1979; NATHANSON and HUNNICUTT 1979a, b). This enzyme is activated by concentrations of octopamine as low as 10^{-7} *M*, has a K_a of from 5 to 15×10^{-6} *M*, and has a V_{max} showing a 15- to 30-fold stimulation over basal activity. Tissue distribution studies indicate that the enzyme is selectively concentrated in those abdominal tail segments which contain lantern tissue, and, more specifically, is localized to the lantern tissue itself. While adenylate cyclase in fat, gut, reproductive organs, and ganglia does show some degree of octopamine stimulation, that activation is small compared to the very large stimulation observed in photogenic tissue. Interestingly, the enzyme has also been identified in larval light organs which show a somewhat different histological structure than that found in the adult firefly. In the larval lantern, which glows with a gradual onset and termination but is unable to flash, end cells are absent and afferent nerves end directly on the photocytes. This suggests that in the larval light organ the enzyme may be localized either in tracheoles or in the photocytes themselves.

Biochemical studies (NATHANSON and HUNNICUTT 1979b, unpublished work) show a pH optimum for the octopamine-sensitive adenylate cyclase of around 7.9, which is similar to the pH optimum of the photochemical reaction involving luciferin and luciferase (SELIGER and MCELROY 1964). In this regard, it is of interest that BOWIE et al. (1973) have noted that cyclic AMP is the only nucleotide which mimics ATP-Mg in altering the emission spectrum of a fluorescent active site probe bound to firefly luciferase. (ATP-Mg normally reacts to form the excited enzyme-luciferyl-adenylate complex necessary for light emission.)

Pharmacological characterization of the lantern enzyme reveals a high degree of specificity for octopamine. Unlike many other invertebrate tissues which contain adenylate cyclases sensitive to more than one amine, the lantern appears to contain only an octopamine-activated enzyme. Dopamine, for example, has less than 4% the activity of octopamine; serotonin, histamine, and acetylcholine have no stimulatory effects. The enzyme shows considerable selectivity for para-octopamine as compared to the meta- or ortho- positional isomers. Similarly, the enzyme is 30 times more sensitive to activation by the naturally-occurring stereoisomer, D(−)-octopamine, than by L(−)-octopamine.

Comparison of the relative potencies of various amines in stimulating the firefly octopamine-sensitive adenylate cyclase has shown a good correlation with the relative potencies of these same amines in causing light production in superfused light organs. For example, synephrine, which is equal in potency to octopamine in causing light production, is the only amine yet found which is more potent than octopamine in stimulating the lantern adenylate cyclase. Norepinephrine and tyramine, which differ from octopamine by a single hydroxyl group, are of intermediate potency in both light production and enzyme stimulation. Isoproterenol and serotonin, which have much less effect on light production, cause little enzyme stimulation. The only discrepancy noted has been for dopamine, which is slightly less active biochemically than reported in physiological studies. In general, agonist potency for the octopamine-sensitive adenylate cyclase is enhanced by para- and β-hydroxylation and by N-methylation, and is reduced by α-methylation and by large substituents on the amine group.

Additivity studies between octopamine and other activating amines show no greater stimulation than by octopamine alone. Because synephrine is somewhat more potent than octopamine, the question arises as to whether this N-methylated derivative of octopamine may be the "natural" or endogenous activator of the octopamine-stimulated enzyme. Although octopamine is found in higher concentrations than synephrine in the lantern, this does not necessarily rule out a possible role for the latter amine.

Whether cyclic AMP actually mediates the effects of octopamine or synephrine in stimulating light production in vivo is not yet entirely clear. Consistent with the known time course of cyclic nucleotide-mediated events in other excitable cells, electrophysiological studies (BUCK et al. 1963) have shown that the latency between normal nerve stimulation and lantern flashing is relatively long (approximately 70 ms). High-intensity stimulation creates a "quick" flash of shorter latency (18 ms) which is thought to result from direct depolarization of the photocyte membrane, bypassing the nerve-end organ linkage. The latency of the slow flash is temperature-dependent, whereas that of the quick flash is not. This is consistent with an enzymatic process (such as activation of adenylate cyclase) occurring prior to depolarization of the photocyte membrane.

OERTEL and CASE (1976) have reported that applications of aminophylline and theophylline to isolated larval light organs will, like octopamine, elicit a glow. Although the methyl xanthines are known to inhibit phosphodiesterase and thus increase endogenous cyclic AMP, they can also mobilize calcium. Therefore, these data alone neither support nor refute a cyclic AMP-mediated mechanism. Furthermore, although exogenous cyclic AMP, itself, was reported ineffective in eliciting light production, lipid soluble and phosphodiesterase resistant analogs were not tried, and thus this negative result does not rule out a cyclic AMP-mediated mechanism. In fact, recent experiments using the phosphodiesterase-resistant, lipid-soluble cyclic AMP analog, p-chlorophenyl-thio-cyclic AMP, have shown that this compound is capable of eliciting light emission when injected in the lantern (J. A. NATHANSON, unpublished work).

Although cyclic AMP is normally thought to be the biologically active second messenger resulting from the adenylate cyclase reaction, it is interesting to mention the possibility that pyrophosphate (the other product of the adenylate cyclase reaction) might also play a role in neural control of light emission. Indeed, since the photochemical reaction is subject to product inhibition which can be overcome by the addition of pyrophosphate (DELUCA and MCELROY 1974; GATES and DELUCA 1975), it has been previously postulated that neural control of pyrophosphate metabolism might regulate light production in the firefly (MCELROY et al. 1969). A potent octopamine-stimulated adenylate cyclase could supply this pyrophosphate.

2. Nerve and Muscle

Presumptive octopaminergic neurons have been identified in the ganglia of several insects (HOYLE et al. 1974; HOYLE 1975; HOYLE and BARKER 1975; EVANS and O'SHEA 1977, 1978; CHRISTENSEN and A. D. CARLSON, personal communication; for reviews, see Evans 1980 a, b). Some of these midline, dorsal, unpaired neurons (DUM cells) send axons peripherally to the leg muscles. Several studies indicate that octopamine may affect the spontaneous rhythmic contractions of such muscles and may also modulate the effects of other, non-octopaminergic neurons, in causing nerve-evoked muscle contraction (HOYLE 1974, 1975; EVANS and O'SHEA 1977, 1978; BUCHAN and EVANS 1980). Although there are as yet no biochemical studies identifying an octopamine-sensitive adenylate cyclase in these leg muscles, structure-activity relationships of various octopamine analogs in affecting muscle physiology offer some indirect support for a cyclic nucleotide mechanism (EVANS and O'SHEA 1978). Thus, in the locust, synephrine has been found to be the only amine more potent than octopamine in inhibiting spontaneous muscle contractions. Phenylethanolamine is significantly less potent than octopamine, followed in order (of decreasing potency) by epinephrine, tyramine, normetanephrine, noradrenaline, and dopamine. Phenylethylamine, tyrosine and DOPA have been reported to be without activity. This order of potency is reasonably similar to that seen for the octopamine-sensitive adenylate cyclase in cockroach ganglia and brain (NATHANSON 1976; HARMAR and HORN 1977), and for the octopamine-sensitive adenylate cyclase in the firefly lantern (NATHANSON and HUNNICUTT 1979b, unpublished work).

The effects of octopamine on the locust myogenic rhythm are inhibited much more effectively by chlorpromazine than by metoclopramide (EVANS 1981). This order of potency is similar to that for the same two antagonists in inhibiting octopamine-stimulated cyclase in the firefly light organ (J. A. NATHANSON, unpublished work). In contrast, the effects of octopamine on nerve-evoked muscle twitch tension and rate of relaxation in the locust are both blocked by much lower concentrations of metoclopramide than chlorpromazine (EVANS 1981). On the basis of this, as well as additional data, EVANS (1981) has proposed the existence of multiple octopamine receptors. The receptor mediating the effects of octopamine on the locust myogenic rhythm is designated octopamine$_1$, while the receptors mediating the effects of octopamine on nerve-evoked a) amplitude and b) rate of relaxation of twitch tension, are designated octopamine$_{2A}$ and octopamine$_{2B}$, respectively. On the basis of this classification it would appear that adenylate cyclase is most likely associated with octopamine$_1$ receptors. Whether octopamine$_2$ receptors are associated with adenylate cyclase is not yet clear.

Although most studies have emphasized the peripheral connections of DUM neurons, it is important to mention that these same neurons also ramify within their ganglia and may form synaptic connections centrally. In this regard, it is of interest to note that octopamine-sensitive adenylate cyclase was first identified in invertebrates in cockroach thoracic ganglia (NATHANSON and GREENGARD 1973, 1974) and has been found subsequently as well in the insect brain (HARMAR and HORN 1977; BODNARYK 1979a, b). The enzyme in both brain and thoracic ganglia is activated by concentrations of octopamine as low as 3×10^{-8} *M*, and has a K_a (1.5×10^{-6} *M*) somewhat lower than that found in the firefly. Otherwise, the agonist and antagonist properties of this enzyme (NATHANSON 1976; HARMAR and HORN 1977) appear similar to those found in the octopamine-sensitive adenylate cyclase of the peripheral firefly light organ (NATHANSON and HUNNICUTT, 1979b, unpublished work). In the insect central nervous system, the enzyme is enriched in ganglia as compared to interganglionic connectives, a finding which is consistent with a possible synaptic role. As yet, however, there are no published electrophysiological studies in such ganglia indicating whether or not octopamine may influence membrane conductances as it does in molluscan ganglia.

3. Metabolic Effects

Although the effects of octopamine on insect physiology may be through a direct action on synaptic processes (either pre- or postsynaptic), it is important to mention that octopamine can also affect energy metabolism in these animals. Indeed, ROBERTSON and STEELE (1972) identified one of the first biological effects of octopamine as the activation of phosphorylase in the insect nerve cord, with consequent glycogenolysis. This effect of octopamine is mimicked by the application of cyclic AMP or the phosphodiesterase inhibitor, theophylline (see also HANOKA and TAKAHASHI 1977; GADE and HOLWERDA 1976). In the locust flight muscle, octopamine has been reported to stimulate glucose trehalose oxidation (CANDY 1978) and to increase cyclic AMP levels (WORM 1980). It is possible that octopamine may be located in the insect corpus cardiacum, a neurohemal organ which releases a hyperglycemic factor into the insect hemolymph (STEELE 1961; see also GOLE and DOWNER 1979). Indeed, EVANS (1978) has recently confirmed that high concentrations of octopamine are present in this organ, and thus it is possible that octopamine may be the natural hyperglycemic factor present in the insect.

Such a metabolic role for octopamine in invertebrates is reminiscent of the glycogenolytic action of epinephrine in the vertebrate liver. Thus, similar to the catecholamines, octopamine may have more than one function mediated through cyclic AMP – first, a role in synaptic transmission, and, second, a role in energy metabolism. Like the catecholamines, other humoral roles for octopamine in the invertebrate are also likely. [Recent experiments in crustacea (below) support this possibility.] NATHANSON (1976) has speculated that octopamine may, in fact, function in invertebrates as a substitute for the catecholamines, perhaps reflecting an evolutionary divergence. In this regard, JUORIO and ROBERTSON (1977) have found that the concentration of octopamine in echinoderm tissues is less than that found in many other invertebrates, and that the ratio of norepinephrine to octopamine is higher. Since the echinoderm is a member of the *Deuterostomia*, to which the chordates also belong, this is in keeping with the possibility that epinephrine and norepinephrine may be the major phenylethylamine neurotransmitters in this evolutionary branch whereas octopamine (and possibly synephrine, tyramine and phenylethanolamine) may be the major phenylethylamine transmitters in the *Protostomia*, which include the arthropods, annelids, molluscs and flatworms.

4. Relationship to Pesticide Action

The formamidine pesticide, chlordimeform (CDM), and its N-monodimethyl derivative, (DCDM), are known to cause marked behavioral abnormalities in susceptible arthropods, suggesting that part of their pesticidal activity is through a neurotoxic effect (MATSUMURA and BEEMAN 1976). Both CDM and DCDM have been reported to mimic the effects of octopamine in stimulating light emission in the firefly lantern (HOLLINGWORTH and MURDOCK 1980) and in affecting nerve-evoked muscle responses in the locust leg (EVANS and GEE 1980). Although these physiological experiments suggest that the formamidines may affect octopamine receptors, the known action of the formamidines as monoamine oxidase inhibitors (AZIZ and KNOWLES 1973), makes it difficult to determine with certainty, from intact tissue preparations, whether the formamidines are acting directly or indirectly.

Recent experiments, examining the biochemical effects of the formamidines on octopamine-sensitive adenylate cyclase in particulate preparations of the firefly light organ, suggest that these pesticides are potent octopaminergic compounds

(NATHANSON and HUNNICUTT 1981). In the lantern preparation, DCDM was found to be a partial agonist (70% of octopamine V_{max}) and was 6-fold more potent ($K_a = 2.2 \times 10^{-6}$ *M*) than octopamine ($K_a = 1.4 \times 10^{-5}$ *M*) in activating adenylate cyclase activity. At high concentrations ($IC_{50} = 3 \times 10^{-4}$ *M*), DCDM caused a 30% inhibition of octopamine stimulation. Activation by DCDM was reversible, non-additive to that due to octopamine, and could be competitively inhibited by several receptor antagonists, including cyproheptadine ($K_i = 2 \times 10^{-6}$ *M*), clozapine ($K_i = 4 \times 10^{-6}$ *M*), fluphenazine ($K_i = 6 \times 10^{-6}$ *M*), phentolamine ($K_i = 1.8 \times 10^{-5}$ *M*), and propranolol ($K_i = 4.7 \times 10^{-5}$ *M*). These inhibitory constants correlate well with those for inhibiting octopamine stimulation. The agonist activity of DCDM was specific for tissue containing an octopamine-activated adenylate cyclase; enzyme activity in the rat caudate nucleus (activated by dopamine) and in the heart and liver (activated by isoproterenol) was little affected by DCDM.

In contrast to DCDM, CDM was a weak octopamine agonist ($K_a = 3 \times 10^{-5}$ *M*; 9% of octopamine V_{max}) in the light organ. At higher concentrations ($IC_{50} =$ 3–10 $\times 10^{-4}$ *M*), CDM was an octopamine antagonist, causing nearly complete inhibition of octopamine stimulation at 1–3 $\times 10^{-3}$ *M*. This inhibitory effect of CDM was reversible, pH dependent, and non-competitive with octopamine. It was also non-selective, since CDM inhibited dopamine-sensitive, beta-adrenergic-sensitive, and non-hormone dependent adenylate cyclases in mammalian brain and liver.

These results indicate that, at low concentrations, DCDM can bind specifically and reversibly to octopamine receptors with a resultant activation of adenylate cyclase. CDM, on the other hand, has little direct effect on octopamine receptors; its octopaminergic actions in vivo are a probable result of its conversion to DCDM. At high, non-pharmacological doses, CDM exerts non-competitive and non-receptor-specific inhibitory effects on adenylate cyclase.

III. Crustacea

KRAVITZ and associates have reported the presence of octopamine within the second roots of lobster thoracic ganglia (BARKER et al. 1972; WALLACE et al. 1974). Some release of octopamine into the hemolymph has been detected near the thoracic root (EVANS et al. 1975, 1976a, b) and much more from the pericardial organs, which lie within the pericardial sinus (EVANS et al. 1975, 1976a, b; SULLIVAN et al. 1977). Recent electronmicroscopic autoradiographic studies of tyramine uptake in the neurosecretory region of the thoracic roots suggest that octopamine is synthesized in nerve terminals morphologically distinct from those which synthesize serotonin (LIVINGSTONE et al. 1981). The location of the presumptive octopamine-containing cell bodies which contribute to the octopamine release from these nerve terminals is not yet entirely clear. The neurons may be present in the thoracic roots or in the thoracic ganglion, itself. Physiological studies have indicated that octopamine can affect the clotting reaction of lobster hematocytes as well as alter cardiac and peripheral muscle contraction (EVANS et al. 1975; BATTELLE and KRAVITZ 1978). [Octopamine at high doses (several mg) also elicits a behavioral motor response when injected systemically (LIVINGSTONE et al. 1980).] Because octopamine also stimulates cyclic AMP production in these same tissues, the possibility exists that octopamine's physiological actions may be mediated through activation of adenylate cyclase. The data supporting this possibility are best described for the lobster hematocytes. In these cells, octopamine causes an accumulation of cyclic AMP with an apparent K_a for octopamine of about 10^{-7} *M*. Synephrine is more potent than octopamine, and alpha-methyloctopamine is about 10 times less potent. Phenylethanolamine, norepinephrine, and tyramine are reported to be considerably less potent; and serotonin, dopamine and histamine are without activity. This order of potency is similar to that for the firefly octopamine-sensitive adenylate cyclase with the exception that, in the firefly, alpha-methyloctopamine is much less potent (NATHANSON and HUNNICUTT 1979b). In the lobster, as in the firefly, octopamine activation is blocked by low concentrations of phentolamine and chlorpromazine. The effects of the various agonists in accelerating hemolymph clotting is similar to their effects on cyclic AMP production with the exception, again, of alpha-methyloctopamine. Taken together, these data offer some support for a possible cyclic AMP mediation of octopamine's action on hemolymph clotting.

IV. Arachnids

An octopamine-activated adenylate cyclase has been reported in the protocerebrum and circumesophageal ring of the horseshoe crab, *Limulus polyphemus* (ATKINSON et al. 1977). As in the insect, phentolamine inhibits octopamine stimulation in a competitive manner.

In the tarantula spider, *Eurypelma marxi*, several monoamines, including octopamine (which is the most effective) have been reported to increase the amplitude of nerve-evoked contractions in the leg muscle (GREGA 1978). These same amines increased cyclic AMP levels in the muscle, and dibutyryl cyclic AMP mimicked the effect of the amines in enhancing nerve-evoked contraction.

D. Dopamine-Cyclic Nucleotide Interactions

As is the case for the other two principle invertebrate biogenic amines (serotonin and octopamine), there is evidence for both a neurotransmitter and a neurohormonal role for dopamine in invertebrate organisms (reviews by WOODRUFF 1971; GERSCHENFELD 1973; KEHOE and MARDER 1976). Also, as with the vertebrates, at least some dopamine receptors appear to activate adenylate cyclase. However, as yet, it is not clear to what extent the electrophysiological or mechanical effects produced by dopamine on nerve and muscle preparations involve elevations in intracellular cyclic AMP.

I. Molluscs

1. Nerve Tissue

Several studies have characterized responses of molluscan neurons to iontophoretic or bath application of dopamine (WOODRUFF and WALKER 1969; WALKER et al. 1968; ASCHER 1972; MACDONALD and BERRY 1978; GOSPE and WILSON 1980,

1981). Some neurons show a hyperpolarizing response due to a potassium conductance increase, while others demonstrate a depolarizing response presumably involving a conductance increase to sodium or possibly to calcium. On some neurons, these responses can occur together, yielding potentials that are composites of the two. When dopamine is applied to R 15 of *Aplysia*, the cell hyperpolarizes (ASCHER 1972) and spontaneous activity is terminated. This is associated with a loss of the negative-resistance region of the current-voltage relation and has been ascribed to a decrease in the voltage-dependent conductance responsible for burst generation (GOSPE and WILSON 1980, 1981). This last dopamine response has been extensively characterized (GOSPE and WILSON 1981). Depolarizing responses to dopamine are blocked by curare and strychnine. Since these latter agents also affect serotonin and acetylcholine depolarizing responses (KEHOE 1972; GERSCHENFELD and PAUPARDIN-TRITSCH 1974), it is fortunate that depolarizing responses to dopamine occur on cells insensitive to serotonin and acetylcholine. The presence of both dopamine responses on the same neurons and the pharmacological similarity of some dopamine responses to responses activated by other agents complicates pharmacological investigations and, as has been pointed out (ASCHER and KEHOE 1975), this problem has been frequently ignored.

Although CEDAR and SCHWARTZ (1972) indicated that dopamine can produce an increase in cyclic AMP in whole ganglia of *Aplysia*, the pharmacological and amine specificity of this activation was not examined. Subsequently, a dopamine activation of adenylate cyclase was demonstrated in homogenates of the central ganglia of the snail, *Helix pomatia* (OSBORNE 1977). 50% activation occurred at about 5×10^{-5} *M* for dopamine and 1.8×10^{-4} *M* for apomorphine. No attempt was made, however, to distinguish dopamine-sensitive cyclases from other amine-sensitive cyclases. The activation of adenylate cyclase by 1.2×10^{-4} *M* dopamine was substantially reduced (greater than 50% reduction) by 10^{-4} *M* curare, 10^{-4} *M* haloperidol or 5×10^{-6} *M* fluphenazine. 10^{-4} *M* strychnine and 10^{-4} *M* chlorpromazine produced some reduction (about 20%) while propranolol and ergometrine were ineffective.

A more recent study examining the effects of both serotonin and dopamine on adenylate cyclase activity in homogenates from *Aplysia* ganglia found that only high concentrations of dopamine stimulated enzyme activity (DRUMMOND et al. 1980b). This dopamine stimulation was thought to be due to an interaction with the serotonin receptor since simultaneous stimulation with high concentrations of dopamine and serotonin showed no additivity. Although failure to demonstrate stimulation in homogenates does not preclude the existence of a specific dopamine-sensitive adenylate cyclase in the tissue, it does raise questions concerning previous investigations on intact ganglia or on homogenates which did not examine the amine specificity of the cyclase stimulation.

Despite the above uncertainties, the reported effectiveness of haloperidol and fluphenazine in reducing dopamine-activated adenylate cyclase does correlate with studies in which haloperidol and fluphenazine at concentrations of $1\text{–}10 \times 10^{-5}$ *M* were shown to reduce both depolarizing and hyperpolarizing responses to dopamine on *Aplysia* neurons (HEISS and HOYER 1974; HEISS et al. 1976). In the latter study applications of up to 1 h were required for neuroleptics to produce full reduction of dopamine responses and, similarly, slow recoveries were observed.

In the water snail, *Planorbis*, concentrations of $1\text{–}10 \times 10^{-5}$ *M* haloperidol and fluphenazine were also effective in reducing or abolishing depolarizing and hyperpolarizing responses either to iontophoretically applied dopamine or to electrical stimulation of a dopaminergic neuron (MACDONALD and BERRY 1978). As in *Aplysia*, long drug applications were required, in contrast to the rapid action of drugs such as curare and strychnine. Neither serotonin nor acetylcholine responses were affected by the two neuroleptics (HEISS et al. 1976).

It is of interest to compare the above physiological results to the effects of neuroleptics on an LSD binding site, in *Helix* ganglia, characterized by greater affinity for dopamine than serotonin (discussed in greater detail below). LSD binding to this site, which is claimed to be a dopamine receptor, is more sensitive to displacement by ergot derivatives than by neuroleptics (DRUMMOND et al. 1978). Furthermore, 50% reductions in LSD binding occur at neuroleptic concentrations (4–100 n*M*) at least two orders of magnitude less than those effective in reducing dopamine iontophoretic responses on molluscan neurons ($10^{-5}-10^{-4}$ *M*). Thus, the high concentrations required for physiological effects in intact ganglia may indicate the presence of substantial penetration barriers, or, alternatively, point out differences between the LSD binding sites and the dopamine receptor mediating the physiological responses.

A study of the effect of dopaminergic agonists on adenylate cyclase activation in *Helix aspersa* and rat striatal homogenates (MUNDAY et al. 1976) points out additional problems in the pharmacological correlation of the dopamine-sensitive adenylate cyclase and the depolarizing responses to dopamine in molluscan neurons. Ergometrine, a partial agonist and blocker of the hyperpolarizing response to dopamine, produces a stimulation of adenylate cyclase activity 63% of maximal (10^{-4} *M* dopamine) at 10^{-5} *M*. This result is hard to reconcile with the possible association of adenylate cyclase with the depolarizing dopamine response. However, since ergometrine is also known to produce some blockade of the dopaminergic depolarizing response at high concentrations, this effect on the cyclase could result from an interaction with the depolarizing receptor. Alternatively, ergometrine may interact with a serotonin-sensitive cyclase.

As pointed out above, the concentrations of drugs effective in reducing dopamine-sensitive LSD binding are quite discordant with concentrations effective against physiological dopamine responses (HEISS et al. 1976; MACDONALD and BERRY 1978). Yet, the apparent ability of some neuroleptic drugs to inhibit adenylate cyclase activation by dopamine in molluscan tissues (OSBORNE 1977) does correlate fairly well with their effectiveness in reducing physiological responses. Although access of agents to receptor sites in intact tissues may make it difficult to assess the concentrations of antagonists required to block physiological responses, another problem also exists. Doses of dopamine necessary to produce measurable membrane potential changes may be saturating for activation of the physiological effect over a substantial area of membrane. In fact, dopamine receptors are located deeply buried in the neuropile of molluscan ganglia and one of the factors determining the slow time course of iontophoretic potentials may be diffusion of agonist (as demonstrated for serotonin activated responses in *Aplysia* (GERSCHENFELD and PAUPARDIN-TRITSCH 1974)). If receptors are present in substantial excess of that necessary for activation of maximal physiological responses, blockade of a substantial percentage of receptors may only shift the dose-response curve of the physiological response along the plateau of the maximal response. In the absence of dose-response information concerning the physiological responses to dopamine application, or information concerning the distribution or density of receptors, it is difficult to correlate the action of pharmacological agents on binding sites, adenylate cyclase activation, and physiological responses.

Definitive proof that a dopamine-activated adenylate cyclase is involved in the synaptically-mediated effects of dopamine within molluscan ganglia remains to be demonstrated. In the central ganglia of the water snail, *Planorbis corneus*, a dopaminergic neuron is known to make both inhibitory and excitatory connections with other neurons (BERRY and COTTRELL 1975). Inhibitory responses are blocked by ergometrine and depolarizing responses by curare in accord with results from dopamine iontophoresis. At high concentrations, ergometrine also reduces the depolarizing responses to dopamine. Caffeine (5 m*M*), theophylline (5 m*M*), and dibutyryl-cyclic AMP (0.5 m*M*) have been reported to enhance inhibitory responses resulting from stimulation of the dopaminergic neuron (PENTREATH and BERRY 1976). However, in the absence of stimulation, exogenously applied dibutyryl-cyclic AMP or cyclic AMP, itself, did not mimic dopamine-produced hyperpolarization. In these experiments, the methylxanthines first reduced inhibitory responses to iontophoretically applied dopamine, prior to potentiation of dopamine responses during washout. The enhancement of the dopaminergic synaptic inhibition could have resulted from either a pre- or postsynaptic site of action.

2. Gill

Peripheral effects of dopamine in molluscan tissue have also been described. Dopamine is present in the gill of *Aplysia* and produces neuromodulatory effects on gill neuromuscular preparations (CARPENTER et al. 1971; SWANN et al. 1978). In gill tissue slices, dopamine produces an increase in cyclic AMP which is additive with that produced by serotonin (KEBABIAN et al. 1979). (It should be borne in mind that additivity experiments in intact tissues may be limited by antagonistic or synergistic effects that would not occur in homogenates.) Half-maximal increases in gill cyclic AMP content have been reported to occur at about 1.5×10^{-5} *M* dopamine and 3×10^{-5} *M* serotonin.

Among various agents tested in the gill, none has been found which effectively discriminates between the dopamine- and serotonin-produced increases in cyclic AMP. Bromo-LSD blocks accumulations stimulated by either amine. In addition, ergot derivatives, including ergonovine, ergotamine, methergoline, and methergine, produce increases in cyclic AMP which, in the case of ergonovine, is as great as that produced by either amine. Fluphenazine (10^{-4} *M*) causes more than a 50% reduction in the cyclic AMP increase elicited by either dopamine or serotonin. These results are in contrast to studies on molluscan neurons in which ergot derivative-sensitive dopamine responses, in general, are not thought to involve an adenylate cyclase. The results in the gill again point out the apparent lack of specificity in invertebrates of many agents thought to have some pharmacological specificity in vertebrate systems; for example, fluphenazine is unable to distinguish between serotonin- and dopamine-sensitive responses in the gill. It is of interest, in this regard, that in a comparison of serotonin-sensitive adenylate cyclase from rat hypothalamus and dopamine-sensitive adenylate cyclase from rat striatum, both cyclases were found to be competitively inhibited by serotoninergic antagonists and neuroleptic agents (ENJALBERT et al. 1978).

3. Muscle

In another molluscan peripheral system, that of the anterior byssus retractor muscle or catch muscle of *Mytilus*, both serotonergic and dopaminergic innervation to this muscle have been described (TWAROG 1976). Evidence discussed elsewhere (Sect. B.I.5) has suggested that the effects of serotonin may be cyclic nucleotide-mediated. Although dopamine can produce a slight elevation in cyclic AMP content in this muscle (KOHLER and LINDL 1980), this is most likely the result of an interaction with the serotonin receptor. Methysergide abolishes cyclic AMP increases to either amine. Clearly, the apparent lack of pharmacological specificity of many amine responses suggests that caution is necessary in evaluating results on amine-activated cyclases for which specificity of amine action is not clearly defined.

II. Insects

1. Salivary Gland

a) Tick

Many studies have examined the role of tick salivary glands in the regulation of internal volume and composition of body fluids during active feeding (KAUFMAN and PHILLIPS 1973a, b, c). In conjunction with such studies on ixodid ticks, some experiments have examined the possible role of biogenic amines and cyclic AMP in influencing the secretion process (KAUFMAN and PHILLIPS 1973b; NEEDHAM and SAUER 1975; KAUFMAN 1976).

A variety of agents, including pilocarpine, cholinesterase inhibitors, dopamine, epinephrine, norepinephrine, and serotonin, have been observed to activate salivary gland fluid secretion in vivo (TATCHELL 1967; MEGAW 1974). In isolated salivary glands, however, only the biogenic amines have been found effective, suggesting that the effects of cholinergic agents are indirect (KAUFMAN and PHILLIPS 1973b; NEEDHAM and SAUER 1975). Of the amines, dopamine ($K_a = 5 \times 10^{-8}$ *M*) is somewhat more potent than epinephrine or norepinephrine ($K_a = 5 \times 10^{-7}$ *M*), which are more effective than serotonin in activating secretion. An as yet unidentified substance from nervous tissue but not other tissues or hemolymph has also been found to activate secretion (KAUFMAN 1976). This observation, coupled with the evidence that the glands are innervated (COONS and ROSHDY 1973), has suggested that secretion is neurally controlled.

In contrast to the effects of serotonin on blowfly salivary glands (Sect. B.II), the secretion rate in response to amine application in the tick slowly increases over many minutes (up to 30 min in one protocol) and slowly decreases following washout (NEEDHAM and SAUER 1975). The reasons for the slow time course of secretion are not known, but the culture medium used for the isolated gland studies appears to be influential (KAUFMAN 1976), and access of amines to salivary gland cells may be slow. Additionally, the high concentration (1–15 m*M*) of L-glutamate used in some tick salines may be important since glutamate is a potential neuroactive agent (KAUFMAN 1976). In fact, in these glands, although 1 mM glutamate is not effective in activating fluid secretion itself, it appears to produce some inhibition of resting chloride uptake, which is thought to be a measure of secretory activity (SAUER et al. 1974). Effects of glutamate on amine-activated secretion have not been examined.

Attempts to activate fluid secretion directly with cyclic AMP or its dibutyryl derivative have been unsuccessful (KAUFMAN and PHILLIPS 1973b; NEEDHAM and SAUER 1975). However, after prior incubation of salivary glands with a catecholamine, either theophylline or cyclic AMP will further activate fluid secretion (NEEDHAM and SAUER 1975). Determination of phosphodiesterase activity during the normal feeding cycle of the tick has demonstrated that enzyme activity drops significantly during the early stages of the feeding process (MCMULLEN and SAUER 1978). A factor found in homogenates from actively feeding ticks has been found to inhibit phosphodiesterase activity when added to homogenates from slowly feeding ticks. On the other hand, preincubation of salivary glands with dopamine produces an activation of phosphodiesterase activity at all stages of feeding. What these data mean is difficult to say, except that they raise the possibility that phosphodiesterase may be regulated during the feeding cycle.

The effect of amines and cyclic AMP on [^{36}Cl] uptake in tick salivary glands has also been examined (SAUER et al. 1974). In glands from non-feeding animals, cyclic AMP and theophylline produce negligible effects on chloride uptake. In isolated glands from feeding ticks, dopamine, epinephrine, norepinephrine, and serotonin all increase chloride uptake. In addition, cyclic AMP and theophylline elevate chloride uptake, while, as mentioned above, glutamate shows a tendency to diminish chloride uptake. Hemolymph is without effect. On glands from non-feeding ticks, only serotonin has been examined and is without effect. It has been shown that the activation of secretion by amines is dependent upon the feeding stage of the tick; that is, secretion is more copious during active feeding stages. Whether this change reflects a change in sensitivity to amines or some other physiological change in gland function is not clear. If a role for catecholamines in the activation of fluid secretion is to be demonstrated, sensitivity of glands to catecholamines at a time corresponding to the onset of feeding must be shown. Alternatively, dopamine or another amine might only serve to modify the activation initiated by some other agent or process.

Recently, 10^{-5} M dopamine has been shown to produce a 2–4 fold increase in adenylate cyclase activity of isolated salivary glands (SCHMIDT et al. 1980). The pharmacology and amine specificity of this cyclase has not yet been described. The enhancement of fluid secretion evoked by low dopamine concentrations in the presence of theophylline supports the idea that a dopamine-activated cyclase is involved in the regulation of secretion. The mechanisms of this secretion process are little understood and thus the possible sites of action for the observed increases in cyclic AMP are only speculative. Of interest, though, an increase in Na^+-K^+-ATPase activity during feeding has been described (KAUFMAN et al. 1976), and ouabain has been observed to inhibit fluid secretion (KAUFMAN and PHILLIPS 1973b; NEEDHAM and SAUER 1975). Additionally, harmaline, which is thought to compete for the Na^+ site in its inhibition of ATPase activity of epithelial tissues (CANESSA et al. 1973), reversibly inhibits fluid secretion from tick glands (NEEDHAM and SAUER 1975). This role of ATPase in secretory activity has led to the as yet unsupported suggestion that a dopamine-activated adenylate cyclase may regulate the activity of the ATPase, thus enhancing the secretory rate.

The overall status of the work on the tick salivary gland indicates that cyclic AMP may be involved in mediating part of the action of amines on this preparation. Thus, it has been shown that (1) cyclic AMP can mimic the effect of amines in enhancing secretion, (2) inhibition of phosphodiesterase enhances secretion, and (3) an amine-activated adenylate cyclase is present. There is no evidence as yet concerning the role of amines in the natural activation of secretion, what amine may be involved, or what cellular processes underlie the amine enhancement of the secretory process. In addition, because of the heterogeneity of cell types in the tick salivary gland preparation, even the site of amine action remains uncertain.

b) Cockroach

The cockroach salivary gland has been used to investigate the pharmacological and electrophysiological properties of a neuroglandular aminergic synapse. Fluid secretion from the gland is activated by dopamine (and other catecholamines) and by serotonin. Further pharmacological studies have shown that the receptors to serotonin and dopamine can be distinguished (HOUSE et al. 1973; BOWSER-RILEY et al. 1978). For example, the secretory response to serotonin shows substantial desensitization, but during this period of insensitivity both nerve- and dopamine-evoked responses are only slightly diminished. In addition, although phentolamine is effective in reducing electrical responses to both catecholamines and serotonin, the inhibitory constant of phentolamine for catecholamine-evoked electrical responses is much lower than that for serotonin. Other pharmacological studies have raised questions concerning the equivalence of the dopamine receptor mediating fluid secretion and that mediating the electrical effect of dopamine. Both ergometrine and methysergide block the hyperpolarizing responses to either catecholamines or nerve stimulation. However, at similar concentrations, neither agent blocks dopamine-activated or nerve-activated fluid secretory responses. Ergometrine, itself, is effective in activating fluid secretion in a dose-dependent manner.

Dopamine is known to be present in the cockroach salivary gland (FRY et al. 1974), and catecholamine-containing terminals have been demonstrated histochemically (BLAND et al. 1973). Both nerve-evoked and dopamine-activated hyperpolarizations have been shown to involve potassium conductance increases (HOUSE 1973; GINSBORG et al. 1974, 1976; HOUSE and SMITH 1978). Several agents, including the neuroleptic, alpha-flupenthixol, have been found effective in blocking both the nerve-evoked and dopamine-activated hyperpolarization of salivary gland cells (HOUSE and GINSBORG 1976; GINSBORG et al. 1976; BOWSER-RILEY et al. 1978). An analysis of the time course of the dopamine-evoked and nerve-evoked potential changes indicates that the latency and slow time course of the potentials cannot be accounted for by either diffusion of agonist or slow receptor activation kinetics, suggesting that some step subsequent to receptor activation may determine the time course of the responses (BLACKMAN et al. 1979a, b). Although not yet demonstrated experimentally, the cockroach salivary gland would appear to be a likely candidate for containing a dopamine-sensitive adenylate cyclase.

2. Other Tissues

Dopamine has been found in high concentrations in the brain of the locust (ROBERTSON 1976), and a dopamine-sensitive adenylate cyclase exists in the thoracic ganglia and brain of the cockroach (NATHANSON and GREENGARD 1973, 1974; HARMAR and HORN 1977). By additivity criteria, the dopamine-sensitive enzyme appears separable from adenylate cyclase (present in the same tissues) activated by octopamine and serotonin. However, low concentrations ($<10^{-6}$ *M*) of several neuroleptics, thought to be relatively specific blockers of dopamine-activated adenylate cyclase in vertebrates, are also effective in reducing octopamine-sensitive adenylate cyclase activation (HARMAR and HORN 1977). Thus, although certain actions of dopamine in insect ganglia may be mediated by cyclic nucleotides, further pharmacological and physiological characterization needs to be done.

III. Crustacea

1. Nerve Tissue

Dopamine is known to be present in several parts of the crustacean nervous system, including a portion of the brain (ELOFFSON et al. 1966), a plexus of nerve fibers around the hindgut (ELOFFSON et al. 1968), the neurosecretory pericardial organs (COOKE and GOLDSTONE 1970; SULLIVAN et al. 1976), and in cell bodies and processes of neurons of the paired commissural ganglia (GOLDSTONE and COOKE 1971; BARKER et al. 1979; KUSHNER and MAYNARD 1977). Little is known concerning the physiological role of dopamine in the brain or hindgut, but some information is available concerning the possible roles of pericardial organ dopamine (see Sect. III.2) and dopamine in the commissural ganglia.

The presence of dopamine in several neurons of the paired commissural ganglia thar rest on either side of the esophagus in the decapods has been demonstrated by histofluorescence methods for the crab (GOLDSTONE and COOKE 1971) and by both biochemical and histofluorescence methods for the spiny lobster, *Panulirus interruptus* (BARKER et al. 1979; KUSHNER and MAYNARD 1977). Some of these neurons send fibers to the stomatogastric ganglion. Subgroups of the approximately 30 neurons of the stomatogastric ganglion produce rhythmic output patterns that drive the activity of muscles involved in masticating food ingested into the foregut (SELVERSTON et al. 1976). One of these rhythms, the pyloric rhythm, is thought to be driven by a group of electrically coupled bursting pacemaker neurons. In the absence of activity from the anterior inputs from the commissural ganglia, the pyloric rhythm and the activity of the bursting neurons is slower (RUSSELL 1979). Subsequent bath application of dopamine produces an activation of the pyloric rhythm that mimics many features of the intact preparation (ANDERSON and BARKER 1977; RAPER 1979). Since muscarinic agonists such as pilocarpine also produce activation of the pyloric rhythm (MARDER and PAUPARDIN-TRITSCH 1978), and serotonin and octopamine also produce alterations in the burst pattern (E. MARDER, unpublished work), it is not known to what extent dopamine is involved in the normal activation of the ganglion.

Although both depolarizing and hyperpolarizing responses to dopamine can be elicited by iontophoresis directly on stomatogastric ganglion neurons (E. MARDER, unpublished work), effects of bath-applied dopamine on the whole ganglion could result from either actions on ganglionic neurons or via effects on presynaptic terminals. Despite this problem, the preparation has been used to examine the possibility that dopamine may activate conductances appropriate for generation of bursting activity in pacemaker neurons through a cyclic AMP-mediated process (EWALD 1978, unpublished work). Theophylline (1 m*M*) enhances the increase in bursting frequency of the pyloric rhythm produced by 4×10^{-5} *M* dopamine. IBMX (0.2 m*M*) is able to increase burst frequency and produce approximately additive effects when applied together with dopamine. In contrast, at concentrations of 0.2–1 m*M*, RO-20-1724, a non-methylxanthine phosphodiesterase inhibitor, slows the frequency of pyloric bursting. Yet, 1 m*M* RO-20-1724 in combination with 2×10^{-5} *M* dopamine produces a greater increase in burst frequency than 2×10^{-5} *M* dopamine alone. Direct effects of the methylxanthine inhibitors on cellular calcium metabolism may account for the differences between the methylxanthines and RO-20-1724. However, interpretation of these results is further complicated by the simultaneous presence of several dopamine responses on stomatogastric neurons. Although 10^{-4} *M* octopamine has been reported to elevate cyclic AMP levels in isolated stomatogastric ganglia (SULLIVAN and BARKER 1975), the effect of dopamine on cyclic AMP levels has not been examined.

2. Muscle

a) Lobster

The presence of dopamine in the pericardial neurosecretory structures adjacent to the decapod heart (COOKE and GOLDSTONE 1970; SULLIVAN et al. 1976) raises the possibility that dopamine may also act as a circulating neurohormone in these animals. Although the targets for circulating dopamine remain unclear, at least four potential sites of action have been examined. These include the limb muscles, foregut muscles, heart and eyestalk.

In the case of limb muscles, concentrations of dopamine above 10^{-5} *M* produce a relaxation and a small increase in evoked contractions in the opener muscle of *Homarus* (BATELLE and KRAVITZ 1978), as well as a small increase in cyclic AMP content. Since serotonin and octopamine also elevate cyclic AMP in this preparation, it is as yet unclear whether these effects of dopamine are due to the activation of a specific dopamine receptor or adenylate cyclase.

In several muscles in the foregut of the spiny lobster, *Panulirus interruptus*, dopamine activates adenylate cyclase activity in broken cell preparations. In homogenates from the p1, gm6b, and cpv 1 a, 1 b muscles, dopamine stimulates adenylate cyclase activity 3- to 12-fold (J. A. NATHANSON, C. LINGLE and E. MARDER, unpublished work). These muscles receive either glutamatergic or cholinergic innervation (MARDER 1976; LINGLE 1980), and no dopaminergic innervation to these muscles is known. However, the muscles are situated just anterior to the dopamine-containing pericardial neurosecretory structures of the heart (SULLIVAN et al. 1976). Although, in some muscles, slight stimulation of adenylate cyclase activity is produced by serotonin or octopamine, this stimulation is not additive to that produced by dopamine. The K_a of the dopamine-sensitive cyclase is about 10^{-6} *M*, with some stimulation occurring at 10^{-7} *M*. Neither fat tissue, opener muscle, or abdominal fast flexor muscle from the same animal shows an activation of adenylate cyclase by dopamine.

On the same foregut preparations which contain dopamine-sensitive adenylate cyclase, dopamine produces potent neuromodulatory effects. At concentrations as low as 10^{-8} *M*, dopamine produces an enhancement of neurally evoked contractions in these same three muscles, the p1, the gm6b, and the cpv 1a, 1b (LINGLE 1979a, b). Maximal responses to dopamine occur above 10^{-5} *M*. The physiological effects of dopamine appear to result from an increase in the amplitude of intracellular excitatory junctional potentials, which can be at least partly accounted for by a dopamine-produced increase in muscle fiber membrane resistance (LINGLE 1981). Whether the effects of dopamine on muscle fiber electrical properties can be accounted for by the activation of the dopamine-sensitive adenylate cyclase remains to be demonstrated. The possibility of multiple dopamine receptors in this system must also be addressed.

Dopamine has also been reported to increase the frequency and amplitude of contractions of isolated, perfused crustacean hearts (BERLIND et al. 1970; FLOREY and RATHMAYER 1978), although the physiological significance of these effects is unclear. Since both serotonin and octopamine are also known to produce effects on crustacean hearts which are to some extent similar to the action of dopamine, information concerning the specificity of these different apparent amine receptors would be useful. One study has compared the effectiveness of dopamine in increasing the frequency of heart rate relative to the action of the two other amines and has observed a species dependency of the relative effectiveness (FLOREY and RATHMAYER 1978). These authors also report that methysergide blocks the action of both dopamine and serotonin on *Astacus* heart again raising some question as to the specificity of the receptors activated by these amines. Yet certainly the low concentrations of dopamine required to produce increases in heart rate suggest that the heart must be considered a candidate for a site of action of dopamine.

As described previously (Sect. B.III.2), serotonin may play a role in the control of release of red-pigment dispersing hormone from the sinus gland of the eyestalk of the fiddler crab (RAO and FINGERMAN 1970; FINGERMAN and RAO 1970; FINGERMAN and FINGERMAN 1975). Investigations from these workers have also indicated that dopamine may play an antagonistic role to that of serotonin by controlling the release of red-pigment concentrating hormone (FINGERMAN et al. 1981). Initial observations on the pharmacology of these effects indicate that the dopamine receptor agonist, ADTN, mimics the effects of dopamine while the neuroleptic, spiroperidol, a dopamine antagonist in the vertebrates, antagonizes the effects attributed to dopamine in concentrating pigment. Although these results were taken as evidence for a possible neurotransmitter role for dopamine, the possibility that pigment hormone release could be controlled by circulating amines must also be considered. The role of cyclic nucleotides in these actions of amines on eyestalk hormone remains to be addressed.

b) Barnacle

Barnacle muscle fibers have been used as a model for the study of the regulation of ionic fluxes. Both cyclic AMP and cyclic GMP have been implicated in activating a ouabain-insensitive sodium efflux (BITTAR et al. 1974, 1976; BITTAR and BEN-

JAMIN 1978), a chloride efflux (BORON et al. 1978), and a calcium efflux (CHENG and CHEN 1975). The interaction of these ionic systems has not been addressed. Little is known concerning agents that might regulate nucleotide levels in barnacle fibers, but recently it has been reported that insulin increases cyclic GMP levels and decreases cyclic AMP levels (BAKER and CARRUTHERS 1980). Insulin was also found to increase glucose uptake into the barnacle muscle fibers. It is not known whether barnacles or other crustaceans have an insulin-like substance, although insulin-like immunoreactivity has been demonstrated in insects (TAGER et al. 1976). Cyclic GMP levels in barnacle muscle are also increased by either application of high potassium salines or by nerve stimulation (BEAM et al. 1977). The effect of KCl does not occur in calcium-free saline suggesting that the increase in cyclic GMP may result from an increase in intracellular calcium during the potassium-induced or nerve-evoked contracture rather than simply resulting from depolarization of the muscle fibers. Little effect on cyclic AMP content has been observed.

E. Peptide – Cyclic Nucleotide Interactions

A rapidly increasing number of studies have been published concerning the presence and possible physiological roles of peptide substances in invertebrate neural and neurosecretory tissues. Several recently published articles have reviewed various aspects of the role of peptides in invertebrates (HAYNES 1980; GREENBERG and PRICE 1980; COOKE 1977; COOKE and SULLIVAN 1981). Some of the effects produced by peptides on neural and non-neural tissues appear to be correlated with alterations in cyclic nucleotides. However, as with many of the studies on amine-cyclic nucleotide interaction described above, it is not yet clear whether activation of a nucleotide cyclase is essential for the physiological effects produced by peptides or is merely an epiphenomenon. The following discussion of peptide-cyclic nucleotide interaction is not meant to be a thorough survey of this rapid growth area; instead, we have chosen to point out briefly a few preparations where cyclic nucleotide involvement in the action of a given peptide is most strongly implicated.

I. Molluscs

FMRFamide (Phe-Met-Arg-Phe-amide) is a neuropeptide isolated and purified from extracts of bivalve ganglia (PRICE and GREENBERG 1977; GREENBERG and PRICE 1979). In general, this peptide increases the amplitude and frequency of the heart beat in bivalve molluscs, although species-dependent inhibition of heart rate has been observed at certain concentrations of FMRFamide (GREENBERG and PRICE 1980). The cardioacceleratory effect of the peptide bears some similarity to the action of serotonin on bivalve hearts (PRICE and GREENBERG 1980); however, it differs in that methysergide blocks the effects of serotonin without modifying the action of FMRFamide. Both FMRFamide and serotonin have been shown to increase cyclic AMP levels in intact clam hearts and to activate adenylate cyclase activity in crude homogenates (HIGGINS and GREENBERG 1974; HIGGINS et al. 1978). As in intact preparations, methysergide prevents the activation of adenylate cyclase by serotonin but not by FMRFamide. The magnitude of adenylate cyclase stimulation by saturating FMRFamide concentrations is equivalent to the stimulatory effect of saturating concentrations of serotonin. However, in the presence of simultaneous saturating concentrations of both agents, the activation of adenylate cyclase is no greater than that produced by saturating concentrations of either agent alone. This raises the possibility that serotonin and FMRFamide may be acting on the same cell population or metabolic pool of cyclic AMP.

A number of other peptides are known to produce effects on the spontaneous activity of molluscan neurons (BARKER and GAINER 1974; IFSHIN et al. 1975; LEVITAN and TRIESTMAN 1977; LEVITAN et al. 1979; MAYERI et al. 1979a, b). Additionally, peptides may mediate some slow synaptic events in molluscs (MAYERI et al. 1979a, b). The possibility that cyclic nucleotides might be involved in the actions of peptides on these preparations has been addressed by two types of experiments: first, an examination of the ability of nucleotides or phosphodiesterase inhibitors to mimic the actions of the peptide, and, second, an examination of the ability of the peptide or peptide-containing extract to activate nucleotide cyclases.

In neuron F1 from *Helix*, R15 from *Aplysia*, and neuron 11 from *Otala*, the vertebrate neurohypophysial peptide hormones, vasopressin and oxytocin, and a peptide-containing extract (PE) from molluscan nervous tissue produce an alteration in the normal endogenous bursting activity of these neurons (BARKER and GAINER 1974; IFSHIN et al. 1975; LEVITAN and TRIESTMAN 1977; TRIESTMAN and LEVITAN 1976; LEVITAN et al. 1979). This alteration consists of an increase in the frequency and number of action potentials within a burst as well as an increase in the duration and magnitude of hyperpolarizations between bursts.

The physiological action of the above peptides has been compared to the effects of cyclic nucleotide analogs on the bursting activity of these neurons. The cyclic AMP analogs, 8-(4-amino-butyl-amino)-cyclic AMP and 8-benzylthio-cyclic AMP, produce alterations in bursting activity similar to the effects of the peptides (TRIESTMAN and LEVITAN 1976). More recently, the activity of R15 has been shown to be differentially influenced by alterations in the intracellular concentrations of either cyclic GMP or cyclic AMP analogs (LEVITAN and NORMAN 1980), suggesting that both nucleotides may play a role in the regulation of neuronal activity.

The ability of oxytocin, vasopressin, and PE to stimulate cyclic AMP accumulation in intact ganglia and to activate adenylate cyclase in membrane preparations has also been examined. Both vertebrate peptides and PE increase the cyclic AMP content of intact *Helix* ganglia. In addition, PE produces a GTP-independent stimulation of adenylate cyclase in ganglion membrane preparations (LEVITAN and TRIESTMAN 1977) and an increase in the cyclic AMP content in single, isolated cell bodies of neurons F1 and R15 (LEVITAN 1978). In these studies, oxytocin and vasopressin were reported to have no effect on adenylate cyclase activity in membranes (LEVITAN et al. 1978), suggesting that the ability of these latter peptides to stimulate cyclic AMP accumulation in intact tissues might represent an indirect action (or, alternatively, that appropriate assay conditions were not established).

II. Insects

In silkmoths, eclosion, the process by which an adult moth hatches from the pupal cuticle, occurs under hormonal control (TRUMAN 1976). This behavioral response appears to be initiated by the nervous system, since, in the isolated nervous system, eclosion hormone can trigger the neuronally-generated motor patterns associated with eclosion (TRUMAN 1978). TRUMAN et al. (1979) showed that treatment of the isolated central nervous system of the silkworm with eclosion hormone produces a doubling in the levels of cyclic GMP. Additionally, in at least some animals, treatments with phosphodiesterase inhibitors or cyclic GMP seemed to potentiate or mimic the effects of the eclosion hormone. As the authors point out, these effects will be easier to study when eclosion hormone has been purified and characterized.

A pentapeptide, proctolin (STARRATT and BROWN 1975; BROWN and STARRATT 1975), is present in the nervous system of a variety of insects (BROWN 1976). In the cockroach, *Periplaneta*, proctolin is thought to be an excitatory transmitter to the proctodeum. In brain homogenates from adult (but not larval) locusts, 10^{-8} *M* proctolin produces a maximal 40% increase in adenylate cyclase activity with smaller increases at higher concentrations (HIRIPI et al. 1979). At similar concentrations, there is a slight decrease (less than 25%) in guanylate cyclase activity.

III. Crustacea

In the Crustacea, a cardioacceleratory peptide or peptides are present in the pericardial neurosecretory structures (COOKE 1964; BELAMARICH and TERWILLIGER 1966; BERLIND and COOKE 1970). One of these peptides is closely related to, or identical with, proctolin (SULLIVAN 1979). No information is available concerning the effects of proctolin on cyclic nucleotide levels in crustacean tissues. However, a recent study has examined the effects of peptide-containing pericardial organ extracts (XPO) on cyclic AMP levels in cardiac ganglia (LEMOS and BERLIND 1981). These extracts, which contain inconsequential quantities of biogenic amines, produce increases in cardiac ganglion burst frequency and burst duration. The effects are mimicked by the applications of cyclic AMP or phosphodiesterase inhibitors but not by serotonin. XPO extracts produce an increase in cyclic AMP levels in intact cardiac ganglia. The results suggest that there is a cardioacceleratory peptide in the pericardial organs whose effects may be mediated by an elevation of cyclic AMP levels in cardiac ganglion cells. However, since the cyclic AMP-producing peptide of LEMOS and BERLIND is trypsin-sensitive, while proctolin is trypsin-insensitive (SULLIVAN 1979), the above effects can not readily be attributed to proctolin.

F. Other Roles for Cyclic Nucleotides in Invertebrates

The presence of adenylate and guanylate cyclase systems have been described for several other invertebrate organisms. In general, although the existence of such enzyme is well established, little is yet known concerning the physiological significance of cyclic nucleotides in these organisms.

I. Sponges

A role for cyclic AMP in controlling the release from dormancy of gemmules of the freshwater sponge, *Spongilla lacustris*, has been described (SIMPSON and RODAN

1976). Dormant gemmules are induced to germinate by raising the incubation temperature from 4 °C to 20 °C. A significant decrease in the cyclic AMP content of gemmules occurs during the first two hours after germination. If agents which are known to inhibit gemmule phosphodiesterase activity, such as aminophylline and IBMX, are applied during the germination process, the cyclic AMP content does not decrease and the germination process is arrested. Direct pretreatment of gemmules with 1 m*M* cyclic AMP inhibits germination by 100%, while 10^{-4} *M* cyclic AMP prevents germination by 50%.

II. Coelenterates

In two coelenterates, *Hydra attenuata* (Cobb et al. 1980) and the sea anemone, *Anthopleura elegantissima* (Gentleman and Mansour 1974), glutathione activates a feeding response. In the anemone, homogenates from the oral disc, but not orther portions of the animals, have been shown to contain a membrane-bound adenylate cyclase activated by glutathione. Also, incubation of whole *Hydra* with glutathione produces increases in the levels of both cyclic GMP and cyclic AMP. However, the time course of the increases in nucleotide levels does not correlate well with the activation of the feeding response.

III. Nematodes

In nematodes, both cyclic AMP and cyclic GMP have been found to be present in whole animal homogenates of the free living worm, *Panagellus redivivus* (Willett and Rahim 1978a, b). Nucleotide cyclase activity and its hormone dependence have not been examined. In studies of the chemotactic behavior of *Caenorhabitis elegans*, 1 m*M* cyclic AMP has been found to attract the nematode (Ward 1973), even in mutants selected for defective attraction by other agents, including NaCl (Dusenberry 1976).

IV. Annelids

In annelids, the role of cyclic AMP both in regeneration processes and in hormone action has been examined. In the polychaete, *Owenia fusiformi*, following anterior amputation, regenerating cells become synchronized in their cell division cycle (Marilley and Thouveny 1978). Adenylate cyclase activity in homogenates from the regenerating zone has been found to undergo periodic fluctuations related to the particular stage of the cell cycle (see Friedman, this volume). There is also a smaller diurnal rhythm (Coulon and Marilley 1978). Adenylate cyclase activity in homogenates from control animals is stimulated by epinephrine, norepinephrine, serotonin, and GABA. The specificity of this stimulation or its involvement in regeneration has not been determined.

In the marine polychaete, *Glycera alba*, cychc AMP has been shown to stimulate phosphofructokinase activity in a fashion similar to that found in the liver fluke (Blackstock 1978).

In the earthworm, *Lumbricus terrestris*, both serotonin- and octopamine-activated adenylate cyclases have been reported (Robertson and Osborne 1979). Dopamine, adenosine, glutamate, glycine, and GABA were without effect. LSD was found to reduce activation of both serotonin- and octopamine-sensitive cyclases.

Acknowledgements. C. J. L. is a recipient of a Muscular Dystrophy Association postdoctoral fellowship. E. M. is supported by NSF grant BNS78-15399, by a grant from the Scottish Rite, and by a McKnight Scholars Award. J. A. N. is supported by NIH grant NS16356, by a McKnight Scholars Award, and by a PMAF Faculty Development Award in Clinical Pharmacology. We thank E. HUNNICUTT and C. OWEN for their assistance in proofreading this chapter.

References

Abrahams SL, Northup JK, Mansour TE (1976) Adenosine cyclic 3′,5′-monophosphate in the liver fluke, *Fasciola hepatica* I. activation of adenylate cyclase by 5-hydroxytryptamine. Mol Pharmacol 12:49–58

Ambron RT, Goldman JE, Shkolnik LJ, Schwartz JH (1980) Synthesis and axonal transport of membrane glycoproteins in a identified serotonergic neuron of *Aplysia*. J Neurophysiol 43:929–944

Anderson WW, Barker DL (1977) Activation of a stomatogastric motor pattern generator by dopamine and L-DOPA. Neurosci Abstr 3:171

Ascher P (1972) Inhibitory and excitatory effects of dopamine on *Aplysia* neurones. J Physiol (Lond) 255:173–205

Ascher P, Kehoe JS (1975) Amine and amino acid receptors in gastropod neurons. In: Handbook of psychopharmacology, Raven Press, New York, vol 4:265–310

Atkinson MM, Herman WS, Sheppard JR (1977) An octopamine-sensitive adenylate cyclase in the central nervous system of *Limulus polyphemus*. Comp Biochem Physiol 58C:107–110

Aziz SA, Knowles CO (1973) Inhibition of monamine oxidase by the pesticide chlordimeform and related compounds. Nature 242:417–418

Bailey CH, Hawkins RD, Chen MC, Kandel ER (1981) Interneurons involved in mediation and modulation of gill-withdrawal reflex in Aplysia. IV. Morphological basis of presynaptic facilitation. J Neurophysiol 45:340–360

Baker PF, Carruthers A (1980) Insulin stimulates sugar transport in giant muscle fibres of the barnacle. Nature 286:276–278

Bandle EF, Levitan IB (1977) Cyclic AMP-stimulated phosphorylation of a high molecular weight endogenous protein substrate in sub-cellular fractions of molluscan nervous system. Brain Res 125:325–331

Barker DL, Molinoff PB, Kravitz EA (1972) Octopamine in the lobster nervous system. Nature New Biol 236:61–62

Barker DL, Kushner PD, Hooper NK (1979) Synthesis of dopamine and octopamine in the crustacean stomatogastric nervous system. Brain Res 161:99–113

Barker J, Gainer H (1974) Peptide regulation of bursting pacemaker activity in a molluscan neurosecretory cell. Science 184:1371–1373

Batta S, Walker RJ, Woodruff GN (1979) Pharmacological studies on *Helix* neuron octopamine receptors. Comp Biochem Physiol 64C:43–51

Battelle BA, Kravitz EA (1978) Targets of octopamine action in the lobster: cyclic nucleotide changes and physiological effects in hemolymph, heart and exoskeletal muscle. J Pharmacol Exp Ther 205:438–448

Bauchau AG, Mengeot JC (1968) Action de la serotonine et de l'hormone diabetogenie des crustaces sur la phosphorylase musculaire. Gen Comp Endocrinol 11:132–138

Beam KG, Nestler EJ, Greengard P (1977) Increased cyclic GMP levels associated with contraction in muscle fibres of the giant barnacle. Nature 267:534–536

Beams HW, Anderson E (1955) Light and electron microscope studies on the light organ of the firefly *(Photinus pyralis)*. Biol Bull 109:375–393

Belamarich FA, Terwilliger RC (1966) Neurosecretion in invertebrates other than insects. I. The nature and localization of neurosecretory substances. Isolation and identification of cardio-excitor hormone from the pericardial organs of *Cancer borealis*. Am Zool 6:101–106

Berlind A (1977) Neurohumoral and reflex control of scaphognathite beating in the crab *Carcinus maenas*. J Comp Physiol 116:77–90

Berlind A, Cooke IM (1970) Release of a neurosecretory hormone as peptide by electrical stimulation of crab pericaridal organs. J Exp Biol 53:679–686

Berlind A, Cooke IM, Goldstone MW (1970) Do the monoamines in crab pericardial organsplay a role in peptide neurosecretion. J Exp Biol 53:669–677

Berridge MJ (1970) The role of 5-hydroxytryptamine and cyclic AMP in the control of fluid secretion by isolated salivary glands. J Exp Biol 53:171–186

Berridge MJ (1972) The mode of action of 5-hydroxytryptamine. J Exp Biol 56:311–321

Berridge MJ (1973) The effects of derivatives of adenosine 3′,5′-monophosphate on fluid secretion by the salivary glands of *Calliphora*. J Exp Biol 59:595–606

Berridge MJ, Fain JN (1979) Inhibition of phosphatidylinositol synthesis and the inactivation of calcium entry after prolonged exposure of the blowfly salivary gland to 5-hydroxytryptamine. Biochem J 178:59–69

Berridge MJ, Lipke H (1979) Changes in calcium transport across *Calliphora* salivary glands induced by 5-hydroxytryptamine and cyclic nucleotides. J Exp Biol 78:137–148

Berridge MJ, Patel NG (1968) Insect salivary glands: stimulation of fluid secretion by 5-hydroxytryptamine and adenosine 3′,5′-monophosphate. Science 162:462–463

Berridge MJ, Prince WT (1971) The electrical response of isolated salivary glands during stimulation with 5-hydroxytryptamine and cyclic AMP. Philos Trans R Soc Lond [Biol] 262:111–120

Berridge MJ, Prince WT (1972a) The role of cyclic AMP in the control of fluid secretion. Adv Cyclic Nucleotide Res 1:137–147

Berridge MJ, Prince WT (1972b) The role of cyclic AMP and calcium in hormone action. Adv Insect Physiol 12:1–49

Berridge MJ, Prince WT (1972c) Transepithelial potential changes during stimulation of isolated salivary glands with 5-hydroxytryptamine and cyclic AMP. J Exp Biol 56:139–153

Berridge MJ, Prince WT (1974) The nature of the binding between LSD and a 5-HT receptor: a possible explanation for hallucinogenic activity. Br J Pharmacol 51:269–278

Berridge MJ, Lindley BD, Prince WJ (1975a) Membrane permeability changes during stimulation of isolated salivary glands of *Calliphora* by 5-hydroxytryptamine. J Physiol (Lond) 244:549–567

Berridge MJ, Lindley BD, Prince WT (1975b) Stimulus-secretion coupling in an insect salivary gland: cell activation by elevated potassium concentrations. J Exp Biol 62:629–636

Berridge MJ, Lindley BD, Prince WT (1976) Studies on the mechanism of fluid secretion by isolated salivary glands of *Calliphora*. J Exp Biol 64:311–322

Berry MS, Cottrell GA (1975) Excitatory, inhibitory, and biphasic synaptic potentials mediated by an identified dopamine-containing neurone. J Physiol (Lond) 244:589–612

Bittar EE, Benjamin H (1978) Mode of action of theophylline on sodium efflux in barnacle muscle fibers. J Membr Biol 39:57–73

Bittar EE, Hift H, Huddart H, Tong E (1974) The effects of caffeine on sodium transport, membrane potential, mechanical tension and ultrastructure in barnacle muscle fibres. J Physiol (Lond) 242:1–34

Bittar EE, Chambers G, Schultz R (1976) Mode of stimulation by adenosine 3′,5′-cyclic monophosphate of the sodium efflux in barnacle muscle fibres. J Physiol (Lond) 257:561–579

Blackman JG, Ginsborg BL, House CR (1979a) On the effect of iontophoretically applied dopamine in salivary gland cells of *Nauphoeta cinerea*. J Physiol (Lond) 287:67–80

Blackman JG, Ginsborg BL, House CR (1979b) On the time course of the electrical response of salivary gland cells of *Nauphoeta cinerea* to iontophoretically applied dopamine. J Physiol (Lond) 287:81–92

Blackstock J (1978) Phosphofructokinase in the polychaete worm, *Glycera alba* (Muller) exposed to low oxygen concentrations: effect of adenosine 3′,5′-cyclic monophosphate activities observed in vitro. Biochem Soc Trans 6:414–416

Bland KP, House CR, Ginsborg BL, Laszlo I (1973) Catecholamine transmitter for salivary secretion in the cockroach. Nature New Biol 244:26–27

Bodnaryk RP (1979a) Basal, dopamine- and octopamine-stimulated adenylate cyclase activity in the brain of the moth, *Mamestra configurata*, during its metamorphosis. J Neurochem 33:275–282
Bodnaryk RP (1979b) Characterization of an octopamine-sensitive adenylate cyclase from insect brain *(Mamestra configurata Wik.)*. Can J Biochem 57:226–232
Boron WF, Russell JM, Brodwick MS (1978) Influence of cyclic AMP on intracellular pH regulation and chloride fluxes in barnacle muscle fibres. Nature 276:511–513
Borowitz JL, Kennedy JR (1968) Actions of sympathomimetic amines on the isolated light organ of the firefly *Photinus pyralis*. Arch Int Pharmacodyn Ther 171:81–92
Bowie LJ, Irwin R, Loken M, DeLuca M, Brand L (1973) Excited-state proton transfer and the mechanism of action of firefly luciferase. Biochemistry 12:1852–1857
Bowser-Riley F, House CR, Smith RK (1978) Competitive antagonism by phentolamine of responses to biogenic amines and the transmitter at a neuroglandular junction. J Physiol (Lond) 279:473–489
Brown BE (1975) Proctolin: a peptide transmitter candidate in insects. Life Sci 17:1241–1252
Brown BE (1976) Occurrence of proctolin in six orders of insects. J Insect Physiol 23:861–864
Brown BE, Starratt AN (1975) Isolation of protolin, a myotropic peptide from *Periplaneta Americana*. J Insect Physiol 21:1879–1881
Brownstein MJ, Saavedra JM, Axelrod J, Zeman GH, Carpenter DO (1974) Coexistence of several putative neurotransmitters in single identified neurons of *Aplysia*. Proc Natl Acad Sci USA 71:4662–4665
Brunelli M, Castellucci V, Kandel ER (1976) Synaptic facilitation and behavioral sensitization in *Aplysia:* possible role of serotonin and cyclic AMP. Science 194:1178–1181
Buchan PB, Evans PD (1980) Use of an operational amplifier signal differentiator reveals that octopamine increases the rate of development of neurally evoked tension in insect muscle. J Exp Biol 85:349–352
Buck JB (1947) The anatomy and physiology of the light organ in fireflies. Ann NY Acad Sci 149:397–483
Buck J, Case JF (1961) Control of flashing in fireflies. I. The lantern as a neuroeffector organ. Biol Bull 121:234–256
Buck J, Case JF, Hanson FE Jr (1963) Control of flashing in fireflies. III. Peripheral excitation. Biol Bull 125:251–269
Candy DJ (1978) The regulation of locust flight muscle metabolism by octopamine and other compounds. Insect Biochem 8:177–181
Canessa M, Jainovich E, De La Fuente M (1973) Harmaline: a competitor of Na ion in the $(Na^+\text{-}K^+)$-ATPase system. J Membr Biol 13:263–282.
Carlson AD (1968a) Effect of adrenergic drugs on the lantern of the larval *Photinis* firefly. J Exp Biol 48:381–387
Carlson AD (1968b) Effects of drugs on luminescence in larval fireflies. J Exp Biol 49:195–199
Carlson AD (1969) Neural control of firefly luminescence. Adv Insect Physiol 6:51–96
Carlson AD (1972) A comparison of transmitter and synephrine on luminescence induction in the firefly larva. J Exp Biol 57:737–743
Carpenter DO, Gaubatz GL (1974) Octopamine receptors on *Aplysia* neurones mediate hyperpolarization by increasing membrane conductance. Nature 252:483–485
Carpenter DO, Breese G, Schanberg S, Kopin I (1971) Serotonin and dopamine: distribution and accumulation in *Aplysia* nervous and non-nervous tissues. Int J Neurosci 2:49–56
Case JF, Buck J (1963) Control of flashing in fireflies. II. Role of central nervous system. Biol Bull 125:234–250
Castellucci VF, Kandel ER (1976) Presynaptic facilitation as a mechanism for behavioral sensitization in *Aplysia*. Science 194:1176–1178
Castellucci VF, Kandel ER, Schwartz JH, Wilson FD, Nairn AC, Greengard P (1980) Intracellular injection of the catalytic subunit of cyclic AMP-dependent protein kinase stimulates facilitation of transmitter release underlying behavioral sensitization in *Aplysia*. Proc Natl Acad Sci USA 77:7492–7496

Cedar H, Schwartz JH (1972) Cyclic adenosine monophosphate in the nervous system of *Aplysia californica.* J Gen Physiol 60:570–587
Cheng S-C, Chen SS (1975) Stimulation by cyclic nucleotides of calcium efflux in barnacle muscle fibers. Life Sci 16:1711–1716
Cobb MH, Heagy W, Danner J, Lenhoff HM, Marshall GR (1980) Effect of glutathione on cyclic nucleotide levels in *Hydra attenuta.* Comp Biochem Physiol 65C:111–115
Cohen JL, Weiss KR, Kupfermann I (1978) Motor control of buccal muscles in *Aplysia.* J Neurophysiol 41:157–180
Cole RA, Twarog BM (1972) Relaxation of catch in a molluscan smooth muscle. I. Effects of drugs which act on the adenyl cyclase system. Comp Biochem Physiol 43A:321–330
Collins C, Miller T (1977) Studies on the action of biogenic amines on cockroach heart. J Exp Biol 67:1–15
Cooke IM (1964) Electrical activity and release of neurosecretory material in crab pericardial organs. Comp Biochem Physiol 13:353–366
Cooke IM (1966) The sites of action of pericardial organ extract and 5-hydroxytryptamine in the decapod crustacean heart. Am Zool 6:107–121
Cooke IM (1977) Electrical activity of neurosecretory terminals and control of peptide hormone release. In: Gainer H (ed) Peptides in neurobiology. Plenum, New York, pp 345–374
Cooke IM, Goldstone MW (1970) Fluorescence localization of monoamines in crab neurosecretory structures. J Exp Biol 53:651–668
Cooke IM, Hartline DK (1975) Neurohormonal alteration of integrative properties of the cardiac ganglion of the lobster *Homarus americanus.* J Exp Biol 63:33–52
Cooke IM, Sullivan RE (1981) Crustacean neurohormones. In: Atwood H (ed) Biology of Crustacea. Academic Press, New York London
Coons LB, Roshdy MA (1973) Fine structure of the salivary glands of unfed male *Dermacentor variabilis* (Say) (Ixodoidea, Ixodidae). J Parasitol 59:900–912
Cottrell GA (1977) Identified amine-containing neurones and their synaptic connections. Neuroscience 2:1–18
Cottrell GA, Powell B (1971) Formation of serotonin by isolated serotonin containing neurons and by isolated non-amine containing neurons. J Neurochem 18:1695–1697
Coulon J, Marilley M (1978) Fluctuations of adenylate cyclase activity during anterior regeneration in *Owenia fusiformis* (Polychaete Annelid). J Embryol Exp Morphol 48:73–78
DeLuca M, McElroy WD (1974) Kinetics of the firefly luciferase catalyzed reactions. Biochemistry 13:921–925
Deterre P, Paupardin-Tritsch D, Bockaert J, Gerschenfeld HM (1981) Role of cyclic AMP in a serotonin-evoked slow inward current in snail neurons. Nature 290:783–785
Dougan DFH, Wade DN (1978a) Action of octopamine agonists and stereo-isomers at a specific octopamine receptor. Clin Exp Pharmacol Physiol 5:333–339
Dougan DFH, Wade DN (1978b) Differential blockade of octopamine and dopamine receptors by analogues of clozapone and metaclopramide. Clin Exp Pharmacol Physiol 5:341–349
Drummond AH, Bucher F, Levitan IB (1978) LSD labels a novel dopamine receptor in molluscan nervous tissue. Nature 272:368–370
Drummond AH, Bucher F, Levitan IB (1980a) Distribution of serotonin and dopamine receptors in *Aplysia* tissues: analyses by (^{3}H) LSD binding and adenylate cyclase stimulation. Brain Res 184:163–177
Drummond AH, Bucher F, Levitan IB (1980b) d-(^{3}H)-Lysergic acid diethylamide binding to serotonin receptors in the molluscan nervous system. J Biol Chem 255:6679–6686
Drummond AH, Benson JA, Levitan IB (1980c) Serotonin-induced hyperpolarization of an identified *Aplysia* neuron is mediated by cyclic AMP. Proc Natl Acad Sci USA 77:5013–5017
Dudel J (1965) 5-hydroxytryptamine on the crayfish neuromuscular junction. Naunyn Schmiedebergs Arch Pharmacol 249:515–528
Dusenberry DB (1976) Chemotactic behavior of mutants of the nematode *Caenorhabitis elegans* that are defective in their attraction to NaCl. J Exp Zool 198:343–352

Eloffson R, Kauri T, Nielsen SO, Stromberg JO (1966) Localization of monoaminergic neurons in the central nervous system of *Astacus astacus* L. (Crustacea), Z Zellforsch Mikrosk Anat 74:464–473
Eloffson R, Kauri T, Nielson SO, Stromberg JO (1968) Catecholamine-containing nerve fibers in the hindgut of *Astacus astacus* L. (Crustacea, Decapoda). Experientia 24:1159–1160
Enjalbert A, Hamon M, Bourgoin S, Bockaert J (1978) Postsynaptic serotonin sensitive adenylate cyclase in the central nervous system II. comparison with dopamine- and isoproterenol-sensitive adenylate cyclases in rat brain. Mol Pharmacol 14:11–23
Evans PD (1978) Octopamine distribution in the insect nervous system. J Neurochem 30:1009–1013
Evans PD (1980a) Biogenic amines in the insect nervous system. Adv Insect Physiol 15:317–473
Evans PD (1980b) Octopamine receptors in insects. In: Sattelle DB, Hall LM, Hildebrand JH (eds) Receptors for neurotransmitters, hormones and pheromones in insects. Elsevier, Amsterdam Oxford New York, pp 245–258
Evans PD (1981) Multiple receptor types for octopamine in the locust. J Physiol (Lond) 318:99–122
Evans PD, Gee JD (1980) Action of formamidine pesticides on octopamine receptors. Nature 287:60–62
Evans PD, O'Shea M (1977) An octopaminergic neurone modulates neuromuscular transmission in the locust. Nature 270:257–259
Evans PD, O'Shea M (1978) The identification of an octopaminergic neurone and the modulation of a myogenic rhythm in the locust. J Exp Biol 73:235–260
Evans PD, Talamo BR, Kravitz EA (1975) Octopamine neurons: morphology, release of octopamine and possible physiological role. Brain Res 90:340–347
Evans PD, Kravitz EA, Talamo BR (1976a) Octopamine release at two points along lobster nerve trunks. J Physiol (Lond) 262:71–89
Evans PD, Kravitz EA, Talamo BR, Wallace BG (1976b) The association of octopamine with specific neurons along lobster nerve trunks. J Physiol (Lond) 262:51–71
Ewald DA (1978) Dopaminergic modulation of a bursting pacemaker oscillation: potentiation by theophylline. Neurosci Abstr 4:295
Fain JN, Berridge MJ (1979) Relationship between hormonal activation of phosphatidylinositol hydrolysis, fluid secretion and calcium flux in the blowfly salivary gland. Biochem J 178:45–58
Farnham PJ, Novak RA, McAdoo DJ (1978) A re-examination of the distributions of octopamine and phenylethanolamine in the *Aplysia* nervous system. J Neurochem 30:1173–1176
Fingerman M, Fingerman SW (1975) The effects of 5-hydroxytryptamine depletors and monoamine oxidase inhibitors on color changes of the fiddler crab, *Uca pugilator;* further evidence in support of the hypothesis that 5-hydroxytryptamine controls the release of red-pigment dispersing hormone. Comp Biochem Physiol 52C:55–59
Fingerman M, Rao KR (1970) Action of biogenic amines on crustacean chromatophores. III. Antagonism by lysergic acid diethylamide on the effect of serotonin and colour changes in the fiddler crab, *Uca pugilator*. Comp Gen Pharmacol 1:341–348
Fingerman M, Julian WE, Spirtes MA, Kostrazewa BM (1974) The presence of 5-hydroxytryptamine in the eyestalks and brain of the fiddler crab, *Uca pugilator*, its quantitative modification by pharmacological agents, and possible role as a neurotransmitter in controlling the release of red pigment-dispersing hormone. Comp Gen Pharmacol 5:299–303
Fingerman M, Hanumante MM, Fingerman SW (1981) The effects of biogenic amines on color changes of the fiddler crab, *Uca pugilator:* further evidence for roles of 5-hydroxytryptamine and dopamine as neurotransmitters triggering release of erythrophorotrophic hormones. Comp Biochem Physiol 68C:205–211
Florey E, Rathmayer M (1978) The effects of octopamine and other amines on the heart and on neuromuscular transmission in decapod crustaceans: further evidence for a role as neurohormone. Comp Biochem Physiol 61C:229–237

Franquinet R, Stengel D, Hanoune J (1976) The adenylate cyclase system in a freshwater planarian *(polycelis tenuis iijima)*. Comp Biochem Physiol 53B:329–333

Franquinet R, Le Moigne A, Hanoune J (1978) The adenylate cyclase system of *Planaria polycelis tenuis*. Activation by serotonin and guanine nucleotides. Biochim Biophys Acta 539:88–97

Fry JP, House CR, Sharman DF (1974) An analysis of the catecholamine content of the salivary gland of the cockroach. Br J Pharmacol 51:116P–117P

Gade G, Holwerda DA (1976) Involvement of cyclic AMP in lipid mobilization in *Locusta migratoria*. Insect Biochem 6:535–540

Gates BJ, DeLuca M (1975) The production of oxyluciferin during the firefly luciferase light reaction. Arch Biochem Biophys 169:616–621

Gentleman S, Mansour TE (1974) Adenylate cyclase in a sea anemone: implication for chemoreception. Biochim Biophys Acta 343:469–479

Gentleman S, Mansour TE (1977) Control of Ca^{++} efflux and cyclic AMP by 5-hydroxytryptamine and dopamine in abalone gill. Life Sci 20:687–694

Gentleman S, Abrahams SL, Mansour TE (1976) Adenosine cyclic 3′,5′-monophosphate in the liver fluke, *Fasciola hepatica*. Mol Pharmacol 12:59–68

Gerschenfeld HM (1973) Chemical transmission in invertebrate central nervous systems and neuromuscular junctions. Physiol Rev 53:1–119

Gerschenfeld HM, Paupardin-Tritsch D (1974) Ionic mechanisms and receptor properties underlying the responses of molluscan neurones to 5-hydroxytryptamine. J Physiol (Lond) 243:426–456

Gerschenfeld HM, Hamon M, Paupardin-Tritsch D (1978) Release of endogenous serotonin from two identified serotonin-containing neurones and the physiological role of serotonin re-uptake. J Physiol (Lond) 274:265–278

Ginsborg BL, House CR, Silinsky EM (1974) Conductance changes associated with the secretory potential in the cockroach salivary gland. J Physiol (Lond) 236:723–731

Ginsborg BL, Turnbull KW, House CR (1976) On the actions of compounds related to dopamine at a neurosecretory synapse. Br J Pharmacol 57:133–140

Glusman S, Kravitz EA (1978) Serotonin (5-HT) modulatory action at the lobster neuromuscular junction. Mechanism of facilitation of transmitter release. Neurosci Abstr 4:369

Goldberg DJ, Goldman JE, Schwartz JH (1976) Alterations in amounts and rates of serotonin transported in an axon of the giant cerebral neurones of *Aplysia californica*. J Physiol (Lond) 259:473–490

Goldberg DJ, Schwartz JH, Sherbany AA (1978) Kinetic properties of normal and perturbed axonal transport of serotonin in a single identified axon. J Physiol (Lond) 281:559–579

Goldman JE, Schwartz JH (1974) Cellular specificity of serotonin storage and axonal transport in identified neurones of *Aplysia californica*. J Physiol (Lond) 242:61–76

Goldman JE, Schwartz JH (1977) Metabolism of (^{3}H) serotonin in the marine mollusc, *Aplysia californica*. Brain Res 137:77–88

Goldman JE, Kim KS, Schwartz JH (1976) Axonal transport of (^{3}H) serotonin in an identified neuron of *Aplysia californica*. J Cell Biol 70:304–318

Goldstone MW, Cooke IM (1971) Histochemical localization of monoamines in the crab central nervous system. Z Zellforsch Mikrosk Anat 116:7–19

Gole JWD, Downer RGH (1979) Elevation of adenosine 3′,5′-monophosphate by octopamine in fat body of the American cockroach *Periplaneta americana*. Comp Biochem Physiol 64C:223–226

Gospe SM, Wilson WA (1980) Dopamine inhibits burst-firing of neurosecretory cell R15 in *Aplysia californica:* establishment of a dose-response relationship. J Pharmacol Exp Ther 214:112–118

Gospe SM, Wilson WA (1981) Pharmacological studies of a novel dopamine-sensitive receptor mediating burst-firing inhibition of neurosecretory cell R15 in *Aplysia californica*. J Pharmacol Exp Ther 216:368–377

Grega DS (1978) The effects of monoamines on tarantula skeletal muscle. Comp Biochem Physiol 61C:337–340.

Greenberg MJ, Price DA (1979) FMRFamide, a cardioexcitatory neuropeptide of molluscs: an agent in search of a mission. Am Zool 19:163–174
Greenberg MJ, Price DA (1980) Cardioregulatory peptide in molluscs. In: Bloom FE (ed) Peptides: integrators of cell and tissue function. Raven, New York, pp 107–126
Hanoka D, Takahashi SY (1977) Adenylate cyclase system and the hyperglycaemic factor in the cockroach, *Periplaneta americana*. Insect Biochem 7:95–99
Hanson FE Jr (1962) Observation on the gross innervation of the firefly light organ. J Insect Physiol 8:105–111
Hanson FE, Miller J, Reynolds GT (1969) Subunit coordination in the firefly light organ. Biol Bull 137:447–464
Harmar AJ, Horn AS (1977) Octopamine-sensitive adenylate cyclase in cockroach brain: effects of agonists, antagonists and guanylyl nucleotides. Mol Pharmacol 13:512–520
Hawkins RD (1981) Interneurons involved in mediation and modulation of gill-withdrawal reflex in *Aplysia*. III. Identified facilitating neurons increase Ca^{++} current in sensory neurons. J Neurophysiol 45:327–339
Hawkins RD, Castellucci VF, Kandel ER (1981 a) Interneurons involved in mediation and modulation of gill-withdrawal reflex in *Aplysia*. I. Identification and characterization. J Neurophysiol 45:304–314
Hawkins RD, Castellucci VF, Kandel ER (1981 b) Interneurons involved in mediation and modulation of gill-withdrawal reflex in *Aplysia*. II. Identified neurons produce heterosynaptic facilitation contributing to behavioral sensitization. J Neurophysiol 45:315–326
Haynes LW (1980) Peptide neuroregulators in invertebrates. Prog Neurobiol 15:205–245
Heiss W-D, Hoyer J (1974) Dopamine receptor blockade by neuroleptic drugs in *Aplysia* neurones. Experientia 30:1318–1320
Heiss W-D, Hoyer J, Thalhammer G (1976) Antipsychotic drugs and dopamine-mediated responses in *Aplysia* neurons. J Neural Transm 39:187–208
Higashi GI, Kreiner PW, Keirns JJ, Bitensky MW (1973) Adenosine 3′,5′-cyclic monophosphate in *Schistosoma mansoni*. Life Sci 13:1211–1220
Higgins WJ (1974) Intracellular actions of 5-hydroxytryptamine on the bivalve myocardium I. Adenylate cyclase and guanylate cyclases. J Exp Zool 190:99–110
Higgins WJ (1977) 5-Hydroxytryptamine-induced tachyphylaxis of the molluscan heart and concomitant desensitization of adenylate cyclase. J Cyclic Nucleotide Res 3:293–302
Higgins WJ, Greenberg MJ (1974) Intracellular actions of 5-hydroxytryptamine on the bivalve myocardium. II. Cyclic nucleotide-dependent protein kinases and microsomal calcium uptake. J Exp Zool 190:305–316
Higgins WJ, Price DA, Greenberg MJ (1978) FMRFamide increases the adenylate cyclase activity and cyclic AMP levels of molluscan heart. Eur J Pharmacol 48:425–430
Hiripi L, Rozsa KS, Miller TA (1979) The effect of proctolin on the adenylate and guanylate cyclases in the Locusta brain at various developmental stages. Experientia 35:1287–1288
Hollingworth RM, Murdock LL (1980) Formamide pesticides: octopamine-like actions in a firefly. Science 208:74–76
House CR (1973) An electrophysiological study of neuroglandular transmission in the isolated salivary glands of the cockroach. J exp Biol 58:29–43
House CR, Ginsborg BL (1976) Action of a dopamine analogue and a neuroleptic at a neuroglandular synapse. Nature 261:332–333
House CR, Smith CK (1978) On the receptors involved in the nervous control of salivary secretion by *Nauphoeta cinerea* Olivier. J Physiol (Lond) 279:457–471
House CR, Ginsborg BL, Silinsky EM (1973) Dopamine receptors in cockroach salivary gland cells. Nature New Biol 245:63
Hoyle G (1974) A function for neurons (DUM) neurosecretory on skeletal muscle of insects. J Exp Zool 189:401–406
Hoyle G (1975) Evidence that insect dorsal unpaired median (DUM) neurons are octopaminergic. J Exp Zool 193:425–431
Hoyle G, Barker DL (1975) Synthesis of octopamine by insect dorsal median unpaired neurons. J Exp Zool 193:433–439

Hoyle G, Dagan D, Moberly B, Colquhoun W (1974) Dorsal unpaired median insect neurons make neurosecretory endings on skeletal muscle. J Exp Zool 187:157–165
Hoyle G, Colquhoun W, Williams M (1980) Fine structure of an octopaminergic neuron and its terminals. J Neurobiol 11:103–126
Ifshin MS, Gainer H, Barker JC (1975) Peptide factor extracted from molluscan ganglia that modulates bursting pacemaker activity. Nature 254:72–74
Irisawa H, Wilkens LA, Greenberg MJ (1972) Increase in membrane conductance by 5-hydroxytryptamine and acetylcholine on the hearts of *Modiolus demissus* and *Mytilus edulis (Mytilidae bivalva)*. Comp Biochem Physiol 45A:653–666
Juorio AV, Robertson HA (1977) Identification and distribution of some monoamines in tissues of the sunflower star *Pycnopodia helianthoides (echinodermata). J. Neurochem 28:573–579*
Kaczmarek LK, Jennings K, Strumwasser F (1978) Neurotransmitter modulation, phosphodiesterase inhibitory effects, and cyclic AMP correlates of afterdischarge in peptidergic neurites. Proc Natl Acad Sci USA 75:5200–5204
Kaczmarek LK, Jennings K, Strumwasser F, Nairn AC, Walter U, Wilson FD, Greengard P (1980) Microinjection of catalytic subunit of cyclic AMP-dependent protein kinase enhances calcium action potentials of bag cell neurons in cell culture. Proc Natl Acad Sci USA 77:7487–7491
Kandel ER (1979) Behavioral biology of Aplysia. Freeman, San Francisco
Kandel ER, Tauc L (1975) Mechanism of heterosynaptic facilitation in the giant cell of the abdominal ganglion in *Aplysia depilans*. J Physiol (Lond) 181:28–47
Kandel ER, Klein M, Bailey CH, Hawkins RD, Castellucci VF, Lubit BW, Schwartz JH (1981) Serotonin, cyclic AMP and the modulation of the calcium current during behavioral arousal. Princeton Symposium
Kaufman W (1976) The influence of various factors on fluid secretion by in vitro salivary glands of ixodid ticks. J Exp Biol 64:727–742
Kaufman WR, Phillips TE (1973a) Ion and water balance in the ixodid tick *Dermacentor andersoni*. I. Routes of ion and water excretion. J Exp Biol 58:523–536
Kaufman WR, Phillips TE (1973b) Ion and water balance in the ixodid tick *Dermacentor andersoni*. II. Mechanisms and control of salivary secretion. J Exp Biol 58:537–547
Kaufman WR, Phillips TE (1973c) Ion and water balance in the ixodid tick *Dermacentor andersoni*. III. Influence of monovalent ions and osmotic pressure on salivary secretion. J Exp Biol 58:549–564
Kaufman W, Diehl PA, Aeschlimann AA (1976) Na,K-ATPase in the salivary gland of the ixodid tick Amblyomma hebraeum (Koch) and its relation to the process of fluid secretion. Experientia 32:986
Kebabian PR, Kebabian JW, Carpenter DO (1979) Regulation of cyclic AMP in heart and gill of *Aplysia* by the putative neurotransmitters dopamine and serotonin. Life Sci 24:1757–1764
Kehoe JS (1972) Three acetylcholine receptors in *Aplysia* neurones. J Physiol (Lond) 225:115–146
Kehoe JS, Marder E (1976) Identification and effects of neural transmitters in invertebrates. Annu Rev Pharmacol Toxicol 16:245–268
Keller R (1965) Über eine hormonale Kontrolle des Polysaccharid-Stoffwechsels beim Flußkrebs *Cambarus affinis* Say. Z vergl Physiol 51:49–59
Keller R (1966) Über eine hormonale Regulation der Glykogen-Synthese beim Flußkrebs *Orconectes limosius* Rafinesque (*Cambarus affinis* Say). Verh Zool Ges Göttingen 272–279
Keller R, Andrew EM (1973) The site of action of crustacean hyperglycemic hormone. Gen comp Endocr 20:572–578
Keller R, Beyer J (1968) Zur hyperglykämischen Wirkung von Serotonin und Augenstielextrakt beim Flußkrebs *Orconectes limosus*. Z. Vgl Physiol 59:78–85
Klein M, Kandel ER (1978) Presynaptic modulation of voltage-dependent Ca^{++}-current: mechanism for behavioral sensitization in *Aplysia californica*. Proc Natl Acad Sci USA 75:3512–3516

Klein M, Kandel ER (1980) Mechanism of calcium current modulation underlying presynaptic facilitation and behavioral sensitization in *Aplysia.* Proc Natl Acad Sci USA 77:6912–6916

Kleinholz LH, Kimball F, McGarvey M (1967) Initial characterization and separation of hyperglycemic (diabetogenic) hormone from the crustacean eyestalk. Gen Comp Endocrinol 8:75–81

Klemm N (1972) Monoamine-containing nervous fibers in foregut and salivary glands of the desert locust, *Shistocerca gregaria* Forskal. Comp Biochem Physiol 43A:207–211

Klemm N, Axelsson S (1973) Detection of dopamine, noradrenaline and 5-hydroxytryptamine in the cerebral ganglion of the desert locust, *Schistocerca gregaria* Forsk. (Insecta, Orthoptera). Brain Res 57:289–298

Kluss BC (1958) Light and electron microscope observations on the photogenic organ of the firefly, *Photuris pennsylvanica* with special reference to the innervation. J Morphol 103:159–185

Kobayashi M, Muneoka Y (1980) Modulatory actions of octopamine and serotonin on the contraction of buccal muscles in *Rapana thomasiana* I. Enhancement of contraction in radular protractor. Comp Biochem Physiol 65C:73–79

Koester J, Mayeri E, Liebeswar G, Kandel ER (1973) Cellular regulation of homeostasis: neuronal control of the circulation in *Aplysia.* Fed Proc 32:2179–2187

Kohler G, Lindl T (1980) Effects of 5-hydroxytryptamine, dopamine, and acetylcholine on accumulation of cyclic AMP and cyclic GMP in the anterior byssus retractor muscle of *Mytilus edulis* L. (Mollusca). Pfluegers Arch 383:257–262

Kravitz EA, Glusman S, Harris-Warrick RM, Livingstone MS, Schwarz T, Goy MF (1980) Amines and a peptide as neurohormones in lobsters: actions on neuromuscular preparations and preliminary studies. J Exp Biol 89:159–176

Kushner PD, Maynard EA (1977) Localization of monoamine fluorescence in the stomatogastric nervous system of lobsters. Brain Res 129:13–28

LeMay A, Jarett L (1975) Pitfalls in the use of lead nitrate for the histochemical demonstration of adenylate cyclase activity. J Cell Biol 65:39–50

Lemos JR, Berlind A (1981) Cyclic adenosine monophosphate mediation of peptide neurohormone effects on the lobster cardiac ganglion. J Exp Biol 90:307–326

Levitan IB (1978) Adenylate cyclase in isolated *Helix* and *Aplysia* neuronal cell bodies: stimulation by serotonin and peptide-containing extract. Brain Res 154:404–408

Levitan IB, Barondes SH (1974) Octopamine- and serotonin-stimulated phosphorylation of specific protein in the abdominal ganglion of *Aplysia californica.* Proc Natl Acad Sci USA 71:1145–1148

Levitan IB, Norman J (1980) Different effects of cyclic AMP and cyclic GMP derivatives on the activity of an identified neuron: biochemical and electrophysiological analysis. Brain Res 187:415–429

Levitan IB, Treistman SN (1977) Modulation of electrical activity and cyclic nucleotide metabolism in molluscan nervous system by a peptide-containing nervous system extract. Brain Res 136:307–317

Levitan IB, Madsen CJ, Barondes SH (1974) Cyclic AMP and amine effects on phosphorylation of specific protein in abdominal ganglion of *Aplysia californica;* localization and kinetic analysis. J Neurobiol 5:511–525

Levitan IB, Bergstroem E, Simonet M (1978) Adenylate cyclase in *Helix* and *Aplysia* ganglia: characteristics of its stimulation by a peptide-containing nervous system extract. J Neurochem 31:1353–1369

Levitan IB, Harmar AJ, Adams WB (1979) Synaptic and hormonal modulation of a neuronal oscillator: a search for molecular mechanisms. J Exp Biol 81:131–151

Liebeswar G, Goldman JE, Koester J, Mayeri E (1975) Neural control of circulation *Aplysia.* III. Neurotransmitters. J Neurophysiol 38:767–779

Lingle CJ (1979a) The effects of acetylcholine, glutamate, and biogenic amines on muscles and neuromuscular transmission in the stomatogastric system of the spiny lobster, *Panulirus interruptus.* PhD thesis, University of Oregon, Eugene

Lingle CJ (1979b) Dopamine modulatory actions at neuromuscular junctions of lobster stomatogastric system. Neurosci Abstr 5:341

Lingle C (1980) The sensitivity of decapod foregut muscles to acetylcholine and glutamate. J Comp Physiol 138:187–199

Lingle C (1981) The modulatory action of dopamine on crustacean foregut neuromuscular preparations. J Exp Biol 94:285–299

Livingstone MS, Harris-Warrick RM, Kravitz EA (1980) Serotonin and octopamine produce opposite postures in lobsters. Science 208:76–79

Livingstone MS, Schaeffer SF, Kravitz EA (1981) Biochemistry and ultrastructure of serotonergic nerve endings in the lobster: serotonin and octopamine are contained in different nerve endings. J Neurobiol 12:27–54

Loveland RE (1963) 5-hydroxytryptamine, the probable mediator of excitation in the heart of *Mercenaria*. Comp Biochem Physiol 9:95–104

Lloyd PE (1980a) Modulation of neuromuscular activity by 5-hydroxytryptamine and endogenous peptides in the snail, *Helix aspersa*. J Comp Physiol 139:333–339

Lloyd PE (1980b) Mechanisms of actin of 5-hydroxytryptamine and endogenous peptides on a neuromuscular preparation in the snail, *Helix aspersa*. J Comp Physiol 139:341–347

MacDonald JF, Berry RS (1978) Further identification of multiple responses mediated by dopamine in the CNS of *Planorbis corneus*. Can J Physiol Pharmacol 56:7–18

Maddrell SHP, Pilcher D, Gardiner B (1971) Pharmacology of the Malpighian tubules of *Rhodnius* and *Carausius*: the structure-activity relationship of tryptamine analogues and the role of cAMP. J Exp Biol 54:779–804

Mandelbaum DE, Koester J, Schonberg M, Weiss KR (1979) Cyclic AMP mediation of the excitatory effect of serotonin in the heart of *Aplysia*. Brain Res 177:388–394

Mansour TE (1957) The effect of lysergic acid diethylamide, 5-hydroxytryptamine, and related compounds on the liver fluke *Fasciola hepatica*. Br J Pharmacol 12:406–408

Mansour TE (1959) Studies on the carbohydrate metabolism of the liver fluke *Fasciola hepatica*. Biochim Biophys Acta 34:456–464

Mansour TE, Lago AD (1958) Biochemical effects of serotonin on *Fasciola hepatica*. J Pharmacol Exp Ther 122:43A

Mansour TE, Mansour JM (1962) Effects of serotonin (5-hydroxytryptamine) and adenosine 3′,5′-phosphate on phosphofructokinase from the liver fluke *Fasciola hepatica*. J Biol Chem 237:629–634

Mansour TE, Mansour JM (1977) Phosphodiesterase in the liver fluke, *Fasciola Hepatica*. Biochem Pharmacol 26:2325–2330

Mansour TE, Stone DB (1970) Biochemical effects of lysergic acid diethylamide on the liver fluke, *Fasciola hepatica*. Biochem Pharmacol 19:1137–1146

Mansour TE, Sutherland EW, Rall JW, Bueding E (1960) The effects of serotonin (5-hydroxytryptamine) on the formation of adenosine 3′,5′-phosphate by tissue particles from the liver fluke, *Fasciola hepatica*. J Biol Chem 235:466–470

Marder E (1976) Cholinergic motor neurones in the stomatogastric system of the lobster. J Physiol (Lond) 257:63–86

Marder E, Paupardin-Tritsch D (1978) The pharmacological properties of some crustacean neuronal acetylcholine, gamma-aminobutyric acid, and l-glutamate responses. J Physiol (Lond) 280:213–236

Marilley M, Thouveny Y (1978) DNA synthesis during the first stages of anterior regeneration in the Polychaete annelid *Owenia fusiformis* (dedifferentiation and early phases of differentiation). J Embryol Exp Morphol 44:81–92

Matsumura F, Beeman RW (1976) Biochemical and physiological effects of chlordimeform. Environ Health Perspect 14:71–82

Mayeri E, Koester J, Kupfermann I, Liebeswar G, Kandel ER (1974) Neural control of circulation in *Aplysia*. I. Motoneurons. J Neurophysiol 37:458–475

Mayeri E, Brownell P, Branton WD (1979a) Multiple, prolonged actions of neuroendocrine bag cells on neurons in *Aplysia*. II. Effects on beating pacemaker and silent neurons. J Neurophysiol 42:1185–1197

Mayeri E, Brownell P, Branton WD, Simon SB (1979b) Multiple, Prolonged actions of neuroendocrine bag cells on neurons in *Aplysia*. I. Effects on bursting pacemaker neurons. J Neurophysiol 42:1165–1183

Maynard DM, Welsh JH (1959) Neurohormones of the pericardial organs of brachyuran Crustacea. J Physiol (Lond) 149:215–227
McCaman MW, McCaman RE (1978) Octopamine and phenylethanolamine in *Aplysia* ganglia and in individual neurons. Brain Res 141:347–352
McElroy WD, Seliger HH, White EH (1969) Mechanism of bioluminescence, chemiluminescence and enzyme function in the oxidation of firefly luciferin. Photochem Photobiol 10:153–170
McMullen HL, Sauer JR (1978) The relationship of phosphodiesterase and cyclic AMP to the process of fluid secretion in the salivary gland of the ixodid tick *Amblyomma americanum*. Experientia 34:1030–1031
Megaw MWJ (1974) Studies on the water balance mechanism of the tick, *Boophilus microplus Canestrini*. Comp Biochem Physiol 48A:115–125
Moraczewski J, Duma A (1978) Ultrastructural localization of adenylate cyclase activity in neoblasts of turbellarian *Dugesia lugubris* (Schmidt O). J Exp Zool 203:491–496
Munday KA, Poat JA, Woodruff GN (1976) Structure activity studies on dopamine receptors; a comparison between rat striatal adenylate cyclase and *Helix aspersa* neurones. Proc Br Physiol Soc 1:452P–453P
Muneoka Y, Kobayashi M (1980) Modulatory actions of octopamine and serotonin on the contraction of buccal muscles in *Rapana thomasiana*. II. Inhibition on contraction in radular retractor. Comp Biochem Physiol 65C:81–86
Nathanson JA (1976) Octopamine-sensitive adenylate cyclase and its possible relationship to the octopamine receptor. In: Usdin E, Sandler M (eds) Trace amines and the brain. Dekker, New York Basel, pp 161–190
Nathanson JA (1979) Octopamine receptors, adenosine 3′,5′-monophosphate, and neural control of firefly flashing. Science 203:65–68
Nathanson JA, Bloom FE (1975) Lead-induced inhibition of adenyl cyclase. Nature 255:419–420
Nathanson JA, Greengard P (1973) Octopamine-sensitive adenylate cyclase: evidence for a biological role of octopamine in nervous tissue. Science 180:308–331
Nathanson JA, Greengard P (1974) Serotonin-sensitive adenylate cyclase in neural tissue and its similarity to the serotonin receptor: a possible site of action of lysergic acid diethylamide. Proc Natl Acad Sci USA 71:797–801
Nathanson JA, Hunnicutt EJ (1979a) Neural control of light emission in *Photuris* larva: identification of octopamine-sensitive adenylate cyclase. J Exp Zool 208:255–262
Nathanson JA, Hunnicutt EJ (1977b) Octopamine-sensitive adenylate cyclase: properties and pharmacological characterization. Neurosci Abstr 5:346
Nathanson JA, Hunnicutt EJ (1981) N-demethylchlordimeform: a potent partial agonist of octopamine-sensitive adenylate cyclase. Mol Pharmacol 20:68–75
Needham GR, Sauer JR (1975) Control of fluid secretion by isolated salivary glands of the lone star tick. J Insect Physiol 21:1893–1898
Northup JK, Mansour TE (1978a) Adenylate cyclase from *Fasciola hepatica* 1. Ligand specificity of adenylate cyclase-coupled serotonin receptors. Mol Pharmacol 14:804–819
Northup JK, Mansour TE (1978b) Adenylate cyclase from *Fasciola hepatica* 2. Role of guanine nucleotides in coupling of adenylate cyclase and serotonin receptors. Mol Pharmacol 14:820–833
Ochsman JL, Berridge MJ (1970) Structural and functional aspects of salivary fluid secretion in *Calliphora*. Tissue Cell 2:281–310
Oertel D, Case JF (1976) Neural excitation of the firefly photocyte: slow depolarization possibly mediated by a cyclic nucleotide. J Exp Biol 65:213–227
Oertel D, Linberg KA, Case JF (1975) Ultrastructure of the larval firefly light organ as related to control of light emission. Cell Tissue Res 164:27–44
Osborne NN (1977) Adenosine 3′-5′-monophosphate in snail *(Helix pomatia)* nervous system. Analysis of dopamine receptors. Experientia 33:917
Paris CG, Kandel ER, Schwartz JH (1980) Serotonin stimulates phosphorylation of a 137,000 dalton membrane protein in the abdominal ganglion of *Aplysia*. Neurosci Abstr 6:844

Pellmar TC (1980) A transmitter-induced calcium current. Fed Proc 40:2631–2636

Pellmar TC, Carpenter DO (1979) Voltage-dependent calcium current induced by serotonin. Nature 277:483–484

Pellmar TC, Carpenter DO (1980) Serotonin induces a voltage-sensitive calcium current in neurons of *Aplysia californica.* J Neurophysiol 44:423–439

Pellmar TC, Wilson WA (1977) Unconventional serotonergic excitation in *Aplysia.* Nature 269:76–78

Pentreath VW, Berry MS (1976) Potentiation of dopaminergic transmission by phosphodiesterase inhibitors and cyclic nucleotides. J Pharm Pharmacol 28:874–877

Pentreath VW, Cottrell GA (1974) Anatomy of an identified serotonin neurone studied by means of injection of tritiated 'transmitter'. Nature 250:655

Peretz B, Estes J (1974) Histology and histochemistry of the peripheral neural plexus in the *Aplysia* gill. J Neurobiol 5:3–19

Peterson MK (1970) The fine structure of the larval firefly light organ. J Morphol 131:103–116

Peterson MK, Buck J (1968) Light organ fine structure in certain Asiatic fireflies. Biol Bull 135:335–348

Pitman RM (1971) Transmitter substances in insects: a review. Comp Gen Pharmacol 2:347–371

Price DA, Greenberg MJ (1977) Structure of a molluscan cardioexcitatory neuropeptide. Science 197:670–671

Price DA, Greenberg MJ (1980) Pharmacology of the molluscan cardioexcitatory neuropeptide, FMRamide. Gen Pharmacol 11:237–241

Prince WT, Berridge MJ (1972) The effects of 5-hydroxytryptamine and cyclic AMP on the potential profile across isolated salivary glands. J Exp Biol 56:323–333

Prince WT, Berridge MJ (1973) The role of calcium in the action of 5-hydroxytryptamine and cyclic AMP on salivary glands. J Exp Biol 58:361–384

Prince WT, Berridge MJ, Rasmussen H (1972) Role of calcium and adenosine-3′,5′-cyclic monophosphate in controlling fly salivary gland secretion. Proc Natl Acad Sci USA 69:553–557

Prince WT, Rasmussen H, Berridge MJ (1973) The role of calcium in fly salivary gland secretion analyzed with the ionophore A-23187. Biochim Biophys Acta 329:98–107

Ramamurthi R, Mumbach MW, Scheer BT (1968) Endocrine control of glycogen synthesis in crabs. Comp Biochem Physiol 26:311–319

Rao KR, Fingerman M (1970) Action of biogenic amines on crustacean chromophores. II. Analysis of the responses of erythrophores in the fiddler crab *Uca pugilator* to indolealkylamines and an eyestalk hormone. Comp Gen Pharmacol 1:117–126

Raper JA (1979) Non-impulse-mediated synaptic transmission during the generation of a cyclic motor program. Science 205:304–306

Rasmussen H, Goodman DBP (1977) Relationships between calcium and cyclic nucleotides in cell activation. Physiol Rev 57:421–509

Robertson HA (1975) The innervation of the salivary gland of the moth, evidence that dopamine is the transmitter. J Exp Biol 63:413–420

Robertson HA (1976) Octopamine, dopamine, and noradrenaline content of the brain of the locust, *Schistocerca gregaria.* Experientia 32:552–553

Robertson HA, Carlson AD (1976) Octopamine: presence in firefly lantern suggests a transmitter role. J Exp Zool 195:159–164

Robertson HA, Osborne NN (1979) Putative neurotransmitters in the Annelid central nervous system: presence of 5-hydroxytryptamine and octopamine-stimulated adenylate cyclases. Comp Biochem Physiol 64C:7–14

Robertson HA, Steele JE (1972) Activation of insect nerve cord phosphorylase by octopamine and adenosine 3′,5′-monophosphate. J Neurochem 19:1603–1606

Russell DF (1979) CNS control of pattern generators in the lobster stomatogastric ganglion. Brain Res 177:598–602

Saavedra JM, Brownstein MJ, Carpenter DO, Axelrod J (1974) Octopamine: presence in single neurons of *Aplysia* suggests neurotransmitter function. Science 185:364–365

Samaranayaka M (1976) Possible involvement of monoamines in the release of adipokinetic hormone in the locust *Schistocerca gregaria*. J Exp Biol 65:415–425
Sauer JR, Frick JM, Hair JA (1974) Control of ^{36}Cl uptake by isolated salivary glands of the lone star tick. J Insect Physiol 20:1771–1778
Schmidt SP, Essenberg RC, Sauer JR (1980) Dopamine-stimulated adenylate cyclase from the salivary glands of an ixodid tick. Fed Proc Abstr 39:2107
Schwartz JH, Shkolnik LJ, Goldberg DL (1979) Specific association of neurotransmitters with somatic lysosomes in an identified serotonergic neuron of *Aplysia californica*. Proc Natl Acad Sci USA 76:5967–5971
Seliger HH, McElroy WD (1964) The colors of firefly bioluminescence: enzyme configuration and species specificity. Proc Natl Acad Sci USA 52:75–81
Selverston AI, Russell DF, Miller JP, King DG (1976) The stomatogastric nervous system: structure and function of a small neural network. Prog Neurobiol 7:215–290
Shapiro E, Castellucci VF, Kandel ER (1980) Presynaptic inhibition in *Aplysia* involves a decrease in the Ca^{++} current of the presynaptic neuron. Proc Natl Acad Sci USA 77:1185–1189
Shimahara T, Tauc L (1975) Heterosynaptic facilitation in the giant cell of *Aplysia*. J Physiol (Lond) 247:321–341
Shimahara T, Tauc L (1976) Identification of a neuron inducing heterosynaptic facilitation on a specific synapse in *Aplysia*. Brain Res 118:142–146
Shimahara T, Tauc L (1977) Cyclic AMP induced by serotonin modulates the activity of an identified synapse in *Aplysia* by facilitating the active permeability to calcium. Brain Res 127:168–172
Shkolnik LJ, Schwartz JH (1980) Genesis and maturation of serotonergic vesicles in identified giant cerebral neuron of *Aplysia*. J Neurophysiol 43:945–967
Simpson TL, Rodan GA (1976) Role of cAMP in the release from dormancy of freshwater sponge gemmules. Dev Biol 49:544–547
Smalley KN (1965) Adrenergic transmission in the light organ of the firefly, *Photinus pyralis*. Comp Biochem Physiol 16:467–477
Smith DS (1963) The organization and innervation of the luminescent organ in a firefly, *Photuris pennsylvanica* (Coleoptera). J Cell Biol 16:323–359
Spindler K-D, Willing A, Keller R (1976) Cyclic nucleotides and crustacean blood glucose levels. Comp Biochem Physiol 54A:301–304
Starratt AM, Brown BE (1975) Structure of the pentapeptide, proctolin, a proposed neurotransmitter in insects. Life Sci 17:1253–1256
Steele JE (1961) Occurrence of a hyperglycemic factor in the corpus cardiacum of an insect. Nature 192:680–681
Stefani E, Gerschenfeld HM (1969) Comparative study of acetylcholine and 5-hydroxytryptamine receptors on single snail neurons. J Neurophysiol 32:61–74
Stone DB, Mansour TE (1967) Phosphofructokinase from the liver fluke *Fasciola hepatica* 1. Activation by adenosine 3′,5′-phosphate and by serotonin. Mol Pharmacol 3:161–176
Sullivan RE (1978) Stimulus-coupled release from identified neurosecretory fibers in the spiny lobster, *Panulirus interruptus*. Life Sci 22:1429–1438
Sullivan RE (1979) A proctolin-like peptide in crab pericardial organs. J Exp Zool 210:543–552
Sullivan RE, Barker DL (1975) Octopamine increases cyclic AMP content of crustacean ganglia and cardiac muscle. Neurosci Abstr 1:354
Sullivan RE, Friend B, McCaman RE (1976) Endogenous levels of octopamine, serotonin, dopamine and acetylcholine in spiny lobster pericardial organs. Neurosci Abstr 2:335
Sullivan RE, Friend BJ, Barker DL (1977) Structure and function of spiny lobster ligamental nerve plexures: evidence for synthesis, storage, and secretion of biogenic amines. J Neurobiol 8:581–605
Swann J, Sinback CN, Carpenter DO (1978) Dopamine-induced muscle contractions and modulation of neuromuscular transmission in *Aplysia*. Brain Res 157:169–172
Tager HS, Markese J, Kramer KJ, Speirs RD, Childs CN (1976) Glucagon-like and insulin-like hormones of the insect neurosecretory system. Biochem J 156:515–520
Tatchell RJ (1967) A modified method for obtaining tick oral secretion. J Parasitol 53:1106–1107

Treistman SN, Drake PF (1979) The effects of cyclic nucleotide agents in *Aplysia*. Brain Res 168:643–647
Treistman SN, Levitan IB (1976) Alteration of electrical activity in molluscan neurons by cyclic nucleotides and peptide factors. Nature 261:62–64
Truman JW (1976) Hormonal release of differential behavior patterns. In: Fentress JC (ed) Simpler networks and behavior. Sinauer, Sunderland, Mass, pp 111–120
Truman JW (1978) Hormonal release of stereotyped motor programmes from the isolated nervous system of the cecropia silkmoth. J Exp Biol 74:151–173
Truman JW, Mumby SM, Welch SK (1979) Involvement of cyclic GMP in the release of stereotyped behavior patterns in moths by a peptide hormone. J Exp Biol 84:201–212
Twarog BM (1954) Responses of a molluscan smooth muscle to acetylcholine and 5-hydroxytryptamine. J Cell Comp Physiol 44:141–163
Twarog BM (1976) Aspects of smooth muscle function in molluscan catch muscle. Physiol Rev 56:829–838
Twarog BM, Cole RA (1972) Relaxation of catch in a molluscan smooth muscle. II. Effects of serotonin, dopamine, and related compounds. Comp Biochem Physiol 43A:331–335
Walker RJ, Woodruff GN, Glaizner D, Sedden CB, Kerkut GA (1968) The pharmacology of *Helix* dopamine receptors of specific neurones in the snail *Helix aspersa*. Comp Biochem Physiol 24:453–469
Walker RJ, Ramage AG, Woodruff GN (1972) The presence of octopamine in the brain of *Helix aspersa* and its action on specific snail neurones. Experientia 28:1173–1174
Wallace BG, Talamo BR, Evans PD, Kravitz EA (1974) Octopamine: selective association with specific neurons in the lobster nervous system. Brain Res 74:349–355
Ward SN (1973) Chemotaxis by the nematode *Caenorhabditus elegans:* identification of attractants and analysis of the response by use of mutants. Proc Natl Acad Sci USA 70:817–832
Weinreich D, McCaman MW, McCaman RE, Vaughn JE (1973) Chemical, enzymatic, and ultrastructural characterization of 5-hydroxytryptamine containing neurons from the ganglia of *Aplysia californica* and *Tritonia diomedia*. J Neurochem 20:969–976
Weiss KR, Cohen J, Kupfermann I (1975) Potentiation of muscle contraction: a possible modulatory function of an identified serotonergic cell in *Aplysia*. Brain Res 99:381–386
Weiss KR, Cohen JL, Kupfermann I (1978a) Modulatory control of buccal musculature by a serotonergic neuron (metacerebral cell) in *Aplysia*. J Neurophysiol 41:181–203
Weiss KR, Schonberg M, Mandelbaum DE, Kupfermann I (1978b) Activity of an individual serotonergic neurone in *Aplysia* enhances synthesis of cyclic adenosine monophosphate. Nature 272:727–728
Weiss KR, Mandelbaum DE, Schonberg M, Kupferman I (1979) Modulation of buccal muscle contractility by serotonergic metacerebral cells in *Aplysia:* evidence for a role of cyclic adenosine monophosphate. J Neurophysiol 42:791–803
Welsh JH (1971) Neurohumoral regulation and the pharmacology of a molluscan heart. Comp Gen Pharmacol 2:423–432
Wilkens LA, Greenberg MJ (1972) Effects of acetylcholine and 5-hydroxytryptamine and their ionic mechanisms of action on the electrical and mechanical activity of molluscan heart smooth muscle. Comp Biochem Physiol 45A:637–651
Willett JD, Rahim I (1978a) Determination of adenosine 3′,5′-cyclic monophosphate levels in tissues of the free living nematode, *Panagrellus redivivus*. Comp Biochem Physiol 60B:403–405
Willett JD, Rahim I (1978b) Determination of guanosine 3′,5′-cyclic-monophosphate in tissues of the free living nematode, *Panagrellus redivivus*. Comp Biochem Physiol 61B:243–246
Wollemann M, S-Rozsa K (1975) Effects of serotonin and catecholamines on the adenylate cyclase of molluscan heart. Comp Biochem Physiol 51C:63–66
Woodruff GN (1971) Dopamine receptors: A review. Comp Gen Pharmacol 2:439–455
Woodruff GN, Walker RJ (1969) The effects of dopamine and other compounds on the activity of neurons of *Helix aspersa:* Structure-activity relationships. Int J Neuropharmacol 8:279–289
Worm RAA (1980) Involvement of cyclic nucleotides in locust flight muscle metabolism. Comp Biochem Physiol 67C:23–27

Subject Index

Handbook of Experimental Pharmacology

Continuation of "Handbuch der experimentellen Pharmakologie"

Volume 16
Erzeugung von Krankheitszuständen durch das Experiment/Experimental Production of Diseases

Part 1
Blut (In Preparation)

Part 2
Atemwege

Part 3
Heart and Circulation

Part 4
Niere, Nierenbecken, Blase

Part 5
Liver

Part 6
Schilddrüse
(In Preparation)

Part 7
Zentralnervensystem

Part 8
Stütz- und Hartgewebe

Part 9
Infektionen I

Part 10
Infektionen II

Part 11 A
Infektionen III

Part 11 B
Infektionen IV

Part 12
Tumoren I

Part 13
Tumoren II

Part 14
Tumoren III
(In Preparation)

Part 15
Kohlenhydratstoffwechsel, Fieber/ Carbohydrate Metabolism, Fever

Volume 17
Ions alcalino-terreux

Part 1
Systèmes isolés

Part 2
Organismes entiers

Volume 18
Histamine and Anti-Histaminics

Part 1
Histamine. Its Chemistry, Metabolism and Physiological and Pharmacological Actions

Part 2
Histamine II and Anti-Histaminics

Volume 19
5-Hydroxytryptamine and Related Indolealkylamines

Volume 20: Part 1
Pharmacology of Fluorides I

Part 2
Pharmacology of Fluorides II

Volume 21
Beryllium

Volume 22: Part 1
Die Gestagene I

Part 2
Die Gestagene II

Volume 23
Neurohypophysial Hormones and Similar Polypeptides

Volume 24
Diuretica

Volume 25
Bradykinin, Kallidin and Kallikrein

Volume 26
Vergleichende Pharmakologie von Überträgersubstanzen in tiersystematischer Darstellung

Volume 27
Anticoagulantien

Springer-Verlag
Berlin
Heidelberg
New York

Handbook of Experimental Pharmacology

Continuation of "Handbuch der experimentellen Pharmakologie"

Volume 28: Part 1
Concepts in Biochemical Pharmacology I

Part 3
Concepts in Biochemical Pharmacology III

Volume 29
Oral wirksame Antidiabetika

Volume 30
Modern Inhalation Anesthetics

Volume 32: Part 1
Insulin I

Part 2
Insulin II

Volume 34
Secretin, Cholecystokinin, Pancreozymin and Gastrin

Volume 35: Part 1
Androgene I

Part 2
Androgens II and Antiandrogens/Androgene II und Antiandrogene

Volume 36
Uranium - Plutonium - Transplutonic Elements

Volume 37
Angiotensin

Volume 38: Part 1
Antineoplastic and Immunosuppressive Agents I

Part 2
Antineoplastic and Immunosuppressive Agents II

Volume 39
Antihypertensive Agents

Volume 40
Organic Nitrates

Volume 41
Hypolipidemic Agents

Volume 42
Neuromuscular Junction

Volume 43
Anabolic-Androgenic Steroids

Volume 44
Heme and Hemoproteins

Volume 45: Part 1
Drug Addiction I

Part 2
Drug Addiction II

Volume 46
Fibrinolytics and Antifibrinolytics

Volume 47
Kinetics of Drug Action

Volume 48
Arthropod Venoms

Volume 49
Ergot Alkaloids and Related Compounds

Volume 50: Part 1
Inflammation

Part 2
Anti-Inflammatory Drugs

Volume 51
Uric Acid

Volume 52
Snake Venoms

Volume 53
Pharmacology of Ganglionic Transmission

Volume 54: Part 1
Adrenergic Activators and Inhibitors I

Part 2
Adrenergic Activators and Inhibitors II

Volume 55: Part 1
Antipsychotics and Antidepressants I

Part 2
Antipsychotics and Antidepressants II

Part 3
Alcohol and Psychotomimeitic, Psychotropic Effects of Central Acting Drugs

Volume 56 I/II
Cardiac Glycosides
(In Preparation)

Volume 57
Tissue Growth Factors

Volume 58: Part 1:
Biochemistry

Springer-Verlag
Berlin
Heidelberg
New York

GPSR Compliance

The European Union's (EU) General Product Safety Regulation (GPSR) is a set of rules that requires consumer products to be safe and our obligations to ensure this.

If you have any concerns about our products, you can contact us on ProductSafety@springernature.com

In case Publisher is established outside the EU, the EU authorized representative is:

Springer Nature Customer Service Center GmbH
Europaplatz 3
69115 Heidelberg, Germany

Batch number: 10838053

Printed by Printforce, the Netherlands